Computer Aided Diagnosis Sensors

Computer Aided Diagnosis Sensors

Editors

Ayman El-Baz
Guruprasad A. Giridharan
Ahmed Shalaby
Ali H. Mahmoud
Mohammed Ghazal

MDPI

Basel • Beijing • Wuhan • Barcelona • Belgrade • Novi Sad • Cluj • Manchester

Editors

Ayman El-Baz
Bioengineering Department,
University of Louisville
Louisville, KY, USA

Guruprasad A. Giridharan
Bioengineering Department,
University of Louisville
Louisville, KY, USA

Ahmed Shalaby
Bioengineering Department,
University of Louisville
Louisville, KY, USA

Ali H. Mahmoud
Bioengineering Department,
University of Louisville
Louisville, KY, USA

Mohammed Ghazal
Department of Electrical,
Computer, and Biomedical
Engineering,
Abu Dhabi University
Abu Dhabi,
United Arab Emirates

Editorial Office
MDPI
St. Alban-Anlage 66
4052 Basel, Switzerland

This is a reprint of articles from the Special Issue published online in the open access journal *Sensors* (ISSN 1424-8220) (available at: https://www.mdpi.com/journal/sensors/special_issues/CADS).

For citation purposes, cite each article independently as indicated on the article page online and as indicated below:

Lastname, A.A.; Lastname, B.B. Article Title. *Journal Name* **Year**, *Volume Number*, Page Range.

ISBN 978-3-0365-9532-0 (Hbk)
ISBN 978-3-0365-9533-7 (PDF)
doi.org/10.3390/books978-3-0365-9533-7

Contents

About the Editors

Ayman El-Baz

Ayman El-Baz is a Distinguished Professor at the University of Louisville, Kentucky, United States, and University of Louisville at Alamein International University (UofL-AIU), New Alamein City, Egypt. Dr. El-Baz earned his B.Sc. and M.Sc. degrees in electrical engineering in 1997 and 2001, respectively. He earned his Ph.D. in electrical engineering from the University of Louisville in 2006. He has two decades of hands-on experience in the fields of bio-imaging modeling and non-invasive computer-assisted diagnosis systems. Dr. El-Baz was named as a Fellow of IEEE, BMES, Coulter, AIMBE and NAI for his contributions to the field of biomedical translational research. He has authored or coauthored more than 700 technical articles.

Guruprasad A. Giridharan

Guruprasad A. Giridharan is a Professor in the Bioengineering Department at the University of Louisville, Kentucky, United States. He received his B.Tech in chemical engineering from the University of Madras, India, in 1998 and M.S. and Ph.D. degrees in chemical engineering from the University of Utah, Salt Lake City, UT, in 2002. He joined the Bioengineering Department at the University of Louisville in 2006. His current research foci include biomedical device development and testing, physiologic control systems, mechanical circulatory support for Fontan circulation, and myocardial recovery strategies. In the past 6 years, Dr. Giridharan has generated over USD 20 million in research funding, which includes grant awards from the American Heart Association, NIH R01, NIH R15, and NIH SBIR programs. He has published 53 peer-reviewed manuscripts, 83 abstracts, 3 book chapters, and 19 patents and disclosures.

Ahmed Shalaby

Ahmed Shalaby is a Research Scientist in the Bioengineering Department at the University of Louisville, Kentucky, United States. He received his B.S. and M.S. degrees in electrical engineering from Alexandria University, Egypt, in 2003 and 2009, respectively. He received his PhD degree in electrical engineering from the University of Louisville in 2014. Dr. Shalaby's research interests include computer vision, image processing, robotics, machine learning, object detection, tracking and medical imaging. Dr. Shalaby works on several projects that use state-of-the-art machine learning techniques for the early diagnosis of brain, kidney and lung disorders.

Ali H. Mahmoud

Ali H. Mahmoud is a Research Scientist in the Bioengineering Department at the University of Louisville, Kentucky, United States. He received his B.S. and M.S. degrees in electrical engineering from Alexandria University, Egypt, in 2005 and 2009, respectively. He received his Ph.D. degree in electrical engineering from the University of Louisville in 2014. Dr. Mahmoud's research interests include computer vision, image processing, robotics, machine learning, object detection, tracking and medical imaging. Dr. Mahmoud works on several projects that use state-of-the-art machine learning techniques for the early diagnosis of brain, kidney and lung disorders.

Mohammed Ghazal

Mohammad Ghazal is a Professor and Chairman of the Department of Electrical, Computer, and Biomedical Engineering at the College of Engineering, Abu Dhabi University, Abu Dhabi, United Arab Emirates. He earned his Ph.D. and M.Sc. in Electrical and Computer Engineering (ECE) from

Concordia University, Canada, in 2010 and 2006, respectively, and was awarded an Alexander Graham Bell Fellowship from NSERC and QFRNT from the Government of Quebec. He earned his B.Sc. in Computer Engineering from the American University of Sharjah, where he received the President's Cup and the Ministry of Education's Shield for Creative Thinking. Dr. Ghazal's current research interests include AI in bioimaging, genomics, and smart systems. He is a senior member of IEEE and a member of ACM and BMES as well as an ABET program evaluator for the Engineering Accreditation Commission. Dr. Ghazal has received several awards, including DHS 1,000,000 from the UAE Prime Minister's Office for an innovative mobile app during the 2015 Government Summit, the distinguished Faculty Award from Abu Dhabi University in 2014 and 2016, and the Abu Dhabi University Research Fellow in 2018. He was also inducted into the American University of Sharjah Hall of Fame by Sheikh Sultan Al Qasimi in 2018. He is the author of over 200 publications in journals and international conferences.

Preface

Sensors used to diagnose, monitor or treat diseases in the medical domain are known as medical sensors. There are several types of medical sensors that can be utilized for various applications, such as temperature probes, force sensors, pressure sensors, oximeters, electrocardiogram sensors that measure the electrical activity of the heart, heart rate sensors, electroencephalogram sensors that measure the electrical activity of the brain, electromyogram sensors that record electrical activity produced by skeletal muscles, and respiration rate sensors that count how many times the chest rises in a minute. The output of these sensors used to be interpreted by humans, which was time consuming and tedious; however, such interpretations became easy with advances in artificial intelligence (AI) techniques and the integration of the sensor outputs into computer-aided diagnostic (CAD) systems.

This reprint highlights several studies that present state-of-the-art AI approaches used to diagnose different diseases and disorders based on the data collected from different medical sensors. This works towards developing comprehensive and automated computer-aided diagnosis by focusing on the different machine learning algorithms that can be used for this purpose as well as novel applications in the medical field.

Ayman El-Baz, Guruprasad A. Giridharan, Ahmed Shalaby, Ali H. Mahmoud, and Mohammed Ghazal
Editors

sensors

MDPI

Editorial

Special Issue "Computer Aided Diagnosis Sensors"

Ayman El-Baz [1,*], Guruprasad A. Giridharan [1], Ahmed Shalaby [1], Ali H. Mahmoud [1] and Mohammed Ghazal [2]

[1] Bioengineering Department, University of Louisville, Louisville, KY 40292, USA
[2] Electrical, Computer, and Biomedical Engineering Department, Abu Dhabi University, Abu Dhabi 59911, United Arab Emirates
[*] Correspondence: aselba01@louisville.edu

1. Introduction

Sensors used to diagnose, monitor or treat diseases in the medical domain are known as medical sensors. There are several types of medical sensors that can be utilized for various applications, such as temperature probes; force sensors; pressure sensors; oximeters; electrocardiogram sensors which measure the electrical activity of the heart; heart rate sensors; electroencephalogram sensors, which measure the electrical activity of the brain; electromyogram sensors that record electrical activity produced by skeletal muscles; and respiration-rate sensors that count how many times the chest rises in a minute. The output of these sensors used to be interpreted by humans, which was time consuming and tedious; however, interpretation became easy with the advance in artificial intelligence (AI) techniques and the integration of the sensor outputs into computer-aided diagnostic (CAD) systems.

This Special Issue has accepted 34 papers that present some of the state-of-the-art AI approaches used to diagnose different diseases and disorders based on the data collected from different medical sensors. This contributes towards achieving our goal, which is to develop comprehensive and automated computer-aided diagnosis tools by focusing on the different machine learning algorithms that can be used for this purpose as well as novel applications in the medical field.

Citation: El-Baz, A.; Giridharan, G.A.; Shalaby, A.; Mahmoud, A.H.; Ghazal, M. Special Issue "Computer Aided Diagnosis Sensors". *Sensors* **2022**, 22, 8052. https://doi.org/10.3390/s22208052

Received: 12 October 2022
Accepted: 19 October 2022
Published: 21 October 2022

Publisher's Note: MDPI stays neutral with regard to jurisdictional claims in published maps and institutional affiliations.

2. Overview of Contribution

Fraiwan and Faouri [1] used deep transfer learning for the automatic detection and classification of skin cancer. Al Mudawi and Alazeb [2] presented an astute way to predict cervical cancer with machine learning (ML) algorithms. AlSaeed and Omar [3] proposed a pre-trained convolutional neural network (CNN) deep learning model (ResNet50) as an automatic feature extraction method for diagnosing Alzheimer's disease from magnetic resonance imaging (MRI). Yasser et al. [4] described a novel framework that can detect diabetic retinopathy (DR) from optical coherence tomography angiography (OCTA) based on capturing the appearance and morphological markers of the retinal vascular system. Holubiac et al. [5] discussed the effect of a strength-training protocol on bone mineral density for postmenopausal women with osteopenia/osteoporosis assessed by dual-energy X-ray absorptiometry (DEXA). Ayyad et al. [6] proposed a new framework for the precise identification of prostatic adenocarcinoma from two imaging modalities.

Tariq et al. [7] proposed a novel feature-based fusion network called FDC-FS for classifying heart and lung sounds. ElNakieb et al. [8] provided a thorough study of implementing feature engineering tools to find discriminant insights from brain imaging of white-matter connectivity and using a machine learning framework for the accurate classification of autistic individuals. Diab et al. [9] presented a brain strategy algorithm for multiple-object tracking based on merging semantic attributes and appearance features. Fraiwan et al. [10] presented a non-contact spirometry using a mobile thermal camera and

AI regression. Ramesh et al. [11] proposed the design and implementation of an explainable deep learning 1D-CNN model for use in smart healthcare systems with general-purpose devices such as smart wearables and smartphones. Liang et al. [12] developed a new flow sensor-based suction index from a measured pump flow (SIMPF) control strategy for rotary left ventricular assist devices (LVADs) to provide adequate cardiac output and prevent left ventricle (LV) suction.

Al-Mohannadi et al. [13] proposed a deep-learning-based approach to apply semantic segmentation for the intima-media complex (IMC) and to calculate the cIMT measurement. Alshboul and Fraiwan [14] developed an algorithm to count the number of chews in eating video recordings using discrete wavelet decomposition and low pass filtration. Hammouda et al. [15] introduced a deep learning-based CAD system to classify the grade groups (GG) system using digitized prostate biopsy specimens (PBSs) using pyramidal CNN, with patch- and pixel-wise classifications. Ahmad et al. [16] provided proof-of-principle for an optical-based, quick, simple, and sensitive screening technology for the detection of SARS-CoV-2, utilizing antigen-antibody binding interactions. Fournelle et al. [17] developed a new mobile ultrasound device for long-term and automated bladder monitoring without user interaction consisting of 32 transmit and receive electronic components as well as a 32-element, phased array, 3 MHz transducer. Khasawneh et al. [18] customized and pre-trained deep learning models based on convolutional neural networks were used to detect pneumonia caused by COVID-19 respiratory complications. Al Ahmad et al. [19] presented a novel immunophenotyping technique using electrical characterization to differentiate between the following two most important cell types of the innate immune system: dendritic cells (DCs) and macrophages (MACs).

Haweel et al. [20] proposed a novel CAD framework to classify 50 autism spectrum disorder (ASD) and 50 typically developed toddlers with the adoption of CNN deep networks. The CAD system includes both local and global diagnosis in a response to speech task. Sharafeldeen et al. [21] presented a new segmentation technique for delineating the lung region in 3D computed tomography (CT) images. To accurately model the distribution of Hounsfield scale values within both chest and lung regions, a new probabilistic model is developed that depends on a linear combination of Gaussians (LCG). Haggag et al. [22] proposed a novel framework for the automatic quantification of the vitreous on optical coherence tomography (OCT) with application for use in the grading of vitreous inflammation. The proposed pipeline consists of two stages, vitreous region segmentation followed by a neural network classifier. In the first stage, the vitreous region is automatically segmented using a U-net CNN (U-CNN). El-Gamal et al. [23] developed a personalized, cortical region-based CAD system that helps visualize the severity of Alzheimer's disease (AD) in different local brain regions. Shehata et al. [24] developed a comprehensive CAD system for the early assessment of renal cancer tumors. The CAD system identifies and integrates the optimal discriminating morphological, textural, and functional features that best describe the malignancy status of a given renal tumor. Alwateer et al. [25] introduced a novel approach for processing healthcare data and predicting useful information with minimum computational cost, using a hybrid algorithm that consists of two phases.

Wagner et al. [26] compared a medical-grade electrocardiography (ECG) system with an ECG sensor of the low-cost DiY (Do-it-Yourself) hardware toolkit BITalino. Their results showed that the BITalino system can be considered as an equivalent recording device for stationary ECG recordings in psychophysiological experiments. Naglah et al. [27] proposed a novel multimodal MRI-based CAD system that differentiates malignant from benign thyroid nodules, based on a novel CNN-based texture learning architecture. Alyoubi et al. [28] proposed a screening system for DR fundus image classification and lesions Localization to help ophthalmologists determine the patients' DR stage. Abdelmaksoud et al. [29] developed a CAD system that detects and identifies prostate cancer from diffusion-weighted imaging (DWI). The identification of prostate cancer was achieved using two previously trained CNN models (AlexNet and VGGNet) that were fed with the estimated ADC maps of the segmented prostate regions. Jo et al. [30] introduced a novel customized optical imaging system for human conjunctiva with deep learning-based segmentation and motion correction. The image segmentation process was performed by the Attention-UNet structure to achieve high-performance segmentation results in conjunctiva images with motion blur.

Dghim et al. [31] evaluated two different strategies of the automatic detection and recognition of Nosema cells from microscopic images and achieved the identification of a robust and successful methodology for automated identification and recognition of Nosema cells versus the other existing objects in the same microscopic images. Hasnul et al. [32] presented a review on emotion recognition research that adopted electrocardiograms as a unimodal approach as well as part of a multimodal approach for emotion-recognition systems. Ayyad et al. [33] presented a literature review of the use of histopathology images and its challenges in detecting prostate cancer, studying different steps of the histopathology image analysis methodology. Santos et al. [34] proposed a new approach based on image-processing techniques, data augmentation, transfer learning, and deep neural networks to assist in the medical diagnosis of fundus lesions.

We express our heartfelt thanks to all the authors for their contributions. We also thank the reviewers for volunteering their time to provide insightful comments and criticism on the submissions. Finally, we appreciate the support of the Editorial Board and Editorial Office of *MDPI Sensors* for making this Special Issue possible.

Funding: This research received no external funding.

Institutional Review Board Statement: Not applicable.

Informed Consent Statement: Not applicable.

Data Availability Statement: Not applicable.

Conflicts of Interest: The authors declare no conflict of interest.

References

1. Fraiwan, M.; Faouri, E. On the Automatic Detection and Classification of Skin Cancer Using Deep Transfer Learning. *Sensors* **2022**, *22*, 4963. [CrossRef] [PubMed]
2. Al Mudawi, N.; Alazeb, A. A Model for Predicting Cervical Cancer Using Machine Learning Algorithms. *Sensors* **2022**, *22*, 4132. [CrossRef] [PubMed]
3. AlSaeed, D.; Omar, S.F. Brain MRI Analysis for Alzheimer's Disease Diagnosis Using CNN-Based Feature Extraction and Machine Learning. *Sensors* **2022**, *22*, 2911. [CrossRef]
4. Yasser, I.; Khalifa, F.; Abdeltawab, H.; Ghazal, M.; Sandhu, H.S.; El-Baz, A. Automated Diagnosis of Optical Coherence Tomography Angiography (OCTA) Based on Machine Learning Techniques. *Sensors* **2022**, *22*, 2342. [CrossRef]
5. Holubiac, I.Ş.; Leuciuc, F.V.; Crăciun, D.M.; Dobrescu, T. Effect of Strength Training Protocol on Bone Mineral Density for Postmenopausal Women with Osteopenia/Osteoporosis Assessed by Dual-Energy X-ray Absorptiometry (DEXA). *Sensors* **2022**, *22*, 1904. [CrossRef] [PubMed]
6. Ayyad, S.M.; Badawy, M.A.; Shehata, M.; Alksas, A.; Mahmoud, A.; Abou El-Ghar, M.; Ghazal, M.; El-Melegy, M.; Abdel-Hamid, N.B.; Labib, L.M.; et al. A New Framework for Precise Identification of Prostatic Adenocarcinoma. *Sensors* **2022**, *22*, 1848. [CrossRef] [PubMed]
7. Tariq, Z.; Shah, S.K.; Lee, Y. Feature-Based Fusion Using CNN for Lung and Heart Sound Classification. *Sensors* **2022**, *22*, 1521. [CrossRef] [PubMed]
8. ElNakieb, Y.; Ali, M.T.; Elnakib, A.; Shalaby, A.; Soliman, A.; Mahmoud, A.; Ghazal, M.; Barnes, G.N.; El-Baz, A. The Role of Diffusion Tensor MR Imaging (DTI) of the Brain in Diagnosing Autism Spectrum Disorder: Promising Results. *Sensors* **2021**, *21*, 8171. [CrossRef] [PubMed]
9. Diab, M.S.; Elhosseini, M.A.; El-Sayed, M.S.; Ali, H.A. Brain Strategy Algorithm for Multiple Object Tracking Based on Merging Semantic Attributes and Appearance Features. *Sensors* **2021**, *21*, 7604. [CrossRef] [PubMed]
10. Fraiwan, L.; Khasawneh, N.; Lweesy, K.; Elbalki, M.; Almarzooqi, A.; Abu Hamra, N. Non-Contact Spirometry Using a Mobile Thermal Camera and AI Regression. *Sensors* **2021**, *21*, 7574. [CrossRef] [PubMed]
11. Ramesh, J.; Solatidehkordi, Z.; Aburukba, R.; Sagahyroon, A. Atrial Fibrillation Classification with Smart Wearables Using Short-Term Heart Rate Variability and Deep Convolutional Neural Networks. *Sensors* **2021**, *21*, 7233. [CrossRef] [PubMed]
12. Liang, L.; Qin, K.; El-Baz, A.S.; Roussel, T.J.; Sethu, P.; Giridharan, G.A.; Wang, Y. A Flow Sensor-Based Suction-Index Control Strategy for Rotary Left Ventricular Assist Devices. *Sensors* **2021**, *21*, 6890. [CrossRef] [PubMed]

13. Al-Mohannadi, A.; Al-Maadeed, S.; Elharrouss, O.; Sadasivuni, K.K. Encoder-Decoder Architecture for Ultrasound IMC Segmentation and cIMT Measurement. *Sensors* **2021**, *21*, 6839. [CrossRef]
14. Alshboul, S.; Fraiwan, M. Determination of Chewing Count from Video Recordings Using Discrete Wavelet Decomposition and Low Pass Filtration. *Sensors* **2021**, *21*, 6806. [CrossRef] [PubMed]
15. Hammouda, K.; Khalifa, F.; El-Melegy, M.; Ghazal, M.; Darwish, H.E.; Abou El-Ghar, M.; El-Baz, A. A Deep Learning Pipeline for Grade Groups Classification Using Digitized Prostate Biopsy Specimens. *Sensors* **2021**, *21*, 6708. [CrossRef] [PubMed]
16. Ahmad, M.A.; Mustafa, F.; Panicker, N.; Rizvi, T.A. Optical Detection of SARS-CoV-2 Utilizing Antigen-Antibody Binding Interactions. *Sensors* **2021**, *21*, 6596. [CrossRef]
17. Fournelle, M.; Grün, T.; Speicher, D.; Weber, S.; Yilmaz, M.; Schoeb, D.; Miernik, A.; Reis, G.; Tretbar, S.; Hewener, H. Portable Ultrasound Research System for Use in Automated Bladder Monitoring with Machine-Learning-Based Segmentation. *Sensors* **2021**, *21*, 6481. [CrossRef]
18. Khasawneh, N.; Fraiwan, M.; Fraiwan, L.; Khassawneh, B.; Ibnian, A. Detection of COVID-19 from Chest X-ray Images Using Deep Convolutional Neural Networks. *Sensors* **2021**, *21*, 5940. [CrossRef]
19. Al Ahmad, M.; Nasser, R.A.; Olule, L.J.A.; Ali, B.R. Electrical Detection of Innate Immune Cells. *Sensors* **2021**, *21*, 5886. [CrossRef]
20. Haweel, R.; Seada, N.; Ghoniemy, S.; Alghamdi, N.S.; El-Baz, A. A CNN Deep Local and Global ASD Classification Approach with Continuous Wavelet Transform Using Task-Based FMRI. *Sensors* **2021**, *21*, 5822. [CrossRef]
21. Sharafeldeen, A.; Elsharkawy, M.; Alghamdi, N.S.; Soliman, A.; El-Baz, A. Precise Segmentation of COVID-19 Infected Lung from CT Images Based on Adaptive First-Order Appearance Model with Morphological/Anatomical Constraints. *Sensors* **2021**, *21*, 5482. [CrossRef] [PubMed]
22. Haggag, S.; Khalifa, F.; Abdeltawab, H.; Elnakib, A.; Ghazal, M.; Mohamed, M.A.; Sandhu, H.S.; Alghamdi, N.S.; El-Baz, A. An Automated CAD System for Accurate Grading of Uveitis Using Optical Coherence Tomography Images. *Sensors* **2021**, *21*, 5457. [CrossRef]
23. El-Gamal, F.E.-Z.A.; Elmogy, M.; Mahmoud, A.; Shalaby, A.; Switala, A.E.; Ghazal, M.; Soliman, H.; Atwan, A.; Alghamdi, N.S.; Barnes, G.N.; et al. A Personalized Computer-Aided Diagnosis System for Mild Cognitive Impairment (MCI) Using Structural MRI (sMRI). *Sensors* **2021**, *21*, 5416. [CrossRef] [PubMed]
24. Shehata, M.; Alksas, A.; Abouelkheir, R.T.; Elmahdy, A.; Shaffie, A.; Soliman, A.; Ghazal, M.; Abu Khalifeh, H.; Salim, R.; Abdel Razek, A.A.K.; et al. A Comprehensive Computer-Assisted Diagnosis System for Early Assessment of Renal Cancer Tumors. *Sensors* **2021**, *21*, 4928. [CrossRef]
25. Alwateer, M.; Almars, A.M.; Areed, K.N.; Elhosseini, M.A.; Haikal, A.Y.; Badawy, M. Ambient Healthcare Approach with Hybrid Whale Optimization Algorithm and Naïve Bayes Classifier. *Sensors* **2021**, *21*, 4579. [CrossRef] [PubMed]
26. Wagner, R.E.; Plácido da Silva, H.; Gramann, K. Validation of a Low-Cost Electrocardiography (ECG) System for Psychophysiological Research. *Sensors* **2021**, *21*, 4485. [CrossRef]
27. Naglah, A.; Khalifa, F.; Khaled, R.; Abdel Razek, A.A.K.; Ghazal, M.; Giridharan, G.; El-Baz, A. Novel MRI-Based CAD System for Early Detection of Thyroid Cancer Using Multi-Input CNN. *Sensors* **2021**, *21*, 3878. [CrossRef] [PubMed]
28. Alyoubi, W.L.; Abulkhair, M.F.; Shalash, W.M. Diabetic Retinopathy Fundus Image Classification and Lesions Localization System Using Deep Learning. *Sensors* **2021**, *21*, 3704. [CrossRef] [PubMed]
29. Abdelmaksoud, I.R.; Shalaby, A.; Mahmoud, A.; Elmogy, M.; Aboelfetouh, A.; Abou El-Ghar, M.; El-Melegy, M.; Alghamdi, N.S.; El-Baz, A. Precise Identification of Prostate Cancer from DWI Using Transfer Learning. *Sensors* **2021**, *21*, 3664. [CrossRef]
30. Jo, H.-C.; Jeong, H.; Lee, J.; Na, K.-S.; Kim, D.-Y. Quantification of Blood Flow Velocity in the Human Conjunctival Microvessels Using Deep Learning-Based Stabilization Algorithm. *Sensors* **2021**, *21*, 3224. [CrossRef]
31. Dghim, S.; Travieso-González, C.M.; Burget, R. Analysis of the Nosema Cells Identification for Microscopic Images. *Sensors* **2021**, *21*, 3068. [CrossRef] [PubMed]
32. Hasnul, M.A.; Aziz, N.A.A.; Alelyani, S.; Mohana, M.; Aziz, A.A. Electrocardiogram-Based Emotion Recognition Systems and Their Applications in Healthcare—A Review. *Sensors* **2021**, *21*, 5015. [CrossRef]
33. Ayyad, S.M.; Shehata, M.; Shalaby, A.; Abou El-Ghar, M.; Ghazal, M.; El-Melegy, M.; Abdel-Hamid, N.B.; Labib, L.M.; Ali, H.A.; El-Baz, A. Role of AI and Histopathological Images in Detecting Prostate Cancer: A Survey. *Sensors* **2021**, *21*, 2586. [CrossRef] [PubMed]
34. Santos, C.; Aguiar, M.; Welfer, D.; Belloni, B. A New Approach for Detecting Fundus Lesions Using Image Processing and Deep Neural Network Architecture Based on YOLO Model. *Sensors* **2022**, *22*, 6441. [CrossRef] [PubMed]

sensors

MDPI

Review

Role of AI and Histopathological Images in Detecting Prostate Cancer: A Survey

Sarah M. Ayyad [1], Mohamed Shehata [2], Ahmed Shalaby [2], Mohamed Abou El-Ghar [3], Mohammed Ghazal [4], Moumen El-Melegy [5], Nahla B. Abdel-Hamid [1], Labib M. Labib [1], H. Arafat Ali [1] and Ayman El-Baz [2,*]

1 Computers and Systems Department, Faculty of Engineering, Mansoura University, Mansoura 35511, Egypt; sarah.aiyad@gmail.com (S.M.A.); nahla_bishri@mans.edu.eg (N.B.A.-H.); labibm@hotmail.com (L.M.L.); h.arafat_ali@mans.edu.eg (H.A.A.)
2 BioImaging Laboratory, Bioengineering Department, University of Louisville, Louisville, KY 40292, USA; mohamed.shehata@louisville.edu (M.S.); ahmed.shalaby@louisville.edu (A.S.)
3 Department of Radiology, Urology and Nephrology Center, Mansoura University, Mansoura 35516, Egypt; maboelghar@yahoo.com
4 Department of Electrical and Computer Engineering, College of Engineering, Abu Dhabi University, Abu Dhabi 59911, United Arab Emirates; mohammed.ghazal@adu.ac.ae
5 Department of Electrical Engineering, Assiut University, Assiut 71511, Egypt; moumen@aun.edu.eg
* Correspondence: aselba01@louisville.edu

Abstract: Prostate cancer is one of the most identified cancers and second most prevalent among cancer-related deaths of men worldwide. Early diagnosis and treatment are substantial to stop or handle the increase and spread of cancer cells in the body. Histopathological image diagnosis is a gold standard for detecting prostate cancer as it has different visual characteristics but interpreting those type of images needs a high level of expertise and takes too much time. One of the ways to accelerate such an analysis is by employing artificial intelligence (AI) through the use of computer-aided diagnosis (CAD) systems. The recent developments in artificial intelligence along with its sub-fields of conventional machine learning and deep learning provide new insights to clinicians and researchers, and an abundance of research is presented specifically for histopathology images tailored for prostate cancer. However, there is a lack of comprehensive surveys that focus on prostate cancer using histopathology images. In this paper, we provide a very comprehensive review of most, if not all, studies that handled the prostate cancer diagnosis using histopathological images. The survey begins with an overview of histopathological image preparation and its challenges. We also briefly review the computing techniques that are commonly applied in image processing, segmentation, feature selection, and classification that can help in detecting prostate malignancies in histopathological images.

Keywords: prostate cancer; image processing; histopathology images; digital image analysis; computational pathology; artificial intelligence

Citation: Ayyad, S.M.; Shehata, M.; Shalaby, A.; Abou El-Ghar, M.; Ghazal, M.; El-Melegy, M.; Abdel-Hamid, N.B.; Labib, L.M.; Ali, H.A.; El-Baz, A. Role of AI and Histopathological Images in Detecting Prostate Cancer: A Survey. *Sensors* **2021**, *21*, 2586. https://doi.org/10.3390/s21082586

Academic Editor: Evangelia I. Zacharaki

Received: 5 February 2021
Accepted: 4 April 2021
Published: 7 April 2021

1. Introduction

Prostate cancer is one of the most common cancers all over the world and considered the second cause of cancer deaths in several countries [1,2]. Nearly one in seven men will be identified to have prostate cancer throughout his life [3,4]. In recent times, statistics show the number of new patients only identified in the United States for 2021 with prostate cancer is nearly 248,530 and the number of deaths is nearly 34,130 [5], so prostate cancer represents a serious healthcare problem in the United States as in many countries. Most tumors do not induce serious clinical symptoms, hence early detection, and localization of prostate cancer at a curable stage is significant for making a medical decision in men with prostate cancer [6].

Because of the lack of progress in the medical field, prostate cancer is increasing as one of the most endemic diseases in the world. The large developments in computing technologies and hardware abilities offer the capability of using computing to tackle issues in many areas. The medical domain is one such area where nowadays a judicious use of technology can assist in improving people's health and to help in tasks including diagnosis. Medical imaging techniques such as computed tomography (CT), X-rays, magnetic resonance imaging (MRI) and ultrasound imaging (sonography) are great models of computing applications reliant on images, some examples of medical images are displayed in Figure 1. In addition to all of these types of images, histopathology images (HI) are another type of medical image that considered a golden standard to detect cancer and we will focus on it in this survey. HI can be obtained by tissue microscopy from biopsies that help pathologists analyze the characteristics of tissues in a cell basis and study cancer growth [7]. In recent years, many studies have been conducted to capture the entire slide with a scanner and save it as a digital image [8]. The word histopathology derives from the Greek *histos* (web [in this case, of tissue]), *pathos* (suffering or disease), and *logos* (study) [9].

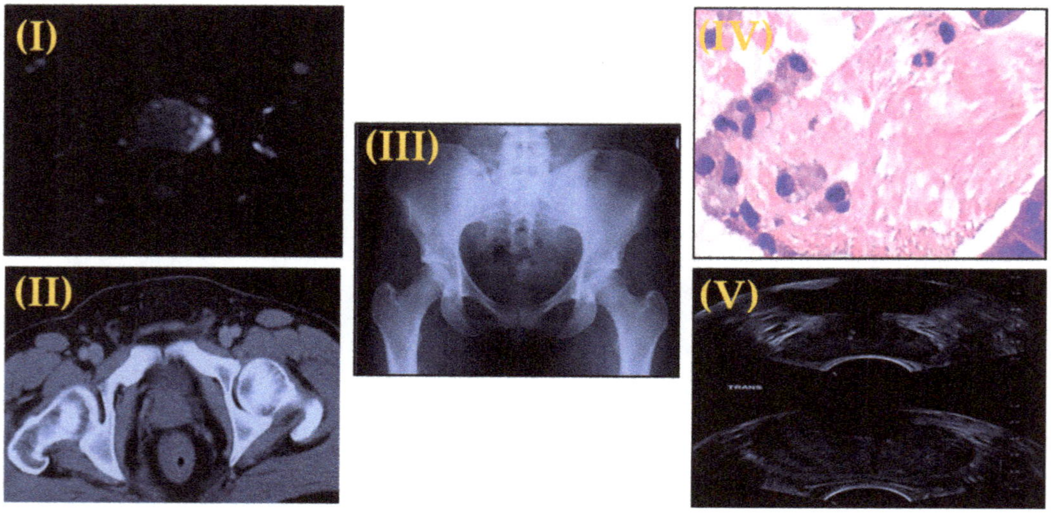

Figure 1. Different Types of Medical Images (**I**) MRI image of prostate, (**II**) CT image of prostate, (**III**) X-Ray image of prostate pelvic area, (**IV**) Histopathological image of prostate tissue, and (**V**) Ultrasound for prostate biopsy.

In recent years, computer-aided diagnosis (CAD) has become the main player in radiological detection, diagnosis, and management of diseases [8,10]. Nowadays, computer-aided diagnosis has become a factor of common clinical diagnosis procedures for cancer detection through the use of histopathological images at medical centers and consequently it has become one of the most major topics in histopathological imaging and diagnosis process [11]. There is a substantial requirement for CAD systems to reduce human errors. Human errors happen because of many reasons including lack of expertise or errors caused from image overlapping, blurring, noise, and weak edge detection. Furthermore, observation of the cells specifically composed of visualizing tiny structures, functions, composition, cellular distribution, and cellular morphology across the tissue, which assists pathologists to make a decision of whether the cells are normal and cancerous [11]. This manual process is very time-consuming, difficult, requires a great deal of experience, and leads to variability in diagnosis. Therefore, CAD is a good choice for pathologists for the development in the improvement of histopathological image precision, segmentation of tumor parts, and classification of disease [11]. The literature shows a plethora of CAD systems applied to histopathological images.

In general, artificial intelligence (AI) has shown a significant growth in medical health applications and in histopathology imagery provides a breeding ground for the expansion of CAD systems [12]. AI and CAD systems will continue to grow among researchers and clinicians to constitute a prognostic set of tools to enable them to detect patients that are susceptible to a specific disease and provide accurate, cheap, and fast technologies [12,13]. AI is an umbrella term encompassing both traditional machine learning (ML), and deep learning (DL). The research we consider in our study is largely categorized as ML-based techniques and DL-based techniques. Conventional machine learning techniques applied in HI analysis typically involve several preprocessing steps, including feature selection, image segmentation and classification. ML techniques have been reviewed extensively in the literature, for instance in [2,14–22]. In the last decade, researchers have turned their focus towards the development of new deep learning techniques as they outperform conventional machine learning techniques in diverse fields and not only HI image analysis. To date, many of these ML techniques have been supplanted by DL, and an abundance of work has evaluated the use of deep learning techniques on HI of prostate cancer [23–33]. Moreover, studies that employ an ensemble of DL techniques and ML techniques gave better results [34]. Table 1 summarizes reviewed papers on prostate cancer detection and diagnosis. One of the main constraints in conventional ML techniques is their training with a limited number of features, which has been overcome in DL techniques where hundreds to thousands of features can be selected from digital images for classification; however, this process requires significant amount of training time [35]. Some of these problems are solved in ensemble techniques as the feature extraction stage is done using pretrained deep networks and samples classified using conventional ML classifiers [35].

Table 1. A brief comparison between previous studies that proposed techniques for prostate histopathology images.

Reference	Study Aim	Year	Strength	Weakness	Number of Patients
[2]	Automated classification using AdaBoost-based Ensemble Learning	2016	They integrated various feature descriptors, different color channels, and classifiers.	The algorithm able to discover only the critical regions on the digital slides	50
[14]	A novel technique of labeling individual glands as malignant or benign was proposed.	2013	The technique can detect individual malignant gland units without relying on the neighboring histology and/or the spatial extent of the cancer.	It applied on a small number of radical prostatectomy patients	8
[15]	Methodology for automated gland and nuclei segmentation	2008	They incorporate low-, high-level knowledge, and structural constraints imposed via domain knowledge.	They focused on a smaller cohort of cancer images and the dataset is private	44
[16]	A new automated method for gland segmentation	2017	This method texture- and gland structure-based methods	The method failed in the images with the cribriform pattern. They validated data using 2-fold cross validation	10
[17]	Multistage Segmentation Using Sample Entropy Texture Analysis	2020	An added advantage of performing multistage segmentation using sample entropy values is that one could easily separate epithelial nuclei from the stroma nuclei in standard H&E stained images without using any additional immunohistochemical (IHC) markers.	It requires identifying sample entropy features	25

Table 1. *Cont.*

Reference	Study Aim	Year	Strength	Weakness	Number of Patients
[18]	A new approach to identify prostate cancer areas in complex	2014	It utilizes the differential information embedded in the intensity characteristics of H&E images to quickly classify areas of the prostate tissue	Classification performance is tested using only KNN algorithm	20
[19]	Ensemble based system for feature selection and classification	2011	They addressed the possibility of missing tumor regions through the use of tile-based probabilities and heat maps.	They focused only on texture feature selection and not used a voting schema for the ensemble classifier to enhance the probability scores	14
[20]	A novel fully automated CAD system	2006	The proposed system represents the first attempt to automatically analyse histopathology across multiple scales	Their system trained using only 3 images	6
[21]	A new multiclass approach	2018	It obtained improved grading results	It was evaluated based on its impact on the performance of the ensemble framework only	213
[22]	A bag-of-words approach to classify images using SpeededUp Robust Features (SURF)	2016	The drawbacks of scale-invariant feature transform descriptor is overcome by the SURF descriptors causing an enhanced output accuracy	More features needed to be integrated with their feature extraction process to enhance accuracy of the classification	75
[23]	An automatic method for segmentation and classification (Integration of Salp Swarm Optimization Algorithm and Rider Optimization Algorithm)	2019	Less time complexity	The maximal accuracy, sensitivity, and specificity does not exceed 90%	20
[24]	A new region-based convolutional neural network framework for multi-task prediction	2018	The model achieved a detection accuracy 99.07% with an average area under the curve of 0.998	They didn't have patient-level information with which to perform a more rigorous patient-level stratification.	40
[25]	An approach to nuclei segmentation using a conditional generative adversarial network	2019	It enforces higher-order consistency and captures better results when compared to conventional CNN models.	The model trained on small annotated patches	34
[26]	Deep neural network algorithm for segmentation of individual nuclei	2019	A simple, fast, and parameter-free postprocessing procedure is done to get the final segmented nuclei as one 1000 × 1000 image can be segmented in less than 5 s.	The model is trained on a small number of images and has been tested on the images that may have different appearances	30

Table 1. *Cont.*

Reference	Study Aim	Year	Strength	Weakness	Number of Patients
[27]	Two novel approaches (combination of 4 types of feature descriptors, advanced machine-learning classifiers) to automatically identify prostate cancer	2019	They apply for the first time on prostate segmented glands, deep-learning algorithms modifying the popular VGG19 neural network.	The hand-driven learning approach employs SVM, where selecting the suitable kernel function could be tricky	35
[28]	Automated Gleason grading via deep learning	2018	The study showed promising results especially for cases with heterogeneous Gleason patterns	The model trained on small mini patches at each iteration	886
[29]	A deep learning system using the U-Net	2019	The system outperformed 10 out of 15 pathologists	The system was built upon three pretrained preprocessing modules, each of which still required pixel-wise annotations.	1243
[30]	Predicting Gleason Score Using OverFeat Trained Deep CNN as feature extractor	2016	It is quite effective, even without from-scratch training on WSI tiles. Processing time is low	Small size of patches	213
[31]	CNN to idiomatically identify the features	2016	The system is not constrained to H&E stained images and could easily be applied to immunohistochemistry	Some detection errors happen at the boundaries of the tissue	254
[32]	DL model to detect cancer based on NASNetLarge architecture and high-quality annotated training dataset	2020	The model demonstrated its strong ability in prediction as accuracy attained 98%	The availability of fully digitalized cohorts represents a bottleneck	400
[33]	A novel benchmark was designed for measuring and comparing the performances of different CNN models with the proposed PROMETEO	2021	Average processing time is less compared to other architectures	The network validated on 3-fold cross-validation method	470
[34]	Novel features that include spatial inter-nuclei statistics and intra-nuclei properties for discriminating high-grade prostate cancer patterns	2018	The system tackled the inter-observer variability in prostate grading and can lead to a consensus-based training that improves both classification	lack examples of the highest grades of disease	56

Many surveys have been published in recent years reviewing histopathological image analysis covering its history, and detailed information of general artificial intelligence techniques [7,8,12,31,36–42]; the main limitation is the lack of comprehensive surveys of histopathological image analysis that focus on prostate cancer [1,43,44]. Accordingly, in this survey we present more prostate histopathology from an image analysis point of view. The main goal of this survey is providing readers a comprehensive overview of the state-of-the-art in terms of image analysis and artificial intelligence techniques i.e., machine learning, and deep learning being tailored specifically for histopathology images in prostate cancer, and its challenges specific to histopathology images analysis, and the future scope. This survey mentions 113 related works, comprising 63 papers that concentrate on prostate cancer. Figure 2 depicts a statistical distribution of studies used in this survey.

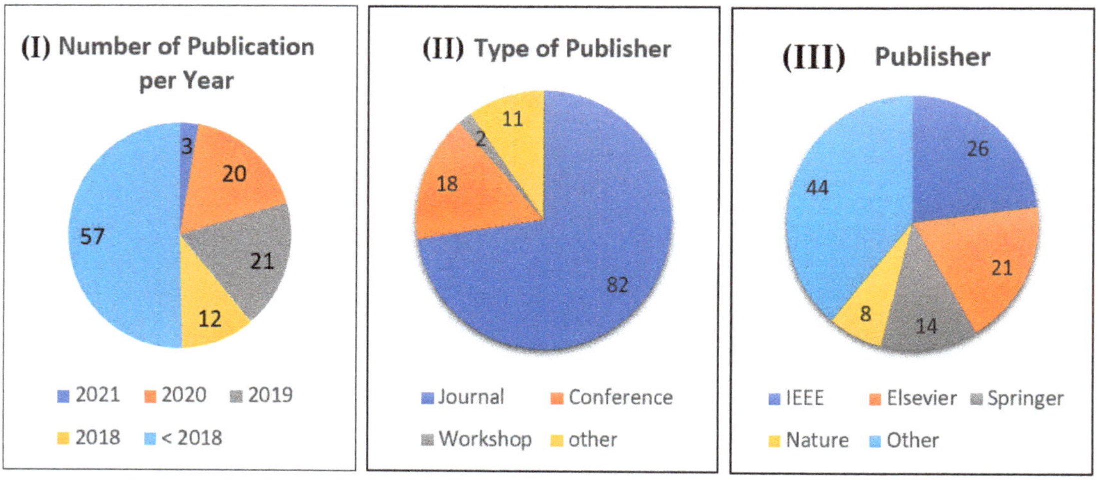

Figure 2. Statistical distribution of studies used in this survey. (**I**) Number of studies per year; (**II**) Type of Publisher, where other denotes a preprint or URL; (**III**) Publisher, where other includes MDPI, Frontiers, AVES, etc.

The selection methodology of our survey was conducted using the well-known academic search engines including IEEE Xplore, Google Scholar, Science Direct, Springer, ACM Digital Library, and ResearchGate. We have employed the following criteria: (I) The paper must be highly related to the research area; (II) papers published in highly rank journals and conferences of relevant domain, such as *Scientific Reports, Expert Systems with Applications, IEEE Transactions on Medical Imaging, Neurocomputing, Journal of Pathology Informatics*, etc. and conferences, such as the International Symposium on Biomedical Imaging, IEEE International Symposium on Biomedical Imaging, International Conference on Machine Vision, etc. (III) Top cited papers are preferred. (IV) Papers that were published within the last 5 years, although we also include papers published before that time if the paper is of high quality. Meanwhile, we ignored many papers that have inadequate criteria including low-quality papers, non-English written papers, and white papers.

This survey is organized as follows: Section 2 introduces a background of histopathology images, their preparation, and challenges. Section 3 focuses on the whole histopathology image analysis methodology and highlights the various methods used for this methodology. Finally, we provide some concluding remarks and present some future possibilities in Section 4.

2. Histopathology Images Background

Histopathology is a significant branch of biology that covers the investigation of the cell anatomy and tissues of organisms at a microscopic level by a histopathologist [45]. Histopathological images are very influential for the final decision procedure of effective therapeutics; these images are essential to investigate the status of a certain biological structure and to diagnose diseases like cancer [39,45]. Digital histopathology represents a significant evolution in modern medicine [46]. It often uses machine vision techniques as a basis. Nevertheless, because of the special properties of digital histopathology images and their processing tasks, specific processing approaches are usually needed. In this survey, we describe the application of histopathology image analysis employing machine learning and deep learning techniques.

Uropathologists use different screening methods to determine the various tumor histology in the prostate in a good quality. Typical tissue of prostate incorporates glands and stroma. The gland is the basic anatomical structural unit of the prostate. The stroma is the fibromuscular tissue around glands [14]. Each gland unit consists of a lumen and rows of epithelial layers surrounding the lumen. The stroma keeps the gland units together. When cancer is in high-grade, stroma and lumen are both replaced by epithelial cells [24]. Once the slides are stained using a hematoxylin and eosin (H&E) solution, the nuclei become dark blue and the epithelial layer and stroma become several shades of purple to pink [14].

To date, one of the most effective ways to measure aggressiveness of prostate cancer is using the Gleason grading system [24,43,47]. The Gleason grading system is completely founded on architectural arrangements of prostatic carcinoma, and a substantial parameter to a therapeutic final decision. Gleason grading has five grade groups from grade 1 (G1) to grade 5 (G5), with a grade of G1 refers to tissue with a maximum grade of resemblance to normal tissue and outstanding prognosis, and a grade of G5 refers to poorly differentiated tissue and the worst prediction [24,29]. Artificial intelligence has the ability to improve the quality of Gleason grading. Abundant automated Gleason grading systems were proposed and have led to increased consistency [28–30,34,48–51].

Histopathology images can be acquired by using specialized cameras with a microscope wherein an automated computerized approach can be carried out [9]. To study various architecture and constituent of tissues under a microscope, the biopsy specimen is embedded in wax and dyed with one or more stains. Staining procedures are used by pathologists for cellular components separation for structural in addition to component visualization of tissue for diagnosis [38]. Stages of the preparation process of the tissue slides are as presented in Figure 3. It consists of five operations, and each of them can affect the quality of the final image [38,45]. (I) Fixation: Samples of biological tissues are fixed with chemical fixation. There are many ways of fixation, but the commonly applied way in the biomedical field is fixation with formaldehyde or glutaraldehyde solution to protect the cells [51]. This is a critical step in tissue preparation and aims to prevent tissue autolysis and putrefaction; (II) Processing: Tissue processing is a crucial step and involves two main processes: dehydration and clearing. Dehydration is used to extract water from the gross tissue and substitute it with a certain concentration of alcohol which solidifies it [52]. This process helps incise superfine sections of the specimen. Clearing consists of removing the dehydrator with a material that will be the solvent in both the embedding paraffin and the dehydrating agent; (III) Tissue Embedding: Thus is the process wherein tissues are carefully positioned in a medium such as wax [51], so when solidified, it will provide enough external support to allow very thin sectioning. This process is essential as the proper tissue orientation is necessary for precise microscopic evaluation; (IV) Sectioning: this process is required to generate superfine slices of tissue samples sufficient such that the details of the microstructure characterization of the cells can be obviously noticed using microscopy methods. After that, carry the superfine slices of sample onto a clean glass slide [38]; (V) Staining: The final step in preparing tissue for light microscopy is to stain it and mount it on the slide. Staining increases contrast to the tissue and, also highlights some specific features which would otherwise be practically invisible in the microscope [38]. There are many types of stain but the most common type of staining for histology is H & E.

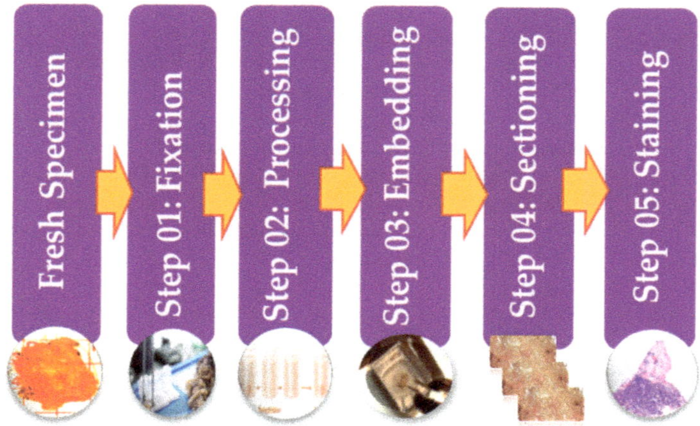

Figure 3. Illustrative figure showing the different preparation steps of histology slides.

2.1. Diagnostic Challenges Using Histopathological Images

Automated prostate cancer diagnosis using histopathology images is deemed to offer great promise for advanced cancer therapy, however, it is not a simple task, as several open scientific challenges have to be overcome before the CAD system of histopathology images can become part of the routine healthcare diagnostic pipeline. These challenges occur because of the numerous technical and computational variabilities and artifacts incurred due to differences in slide preparation and because of the complicated structure of the tumor tissues architecture [41]. Image analysis techniques are substantially reliant on the quality of the digital slide images. In the following paragraphs, we will discuss the different challenges of histopathology image analysis and computational techniques to deal with them.

2.1.1. Extremely Large Image Size

These days, one of the growing challenges is how to handle the extremely large size of histopathology image datasets [53]. Whenever images, for example, cars, humans, or animals are classified using artificial intelligence techniques, small images such as 512×512 pixels are usually applied as an input [54,55]. Large-sized images usually have to be rescaled into a smaller size, which is adequate for differentiation, as increasing the size of the input image will result in increased computational complexity, thus making the analysis process more challenging and time-consuming. On the contrary, histopathology images contain as many as hundreds of thousands to millions of pixels, which is generally laborious to analyze as is. Nevertheless, rescaling the whole image to a lower dimension such as 512×512 may cause loss of information at the cellular level, which leads to a marked drop of the identification accuracy. Thus, the whole histopathology image is often divided into partial regions of about 1024×1024 pixels called patches, where each patch is examined apart, such as detecting region-of-interests [56]. Thus, many studies such as [16,24–27,48,57,58] presented in this survey, especially those dealing with deep learning applied patching technique to overcome the extremely large histopathological images.

2.1.2. Insufficient Labeled Images

Perhaps the biggest challenge in analyzing histopathological images is that only a limited number of training set data is available. As healthcare image datasets often have a considerably lower size than a natural view of images, this causes direct application of many conventional artificial intelligence techniques not suitable for medical image datasets [53]. One of the important keys of success of DL in common image recognition tasks is the abundance of training data. Label information at a pixel level or a patch level is essential in histopathology image tasks such as diagnosis. Label information could be collected easily in common image processing from the internet and it is also possible to use crowdsourced labeling since the human brain is able to identify objects and perform labelling work while ignoring artifacts [59]. Nevertheless, only highly qualified pathologists can manually label histopathological images properly, and this process at the regional level in a large histopathology image needs a long time and is tedious. Therefore, the paramount limitation in designing high-quality histopathology image analysis techniques lies in the paucity of freely public annotated datasets [24,60]. Many researchers have attempted to alleviate such a problem of insufficient amount labeled images. Most of these solutions fall under one of the following categories: (I) increasing the number of labeled data, such in [25,30], (II) predicting the labels of test images or self-taught learning, such as applying transfer learning [24,61], or (III) utilizing of weak label or unlabeled data [62].

2.1.3. Artifacts and Color Variation

Another major challenge is the presence of artifacts and color variation [8,11,36,59,63,64]. Histopathology images are captured through several stages as previously mentioned. At each stage, unwanted anomalies that are unassociated with the underlying biological factors, could be represented by differences in specimen preparation, staining, and even scanning with equipment from different vendors. For instance, when specimen sections are placed onto the slides, they may be folded and rumpled; dust may besmear the slides during scanning process; loss of microscope focus leads to blurred regions, noise, and shadows; and occasionally tissue regions are marked by color markers or chromatic aberrations [8,41]. Learning without considering these artifacts, as shown in Figure 4, may deteriorate the performance of decision support algorithms. When digital images are produced, the slides should be uniformly illuminated by the light source. Tissue autofluorescence differences in microscopic setup, staining protocol, and organ size could generate irregular lighting across the tissue samples. Additionally, the scanner's sensitivity varies for different wavelengths of the light spectrum [41]. Large variations in light are considered an important factor for the precise prostate cancer diagnosis. These variations need to be handled earlier before employing image processing techniques [63,64].

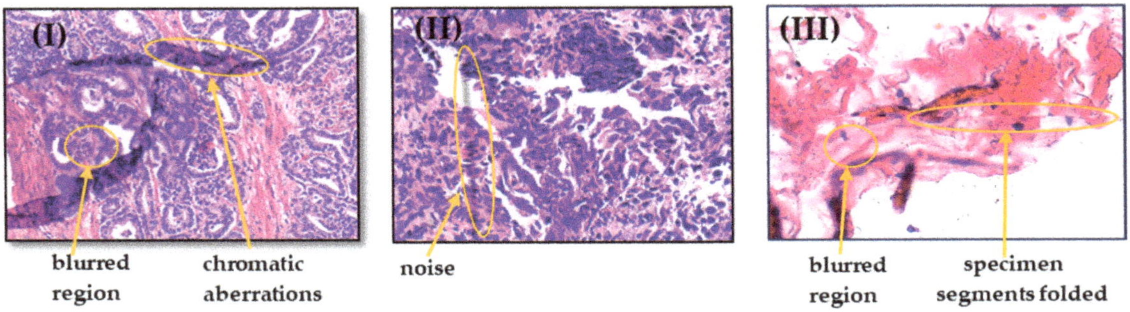

Figure 4. Examples of possible artifacts in histopathological images, where (**I**) contains chromatic aberrations and blurred regions; (**II**) contains noise, and (**III**) contains specimen segments folded and blurred regions.

To tackle these problems, many different techniques have been designed, including conversion to grayscale [65,66], color normalization [67,68], and color augmentation [69]. One of the simplest methods is the conversion of colored histopathology images to grayscale, however, it disregards the significant information concerning the color representation used by pathologists since the beginning. On the contrary, the color normalization method attempts to adapt the color values of images on a pixel-by-pixel basis so that the color distribution of the source image matches a reference image. Color separation and stain normalization were applied on the histopathology images for the first time in [70]. Afterwards several distinct color and stain normalization techniques have been used as a preprocessing step in several techniques for histopathological image analysis.

2.1.4. Multi-Level Magnification Led to Multi-Level Information

Magnification is the phenomenon of enlarging the proportion of biological structures that are apparent under the microscope based on different objective lenses [39]. Traditional microscopes have a standard set of objectives with 2X, 8X, 40X, 200X, and 400X power [39]. Tissues generally consist of cells and fibers, where each tissue shows specific cellular features. Information concerning cell shapes is taken accurately under a high power objective and images are more deterministic and informative to predict disease outcome, but structural information such as a glandular structure that are made of many cells are better taken under a lower magnification, so that images cover a wider field of view. Because malignant tissues exhibit both cellular and structural abnormalities, each of the images captured at different magnifications could provide significant information. Even in AI, researchers employing image datasets with different levels of magnifications, such as in [71,72]. As already pointed out, it is challenging to process the images at its original resolution directly, images are usually rescaled to adapt different magnifications and configured to be input for processing. Regarding diagnosis, the most informative magnification remains a subject of controversy, whereas efficiency enhancement is sometimes attained by entering both low and high magnification images simultaneously as input, probably depending on the applied AI technique or type of disease. Moreover, the status of histopathological images does not need to be determined by the cells, images with different levels of magnification are adopted to learn distinctive features [71].

As depicted in Figure 5, histopathological images with multiple levels of magnification can depict various types of information. When the histopathological images are with low magnification, cells will be difficult to detect, while the high magnification image shows more fine-grained details.

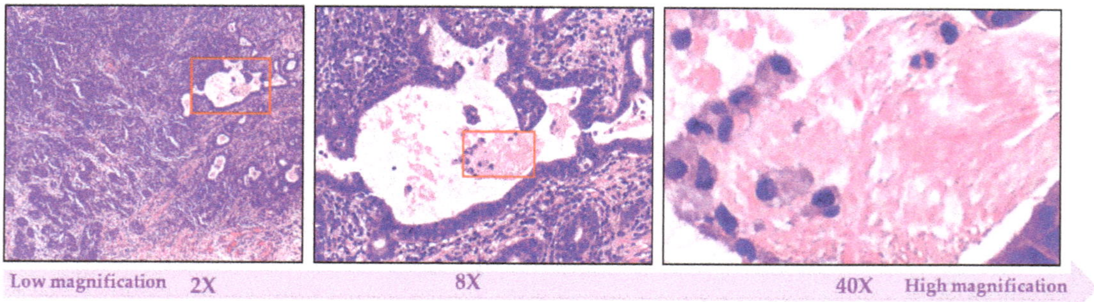

Figure 5. Illustrative figure showing the different levels of magnification (starting from 2× up to more than 40×) that might be applied on histopathological images.

3. Histopathology Image Analysis Methodology

Digitized histopathology is a current direction that makes huge numbers of images available for automated analysis. It enables visualization and interpretation of pathology cells and tissue samples in a great resolution images and with the assistance of software tools [36,37]. This opens a new era to design image analysis techniques that assist clinicians and promote their image descriptions (e.g., grading, staging) with the purpose of image features quantification. In that respect, the computer-aided diagnosis of histological image analysis is a newly challenging domain for biomedical image analysis. CAD can be defined as detecting cancer within the examined tissue using computer software [60,73,74], which is the main mission of the pathologist [8]. The combination of conventional diagnosis techniques with computational AI techniques provides a good possibility to decrease the workload of pathologists while preserving performance. There is a need for a precise CAD system that minimizes reading interpretation times, lowers necessary experience in anatomic pathology, and provides a consistent risk evaluation of cancer existence in prostate histopathology images without additional burden to pathologists. Such a CAD system would automatically find out suspected lesions in prostate histopathology images to assist screen for prostate cancer in large patient populations. A typical CAD system for detecting prostate cancer receives raw histopathological images, preprocesses them, and produces a particular diagnostic result [10].

Over the last two decades, numerous research papers on CAD systems were published. Automated systems for digital histopathological imaging can maintain reproducibility and consistency using suitable image processing techniques [41]. In fact, there are many research perspectives for CAD systems applied in the histopathological domain, including: (I) cancer detection in the given tissue, (II) automatic grading to correctly quantify the level of the malignancy, which can offer more insights into disease characterization, (III) cell/nuclei/gland segmentation that discovers and separates these regions from images, and (IV) multi-class classification for the different subtypes of a specific type of cancer.

CAD systems can be broadly subdivided into two groups. The first uses handcrafted features and relies on conventional machine learning techniques, while the second uses deep learning techniques. For this reason, we will discuss these two groups separately in Sections 3.2 and 3.3, below. Figure 6 displays the process model for handcrafted features based on machine learning techniques versus deep learning techniques of histopathological image analysis. The process model of the two groups of analysis passes through a number of stages that highlight specific structures in the image analysis methodology. There are two common components that are shared by the process model, which are image acquisition and image preprocessing.

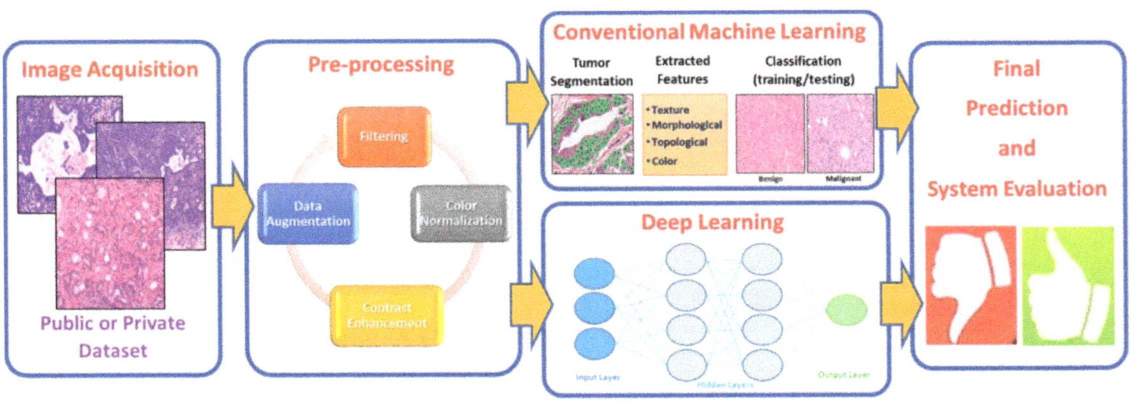

Figure 6. An illustrative block diagram of a typical prostate CAD System starting from the image acquisition until obtaining the final diagnosis.

3.1. Image Acquisition

In the first phase, histopathology images can be acquired from a public dataset or a private dataset. The choice of a dataset is a dominant factor to establish for any experimental setup. One of the main challenges when dealing with prostate histopathology images is the lack of representative public image datasets annotated by multiple pathologists with high quality. Most research dealing with prostate histopathology images work with private datasets. As shown in Table 2, we provide list of the publicly available datasets [75–79]. It is noted that PANDA challenge [78] provides the largest public histopathology image dataset in prostate cancer.

Table 2. Details of publicly available datasets containing prostate histopathology images.

Dataset	URL	Magnification	Year	Dataset Size	Number of Patients
Annotated dataset	[75]	40×	2017	4 images for training and 2 for validation	6
Prostate Fused-MRI-Pathology	[76]	20×	Last modified 2021	comprises a total of 28 3 Tesla T1-weighted, T2-weighted, Diffusion weighted and Dynamic Contrast Enhanced prostate MRI along with accompanying digitized histopathology images	28
TCGA-PRAD project	[77]	40×	Last modified 2020	It includes includes 368 digitized prostate pathology slides	14
Prostate cANcer graDe Assessment (PANDA) Challenge	[78]	20×	2020	It consists of 11.000 cases for training, 400 cases for public test set, and 400 cases for private test set	NA
PESO dataset	[79]	10×	2019	It consists of 62 case for the training set and 40 case for the testing set	102

3.2. Image Preprocessing

Preprocessing is a basic stage of most automated CAD systems [35]. In the preprocessing stage, raw data are processed to normalize the image or to transform the image to a domain where cancer can be easily diagnosed [10]. Preprocessing can enhance histopathology images and ameliorate the interpretability for human viewers since the acquired images contain different types of noises or artifacts and may not have adequate contrast or illumination due to the scanning [36,46]. It is necessary that the acquired images be of good quality to generate the intended result [40]. Appropriate image pre-processing methods could compensate for these differences between images. Various existing preprocessing methods are commonly used to boost the results of the analysis process can be grouped as illustrated in the following subsections and summarized in Figure 7.

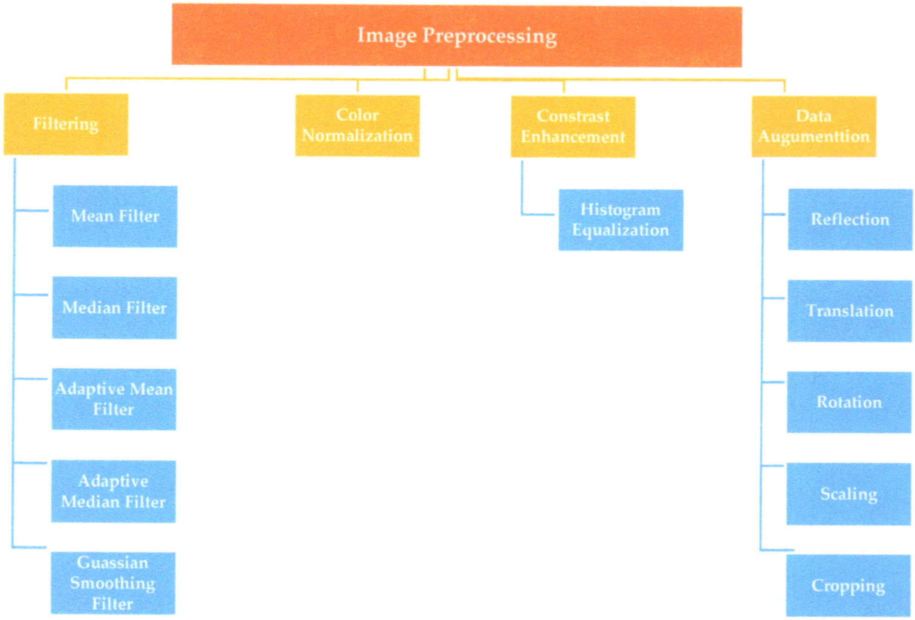

Figure 7. Taxonomy of different image preprocessing methods.

3.2.1. Filtering

There are various methods for enhancing images. The basic and simple methods can be classified as filtering. Filtering is used to eradicate unwanted variation (noise) from images. There are different noise eliminating filters used for removing undesirable information from images, i.e., mean filters, median filters, adaptive mean filters, adaptive median filters, and Gaussian smoothing filters. The mean filter is the simplest linear filter [80]. It eliminates the noise, blur images, and reduces sharp edges [81]. Similarly, the median filter has also been employed to eliminate noise from histopathology images [40]. The median filter is a nonlinear digital filtering method. It is commonly used in digital image processing because under certain conditions, it maintains edges whilst removing noise [82]. Adaptive filtering is used to remove noise from images without degradation. It involves a tradeoff between smoothing efficiency, preservation of discontinuities, and the generation of artifacts. Gaussian filtering is a smoothing filter method. It has been applied for smoothing the images, to overcome the variations in staining, as well to reduce noise [40]. The Gaussian filter is a very good filter for removing noise expressed in a normal distribution [80].

3.2.2. Color Normalization Techniques

In histopathology CAD systems, color normalization plays a significant role because the perception of information in images could negatively affected by color and concentration differences [83,84]. Two issues have made the color normalization process a challenging task [83]: (I) the presence of diagnostically significant but visually subtle details in color images. (II) the heterogeneous nature of tissue composition. Among the image preprocessing techniques, color normalization was the most common. In the last two decades, many color normalization techniques to histopathology image analysis have been proposed. In [85], authors developed a reliable color-based segmentation approach for histological structures that applied image gradients estimated in the LUV color space instead of RGB color space to handle matters relating to stain variability. Another approach presented in [84], founded on using of nine common color filters selected for histology H & E stained slides. The authors conducted two experiments, and results showed that pathologists became more sensitive to the color of the image than before. While in [86], a new color correction technique is proposed and developed in the linear RGB color space. This technique can easily be integrated to the slide scanning process. The technique is also handy in the sense that the data needed for color correction are extracted from the color calibration slide wherein nine reference color patches embedded on the glass slide, and the spectral properties of these patches are known beforehand.

3.2.3. Histogram Equalization

The histogram of an image is a mathematical graph representing frequencies of occurrence of distinct color intensities in that image. It summarizes the image with respect to quality, contrast, and brightness [40]. Histogram equalization of the image is a popular and simple ways for enhancing image contrast to normalize the distribution of probability of occurrence of intensities in the image and used for removing color variations due to illumination conditions and staining process [40]. There are many previous works published in histogram equalization. In [87], the authors tried to overcome the problem of changing the brightness of an image when applying traditional histogram equalization. They introduced a novel extension of bi-histogram equalization technique. It effectively separates the objects from the background. Another novel method for histopathology images was introduced in [88], is a fully automated stain normalization technique to minimize batch effects and thus help improving analysis of digitalized pathology images. Among the different histogram techniques, one paper applied multi-objective histogram equalization by using particle swarm optimization (PSO) [89]. The proposed technique works by segmenting the histogram of the image into two sub-images. Then, a number of optimized constraints are employed. PSO used to explore the optimal constraints. This technique preserves the brightness of the image while enhancing the contrast.

3.2.4. Data Augmentation

In the artificial intelligence domain, the model efficiency always enhances with the amount of the training data that has been used. Data augmentation (DA) is a strategy used to artificially enlarge the size of the training data without introducing labeling costs [90–94]. DA has already been used in many domains, including image processing and audio classification. The most common means of data augmentation in image analysis include reflection, translation, rotation, scaling, and cropping [90]. Applying conventional data augmentation methods is one popular way to increase both the number and diversity of images in small datasets. Nevertheless, it is not always used in all problems. A significant amount of DA techniques on specific problem-dependent are proposed can also be applied to expand small datasets. One of the powerful and common methods used in data augmentation is generative adversarial networks (GANs) [91]. GANs are based on competition between two neural networks. GANs consist of a discriminator and a generator, two neural networks trained as adversaries, therefore its name is adversarial. Over the past years, there have been many attempts in exploring the use of GANs in generating synthetic data for data augmentation given limited or imbalanced datasets. One variant of GANs is proposed in [92]. It is used to enhance generalizability in CT segmentation tasks. Another variant of GANs used in histopathology images proposed in [93]. But applying these techniques always require a relatively high effort. Moreover, there exist lots of excellent studies for data augmentation. In [94], the authors proposed a novel technique capable of augmenting histopathology images and distributing the variance between patients through image blending using the Gaussian-Laplacian pyramid. This technique produces new training images composed of half images of different patients. This method tries to prevent that a model learns color representations of patients, which related but to the staining process. Some studies aim to enhance the overfitting problem caused by the lack of samples by employing different data augmentation techniques. For example, in [26] authors used five DA techniques (rotation, flipping, shifting, rescaling, and random elastic transformation). Experimental results showed the effectiveness of applying different DA methods in the nuclei segmentation task.

3.3. *Traditional Machine Learning Techniques*

Machine learning (ML) is an automated learning process of machines to categorize and recognize different data such as text, images, and videos. ML employs algorithmic techniques to analyze, learn, and make decisions from the input data [95]. ML has been widely employed in many applications, including image processing, specifically in our study in histopathological image analysis. Traditional machine learning techniques typically involve several steps to deal with histopathology images including segmentation, feature extraction, and classification, as represented in Figure 6. Each step is described in the following subsections.

3.3.1. Image Segmentation

Segmentation process is one of the main research efforts in histopathology image analysis. It is the process of separating objects in an image that are of interest to the developed application by using various methods [40]. It can make anatomical structures like glands, nuclei and so on more obvious for a subsequent automatic or manual image classification [7]. The various morphological features of these structures like size, shape, extent, and color intensity, are also important factors for existence of prostate cancer. To analyse all these indicators, images need to be segmented first [38]. Prostate segmentation is a challenging process. It is difficult to determine the boundary between the prostate and the surrounding tissues. Even for experienced pathologists, the interobserver variability of manual prostate segmentation is large [10]. A precise prostate cancer segmentation may help effectively in guiding radiation therapy and biopsy therapy as well as its application in diagnosis [10].

Many researchers have applied various segmentation techniques in their research, which can be broadly classified into classical techniques and machine learning techniques, as represented in Figure 8. However, there is no general segmentation technique proven to be effective for all kind of images. In [23], the segmentation task in prostate cancer is carried out using the color space transformation and thresholding techniques. This process aids to form the gland region, which is subjected to feature extraction by applying multiple-kernel scale-invariant feature transform method. In [15], authors presented a new automatic nuclei and gland segmentation technique for prostate histopathology which incorporates an integration of high-level, low-level, and domain-specific information. The segmentation technique is utilized for three different applications: (I) classifying intermediate grades of prostate cancer, (II) identifying cancer from normal regions, and (III) discriminating Bloom-Richardson high-grade cancer from low-grade cancer. In [16], authors proposed an automated technique for gland segmentation in prostate cancer using histopathology images using machine learning and image processing methods. This technique outperforms structure and texture-based techniques. However, this technique fails in the images with the cribriform pattern, resulting in inaccurate segmentation. Another study [96] tried to overcome the necessary condition of the conventional thresholding segmentation method to give accurate results, where the nuclei must have a wide range of intensities to be easy differentiated from the background. Their adaptive thresholding technique passes through four different stages: (I) detecting the nuclei, (II) optimizing the primary contours through a rough texture segmentation, (III) optimizing the convergence, and finally (IV) splitting the overlapping segmentation masks.

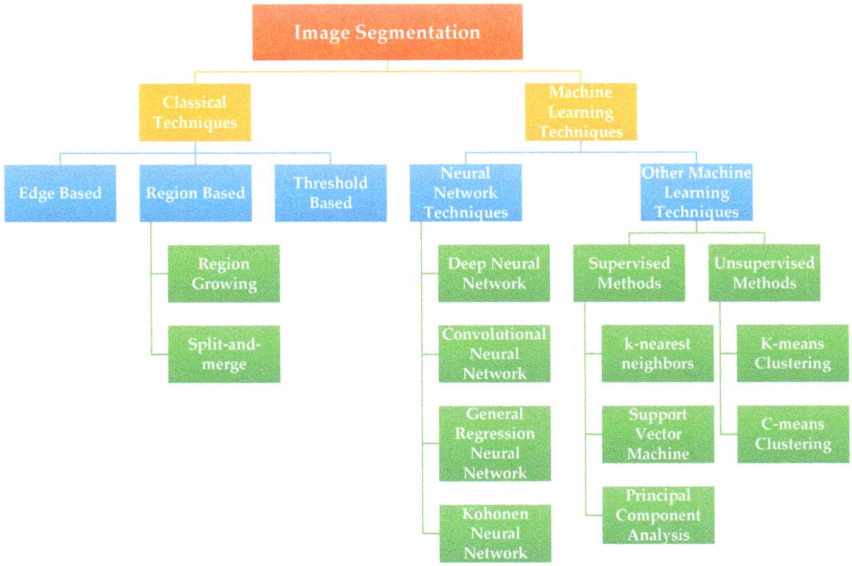

Figure 8. Image segmentation taxonomy compromising different techniques that are used to segment histopathological images.

Other methods such as [17] used two-stage segmentation. Firstly, the mean-shift (MS) algorithm is used to perform the coarse segmentation to split the tissue constituents in four parts. After that, wavelet filters are used to perform fine segmentation of glandular tissue. Although, there exists other studies that segment each individual cell. for example, an early study [97], where authors focused on dynamic segmentation of live cells for the purpose of quantification of different modalities. Their technique can identify the cell boundary no matter how many times it is used in the system.

There exist few studies that focus on utilizing cell nucleus and blue mucin. In [98], authors depend in their segmentation on the structure of glands to separate them from the background by analyzing the color space of histopathology image. Another segmentation technique, proposed in [99], combined the similarity of morphological characteristics related to the appearance of lumen components. It operated in three stages: (I) classification of pixels, (II) extraction of inner gland boundary, and finally (III) complete gland construction. The performance of the abovementioned techniques is constrained by the size and the characteristics of labelled datasets and the variation needed in the images to model the distribution of relevant tissue features.

3.3.2. Feature Selection

Feature selection refers to eliciting the best feature subset that can accurately label images from a dataset as belonging to one or more classes [100,101]. This has now been a significant domain to researchers with new advancements in histopathological image analysis. Just a few applications produce their data already in a form that classifiers can construe and do not need a feature selection process. However, histopathology images require representing characteristics of the tumor cells or tissues in a quantitative way [7,41]. The extracted features should be identifiable and distinct to an extent to be able to automatically classify normal and malignant tissues and to grade them correspondingly [41]. In HI, selecting which distinctive features will be feeding the classifier is more essential than picking the classifier itself, and when feature selection is applied, classification accuracy will be improved as many features are selected from all features [10]. Selecting distinctive features from targets of interest is a challenging task in an effective CAD system. Common features for HI comprise size, shape, histogram, texture, intensity, and multiple features. Feature descriptors to be selected in HI can be categorized into four groups: texture-based features, topological-based features, morphological-based features, color-based features, and other features [38,39,45,46]. Table 3 provides a brief view for the feature extraction publications suggested in HI of prostate cancer. The following paragraphs detail the different features selection procedures that have been employed for classifying histological images.

Table 3. Summary of publications focused on feature selection of prostate histopathology images.

Features Type	Reference	Year	Accuracy Result
Texture	[56]	2011	The AUC value is 0.91 for the first database and 0.96 for the second database.
	[102]	2015	The proposed method outperforms the classic SVM-RFE in accuracy and reducing redundancy.
	[103]	2018	The proposed method attained a classification accuracy around 99%.
Topological	[13]	2011	The model attainted an average accuracy 90%.
	[50]	2011	The test classification results have an average of 96.76%
	[49]	2017	The developed way achieved 93.0% training accuracy and 97.6% testing accuracy, for the tested cases.
Morphological	[15]	2007	Average accuracy for prostate cancer classification was 92.48%
	[104]	2011	The system achieved 0.55 under the precision recall curve measure
	[58]	2019	The prediction model resulted an average accuracy of 90.2%
Color	[98]	2012	The proposed method attained an average of 86% accuracy in classifying a tissue pattern into different classes.
	[105]	2006	They achieved accuracy of 91.3%
Color & Texture	[106]	2012	The algorithm achieved an average of 86% and 93% of classification accuracy.
	[107]	2012	Classification accuracies are 97.6%, 96.6% and 87.3% when differentiating Gleason 4 versus Gleason 3, Gleason 5 versus Gleason 3, and Gleason 5 versus Gleason 4.
Topological & Morphological & Texture	[48]	2007	SVM classifier applied to test the accuracy of the extracted features and achieved about 93% when differentiating among Gleason grade 3 and stroma, 92.4% among epithelium and stroma, and 76.9% among Gleason 4 and 3.
	[27]	2019	The proposed model using hand-crafted features achieved an average accuracy of 94.6%.

Texture-based features are related to the spatial distribution of repetitive intensities inside the tissue [9]. Examination texture features of each tissue components gives a valuable discriminative information in the diagnosis and grading systems of prostate cancer. In [56], authors applied a quantitative texture feature selection, for example, gland density, gland size, and gland circularity, and evaluated the accuracy of these features in discriminating normal from cancer glands using the ROC curve. The model achieved an average of 0.94 of AUC. In [102], a new method was proposed to overcome redundancy among features and that considered one of the most important reasons for weakness of SVM-RFE. The main purpose of their proposed feature selection method is to merge the SVMRFE with filter measure to extract the least features and enhance the classification accuracy of the model. Another work [103] focused on a type of texture-based features, called local binary pattern (LBP), and introduced a new modified version called multispectral multiscale LBP (MMLBP). This algorithm varies from the standard LBP in which it takes into consideration the joint information within spectral and spatial directions of the image. MMLBP attained a classification accuracy of around 99%.

Topological-based features enable characterization of cellular structure in histopathology images. These features apply the theories of algebraic topology and this is especially beneficial to the segmentation task [13,39]. In [13], 50 topological-based features were selected for designing a new data fusion algorithm in prostate histopathology images, incorporating 25 nearest-neighbor and 25 graph-based features. A pioneering effort on the use of topological features for automated scoring of prostate cancer using histopathological images was done in [50], where the authors introduced a new class of topological features that make use of network cycle structure. Another work [49] selected a set of visually significative features for the purpose of differentiation between different grades in prostate cancer using topological-based features. It based on computing the shortest path from the nuclei to their closest luminal spaces.

Morphological-based features give information about shape, color, structure, and size of the cells in HI [39]. Morphological features are useful to provide details for form and structure of abnormal cells of prostate cancer [9]. Many studies showed the viability of this type of features to help characterization of the histopathological prostate images. In [15], they presented a new automatic gland and nuclei segmentation system for prostate histopathology images and utilize an accurate extraction of various morphological features. In [104], the authors presented a content-based image retrieval system that takes advantage of a novel set of morphological attributes called explicit shape descriptors that properly depict the similarity between the morphology of objects of interest. A recent study [58], proposed a new machine learning classification method to classify Gleason grade groups of histopathology images for prostate cancer using new proposed morphological features.

Color-based features provide information of the grey level or color of pixels provided in the region of interest. Feature selection based on this type of features utilizes different color spaces. In [98], authors introduced a novel technique for grading prostate malignancy using digitized histopathological specimens of the prostate tissue. The color space that represents the tissue image is the Lab color space. The Lab color space is preferable than RGB since it is designed to approximate the color perception in human visual system. Also, in [14] classification is based on the lab color space. In [105], authors presented a wavelet-based color feature selection technique utilizing CIELAB color space. They compared CIELAB in their experiments with many color spaces e.g., RGB, KLT and HSV. CIELAB attained the highest accuracy.

However, most of the research that focus on feature selection apply a combination of different types of feature selection to improve the performance. The work presented in [106] introduced a new content-based microscopic image. The authors applied a hybrid color and texture feature selection method. They used RGB and HSV color spaces for color-based feature selection and for each image, an overall of 80 texture features were selected. The performance of the retrieval system was evaluated for various histopathology image types and the best retrieval performance was obtained for prostate images. In [107], the authors proposed an integrated feature set that combines color and morphological features to design new CAD system to automatic grade prostatic carcinoma biopsy images. Another CAD system was introduced in [50] to automatic grade of prostate cancer. The research used a total of 102 topological-based, morphological-based, and texture-based selected features from each tissue patch so that quantifying the arrangement of glandular and nuclei structures within histopathological images of prostate cancer tissues. Another recent research in [27], provided an automatic system able to accurately detect specific areas susceptible to be cancerous through presenting a novel method, a combination of topological-based, morphological-based, and texture-based feature selection for addressing the hand-crafted feature selection stage.

3.3.3. Classification

Classification is one of the important data analysis domains, which focuses on assigning a sample to one of a set of classes, based on its features [108,109]. For histopathological images, choosing the appropriate classifier is very significant to cope with huge, high visual complexity datasets. After segmentation and feature selection, the selected optimal classifier is applied to classify images for detecting malignancy in HI. In this step, a cell or tissue is assigned to one of the classes and then it can also be classified for malignancy level e.g., grading of tumor or type of the tumor [38]. Machine learning classifiers operate in two modes: learning mode and classification mode. In the learning mode, the selected features from annotated histopathological images are used to train the classifier. Afterwards, the classifier is used in classification mode on cases without knowledge of true annotation [10,41]. The different selected features from HI are used to classify the new images as normal or malignant. Constructing automated classifier systems of histopathological images is a challenge task in machine learning as histopathological images do not hold the same morphologic structure of macroscopic images such as human faces, trucks, text, or animals [94]. Numerous classification methods have been developed for histopathological images employing machine learning algorithms like k-nearest neighbors (KNN), support vector machine (SVM), logistic regression method, random forests (RF), decision trees, fuzzy systems, etc. The details regarding the developed classifiers dealt with classifying histopathological prostate images have been summarized in Table 4.

Table 4. Summary of publications focused on Prostate histopathology image classification.

Classifier	Reference	Year	AUC	Accuracy	Specificity	Sensitivity
KNN	[66]	2003	-	0.917	-	-
	[18]	2014	-	0.76	-	-
SVM	[48]	2007	-	0.876	-	-
	[14]	2013	0.75	-	0.83	0.81
	[13]	2019	0.98 ± 0.011 for artefacts versus glands 0.92 ± 0.04 for benign versus pathological	0.95 ± 0.02 for artefacts versus glands 0.88 ± 0.07 for benign versus pathological	0.95 ± 0.03 for artefacts versus glands 0.87 ± 0.07 for benign versus pathological	0.94 ± 0.01 for artefacts versus glands 0.80 ± 0.06 for benign versus pathological
	[58]	2019	-	0.655 (one-shot classification) 0.92 (Binary classification)	-	-
Bag-of-Words	[22]	2016	-	0.901	0.905	0.79
MLA	[21]	2018	-	0.883	0.94	0.876
Boosting Cascade	[20]	2006	-	0.88	-	-
SVM and Random Forest	[19]	2011	0.95	-	0.91	0.89
Fuzzy Set Theory + Genetic Algorithm	[110]	2013	0.824	-	0.95714	0.7097
Adaboost	[2]	2016	-	0.978	-	-

KNN is one of the simplest, versatile, and efficient methods used for image classification [99]. For instance, the authors in [66] applied KNN to classify HI into four grades of cancer ranked from 2 to 5. They used different K, e.g., 1, 3, 5, 7 and compared the results. With K = 1, achieved the highest performance of classification. Another work [18] applied a KNN classifier with K = 3 to develop an analytical framework to differentiate between stroma and glands in histopathological images of radical prostatectomies and to differentiate different Gleason grades. The proposed framework can be used firstly before quantifying and stratifying anatomic tissue structures.

In theory, a support vector machine (SVM) algorithm could obtain a high performance because it can maximize the margin between normal and cancerous training samples [10]. There exist many works that make use of SVM classifiers in prostate cancer histopathological images [13–15,48,58,103,106,107]. In [14], a novel methodology was proposed for labelling individual glands as normal or cancerous. They applied SVM classifier. SVM is trained by a linear kernel function to filter out the non-nuclei objects. In [13], the authors addressed the classification stage using a hand-crafted method that make use of two widely known classifiers. Specifically, they optimized SVM classifier and used a quadratic kernel to handle the multi-class classification from a nonlinear method. They achieved promising results. In [58], the authors developed an automated grading system for histopathological images of prostate cancer using SVM. After several experiments to compare between SVM and multilayer perceptron classification method (MLP), they reached to that SVM attained better results than MLP. Another study introduced a new system for quantitative and automated grading of prostate biopsy samples [48]. This work used a SVM classifier to differentiate between four categories of tissue patterns and they used cross-validation to get the best parameters for the classifier.

Inspired by the bag-of-words (BoW) model extensively used in natural language processing, the authors in [22] developed a new CAD system for prostate cancer using speeded-up robust features (SURF). In [21], a new method named multi-level learning architecture (MLA) is proposed. It depends on the divide-and-conquer algorithm by assigning each binary task into two different subtasks e.g., (strong and weak).

Multi-classifier systems or ensemble-based combine accuracies of different similar classifiers for improving the predictions for a problem [7,36]. Early research [20] employed a modified version of the popular ensemble classifier AdaBoost. To the best of our knowledge, their research is the first attempt at automatically analyzing prostatic adenocarcinoma across multiple scales. Some researchers tried to propose a classification technique to work in multiclass problems. In [19], another ensemble method (SVM plus random forests) was used to adapt to various imaging modalities, image features, and histological decisions. They employed statistical analysis using the Friedman test to rank the results of classifiers on datasets. To the best of our knowledge [110] is the only example that applied a fuzzy system to HI of prostate cancer, where the authors designed membership functions of the fuzzy system by using a genetic algorithm. In [2], the authors presented an adaptive boosting algorithm to support automated Gleason grading of prostate adenocarcinoma (PRCA). They prepared a pool of classifiers (SVM with linear and radial basis function kernels, adaptive boosting algorithm, decision tree, RF, linear discriminant analysis (DA) and quadratic DA). Results of all classifiers were combined using an adaptive boosting classifier.

3.4. Deep Learning-Based Techniques

Recently, adoption of deep learning (DL) techniques in biomedical imaging has had a positive impact on a broad range of tasks including automatic analysis of histopathology images [34,36]. DL creates new clinical tools that outperform the aforementioned classical machine learning techniques with handcrafted features in terms of accuracy, objectivity, consistency, and reproducibility. It also provides new insights to clinicians and researchers [59]. DL techniques are currently the most frequently studied in prostate cancer histopathology imaging and studies [28,34] have proven that DL models can accurately detect cancer in histopathological images. DL techniques takes original digital images as input, with a minimum preprocessing, and have the benefit of learning features instead of the conventional selection of handcrafted features, which may be not sufficient or not accurate [34]. Deep learning techniques learn salient features from data, so a large number of input images is of great value to the training process. Deep learning cannot be regarded as a singular technique; it can nearly be considered as adaptation of multi-layer artificial neural networks to a large variety of challenges, from natural language processing, fraud detection to computer vision [31]. Neural networks consist mainly of an input layer, a number of hidden layers, and an output layer, where each layer is composed of neurons. The input layer firstly takes input data, then the hidden layers execute some mathematical computations on those input data [111]. The output values of the network are predicated on the adjustment of internal weights [36]. These weights are computed by the network through iterative forward or backward propagation of the training data and error back-propagation respectively [36]. This process takes less effort to code than the conventional machine learning.

The main obstacle of any deep learning technique is its need for a substantial training set. Fortunately, histopathology images contain a great deal of information at small scales. Accordingly, a single slide can produce considerable amount of training patches [34]. Patches generate the effect of extracting portions of an image with the same structure but relate to images belonging to different classes [7]. Patches are commonly square portions having dimensionality that ranges from 32×32 pixels to $10{,}000 \times 10{,}000$ pixels [59]. Another obstacle of deep learning is the inadequacy of interpreting features and this may slow the development of CAD systems [34]. In the last decade, neural network architectures like convolution neural network (CNN), fully convolutional network (FCN), deep neural networks (DNN), and generative adversarial networks (GAN) are attracting the attention from the research community because of its recently impressed results on large datasets. A considerable amount of effort is done on prostate cancer histopathological images using the different neural networks.

A particular neural network subtype, convolutional neural network; has made sound advancements in image processing [31,112]. Convolutional networks have the ability to identify visual patterns with less processing and is persistent in existence of variations and distortions in pattern [36]. The basic CNN structure is comprised of convolutional, pooling, activation, classification, and fully connected layers [36,90]. The Histopathology imagery domain is rapidly adjusting this architecture to enhance a wide range of challenges. In [31], authors investigated the general applicability of CNN for increasing the performance of prostate and breast cancer detection in histopathology images. They used fully connected CNN to get cancer maps for each pixel and make segmentation in the whole slide images. Results proved that DL has great potential for increasing the performance of detecting malignancies in H & E images as AUC ranges from 0.88 to 0.99. As far as we know, researchers in [54] were the first to use images of the entire prostate gland as an input to the network, instead of using image patches or regions with gland information. They designed a new CNN architecture that comprises feature selection stage, characterized by the compound of four convolutional blocks, and the classification phase compound of two fully connected layers.

Various papers have applied CNN to automatic Gleason grading to perform better than systems that use conventional machine learning methods. The first attempt to apply convolutional networks to Gleason score grading prediction is [30], where the authors applied a pre-trained CNN. The classification stage in CNN was excluded and replaced with RF and SVM algorithms to classify the feature vectors selected from the network. In [28], the authors trained different variants of CNN as Gleason score annotator and utilized the prediction of the model to assign patients into low, medium, and high levels of risk, attaining pathology stratification results at expert level. Their experiments shown improved efficacy regarding the applicability of CNN reaching more reproducible and consistent prostate cancer grading, specifically for cases with heterogeneous Gleason patterns. Recently, a fully automated grading system using the U-Net was proposed in [29], where the authors adopted the conventional U-Net architecture, however after several experiments, they made the network deeper to be composed of six levels as they added additional skip connections within each layer block. Their model attained a high agreement with pathologists.

Aside from CNN, many authors have tried to utilize different techniques in histopathology imagery in prostate cancer, for example, the authors in [23] proposed a new deep learning technique that combines the multi-model neural network, ride NN and optimization algorithm, Salp–Rider algorithm (SRA), generating the new technique SSA-RideNN. The experiments showed that SSA-RideNN attained a maximal accuracy, specificity, and sensitivity.

Since the comparison of different techniques is difficult, some studies like [34] tried to compare different classifiers and deep learning algorithm for automatic grading of prostate cancer in HI on their new CAD system. Specifically, they have evaluated the performance of SVM, random forest with several number of trees, logistic regression, and linear discriminant analysis, and they also estimated the performance of a convolutional neural network (CNN) on the same training and testing subsets. They used Cohen's kappa coefficient to evaluate the performance. The highest value attained is 0.52 by logistic regression, while 0.37 is attained by using CNN. More recently, the authors in [113] tried to compare different architectures of CNN—EfficientNet, DenseNet, and U-Net—on two datasets of prostate cancer HI. Experiments were performed on three-fold cross-validation and U-Net attained the best results.

Some researchers have studied on the use of DL techniques for automated segmentation of prostate cancer on histopathology images. In [25], the authors tried to overcome the struggles of CNN to distinguish overlapping segmentation instances. The study presented a new nuclei segmentation technique that utilized the conditional generative adversarial network (cGAN). Their proposed technique enforces a higher consistency when compared with traditional CNN architectures. In [26], the authors proposed a new nuclei boundary (NB) segmentation technique using CNN. The technique was proved to be efficient and faster than other traditional techniques, as one image of dimension 1000×1000 pixel can be segmented in less than five seconds. It works in the following way: firstly, the images are normalized into the same color space. Secondly, images are split into overlapping patches to tackle the extremely large image challenge. Thirdly, they proposed a new nucleus segmentation technique to identify nuclei and boundaries on each patch. Finally, the predictions of all the patches are combined to get the final prediction result of the whole image. Driven by the success of region-based CNN (RCNN) and its extensions, authors in [24] applied RCNN for detection epithelial cells employing grading network head (GNH). They applied a ResNet in their network for feature selection. Then, they employed GNH for detecting the class. They added a branch that produces an epithelial cell score using GNH. Since the proposed network was inspired by Mask RCNN, it was named Path R-CNN. The details regarding deep learning methods for prostate histopathology images have been summarized in Table 5.

Table 5. Summary of publications focused on applying deep learning methods for prostate histopathology images.

Method		Reference	Year	Accuracy Result	Software
CNN		[31]	2016	AUC ranges from 0.88 to 0.99.	N/A
CNN built upon VGG19		[27]	2019	Average accuracy of classifying Artefacts vs. Glands is 95.4%, average accuracy of classifying Benign vs. Pathological is 88.3%, Average accuracy of Multi-class classification is 87.6%	Matlab 2018b + Python 3.5 with Keras library and Tensorflow as backend.
Pretrained CNN		[30]	2016	The classification accuracy per image patch is 81%, while for the whole images, the classification accuracy is 89%.	N/A
Different CNN Architectures	ResNet-50	[28]	2018	They evaluated their results using test cohort and they observed that MobileNet attained the best performance on the validation set	Python 3 with Keras library and tensorflow as backend. Some analysis was done in R by the help of using survminer and survival packages.
	MobileNet				
	Inception-V3				
	DenseNet-121				
	VGG-16				
U-Net		[29]	2020	The developed model achieved accuracy of 99% for biopsies containing tumor and a specificity of 82%.	Tensorflow and Keras
SSA-RideNN		[23]	2019	The technique achieved maximal accuracy of 89.6% and sensitivity of 89.1%, and specificity of 85.9%	Matlab
SVM		[34]	2018	They used Cohen's kappa coefficient to evaluate the performance. The highest value attained is 0.52 by logistic regression, while 0.37 is attained by using CNN.	Matlab
Random forest					
linear discriminant analysis					
logistic regression					
CNN					
Different CNN Architectures	EfficientNet	[113]	2020	UNet attained the best result of AUC about 0.98	N/A
	DenseNet				
	U-Net				
cGAN		[25]	2018	The proposed technique achieved F1-score 85.7% for prostate dataset	Pytorch 0.4
NB that utilizes CNN		[26]	2019	Their proposed model achieves 81.3% precision, 91.4% in recall, and 85.4% in F1.	Python 2.7 with Keras library and Tensorflow
Path RCNN		[24]	2019	Path RCNN attained accuracy of 99% and a mean of area under the curve of 0.99.	Python and Tensorflow backend

4. Conclusions and Future Perspectives

More than 28% of cancers in men arise in the prostate gland, causing prostate cancer, and detection of this type has a high priority in cancer research. Histopathology images may enhance the early diagnosis and treatment of prostate cancer patients through providing functional and morphological data about the prostate. Histology is nothing but examining the stained sample on the slide glass under a microscope. In this survey, we presented a literature review of the use of histopathology images and its challenges. We studied different steps of histopathology image analysis methodology. This automatic process assists pathologists and clinicians in diagnosis and lowers the time spent for examining large number of tissues. The survey revealed a greater utilization of deep learning techniques and a constant use of conventional machine learning techniques. It also revealed that the histopathology image analysis is a topic of increasing interest. Our findings reveal that there is still room for improvement as CAD systems of histology images composed of complicated combination of image processing, feature selection, image segmentation, and classification stage. Moreover, the image processing techniques mentioned in this survey is not applicable for prostate histopathology image analysis only, but also applicable in many image analysis domains. This research is an attempt to summarize the most common and recent developments in prostate cancer CAD systems using histopathology images and to give an outline on the performance and efficacy of different techniques.

The domain of histopathology image processing of prostate cancer detection is very vast. According to the challenges to this type of images and disease characteristics, research in this domain is still being unlocked and many opportunities and future perspectives remain to study and analyze including: (I) the ability of enhanced interaction with images from various scanners and across pathologies, in addition to the development of new techniques that can learn from unlabeled or weakly labeled data; (II) allowing online consultations; (III) providing accessible histopathology analysis services in remote areas with limited pathology assist; (IV) developing of new data fusion techniques for integrating radiologic and histologic measurements for improved disease diagnosis with the functionality of real-time image processing and finally (V) applications and computerized software for histopathological image processing techniques may be incorporated into microscopes with small size chips. It is therefore expected from those opportunities and future perspective that we are standing at the threshold of an era that will transform the personalized diagnosis into better diagnostic systems to decrease the workload of pathologists.

Author Contributions: Conceptualization, S.M.A., M.S., M.A.E.-G., M.E.-M., H.A.A. and A.E.-B.; methodology, S.M.A., M.S., A.S. and A.E.-B.; validation, M.A.E.-G., M.E.-M., M.G., N.B.A.-H., L.M.L., H.A.A. and A.E.-B.; formal analysis, S.M.A., M.S., H.A.A. and A.E.-B.; investigation, S.M.A., M.S., A.S., M.G., N.B.A.-H., L.M.L., H.A.A. and A.E.-B.; resources, M.A.E.-G., M.G., M.E.-M. and A.E.-B.; data curation, M.A.E.-G., M.E.-M., M.G. and A.E.-B.; writing—original draft preparation, S.M.A., M.S. and A.E.-B.; figures preparation, S.M.A., M.S. and A.S.; writing—review and editing, S.M.A., M.S., A.S., N.B.A.-H., L.M.L., H.A.A. and A.E.-B.; supervision, N.B.A.-H., L.M.L., H.A.A. and A.E.-B.; project administration, A.E.-B. All authors have read and agreed to the published version of the manuscript.

Funding: This research received no external funding.

Institutional Review Board Statement: The study was conducted according to the guidelines of the Declaration of Helsinki, and approved by the Institutional Review Board of Mansoura University (R.21.04.1289).

Informed Consent Statement: Informed consent was obtained from all subjects involved in the study.

Data Availability Statement: No data available.

Acknowledgments: Authors like to acknowledge the support of the Academy of Scientific Research and Technology in Egypt in this work.

Conflicts of Interest: The authors declare no conflict of interest.

References

1. Harmon, S.A.; Tuncer, S.; Sanford, T.; Choyke, P.L.; Turkbey, B. Artificial intelligence at the intersection of pathology and radiology in prostate cancer. *Diagn. Interv. Radiol.* **2019**, *25*, 183–188. [CrossRef] [PubMed]
2. Huang, C.-H.; Kalaw, E.M. Automated classification for pathological prostate images using AdaBoost-based Ensemble Learning. In Proceedings of the 2016 IEEE Symposium Series on Computational Intelligence (SSCI), Athens, Greece, 6–9 December 2017; pp. 1–4. [CrossRef]
3. Reda, I.; Ayinde, B.O.; Elmogy, M.; Shalaby, A.; El-Melegy, M.; El-Ghar, M.A.; El-Fetouh, A.A.; Ghazal, M.; El-Baz, A. A new CNN-based system for early diagnosis of prostate cancer. In Proceedings of the 2018 IEEE 15th International Symposium on Biomedical Imaging (ISBI 2018), Washington, DC, USA, 4–7 April 2018; pp. 207–210.
4. Ried, K.; Tamanna, T.; Matthews, S.; Eng, P.; Sali, A. New Screening Test Improves Detection of Prostate Cancer Using Circulating Tumor Cells and Prostate-Specific Markers. *Front. Oncol.* **2020**, *10*, 582. [CrossRef] [PubMed]
5. American Cancer Society. Key Statistics for Prostate Cancer. Available online: http://www.cancer.org/cancer/prostate-cancer/about/key-statistics.html (accessed on 29 January 2021).
6. Hoogland, A.M.; Kweldam, C.F.; Van Leenders, G.J.L.H. Prognostic Histopathological and Molecular Markers on Prostate Cancer Needle-Biopsies: A Review. *BioMed Res. Int.* **2014**, *2014*, 1–12. [CrossRef] [PubMed]
7. de Matos, J.; Britto, A.D.S., Jr.; Oliveira, L.E.; Koerich, A.L. Histopathologic image processing: A review. *arXiv* **2019**, arXiv:1904.07900. Available online: https://arxiv.org/abs/1904.07900 (accessed on 5 January 2021).
8. Komura, D.; Ishikawa, S. Machine Learning Methods for Histopathological Image Analysis. *Comput. Struct. Biotechnol. J.* **2018**, *16*, 34–42. [CrossRef]
9. Aswathy, M.; Jagannath, M. Detection of breast cancer on digital histopathology images: Present status and future possibilities. *Inform. Med. Unlocked* **2017**, *8*, 74–79. [CrossRef]
10. Wang, S.; Burtt, K.; Turkbey, B.; Choyke, P.; Summers, R.M. Computer Aided-Diagnosis of Prostate Cancer on Multiparametric MRI: A Technical Review of Current Research. *BioMed Res. Int.* **2014**, *2014*, 1–11. [CrossRef]
11. Anuranjeeta; Shukla, K.K.; Tiwari, A.; Sharma, S. Classification of Histopathological Images of Breast Cancerous and Non Cancerous Cells based on Morphological Features. *Biomed. Pharmacol. J.* **2017**, *10*, 353–366. [CrossRef]
12. Serag, A.; Ion-Margineanu, A.; Qureshi, H.; McMillan, R.; Saint Martin, M.J.; Diamond, J.; O'Reilly, P.; Hamilton, P. Translational AI and Deep Learning in Diagnostic Pathology. *Front. Med.* **2019**, *6*, 185. [CrossRef]
13. Madabhushi, A.; Agner, S.; Basavanhally, A.; Doyle, S.; Lee, G. Computer-aided prognosis: Predicting patient and disease outcome via quantitative fusion of multi-scale, multi-modal data. *Comput. Med. Imaging Graph.* **2011**, *35*, 506–514. [CrossRef]
14. Rashid, S.; Fazli, L.; Boag, A.; Siemens, R.; Abolmaesumi, P.; Salcudean, S.E. Separation of Benign and Malignant Glands in Prostatic Adenocarcinoma. In Proceedings of the International Conference on Medical Image Computing and Computer-Assisted Intervention, Nagoya, Japan, 22–26 September 2013; Springer International Publishing: Berlin/Heidelberg, Germany, 2013; pp. 461–468.
15. Naik, S.; Doyle, S.; Agner, S.; Madabhushi, A.; Feldman, M.; Tomaszewski, J. Automated gland and nuclei segmentation for grading of prostate and breast cancer histopathology. In Proceedings of the 2008 5th IEEE International Symposium on Biomedical Imaging: From Nano to Macro, Paris, France, 14–17 May 2008; pp. 284–287.
16. Singh, M.; Kalaw, E.M.; Giron, D.M.; Chong, K.-T.; Tan, C.L.; Lee, H.K. Gland segmentation in prostate histopathological images. *J. Med. Imaging* **2017**, *4*, 027501. [CrossRef] [PubMed]
17. Ali, T.; Masood, K.; Irfan, M.; Draz, U.; Nagra, A.; Asif, M.; Alshehri, B.; Glowacz, A.; Tadeusiewicz, R.; Mahnashi, M.; et al. Multistage Segmentation of Prostate Cancer Tissues Using Sample Entropy Texture Analysis. *Entropy* **2020**, *22*, 1370. [CrossRef]
18. Salman, S.; Ma, Z.; Mohanty, S.; Bhele, S.; Chu, Y.-T.; Knudsen, B.; Gertych, A. A Machine Learning Approach to Identify Prostate Cancer Areas in Complex Histological Images. In *Intelligent and Fuzzy Techniques in Big Data Analytics and Decision Making*; Springer Science and Business Media LLC: Berlin/Heidelberg, Germany, 2014; Volume 283, pp. 295–306.
19. DiFranco, M.D.; O'Hurley, G.; Kay, E.W.; Watson, R.W.G.; Cunningham, P. Ensemble based system for whole-slide prostate cancer probability mapping using color texture features. *Comput. Med. Imaging Graph.* **2011**, *35*, 629–645. [CrossRef]
20. Doyle, S.; Madabhushi, A.; Feldman, M.; Tomaszeweski, J. A Boosting Cascade for Automated Detection of Prostate Cancer from Digitized Histology. In Proceedings of the International Conference on Medical Image Computing and Computer-Assisted Intervention, Copenhagen, Denmark, 1–6 October 2006; Springer Science and Business Media LLC: Berlin/Heidelberg, Germany, 2006; Volume 9, pp. 504–511.
21. Albashish, D.; Sahran, S.; Abdullah, A.; Adam, A.; Alweshah, M. A hierarchical classifier for multiclass prostate histopathology image gleason grading. *J. Inf. Commun. Technol.* **2018**, *17*, 323–346. [CrossRef]
22. Sanghavi, F.M. Automated classification of histopathology images of prostate cancer using a Bag-of-Words approach. In *Mobile Multimedia/Image Processing, Security, and Applications 2016*; SPIE: Bellingham, WA, USA, 2016; Volume 9869, p. 98690. [CrossRef]
23. Gurav, S.B.; Kulhalli, K.V.; Desai, V.V. Prostate cancer detection using histopathology images and classification using improved RideNN. *Biomed. Eng. Appl. Basis Commun.* **2019**, *31*. [CrossRef]
24. Li, W.; Li, J.; Sarma, K.V.; Ho, K.C.; Shen, S.; Knudsen, B.S.; Gertych, A.; Arnold, C.W. Path R-CNN for Prostate Cancer Diagnosis and Gleason Grading of Histological Images. *IEEE Trans. Med. Imaging* **2019**, *38*, 945–954. [CrossRef]
25. Mahmood, F.; Borders, D.; Chen, R.J.; McKay, G.N.; Salimian, K.J.; Baras, A.; Durr, N.J. Deep Adversarial Training for Multi-Organ Nuclei Segmentation in Histopathology Images. *IEEE Trans. Med. Imaging* **2020**, *39*, 3257–3267. [CrossRef] [PubMed]

26. Cui, Y.; Zhang, G.; Liu, Z.; Xiong, Z.; Hu, J. A deep learning algorithm for one-step contour aware nuclei segmentation of histopathology images. *Med. Biol. Eng. Comput.* **2019**, *57*, 2027–2043. [CrossRef]
27. García, G.; Colomer, A.; Naranjo, V. First-Stage Prostate Cancer Identification on Histopathological Images: Hand-Driven versus Automatic Learning. *Entropy* **2019**, *21*, 356. [CrossRef] [PubMed]
28. Arvaniti, E.; Fricker, K.S.; Moret, M.; Rupp, N.; Hermanns, T.; Fankhauser, C.; Wey, N.; Wild, P.J.; Rüschoff, J.H.; Claassen, M. Automated Gleason grading of prostate cancer tissue microarrays via deep learning. *Sci. Rep.* **2018**, *8*, 1–11. [CrossRef] [PubMed]
29. Bulten, W.; Pinckaers, H.; van Boven, H.; Vink, R.; de Bel, T.; van Ginneken, B.; van der Laak, J.; de Kaa, C.H.; Litjens, G. Automated gleason grading of prostate biopsies using deep learning. *arXiv* **2019**, arXiv:1907.07980. Available online: https://arxiv.org/abs/1907.07980 (accessed on 10 January 2021).
30. Kallen, H.; Molin, J.; Heyden, A.; Lundstrom, C.; Astrom, K. Towards grading gleason score using generically trained deep convolutional neural networks. In Proceedings of the 2016 IEEE 13th International Symposium on Biomedical Imaging (ISBI), Prague, Czech Republic, 13–16 April 2016; pp. 1163–1167.
31. Litjens, G.; Sánchez, C.I.; Timofeeva, N.; Hermsen, M.; Nagtegaal, I.; Kovacs, I.; Van De Kaa, C.H.; Bult, P.; Van Ginneken, B.; Van Der Laak, J. Deep learning as a tool for increased accuracy and efficiency of histopathological diagnosis. *Sci. Rep.* **2016**, *6*, 26286. [CrossRef] [PubMed]
32. Tolkach, Y.; Dohmgörgen, T.; Toma, M.; Kristiansen, G. High-accuracy prostate cancer pathology using deep learning. *Nat. Mach. Intell.* **2020**, *2*, 1–8. [CrossRef]
33. Duran-Lopez, L.; Dominguez-Morales, J.; Rios-Navarro, A.; Gutierrez-Galan, D.; Jimenez-Fernandez, A.; Vicente-Diaz, S.; Linares-Barranco, A. Performance Evaluation of Deep Learning-Based Prostate Cancer Screening Methods in Histopathological Images: Measuring the Impact of the Model's Complexity on Its Processing Speed. *Sensors* **2021**, *21*, 1122. [CrossRef]
34. Nir, G.; Hor, S.; Karimi, D.; Fazli, L.; Skinnider, B.F.; Tavassoli, P.; Turbin, D.; Villamil, C.F.; Wang, G.; Wilson, R.S.; et al. Automatic grading of prostate cancer in digitized histopathology images: Learning from multiple experts. *Med. Image Anal.* **2018**, *50*, 167–180. [CrossRef]
35. Tariq, M.; Iqbal, S.; Ayesha, H.; Abbas, I.; Ahmad, K.T.; Niazi, M.F.K. Medical image based breast cancer diagnosis: State of the art and future directions. *Expert Syst. Appl.* **2021**, *167*, 114095. [CrossRef]
36. Jimenez-del-Toro, O.; Otálora, S.; Andersson, M.; Eurén, K.; Hedlund, M.; Rousson, M.; Atzori, M. Analysis of histopathology images: From traditional machine learning to deep learning. In *Biomedical Texture Analysis*; Academic Press: Cambridge, MA, USA, 2017; pp. 281–314.
37. Madabhushi, A.; Lee, G. Image analysis and machine learning in digital pathology: Challenges and opportunities. *Med. Image Anal.* **2016**, *33*, 170–175. [CrossRef] [PubMed]
38. Belsare, A. Histopathological Image Analysis Using Image Processing Techniques: An Overview. *Signal Image Process. Int. J.* **2012**, *3*, 23–36. [CrossRef]
39. Arevalo, J.; Cruz-Roa, A.; González, F.A. Histopathology image representation for automatic analysis: A state-of-the-art review. *Rev. Med.* **2014**, *22*, 79–91. [CrossRef]
40. Jothi, J.A.A.; Rajam, V.M.A. A survey on automated cancer diagnosis from histopathology images. *Artif. Intell. Rev.* **2017**, *48*, 31–81. [CrossRef]
41. Das, A.; Nair, M.S.; Peter, S.D. Computer-Aided Histopathological Image Analysis Techniques for Automated Nuclear Atypia Scoring of Breast Cancer: A Review. *J. Digit. Imaging* **2020**, *33*, 1–31. [CrossRef]
42. Madabhushi, A. Digital pathology image analysis: Opportunities and challenges. *Imaging Med.* **2009**, *1*, 7–10. [CrossRef]
43. Humphrey, P.A. Histopathology of Prostate Cancer. *Cold Spring Harb. Perspect. Med.* **2017**, *7*, a030411. [CrossRef]
44. Mosquera-Lopez, C.; Agaian, S.; Velez-Hoyos, A.; Thompson, I. Computer-Aided Prostate Cancer Diagnosis from Digitized Histopathology: A Review on Texture-Based Systems. *IEEE Rev. Biomed. Eng.* **2015**, *8*, 98–113. [CrossRef]
45. Li, C.; Chen, H.; Li, X.; Xu, N.; Hu, Z.; Xue, D.; Qi, S.; Ma, H.; Zhang, L.; Sun, H. A review for cervical histopathology image analysis using machine vision approaches. *Artif. Intell. Rev.* **2020**, *53*, 4821–4862. [CrossRef]
46. Krithiga, R.; Geetha, P. Breast Cancer Detection, Segmentation and Classification on Histopathology Images Analysis: A Systematic Review. *Arch. Comput. Methods Eng.* **2020**, *10*, 1–13. [CrossRef]
47. Van Booven, D.J.; Kuchakulla, M.; Pai, R.; Frech, F.S.; Ramasahayam, R.; Reddy, P.; Parmar, M.; Ramasamy, R.; Arora, H. A Systematic Review of Artificial Intelligence in Prostate Cancer. *Res. Rep. Urol.* **2021**, *13*, 31–39. [CrossRef] [PubMed]
48. Doyle, S.; Hwang, M.; Shah, K.; Madabhushi, A.; Feldman, M.; Tomaszeweski, J. Automated grading of prostate cancer using architectural and textural image features. In Proceedings of the 2007 4th IEEE International Symposium on Biomedical Imaging: From Nano to Macro, Arlington, VA, USA, 12–15 April 2007; pp. 1284–1287. [CrossRef]
49. Niazi, M.K.K.; Yao, K.; Zynger, D.L.; Clinton, S.K.; Chen, J.; Koyuturk, M.; LaFramboise, T.; Gurcan, M. Visually Meaningful Histopathological Features for Automatic Grading of Prostate Cancer. *IEEE J. Biomed. Health Inform.* **2017**, *21*, 1027–1038. [CrossRef] [PubMed]
50. Khurd, P.; Bahlmann, C.; Maday, P.; Kamen, A.; Gibbs-Strauss, S.; Genega, E.M.; Frangioni, J.V. Computer-aided Gleason grading of prostate cancer histopathological images using texton forests. In Proceedings of the 2010 IEEE International Symposium on Biomedical Imaging: From Nano to Macro, Rotterdam, The Netherlands, 14–17 April 2010; pp. 636–639. [CrossRef]
51. Slaoui, M.; Fiette, L. Histopathology Procedures: From Tissue Sampling to Histopathological Evaluation. In *Methods in Molecular Biology*; Springer: Berlin/Heidelberg, Germany, 2010; Volume 691, pp. 69–82.

52. Cahill, L.C.; Fujimoto, J.G.; Giacomelli, M.G.; Yoshitake, T.; Wu, Y.; Lin, D.I.; Ye, H.; Carrasco-Zevallos, O.M.; Wagner, A.A.; Rosen, S. Comparing histologic evaluation of prostate tissue using nonlinear microscopy and paraffin H&E: A pilot study. *Mod. Pathol.* **2019**, *32*, 1158–1167. [CrossRef] [PubMed]
53. Xu, Y.; Jia, Z.; Wang, L.-B.; Ai, Y.; Zhang, F.; Lai, M.; Chang, E.I.-C. Large scale tissue histopathology image classification, segmentation, and visualization via deep convolutional activation features. *BMC Bioinform.* **2017**, *18*, 1–17. [CrossRef]
54. Zangeneh, E.; Rahmati, M.; Mohsenzadeh, Y. Low resolution face recognition using a two-branch deep convolutional neural network architecture. *Expert Syst. Appl.* **2020**, *139*, 112854. [CrossRef]
55. Kramberger, T.; Potočnik, B. LSUN-Stanford Car Dataset: Enhancing Large-Scale Car Image Datasets Using Deep Learning for Usage in GAN Training. *Appl. Sci.* **2020**, *10*, 4913. [CrossRef]
56. Peng, Y.; Jiang, Y.; Eisengart, L.; Healy, M.A.; Straus, F.H.; Yang, X.J. Computer-aided identification of prostatic adenocarcinoma: Segmentation of glandular structures. *J. Pathol. Inform.* **2011**, *2*, 33. [CrossRef] [PubMed]
57. Zhu, C.; Song, F.; Wang, Y.; Dong, H.; Guo, Y.; Liu, J. Breast cancer histopathology image classification through assembling multiple compact CNNs. *BMC Med. Inform. Decis. Mak.* **2019**, *19*, 1–17. [CrossRef] [PubMed]
58. Bhattacharjee, S.; Park, H.-G.; Kim, C.-H.; Prakash, D.; Madusanka, N.; So, J.-H.; Cho, N.-H.; Choi, H.-K. Quantitative Analysis of Benign and Malignant Tumors in Histopathology: Predicting Prostate Cancer Grading Using SVM. *Appl. Sci.* **2019**, *9*, 2969. [CrossRef]
59. Dimitriou, N.; Arandjelović, O.; Caie, P.D. Deep Learning for Whole Slide Image Analysis: An Overview. *Front. Med.* **2019**, *6*, 264. [CrossRef]
60. Veta, M.M.; Pluim, J.P.W.; Van Diest, P.J.; Viergever, M.A. Breast Cancer Histopathology Image Analysis: A Review. *IEEE Trans. Biomed. Eng.* **2014**, *61*, 1400–1411. [CrossRef]
61. Şerbănescu, M.-S.; Manea, N.C.; Streba, L.; Belciug, S.; Pleşea, I.E.; Pirici, I.; Bungărdean, R.M.; Pleşea, R.M. Automated Gleason grading of prostate cancer using transfer learning from general-purpose deep-learning networks. *Rom. J. Morphol. Embryol. Rev. Roum. Morphol. Embryol.* **2020**, *61*, 149–155. [CrossRef]
62. Arvaniti, E.; Claassen, M. Coupling weak and strong supervision for classification of prostate cancer histopathology images. *arXiv* **2018**, arXiv:1811.07013. Available online: https://arxiv.org/abs/1811.07013 (accessed on 2 January 2021).
63. A Sharif, S.M.; Naqvi, R.A.; Biswas, M. Learning Medical Image Denoising with Deep Dynamic Residual Attention Network. *Mathematics* **2020**, *8*, 2192. [CrossRef]
64. Çelik, G.; Talu, M.F. Resizing and cleaning of histopathological images using generative adversarial networks. *Phys. A Stat. Mech. Its Appl.* **2020**, *554*, 122652. [CrossRef]
65. Arif, M.; Rajpoot, N. Classification of potential nuclei in prostate histology images using shape manifold learning. In Proceedings of the 2007 International Conference on Machine Vision, Isalambad, Pakistan, 28–29 December 2007; pp. 113–118.
66. Jafari-Khouzani, K.; Soltanian-Zadeh, H. Multiwavelet grading of pathological images of prostate. *IEEE Trans. Biomed. Eng.* **2003**, *50*, 697–704. [CrossRef]
67. Li, X.; Plataniotis, K.N. A Complete Color Normalization Approach to Histopathology Images Using Color Cues Computed From Saturation-Weighted Statistics. *IEEE Trans. Biomed. Eng.* **2015**, *62*, 1862–1873. [CrossRef] [PubMed]
68. Piórkowski, A. Color Normalization-Based Nuclei Detection in Images of Hematoxylin and Eosin-Stained Multi Organ Tissues. In Proceedings of the International Conference on Image Processing and Communications, Bydgoszcz, Poland, 11–13 September 2019; pp. 57–64.
69. Xiao, Y.; Decenciere, E.; Velasco-Forero, S.; Burdin, H.; Bornschlogl, T.; Bernerd, F.; Warrick, E.; Baldeweck, T. A New Color Augmentation Method for Deep Learning Segmentation of Histological Images. In Proceedings of the 2019 IEEE 16th International Symposium on Biomedical Imaging (ISBI 2019), Venice, Italy, 8–11 April 2019; pp. 886–890. [CrossRef]
70. Vicory, J.; Couture, H.D.; Thomas, N.E.; Borland, D.; Marron, J.; Woosley, J.; Niethammer, M. Appearance normalization of histology slides. *Comput. Med. Imaging Graph.* **2015**, *43*, 89–98. [CrossRef] [PubMed]
71. Gu, Y.; Yang, J. Multi-level magnification correlation hashing for scalable histopathological image retrieval. *Neurocomputing* **2019**, *351*, 134–145. [CrossRef]
72. Campanella, G.; Hanna, M.G.; Geneslaw, L.; Miraflor, A.; Silva, V.W.K.; Busam, K.J.; Brogi, E.; Reuter, V.E.; Klimstra, D.S.; Fuchs, T.J. Clinical-grade computational pathology using weakly supervised deep learning on whole slide images. *Nat. Med.* **2019**, *25*, 1301–1309. [CrossRef] [PubMed]
73. McClure, P.; Elnakib, A.; El-Ghar, M.A.; Khalifa, F.; Soliman, A.; El-Diasty, T.; Suri, J.S.; Elmaghraby, A.; El-Baz, A. In-Vitro and In-Vivo Diagnostic Techniques for Prostate Cancer: A Review. *J. Biomed. Nanotechnol.* **2014**, *10*, 2747–2777. [CrossRef] [PubMed]
74. Reda, I.; Khalil, A.; Elmogy, M.; El-Fetouh, A.A.; Shalaby, A.; El-Ghar, M.A.; Elmaghraby, A.; Ghazal, M.; El-Baz, A. Deep Learning Role in Early Diagnosis of Prostate Cancer. *Technol. Cancer Res. Treat.* **2018**, *17*, 1533034618775530. [CrossRef] [PubMed]
75. Kumar, N.; Verma, R.; Sharma, S.; Bhargava, S.; Vahadane, A.; Sethi, A. A Dataset and a Technique for Generalized Nuclear Segmentation for Computational Pathology. *IEEE Trans. Med. Imaging* **2017**, *36*, 1550–1560. [CrossRef]
76. Prostate Fused-MRI-Pathology. Available online: https://wiki.cancerimagingarchive.net/display/Public/Prostate+Fused-MRI-Pathology (accessed on 27 March 2021).
77. TCGA-PRAD. Available online: https://wiki.cancerimagingarchive.net/display/Public/TCGA-PRAD (accessed on 27 March 2021).
78. Prostate cANcer graDe Assessment (PANDA) Challenge. Available online: https://www.kaggle.com/c/prostate-cancer-grade-assessment/data (accessed on 27 March 2021).

79. PESO: Prostate Epithelium Segmentation on H&E-Stained Prostatectomy Whole Slide Images. Available online: https://zenodo.org/record/1485967#.YF945q8zbIU (accessed on 27 March 2021).
80. Jain, R.; Kasturi, R.; Schunck, B.G. *Machine Vision*; McGraw-Hill International Edition: New York, NY, USA, 1995.
81. Hoshyar, A.N.; Al-Jumaily, A.; Hoshyar, A.N. The Beneficial Techniques in Preprocessing Step of Skin Cancer Detection System Comparing. *Procedia Comput. Sci.* **2014**, *42*, 25–31. [CrossRef]
82. Patidar, P.; Gupta, M.; Srivastava, S.; Nagawat, A.K. Image De-noising by Various Filters for Different Noise. *Int. J. Comput. Appl.* **2010**, *9*, 45–50. [CrossRef]
83. Lee, G.; Singanamalli, A.; Wang, H.; Feldman, M.D.; Master, S.R.; Shih, N.N.C.; Spangler, E.; Rebbeck, T.; Tomaszewski, J.E.; Madabhushi, A. Supervised multi-view canonical correlation analysis (sMVCCA): Integrating histologic and proteomic features for predicting recurrent prostate cancer. *IEEE Trans. Med Imaging* **2014**, *34*, 284–297. [CrossRef] [PubMed]
84. Gurcan, M.N.; Boucheron, L.E.; Can, A.; Madabhushi, A.; Rajpoot, N.M.; Yener, B. Histopathological Image Analysis: A Review. *IEEE Rev. Biomed. Eng.* **2009**, *2*, 147–171. [CrossRef] [PubMed]
85. Yang, L.; Meer, P.; Foran, D.J. Unsupervised segmentation based on robust estimation and color active contour models. *IEEE Trans. Inf. Technol. Biomed.* **2005**, *9*, 475–486. [CrossRef]
86. Bautista, P.A.; Hashimoto, N.; Yagi, Y. Color standardization in whole slide imaging using a color calibration slide. *J. Pathol. Inform.* **2014**, *5*, 4. [CrossRef]
87. Zuo, C.; Chen, Q.; Sui, X. Range Limited Bi-Histogram Equalization for image contrast enhancement. *Optik* **2013**, *124*, 425–431. [CrossRef]
88. Tam, A.; Barker, J.; Rubin, D.L. A method for normalizing pathology images to improve feature extraction for quantitative pathology. *Med. Phys.* **2016**, *43*, 528–537. [CrossRef]
89. Shanmugavadivu, P.; Balasubramanian, K. Particle swarm optimized multi-objective histogram equalization for image enhancement. *Opt. Laser Technol.* **2014**, *57*, 243–251. [CrossRef]
90. Nanni, L.; Brahnam, S.; Ghidoni, S.; Maguolo, G. General purpose (GenP) bioimage ensemble of handcrafted and learned features with data augmentation. *arXiv* **2019**, arXiv:1904.08084. Available online: https://arxiv.org/abs/1904.08084 (accessed on 30 January 2021).
91. Shin, H.-C.; Tenenholtz, N.A.; Rogers, J.K.; Schwarz, C.G.; Senjem, M.L.; Gunter, J.L.; Andriole, K.P.; Michalski, M. Medical Image Synthesis for Data Augmentation and Anonymization Using Generative Adversarial Networks. In *Tools and Algorithms for the Construction and Analysis of Systems*; Springer Science and Business Media LLC: Berlin/Heidelberg, Germany, 2018; pp. 1–11.
92. Sandfort, V.; Yan, K.; Pickhardt, P.J.; Summers, R.M. Data augmentation using generative adversarial networks (CycleGAN) to improve generalizability in CT segmentation tasks. *Sci. Rep.* **2019**, *9*, 16884. [CrossRef]
93. Liu, S.; Shah, Z.; Sav, A.; Russo, C.; Berkovsky, S.; Qian, Y.; Coiera, E.; Di Ieva, A. Isocitrate dehydrogenase (IDH) status prediction in histopathology images of gliomas using deep learning. *Sci. Rep.* **2020**, *10*, 7733. [CrossRef]
94. Ataky, S.T.M.; De Matos, J.; Britto, A.D.S.; Oliveira, L.E.S.; Koerich, A.L. Data Augmentation for Histopathological Images Based on Gaussian-Laplacian Pyramid Blending. In Proceedings of the 2020 International Joint Conference on Neural Networks (IJCNN), Glasgow, UK, 19–24 July 2020; pp. 1–8. [CrossRef]
95. Chauhan, N.K.; Singh, K. A Review on Conventional Machine Learning vs Deep Learning. In Proceedings of the 2018 International Conference on Computing, Power and Communication Technologies (GUCON), Greater Noida, India, 28–29 September 2018; pp. 347–352.
96. Nielsen, B.; Albregtsen, F.; Danielsen, H.E. Automatic segmentation of cell nuclei in Feulgen-stained histological sections of prostate cancer and quantitative evaluation of segmentation results. *Cytom. Part A* **2012**, *81*, 588–601. [CrossRef]
97. Simon, I.; Pound, C.R.; Partin, A.W.; Clemens, J.Q.; Christens-Barry, W.A. Automated image analysis system for detecting boundaries of live prostate cancer cells. *Cytometry* **1998**, *31*, 287–294. [CrossRef]
98. Nguyen, K.; Sabata, B.; Jain, A.K. Prostate cancer grading: Gland segmentation and structural features. *Pattern Recognit. Lett.* **2012**, *33*, 951–961. [CrossRef]
99. Nguyen, K.; Jain, A.K.; Allen, R.L. Automated Gland Segmentation and Classification for Gleason Grading of Prostate Tissue Images. In Proceedings of the 2010 20th International Conference on Pattern Recognition, Istanbul, Turkey, 23–26 August 2010; pp. 1497–1500.
100. Ayyad, S.M.; Saleh, A.I.; Labib, L.M.; Aiyad, S.M. A new distributed feature selection technique for classifying gene expression data. *Int. J. Biomath.* **2019**, *12*. [CrossRef]
101. Ayyad, S.M.; Saleh, A.I.; Labib, L.M. Gene expression cancer classification using modified K-Nearest Neighbors technique. *Biosystems* **2019**, *176*, 41–51. [CrossRef]
102. Albashish, D.; Sahran, S.; Abdullah, A.; Adam, A.; Shukor, N.A.; Pauzi, S.H.M. Multi-scoring feature selection method based on SVM-RFE for prostate cancer diagnosis. In Proceedings of the 2015 International Conference on Electrical Engineering and Informatics (ICEEI), Denpasar, Indonesia, 10–11 August 2015; pp. 682–686.
103. Peyret, R.; Bouridane, A.; Khelifi, F.; Tahir, M.A.; Al-Maadeed, S. Automatic classification of colorectal and prostatic histologic tumor images using multiscale multispectral local binary pattern texture features and stacked generalization. *Neurocomputing* **2018**, *275*, 83–93. [CrossRef]
104. Sparks, R.; Madabhushi, A. Content-based image retrieval utilizing explicit shape descriptors: Applications to breast MRI and prostate histopathology. *SPIE Med. Imaging* **2011**, *7962*, 79621. [CrossRef]

105. Tabesh, A.; Teverovskiy, M. Tumor Classification in Histological Images of Prostate Using Color Texture. In Proceedings of the 2006 Fortieth Asilomar Conference on Signals, Systems and Computers, Pacific Grove, CA, USA, 29 October–1 November 2006; pp. 841–845.
106. Akakin, H.C.; Gurcan, M.N. Content-Based Microscopic Image Retrieval System for Multi-Image Queries. *IEEE Trans. Inf. Technol. Biomed.* **2012**, *16*, 758–769. [CrossRef]
107. Lopez, C.M.; Agaian, S.; Sanchez, I.; Almuntashri, A.; Zinalabdin, O.; Al Rikabi, A.; Thompson, I. Exploration of efficacy of gland morphology and architectural features in prostate cancer gleason grading. In Proceedings of the 2012 IEEE International Conference on Systems, Man, and Cybernetics (SMC), Seoul, Korea, 14–17 October 2012; pp. 2849–2854.
108. Shaban, W.M.; Rabie, A.H.; Saleh, A.I.; Abo-Elsoud, M. A new COVID-19 Patients Detection Strategy (CPDS) based on hybrid feature selection and enhanced KNN classifier. *Knowl. -Based Syst.* **2020**, *205*, 106270. [CrossRef] [PubMed]
109. Ayyad, S.M.; Saleh, A.I.; Labib, L.M. Classification techniques in gene expression microarray data. *Int. J. Comput. Sci. Mob. Comput.* **2018**, *7*, 52–56.
110. Castanho, M.; Hernandes, F.; De Ré, A.; Rautenberg, S.; Billis, A. Fuzzy expert system for predicting pathological stage of prostate cancer. *Expert Syst. Appl.* **2013**, *40*, 466–470. [CrossRef]
111. Shaban, W.M.; Rabie, A.H.; Saleh, A.I.; Abo-Elsoud, M. Detecting COVID-19 patients based on fuzzy inference engine and Deep Neural Network. *Appl. Soft Comput.* **2020**, *99*, 106906. [CrossRef] [PubMed]
112. Khan, S.; Yong, S.-P. A comparison of deep learning and hand crafted features in medical image modality classification. In Proceedings of the 2016 3rd International Conference on Computer and Information Sciences (ICCOINS), Kuala Lumpur, Malaysia, 15–17 August 2016; pp. 633–638.
113. Swiderska-Chadaj, Z.; De Bel, T.; Blanchet, L.; Baidoshvili, A.; Vossen, D.; Van Der Laak, J.; Litjens, G. Impact of rescanning and normalization on convolutional neural network performance in multi-center, whole-slide classification of prostate cancer. *Sci. Rep.* **2020**, *10*, 1–14. [CrossRef] [PubMed]

sensors

MDPI

Article

Analysis of the Nosema Cells Identification for Microscopic Images

Soumaya Dghim [1], Carlos M. Travieso-González [1,*] and Radim Burget [2]

[1] Signals and Communications Department (DSC), Institute for Technological Development and Innovation in Communications (IDeTIC), University of Las Palmas de Gran Canaria (ULPGC), Las Palmas de Gran Canaria, 35001 Canary Islands, Spain; soumaya.dghim101@alu.ulpgc.es
[2] Department of Telecommunications, Faculty of Electrical Engineering and Communication, Brno University of Technology (BUT), 61600 Brno, Czech Republic; burgetrm@vutbr.cz
* Correspondence: carlos.travieso@ulpgc.es

Abstract: The use of image processing tools, machine learning, and deep learning approaches has become very useful and robust in recent years. This paper introduces the detection of the Nosema disease, which is considered to be one of the most economically significant diseases today. This work shows a solution for recognizing and identifying Nosema cells between the other existing objects in the microscopic image. Two main strategies are examined. The first strategy uses image processing tools to extract the most valuable information and features from the dataset of microscopic images. Then, machine learning methods are applied, such as a neural network (ANN) and support vector machine (SVM) for detecting and classifying the Nosema disease cells. The second strategy explores deep learning and transfers learning. Several approaches were examined, including a convolutional neural network (CNN) classifier and several methods of transfer learning (AlexNet, VGG-16 and VGG-19), which were fine-tuned and applied to the object sub-images in order to identify the Nosema images from the other object images. The best accuracy was reached by the VGG-16 pre-trained neural network with 96.25%.

Keywords: image processing; Nosema disease; machine learning; deep learning; image; disease detection

Citation: Dghim, S.; Travieso-González, C.M.; Burget, R. Analysis of the Nosema Cells Identification for Microscopic Images. *Sensors* **2021**, *21*, 68. https://doi.org/10.3390/s21093068

Academic Editor: Ayman El-baz

Received: 16 March 2021
Accepted: 26 April 2021
Published: 28 April 2021

1. Introduction

Several deadly diseases endanger honeybees. Possibly one of the best known is Nosema. Nosema, which is also called Nosemiasis or Nosemosi [1], is caused by two species of microsporidia, *Nosema apis* (*N. apis*) and Nosema ceraena (*N. ceraena*) [2]. Several works were published regarding the impact of Nosema disease on commerce, society and food, as shown in [3,4], and the disease is currently of one the major economic importance worldwide [5]. The health of the two species of bees is a particular interest of biologists, not only because of their significant role in the economy and food production but also because of the vital role they give in the pollination of agricultural and horticultural crops. Many biological descriptions of its DNA and its behavior can be found in literature, for example in [6,7]. Furthermore, several recent works try to treat this disease using a chemical simulation, as presented in [8,9].

Furthermore, from a computer science point of view, honeybees are of significant interest. Several works were, for example, involved in bees and controlling their behavior [10]. The study presented monitoring the behavior of bees to help people associated with beekeeping to manage their honey colonies and discover the bee disturbance caused by a pathogen, Colony Collapse Disorder (CCD) or colony health assessment. In [11], many tools of image analysis were explored to study the honeybee auto grooming behavior. Chemical and gas sensors were used for measurement. Destructor infestations are applied inside the honeybee colony to detect disease. The study was based on measurements of the atmosphere of six beehives using six types of solid-state gas sensors during a 12-h experiment [12]. Regarding the image processing of Nosema disease part, there are currently two major works. In [13], the authors used the Scale Invariant Feature Transform to extract features from cell images. It is a technique that transforms image data into scale-invariant coordinates relative to local features. A segmentation technique and a support vector machine algorithm were then applied to microscopic processed images to automatically classify *N. apis* and *N. ceranae* microsporidia. In [14], the authors used the image processing techniques to extract the most valuable features from Nosema microscopic images and apply an Artificial Neural Network (ANN) for the recognition, which was statistically evaluated using the cross-validation technique. The last two works used image processing tools for feature extraction and Support Vector Machine (SVM) and ANN for classification. Today the traditional tools of machine learning like ANN, Convolutional Neural Network (CNN), and SVM are frequently used in human disease detection [15], especially in medical image classification of Heart diseases [16], Alzheimer disease [17] and Thorax diseases [18]. Deep learning approaches were used in [19] for semantic images segmentation. This work used the Atrous convolutional Neural Network for segmentation and some pre-trained NN for validation like PASCAL-Context, PASCAL-Person-Part and CityscapesDeep. In [20], a method using a 2D overlapping ellipse was implemented using the tools of image processing and applied to the problem of segmenting potentially overlapping cells in fluorescence microscopy images. Deep learning is an end-to-end machine learning process that trains feature extraction together with the classification itself. Instead of organizing statistics to run through predefined equations, deep learning uses multiple layers of processing data and setting fundamental parameters on knowledge records, and it trains the computer to analyze and recognize data. Deep learning approaches are widely applied in the analysis of microscopic images in many fields: human microbiota [21], material sciences [22], microorganism detection [23], cellular image processing [24] and many other important works in this field. Deep learning techniques have accelerated with transfer learning the ability to recognize and classify several diseases. The objective of this paper is to validate this hypothesis.

All the methods of Nosema detection and recognition presented by the biologists in the literature were either molecular detections or genetic descriptions. This paper evaluates two different strategies for automatic identification of the Nosema cell disease based on the microscopic images. First, images of Nosema cells and the existing objects have been cropped from the principal microscopic images. Using these images, the first dataset has been built. Then, the obtained images were processed again and several different features have been extracted. These features were used to create a second dataset. The obtained databases were used for the evaluation recognition of the Nosema cells. The first approach uses a model, which uses the extracted features by an ANN and an SVM. The second approach uses the deep learning and transfer learning methods: first, CNN, and then pre-trained networks AlexNet, VGG-16 and VGG-19. The tools of transfer learning used by authors reached notable results as this is the first time they have been used for the purpose of Nosema cell recognition.

The main innovation of this paper is the evaluation of two different strategies of automatic detection and recognition Nosema cells from microscopic images and identification of the robust and successful approach as a robust methodology for automated identifying and recognizing Nosema cells versus the other existing objects in the same microscopic images.

The rest of the paper is organized as follow: Section 2 describes the dataset preparation. In Section 3 is described dataset, segmentation, features extraction, ANN training, the use of SVM, CNN, the use of Alex Net, VGG-16 and VGG-19. The experiments are described in Section 4. Section 5 discusses the obtained results. Finally, the paper is concluded.

2. Materials: Preparation of The Dataset

For the experiment, Nosema microscopic images were used. So far, it is not known whether these images contain a sufficient amount of information for accurate detection and recognition of the disease cells. It was only known that the important information was diffused all over the image and behind the majority of unimportant data. The used images in this work are 400 RGB images, encoded with JPEG and with a resolution of 2272 × 1704 pixels. Each sample was labelled by one of the 7 classes, according to the severity of the disease or the number of disease cells present in the microscopic image. From these 400 RGB images, a set of sub-images have been extracted. To do that, each microscopic image was divided into many smaller images forming subdivisions of the existing and clear objects. This first phase was done manually due to the low quality of input images by cropping the object of interest (i.e., cells). All the existing objects in the microscopic images were extracted as sub-images and labelled whether they stand for: Nosema(N) and not Nosema cells (n-N), see Figure 1. The area chosen was as small as possible, where an isolated and clear microscopic cell is located. Then, in the second automatic phase, the selected objects are processed to prepare them for the segmentation process (see Figure 1).

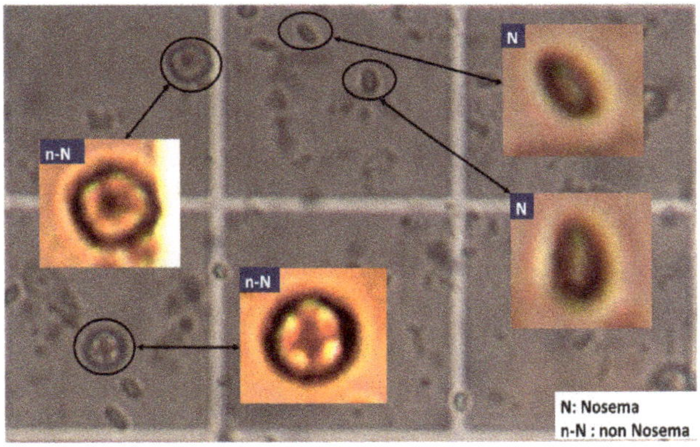

Figure 1. Example of extraction of Nosema cells and other existing objects in a part of one microscopic image.

Based on the steps described above, a dataset containing 2000 sample images in total was created. It consists of 1000 Nosema cells samples and 1000 images, which are not Nosema cells, i.e., any other existing objects in the microscopic images. Table 1 below shows information about the extracted sub-images for dataset construction.

Table 1. Dataset of extracted sub-images.

Images	Number	Color	Type	Resolution
Nosema sub-images	1000	RGB	JPEG	229 × 161
Non-Nosema sub-images	1000	RGB	JPEG	450 × 257

The microscopic sub-images were examined using two strategies:

- The first strategy is based on an image processing approach, where features were extracted manually.
- The second set of strategies is based on the use of the whole sub-image and the deep learning.

Figure 2 shows strategies covered in the paper.

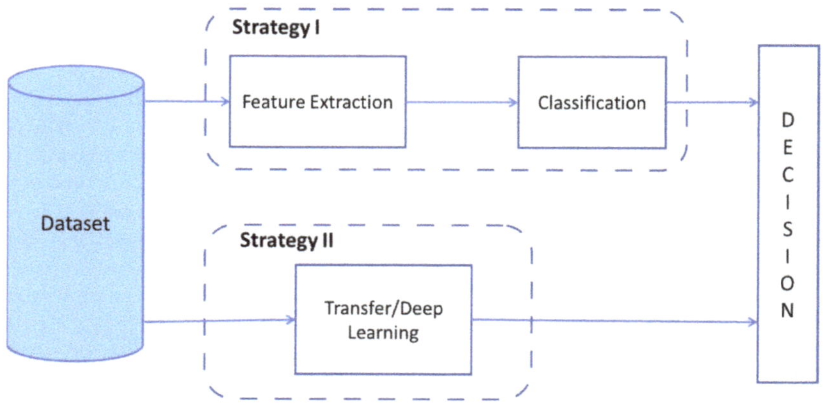

Figure 2. Implemented Strategies for Nosema Recognition.

3. Methods

In the scope of this study, two different strategies were implemented. All the methods are shown according to both of the strategies. The methods are working on the dataset of sub-images (2000 images).

3.1. *Strategy 1: Nosema Cells Recognition with Image Processing and Machine Learning*

This subsection is divided into two parts. The first part describes how the features were extracted and prepared for the training of a model. The second part shows the proposed classification systems.

3.1.1. Preprocessing for Feature Extraction

A preprocessing stage is necessary before extraction of the features. The initial point is an RGB image. The first step is to convert the image from RGB to a grayscale image. The second step consists of binarization of the image by the thresholding using the Otsu method [25]. In the third step, the flood-fill operation was used on background pixels of the input binary image to fill the object hole from its specific locations and then to ignore all smaller existing objects in the image of the desired object. As the final step, the object perimeter is enhanced using the dilatation method [26]. So, the desired shape of the object is obtained by calculating the difference between the two images, before and after perimeter enhancement. The result of the final step is a shape image, which was extracted from the sub-image of the dataset (see Figure 3).

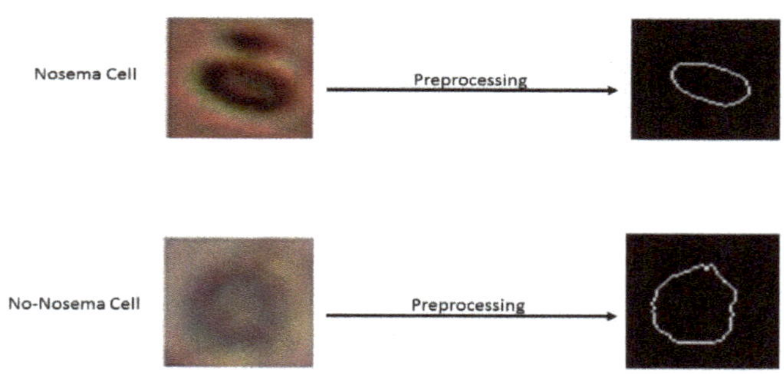

Figure 3. Shape results of two examples before and after preprocessing. The first sample is Nosema and the second is non Nosema object.

From the shape image, in total 9 features were extracted. They describe the structure of the Nosema cell and consist of 6 geometric and 3 statistic features. Furthermore, from the extracted sub-images, 6 texture features and 4 Gray Level Co-occurrence Matrices (GLCM) color features were calculated.

Geometric Features Extraction

The geometric features describe basic characteristics of geometric form. They are also the most significant for us because, after several experiments, the best results were achieved using them. These parameters were used and defined in [14] respectively:

- The size/the perimeter: given that the shape of the Nosema cell is similar to an ellipse form and the other objects have different rounds shapes, perimeter formula of an ellipse adopted have been adopted in this study. This calculation is based on a and b variables where a is the semi-major axis and b is the semi-minor axis. Perimeter P is given by the following equation:

$$P = \pi \cdot \sqrt{2 \cdot (a^2 + b)^2} \tag{1}$$

- Area A is given by the following formula:

$$\mathrm{A} = \pi \cdot a \cdot b \tag{2}$$

- Relation R is the dividing quotient of the height (H) and width (W) of the shape.

$$\mathrm{R} = \mathrm{H}/\mathrm{W} \tag{3}$$

- The equivalent diameter (D), which is the diameter of the circle with the same area of the object,

$$\mathrm{D} = \sqrt{4 \times \frac{\mathrm{A}}{\pi}} \tag{4}$$

- The solidity (S): it is the portion of the area of the convex region contained in the object,

$$\mathrm{S} = \frac{\mathrm{A}}{\text{convex area}} \tag{5}$$

- The eccentricity (E): it is the relation between the distance of the focus of the ellipse and the length of the principal axis. Let $f = 1 - \frac{a}{b}$ in which a is the semi-major axis and b is the semi-minor axis of the ellipse.

$$\mathrm{E} = \sqrt{f \times (2 - f)} \tag{6}$$

Statistic Features Extraction

The remaining features 7, 8 and 9 were calculated using the polar coordinates of the object, in particular, the polar coordinates of a Cartesian point (x, y). Let us say that a point M is at such a distance (r) and such a direction (θ) of the point of origin (o) of the reference point. It is a projection or a one-dimensional representation of the boundary. This is found by computing the distances from the centroid (center of "mass") of the object to the boundary as a function of angles in any chosen increment. The resulting set of distances, when properly scaled, was the vector needed as distances of the angle to the boundary pixel.

After that, a value for these distances is truncated, which are the nearest integers to a value to calculate the last three respective parameters.

- The standard deviation of these distances have been calculated and which is the feature number 7, the standard deviation is a measure of variability, or what the range of values is, it normalizes the elements of N along the first array dimension whose size does not equal to 1; where P can be a vector or a matrix and in this case is a vector of the radius values of polar coordinates of the studied object, and E is its mean. It is given by Equation (7):

$$Std.deviation\ (\sigma) = \sqrt{\frac{1}{N} \cdot \sum_{j=1}^{N} (P_{ij} - E_i)^2} \quad (7)$$

- The Variance σ^2 is the mean of the squared distances between a value and the mean of those values: it normalizes Y by $n - 1$ if $n > 1$, where n is the sample size or pixels shape number. This is an unbiased estimator of the variance of the population from which x is drawn, as long as x consists of independent, distributed distances. For $n = 1$, Y is normalized by n with μ is the average of all x values. In this case, the variance is calculated as the normalized distances between the centroid and every single pixel in the object shape.

$$\sigma^2 = \frac{(x_1 - \mu)^2 + (x_2 - \mu)^2 + (x_3 - \mu)^2 + \ldots + (x_n - \mu)^2}{n} \quad (8)$$

- The Variance derivate is the derivate that calculates the difference and the approximate derivative of the variance (X), for a vector X, is [X(2) − X(1) X(3) − X(2) . . . X(n) − X(n−1)]. It is given by the following equation:

$$f'(\sigma^2) = -n^{-2}\left[(x_1 - \mu)^2 + (x_2 - \mu)^2 + (x_3 - \mu)^2 + \ldots + (x_n - \mu)^2\right] \quad (9)$$

Features Extraction: Texture and GLCM

The next step consists of the use of the RGB object image to extract more information about texture and color. Nevertheless, before that, it is needed to separate the object from its background in the image; to do that: individual Hue (V), saturation (S) and Value (V) channels have been extracted after converting the image from RGB to HSV color spice image, then authors look for the vivid color by thresholding the V mask, after that, authors set the H and S masks to 0 and the V mask to 1 and concatenate the three new HSV channels. Finally, the authors convert back the image to RGB color image to have the object without it's background, as shown in Figure 4:

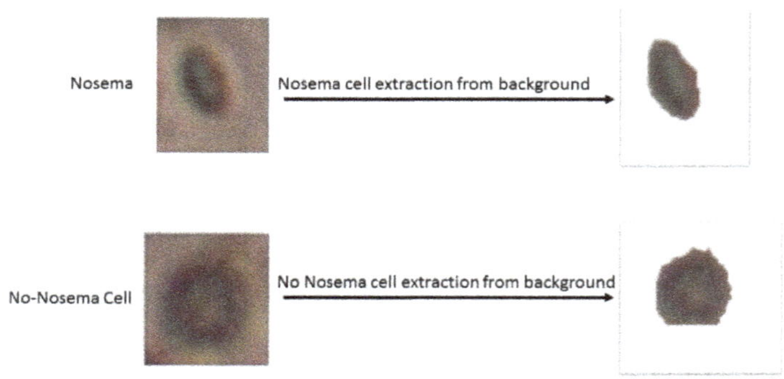

Figure 4. Example of a Nosema cell and non-Nosema object extraction from its backgrounds.

The number of texture parameters is 6 and they are the measurement of the entropy of RGB and HSV channels; it can be defined as a logarithmic measurement of the number of states with a significant probability of being occupied. The input intensity images are the blue, red, green and yellow channels. Furthermore, the Hue and saturation masks' randomness is calculated. The value/lightness channel was dropped since it does not give any extra information. Suppose x_i is the set of pixels with the color/channel i of the image and $p(x_i)$ is its probability. The 6 entropy parameters are calculated by the same equation 10 above:

$$E(x_i) = \sum_{i=1}^{N} P(x_i) \cdot log_2(p(x_i)). \quad (10)$$

As mentioned before, the Nosema cells look to be more yellow inside, that is the way a Grey Level Co-occurrence Matrix was applied to the yellow mask to extract more texture information about this color. The GLCM is very widely used as a statistical method of extracting a textural feature from images. It was used in several works of feature extraction, like in features skin extraction [27] or plant disease feature extraction [28]. GLCM is widely used to extract useful information from medical images, that is why GLCM is developed to overcome the limitations of the available extracted features and to be more accurate as indicated in [29], a novel strategy to compute the GLCM called HaraliCU can offload the computations into the Graphics Processing Units (GPU) cores, thus allowing to drastically reduce the running time required by the execution on Central Processing Units (CPUs). In [30], a developed method called CHASM exploits the HaraliCU method mentioned previously, a GPU-enabled approach, capable of overcoming the issues of existing tools by effectively computing the feature maps for high-resolution images with their full dynamics of grayscale levels, and CUDA-SOM, a GPU-based implementation of the SOMs for the identification of clusters of pixels in the image. The general rule in the statistical texture calculator says that these are calculated from the statistical distribution of combinations of intensities observed at specified positions relative to each other in the image. Based on the number of pixels in each combination, statistics are categorized into first-order, second-order, and higher-order statistics. The GLCM is a method of extracting the second-order statistical texture characteristics. Third-order and higher-order textures are theoretically possible but not commonly implemented due to computation time demands and difficulty to interpret them [31]. The GLCM is considered a greyscale image I defined in Z. The grey level co-occurrence matrix is defined to be a square matrix G_d of size N where, N is the total number of grey levels in the image. The (i, j) th entry of G_d represents the number of times a pixel X with intensity value i is separated from a pixel Y with intensity value j at a particular distance k in a particular direction d. Where the distance k is a non-negative integer and the direction d is specified by $d = (d_1, d_2, d_3, \ldots d_n)$, where $d_i \in \{0, k, -k\}$ $\forall i = 1, 2, 3, \ldots, n$ [32]. Four features were extracted from the Haralick GLCM applied to the image of the yellow channel: contrast, correlation, energy, and homogeneity, the most significant features given by the GLCM.

$$Contrast = \sum_{n=0}^{Ng-1} n^2 \cdot \left[\sum_{i=1}^{Ng} \sum_{j=1}^{Ng} p(i,j) \right] \quad (11)$$

Correlation measures the linear dependency of grey levels of neighboring pixels:

$$Correlation = \frac{1}{(\sigma i.\sigma j)} \cdot \sum_i \sum_j (i - \mu i) \cdot (j - \mu j) \cdot P_{i,j}\,. \quad (12)$$

It is also called Angular Second Moment (ASM), and it is of high value when two neighbor pixels are very similar:

$$Energy = \sum_{i=0}^{Ng-1} \sum_{j=0}^{Ng-1} p(i,j)^2 \quad (13)$$

Homogeneity is high when a local grey level is uniform:

$$Homogeneity = \sum_i \sum_j P(i,j) \cdot \frac{1}{1 + (i-j)^2}\,. \quad (14)$$

Segmentation Diagram Block and Recognition

The automatic approach of this part of work is to study the existing objects in the microscopic images of Nosema disease; to study both Nosema cells and other types of cells present in microscopic images, the desired objects are detected, useful features are extracted (geometric, texture and statistic features) by an automatic segmentation method, and the result is a vector of 19 features. Then, a multilayer Neural Network system is used as a classifier, the set of features in order to recognize the Nosema disease cells vs. the other objects in the images.

Once the features of the different object were extracted, the feature dataset is generated: it consists of 19 features for 2000 objects, i.e., a 38,000 value divided equally between two kind of objects: one for the calculated features of the objects of interest (Nosema cells), and the other for other existed object in the microscopic images. This part of the work was significantly computationally demanding since the extraction of 2000 sub-images as well as the calculation of 19 features for each image cost many days of computations, using a CPU, in particular, PcCom Basic Elite Pro Intel Core i7-9700/8GB/240SSD.

In this part of the paper, neural networks were used for the automatic detection of Nosema diseases in honeybees. The neural networks proved their quality in many real-world applications as well as for classification tasks. Usually, a neural network is made up of two parts which constitute the set of learning functionalities used to train the NN model, while a set of testing functionality is used to verify the correctness of the trained NN model. The appropriate network design should be configured, including network type, learning method and with one or two hidden layers. In the learning phase, the connection weights were always updated until they reached the defined iteration number or the acceptable error. Therefore, the ability of the ANN model to respond accurately was ensured by using the mean squared error (MSE) criterion to emphasize the validity of the model between input and network output. Furthermore, the network calculates the outputs and automatically adjusts the weights to reduce errors and recognize the objects.

For the experiment, the dataset was divided into a learning part of the model and another part for testing and validation. During the proposed approach, two types of experiments were conducted: in the first one, the model was tested with only the 15 geometric, statistic and texture features without counting the yellow color features calculated with the GLCM. The second experiment was implemented by concatenating all the 19 features. Furthermore, these two experiments were done to prove the strong presence of yellow color in the cell of Nosema. The experiments were done by applying different precision of the data division between data for training and the data for testing. The experiment was conducted with several different neural network architectures—in particular, it has experimented with the number of neurons in the hidden layer. Each test was repeated at least 30 times to obtain the optimal value of success recognition accuracy. First of all, the program was tested with a number of neurons equal to the number of input features extracted from the images (15 or 19) in which the weight is added randomly, and after that, the number of neurons was increased in the hidden layer by 50 in every new experiment (see Table 2).

3.1.2. The Use of Support Vector Machine: SVM

Support vector machines SVM is a supervised learning algorithm used for classification and regression problems [33]. To ensure that SVM will give the optimal result, the parameters of the classifier were optimized. The optimized options have been the cost "C", also called error term or regularization parameter and the kernel trick function, which calculates the dot product of two vectors in the space of very large characteristics. Different kernel functions can be specified for the decision function and the radial basis function (RBF) is commonly used, especially for nonlinear hyperplanes. RBF kernel for the SVM has been chosen, which is in the following form:

$$K(X_1, X_2) = exponent\left(-\gamma\cdot||X_{1-}X_2||^2\right) \tag{15}$$

where $||X_1 - X_2||$ is the Euclidean distance between X_1 and X_2, and γ: gamma is used only for RBF kernel. The non-regularization of the values of "γ" and "C" will cause overfitting or an underfitting of the model. The SVM has been configured with $C = 3$ and $\gamma = 5 \times 10^{-5}$ as the architecture with the best result. In this case, the SVM model will classify two classes corresponding to Nosema cells and non-Nosema cells (or other objects).

Figure 5 shows the diagram block of the processing model for ANN and SVM classification systems for the first implemented strategy.

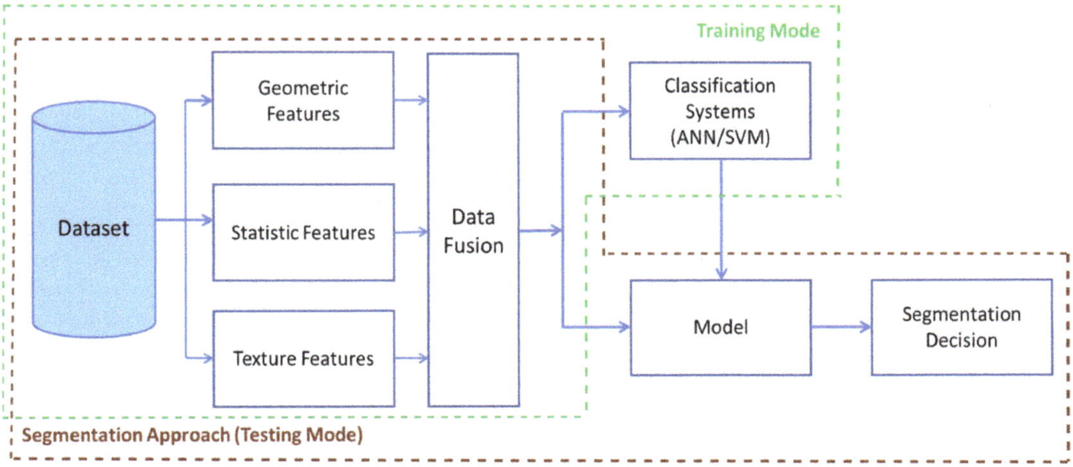

Figure 5. The Segmentation Diagram Block of the first strategy in Nosema detection: The Training Mode consists of the part of dataset construction, features extraction, and their fusion to be trained with ANN and SVM. The Testing Mode consists of data preparation for testing the model and decision making.

3.2. Strategy 2: Nosema Cells Recognition Using Deep Learning Approaches

3.2.1. Nosema Recognition with the Implemented CNN

A convolutional neural network CNN is a network architecture for deep learning which learns directly from data. They are used to classify images or to predict continuous data. In the scope of this paper, a new CNN network was designed, but before entering them into the network, input data and the predictors have been normalized were normalized. Furthermore, batch normalization layers should be used to normalize the outputs of each convolutional and fully connected layer. The architecture of a CNN should contain input layers that define the size and type of input data, the middle layers which contain the main layers of learning and computation, and an output layer that defines the size and type of output data. The experiment is described in detail in Table 3 and its description is in the Experimental Methodology and Result section.

3.2.2. The Use of Transfer Learning

Another approach to work in Deep Learning is using a pre-trained Deep Neural Network. For the first approach, the advantage is its structure; a model of an already existing Deep Neural Network is used by applying a few simple changes. In the latter case, a limited data set is used and knowledge is transferred from this model to a new task. It is also said to transfer the learned characteristics of a pre-trained CNN to a new problem with a limited data set. Transfer learning involves forming a CNN with available labelled source data (called a source learner) and then extracting the inner layers that represent a generic representation of mid-level entities to a target CNN learner. An adaptation layer is added to the target CNN learner to correct for any different conditional distributions between the source and target domains. The experiments are performed on the object image classification, where the average precision is measured as a measure of performance.

The first experiment was performed using the Pascal VOC 2007 dataset as the target and ImageNet 2012 as the source. The second experiment was performed using the Pascal VOC 2012 dataset as the target and ImageNet 2012 as the source. The tests have successfully demonstrated the ability to transfer information from one CNN learner to another [34].

The main advantage of transfer learning is that it does not need a lot of data to give a good accuracy (and this is true in most cases). Transfer learning has proven to be a solution to many real problems. Some of them are; for example [35], the transfer learning techniques were used to improve the global climate by classifying aerosol dust particles. In [36], and in using transfer learning tools, an approach has been proposed to be able to identify low-income areas in developing countries that are important for disaster relief efforts. In [37], transfer learning is used to improve disease prediction. In [38], transfer learning was used to improve the problem of facial recognition using the face image information of a source group to improve the learning of a classifier for a target group. In [39] transfer learning was applied to the field of biology. Therefore, the following concept was applied for the analysis of Nosema disease.

Nosema Recognition with Alexnet Classifier

Several architectures were examined, and AlexNet was one of them. AlexNet is one of the first pre-trained Neural Networks; it is trained using a large image dataset called ImageNet, which in turn contains more than millions of images and 22 thousand visual categories. AlexNet is trained on more than a million images and can classify images into 1000 object categories. This paper used the pre-trained weights of the AlexNet network, which contains 25 layers. Then, the network was fine-tuned for the classification problem by replacing the last three layers of AlexNet pre-trained model with a fully connected layer (layer number 23), a softmax layer (layer number 24) and a classification output layer (layer number 25). The new model was fine-tuned using 2000 input cell images for two classes: Nosema class and Non Nosema Class. Since AlexNet requires exactly 227 $\times$ 227 RGB input images, the images were automatically resized to this dimension during the data augmentation. The augmentation of the data helps prevent the network from overfitting and helps its better generalization capabilities. Furthermore, the data were split into two parts, one for training and the other for validation of results. Each experiment and its results are shown in Table 7, Section 4.

Nosema Recognition VGG-16 and VGG-19 Classifiers

VGG-16 and VGG-19 are another pre-trained neural network models. They are again pre-trained using ImageNet dataset. These two models were chosen because they learned a good representation of low-level characteristics such as space, edges, color, lighting, texture and shapes; and these characteristics are very useful for knowledge transfer and act as a feature extractor for new images. Since the images in this work belong to completely different categories from the source dataset, but the pre-trained model should still be able to extract relevant features from these images based on transfer learning principles. These pre-trained models—VGG-16 and VGG-19 were transferred again for classification of images of Nosema cells against images of other objects.

VGG-16 pre-trained network contains 41 layers and VGG-19 contains 47 layers. The last three layers of VGG-16 and the number of layers 45 and 47 for VGG-19 were replaced with fully connected layers and trained with 1000 Nosema images and 1000 non-Nosema images. The network expects 224 $\times$ 224 RGB or grayscale input images, so the input images were resized. The dataset was split into learning and validation parts regarding different average of data division. Figure 6 shows the used model for modification of the pre-trained transfer learning models used in this paper.

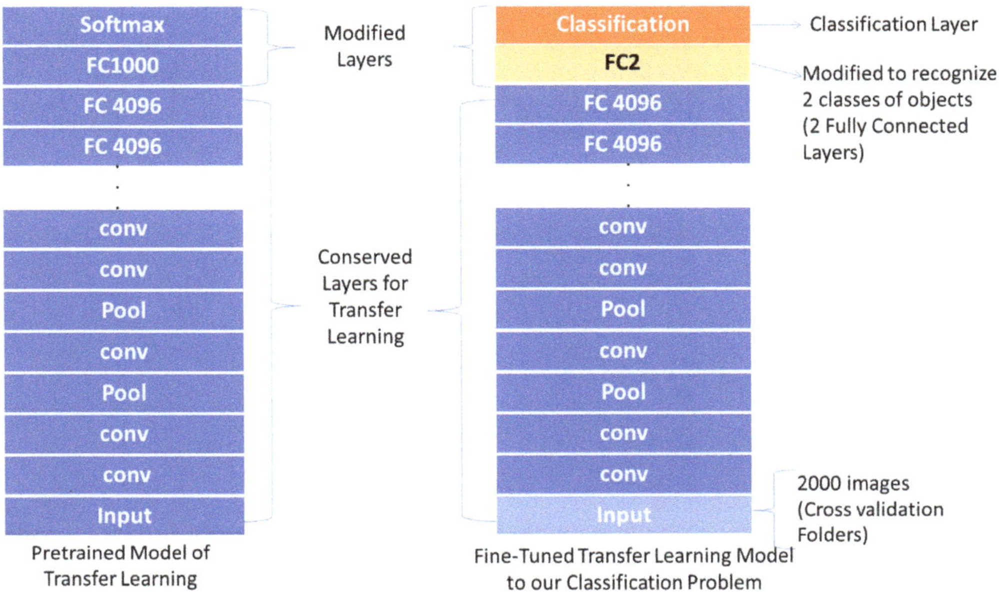

Figure 6. Modifying Transfer Learning Models for This Proposal.

4. Experimental Methodology and Results

For the statistical evaluation, the 10-fold cross-validation strategy was followed between 10% and 90%. Accuracy is used as a quality measure here. The experiments have been designed for machine learning approaches (SVM and ANN), transfer learning approaches (AlexNet, VGG-16 and VGG-19), and deep learning method with CNN.

The first experiment was done for ANN and SVM. For ANN, just a single hidden layer was used and only the number of neurons in the hidden layer was adjusted, using 15 or 19 neurons for the input layer and 1 neuron for the output layer (see Table 2).

Table 2. Results for experiments with ANN and SVM.

Number of Features	Classifier	Accuracy	Observation
15 Features	ANN	79.00%	For 1400 neurons in the hidden layer
	SVM	81.00%	Using kernel RBF
19 Features	ANN	83.20%	For 1400 neurons in the hidden layer
	SVM	83.50%	Using kernel RBF

The next experiment used the deep learning method, in particular deep CNN classifier. The architecture of CNN had 3 convolutional blocks, which have been stacked with 3 × 3 filters followed by a 2 × 2 subsampling layer (max_pooling). In this way, increasing the number of filters increases the depth of the network, and a kind of cone is formed with increasingly reduced but more relevant characteristics. It should be noted that in convolutional layers, padding is used to ensure that the height and width of the output feature maps match the inputs. Finally, each layer will use the ReLU activation function. Additionally, dropout layers have been added that implement regularization. The dropout technique is a simple technique that will randomly remove nodes from the network and has the effect of regularization as the remaining nodes must adapt to compensate for the slack of the removed nodes and a layer of batch normalization. Batch normalization (batch_normalization) is a technique designed to automatically standardize inputs to a layer in a deep learning neural network and has the effect of speeding up the process of training a neural network and, in some cases, improving the performance of the model. Once the above has been commented on, in Table 3, the architecture used for an 80 × 80 input image with three RGB channels is shown. The accuracy reached 92.50%.

Table 3. CNN architecture for an 80 × 80 input image.

Layer Type	Output Shape	Number of Parameters
conv2d (Conv2D)	(None, 80, 80, 32)	896
batch_normalization (BatchNo)	(None, 80, 80, 32)	128
conv2d_1 (Conv2D)	(None, 80, 80, 32)	9248
batch_normalization_1 (Batch)	(None, 80, 80, 32)	128
max_pooling2d (MaxPooling2D)	(None, 80, 80, 32)	0
dropout (Dropout)	(None, 80, 80, 32)	0
conv2d_2 (Conv2D)	(None, 80, 80, 64)	18,496
batch_normalization_2 (Batch)	(None, 40, 40, 64)	256
conv2d_3 (Conv2D)	(None, 40, 40, 64)	36,928
batch_normalization_3 (Batch)	(None, 40, 40, 64)	256
max_pooling2d_1 (MaxPooling2)	(None, 40, 40, 64)	0
dropout_1 (Dropout)	(None, 40, 40, 64)	0

Finally, the last experiment was for transfer learning approaches. AlexNet is known for its simplicity, but in the case of this experiment, it does not give an encouraging result. SGDM was the default and chosen optimizer for AlexNet. AlexNet does not require many options to work well, and the default training options were reserved. Sixty-four is the size of mini-bach and the initial learning rate was chosen as 0.001. The maximum number of epochs is fixed to 20; this chosen training options made the experiment faster (see Table 4). Table 5 describes the four cross-validation folders experiments and given accuracy by each one. As is shown in Table 5, the third experiments in which the data were split between 70% for training and 30% for test and validation, give the best accuracy (87.48%) by 6 epochs number.

Table 4. Experimental training parameters for AlexNet, VGG-16 and VGG-19.

Model	Parameters	Setting Values
AlexNet	Learning algorithm	Sgdm
	Initial Learning Rate	0.001
	Mini-batchsize	64
	Maximum epochs	0
VGG-16 and VGG-19	Learning algorithm	Adam
	Initial Learning rate	0.0004
	Mini-batch size	10
	Maximum epochs	25
	Validation Frequency	3
	Validation Information	Test-Images

Table 5. Cross-validation and simulation results for Alex-Net classifier.

Experiment (Trained Data, the Rest for Validation)	Accuracy	Epochs Number
0.5	84.58%	6
0.6	83.98%	6
0.7	86.98%	6
0.8	85.28%	6

Only the last three layers of VGG-16 and VGG19 were modified to make them fit the target domain. The fully connected layer (FC) in both models has been changed to a new FC layer with an output size of 2 according to the 2 classes, which were needed to classify. Adam was the chosen optimizer, given his good learning rate and the specific adaptive nature of the learning rate parameters. For Adam, the initial learning rate was chosen as 0.0004; a small valor is a good option to increase the training time. The size of the mini-batch was fixed at 10. The validation information of the model is that given in the test. Thus, a learning factor of 10 is defined. The maximum number of epochs was fixed to 25 but during the simulation process, the number was variable according to the experiments carried out, but it was initialized in the first experiment to 6. Finally, a validation frequency set to 3. The trained options of the experiment are listed in Table 4.

Detailed results for VGG-16 and VGG-19 neural networks are shown in Table 4, and while the best simulation accuracy is given by VGG-16, Figure 7 describes the followed steps using VGG16 to identify the Nosema and Figure 8 shows the best accuracy. Three experiments have been implemented, but only those that gave good results with a similar number of epochs for the two pre-trained networks have been described in Table 6. The data was split between training and validation, the experiments were conducted 30 times, following a 10-fold cross-validation process. The three last experiments gave the best accuracy; the first one took 70% of data for training and the 30% were for validation and the best accuracy was given by 6 epochs number. In the second experiment, 80% were placed for training, and the rest were for validation, the experiment was repeated several times with increasing the number of epochs and as Table 6 shows, the best accuracy given by VGG-16 is 96.25% with 20 epochs, and for VGG-19, the highest accuracy is 93.50% with 25 epochs, and in the third experiment presented in the result section, the data were divided between 90% for training and 10% for testing, and the results made an accuracy fall.

Table 6. Cross-validation and simulation results for VGG-16 and VGG-19 classifiers.

Experiments	Epochs	Accuracy	
		VGG-16	VGG-19
0.7	6	76.29%	71.95%
08	6	92.50%	93.00%
	12	94.50%	82.00%
	20	96.25%	92.32%
	25	93.00%	93.50%
0.9	6	88.00%	77.00%

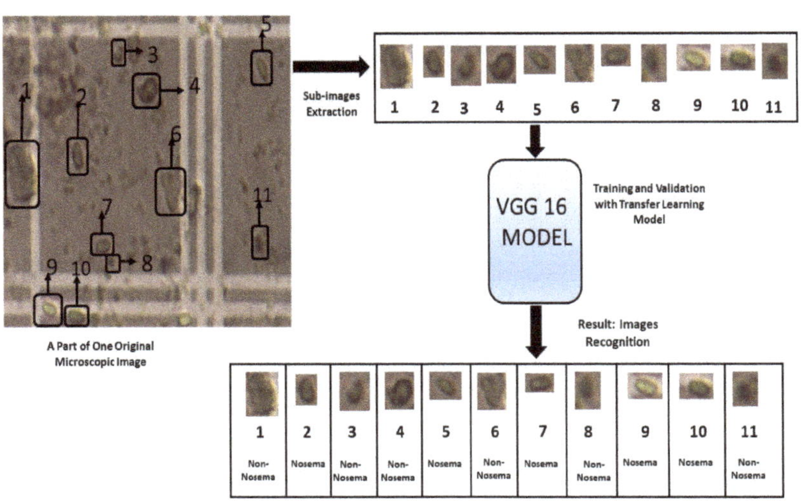

Figure 7. The steps followed for the recognition of Nosema cells using VGG 16 Model.

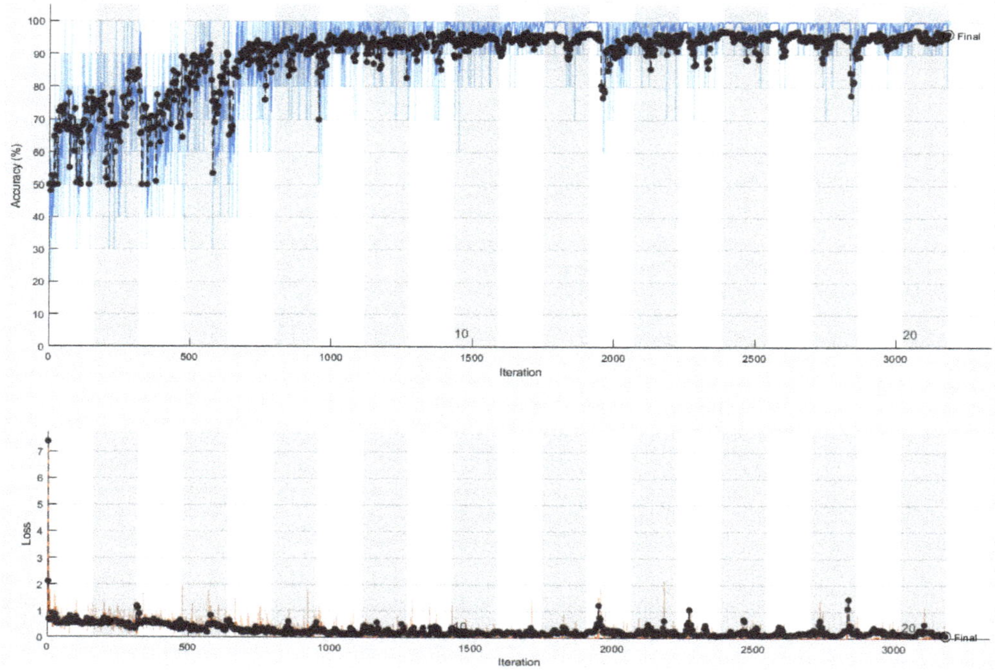

Figure 8. The Accuracy (blue curve) and loss (orange curve) results given by VGG-16 simulation: 96.25% of success accuracy with 20 epochs.

Table 7 summarizes the main results of the different experiments. The best result is reached using VGG-16 with accuracy of 96.25%, and the lowest accuracy is given by ANN (83.20%). Those results will be discussed in the next section.

Table 7. A summary of best results given by the 6 used tools for Nosema classification.

ANN	SVM	CNN	AlexNet	VGG-16	VGG-19
83.20%	83.50%	92.5%	87.48%	96.25%	93.00%

5. Discussion

This section discusses in detail the behavior and features of each experiment and it discusses compromise between accuracy and the robustness of the proposed methods was included. Besides, a comparison vs. the most representative publication on this topic (see Table 8), with comparison vs. a previous work [14], authors increased the dataset from 185 to 2000 images and the extracted features number from 9 to 19, and those features for the Nosema cell are related to several aspects of the image cell: geometric shape, statistical characteristics, texture and color features given by GLCM. Two strategies were followed to recognize Nosema; while only one was followed (ANN) in [14]; the first strategy consists of the use of calculated characteristics by an ANN and an SVM and the second is based on sub-images extracted from treated microscopic images using an implemented CNN and the tools of transfer Learning. ANN used in [14] gave a success rate of 91.1% in Nosema recognition. SVM also was used in [13] to classify the two types of Nosema and other objects. The experiments reached relative and accurate values.

Table 8. Results from other references for Nosema recognition.

Reference	Data Size	Method	Accuracy
[14]	185 images (1655 extracted features)	ANN	91.10%
This work	2000 images	ANN	83.20%
This work	2000 images	SVM	83.50%
This work	2000 images	CNN	92.50%
This work	2000 images	AlexNet	87.48%
This work	2000 images	VGG-16	96.25%
This work	2000 images	VGG-19	93.50%

From Tables 2–6, it can be concluded that whether it is the largest dataset or the smallest dataset, the level of learning of the network with transfer learning models is obviously better than the traditional models, especially ANNs are examined in this study and SVM which brought near results. Furthermore, one notes a clear rate of convergence of the transfer model VGG-16 and VGG-19 at the level of the provided results. In addition, these transfer models are a bit faster than ANN and SVM, at least in this case. CNN has demonstrated its effectiveness in this problem of recognizing or classifying Nosema cells as a deep learning model. CNN was almost comparable to VGG-19. On the other hand, it should be said that the training options for the ANNs, as well as the transfer learning algorithms, make a difference in the results.

In front of AlexNet, the VGG-16, VGG-19 and CNN have proven their strong effectiveness in this work in the classification of patterns, cells and objects.

For the features extraction part, several different features from the sub-images were evaluated: geometric, statistic, texture and GLCM features extracted from the yellow channel. This experiment used a large database, the results given by the ANN as well as by the SVM good since it is the first time. The quality of the microscopic images used in this work did not always help to extract clear and sharp objects. By calculating the results with a different number of features (15 and 19), the importance of the data extracted by the GLCM in the resulting amelioration was approved.

6. Conclusions

In order to identify Nosema cells, this experiment examined two strategies of classification: the traditional ones and the deep learning classifiers. Different experiments were implemented for both strategies, despite the noisy quality of the microscopic images used. The best accuracy for the recognition or classification of Nosema is reached by VGG-16, 96.25%, which is compared to state of the art is the most accurate methodology in this area so far.

The innovation of this proposal is to analyze and find the better option for this identification, checking different strategies to implement an automatic identification of Nosema cell, as was shown after experiments, and with good and robust accuracy. It was reached with VGG-16 architecture.

After reviewing the state-of-the-art material, it can be concluded that only a few automatic approaches have been introduced so far. Because of this, we contribute with a variety of explored classification methods and their accuracies. In particular, we would emphasize the difference between shallow ANNs with handcrafted features and end-to-end learning using the deep learning approach using CNN together with several transfer learning architectures.

Author Contributions: Conceptualization, S.D. and C.M.T.-G.; methodology, S.D. and C.M.T.-G.; software, S.D. and C.M.T.-G.; validation, S.D., C.M.T.-G. and R.B.; formal analysis, S.D., C.M.T.-G. and R.B.; investigation, S.D. and C.M.T.-G.; resources, C.M.T.-G.; data curation, S.D. and C.M.T.-G.; writing—original draft preparation, S.D.; writing—review and editing, S.D., C.M.T.-G. and R.B.; visualization, S.D., C.M.T.-G. and R.B.; supervision, C.M.T.-G. and R.B.; project administration, C.M.T.-G.; funding acquisition, C.M.T.-G. All authors have read and agreed to the published version of the manuscript.

Funding: This research received no external funding.

Institutional Review Board Statement: Not applicable.

Informed Consent Statement: Not applicable.

Data Availability Statement: The data presented in this study are available on request from the corresponding author. The data are not publicly available due to starting state of the research.

Conflicts of Interest: The authors declare no conflict of interest.

References

1. Lewis, C.; Denny, J.B.B.; Jarrad, R.P.; Earle, S.R. *Nosema pyrausta*: Its biology, history, and potential role in a landscape of transgenic insecticidal crops. *Biol. Control* **2009**, *48*, 223–231. [CrossRef]
2. Andre, J.B.; Emily, D.J.; Jayre, A.J.; Herman, K.L. North American Propolis Extracts From Upstate New York Decrease Nosema ceranae (Microsporidia) Spore Levels in Honey Bees (*Apis mellifera*). *Front. Microbiol.* **2020**, *11*, 1719.
3. Sinpoo, C.; Paxton, R.J.; Disayathanoowat, T.; Krongdang, S.; Chantawannakul, P. Impact of *Nosema ceranae* and *Nosema apis* on individual worker bees of the two host species (*Apis cerana* and *Apis mellifera*) and regulation of host immune response. *J. Insect Physiol.* **2018**, *105*, 1–8. [CrossRef]
4. Paneka, J.; Paris, L.; Roriz, D.; Mone, A.; Dubuffet, A.; Delbac, F.; Diogon, M.; El Alaoui, H. Impact of the microsporidian *Nosema ceranae* on the gut epithelium renewal of the honeybee, *Apis mellifera*. *J. Invertebr. Pathol.* **2018**, *159*, 121–128. [CrossRef] [PubMed]
5. Calderón, R.A.; Ramírez, F. *Enfermedades de las Abejas Melíferas, con Énfasis en Abejas Africanizadas*; CINAT-UNA: Heredia, Costa Rica, 2010; p. 125.
6. Higes, M.; Hernández, R.M.; Bailón, E.G.; Palencia, P.G.; Meana, A. Detection of infective *Nosema ceranae* (Microsporidia) spores in corbicular pollen of forager honeybees. *J. Invertebr. Pathol.* **2008**, *97*, 76–78. [CrossRef]
7. Higes, M.; Martín, R.; Meana, A. *Nosema ceranae* in Europe: An emergent type C nosemosis. *Apidologie* **2010**, *41*, 375–392. [CrossRef]
8. Suwannapong, G.; Maksong, S.; Phainchajoen, M.; Benbow, M.E.; Mayack, C. Survival and health improvement of *Nosema* infected *Apis florea* (Hymenoptera: Apidae) bees after treatment with propolis extract. *J. Asia Pac. Entomol.* **2018**, *21*, 437–444. [CrossRef]
9. Mura, A.; Pusceddu, M.; Theodorou, P.; Angioni, A.; Flori, I.; Paxton, R.J.; Satta, A. Propolis Consumption Reduces *Nosema ceranae* Infection of European Honey Bees (*Apis mellifera*). *Insects* **2020**, *11*, 124. [CrossRef]
10. Tu, G.J.; Hansen, M.K.; Kryger, P.; Ahrendt, P. Automatic behaviour analysis system for honeybees using computer vision. *Comput. Electron. Agric.* **2016**, *122*, 10–18. [CrossRef]
11. Giuffre, C.; Lubkin, S.R.; Tarpy, D.R. Automated assay and differential model of western honey bee (*Apis mellifera*) autogrooming using digital image processing. *Comput. Electron. Agric.* **2017**, *135*, 338–344. [CrossRef]
12. Szczurek, A.; Maciejewska, M.; Bąk, B.; Wilde, J.; Siuda, M. Semiconductor gas sensor as a detector of Varroa destructor infestation of honey bee colonies—Statistical evaluation. *Comput. Electron. Agric.* **2019**, *162*, 405–411. [CrossRef]
13. Alvarez-Ramos, C.M.; Niño, E.; Santos, M. Automatic Classification of *Nosema* Pathogenic Agents through Machine Vision techniques and Kernel-based Vector Machines. In Proceedings of the 2013 8th Computing Colombian Conference (8CCC), Armenia, Colombia, 21–23 August 2013; [CrossRef]
14. Dghim, S.; Travieso, C.M.; Dutta, M.K.; Hernández, L.E. *Nosema* Pathogenic Agent Recognition Based on Geometrical and Texture Features Using Neural Network Classifier. In Proceedings of the International Conference on Contemporary Computing and Applications (IC3A) 2020, Lucknow, India, 5–7 February 2020.
15. Yadav, S.S.; Jadhav, S.M. Deep convolutional neural network based medical image classification for disease diagnosis. *J. Big Data* **2019**, *6*, 113. [CrossRef]
16. Khemphila, A.; Boonjing, V. Heart Disease Classification Using Neural Network and Feature Selection. In Proceedings of the 21st International Conference on Systems Engineering 2011, Las Vegas, NV, USA, 16–18 August 2011.
17. Jain, R.; Jain, N.; Aggarwal, A.; Hemanth, D.J. Convolutional Neural Network Based Alzheimer's Disease Classification from Magnetic Resonance Brain Images. *Cogn. Syst. Res.* **2018**, *57*, 147–159. [CrossRef]
18. Guan, Q.; Huang, Y.; Zhong, Z.; Zheng, Z.; Zheng, L.; Yang, Y. Thorax Disease Classification with Attention Guided Convolutional Neural Network. *Pattern Recognit. Lett.* **2019**, *131*, 38–45. [CrossRef]

19. Chen, L.C.; Papandreou, G.; Kokkinos, I.; Murphy, K.; Yuille, A.L. Deeplab: Semantic image segmentation with deep convolutional nets, atrous convolution, and fully connected crfs. *IEEE Trans. Pattern Anal. Mach. Intell.* **2018**, *40*, 834–848. [CrossRef] [PubMed]
20. Panagiotakis, C.; Argyros, A. Region-Based Fitting of Overlapping Ellipses and Its Application to Cells Segmentation. *Image Vis. Comput.* **2020**, *93*, 103810. [CrossRef]
21. Zieliński, B.; Sroka-Oleksiak, A.; Rymarczyk, D.; Piekarczyk, A.; Brzychczy-Włoch, M. Deep learning approach to describe and classify fungi microscopic images. *PLoS ONE* **2020**, *15*, e0234806. [CrossRef]
22. Ge, M.; Su, F.; Zhao, Z.; Su, D. Deedeep learning analysis on microscopic imaging in materials science. *Mater. Today Nano* **2020**, *11*, 100087. [CrossRef]
23. Zhang, Y.; Jiang, H.; Ye, T.; Juhas, M. Deep Learning for Imaging and Detection of Microorganisms. *Trends Microbiol.* **2021**. [CrossRef]
24. Moen, E.; Bannon, D.; Kudo, T.; Graf, W.; Covert, M.; Valen, D.V. Deep learning for cellular image analysis. *Nat. Methods* **2019**, *16*, 1233–1246. [CrossRef] [PubMed]
25. Miss, H.; Vala, J.; Baxi, A. A Review on Otsu Image Segmentation Algorithm. *Intern. J. Adv. Res. Comp. Eng. Tech.* **2013**, *2*, 387–389.
26. Gonzales, R.C.; Woods, R.E. *Digital Image Processing*, 4th ed.; Pearson: Upper Saddle River, NJ, USA, 2017.
27. Kolkur, S.; Kalbande, D.R. Survey of Texture Based Feature Extraction for Skin Disease Detection. In Proceedings of the International Conference on ICT in Business Industry & Government (ICTBIG) 2016, Indore, India, 18–19 November 2016.
28. Al-Hiary, H.; Ahmad, S.B.; Reyalat, M.; Braik, M.; ALRahamneh, Z. Fast and Accurate Detection and Classification of Plant Diseases. *Inter. J. Comp. Appl.* **2011**, *17*, 31–38. [CrossRef]
29. Rundo, L.; Tangherloni, A.; Galimberti, S.; Cazzaniga, P.; Woitek, R.; Sala, E.; Nobile, M.S.; Mauri, G. HaraliCU: GPU-powered Haralick feature extraction on medical images exploiting the full dynamics of gray-scale levels. In Proceedings of the International Conference on Parallel Computing Technologies 2020, Macau, China, 7–10 December 2020.
30. Rundo, L.; Tangherloni, A.; Cazzaniga, P.; Mistri, M.; Galimberti, S.; Woitek, R.; Sala, E.; Mauri, G.; Nobile, M.S. A CUDA-powered method for the feature extraction and unsupervised analysis of medical images. *J. Supercomput.* **2021**. [CrossRef]
31. Mohanaiah, P.; Sathyanarayana, P.; GuruKumar, L. Image Texture Feature Extraction Using GLCM Approach. *Int. J. Sci. Res. Pub.* **2013**, *3322*, 750–757. [CrossRef]
32. Sebastian, B.; Unnikrishnan, A.; Balakrishnan, K. Grey level co-occurrence matrices: Generalization and some new features. *Int. J. Comput. Sci. Eng. Inf. Technol.* **2012**, *8*, 1463–1465.
33. Tian, Y.; Shi, Y.; Liu, X. Recent Advances on Support Vector Machines Research. *Tech. Econ. Dev. Econ.* **2012**, *18*, 5–33. [CrossRef]
34. Weiss, K.; Khoshgoftaar, T.M.; Wang, D. A survey of transfer learning. *J. Big Data* **2016**, *3*, 9. [CrossRef]
35. Ma, Y.; Gong, W.; Mao, F. Transfer learning used to analyze the dynamic evolution of the dust aerosol. *J. Quant. Spectrosc. Radiat. Transf.* **2015**, *153*, 119–130. [CrossRef]
36. Xie, M.; Jean, N.; Burke, M.; Lobell, D.; Ermon, S. Transfer learning from deep features for remote sensing and poverty mapping. In Proceedings of the 30th AAAI Conference on Artificial Intelligence 2015, Pheonix, AZ, USA, 12–17 February 2015; pp. 1–10.
37. Ogoe, H.A.; Visweswaran, S.; Lu, X.; Gopalakrishnan, V. Knowledge transfer via classification rules using functional mapping for integrative modeling of gene expression data. *BMC Bioinform.* **2015**, *7*, 1–15. [CrossRef]
38. Kan, M.; Wu, J.; Shan, S.; Chen, X. Domain adaptation for face recognition: Targetize source domain bridged by common subspace. *Int. J. Comput. Vis.* **2014**, *109*, 94–109. [CrossRef]
39. Widmer, C.; Ratsch, G. Multitask learning in computational biology. *JMLR* **2012**, *27*, 207–216.

sensors

MDPI

Article

Quantification of Blood Flow Velocity in the Human Conjunctival Microvessels Using Deep Learning-Based Stabilization Algorithm

Hang-Chan Jo [1,2], Hyeonwoo Jeong [1], Junhyuk Lee [1], Kyung-Sun Na [3,*] and Dae-Yu Kim [1,2,4,*]

1 Department of Electrical and Computer Engineering, Inha University, Incheon 22212, Korea; hjofficial@inha.edu (H.-C.J.); dydrl9713@inha.edu (H.J.); jhsky0919@naver.com (J.L.)
2 Center for Sensor Systems, Inha University, Incheon 22212, Korea
3 Department of Ophthalmology & Visual Science, Yeouido St. Mary's Hospital, College of Medicine, The Catholic University of Korea, Seoul 07345, Korea
4 Inha Research Institute for Aerospace Medicine, Inha University, Incheon 22212, Korea
* Correspondence: drna@catholic.ac.kr (K.-S.N.); dyukim@inha.ac.kr (D.-Y.K.); Tel.: +82-02-3779-1520 (K.-S.N.); +82-32-860-7394 (D.-Y.K.)

Abstract: The quantification of blood flow velocity in the human conjunctiva is clinically essential for assessing microvascular hemodynamics. Since the conjunctival microvessel is imaged in several seconds, eye motion during image acquisition causes motion artifacts limiting the accuracy of image segmentation performance and measurement of the blood flow velocity. In this paper, we introduce a novel customized optical imaging system for human conjunctiva with deep learning-based segmentation and motion correction. The image segmentation process is performed by the Attention-UNet structure to achieve high-performance segmentation results in conjunctiva images with motion blur. Motion correction processes with two steps—registration and template matching—are used to correct for large displacements and fine movements. The image displacement values decrease to 4–7 μm during registration (first step) and less than 1 μm during template matching (second step). With the corrected images, the blood flow velocity is calculated for selected vessels considering temporal signal variances and vessel lengths. These methods for resolving motion artifacts contribute insights into studies quantifying the hemodynamics of the conjunctiva, as well as other tissues.

Keywords: blood flow velocity quantification; conjunctival microvessel; deep learning; image processing; motion correction; optical imaging system; vessel segmentation

Citation: Jo, H.-C.; Jeong, H.; Lee, J.; Na, K.-S.; Kim, D.-Y. Quantification of Blood Flow Velocity in the Human Conjunctival Microvessels Using Deep Learning-Based Stabilization Algorithm. *Sensors* **2021**, *21*, 3224. https://doi.org/10.3390/s21093224

Academic Editor: Ayman El-baz

Received: 7 April 2021
Accepted: 1 May 2021
Published: 6 May 2021

1. Introduction

The conjunctiva is a translucent and highly vascularized membrane covering the sclera of the human eye. These properties enable the conjunctiva to be the only tissue observing red blood cell (RBC) shift that can be utilized for measuring the blood flow velocity directly from the surface. Quantitative analysis of the blood flow velocity has been used to estimate the progression of eye diseases, including diabetic retinopathy [1] and dry eye syndrome [2–4]. The diabetic retinopathy patients group had slower blood flow velocities in the conjunctiva than the control group [1]. In the case of dry eye syndrome, the normal group had slow blood flow velocities in the conjunctiva [2–4]. Moreover, patients with unilateral ischemic stroke [5] and high cardiovascular disease risk [6] tend to have slower conjunctival blood flow velocities. These studies demonstrated that quantifying the conjunctival blood flow velocity can contribute to evaluate not only ophthalmic diseases but, also, systemic diseases in critical organs, especially the brain and cardiovascular system.

Conventional methods for quantifying the conjunctival blood flow velocity use functional slit-lamp biomicroscopy [7], a noninvasive optical imaging system (EyeFlow) [8], and orthogonal polarization spectral imaging [9]. These methods can be disturbed by motion artifacts inherited from the image acquisition process due to eye movements. The motion artifacts cause two distinct problems: (1) image displacement and (2) low-quality images.

First, the image displacement problem causes the vessel to be misaligned from the central point. Registration was performed by calculating the difference of the correlation coefficients from the reference frame [10–12]. In another method, the sharpness index of each image was measured by calculating pixel-to-pixel intensity variance, eliminating the inadequate frames below the threshold value [13]. These two methods can compensate for rapid eye movements but have difficulty correcting for fibrillation or respiratory eye movements.

Second, the segmentation, which is the essential step for quantifying the microcirculation, remains challenging for low-quality images of blurry structures and uneven light illumination by subject motions. Various segmentation methods [7,10,14,15] were applied to the conjunctiva images with motion artifacts. The Frangi filter [10,14] is the most commonly used segmentation algorithm and exploits multiscale information from the eigenvalues of the Hessian matrix. The supervised method [16], which uses the Gabor wavelet filter and the Gaussian mixture model (GMM) classifier, was suggested for conjunctiva vessel segmentation [7,15]. These two segmentation methods are efficient in identifying vessels but lack of the ability to identify low-quality vessels.

We solved the image displacement and low-quality image problems caused by motion artifacts by proposing a custom-built optical system with a two-step calibration method and a deep learning-based segmentation model. The custom-built optical system was optimized to acquire human bulbar conjunctival images. The two-step calibration method was motivated by the fact that image displacements can result from sudden eye movements and respiratory movements. The first step, registration, corrects the sudden eye movements. The second step, template matching, eliminates the respiratory movements. Since deep learning-based segmentation is effective with low-quality conjunctival images [17], a custom-built Attention-UNet model was constructed to extract accurate conjunctiva vascular information. The blood flow velocity was measured by generating a spatial–temporal analysis (STA) image from the corrected image sequence and vascular features. With this configured system, we can acquire a conjunctival vascular image set with minimal motion and accurately quantify conjunctival blood flow velocity.

2. Materials and Methods

2.1. Process of Quantifying Blood Flow Velocity

Quantification of the blood flow velocity is performed by the six steps shown in Figure 1. After acquiring image frames for 3 s with 25 fps, image processing, including image registration, feature extraction, and motion correction, provides motion-free image sequences for measuring the blood flow velocity through tracking the position of red blood cells. Detailed explanations of imaging acquisition, registration, and deep learning-based image segmentation and quantification are shown in following sections.

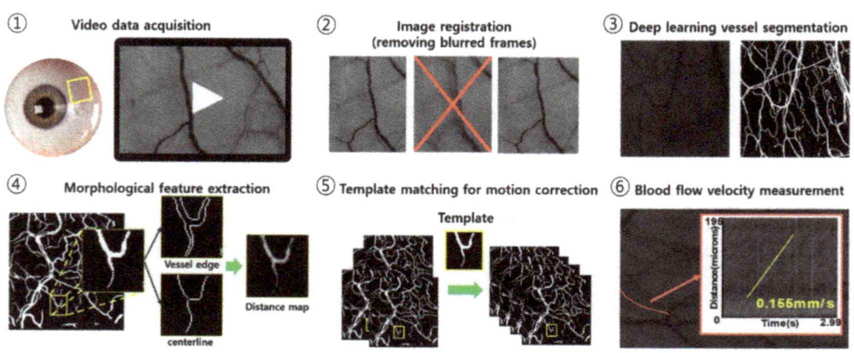

Figure 1. The summary of experimental phase in this study.

2.2. Image Acquisition

The schematic of a customized optical imaging system is depicted in Figure 2. The conjunctival imaging system uses a green LED with a central wavelength of 525 nm and a spectral bandwidth of 5 nm, because hemoglobin and deoxyhemoglobin have high extinction coefficients at a wavelength of 530 nm. Accordingly, the image contrast between the blood vessels and the white sclera can be improved. We illuminate the uniform light using a diffuser (ED1-C50-MD, Thorlabs Inc., Newton, NJ, USA) forward to the LED. The power of the LED at the eye pupil is 300 $\mu W/cm^2$, which is 0.3 times the laser safety standards (ANSI) limits under the condition of 10-min exposure [18].

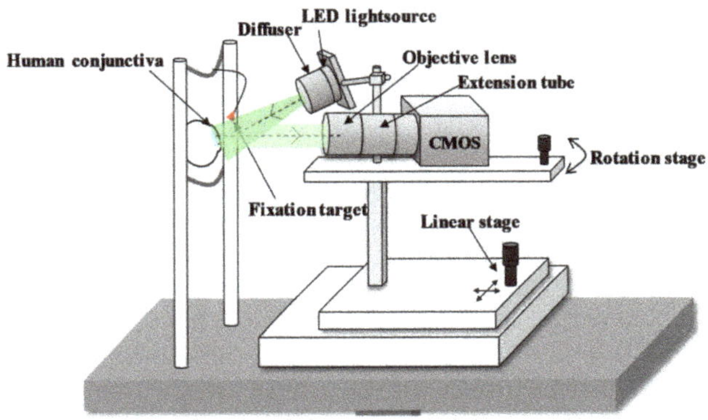

Figure 2. Custom-built optical imaging system for human bulbar conjunctiva.

The diffusely reflected light from the conjunctiva transmits to the complementary metal oxide semiconductor (CMOS) sensor-based camera (UI-3080CP Rev.2, IDS Inc., Obersulm, Germany) with an imaging sensor size of 8.473 mm $\times$ 7.086 mm to acquire a maximum resolution of 2456 $\times$ 2054 pixels. The pixel size on the camera sensor is 3.45 μm $\times$ 3.45 μm. The frame rate is set at 20 fps but is enhanced to 25 fps by binning the image size to 2208 $\times$ 1848 pixels for a more continuous blood flow assessment. The video data are recorded for approximately 3 s with 25 fps.

The magnification of the system is designed to achieve RBC flow imaging. An RBC with an average diameter of 7.5 μm [19] should be imaged by at least 2 pixels on the camera sensor to distinguish the individual RBC particles [20]. Moreover, the magnification for the reliable quantification of RBC flow velocity requires 4 to 5 pixels imaged per RBC [21], corresponding to 2$\times$ in our system. To achieve this magnification, we use a high-magnification zoom lens (MVL6 $\times$ 12Z, Thorlabs Inc., Newton, NJ, USA) with an adjustable magnification between 0.7$\times$ and 6$\times$. An extension tube (MVL20A, Thorlabs Inc., Newton, NJ, USA) with 2$\times$ magnification is connected for additional magnification, for a total range of 1.832$\times$ to 7.5$\times$. An optimized magnification is set at 3.798$\times$ for a field of view of 2.00 mm $\times$ 1.68 mm, thereby sampling each RBC with 8.26 pixels.

2.3. Image Registration

Image registration is the process of eliminating the blurred frames caused by rapid eye motion or blinking. Image sequences are first examined with an image contrast index that can determine the quality of the images. To obtain the contrast index, we apply the Sobel edge algorithm [22,23], a method of quantitatively measuring the contrast of an image [24]. The contrast index is calculated with the Equation (1).

$$Contrast\ Index = \left(\sum_{y=1}^{N} \sum_{x=1}^{M} I_{xy} \right) / (M \cdot N) \quad (1)$$

where M, N are the dimensions of the image, x, y are the pixel indices of each axis, and I_{xy} is the image pixel intensity. The overall image contrast is estimated by the average value of the edge intensity. The blurred frames with low-contrast indices are resolved by extracting only frames with a contrast index greater than 95% of the maximum value. A template frame is then designated based on the highest contrast index. The rest of the consecutive frames are automatically aligned to the template frame using the ImageJ plugin called motion corrector [25]. This algorithm corrects the image translation by maximizing the overlapping region between two images, thereby eliminating the significant displacement caused by rapid eye motions.

2.4. Deep Learning Vessel Segmentation

2.4.1. Dataset

A conjunctival vessel dataset and a high-resolution fundus (HRF) dataset are used to train and evaluate the deep learning model [26]. The HRF dataset has been established by the research team at the Friedrich-Alexander Universität and used to test the effectiveness of the deep learning-based segmentation algorithm [26]. The conjunctival vessel data are collected from the conjunctiva of five healthy human subjects (five males, age = 27 $\pm$ 1) with the custom-built imaging system. This dataset contains 15 conjunctiva images with a size of 2208 $\times$ 1848 pixels. The conjunctiva images used for network learning are randomly selected in the frames extracted from image sequences without motion-blurred images. The HRF dataset comprises 45 color fundus images, equally distributed into three subsets (healthy, diabetic retinopathy, and glaucoma). Each image in the HRF dataset is 3304 $\times$ 2236 pixels. Both datasets have annotated vessel structures in the form of binary images.

2.4.2. Image Preprocessing and Preparation

Preprocessing enhances the contrast of the vessel in the image and removes uneven illuminations that occurred in the image acquisition step. We apply three preprocessing steps. In the first step, we crop the HRF images from the center point to the same size as the conjunctival images and resize both to 1104 $\times$ 924 pixels (0.5$\times$). Figure 3a,e illustrates the raw data of the conjunctival image and resized HRF image. In the second step, we extract the green channel from the HRF images. The green channel has a higher contrast and lower background noise than the other channels. Finally, contrast-limited adaptive histogram equalization (CLAHE) [27] is applied in the green channel of the HRF in Figure 3f and conjunctival images in Figure 3b to enhance the contrast of the images. After preprocessing, two datasets are combined into a single dataset to enhance the generalization ability of the model.

A convolutional neural network (CNN) requires large amounts of training data to prevent overfitting of the network and improve the generalization ability. To train the dataset, we exploit a patch-wise strategy [17,28–30] and data augmentation. The patch-wise strategy is used to learn a small amount of data efficiently and overcome the memory limitations caused by high-image resolution. This strategy randomly extracts patches in the range of 64 to 128 pixels. The patch sizes from 65 $\times$ 65 pixels to 128 $\times$ 128 pixels are resized to 64 $\times$ 64-pixel patches. After resizing the extracted patches, overlapped regions of the conjunctiva in each different-sized patch are recognized as different regions in the network model.

A total of 300,000 patches are obtained by sampling 5000 patches from each image. Figure 3c,g are examples of patch-wise extractions. Figure 3d,h are the corresponding ground-truth images of the patches (Figure 3c,g) for the supervised learning of the convolutional neural network.

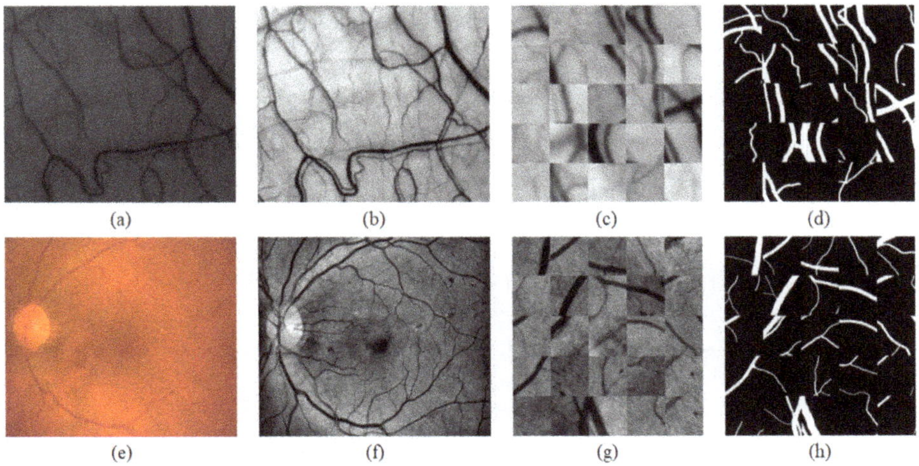

Figure 3. Preparation steps of the conjunctival dataset and the HRF dataset. The conjunctival data preparation step: (**a**) raw data of the conjunctival image, (**b**) CLAHE-adopted image, (**c**) conjunctiva patches, and (**d**) corresponding ground-truth of (**c**). The HRF data preparation step: (**e**) resized HRF image, (**f**) CLAHE-adopted image, (**g**) HRF patches, and the (**h**) corresponding ground-truth of (**g**).

Data augmentation is applied to extract the patches with additional vascular features to improve the CNN generalization ability. We applied data augmentations such as geometrical distortions (rotation, shearing, and transformation) and motion blur. Geometrical distortions can increase the representation of the patches. Motion blur is used to learn the deformed vessel based on the movements that occurred in the image acquisition step. The patches are normalized to the zero mean and unit variance before the training process to reduce the effect of the large intensity variance.

2.4.3. Network Architecture

The Attention-UNet architecture [31] is adopted to learn the vascular features. We customize the Attention-UNet to optimize our datasets. The details of the architecture are described in Figure 4. The architecture is based on a layered CNN, consisting of an encoder–decoder structure with three stages and an attention mechanism.

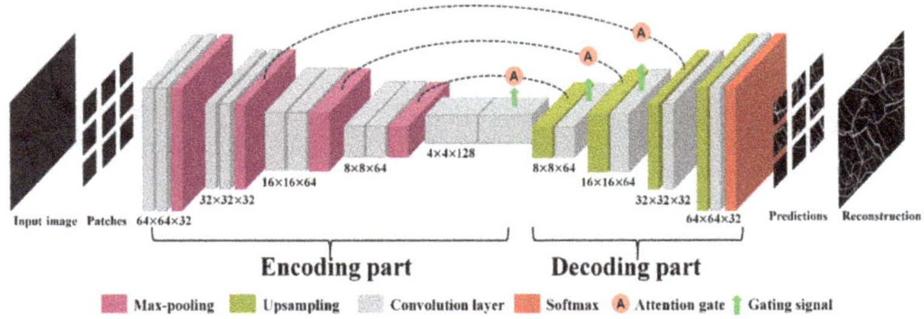

Figure 4. Customized Attention-UNet architecture.

The encoder gradually reduces the spatial dimension of the input to learn a low-resolution feature map. Each stage of the encoder consists of two convolution layers and one max-pooling layer. At the end of the encoder stage, a bottom layer exists without max-pooling. Whenever the stage progresses to the next stage, the filter size of the convolution layer doubles, and the dimensions of the input are halved. Each convolution layer comprises a 3×3 convolution filter with a stride of 1, batch normalization, and a rectified linear unit (ReLU).

The decoder enables precise localization by merging the low-resolution features from the previous layer and high-resolution features from the encoder of the same stage. When the low-resolution features are transported, the upsampling process, which is implemented by transposing a convolution kernel (kernel size = 3 × 3, stride = 2), reconstructs the salient features from the input. Before the encoder transfers the features, an attention gate is used to suppress the irrelevant background of the input and highlight the relevant foreground features. At the end of the 3-stage decoding, the last convolutional kernel (kernel size = 1 × 1) and SoftMax activation function are used for mapping the feature vector and classify the vessel.

2.4.4. Model Training and Testing

The deep learning model using Keras is trained and validated on a CPU (Xeon(R) silver 4112, Intel Corporation, Santa Clara, CA, USA) and a GPU (Quadro P4000, Nvidia Corporation, Santa Clara, CA, USA) operated by Ubuntu (16.04 LTS, Canonical Ltd, London, UK).

In the training process, the complete set of augmented patches is split into 240,000 for training the network and 60,000 for validation. The training process has 150 epochs with the strategy of reducing the learning rate on the plateau. A validation set is used to evaluate the performance of the model in each epoch. If the performance of the model in the validation set does not change in 15 epochs, the strategy will reduce the learning rate by 1/10. The training of the model is progressed by an adaptive moment estimation (Adam) optimizer (initial learning rate = 0.00005) and the Dice coefficient [32] as the loss function.

In conjunctival images, blood vessel information occupies a small portion of the entire image compared to the background region. Therefore, the Dice coefficient is used to solve the class imbalance problem. The Dice coefficient is defined in the Equation (2):

$$Dice\ Coefficient = \frac{2\sum_i^N p_i \cdot q_i}{\sum_I^N {p_i}^2 + \sum_i^N {q_i}^2} \tag{2}$$

where p_i is predicted segmentation map, and q_i is the binary ground-truth image. N denotes the number of pixels in each image, and i is the position of the pixel in the image.

In the test phase, the CNN infers the test image, excluding the training dataset. The test image is generated by averaging 30 frames to distinguish the obscure vessel from the registered conjunctival images. By inferencing the test data using the optimal model for validation, a reference segmentation map is acquired.

2.5. Morphological Feature Extraction

The vessel length and diameter are measured from segmented conjunctival vessel images. Distinguishing the connected vessel segments is necessary to extract these morphological vessel features. The centerline and intersection points of the vessels are required to separate individual vessel segments. The centerline is obtained by a skeleton image using the pixel-wise thinning algorithm [33,34], a method of performing an iterative process until it remains one pixel wide in the segmented vessels. Skeleton segments lower than 20 pixels are removed, because these segments are not recognized as a connected vascular network. The intersection points at bifurcation and crossover are determined by the number of neighbors, a convolution result with a 3 × 3 unity kernel for each pixel of the centerline. The bifurcation points correspond to three in the convolution result, and the crossovers have a result greater than three. By removing these two points, each vessel segment is separated and given identification. We measure the vessel length and the diameter from the identified vessel segment. The length of the vessel is obtained by counting each pixel of the skeletonized vessel along its centerline. Moreover, the vessel diameters are measured in Euclidean distance by calculating the perpendicular distance from the centerline to the nearest background of the binary segmented vessels.

2.6. Template Matching for Motion Correction

The template matching algorithm is used for correcting the fine movements in image sequences caused by respiratory movement. First, the template image is assigned by selecting a template vessel considering the morphological features, including the vessel length and diameter. The template vessel must be contained in all frames and distinguished from other blood vessels. Equation (3) is applied to each vessel segment to select a vessel of the template image with a long length and large diameter.

$$N(L,D) = w_1 \cdot L + w_2 \cdot D \tag{3}$$

$N(L,D)$ is the function for selecting the template vessel, w_1, w_2 are the weight factors, L is the length of the vessel segment, and D is the diameter of the vessel. The vessel length and diameter are normalized to equalize the scales of each parameter. The vessel segment with the highest value of the function is determined as the template vessel.

We generate the template image by cropping the selected template vessel to the minimum bounding box. The template-matching algorithm based on the assigned template image is applied to the target frames, and this algorithm is implemented with the cvMatchTemplate function in the OpenCV library [35]. This function calculates the normalized correlation coefficient $R(x,y)$ at each pixel to search the most similar region with the template image, as shown in the Equation (4):

$$R(x,y) = \frac{\sum_{x',y'}(T(x',y') \cdot I(x+x',y+y'))}{\sqrt{\sum_{x',y'} T(x',y')^2 \cdot \sum_{x',y'} I(x+x',y+y')^2}} \tag{4}$$

where T is the template image, I is a source image to find a match with the template image, x, y is the pixel location of the source image, and x', y' indicates the pixel location of the template image. After finding the most similar region to the template image with the source images, the displacement value is obtained from the center point of the source image. We shift the source images as much as the displacement value, thereby successfully correcting the fine movements.

2.7. Blood Flow Velocity Measurements

Several blood vessels can be observed in motion-corrected conjunctival images, but a RBC shift is not detectable in all blood vessels. Measuring the blood flow velocity requires distinguishing the blood vessels capable of detecting the RBC shift. Generally, vessels with measurable blood flow have high temporal variance in the centerline due to the RBC shifts. Moreover, vessels with longer lengths are more conducive to measuring the blood flow velocity, because the movements of RBC can be observed continuously for a long duration. Considering the temporal variance and vessel length, an index of observability is defined as shown in the Equation (5):

$$Observability\ Index = \alpha \cdot \sigma_t + \beta \cdot L \tag{5}$$

where α, β is the weighting factor, σ_t is the temporal variance, and L is the length of the vessel segments. Vessels with a high index are considered to be capable of measuring the blood flow velocity. We choose 15 vessel segments with the highest observability index to analyze the blood flow velocity.

The blood flow velocity is measured by tracking the RBC movements in the selected vessels centerline, as depicted in Figure 5a. Tracking is performed using the spatial–temporal analysis (STA) method, which demonstrates an alteration of the pixel intensity of the centerline due to the RBC movements. Figure 5b displays an example of an alteration in the pixel intensity of the vessel centerlines as a function of time. We generate the STA image by stacking the centerlines to each column, as depicted in Figure 5c. Frames corresponding to 3.7 s are stacked to form 70 columns. Consequently, the flow of the RBC cluster forms lines consistent with the yellow line in Figure 5c, with the slope on the STA image. The blood flow velocities are measured by calculating the average values of the slopes.

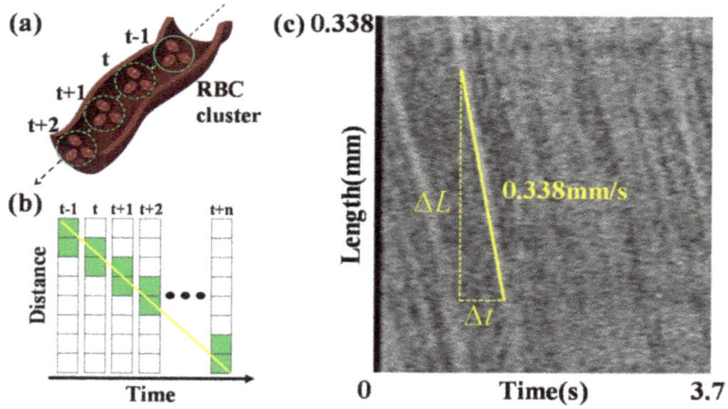

Figure 5. (**a**) The RBC cluster shifts over time in the vessel centerline. (**b**) Pixel intensity of the vessel centerline changes due to the RBC cluster shift. (**c**) Spatial–temporal analysis (STA) image generated by the pixel intensity from the vessel centerline as stacking at each column. The x and y axes indicate the frame time and vessel length, respectively. The yellow line shown in the STA image displays the slope, indicating the blood flow velocity.

3. Results

3.1. Segmentation

We identified blurry, low-contrast conjunctival vessels by constructing a dataset mixed with conjunctiva images and HRF to train the custom-built Attention-UNet model. The segmentation map was obtained using model prediction on the averaged image. Figure 6 illustrates the results of the model prediction. The conjunctival image of Figure 6a is unseen data obtained from healthy subjects. Figure 6b,e,h are additional processed images to show the unseen data of Figure 6a,d,g for readers. Figure 6c results from the model prediction in Figure 6a. Each box with a color boundary in Figure 6a–c represents regions of interest for the low-contrast, blurry vessels. These results demonstrate that Attention-UNet trained with mixed datasets is accurate for low-contrast vascular structures without additional postprocessing.

3.2. Motion Correction

To evaluate the performance of the motion correction processes, we compare the displacement values of 70 frames of the conjunctival microvessels. Figure 7 illustrates the horizontal and vertical axial displacement values of the source images from the first frame. In the uncorrected case (black line), the intense axial motions of the frames are visible. After the correction process, the axial motions are noticeably reduced (red and blue lines). For the horizontal axis depicted in Figure 7a, the mean axial displacement decreased to 2.69 μm from 16.84 μm after the first registration process. After the second process of motion correction, it decreased to 0.9 μm. For the vertical axis depicted in Figure 7b, it also decreased to 0.81 μm from 14 μm. Consequently, most of the displacement values decreased, except for the movements smaller than 1 μm.

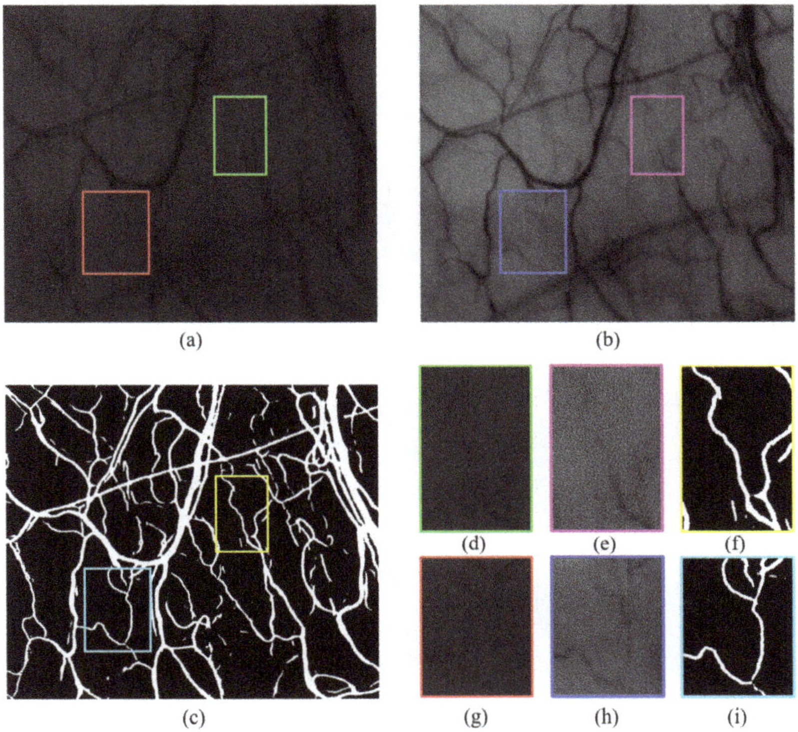

Figure 6. (**a**) Averaged conjunctival image. (**b**) Brightness and contrast-adjusted (**a**) by Image J (set display range: 25–115). (**c**) Attention-UNet segmentation results. (**d**,**g**) Cropped images from the low-contrast, blurry areas of (**a**). (**e**,**h**) Cropped images from (**b**). (**f**,**i**) Corresponding to the prediction results of (**d**,**g**). Brightness and contrast-adjusted images (**b**,**e**,**h**) were placed to provide easier visibility for the reader.

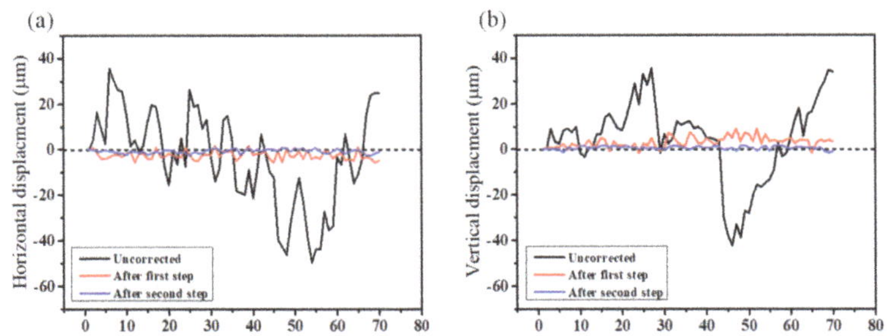

Figure 7. Comparison of the displacement values between uncorrected (black line) and motion-corrected (red and blue lines) image sequence. Red line indicates the displacement values after the first registration step, and the blue line represents after the second motion correction step. (**a**) Horizontal displacement values. (**b**) Vertical displacement values.

Furthermore, we compared before and after the motion correction of the spatial–temporal analysis (STA) images, which are crucial to quantifying the blood flow velocity. The red line in Figure 8a displays a target vessel to analyze the blood flow velocity. Figure 8b illustrates an STA image before motion correction. In this STA image, the slope required to calculate the blood flow velocity cannot be verified because of the motion artifacts. In contrast, the clear edges of the slope displayed by the yellow line in Figure 8c are observed in the STA image after motion correction. Finally, the blood flow velocity obtained from the average values of the yellow slopes is 0.338 mm/s.

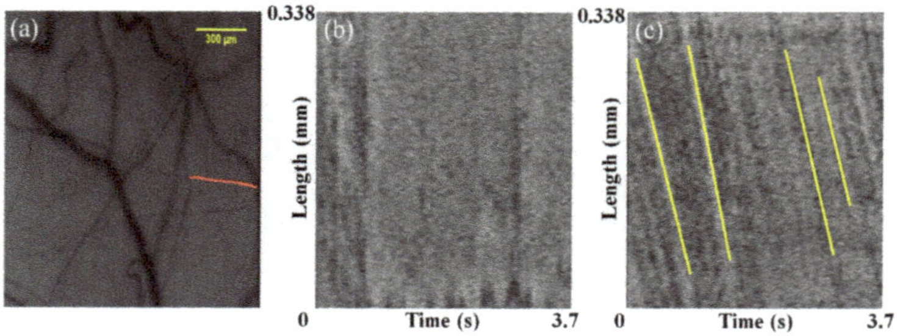

Figure 8. (**a**) Vessel used to generate the STA image (red line). (**b**) STA image before motion correction. (**c**) STA image after motion correction. Yellow lines represent slopes, which indicate blood flow velocity.

Table 1 illustrates the characteristics of conjunctival microvessels, including diameter, length, and blood flow velocity. These characteristics are measured in the selected vessel segments with the highest observability indices. Starting with V1, 10 blood vessels with a high observability index are sequentially arranged. The minimum and Table 1 illustrate the characteristics of the conjunctival microvessels, including diameter, length, and blood flow velocity. These characteristics are measured in the selected vessel segments with the highest observability indices. Starting with V1, 10 blood vessels with a high observability index are sequentially arranged. The minimum and maximum blood vessel diameters are 8.172 and 15.62 μm. The blood flow velocity ranges between 0.078 and 0.338 mm/s, similar to the values in a previous study, were measured with other equipment [36].

Table 1. Diameter, length, and blood flow velocity of conjunctival microvessels.

Vessel	Diameter (μm)	Length (mm)	Blood Flow Velocity (mm/s)
V1	13.158	0.414	0.086
V2	15.282	0.356	0.097
V3	8.172	0.338	0.338
V4	9.878	0.330	0.090
V5	10.170	0.318	0.270
V6	8.682	0.220	0.141
V7	9.574	0.250	0.078
V8	15.422	0.246	0.137
V9	15.620	0.128	0.114
V10	9.934	0.214	0.153

4. Discussion

In this paper, we introduced a system that can accurately quantify the conjunctival blood flow velocity by overcoming motion artifacts. First, Attention-UNet was implemented to precisely segment the low-quality vessel images. The Attention-UNet trained with a retinal dataset was used to segment conjunctival vessels with low-contrast, blurry structures [17]. This study inferred that Attention-UNet has a high generalization ability to learn the vascular structure.

Second, we conducted a two-step correction process to solve the problem of changing local information. Fine movements are critical to high magnification imaging to track red blood cells (RBC) for measuring the blood flow. Although we corrected a large motion through the registration process, 4–7 μm of the displacement remained. An additional correction process was essential to obtain an accurate blood flow velocity by tracking RBC particles of approximately 7.5 μm in diameter [19]. Therefore, we implemented an additional motion correction algorithm, template matching, by considering the vessel features, including diameter and length. The displacements of the conjunctival microvasculature images are reduced to the order of 1 μm while minimizing the frame loss.

We construct a custom-built optical system to image the human conjunctiva and acquire the conjunctival images from five healthy subjects. Conjunctival datasets have a risk of overfitting due to a lack of images, which we avoided by adding a retinal dataset with a similar domain to the conjunctival images. The high-resolution fundus (HRF) dataset was selected as an additional dataset because of the vessel size similar to our conjunctival image. The model trained by the mixed dataset achieved more accurate segmentation results than the conjunctival dataset only.

Furthermore, our motion correction process can produce insights in observing blood flow velocity for an extended period by correcting their fine control movements. When the human eye gazes at a fixed object, the dwelling time ranges from 90 to 900 ms [37]. After the dwelling time, the fixated eyes start vibrating. Due to eye movements caused by the short dwelling time, conjunctival hemodynamics were observed for only 0.3 s in a previous study [10].

However, the velocity pulse period (VPP), which is the time varying the blood flow velocity, due to the cardiac impulse is 940 ms [38], longer than the dwelling time. Consequently, it is necessary to observe the blood flow velocity for a more extended period than the VPP. Since we compensate for the motion above the VPP, the blood flow velocity is quantified above three seconds through the STA image. We created an opportunity for quantifying the long-term blood flow assessment, limited by a dwelling time shorter than the cardiac cycle time.

A limitation in the current configuration is that it can be difficult to compensate for the motion blur caused by movements that are faster than the frame rates. This type of image can be blurred, even if the location is not changed. One way to mitigate this problem is to reduce the exposure time and increase the frame rate. However, such an approach would inevitably decrease the contrast of the image. We overcame this limitation by comparing the contrast index assigned during registration, thereby removing the blurred frames with low-contrast values.

This study adopted several capabilities, including image registration, deep learning vessel segmentation, and template matching for motion correction, to quantify the microcirculation of the human conjunctiva. Using these methods, we acquired a blood flow velocity of 0.078 to 0.338 mm/s in the conjunctiva vessels. Although we could not perfectly control the factors affecting the blood flow velocity, we could confirm that our results partially corresponded to a previous study measuring the conjunctiva blood flow range as 0.19 to 0.33 mm/s [36].

As further works, our image processing method could provide blood flow velocity in the retina, wrists, lips, and fingernails. In addition, when significant correlations of conjunctival hemodynamics with cardiovascular diseases, as well as diabetes, are demonstrated, the developed imaging system and processing method can be used as one of the methods providing pre-diagnostic factors for systemic diseases [1,39].

5. Conclusions

We demonstrate a system that resolves motion artifacts to quantify the conjunctival blood flow velocity. Deep learning-based segmentation and motion correction techniques are used to solve the motion artifacts during image acquisition. We evaluated the system performance by analyzing conjunctival images from five healthy volunteers. The system segment low-contrast vessels reduced the image displacement to less than 1 to 2 μm. Pathways of red blood cells could be tracked free from the motion artifacts, resulting in quantifying the blood flow velocity. The range of quantifying the conjunctival blood flow velocity is 0.078~0.338 mm/s in a healthy subject. This conjunctival imaging instrument is applicable for imaging subjects with limited forward-looking capabilities or an unsteady fixation.

Author Contributions: Conceptualization, H.-C.J. and D.-Y.K.; methodology, H.-C.J., J.L. and D.-Y.K.; software, H.J.; resources, K.-S.N.; writing—original draft preparation, H.J. and J.L.; writing—review and editing, H.-C.J. and D.-Y.K.; supervision, D.-Y.K.; and project administration, D.-Y.K. All authors have read and agreed to the published version of the manuscript.

Funding: This work was supported by the National Research Foundation of Korea (NRF), the Ministry of Education, through the Basic Science Research Program under grant no. 2018R1A6A1A03025523, by the Ministry of Science and ICT under grant no. 2019R1A2C1006814, by the National Research Foundation of Korea (NRF) under grant no. 2019R1F1A1061421, and by the grant of the Catholic University Yeouido St.Mary's Hospital made in the program year of 2020.

Institutional Review Board Statement: This study was conducted according to the guidelines of the Declaration of Helsinki and approved by the Institutional Review Board of Yeouido St. Mary's Hospital (CMC IRB_SC19DESE0067, 23 September 2019).

Informed Consent Statement: Informed consent was obtained from all subjects involved in the study. Written informed consent was obtained from the patient(s) to publish this paper.

Data Availability Statement: In this paper, both publicly available datasets and custom datasets were used. Publicly available datasets were analyzed in this study. This data can be found here: https://www5.cs.fau.de/research/data/fundus-images/, accessed on 3 May 2021. The custom data presented in this study are available on request from the corresponding author. The data are not publicly available due to privacy.

Conflicts of Interest: The authors declare no conflict of interest.

References

1. Khansari, M.M.; Wanek, J.; Tan, M.; Joslin, C.E.; Kresovich, J.K.; Camardo, N.; Blair, N.P.; Shahidi, M. Assessment of conjunctival microvascular hemodynamics in stages of diabetic microvasculopathy. *Sci. Rep.* **2017**, *7*, 1–9. [CrossRef] [PubMed]
2. Chen, W.; Batawi, H.I.M.; Alava, J.R.; Galor, A.; Yuan, J.; Sarantopoulos, C.D.; McClellan, A.L.; Feuer, W.J.; Levitt, R.C.; Wang, J. Bulbar conjunctival microvascular responses in dry eye. *Ocul. Surf.* **2017**, *15*, 193–201. [CrossRef] [PubMed]
3. Wang, J.; Jiang, H.; Tao, A.; DeBuc, D.; Shao, Y.; Zhong, J.; Pineda, S. Limbal capillary perfusion and blood flow velocity as a potential biomarker for evaluating dry eye. *Investig. Ophthalmol. Vis. Sci.* **2013**, *54*, 4335.
4. Chen, W.; Deng, Y.; Jiang, H.; Wang, J.; Zhong, J.; Li, S.; Peng, L.; Wang, B.; Yang, R.; Zhang, H. Microvascular abnormalities in dry eye patients. *Microvasc. Res.* **2018**, *118*, 155–161. [CrossRef]
5. Valeshabad, A.K.; Wanek, J.; Mukarram, F.; Zelkha, R.; Testai, F.D.; Shahidi, M. Feasibility of assessment of conjunctival microvascular hemodynamics in unilateral ischemic stroke. *Microvasc. Res.* **2015**, *100*, 4–8. [CrossRef]
6. Karanam, V.C.; Tamariz, L.; Batawi, H.; Wang, J.; Galor, A. Functional slit lamp biomicroscopy metrics correlate with cardiovascular risk. *Ocul. Surf.* **2019**, *17*, 64–69. [CrossRef]
7. Jiang, H.; Zhong, J.; DeBuc, D.C.; Tao, A.; Xu, Z.; Lam, B.L.; Liu, C.; Wang, J. Functional slit lamp biomicroscopy for imaging bulbar conjunctival microvasculature in contact lens wearers. *Microvasc. Res.* **2014**, *92*, 62–71. [CrossRef]
8. Shahidi, M.; Wanek, J.; Gaynes, B.; Wu, T. Quantitative assessment of conjunctival microvascular circulation of the human eye. *Microvasc. Res.* **2010**, *79*, 109–113. [CrossRef]
9. van Zijderveld, R.; Ince, C.; Schlingemann, R.O. Orthogonal polarization spectral imaging of conjunctival microcirculation. *Graefe's Arch. Clin. Exp. Ophthalmol.* **2014**, *252*, 773–779. [CrossRef]
10. Khansari, M.M.; Wanek, J.; Felder, A.E.; Camardo, N.; Shahidi, M. Automated assessment of hemodynamics in the conjunctival microvasculature network. *IEEE Trans. Med Imaging* **2015**, *35*, 605–611. [CrossRef]
11. Wang, L.; Yuan, J.; Jiang, H.; Yan, W.; Cintrón-Colón, H.R.; Perez, V.L.; DeBuc, D.C.; Feuer, W.J.; Wang, J. Vessel sampling and blood flow velocity distribution with vessel diameter for characterizing the human bulbar conjunctival microvasculature. *Eye Contact Lens* **2016**, *42*, 135. [CrossRef]
12. Goobic, A.P.; Tang, J.; Acton, S.T. Image stabilization and registration for tracking cells in the microvasculature. *IEEE Trans. Biomed. Eng.* **2005**, *52*, 287–299. [CrossRef]
13. Brennan, P.F.; McNeil, A.J.; Jing, M.; Awuah, A.; Finlay, D.D.; Blighe, K.; McLaughlin, J.A.; Wang, R.; Moore, J.; Nesbit, M.A. Quantitative assessment of the conjunctival microcirculation using a smartphone and slit-lamp biomicroscope. *Microvasc. Res.* **2019**, *126*, 103907. [CrossRef]
14. Frangi, A.F.; Niessen, W.J.; Vincken, K.L.; Viergever, M.A. Multiscale vessel enhancement filtering. In Proceedings of the International Conference on Medical Image Computing and Computer-Assisted Intervention, MICCAI 98, Cambridge, MA, USA, 11–13 October 1998; pp. 130–137.
15. Doubal, F.; MacGillivray, T.; Patton, N.; Dhillon, B.; Dennis, M.; Wardlaw, J. Fractal analysis of retinal vessels suggests that a distinct vasculopathy causes lacunar stroke. *Neurology* **2010**, *74*, 1102–1107. [CrossRef]

16. Soares, J.V.; Leandro, J.J.; Cesar, R.M.; Jelinek, H.F.; Cree, M.J. Retinal vessel segmentation using the 2-D Gabor wavelet and supervised classification. *IEEE Trans. Med. Imaging* **2006**, *25*, 1214–1222. [CrossRef]
17. Luo, Z.; Zhang, Y.; Zhou, L.; Zhang, B.; Luo, J.; Wu, H. Micro-vessel image segmentation based on the AD-UNet model. *IEEE Access* **2019**, *7*, 143402–143411. [CrossRef]
18. Delori, F.C.; Webb, R.H.; Sliney, D.H. Maximum permissible exposures for ocular safety (ANSI 2000), with emphasis on ophthalmic devices. *JOSA A* **2007**, *24*, 1250–1265. [CrossRef]
19. Persons, E.L. Studies on red blood cell diameter: III. The relative diameter of immature (reticulocytes) and adult red blood cells in health and anemia, especially in pernicious anemia. *J. Clin. Investig.* **1929**, *7*, 615–629. [CrossRef]
20. Webb, R.H.; Dorey, C.K. The pixilated image. In *Handbook of Biological Confocal Microscopy*; Springer: Boston, MA, USA, 1995; pp. 55–67.
21. Deneux, T.; Takerkart, S.; Grinvald, A.; Masson, G.S.; Vanzetta, I. A processing work-flow for measuring erythrocytes velocity in extended vascular networks from wide field high-resolution optical imaging data. *Neuroimage* **2012**, *59*, 2569–2588. [CrossRef]
22. Vincent, O.R.; Folorunso, O. A descriptive algorithm for sobel image edge detection. In Proceedings of the Informing Science & IT Education Conference (InSITE 2009), Macon, GA, USA, 12–15 June 2009; pp. 97–107.
23. Wang, Z.; Feng, C.; Ang, W.T.; Tan, S.Y.M.; Latt, W.T. Autofocusing and polar body detection in automated cell manipulation. *IEEE Trans. Biomed. Eng.* **2016**, *64*, 1099–1105. [CrossRef]
24. Shih, L. Autofocus survey: A comparison of algorithms. In Proceedings of the Digital Photography III, Electronic Imaging 2007, San Jose, CA, USA, 28 January–1 February 2007; p. 65020B.
25. Dubbs, A.; Guevara, J.; Yuste, R. moco: Fast motion correction for calcium imaging. *Front. Neuroinformatics* **2016**, *10*, 6. [CrossRef] [PubMed]
26. Odstrcilik, J.; Kolar, R.; Budai, A.; Hornegger, J.; Jan, J.; Gazarek, J.; Kubena, T.; Cernosek, P.; Svoboda, O.; Angelopoulou, E. Retinal vessel segmentation by improved matched filtering: Evaluation on a new high-resolution fundus image database. *IET Image Process.* **2013**, *7*, 373–383. [CrossRef]
27. Pizer, S.M.; Amburn, E.P.; Austin, J.D.; Cromartie, R.; Geselowitz, A.; Greer, T.; ter Haar Romeny, B.; Zimmerman, J.B.; Zuiderveld, K. Adaptive histogram equalization and its variations. *Comput. Vis. Graph. Image Process.* **1987**, *39*, 355–368. [CrossRef]
28. Yamanakkanavar, N.; Lee, B. Using a Patch-Wise M-Net Convolutional Neural Network for Tissue Segmentation in Brain MRI Images. *IEEE Access* **2020**, *8*, 120946–120958. [CrossRef]
29. Wang, C.; Zhao, Z.; Ren, Q.; Xu, Y.; Yu, Y. Dense U-net based on patch-based learning for retinal vessel segmentation. *Entropy* **2019**, *21*, 168. [CrossRef] [PubMed]
30. Yan, Z.; Yang, X.; Cheng, K.-T. Joint segment-level and pixel-wise losses for deep learning based retinal vessel segmentation. *IEEE Trans. Biomed. Eng.* **2018**, *65*, 1912–1923. [CrossRef]
31. Oktay, O.; Schlemper, J.; Folgoc, L.L.; Lee, M.; Heinrich, M.; Misawa, K.; Mori, K.; McDonagh, S.; Hammerla, N.Y.; Kainz, B. Attention u-net: Learning where to look for the pancreas. *arXiv* **2018**, arXiv:1804.03999.
32. Zou, K.H.; Warfield, S.K.; Bharatha, A.; Tempany, C.M.; Kaus, M.R.; Haker, S.J.; Wells III, W.M.; Jolesz, F.A.; Kikinis, R. Statistical validation of image segmentation quality based on a spatial overlap index1: Scientific reports. *Acad. Radiol.* **2004**, *11*, 178–189. [CrossRef]
33. Lee, T.-C.; Kashyap, R.L.; Chu, C.-N. Building skeleton models via 3-D medial surface axis thinning algorithms. *Cvgip Graph. Models Image Process.* **1994**, *56*, 462–478. [CrossRef]
34. Klingler, J.W.; Vaughan, C.L.; Fraker, T.; Andrews, L.T. Segmentation of echocardiographic images using mathematical morphology. *IEEE Trans. Biomed. Eng.* **1988**, *35*, 925–934. [CrossRef]
35. Bradski, G.; Kaehler, A. *Learning OpenCV: Computer Vision with the OpenCV Library*; O'Reilly Media, Inc.: Newton, MA, USA, 2008.
36. Xiao, P.; Duan, Z.; Wang, G.; Deng, Y.; Wang, Q.; Zhang, J.; Liang, S.; Yuan, J. Multi-modal Anterior Eye Imager Combining Ultra-High Resolution OCT and Microvascular Imaging for Structural and Functional Evaluation of the Human Eye. *Appl. Sci.* **2020**, *10*, 2545. [CrossRef]
37. Duncan, J.; Ward, R.; Shapiro, K. Direct measurement of attentional dwell time in human vision. *Nature* **1994**, *369*, 313–315. [CrossRef]
38. Koutsiaris, A.G.; Tachmitzi, S.V.; Papavasileiou, P.; Batis, N.; Kotoula, M.G.; Giannoukas, A.D.; Tsironi, E. Blood velocity pulse quantification in the human conjunctival pre-capillary arterioles. *Microvasc. Res.* **2010**, *80*, 202–208. [CrossRef]
39. Strain, W.D.; Paldánius, P. Diabetes, cardiovascular disease and the microcirculation. *Cardiovasc. Diabetol.* **2018**, *17*, 1–10. [CrossRef]

sensors

MDPI

Article

Precise Identification of Prostate Cancer from DWI Using Transfer Learning

Islam R. Abdelmaksoud [1,2], Ahmed Shalaby [1], Ali Mahmoud [1], Mohammed Elmogy [2], Ahmed Aboelfetouh [2], Mohamed Abou El-Ghar [3], Moumen El-Melegy [4], Norah Saleh Alghamdi [5,*] and Ayman El-Baz [1]

1 Bioengineering Department, University of Louisville, Louisville, KY 40292, USA; islam-cis@mans.edu.eg (I.R.A.); ahmed.shalaby@louisville.edu (A.S.); ahmahm01@louisville.edu (A.M.); aselba01@louisville.edu (A.E.-B.)
2 Faculty of Computers and Information, Mansoura University, Dakahlia 35516, Egypt; melmogy@mans.edu.eg (M.E.); elfetouh@mans.edu.eg (A.A.)
3 Radiology Department, Urology and Nephrology Center, University of Mansoura, Dakahlia 35516, Egypt; maboelghar@mans.edu.eg
4 Electrical Engineering Department, Assiut University, Assiut 71515, Egypt; moumen@aun.edu.eg
5 College of Computer and Information Science, Princess Nourah Bint Abdulrahman University, Riyadh 11564, Saudi Arabia
* Correspondence: NOSAlghamdi@pnu.edu.sa

Abstract: Background and Objective: The use of computer-aided detection (CAD) systems can help radiologists make objective decisions and reduce the dependence on invasive techniques. In this study, a CAD system that detects and identifies prostate cancer from diffusion-weighted imaging (DWI) is developed. **Methods:** The proposed system first uses non-negative matrix factorization (NMF) to integrate three different types of features for the accurate segmentation of prostate regions. Then, discriminatory features in the form of apparent diffusion coefficient (ADC) volumes are estimated from the segmented regions. The ADC maps that constitute these volumes are labeled by a radiologist to identify the ADC maps with malignant or benign tumors. Finally, transfer learning is used to fine-tune two different previously-trained convolutional neural network (CNN) models (AlexNet and VGGNet) for detecting and identifying prostate cancer. **Results:** Multiple experiments were conducted to evaluate the accuracy of different CNN models using DWI datasets acquired at nine distinct b-values that included both high and low b-values. The average accuracy of AlexNet at the nine b-values was 89.2 ± 1.5% with average sensitivity and specificity of 87.5 ± 2.3% and 90.9 ± 1.9%. These results improved with the use of the deeper CNN model (VGGNet). The average accuracy of VGGNet was 91.2 ± 1.3% with sensitivity and specificity of 91.7 ± 1.7% and 90.1 ± 2.8%. **Conclusions:** The results of the conducted experiments emphasize the feasibility and accuracy of the developed system and the improvement of this accuracy using the deeper CNN.

Keywords: prostate cancer; transfer learning; ALexNet; VGGNet; ADC maps

Citation: Abdelmaksoud, I.R.; Shalaby, A.; Mahmoud, A.; Elmogy, M.; Aboelfetouh, A.; Abou El-Ghar, M.; El-Melegy, M.; Alghamdi, N.S.; El-Baz, A. Precise Identification of Prostate Cancer from DWI Using Transfer Learning. *Sensors* **2021**, *21*, 3664. https://doi.org/10.3390/s21113664

Academic Editor: Loris Nanni

Received: 27 March 2021
Accepted: 18 May 2021
Published: 25 May 2021

1. Introduction

Prostate cancer is a major health problem, especially in western countries. For example, this disease is the second leading cause of mortality among males in the United States [1]. In 2020, the number of new prostate cancer cases and the number of deaths caused by prostate cancer among Americans are expected to be 191,930 and 33,330, respectively [1]. Currently, the definitive technique of diagnosing prostate cancer is transrectal ultrasound (TRUS)-guided biopsy. However, biopsy is an invasive procedure that can miss up to 30% of cancers [2]. In order to minimize the errors of detecting prostate cancer by TRUS-guided biopsy, many alternatives, such as magnetic resonance imaging (MRI)-guided biopsy, have been investigated [3].

Recently, MRI has evolved in its capabilities of detecting prostate cancer in addition to its use in guiding biopsies for better accuracy. Multiple MRI sequences, which include

T2-weighted MRI, diffusion-weighted imaging (DWI), and dynamic contrast-enhanced MRI (DCE-MRI), are used in various clinical tasks, such as active surveillance, localization, and determining the stage of prostate cancer [4,5]. However, detecting and localizing prostate cancer from MRI data is a challenging task. As large volumes of MRI data, from different protocols and sometimes from different scanners, have to be analyzed, these variations can lead to inter-observer differences. Computer-aided detection (CAD) systems can help physicians make objective and fast decisions. These systems can also enhance the quantitative evaluation of prostate cancer.

Developing MRI-based CAD systems for identifying prostate cancer has become a subject of active research [6]. For instance, Viswanath et al. [7] examined the performance of multiple classical classifiers and their bagging and boosting ensembles using a multi-institutional T2-weighed MRI dataset of 85 subjects. These classifiers were fed with radiomic features and their performance was evaluated using the receiver operating characteristic (ROC) curve. The highest average area under the curve (AUC) was obtained by the boosted quadratic discriminant analysis. Riccardo et al. [8] found that the accuracy of targeted biopsy improved by 13.2% in case of combining physician analysis of multiparametric MRI with CAD results. Rampun et al. [9] compared the accuracy of eleven classifiers using a T2-weighed MRI dataset of 45 subjects. Their system employed feature selection on a feature space of size 215 to select the best discriminating features. The highest resulting accuracy was 85.5%. More detailed and profound literature review can be found in the recent survey by Gao et al. [10].

Although existing systems have achieved satisfactory results, these systems base their diagnosis on handcrafted features that are validated on small datasets. The good empirical design of these handcrafted features determines their accuracy. An alternative approach for handcrafted features is to learn the discriminating features automatically.

Deep learning structures, especially convolutional neural networks (CNN), are able to automatically learn multiple levels of features from data in a hierarchical manner [11]. These structures have achieved accurate results in multiple computer vision tasks [12–16] as well as lesions detection tasks [17]. Ishioka et al. [18], developed a prostate cancer CAD algorithm that aimed to reduce the variation in the interpretation of T2-weighted MRI. They used histogram smoothing to convert the 12-bit intensity data from the original T2-weighted MR images into 8-bit images. These images were normalized and subjected to data augmentation to increase the employed training data. The detection of prostate cancer was obtained using a CNN architecture that combined both U-net and ResNet50. Their algorithm resulted in an AUC of 0.65. Mehrtash et al. [19] evaluated the performance of CNN with different MRI modalities. The highest performance achieved by their system in terms of AUC was 0.8. This performance was achieved by including zonal information of tumors with DWI and DCE-MRI. Yang et al. [20] proposed a system for detecting and localizing the presence of prostate cancer from T2-weighted MRI and apparent diffusion coefficient (ADC) images. Their system used an individual CNN for each of the used two modalities to produce a response map indicating the malignancy likelihood of each pixel. An average pooling is performed before the last convolutional layer of each CNN to obtain a feature vector. The feature vectors from each modality are concatenated and used as input into a support vector machine (SVM). A sensitivity of 46% and 97% was achieved at 0.1 and 10 false positives per normal case. Le et al. [21] integrated a similarity cost function with the CNN cost function to better fuse ADCs with T2-weighted MRI. The authors investigated multiple data augmentation techniques, multiple CNN architectures, and multiple fusion schemes to find out the combination that can lead to the best accuracy. The final differentiation between malignant and benign tissues was based on the integration between the results of CNN and the results of handcrafted features using an SVM classifier. An accuracy of 91.5% was achieved. Wang et al. [22] found that optimizing the steps of prostate segmentation, multi-modal registration and cancer localization in a joint manner can reduce the computation burdens of optimizing each step individually. Moreover, this joint optimization improves the accuracy by reducing the accumulation of errors over the different steps. Song et al. [23] developed a patch-based CNN system for differentiating between malignant and benign prostate lesions from multiparametric MRI. Their proposed CNN model consisted of three blocks of layers before the final fully-connected (FC) layers. Each block consisted of three convolutional layers followed by a dropout layer and a max-pooling layer. Their model resulted in sensitivity and specificity of 87% and 90.6%, respectively. Hosseinzadeh et al. [24] developed 2D-UNet model to produce maps of prostate zones. In their system, the inclusion of zonal information improved the average sensitivity at three different false positives by 5%.

Schelb et al. [25] used a dataset of two modalities (T2-weighted MRI and DWI) to train a U-Net classifier. Their system showed that the performance of a U-Net classifier is similar to the clinical assessment. Xu et al. [26] developed a system to detect prostate lesions using a residual network. Their system resulted in an accuracy of 93%. Yuan et al. [27] developed a system for classifying prostate cancer from three MRI modalities. Their systems employed three CNNs. Each CNN was fed with a different modality to learn discriminative features. Their system resulted in an accuracy of 86.9%. Chen et al. [28] tuned two pre-trained CNNs, namely, InceptionV3 and VGG-16, using PROSTATEx challenge dataset. An AUC of 0.83 was obtained using VGG-16. Abbasi et al. [29] tuned a pre-trained CNN model(GoogLeNet) using a prostate cancer MRI dataset. They compared GoogLeNet with other classifiers, such as, decision tree and SVM. They found that GoogLeNet outperformed these conventional classifiers. A recent survey by Wildeboer et al. [30] listed more than 80 CAD systems for diagnosing prostate cancer. In this survey, the different CAD systems were categorized according to the employed imaging modalities and the employed classifiers.

Training deep architectures with huge numbers of parameters from scratch requires large amounts of data. Typically, the amount of data in the medical domain is small when compared to that of natural images used in conventional computer vision applications. Training deep architectures with small amounts of data can lead to overfitting, which means the network can correctly classify the data used for training but is not able to correctly classify new data (i.e., the network does not generalize well). Moreover, if the amount of medical data is sufficient, annotating this data by multiple experts to prepare it for training can be an impeding factor. In order to overcome these limitations, this work modifies previously-trained CNNs and fine-tunes them for detecting and identifying prostate cancer. The process of fine-tuning such deep networks can be done with small datasets.

The main contribution of this work does not depend on which deep learning network is used; the main contribution is representing the input data in a different form (ADC maps) to be more separable to achieve acceptable accuracy, no matter which deep learning network is used. To prove this point, AlexNet, which is a deep learning network that has only five convolutional layers, is used in the beginning. AlexNet achieved an average accuracy of $89.2 \pm 1.5\%$ at the nine b-values. For further validation, VGGNet, which has more layers that increase its learning ability, is then used. VGGNet achieved an average accuracy of $91.2 \pm 1.3\%$ at the nine b-values. The ADC maps used in the proposed system are calculated at both low and high b-values. This enables the proposed system to capture both blood perfusion and water diffusion for an accurate diagnosis of prostate cancer. The b-value is a measure of the degree of diffusion weighting employed to generate diffusion-weighted images. It is a parameter that relies on the timing and strength of the used gradient pulses. The details of this process are discussed in the following sections.

2. Methods and Materials

The DWI datasets used in this work were collected from 37 subjects (16 benign and 21 malignant) using two distinct scanners (1.5 Tesla (T) scanner and 3T scanner) at nine distinct b-values (100, 200, ..., 800, 1000 s/mm^2). The acquisition parameters of the 1.5 T scanner in axial plane were: TE = 84.6 ms, TR = 8000 ms, Bandwidth = 142.86 kHz, FOV = 34 cm, slice thickness = 3 mm, inter-slice gap = 0 mm, voxel size = $1.25 \times 1.25 \times 3.00$ mm^3. The 3T DW images were acquired in the transverse plane. The acquisition parameters of the second 3T scanner were: TR = 4300–4800 ms, TE = 75–88 ms, acquisition matrix = 128×126, reconstruction matrix = 256 × 256, FOV = 20 cm. The scanning was done using full-echo and full-k-space. However, a SENSE acceleration factor of 2 was used, thus skipping over every-other line in k-space. Excitation and read-out were spectral fat-suppressed, standard 2D multi-slice 90–180 spin-echo Stejskal-Tanner DWI, with single-shot echo-planar-imaging read-out. A single diffusion encoding direction of [1,1,1] was used (i.e., X,Y,Z gradient channels were on simultaneously) to obtain minimal TE at the maximum b-value. Each b-value was averaged 7 times. Big delta = 47 ms and little delta = 15 ms. All the cases involved in this study performed MRI when there was a clinical suspicion of malignancy. The final diagnosis of the cases was established by biopsy that was carried out after MRI. Therefore, the ground truth of diagnosis of all subjects was based on the results of the biopsy. From the malignant cases, 234 slices were labelled manually by a radiologist as having malignant tumors. The analysis and labeling of all the cases were performed in a slice-wise manner. A similar number, 236, of DW slices from benign cases were chosen to create a balanced dataset of malignant and benign slices. These slices represent all the DW slices of 13 benign cases in addition to 5 slices from the remaining 3 benign cases. The ADC maps of the DWI datasets were calculated, as will be explained in the following subsection. The corresponding 470 ADC maps of the labelled DW slices were used to train and test the performance of the developed model, as explained in the following sections.

Figure 1 shows the general framework of the developed CAD system for detecting and identifying prostate cancer, which incorporates three main steps: prostate segmentation, identifying discriminatory features, and identifying slices with prostate cancer. Prostate segmentation integrates three types of features using non-negative matrix factorization (NMF) to guide the evolution of a level set model. These features are shape-priors of prostates, intensities of voxels and spatial features of neighboring voxels. The effect of incorporating each of these features into the accuracy of the used segmentation approach is explained in detail in [31]. Appearance, shape and spatial information were extracted for each voxel. NMF was used to reduce and make the combined features more separable. Curvature and Euclidean distances between the reduced features (test subject) to the centroids of NMF classes (calculated from training subjects) were used to estimate the voxel-wise guiding force of the level set. If the voxel belongs to the prostate, the level set grows. Otherwise, the level set shrinks. More details about the used segmentation approach can be found in [31]. The second step was identifying discriminatory features, which can discriminate malignant from benign cases. In this study, ADC volumes of the segmented prostates were estimated and used for this purpose. By nature, the prostate is a small organ compared to other organs. To be sure that the proposed model would capture the features that discriminate between malignant tumors and benign tumors, the ADC features were calculated only from the prostate region. This ensured that the system learned the features related only to prostate cancer. The first two processing steps of the proposed framework are illustrated for two different cases (one benign and one malignant) in Figure 2.

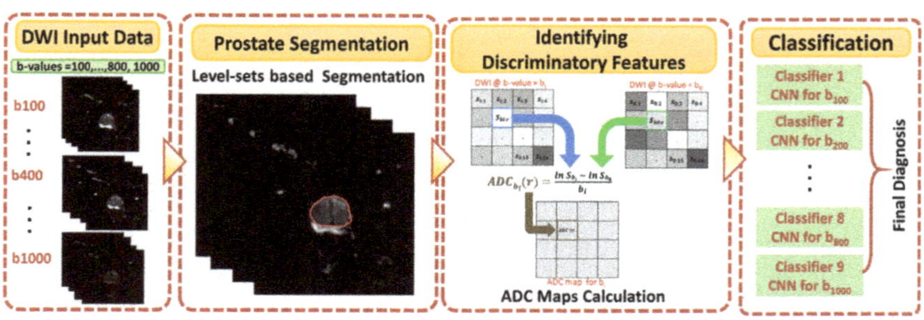

Figure 1. Overall workflow of the proposed model showing the DWI input data at nine b-values and its three basic steps, which are prostate segmentation, calculation of ADC maps as discriminating features, and the identification of slices with tumor using previously-trained CNN models.

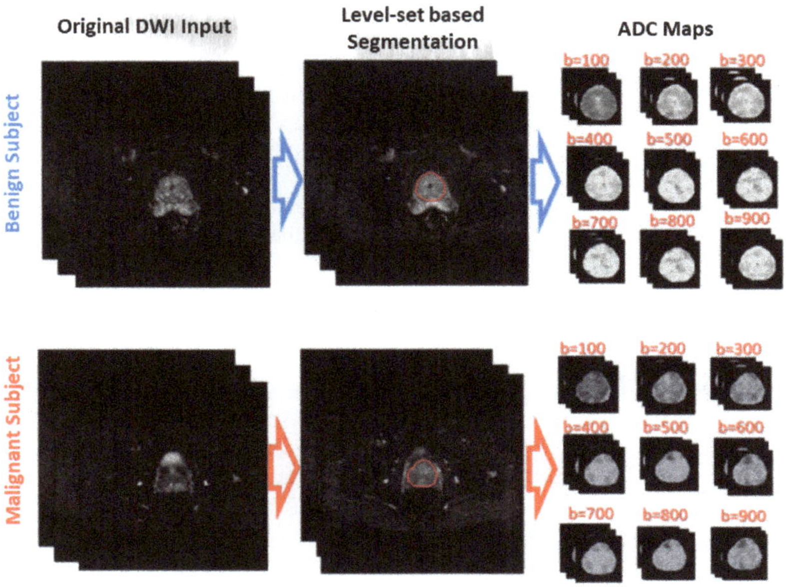

Figure 2. Illustration of the first two processing steps of the proposed framework on two different cases (one benign and one malignant).

The 2D cross sections that constitute these ADC volumes were extracted and used as input to the employed CNN-based model. This process is shown in Figure 3. The final step was identifying slices with tumors using a previously-trained CNN model. In the following subsections, the details of estimating the ADC maps and the use of these maps to fine-tune CNN models for identifying prostate cancer are presented.

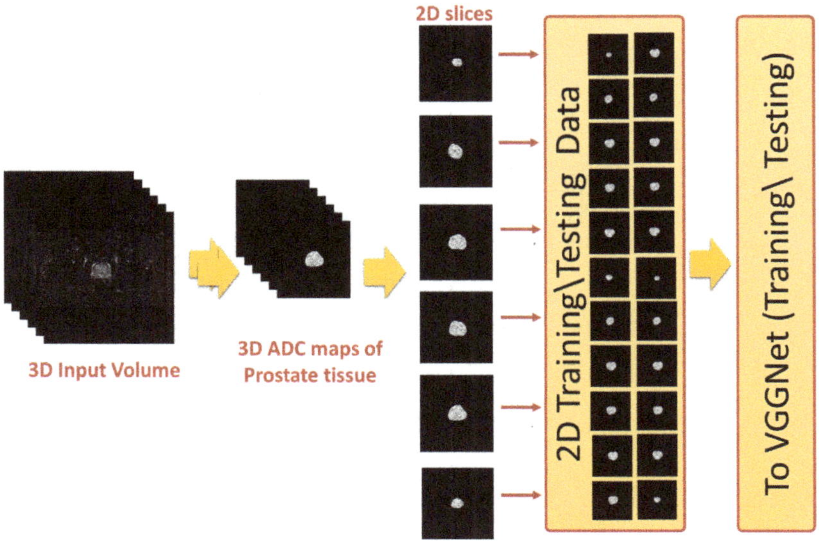

Figure 3. Illustration of slice-wise analysis of ADC volumes.

2.1. Identifying Discriminatory Features

Currently, DWI is one of the promising modalities utilized for the identification of prostate cancer. DWI is a functional MRI modality similar to DCE-MRI. However, what distinguishes DWI is its fast acquisition time, as there are no contrast agents used. The problem with contrast agents is the potential harm they cause to patients who have kidney disorders. DWI depends on the differences in the motion of water molecules inside the body to create images. DW images visualize and quantify this microscopic motion [32]. The molecules' motion is random, and there is a positive correlation between the level of randomness and the loss in the signal, which is given by [33]:

$$S_d \sim e^{-b\times ADC}, \quad (1)$$

where b is a parameter that relies on the timing and strength of the used gradient pulses, and ADC is a measure of the magnitude of water molecules' diffusion within the tissues. The utilization of gradient pulses gives rise to enhanced diffusion sensitivity compared to the steady state gradients [34].

The intensities of pixels in a slice acquired at a specific b-value (S_b) are equal to the intensities of the congruent pixels of the baseline slice (b = 0 s/mm^2) lowered by the signal loss defined in Equation (1). These intensities are given by:

$$S_b = S_0 \times e^{-b\times ADC}. \quad (2)$$

There is a negative relationship between the cellular density of a tissue region and its ADC values, as regions with dense cells restrict the mobility of water molecules. Since the quality of DWI is low, a large number of researchers choose to utilize the quantitative ADC maps computed from DWI to identify prostate cancer. The reason for the discriminating capabilities of ADCs is that malignant prostate tissues have smaller ADC values than healthy or benign tissues. The following equation shows that two DW images are required to calculate an ADC map:

$$ADC = -\frac{lnS_{b_1} - lnS_0}{b_1}. \quad (3)$$

The first image is collected at a specific b-value (b_1 > 0 s/mm^2) while the second is collected at b_0 (b = 0 s/mm^2). Another justification for employing ADC maps in this study is that the calculation of ADC maps is not sensitive to the used magnetic field strength [35]. This is suitable for the DWI datasets used in this study, as they were collected by two scanners that have different magnetic field strengths. Moreover, integrating handcrafted features with the automatically-learned features by CNNs can improve accuracy [36]. Since each ADC map represents the difference between two DW images, these maps are themselves images. Therefore, they can be used as input to the CNN model instead of the DW images. As these maps have better discriminating capabilities, their use improves the accuracy of the system.

2.2. Identification of Prostate Cancer

In this study, two different CNN models were used for prostate cancer identification. There are multiple advantages of using CNN over traditional neural networks. First, CNNs typically contain a larger number of layers than traditional neural networks. Augmenting the number of layers allows CNN to learn high levels of abstraction as the first layers learn primitive components while end layers use these learned primitive features to form the high-level features. The process of learning the features is done automatically by CNNs. Second, CNN takes both 2D images and 3D volumes directly as inputs without the need to convert these inputs into vectors, as in the case of neural networks. This preserves the inputs' spatial information. Third, the network connections and hence the network parameters of CNNs are fewer than the network connections in similar traditional neural networks. This reduction simplifies and expedites the training process of CNNs [37,38].

In this work, DW slices that contained tumors were labeled by a radiologist. The ADC maps that correspond to these labeled DW slices were divided into two groups. The first group contained ADC maps with malignant tumors, and the second group contained ADC maps from benign subjects. The number of ADC maps in the benign group was 236, and the number of ADC maps in the malignant group was 234. These ADC maps were used to train and evaluate two different previously-trained CNN models, which are AlexNet [39] and VGGNet [40].

ALexNet expects an input image of size 227 × 227 × 3, whereas the size of an input image for VGGNet was 224 × 224 × 3. The sizes of the calculated ADC maps were the same as the sizes of the corresponding DW images, which were 256 × 256 for the 1.5T images and 144 × 144 for the 3T images. To make these ADC maps suitable as inputs for the employed CNN models, the ADC maps of the larger sizes were center cropped, while the ADC maps of smaller sizes were zero padded. Then, each of these ADC maps was concatenated along the depth dimension to generate a three-channel image, which was the expected input to each of the employed CNN models.

Since the number of ADC maps is considered small for training and evaluating a CNN model from scratch, as training such deep structures from scratch with a small dataset leads to overfitting, a transfer learning model was adopted in this study. The idea of transfer learning is to modify a network that is trained to solve a certain problem and use it to solve a new problem in a different domain. The training of the original network is typically done with millions of images from the original domain. The advantage of transfer learning is that the adoption of this previously-trained network to solve a new problem requires far fewer images from the new domain. This is done by replacing the last few layers, including the output layer of the original network, with new layers appropriate to the new problem. In this work, the original output layer of either AlexNet or VGGNet, which assigns its input image to one of 1000 categories, was replaced with an output layer that classified its input ADC maps into either benign or malignant (Figure 4).

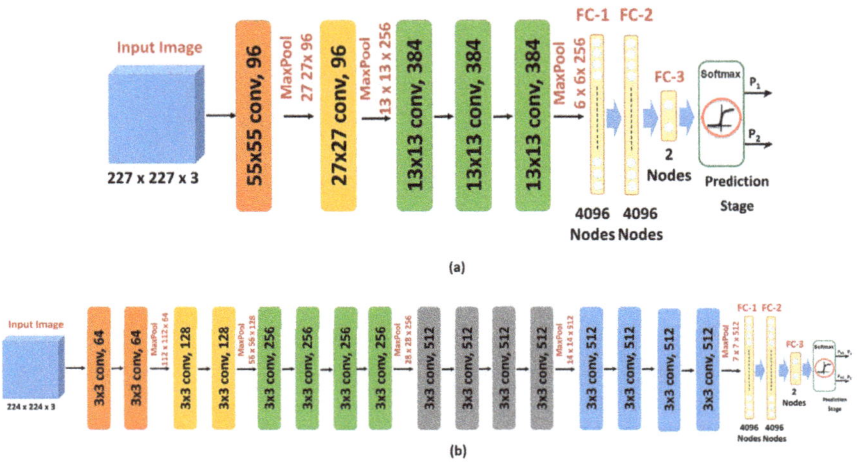

Figure 4. Illustration of the two different CNNs used in this study, (**a**) ALexNet, and (**b**) VGGNet.

The introduction and success of AlexNet have revolutionized the use of CNNs for multiple classification tasks. AlexNet is a CNN that contains five convolutional layers and three FC layers (Figure 4a). The network depth has a remarkable influence on its accuracy as the accuracy of AlexNet drops by 2% in the case of removing any of the five convolution layers. Rectified linear units (ReLUs) [41] are employed as activation functions by AlexNet. There are two main advantages of using ReLUs. First, ReLUs are saturation-free even in case of unnormalized inputs. Second, the training time of CNNs with ReLUs is shorter than the training time of CNNs with saturating activations (e.g., sigmoid). AlexNet is trained with a large dataset of natural images (ImageNet). This dataset contains more than one million images that belong to one thousand categories. To reduce the classification error, AlexNet employs overlapping pooling and response normalization [39]. AlexNet employs dropout [42] and data augmentation to overcome the overfitting issue. Two different forms of data augmentation were used: intensity alteration and transformations (translations and horizontal reflections) [39].

VGGNet is another deep CNN that is trained using ImageNet dataset. The main goal of developing VGGNet is to evaluate the effect of the network depth on the accuracies of CNNs. To achieve this goal, the developers examined five different network architectures with different depths, while the other parameters are fixed for a fair comparison. The input image is processed by a sequence of convolution layers, max-pooling layers [43], FC layers, and a softmax layer. VGGNet uses ReLU non-linearity activation. The number of convolutional layers of the different architectures ranges from 8 to 16 layers. The numbers of pooling layers and FC layers are 5 and 3, respectively. These numbers do not differ across the different architectures. The pooling layers follow some, but not all, of the convolutional layers. The convolution layers use kernels of small fixed receptive fields of 3×3 to lower the number of parameters. The pooling layers use fixed windows of 2×2 and a stride of 2. The number of filters of the first convolutional layer is 64. When a pooling layer is used, the number of filters of the following convolutional layer is doubled until the number of kernels reaches 512 [40].

In this work, the deepest architecture was used. This architecture has 19 layers with weights (16 convolutional layers and 3 FC layers) (Figure 4b). This architecture has 144 million parameters. This large number of parameters increases the training time of VGGNet, especially when compared with other CNNs with smaller numbers of parameters, such as AlexNet (60 million parameters) and GoogLeNet (4 million parameters). However, the performance of VGGNet in many transfer learning tasks is better than GoogLeNet [44]. Both AlexNet and VGGNet were optimized using stochastic gradient descent with momentum and the loss function was cross entropy. The other training parameters were the following: number of epochs = 50, learning rate = 0.0001, momentum = 0.9, mini-batch-size = 10, L_2 regularization = 0.0001. The basic architecture and configuration parameters of both the original and the fine-tuned AlexNet and VGGNet are summarized in Table 1.

Table 1. Basic architecture and configuration parameters of both AlexNet and VGGNet, where Conv. means convolutional, FC means fully-connected, SGDM means stochastic gradient descent with momentum, and cross entr. means cross entropy.

	AlexNet		**VGGNet**	
	Original	**Fine-Tuned**	**Original**	**Fine-Tuned**
No. of training images	>1 million	329–423	>1 million	329–423
Size of input images	227×227	227×227	224×224	224×224
No. of output categories	1000	2	1000	2
No. of Conv. layers	5	5	16	16
FC layers	3	3	3	3
Optimizer	SGDM	SGDM	SGDM	SGDM
Loss function	cross entr.	cross entr.	cross entr.	cross entr.

3. Results

Multiple experiments were conducted to test the performance of the developed system and to compare its performance with other modern machine-learning classifiers. In the first experiment, 70% of the ADC maps of both the malignant and benign cases at each b-value were used for fine-tuning an AlexNet-based model. The other 30%, which represent 71

ADC maps from benign cases and 70 ADC maps with malignant tumors, were employed to evaluate the accuracy of the tuned model. The ADC slices used for training were from different patients to the ADC slices used for testing to avoid any correlation that could exist between ADC slices of the same patient. The results of this experiment at each b-value are shown in Table 2.

Table 2. Performance of AlexNet at 9 b-values using 141 ADC maps.

b-Value	Accuracy%	Sensitivity (Recall)%	Specificity%	Precision%
100 s/mm^2	86.52	84.29	88.73	88.06
200 s/mm^2	90.07	85.71	94.37	93.75
300 s/mm^2	88.65	85.71	91.55	90.91
400 s/mm^2	88.65	88.57	88.73	91.18
500 s/mm^2	91.49	91.43	91.55	91.43
600 s/mm^2	89.36	88.57	90.14	89.86
700 s/mm^2	87.94	85.71	90.14	89.55
800 s/mm^2	90.07	90.00	90.14	90.00
1000 s/mm^2	90.07	87.14	92.96	92.06

In a similar experiment, 80% of the ADC maps were used for tuning an AlexNet-based model. The remaining 20% or 94 ADC maps were used to evaluate the accuracy of the tuned model. The reason behind this 80:20 division of the dataset was to satisfy the Pareto principle. The results of this experiment are reported in Table 3.

Table 3. Performance of AlexNet at 9 b-values using 94 randomly chosen ADC maps.

b-Value	Accuracy%	Sensitivity (Recall)%	Specificity%	Precision%
100 s/mm^2	87.23	87.23	87.23	87.23
200 s/mm^2	90.43	89.36	91.49	91.30
300 s/mm^2	89.36	89.36	89.36	89.36
400 s/mm^2	89.36	91.49	87.23	87.76
500 s/mm^2	90.43	91.49	89.36	89.58
600 s/mm^2	91.49	89.36	93.62	93.33
700 s/mm^2	88.33	89.36	87.23	87.50
800 s/mm^2	91.49	93.62	89.36	89.80
1000 s/mm^2	89.36	93.62	85.11	86.27

Similarly, in another experiment, 70% of the ADC maps of both the benign and malignant cases at each b-value were randomly chosen for tuning an AlexNet-based model. The other 30% of the ADC maps were used to evaluate the accuracy of the tuned model. Since the ADC maps used for evaluating the accuracy of the system at each b-value were chosen randomly, this experiment was repeated 10 times at each b-value. To ensure the stability of the reported results, the mean accuracy of the 10 experiments conducted at each b-value, in addition to the mean sensitivity and the mean specificity, are listed in Table 4.

Table 4. Average Performance of AlexNet at 9 b-values using 141 randomly chosen ADC maps and repeating the experiment 10 times.

b-Value	Accuracy%	Sensitivity%	Specificity%
100 s/mm^2	87.52 ± 0.01	89.14 ± 0.04	85.92 ± 0.04
200 s/mm^2	89.29 ± 0.01	88.71 ± 0.04	89.86 ± 0.03
300 s/mm^2	89.57 ± 0.02	89.00 ± 0.03	90.14 ± 0.03
400 s/mm^2	89.57 ± 0.02	89.71 ± 0.03	89.44 ± 0.04
500 s/mm^2	89.22 ± 0.03	88.29 ± 0.04	90.14 ± 0.04
600 s/mm^2	88.01 ± 0.03	88.00 ± 0.07	88.03 ± 0.05
700 s/mm^2	89.72 ± 0.02	89.29 ± 0.04	90.14 ± 0.03
800 s/mm^2	89.63 ± 0.03	88.57 ± 0.05	90.70 ± 0.03
1000 s/mm^2	90.43 ± 0.02	90.86 ± 0.04	90.00 ± 0.04

In another experiment, 10-fold cross validation was applied using the 470 ADC maps. Each fold contained 47 ADC maps. Nine folds were used for training whereas the remaining fold was used for testing the system. This operation was repeated 10 times with the change of the testing fold each time. The performance of the 10-fold cross validation using AlexNet at the different b-values is reported in Table 5.

Table 5. 10-fold cross validation of AlexNet at 9 b-values.

b-Value	100	200	300	400	500	600	700	800	1000
1st fold	93.62	87.23	93.62	93.62	91.49	89.36	91.49	91.49	87.23
2nd fold	78.72	82.98	78.72	82.98	87.23	82.98	85.11	80.85	78.72
3rd fold	91.49	95.74	91.49	89.36	93.62	93.62	95.74	93.62	91.49
4th fold	95.74	97.87	97.87	93.62	93.62	95.74	97.87	97.87	91.49
5th fold	87.23	89.36	91.49	91.49	89.36	93.62	87.23	91.49	91.49
6th fold	85.11	80.85	82.98	82.98	87.23	80.85	85.11	87.23	89.36
7th fold	91.49	93.62	89.36	97.87	95.74	93.62	93.62	95.74	93.62
8th fold	89.36	87.23	87.23	89.36	89.36	89.36	87.23	89.36	89.36
9th fold	93.62	91.49	91.49	93.62	91.49	93.62	89.36	91.49	91.49
10th fold	82.98	85.11	85.11	87.23	87.23	85.11	87.23	87.23	85.11
Average%	88.94	89.15	88.94	90.21	90.64	89.79	90.00	90.64	88.94

In order to evaluate the effect of the depth of the used CNNs on the resulting accuracy, an experiment was conducted. In this experiment, 70% of the ADC maps were used for tuning a deeper CNN (VGGNet), while the remaining 30% were used to evaluate the trained model. VGGNet has 16 convolutional layers in comparison to five convolutional layers in AlexNet. The performance using VGGNet is listed in Table 6. As can be noticed, the use of the deeper network improves the accuracy at all b-values except for b-value = 500 s/mm^2. The highest improvement in the accuracy is at b-value = 600 s/mm^2. The use of VGGNet leads to an average improvement of 1.97% in the accuracy.

The time required for training VGGNet model is much longer than the time required for training the AlexNet model. For example, the time required for fine-tuning AlexNet in the first experiment was 5 min and 25 s, whereas the time required for fine-tuning the deeper CNN (VGGNet) in the similar experiment was about 97 min. The proposed models were developed using MATLAB 2017b. The training of the proposed model was performed using a workstation with a graphics processing unit (GPU) of type NVIDIA Quadro K1200.

In a similar experiment, 80% of the ADC maps were used for tuning a VGGNet-based model. The remaining 20% or 94 ADC maps were used to evaluate the accuracy of the tuned model. The results of this experiment are reported in Table 7.

Table 6. Performance of VGGNet at 9 b-values using 141 randomly chosen ADC maps.

b-Value	Accuracy%	Sensitivity (Recall)%	Specificity%	Precision%
100 s/mm^2	90.07	88.57	91.55	91.18
200 s/mm^2	92.20	92.86	91.55	91.55
300 s/mm^2	90.07	90.00	90.14	90.00
400 s/mm^2	90.07	90.00	90.14	90.00
500 s/mm^2	90.78	91.43	90.14	90.14
600 s/mm^2	93.62	92.86	94.37	94.20
700 s/mm^2	90.07	92.86	87.32	97.84
800 s/mm^2	92.20	92.86	91.55	91.55
1000 s/mm^2	91.49	92.86	90.14	90.28

Table 7. Performance of VGGNet at 9 b-values using 94 randomly chosen ADC maps.

b-Value	Accuracy%	Sensitivity (Recall)%	Specificity%	Precision%
100 s/mm^2	91.49	87.23	95.74	95.35
200 s/mm^2	90.43	89.36	91.49	91.30
300 s/mm^2	91.49	91.49	91.49	91.49
400 s/mm^2	90.43	87.23	93.62	93.18
500 s/mm^2	92.55	89.36	95.74	95.45
600 s/mm^2	94.68	91.49	97.87	97.73
700 s/mm^2	90.43	87.23	93.62	93.18
800 s/mm^2	92.55	89.36	95.74	95.45
1000 s/mm^2	92.55	93.62	91.49	91.67

In another experiment, 10-fold cross validation is applied using VGGNet at the different b-values. The results of this experiment are reported in Table 8.

Table 8. 10-fold cross validation of VGGNet at 9 b-values.

b-Value	100	200	300	400	500	600	700	800	1000
1st fold	85.11	91.49	89.36	91.49	95.74	95.74	95.74	95.74	95.74
2nd fold	82.98	89.36	89.36	87.23	89.36	89.36	89.36	91.49	87.23
3rd fold	89.36	91.49	85.11	93.62	91.49	91.49	95.74	97.87	91.49
4th fold	93.62	91.49	89.36	93.62	97.87	97.87	97.87	93.62	97.87
5th fold	89.36	93.62	93.62	89.36	89.36	91.49	89.36	91.49	87.23
6th fold	89.36	80.85	87.23	87.23	82.98	85.11	89.36	89.36	82.98
7th fold	80.85	91.49	91.49	95.74	97.87	97.87	93.62	95.74	95.74
8th fold	87.23	97.87	93.62	91.49	97.87	87.23	89.36	93.62	85.11
9th fold	93.62	95.74	97.87	97.87	97.87	95.74	93.62	95.74	93.62
10th fold	78.72	80.85	89.36	82.98	85.11	85.11	80.85	85.11	87.23
Average%	87.02	90.43	90.64	91.06	92.55	91.70	91.49	92.98	90.43

In order to show the merits of CNNs over classical machine-learning classifiers, the performance of CNN is compared to the performance of SVM with both linear and quadratic kernels. The models of SVMs were trained using 70% of the ADC maps and evaluated using the remaining 30% of the ADC maps. The inputs to the SVMs were the same as the inputs to the CNNs. The inputs to the SVMs were the ADC maps (raw data). In order to be used as input to the SVMs, each ADC map has to be transformed into a vector. This vector represents a row in the data matrix used to train the SVM. The results of these SVMs are reported in Table 9. The high performance of the CNN models highlights the importance of the inputs' spatial information that is preserved in the case of CNNs. However, the inputs' spatial information is lost in the case of conventional models such as SVMs.

Table 9. Performance of SVMs with linear kernel (lin. ker.) and quadratic kernel (quad. ker.) at 9 b-values using 141 randomly chosen ADC maps, where Acc. means accuracy, Sen. means sensitivity, and Spec. means specificity.

	SVM with Lin. Ker.			SVM with Quad. Ker.		
b-Value	**Acc. %**	**Sen. %**	**Spec. %**	**Acc. %**	**Sen. %**	**Spec. %**
100 s/mm^2	75.18	65.71	84.51	78.01	71.43	84.51
200 s/mm^2	75.89	72.86	78.87	78.72	78.57	78.87
300 s/mm^2	73.05	58.57	87.32	82.27	77.14	87.32
400 s/mm^2	68.79	75.71	61.97	80.85	88.57	73.24
500 s/mm^2	79.43	82.86	76.06	82.27	81.43	83.10
600 s/mm^2	73.76	68.57	78.87	80.14	77.14	83.10
700 s/mm^2	68.79	71.43	66.20	80.14	80.00	80.28
800 s/mm^2	71.63	74.29	69.01	81.56	87.14	76.06
1000 s/mm^2	73.76	70.00	77.46	81.56	82.86	80.28

The ROC curves of two CNN models (AlexNet and VGGNet) and two variants of SVMs with linear and quadratic kernels are shown in Figure 5. Since the ROC curves of each of these classifiers at the distinct b-values have similar shapes, the ROC curves at only five b-values are displayed to simplify the figures.

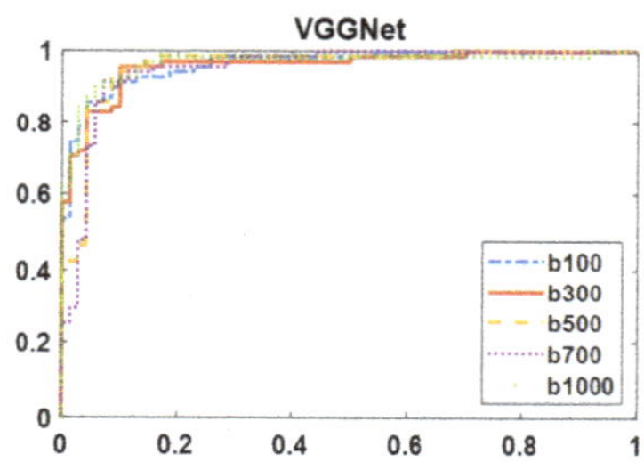

(**a**) ROC curve of VGGNet

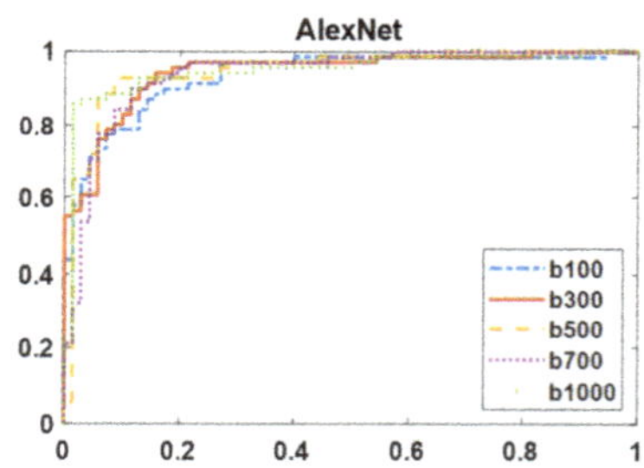

(**b**) ROC curve of AlexNet

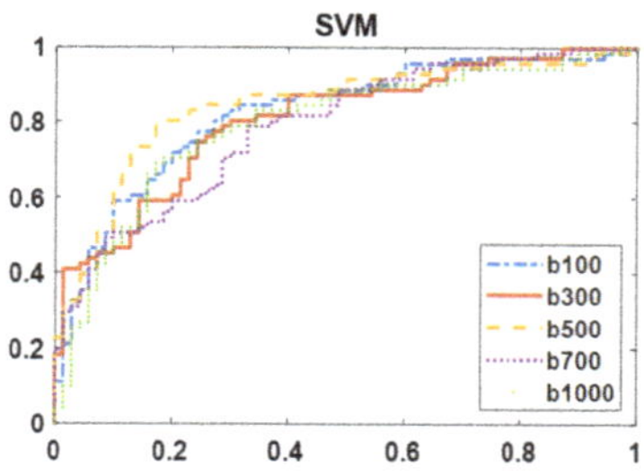

(**c**) ROC curve of support vector machine (SVM) with linear kernel

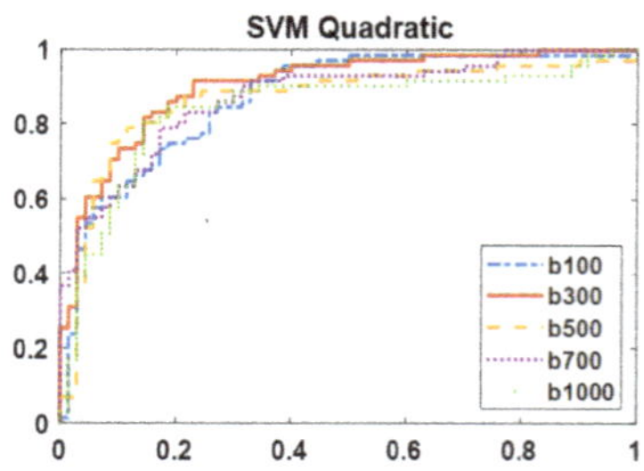

(**d**) ROC curve of SVM with quadratic kernel

Figure 5. ROC curves at five b-values(100, 300, 500, 700, and 1000 s/mm^2) of four different classifiers: (**a**) VGGNet, (**b**) AlexNet, (**c**) SVM with linear kernel, and (**d**) SVM with quadratic kernel. As these figures show, CNN-based models (VGGNet and AlexNet) result in higher AUCs than the two variants of SVMs with linear and quadratic kernels at the distinct b-values.

An experiment was conducted to compare the performance of the proposed approach to one of the state-of-the-art CNNs, which is GoogLeNet [45]. This CNN was the winner of the ImageNet challenge in 2014. This deep network consists of 22 layers. However, the number of its parameters is reduced dramatically due to the use of the Inception module and the removal of the FC layers. The resulting performance of GoogLeNet is listed in

Table 10. The performance results of GoogLeNet are close to the results of both AlexNet and VGGNet. These results boosts the feasibility of the transfer learning in diagnosing prostate cancer.

Table 10. Performance of GoogLeNet at 9 b-values using 141 ADC maps.

b-Value	Accuracy%	Sensitivity%	Specificity%
100 s/mm^2	85.82	85.71	85.92
200 s/mm^2	90.78	85.71	95.77
300 s/mm^2	87.23	85.71	88.73
400 s/mm^2	87.23	82.86	91.55
500 s/mm^2	87.94	90.00	85.92
600 s/mm^2	88.65	88.57	88.73
700 s/mm^2	90.07	91.43	88.73
800 s/mm^2	88.65	85.71	91.55
1000 s/mm^2	89.36	90.00	88.73

4. Discussion

In this study, a transfer learning model is adopted to detect and identify prostate cancer. When the employed CNN models were originally trained using natural images, they used conventional techniques such as, data augmentation and dropout in order to reduce the effect of overfitting. The combination of both conventional overfitting handling techniques and transfer learning can minimize the effect of overfitting.

The proposed system starts with segmentation to limit the region-of-interest (ROI) to the prostate region only. In this system, prostate segmentation is performed using level set due to its capability to provide continuous segmented object. However, any segmentation approach can be integrated with the proposed system, as long as, it provides a continuous segmented object. For example, Comelli et al. [46], presented a fast deep learning network, namely efficient neural network (ENet), for prostate segmentation from T2-weighted MRI. ENet is initially used for image segmentation tasks in self-driving cars where hardware availability is limited and the accuracy is critical for user safety. In this study [46], ENet is trained using a dataset of 85 subjects and results in a dice similarity coefficient of 90.89%.

Several studies suggested that the use of DWI acquired at higher b-values are preferable for accurate detection and diagnosis of prostate cancer [47–51]. This study shows that the use of ADC maps calculated at lower b-values results in an accuracy close to the accuracy of the ADC maps calculated at higher b-values. There is a slight accuracy increase for the ADC maps calculated at higher b-values. This accuracy increase is more obvious in the case of using a less-deeper CNN (AlexNet). One of the advantages of using ADC maps is that they are insensitive to the magnetic field strengths of the used scanners (1.5T or 3T) [35]. The ADC maps used in this study were calculated from DWI acquired with 1.5T and 3T scanners at nine b-values. The results show that the dependence on ADC maps can also mitigate the differences in the accuracy between higher and lower b-values, especially in the case of using deeper CNN models.

The developed approach performs slice-wise analysis. However, the proposed framework is generic and can perform both slice-wise analysis and prostate-zonal analysis based on how the model is trained. Since the system shows good performance in slice-wise analysis, the authors did not investigate it on zonal analysis. Investigating the performance of the system in prostate-zonal analysis is a good potential for future work.

According to the literature, a sensitivity and a positive predictive value of 80% and 87%, have been reported for men with high prostate-specific antigen (PSA) values using positron emission tomography/computed tomography (PET/CT) [52,53].

According to Sun et al. [54], the performance of deep learning networks increases logarithmically based on the size of the training data. One way to improve the performance in the case of limited data is to conduct multiple experiments and choose the best results. In this work, to obtain the best performance, 10-fold cross validation was used to obtain almost the same performance, no matter which fold was used for training and which fold was used for testing.

The use of two different CNN models in this work shows that the depth of the CNN model positively affects the performance of the system. However, much longer processing times are required to train the deeper architectures. The results of this study show that the use of a deeper CNN (VGGNet) increases the accuracy of prostate cancer detection more than the less-deep CNN (AlexNet). However, this accuracy is still far from perfect. Examining the effect of using much deeper CNN models, such as ResNet [55], can be a potential future work. Moreover, in this system, prostate cancer identification from DWI acquired at nine b-values was investigated. This investigation can be extended by performing a statistical analysis of the used b-values to select the best minimal combination of b-values that lead to the best accuracy. Choosing a minimal combination of b-values will reduce both the acquisition time of DWI and the computational complexities. Another area of potential future work could be the use of artificial intelligence optimization techniques on a combination of imaging markers and clinical markers (such as PSA) to optimize prostate cancer management.

5. Conclusions

In conclusion, this paper presents a CAD system for prostate cancer detection and identification from DWI. The identification of prostate cancer is achieved using two previously-trained CNN models (AlexNet and VGGNet) that are fed with the estimated ADC maps of the segmented prostate regions. The conducted experiments show that the use of previously-trained CNN models for detecting prostate cancer is feasible. These previously-trained CNN models learn the discriminatory features automatically. The results section shows that CNN models outperform conventional models. The accuracy of conventional models depends on the good design of the used handcrafted features.

Author Contributions: Conceptualization, I.R.A., A.S., A.M., M.E., A.A., M.A.E.-G., M.E.-M., N.S.A. and A.E.-B.; Formal analysis, I.R.A. and M.E.-M.; Investigation, I.R.A., M.E., A.A., M.A.E.-G., M.E.-M. and A.E.-B.; Methodology, I.R.A., A.S., A.M., M.E., A.A., M.A.E.-G., M.E.-M., N.S.A. and A.E.-B.; Project administration, N.S.A. and A.E.-B.; Software, I.R.A., N.S.A. and A.E.-B.; Supervision, M.E., N.S.A. and A.E.-B.; Validation, M.E.-M.; Visualization, I.R.A. and A.S.; Writing—original draft, I.R.A., A.S., A.M., M.E., A.A., M.A.E.-G., M.E.-M., N.S.A. and A.E.-B.; Writing—review & editing, I.R.A., A.S., A.M., M.E., N.S.A. and A.E.-B. All authors have read and agreed to the published version of the manuscript.

Funding: This research was funded by the Deanship of Scientific Research at Princess Nourah bint Abdulrahman University through the Fast-track Research Funding Program.

Institutional Review Board Statement: The study was conducted according to the guidelines of the Declaration of Helsinki, and approved by the Institutional Review Board of Mansoura University (R.21.04.1289).

Informed Consent Statement: Informed consent was obtained from all subjects involved in the study.

Data Availability Statement: The data that support the findings of this study are available from the corresponding author upon reasonable request.

Conflicts of Interest: The authors declare no conflict of interest.

References

1. American Cancer Society. Key Statistics for Prostate Cancer. 2019. Available online: https://www.cancer.org/cancer/prostate-cancer/about/key-statistics.html (accessed on 10 February 2020).
2. Hricak, H. MR imaging and MR spectroscopic imaging in the pre-treatment evaluation of prostate cancer. *Br. J. Radiol.* **2005**, *78*, S103–S111. [CrossRef]
3. Brown, A.M.; Elbuluk, O.; Mertan, F.; Sankineni, S.; Margolis, D.J.; Wood, B.J.; Pinto, P.A.; Choyke, P.L.; Turkbey, B. Recent advances in image-guided targeted prostate biopsy. *Abdom. Radiol.* **2015**, *40*, 1788–1799. [CrossRef] [PubMed]

4. Hoeks, C.M.; Barentsz, J.O.; Hambrock, T.; Yakar, D.; Somford, D.M.; Heijmink, S.W.; Scheenen, T.W.; Vos, P.C.; Huisman, H.; van Oort, I.M.; et al. Prostate cancer: Multiparametric MR imaging for detection, localization, and staging. *Radiology* **2011**, *261*, 46–66. [CrossRef] [PubMed]
5. Liu, L.; Tian, Z.; Zhang, Z.; Fei, B. Computer-aided detection of prostate cancer with MRI: Technology and applications. *Acad. Radiol.* **2016**, *23*, 1024–1046. [CrossRef] [PubMed]
6. Fei, B. Computer-aided diagnosis of prostate cancer with MRI. *Curr. Opin. Biomed. Eng.* **2017**, *3*, 20–27. [CrossRef] [PubMed]
7. Viswanath, S.E.; Chirra, P.V.; Yim, M.C.; Rofsky, N.M.; Purysko, A.S.; Rosen, M.A.; Bloch, B.N.; Madabhushi, A. Comparing radiomic classifiers and classifier ensembles for detection of peripheral zone prostate tumors on T2-weighted MRI: A multi-site study. *BMC Med. Imaging* **2019**, *19*, 22. [CrossRef] [PubMed]
8. Campa, R.; Del Monte, M.; Barchetti, G.; Pecoraro, M.; Salvo, V.; Ceravolo, I.; Indino, E.L.; Ciardi, A.; Catalano, C.; Panebianco, V. Improvement of prostate cancer detection combining a computer-aided diagnostic system with TRUS-MRI targeted biopsy. *Abdom. Radiol.* **2019**, *44*, 264–271. [CrossRef] [PubMed]
9. Rampun, A.; Zheng, L.; Malcolm, P.; Tiddeman, B.; Zwiggelaar, R. Computer-aided detection of prostate cancer in T2-weighted MRI within the peripheral zone. *Phys. Med. Biol.* **2016**, *61*, 4796. [CrossRef] [PubMed]
10. Gao, J.; Jiang, Q.; Zhou, B.; Chen, D. Convolutional neural networks for computer-aided detection or diagnosis in medical image analysis: An overview. *Math. Biosci. Eng.* **2019**, *16*, 6536. [CrossRef]
11. Srinivas, S.; Sarvadevabhatla, R.K.; Mopuri, K.R.; Prabhu, N.; Kruthiventi, S.S.; Babu, R.V. A Taxonomy of Deep Convolutional Neural Nets for Computer Vision. *Front. Robot AI* **2016**, *2*, 36–48. [CrossRef]
12. Guo, Y.; Liu, Y.; Oerlemans, A.; Lao, S.; Wu, S.; Lew, M.S. Deep learning for visual understanding: A review. *Neurocomputing* **2016**, *187*, 27–48. [CrossRef]
13. Lu, H.; Li, Y.; Uemura, T.; Kim, H.; Serikawa, S. Low illumination underwater light field images reconstruction using deep convolutional neural networks. *Future Gener. Comput. Syst.* **2018**, *82*, 142–148. [CrossRef]
14. Li, Y.; Wang, G.; Nie, L.; Wang, Q.; Tan, W. Distance metric optimization driven convolutional neural network for age invariant face recognition. *Pattern Recognit.* **2018**, *75*, 51–62. [CrossRef]
15. Babaee, M.; Dinh, D.T.; Rigoll, G. A deep convolutional neural network for video sequence background subtraction. *Pattern Recognit.* **2018**, *76*, 635–649. [CrossRef]
16. Sabokrou, M.; Fayyaz, M.; Fathy, M.; Moayed, Z.; Klette, R. Deep-anomaly: Fully convolutional neural network for fast anomaly detection in crowded scenes. *Comput. Vis. Image Underst.* **2018**, *172*, 88–97. [CrossRef]
17. Tajbakhsh, N.; Shin, J.Y.; Gurudu, S.R.; Hurst, R.T.; Kendall, C.B.; Gotway, M.B.; Liang, J. Convolutional Neural Networks for Medical Image Analysis: Full Training or Fine Tuning? *IEEE Trans. Med. Imaging* **2016**, *35*, 1299–1312. [CrossRef] [PubMed]
18. Ishioka, J.; Matsuoka, Y.; Uehara, S.; Yasuda, Y.; Kijima, T.; Yoshida, S.; Yokoyama, M.; Saito, K.; Kihara, K.; Numao, N.; et al. Computer-aided diagnosis of prostate cancer on magnetic resonance imaging using a convolutional neural network algorithm. *BJU Int.* **2018**, *122*, 411–417. [CrossRef] [PubMed]
19. Mehrtash, A.; Sedghi, A.; Ghafoorian, M.; Taghipour, M.; Tempany, C.M.; Wells III, W.M.; Kapur, T.; Mousavi, P.; Abolmaesumi, P.; Fedorov, A. Classification of clinical significance of MRI prostate findings using 3D convolutional neural networks. Medical Imaging 2017: Computer-Aided Diagnosis. *Int. Soc. Opt. Photonics* **2017**, *10134*, 101342A.
20. Yang, X.; Liu, C.; Wang, Z.; Yang, J.; Le Min, H.; Wang, L.; Cheng, K.T.T. Co-trained convolutional neural networks for automated detection of prostate cancer in multi-parametric MRI. *Med. Image Anal.* **2017**, *42*, 212–227. [CrossRef] [PubMed]
21. Le, M.H.; Chen, J.; Wang, L.; Wang, Z.; Liu, W.; Cheng, K.T.T.; Yang, X. Automated diagnosis of prostate cancer in multi-parametric MRI based on multimodal convolutional neural networks. *Phys. Med. Biol.* **2017**, *62*, 6497–6514. [CrossRef]
22. Wang, Z.; Liu, C.; Cheng, D.; Wang, L.; Yang, X.; Cheng, K.T. Automated Detection of Clinically Significant Prostate Cancer in mp-MRI Images Based on an End-to-End Deep Neural Network. *IEEE Trans. Med. Imaging* **2018**, *37*, 1127–1139. [CrossRef]
23. Song, Y.; Zhang, Y.D.; Yan, X.; Liu, H.; Zhou, M.; Hu, B.; Yang, G. Computer-aided diagnosis of prostate cancer using a deep convolutional neural network from multiparametric MRI. *J. Magn. Reson. Imaging* **2018**, *48*, 1570–1577. [CrossRef] [PubMed]
24. Hosseinzadeh, M.; Brand, P.; Huisman, H. Effect of Adding Probabilistic Zonal Prior in Deep Learning-based Prostate Cancer Detection. *arXiv* **2019**, arXiv:1907.12382.
25. Schelb, P.; Kohl, S.; Radtke, J.P.; Wiesenfarth, M.; Kickingereder, P.; Bickelhaupt, S.; Kuder, T.A.; Stenzinger, A.; Hohenfellner, M.; Schlemmer, H.P.; et al. Classification of cancer at prostate MRI: Deep learning versus clinical PI-RADS assessment. *Radiology* **2019**, *293*, 607–617. [CrossRef]
26. Xu, H.; Baxter, J.S.; Akin, O.; Cantor-Rivera, D. Prostate cancer detection using residual networks. *Int. J. Comput. Assist. Radiol. Surg.* **2019**, *14*, 1647–1650. [CrossRef] [PubMed]
27. Yuan, Y.; Qin, W.; Buyyounouski, M.; Ibragimov, B.; Hancock, S.; Han, B.; Xing, L. Prostate cancer classification with multiparametric MRI transfer learning model. *Med. Phys.* **2019**, *46*, 756–765. [CrossRef] [PubMed]
28. Chen, Q.; Xu, X.; Hu, S.; Li, X.; Zou, Q.; Li, Y. A transfer learning approach for classification of clinical significant prostate cancers from mpMRI scans. Medical Imaging 2017: Computer-Aided Diagnosis. *Int. Soc. Opt. Photonics* **2017**, *10134*, 101344F.
29. Abbasi, A.A.; Hussain, L.; Awan, I.A.; Abbasi, I.; Majid, A.; Nadeem, M.S.A.; Chaudhary, Q.A. Detecting prostate cancer using deep learning convolution neural network with transfer learning approach. *Cogn. Neurodyn.* **2020**, *14*, 523–533. [CrossRef]
30. Wildeboer, R.R.; van Sloun, R.J.; Wijkstra, H.; Mischi, M. Artificial intelligence in multiparametric prostate cancer imaging with focus on deep-learning methods. *Comput. Methods Programs Biomed.* **2020**, *189*, 105316. [CrossRef]

31. McClure, P.; Khalifa, F.; Soliman, A.; El-Ghar, M.A.; Gimelfarb, G.; Elmagraby, A.; El-Baz, A. A novel NMF guided level-set for DWI prostate segmentation. *J. Comput. Sci. Syst. Biol.* **2014**, *7*, 209–216. [CrossRef]
32. Kwee, T.C.; Galbán, C.J.; Tsien, C.; Junck, L.; Sundgren, P.C.; Ivancevic, M.K.; Johnson, T.D.; Meyer, C.R.; Rehemtulla, A.; Ross, B.D.; et al. Comparison of apparent diffusion coefficients and distributed diffusion coefficients in high-grade gliomas. *J. Magn. Reson. Imaging* **2010**, *31*, 531–537. [CrossRef]
33. Huisman, T.A.G.M. Diffusion-weighted imaging: Basic concepts and application in cerebral stroke and head trauma. *Eur. Radiol.* **2003**, *13*, 2283–2297. [CrossRef] [PubMed]
34. Hrabe, J.; Kaur, G.; Guilfoyle, D.N. Principles and limitations of NMR diffusion measurements. *J. Med. Phys.* **2007**, *32*, 34–42. [CrossRef] [PubMed]
35. Jeong, D.; Malalis, C.; Arrington, J.A.; Field, A.S.; Choi, J.W.; Kocak, M. Mean apparent diffusion coefficient values in defining radiotherapy planning target volumes in glioblastoma. *Quant. Imaging Med. Surg.* **2015**, *5*, 835–845. [PubMed]
36. Choi, Y.J.; Kim, J.K.; Kim, N.; Kim, K.W.; Choi, E.K.; Cho, K.S. Functional MR imaging of prostate cancer. *Radiographics* **2007**, *27*, 63–75. [CrossRef]
37. LeCun, Y.; Kavukcuoglu, K.; Farabet, C. Convolutional networks and applications in vision. In Proceedings of the 2010 IEEE International Symposium on Circuits and Systems, Paris, France, 30 May–2 June 2010; pp. 253–256. [CrossRef]
38. Gu, J.; Wang, Z.; Kuen, J.; Ma, L.; Shahroudy, A.; Shuai, B.; Liu, T.; Wang, X.; Wang, G.; Cai, J.; et al. Recent advances in convolutional neural networks. *Pattern Recognit.* **2018**, *77*, 354–377. [CrossRef]
39. Krizhevsky, A.; Sutskever, I.; Hinton, G.E. Imagenet classification with deep convolutional neural networks. *Adv. Neural. Inf. Process Syst.* **2012**, *25*, 1097–1105. [CrossRef]
40. Simonyan, K.; Zisserman, A. Very deep convolutional networks for large-scale image recognition. *arXiv* **2014**, arXiv:1409.1556.
41. Nair, V.; Hinton, G.E. Rectified linear units improve restricted boltzmann machines. In Proceedings of the International Conference Mach Learning, Haifa, Israel, 21–24 June 2010; pp. 807–814.
42. Hinton, G.E.O. Improving neural networks by preventing co-adaptation of feature detectors. *arXiv* **2012**, arXiv:1207.0580.
43. Boureau, Y.L.; Ponce, J.; LeCun, Y. A theoretical analysis of feature pooling in visual recognition. In Proceedings of the International Conference Mach Learning, Haifa, Israel, 21–24 June 2010; pp. 111–118.
44. Xu, B.; Fu, Y.; Jiang, Y.G.; Li, B.; Sigal, L. Heterogeneous Knowledge Transfer in Video Emotion Recognition, Attribution and Summarization. *IEEE Trans. Affect. Comput.* **2018**, *9*, 255–270. [CrossRef]
45. Szegedy, C.; Liu, W.; Jia, Y.; Sermanet, P.; Reed, S.; Anguelov, D.; Erhan, D.; Vanhoucke, V.; Rabinovich, A. Going deeper with convolutions. In Proceedings of the 2015 IEEE Conference on Computer Vision and Pattern Recognition, Boston, MA, USA, 7–12 June 2015; pp. 1–9.
46. Comelli, A.; Dahiya, N.; Stefano, A.; Vernuccio, F.; Portoghese, M.; Cutaia, G.; Bruno, A.; Salvaggio, G.; Yezzi, A. Deep Learning-Based Methods for Prostate Segmentation in Magnetic Resonance Imaging. *Appl. Sci.* **2021**, *11*, 782. [CrossRef] [PubMed]
47. Metens, T.; Miranda, D.; Absil, J.; Matos, C. What is the optimal b value in diffusion-weighted MR imaging to depict prostate cancer at 3T? *Eur. Radiol.* **2012**, *22*, 703–709. [CrossRef]
48. Katahira, K.; Takahara, T.; Kwee, T.C.; Oda, S.; Suzuki, Y.; Morishita, S.; Kitani, K.; Hamada, Y.; Kitaoka, M.; Yamashita, Y.; Ultra-high-b-value diffusion-weighted MR imaging for the detection of prostate cancer: Evaluation in 201 cases with histopathological correlation. *Eur. Radiol.* **2011**, *21*, 188–196. [CrossRef] [PubMed]
49. Grant, K.B.; Agarwal, H.K.; Shih, J.H.; Bernardo, M.; Pang, Y.; Daar, D.; Merino, M.J.; Wood, B.J.; Pinto, P.A.; Choyke, P.L.; et al. Comparison of calculated and acquired high b value diffusion-weighted imaging in prostate cancer. *Abdom. Radiol.* **2015**, *40*, 578–586. [CrossRef] [PubMed]
50. Pang, Y.; Turkbey, B.; Bernardo, M.; Kruecker, J.; Kadoury, S.; Merino, M.J.; Wood, B.J.; Pinto, P.A.; Choyke, P.L. Intravoxel incoherent motion MR imaging for prostate cancer: An evaluation of perfusion fraction and diffusion coefficient derived from different b-value combinations. *Magn. Reson. Med.* **2013**, *69*, 553–562. [CrossRef]
51. Rosenkrantz, A.B.; Mannelli, L.; Kong, X.; Niver, B.E.; Berkman, D.S.; Babb, J.S.; Melamed, J.; Taneja, S.S. Prostate cancer: Utility of fusion of T2-weighted and high b-value diffusion-weighted images for peripheral zone tumor detection and localization. *J. Magn. Reson. Imaging* **2011**, *34*, 95–100. [CrossRef] [PubMed]
52. Wallitt, K.L.; Khan, S.R.; Dubash, S.; Tam, H.H.; Khan, S.; Barwick, T.D. Clinical PET imaging in prostate cancer. *Radiographics* **2017**, *37*, 1512–1536. [CrossRef]
53. Tateishi, U.; Morita, S.; Taguri, M.; Shizukuishi, K.; Minamimoto, R.; Kawaguchi, M.; Murano, T.; Terauchi, T.; Inoue, T.; Kim, E.E. A meta-analysis of 18 F-Fluoride positron emission tomography for assessment of metastatic bone tumor. *Ann. Nucl. Med.* **2010**, *24*, 523–531. [CrossRef] [PubMed]
54. Sun, C.; Shrivastava, A.; Singh, S.; Gupta, A. Revisiting unreasonable effectiveness of data in deep learning era. In Proceedings of the IEEE International Conference on Computer Vision (ICCV), Venice, Italy, 22–29 October 2017; pp. 843–852.
55. He, K.; Zhang, X.; Ren, S.; Sun, J. Deep residual learning for image recognition. In Proceedings of the IEEE Conference on Computer Vision and Pattern Recognition, Las Vegas, NV, USA, 27–30 June 2016; pp. 770–778.

sensors

MDPI

Article

Diabetic Retinopathy Fundus Image Classification and Lesions Localization System Using Deep Learning

Wejdan L. Alyoubi [1,*], Maysoon F. Abulkhair [1] and Wafaa M. Shalash [1,2]

[1] Information Technology Department, King Abdulaziz University, Jeddah 21589, Saudi Arabia; mabualkhair@kau.edu.sa (M.F.A.); wshalash@kau.edu.sa (W.M.S.)
[2] Computer Science Department, Faculty of Computers and Artificial Intelligence, Benha University, Benha 13518, Egypt
* Correspondence: walyoubi0016@stu.kau.edu.sa

Abstract: Diabetic retinopathy (DR) is a disease resulting from diabetes complications, causing non-reversible damage to retina blood vessels. DR is a leading cause of blindness if not detected early. The currently available DR treatments are limited to stopping or delaying the deterioration of sight, highlighting the importance of regular scanning using high-efficiency computer-based systems to diagnose cases early. The current work presented fully automatic diagnosis systems that exceed manual techniques to avoid misdiagnosis, reducing time, effort and cost. The proposed system classifies DR images into five stages—no-DR, mild, moderate, severe and proliferative DR—as well as localizing the affected lesions on retain surface. The system comprises two deep learning-based models. The first model (CNN512) used the whole image as an input to the CNN model to classify it into one of the five DR stages. It achieved an accuracy of 88.6% and 84.1% on the DDR and the APTOS Kaggle 2019 public datasets, respectively, compared to the state-of-the-art results. Simultaneously, the second model used an adopted YOLOv3 model to detect and localize the DR lesions, achieving a 0.216 mAP in lesion localization on the DDR dataset, which improves the current state-of-the-art results. Finally, both of the proposed structures, CNN512 and YOLOv3, were fused to classify DR images and localize DR lesions, obtaining an accuracy of 89% with 89% sensitivity, 97.3 specificity and that exceeds the current state-of-the-art results.

Keywords: computer-aided diagnosis; convolutional neural networks; deep learning; diabetic retinopathy; diabetic retinopathy classification; diabetic retinopathy lesions localization; YOLO

Citation: Alyoubi, W.L.; Abulkhair, M.F.; Shalash, W.M. Diabetic Retinopathy Fundus Image Classification and Lesions Localization System Using Deep Learning. *Sensors* **2021**, *21*, 3704. https://doi.org/10.3390/s21113704

Academic Editors: Ayman El-Baz, Guruprasad A. Giridharan, Ahmed Shalaby, Ali H. Mahmoud and Mohammed Ghazal

Received: 17 April 2021
Accepted: 21 May 2021
Published: 26 May 2021

1. Introduction

Diabetic retinopathy (DR) is a common diabetes complication that occurs when the retina's blood vessels are damaged due to high blood sugar levels, resulting in swelling and leaking of the vessels [1]. In an advanced DR stage, the vision may be lost completely. The percentage of blindness worldwide resulting from DR is 2.6% [2]. Therefore, diabetes patients need regular screening of the retina to detect DR early, manage its progression and avoid the risk of blindness.

The leaking blood and fluids appear as spots, called lesions, in the fundus retina image. Lesions can be recognised as either red lesions or bright lesions. Red lesions involve microaneurysms (MA) and haemorrhage (HM), while bright lesions involve soft and hard exudates (EX) as shown in Figure 1. The small dark red dots are called MA and the larger spots are called HM. Hard EX appears as bright yellow spots, while soft EX, also called cotton wool, appears as yellowish-white and fluffy spots caused by nerve fiber damage [3]. The five DR stages depend on the types and numbers of lesions on the retina image, as shown in Table 1. Samples of the various DR stages (no DR, mild DR, moderate DR, severe DR, and proliferative DR) are shown in Figure 2.

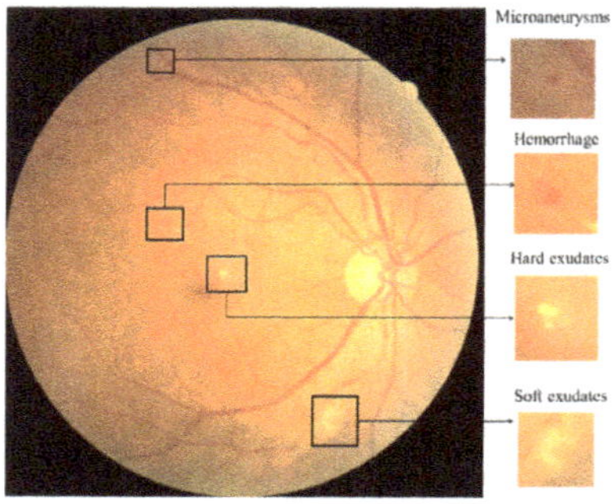

Figure 1. The different types of DR lesions.

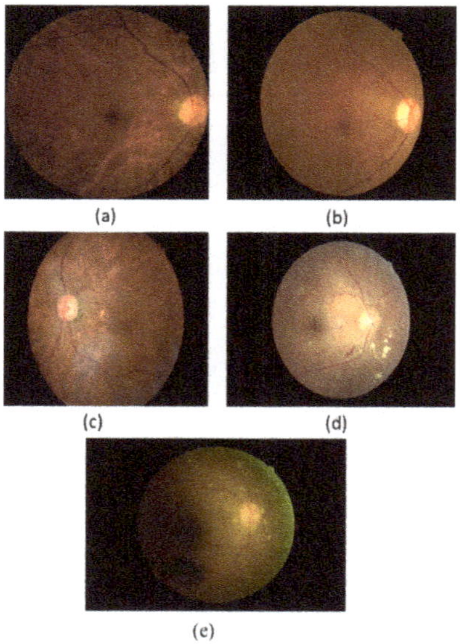

Figure 2. The DR stages: (**a**) No DR (**b**) Mild, (**c**) Moderate, (**d**) Severe, (**e**) Proliferative DR.

Table 1. The DR stages depending on lesions classification [4].

DR Severity Level	Lesions
No DR	No lesions.
Mild DR	MA only.
Moderate DR	More than just MA but less than severe DR.
Severe DR	Any of the following: more than 20 intraretinal HM in each of 4 quadrants; definite venous beading in 2+ quadrants; Prominent intraretinal microvascular abnormalities in 1+ quadrant and no signs of proliferative DR.
Proliferative DR	One or more of the following: neovascularization, pre-retinal HM.

The manual diagnosis of DR by ophthalmologists is time-consuming, requires considerable effort, and is prone to disease misdiagnosis. Therefore, using a computer-aided diagnosis system can avoid misdiagnosis and reduce overall cost, time and effort. During the last decade, deep learning (DL) approach has emerged and been adopted in many fields, including medical image analysis. DL can identify features accurately from input data for classification or segmentation and typically outperforms all traditional image analysis techniques. DL techniques does not need to extract the hand-crafted features while it requires extensive data for training [5]. In contrast, machine learning techniques require extraction of the hand-crafted features, but they do not need extensive data for training. In DR detection, the machine learning techniques need to extract the vessel firstly, as in [6,7]. Then, extract DR lesions' features for classification as in [8]. DL applications include the segmentation, classification, retrieval, detection and registration of the images [9]. Convolutional Neural Network (CNN) is a type of DL method that is a widely used [9], highly effective and successful method for image analysis [10,11].

There has been a considerable number of efforts to automate DR image classification using DL to help ophthalmologists detect the disease in its early stages. However, most of these efforts focused only on detecting DR instead of detecting various DR stages. Moreover, there have been limited efforts to classify and localize all the DR lesions types, which is very helpful in practice, as ophthalmologists can evaluate DR severity and monitor its progression based on the appearance of these lesions. For these reasons, we propose a fully automated screening system using CNN to detect the DR five stages and localize all DR lesion types simultaneously. The proposed system helps ophthalmologists mimic their DR diagnosis method, which localizes DR lesions, identifying its type and determining the DR exact stage. The current study investigates three CNN-based models to classify the DR images into stages. The first model was designed using transfer learning by fine-tuning EfficientNetB0 [12]. The other two models, CNN512 and CNN229, were designed, tuned and trained from scratch. For DR lesions localization and classification, a tuned YOLOv3 [13] model was used. To achieve the best DR stages classification result, the image classification model and the DR lesions localization model were fused. We investigate many CNN structures to classify and localize DR images' lesions until it reaches the best combination of a CNN and YOLOv3 structure to present a fully automatic DR grading and localization system. The present study's main contribution is the promising new design and fusion of two models to construct the proposed screening system. The first structure is the CNN512, a CNN designed, tuned and trained from scratch to classify each image according to one of the DR stages. While the second is a modified YOLOv3 to localize its DR lesions simultaneously. The proposed system shows a promising result.

As far as we know, YOLOv3 has been used in the detection of the red lesion as in [14]. The novelty of the current work is considered the first research used YOLOv3 to detect the different DR lesions.

This paper is structured as follows: Section 2 briefly analyses deep learning based related works on DR stages and lesions detecting, while Section 3 presents the materials and proposed methods. Section 4 describes the experiments and results. The discussion and conclusion are presented in Sections 5 and 6, respectively.

2. Related Works

CNN has been used widely in the classification and localisation of retinal fundus images. The DR detection works using DL can be categorized into three main categories: binary DR classification, multi-level DR classification and hybrid classification. In the following sections, we will summarise the recent efforts in DR classification in these three categories. A comparison between the related works is presented in Table 2.

2.1. Binary Classification

This section looks at the studies that have classified DR images into two categories. Pires et al. [15] proposed a custom CNN to detect referable DR images and non-referable DR images. Their CNN were trained on the Kaggle [16] and achieved an AUC of 98.2% on the Messidor-2 [17]. Jiang et al. [18] created a new dataset to classify DR images to referable DR or not using three pretrained CNNs; Inception-Resnet-V2 [19], Inception V3 [20] and Resnet152 [21]. These CNNs were combined using the Adaboost algorithm. They obtained an AUC of 0.946. Liu et al. [22] created a weighted paths CNN called WP-CNN to classify referable DR images in a private dataset. They reported an accuracy (ACC) of 94.23%.

Das et al. [23] proposed two independent CNN to classify the images into normal or DR images. Their CNNs obtained an ACC of 98.7% on the DIARETDB1 dataset. Although the previous studies achieved good results in detecting DR, they did not take the five DR stages and the various lesions into account. The main drawback of the binary classification method is that it only classifies the DR images into two categories, without considering the five DR stages. The identification of the exact DR stages is essential in selecting a suitable treatment process and preventing retina deterioration.

Table 2. Comparison between the related works that used DL to classify DR Images.

Ref.	Number of Classes	Detect Lesion	Dataset	Performance Measure			
				AUC	ACC	SEN	SP
[15]	2	No	Messidor-2, DR2	98.2% 98%	-	-	-
[22]	2	No	private dataset, STARE	0.9823 0.951	94.23% 90.84%	90.94%	95.74%
[18]	2	No	private dataset	0.946	88.21%	85.57%	90.85%
[23]	2	No	private dataset	-	98.7%	0.996	98.2%
[24]	5	No	Kaggle	-	63.23%	-	-
[25]	5	No	Kaggle	0.978	95.6%	86.4%	97.4%
[26]	4	No	Messidor	-	98.15%	98.94%	97.87%
[27]	4	No	private dataset	-	96.5%	98.1%	98.9%
[28]	5	No	IDRiD	-	90.07%	-	-
[29]	4	No	Messidor	-	96.35	92.35	97.45
[30]	5	No	IDRiD	-	65.1%	-	-
[31]	5	No	APTOS 2019	-	0.77	-	-
[32]	5	No	Messidor, DDR, Kaggle	-	0.8408 0.8569 0.8668	-	-
[33]	5	No	APTOS 2019	-	83.09	88.24	87
[34]	5	No	APTOS 2019	-	82.54	83	-
[35]	3	No	private dataset, EYEPACS	0.955, 0.984, 0.955	-	-	-
[36]	2	Red lesion only	Messidor	0.912	-	0.94	-
[37]	5	Yes	DDR	-	0.8284	-	-
[38]	5	Red lesion only	private dataset, Messidor	- 0.972	92.95 -	99.39% 92.59%	99.93% 96.20%

2.2. Multi-Level Classification

This section reviews the works that have classified DR images into various stages. Wang et al. [24] examined the performance of three pre-trained CNNs in the Kaggle dataset [16] to classify all the stages of the DR images. The three CNN architectures used were InceptionNet V3 [20], AlexNet [39] and VGG16 [40]. The best average ACC of 63.23% was obtained by InceptionNet V3. The work of [25] transferred learning pre-trained AlexNet [39], VggNet [40], GoogleNet [41] and ResNet [21] to detect the different DR stages in the Kaggle dataset [16]. Their results showed that VggNet achieved the higher ACC, with a value of 95.68%. Mobeen-ur-Rehman et al. [26] proposed a simple CNN to detect the DR stages of the Messidor dataset [17]. Their CNN obtained an excellent ACC of 98.15%. Zhang et al. [27] proposed a method to detect the DR stages of their private dataset. They fine-tuned InceptionV3 [20] , ResNet50 [42], Xception [43], InceptionResNetV2 [19], and DenseNets [44] and then combined the strongest CNNs. This method obtained an ACC of 96.5%. Harangi et al. [28] classified the DR stages by integrating hand-crafted features and AlexNet [39]. They used the Kaggle dataset [16] for training and the IDRiD [45] dataset for testing. This method achieved an ACC of 90.07%. Shanthi and Sabeenian [29] used Alexnet [39] to classify the DR stages of the Messidor dataset [17]. Their ACC was 96.35%. Li et al. [30] used ResNet50 [21] with attention modules to classify the stages in the IDRiD dataset [45], resulting in a 65.1% joint ACC. Dekhil et al. [31] transferred learning

VGG16 [40] to classify the DR stages in the APTOS 2019 Kaggle dataset [46], and they achieved an ACC of 77%. He et al. [32] proposed a CABNet network to classify DR images into stages, achieving an ACC of 85.69% in the DDR [37]. Kassani et al. [33] modified Xception model [43] to classify the DR stages in the APTOS 2019 Kaggle dataset [46], resulting in a 83.09% ACC. Bodapati et al. [34] proposed a composite network with gated attention to classify DR images into stages, achieving an ACC of 82.54% in the APTOS 2019 Kaggle dataset [46]. Hsieh et al. [35] trained the modified Inception-v4 [19] and the modified ResNet [21] to detect any DR, proliferative DR and referable DR in their private dataset and the EYEPACS dataset. They obtained an AUC of 0.955, 0.984 and 0.955, respectively in detecting any DR, proliferative DR and referable DR.

These previous studies demonstrated that CNN is effective in classifying DR images. However, localising DR lesions with DR image classification is more efficient for ophthalmologists at diagnosis. Moreover, Alyoubi et al. [47] reported that most of the studies, almost 70%, classified the fundus images using binary classifiers such as DR or non-DR, while only 27% classified the input to one or more stages, as shown in Figure 3.

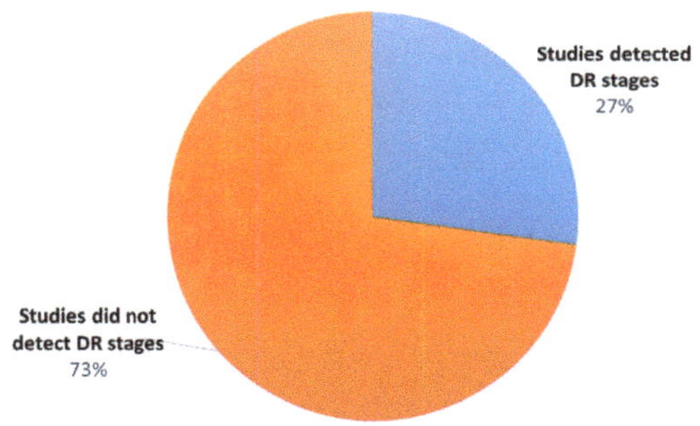

Figure 3. The ratio of studies that classified the DR stages [47].

2.3. Hybrid Classification

This section presents the studies that classified DR images and localised lesions at the same time. Zago et al. [36] used VGG16 [40] to detect red lesion patches of the DR images, and then they classified the image to DR or no-DR based on the detected red lesions. Their best results were achieved in the Messidor dataset [17] with an AUC of 0.912. Li et al. [37] created a dataset called the DDR to classify images into five DR stages and to localise lesions. For the stages classification, they achieved the best ACC of 82.84% using SE-BN-Inception [48], while for localisation, they achieved a mAP of 9.2 using Faster RCNN [49]. Wang et al. [38] used two modified RFCN [50] to detect the stages of DR and localise the MA and HM. Then the results from the two RFCN were merged. In their private dataset, this method achieved a mAP of 92.15 in localizing, while in classification, they achieved a 92.95% ACC.

Many studies, such as those by W. Alyoubi et al. [47] and T. Li et al. [51], show that the main limitation of the DR classification systems is that only a limited number of the studies detected and localized the types of DR lesions on the fundus image, as shown in Figure 4. Furthermore, there are limited studies that detected the DR stages, grading and lesions together. Lesions localization with high accuracy helps with grading the cases and the patients' follow-up, which is considered a critical requirement for DR patients.

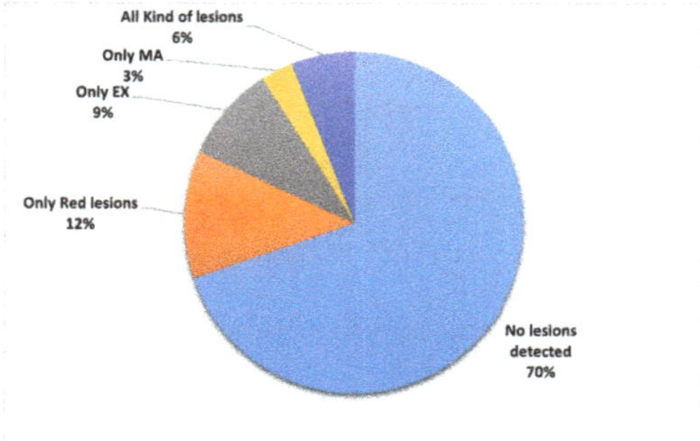

Figure 4. The ratio of studies that classified the DR lesions [47].

3. Materials and Methods

This section presents the datasets and the preprocessing methods used in the current work. Moreover, it explains the two proposed methods, shown in Figure 5, to classify the DR stages and localise the DR lesions types. The first method, called the Image-Based Method, utilises the whole preprocessed RGB retina images as an input for the CNN, while the second method, called Lesion localization method, is based on the lesions detection in order to classify the images into the five DR stages.

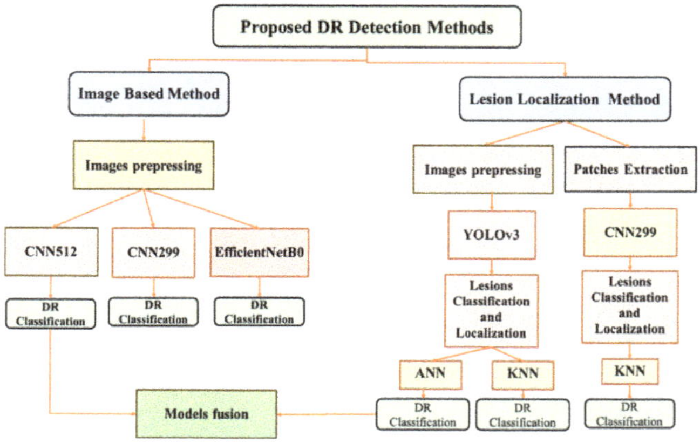

Figure 5. Block diagram of the different proposed models for DR images classification and localization.

3.1. Datasets

Two publicly available fundus retina datasets were used in this work: the DDR [37] and Asia Pacific Tele-Ophthalmology Society (APTOS) 2019 Kaggle [46]. Table 3 shows more details about these datasets.

- The DDR dataset [37] consists of 13673 fundus images acquired at a 45° field of view (FOV). Among these, there are 1151 ungradable images, 6266 normal images, and 6256 DR images. There are 757 images annotated by providing a bounding box for lesions (MA, HM, hard EX, and soft EX) to locate all DR lesion types. The dataset has different image sizes, classified to five DR stages and split into train, valid, and test images. The distribution of the dataset is imbalanced in that the normal images are more than the DR images. The annotated lesions distribution is shown in Table 4.
- The APTOS 2019 Kaggle dataset [46] consists of 3662 retina images with different image sizes. Only the ground truths of the training images are publicly available. The dataset is classified into five DR stages. In addition, 1805 of the images are normal and 1857 are DR images. The distribution of the dataset is imbalanced, with most of the images normal.

Table 3. The DR datasets details.

	DDR	DDR Lesions Annotated	APTOS 2019 Kaggle
Training	10,019 images	606 images	2929 images
Testing	2503 images	149 images	733 images
No DR	6266 images	-	1805 images
Mild	630 images	99 images	370 images
Moderate	4477 images	548 images	999 images
Severe	236 images	34 images	193 images
Proliferative	913 images	74 images	295 images
Image Size	Different image size	Different image size	Different image size
Total	12,522 images	755 images	3662 images

Table 4. The annotated lesions distribution in the DDR dataset.

	MA Number	HM Number	Hard EX Number	Soft EX Number	Total
Training	7824	11,196	21,739	944	41,703
Testing	2556	1342	1920	349	6167
Total	10,380	12,538	23,659	1293	47,870

3.2. Preprocessing

Image preprocessing is important for improving the quality of retinal images, since images with low quality can reduce the network's performance [25] and it is necessary to ensure that all the images are consistent and that the features of the images are enhanced [52,53]. The applied preprocessing methods, shown in Figure 6, are as follows. The result of the preprocessing step is shown in Figure 7.

- Image Enhancement: Two methods were used to enhance the images, the enhance luminosity method [54] and Contrast Limited Adaptive Histogram Equalization (CLAHE). CLAHE [55] is successful in enhancing the contrast of the fundus images [56] and improving the low contrast of medical images [57]. CLAHE is applied to the L channel of the retina images that have a higher contrast [44], with tile size 8×8 and Clip Limit 5.0.
- Image Noise Removal: The CLAHE method can cause some noise in the images [54] and, to remove this noise, we applied the Gaussian filter, as represented in Equation (1).

$$G_0(x,y) = Ae^{\frac{-(x-\mu_x)^2}{2\sigma_x^2} + \frac{-(y-\mu_y)^2}{2\sigma_y^2}} \tag{1}$$

where μ is the mean, A is the amplitude and σ is the standard deviation of each of the variables x and y.

- Image Cropping: The images were cropped to eliminate the unnecessary black pixels around the retina. Thus, the bounding box lesion positions in the annotation files were changed. To fix that, we automated changing the bounding box position of each image based on the number of removed pixels around the retina.
- Colour Normalisation: The retina images were captured from patients of different age, and various ethnicity [58], at different levels of lighting in the fundus image. These conditions have an effect on the value of pixel intensity of each image and create unnecessary variation in the image [58]. To overcome this, the retina images were normalised by normalising each channel of RGB images. For the normalization, we subtract the mean, and after that, divide the variance of the images [25], as shown in Equation (2).

$$z = \frac{(x - u)}{s} \quad (2)$$

where x is training RGB retina images, u is the mean of the RGB retina training images and s is the standard deviation of the training RGB retina images.

- Online data augmentation was adopted to enlarge the training dataset and to improve the generalisation and performance of the CNN. The images were augmented by performing rotation, flipping, shearing, and translation, as well as randomly darkening and brightening them, as shown in Figure 8. The augmentation parameters are presented in Table 5. Finally, the images were resized into a fixed size that varied according to the CNN used.
- Extract Lesions Patches: Some preprocessing methods were applied for Lesion localization Method to extract the lesion patches from each image for the CNN training. First, we cropped the annotated bounding box of each lesion and then padded it by zero if its size was less than (65 × 65); otherwise, we resized the patch to (65 × 65) to standardise the size of the patches.

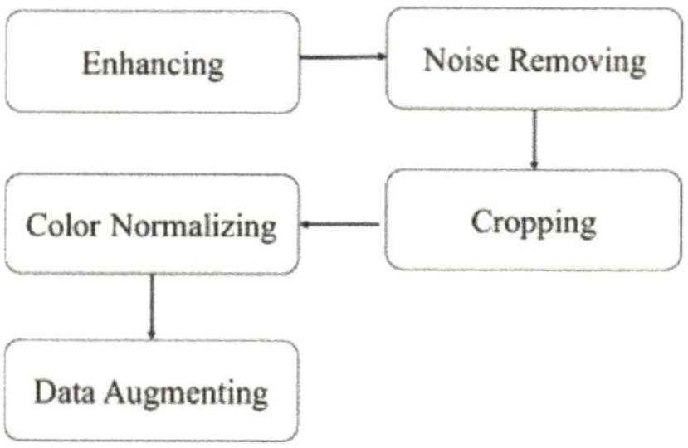

Figure 6. The retina images preprocessing methods.

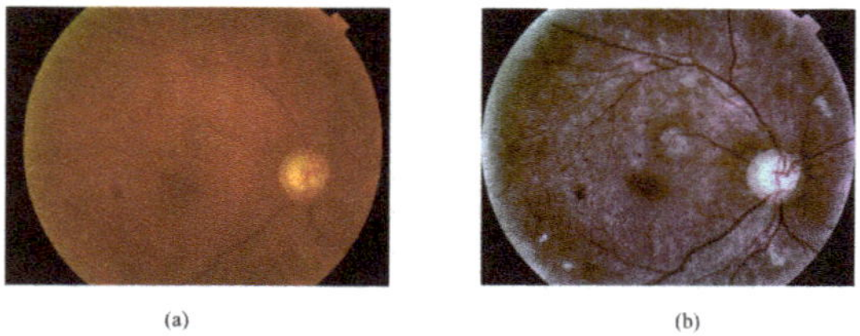

Figure 7. Sample images of the (**a**) original image and (**b**) the preprocessing image.

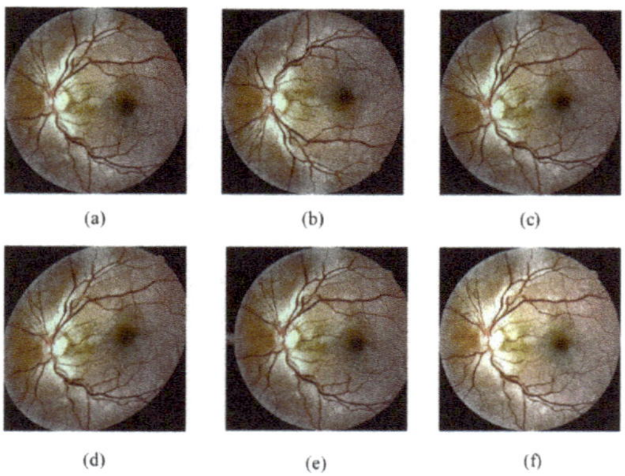

Figure 8. Sample of an image augmentation: (**a**) original image, (**b**) flipped image, (**c**) rotated image, (**d**) sheared image, (**e**) translated image and (**f**) brightened image.

In addition to the above preprocessing methods, we noticed that some of the image annotation files contained duplicate lesions. Thus, we automated the removal of the duplicate lesions in the annotation file as in Algorithm 1. Moreover, the bounding box of each lesion was enlarged by 10 pixels around each lesion to make the lesions clearer for learning. The chosen number was suitable for the resolution used.

Table 5. Data augmentation parameters.

Transformation Type	Description
Rotation	Rotate the image randomly between $(-35°, 35°)$.
Flipping	Horizontal and vertical flip for the images.
Shearing	Randomly Shear images with angle between $-15°$ and $15°$.
Translation	Randomly with shift between -10% and 10% of pixels.
Brightness range	Randomly darken the image and brighten. The values less than 1.0 the image darken whereas values larger than 1.0 brighten the image. The used values (0.25, 1.25).

Algorithm 1: Automate detecting and removing duplicate lesions.

```
Input  : The annotation file of an image.
Ouput: The annotation file of an image without lesions duplication.
box: contain the position values (xmin, xmax, ymin and ymax) of a lesion.
Declare list Box-list.
for each box in annotation file do
    Boxes = [xmin, xmax, ymin, ymax]
    if boxes in Box-list then
        remove box
    else
        append boxes to Box-list
    end
end
```

3.3. *Image Based Method*

This method takes the whole image as input to the CNN. The CNN architecture involves four main layers: convolution layers (CONV), pooling layers, fully connected layers (FC) and classification layer. The CONV layer role is to extract the features of the images by convolving different filters, while the pooling layer reduce the dimensions of the feature maps [59]. The FC layers are a compact feature to describe the whole input image. The Batch Normalisation layer role is to normalise the inputs of a layer during training to increase the training speed and regularise the CNN. We proposed two simple custom CNN models with different image sizes to classify the DR images. Moreover, EfficientNetB0 [12] was fine-tuned to classify the DR images.

3.3.1. Designed CNN Model

We started designing the proposed CNN as similar CNN from related works like [26]. Then, we increased the input layer size to consider the MA lesion and the number of CNN layers were increased gradually to improve the CNN performance. We adjusted the hyperparameter as in Section 4. After many attempts with many CNNs architectures as described in Section 4.3, we improved the DR classification using the proposed CNN.

The first proposed CNN (CNN299) contains one Zero Padding layer with a value of 2, four CONV layers, four Max Pooling layers, six Batch Normalization layers, two FC layers and one SoftMax layer for classification. The second proposed CNN (CNN512) contains one Zero Padding layer with a value of 2, six CONV layers, each followed by Max Pooling layers, eight Batch Normalization layers, two FC layers and one SoftMax layer for classification. The used input size of the CNNs was chosen to be suitable to the available computation power and it was not too small in order to avoid losing small lesions. The input image size was 299 × 299 × 3 for CNN299 and 512 × 512 × 3 for CNN512. The number of parameters of the CNN299 was 28,412,981 and for the CNN512 was 8,211,613. The CNN299 and CNN512 architectures are shown in Figure 9 and Table 6 and 7.

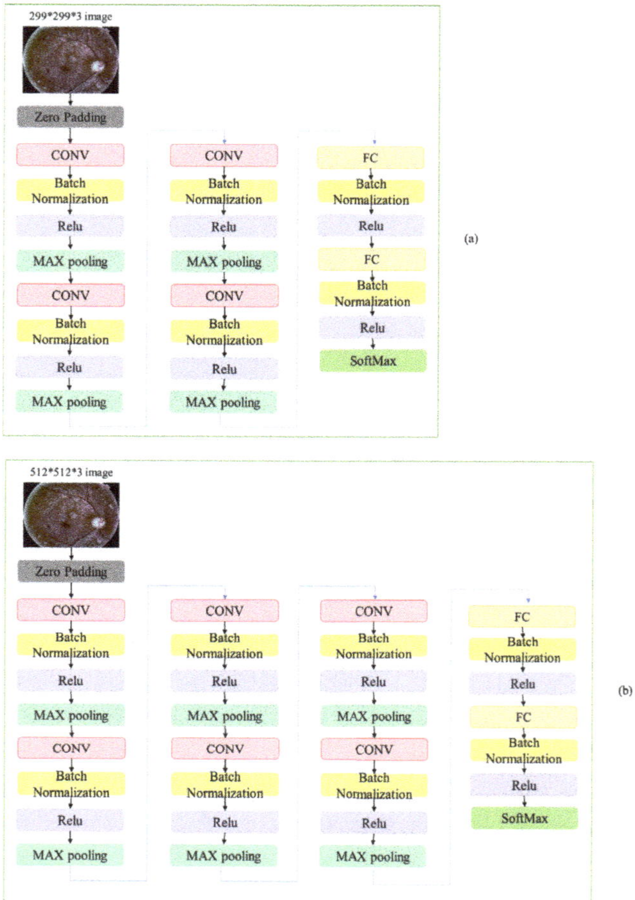

Figure 9. The proposed custom CNN architectures: (**a**) CNN299 and (**b**) CNN512.

Table 6. The proposed CNN299 layers detail.

Layer	Operator	Layer Details
Input Layer	Zero Padding layer	Padding (2,2)
Layer 1	2D CONV layer	Kernel number = 32, kernel size = 3
Layer 2	Batch Normalization layer	-
Layer 3	Relu layer	-
Layer 4	Max Pooling layer	Pooling size (2,2)
Layer 5	2D CONV layer	Kernel number = 64, kernel size = 3
Layer 6	Batch Normalization layer	-
Layer 7	Relu layer	-
Layer 8	Max Pooling layer	Pooling size (2,2)
Layer 9	2D CONV layer	Kernel number = 96, kernel size = 3
Layer 10	Batch Normalization layer	-
Layer 11	Relu layer	-
Layer 12	Max Pooling layer	Pooling size (2,2)

Table 6. *Cont.*

Layer	Operator	Layer Details
Layer 13	2D CONV layer	Kernel number = 96, kernel size = 3
Layer 14	Batch Normalization layer	-
Layer 15	Relu layer	-
Layer 16	Max Pooling layer	Pooling size (2,2)
Layer 17	Flatten layer	-
Layer 18	FC layer	Neurons number = 1000
Layer 19	Batch Normalization layer	-
Layer 20	Relu layer	-
Layer 21	FC layer	Neurons number = 500
Layer 22	Batch Normalization layer	-
Layer 23	Relu layer	-
Layer 24	FC layer	With SoftMax activation

Table 7. The proposed CNN512 layers detail.

Layer	Operator	Layer Details
Input Layer	Zero Padding layer	Padding (2,2)
Layer 1	2D CONV layer	Kernel number = 32, kernel size = 3
Layer 2	Batch Normalization layer	-
Layer 3	Relu layer	-
Layer 4	Max Pooling layer	Pooling size (2,2)
Layer 5	2D CONV layer	Kernel number = 64, kernel size = 3
Layer 6	Batch Normalization layer	-
Layer 7	Relu layer	-
Layer 8	Max Pooling layer	Pooling size (2,2)
Layer 9	2D CONV layer	Kernel number = 96, kernel size = 3
Layer 10	Batch Normalization layer	-
Layer 11	Relu layer	-
Layer 12	Max Pooling layer	Pooling size (2,2)
Layer 13	2D CONV layer	Kernel number = 96, kernel size = 3
Layer 14	Batch Normalization layer	-
Layer 15	Relu layer	-
Layer 16	Max Pooling layer	Pooling size (2,2)
Layer 17	2D CONV layer	Kernel number = 128, kernel size = 3
Layer 18	Batch Normalization layer	-
Layer 19	Relu layer	-
Layer 20	Max Pooling layer	Pooling size (2,2)
Layer 21	2D CONV layer	Kernel number = 200, kernel size = 3
Layer 22	Batch Normalization layer	-
Layer 23	Relu layer	-
Layer 24	Max Pooling layer	Pooling size (2,2)
Layer 25	Flatten layer	-
Layer 26	FC layer	Neurons number = 1000
Layer 27	Batch Normalization layer	-
Layer 28	Relu layer	-
Layer 29	FC layer	Neurons number = 500
Layer 30	Batch Normalization layer	-
Layer 31	Relu layer	-
Layer 32	FC layer	With SoftMax activation

3.3.2. Using Transfer Learning

Transfer learning is a well-known machine learning technique in which a pre-trained neural network is used to solve a problem similar to what the network was initially designed and trained to solve. Transfer learning is a commonly used technique with deep learning as it can overcome many problems associated with deep neural networks. Using transfer learning can reduce the training time and tuning efforts for many hyperparameters [60]. It transfers the knowledge from a pretrained network that was trained on large training data to a target network in which limited training data are available [11]. There are two deep transfer learning strategies: feature extraction of pretrained models and fine-tuning the pretrained models [10]. EfficientNet is a pretrained network [12]. It is a recently proposed model and has achieved state-of-the-art results on the ImageNet dataset. EfficientNetB0 [12] was fine-tuned by initialising its weights with ImageNet weights and re-training all of its layers with the used retina datasets. The top layers of EfficientNetB0 were removed and replaced by new layers which are the Global Average Pooling (GAP) layer, two FC layers and SoftMax layer, as shown in Figure 10. At FC layers, we added Dropout with a rate of 0.5 in all used CNNs to overcome an overfitting problem.

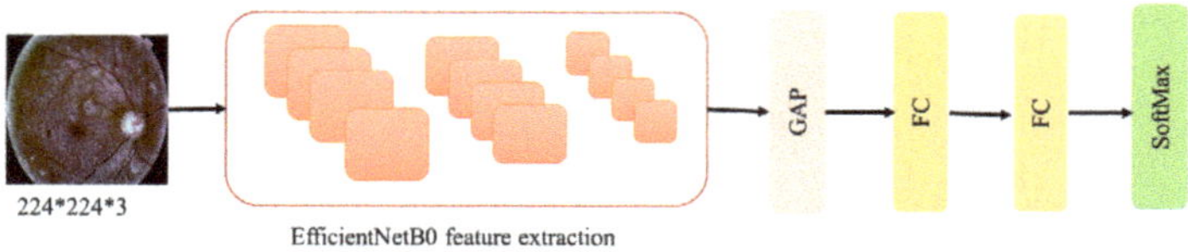

Figure 10. Transfer learning EfficientNetB0.

3.4. Lesion Localization Method

The current work proposed two methods for the lesions localization: fine-tuning YOLOv3 [13] and cropping the images into small and fixed-size patches. YOLOv3 is a publicly available object detector model that predicts object bounding box (localise) and predict its class. YOLOv3 predicts objects from the whole image at three different outputs with three different scales in order to predict the object boxes. YOLOv3 contains 53 CONV layers formed in a network called Darknet-53 [13].

In the first method, all the YOLOv3 [13] layers were fine-tuned and re-trained using the preprocessed images of the DDR dataset, with an input size of 416 × 416 pixels to localise and classify all the DR lesions types. One dropout after layer 79 was added to improve the performance of YOLOv3. The second method to localise lesions is based on cropping the preprocessing images of the size 600 × 600 into 65 × 65 patches and then feeding them to CNN299 to classify them into different lesions types, as shown in Figure 11. The annotated lesions files were used to extract the lesion patches and then preprocess them. After that, these preprocessed patches were used to train the CNN299 from scratch to classify the various DR lesions of the DDR dataset. For detecting the non-lesions patches, we extracted patches from the non-DR images. Figure 11 illustrates the steps of the Lesion Localization method.

Moreover, the performance of classifying the images into DR stages based on the detected number of lesions types from Lesion localization Method was investigated by training three machine learning methods. Three different classifiers were tested to classify the DR stage according to the existence of various DR lesions. These classifiers were the k-nearest neighbors (KNN) [61], artificial neural networks (ANN) and the support vector machine (SVM). The ANN used contains three FC layers, with each FC followed by Batch Normalization layers. The last layer was the SoftMax layer for classification. The classification performance of localization method was compared with the Image Based Method. Finally, the robust classification method was fused with a strong localization method.

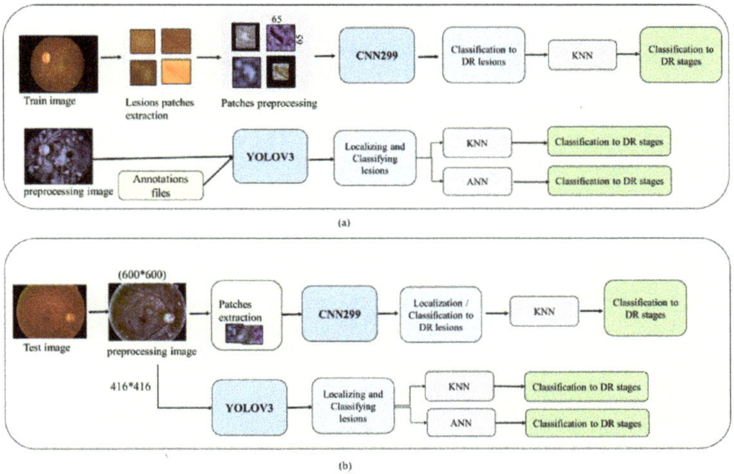

Figure 11. The proposed Lesion Localization method to detect DR stages and locate lesions for (**a**) train and (**b**) test images.

4. Experiments and Results

4.1. Configuration

The proposed system was implemented using the Python language and Keras framework [62] built on top of TensorFlow. All experiments were performed on two GPU resources: NVIDIA Tesla K20 GPU with 5 GB memory and NVIDIA GeForce 930 mx with 2 GB memory. The datasets were split into 80% for training and 20% for testing.

Deep learning network hyperparameters are variables that pre-select by a human designer or tuned via optimizing hyperparameters methods [63]. These methods involve random search [64], grid search [65], and gradient-based optimization [66]. We utilized manual hyperparameters tuning to speed up the process of tuning hyperparameters. The hyperparameter configuration of the used CNN models and YOLOv3 are shown in Tables 8 and 9, respectively.

Table 8. The hyperparameter configuration of CNNs.

Configuration	Values
Optimizer	SGD
Momentum	0.9
Max Learning rate	1×10^{-1} in custom CNNs 1×10^{-2} in EfficientNetB0
Base Learning rate	1×10^{-4}
Mode	triangular
Class weight	auto
Dropout	0.5
Augmentation	20 times

Table 9. The YOLOv3 hyperparameter configuration.

Configuration	Values
Optimizer	SGD and Adam
Momentum	0.9
Learning rate	1×10^{-3}
Anchors number	9
Augmentation	5 times
Input size	(416,416,3)
CNN model	Darknet53
Object threshold	0.45
NMS threshold	0.45
Dropout	0.5

4.2. Performance Metrics

The metrics used to evaluate the performance of CNNs are accuracy (ACC), specificity (SP), sensitivity (SEN), Receiver Operating Characteristic (ROC) curve, Area Under the ROC Curve (AUC), positive predictive value (PPV) (also called Precision), Negative predictive value (NPV) and Disc similarity coefficient (DSC). ACC is the percentage of accurately classified images. SP is the percentage of images accurately classified as normal images, while SEN is the percentage of images accurately classified as DR images. The ratio between SEN and SP is graphically illustrated in the ROC curve and the value computed by ROC AUC. PPV is the percentage of DR images accurately classified as DR images while NPV is the percentage of normal images accurately classified as normal. The metrics used to evaluate the performance of YOLOv3 is Average precision (AP). The mean AP (mAP) is the average of the AP for each class. Each measurement is illustrated as follows.

$$SP = \frac{TN}{(TN + FP)} \tag{3}$$

$$SEN = \frac{TP}{(TP + FN)} \tag{4}$$

$$ACC = \frac{(TN + TP)}{(TN + TP + FN + FP)} \tag{5}$$

$$PPV = \frac{TP}{(TP + FP)} \tag{6}$$

$$NPV = \frac{TN}{(TN + FN)} \tag{7}$$

$$AP = \sum_{n}(R_n - R_{n-1})P_n \tag{8}$$

where false positive (FP) refers to the non-DR images that are classified as DR, while false negative (FN) means the DR images that are classified as non-DR. True positive (TP) refers to the DR images that are classified as DR and true negative (TN) is the non-DR images that are classified as non-DR. R_n and P_n are the recall and the precision at the n threshold.

4.3. Image Based Method Results

Regarding the Image-Based Method, three CNN architectures were built for detecting the five DR stages: two custom CNNs, with different input sizes that were trained from scratch, and one fine-tuned EfficientNetB0. The CNNs were trained and tested on the DDR and the Kaggle APTOS 2019 datasets independently.

In the experiments, the stochastic gradient descent (SGD) algorithm with the Nesterov Momentum was adopted. Moreover, Cyclical Learning Rates [67] with Learning rate range $[1 \times 10^{-4}, 1 \times 10^{-1}]$ and $[1 \times 10^{-4}, 1 \times 10^{-2}]$ were used for the custom CNNs and EfficientNetB0, respectively. The dropout at FC layers of the CNNs was implemented to reduce the overfitting and improve the CNNs' performance. The distribution of all datasets' classes was imbalanced and, to fix that, the class weight parameter was set to "auto". The experiments showed that the CNN512 with the input size of 512 had a better performance than the other CNNs in both datasets. From Tables 10 and 11, we found that the CNN512 with dropout achieved the highest ACC of 0.841 and 0.886 in the APTOS 2019 and the DDR datasets, respectively. The experiments also showed that the enhanced images luminosity method did not improve the classification accuracy when applied to the APTOS 2019 dataset with the CNN299 model, as shown in Table 11. Tables 12 and 13 show the classification results of each DR stage from the APTOS 2019 and the DDR datasets, respectively. The ROC curves and confusion matrixes of the best proposed model results are shown in Figure 12.

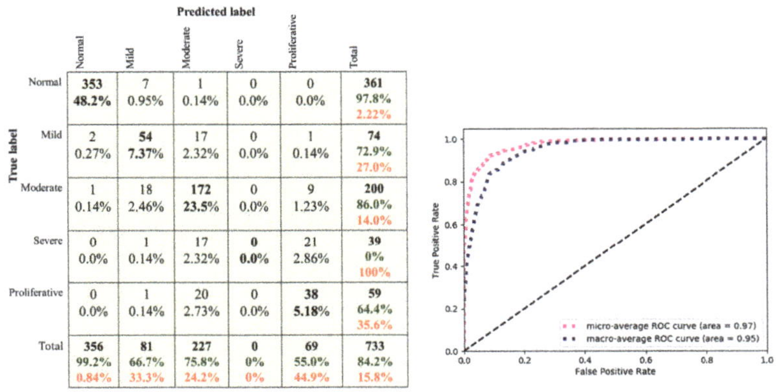

(a)

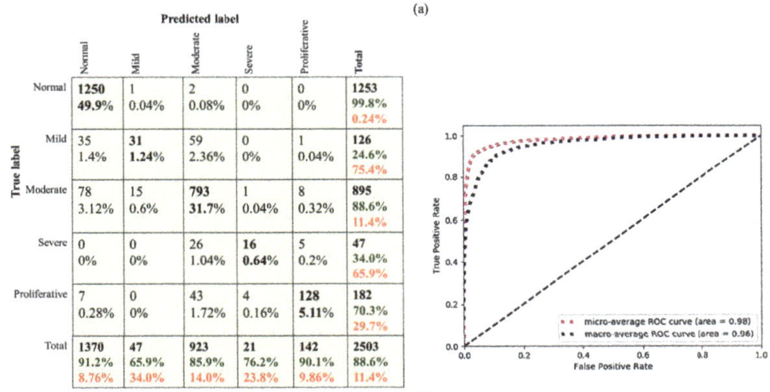

(b)

Figure 12. The ROC curves of the (**a**) APTOS 2019 and (**b**) the DDR datasets on CNN512.

Table 10. Comparison between the proposed models and the state-of-the-art models on the DDR dataset.

Model	Image Size	ACC	SEN	SP	AUC
Tao Li et al. [37]	224	0.828	-	-	-
Along He et al. [32]	512	0.856	-	-	-
CNN299	299	0.800	-	-	-
CNN299 + dropout	299	0.833	-	-	-
CNN512	512	0.858	0.858	0.963	0.975
CNN512 + dropout	512	0.886	0.886	0.971	0.979
EfficientNetB0	224	0.823	-	-	-
EfficientNetB0 + dropout	224	0.822	-	-	-
Models fusion	512	0.890	0.890	0.973	0.970

Table 11. Comparison between the proposed models and the state of-art models on the APTOS 2019 dataset.

Model	Image Size	ACC	SEN	SP	AUC
Omar Dekhil et al. [31]	224	0.77	-	-	-
kassani et al. [33]	600	83.09	88.2	87.0	-
Bodapati et al. [34]	-	82.54	83	-	-
CNN299	299	0.821	-	-	-
CNN299 + dropout	299	0.832	-	-	-
CNN299 + dropout + enhance luminosity	299	0.832	-	-	-
CNN512	512	0.834	0.834	0.957	0.97
CNN512 + dropout	512	0.841	0.841	0.960	0.973
EfficientNetB0	224	0.823	-	-	-
EfficientNetB0 + dropout	224	0.822	-	-	-

Table 12. The performance measures of the DR stages using CNN512 for the APTOS 2019 dataset.

Stage	SEN	SP	PPV	NPV
No DR	0.978	0.991	0.991	0.979
Mild DR	0.730	0.959	0.667	0.969
Moderate DR	0.860	0.897	0.758	0.945
Severe DR	0	100	0	0.947
Proliferative DR	0.644	0.954	0.550	0.968

Table 13. The performance measures of the DR stages using CNN512 for the DDR dataset.

Stage	SEN	SP	PPV	NPV
No DR	0.998	0.904	0.912	0.997
Mild DR	0.246	0.993	0.660	0.961
Moderate DR	0.886	0.919	0.859	0.935
Severe DR	0.340	0.998	0.762	0.988
Proliferative DR	0.703	0.993	0.901	0.977

4.4. Lesion Localization Method Results

YOLOv3 is trained on the DDR dataset to locate all DR lesions types and draws a bounding box around each lesion. YOLOv3 is trained using 608 images and tested using 149 images with 9 anchors. In the experiments, all YOLOv3 layers were retrained on the DDR dataset with a SGD optimizer, 0.9 momentum and fixed 1×10^{-3} learning rate. It was observed through the experiments that YOLOv3 with the learning rate 1×10^{-3} and one dropout after layer 79 had a better performance on the valid DDR dataset. YOLOv3 achieved the highest mAP of 0.216 at localising the DR lesions of the valid set when one dropout and the Adam optimizer were used, as shown in Table 14.

On the other hand, the KNN method obtained the best results for classifying the DR lesions into various DR stages, as in Table 15. The detected lesions by YOLOv3 and CNN299 were fed to the KNN or ANN to classify them into the different DR stages. When YOLOv3 and CNN299 did not detect any lesions, the image was classified as no DR stage. From Table 16, we found that the detected lesions from YOLOv3 with SGD and then classified by the KNN achieved the highest ACC of 0.712 in the valid set of the DDR dataset.

Table 14. Results of YOLOv3 on the DDR Dataset.

Model	mAP
YOLOv3 + SGD	0.110
YOLOv3 + SGD+ dropout	0.171
YOLOv3 + Adam optimizer + dropout	0.216

Table 15. The DR stages classification training results using machine learning.

Model	ACC
KNN	0.985
ANN	0.893
SVM	0.872

Table 16. The results of DR stages classification using Lesion localization Method on the DDR dataset.

Model	Valid Images Number	ACC	SEN	SP	AUC
CNN299 + KNN	250 images	0.62	0.62	0.90	0.762
YOLOv3 + SGD+ dropout + KNN	250 images	0.712	0.712	0.928	0.820
YOLOv3 + Adam+ dropout + KNN	250 images	0.552	0.552	0.888	0.720
YOLOv3 + SGD+ dropout + KNN	2503 images	0.528	0.528	0.882	0.705
YOLOv3 + ADAM+ dropout +ANN	2503 images	0.481	0.481	0.870	0.789

4.5. Comparison against State-of-the-Art Methods

Compared to the state of-the-art methods on the DDR and the APTOS 2019 datasets, our CNN512 achieved high results. Our CNN512 on the DDR dataset achieved a 0.886 ACC, while in the works of [32,37] achieved 0.828 and 0.856 ACC, respectively. In the APTOS 2019 dataset, our CNN512 achieved a 0.841 ACC, which is better than the works of [31,33,34]. The results of the CNNs in both datasets are shown in Tables 10 and 11, respectively.

When compared to the results achieved by YOLOv3 on the DDR dataset with the state-of-the-art methods, YOLOv3 obtained better results. Table 17 shows that YOLOv3 achieved a better mAP on a valid set than the work of [37] that used Faster RCNN.

Table 17. Comparison between the YOLOv3 model and the state of-art models on the DDR dataset.

Model	mAP
Tao li et al. [37]	0.092
YOLOv3 + Adam optimizer + dropout	0.216

4.6. Models Fusion

From the experiments, we found that the proposed CNN512 achieved the best DR stages classification results on the DDR dataset unlike the classification based on the detected DR lesions. Also, YOLOv3 classified and localised lesions on the retina with the best results. Thus, for classifying the retina images to the DR stages and localising DR lesions at the same time with the best results, CNN512 and YOLOv3 were fused. The classification predictions from the CNN512 model and YOLOv3 model with ANN were combined using average voting to fuse models. Average voting takes the average probabilities predicted from the two models as the final prediction result. When compared the results achieved by fused models on the DDR dataset with the state-of-the-art methods, the fused models obtained a 0.890 ACC exceeds the state-of-the-art results as shown in Table 10. Sample images visualization of lesions localising and stages classifying for the ground truth images and predicted images by the fused models are shown in Figure 13. The ROC curves and confusion matrixes of the fused models are shown in Figure 14. The average inference time for the fused models is 6.36 s using NVIDIA Tesla K20 GPU.

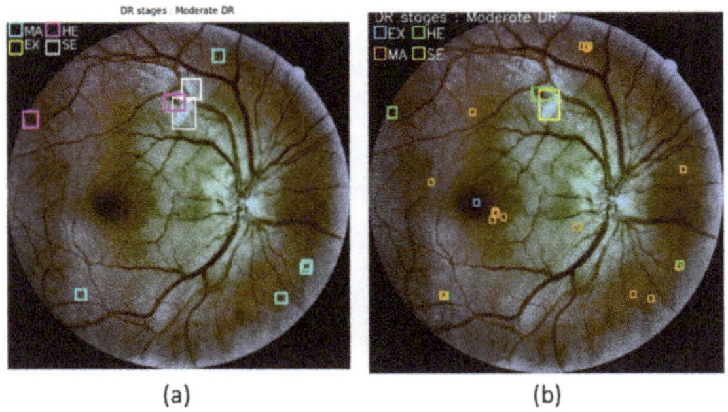

Figure 13. Sample of the DDR images visualization for: (**a**) the ground truth images annotation, (**b**) predicted images by fused model.

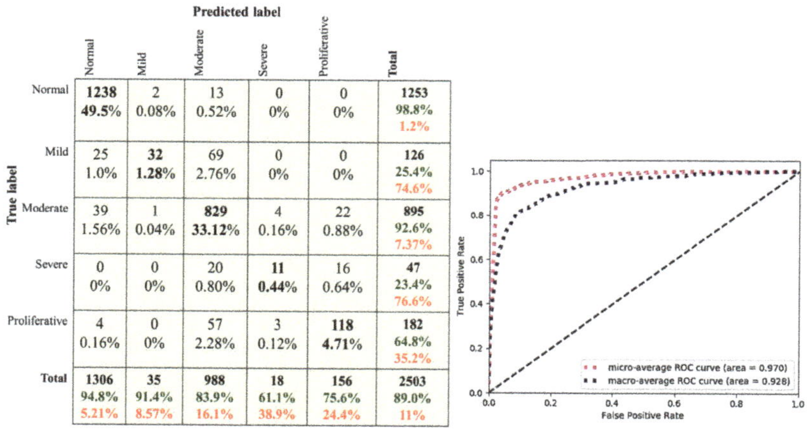

Figure 14. The confusion matrixes and ROC curves of the DDR dataset on fused models.

5. Discussion

Diabetic retinopathy (DR) is one of the most severe diabetes complications, causing non-reversible damage to retina blood vessels. Regular scanning using high-efficiency computer-based systems to diagnose cases early will help diabetes patients to stop or delay the deterioration of sight. This study proposed a DR screening system using the deep learning technique. The proposed screening system provides classification and DR lesions localization for DR images to help ophthalmologists diagnose the patients' DR stage. The experimental results demonstrated that our custom CNN512 model achieved state-of-the-art classification results on the used two datasets.

Furthermore, the fine-tuned YOLOv3 model obtained state-of-the-art localization results on the DDR dataset. CNN512 model and the fine-tuned YOLOv3 model were integrated to classify the DR images into stages and localize all lesion types. As we notice from the results, all of the models are slightly high with the DDR dataset rather than the APTOS dataset, which might result from the larger DDR training set. If a close look is taken on Tables 12 and 13, it will be noticed that the sensitivity for mild and severe DR is lower than other stages; this resulted from the imbalance of the used datasets. For example, the mild class on DDR is less than 5% of the total dataset size; also, the severe stage image size is less than 2% of the DDR dataset. This limits the system performance for both mild and severe classes' diagnoses, and it is reflected on PPV value even when we used the data augmentation technique to increase the data size. We inferred that, as the input image's size increased, the model's accuracy increased but this is limited with the available computing power. Some of the misclassified lesions in the images were examined and we found that spots detected on the retina by YOLOv3 were not in the ground truth lesions. The missed labeling of used images affected the results that the model obtained. Figure 15 shows samples of the incorrectly labeled lesions from the DDR dataset.

Recently, a new trend has appeared in DR which is developing a system that attempts to predict the development and change in DR over time as in [68,69]. In [68], they predicted future DR image using vessel and lesion information, achieving a 0.74 F1-score. In contrast, in [69], they evaluated the changes in DR using optimization algorithm and Support Vector Machines, obtaining a 95.23% ACC.

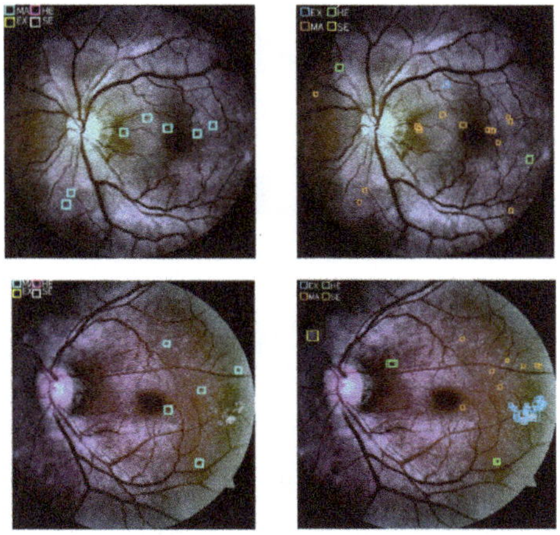

Figure 15. Samples of the miss labeled lesions from the DDR dataset compared to the predicted lesions by YOLOv3.

In the future, we could improve the localization of the lesions by creating a custom object detection model and by improving the performance classification of the CNN512 by adding more layers. Testing and tuning the system on more balanced datasets might improve its performance. In addition, we aim to adopt YOLOv4 and YOLOv5 to detect all DR lesions to obtain their benefits, such as ACC and speed. The current work opens the pathway to building a complete automatic follow-up system for DR. DR is a lifelong disease with a prolonged potential phase, so patients follow-up regularly will prevent patients' blindness and delay sight deterioration. Table 18 Comparing the performance of the proposed models in term of accuracy.

Table 18. The performance comparison among all of the models.

Model	EfficientNetB0 + Dropout		CNN299 + Dropout		CNN512 + Dropout		Model Fusion
Dataset	APTOS	DDR	APTOS	DDR	APTOS	DDR	DDR
ACC	0.822	0.822	0.832	0.833	0.841	**0.886**	**0.890**

6. Conclusions

The prevalence of diabetes is increasing worldwide, and the complication of DR is also increasing. This disorder is threatening diabetes patients' vision if DR is detected in the last stages. Therefore, the detection and treatment of DR in its early stages is essential to decrease the risk of blindness. The manual diagnosis process of DR with the increasing suffering from DR became not sufficiently effective. Therefore, automating DR's diagnosis using computer-aided screening systems (CASS) saves effort, time, and cost.

Additionally, the most critical point for using CASS is to avoid the negative impact of losing eyesight. Recently, the deep learning (DL) method has achieved superior performance in classification and segmentation. The current work provides an effective complete automated screening system to help in DR diagnosis. The quality and balance of the datasets used to build a DR screening system are very critical. In the future, we aim to combine multiple datasets to achieve the balance of the dataset.

Author Contributions: Conceptualization, W.L.A. and W.M.S.; methodology, W.L.A. and W.M.S.; software, W.L.A.; validation, W.L.A.; formal analysis, W.L.A. and W.M.S.; investigation, W.L.A. and W.M.S.; resources, W.L.A.; data curation,W.L.A.; writing—original draft preparation, W.L.A.; writing—review and editing, W.L.A., M.F.A. and W.M.S.; visualization, W.L.A. and W.M.S.; supervision, W.L.A.,

M.F.A. and W.M.S.; project administration, W.L.A. and W.M.S. All authors have read and agreed to the published version of the manuscript.

Funding: This research received no external funding.

Institutional Review Board Statement: Not applicable.

Informed Consent Statement: Not applicable.

Data Availability Statement: Publicly available datasets were used in this study. DDR dataset at https://doi.org/10.1016/j.ins.2019.06.011 accessed 28 August 2019 and APTOS 2019 Blindness Detection at https://www.kaggle.com/c/aptos2019-blindness-detection/overview/evaluation accessed 1January 2020.

Acknowledgments: This work was implemented by the High Performance Computing Center (Aziz Supercomputer) of King Abdul-Aziz University [70].

Conflicts of Interest: The authors declare no conflict of interest.

References

1. American Academy of Ophthalmology-What Is Diabetic Retinopathy. Available online: https://www.aao.org/eye-health/diseases/what-is-diabetic-retinopathy (accessed on 1 January 2019).
2. Bourne, R.R.; Stevens, G.A.; White, R.A.; Smith, J.L.; Flaxman, S.R.; Price, H.; Jonas, J.B.; Keeffe, J.; Leasher, J.; Naidoo, K.; et al. Causes of vision loss worldwide, 1990-2010: A systematic analysis. *Lancet Glob. Health* **2013**, *1*, 339–349. [CrossRef]
3. Taylor, R.; Batey, D. *Handbook of Retinal Screening in Diabetes:Diagnosis and Management*, 2nd ed.; John Wiley & Sons, Ltd., Wiley-Blackwell: Hoboken, NJ, USA, 2012; pp. 1–173. [CrossRef]
4. Wilkinson, C.P.; Ferris, F.L.; Klein, R.E.; Lee, P.P.; Agardh, C.D.; Davis, M.; Dills, D.; Kampik, A.; Pararajasegaram, R.; Verdaguer, J.T.; Lum, F. Proposed international clinical diabetic retinopathy and diabetic macular edema disease severity scales. *Am. Acad. Ophthalmol.* **2003**, *110*, 1677–1682. [CrossRef]
5. Deng, L.; Yu, D. Deep learning: Methods and applications. *Found. Trends Signal Process.* **2014**, *7*, 197–387. [CrossRef]
6. Vega, R.; Sanchez-Ante, G.; Falcon-Morales, L.E.; Sossa, H.; Guevara, E. Retinal vessel extraction using lattice neural networks with dendritic processing. *Comput. Biol. Med.* **2015**, *58*, 20–30. [CrossRef] [PubMed]
7. Al Zaid, E.; Shalash, W.M.; Abulkhair, M.F. Retinal blood vessels segmentation using Gabor filters. In Proceedings of the 2018 1st International Conference on Computer Applications & Information Security (ICCAIS), Riyadh, Saudi Arabia, 4–6 April 2018; pp. 1–6.
8. Sikder, N.; Masud, M.; Bairagi, A.K.; Arif, A.S.M.; Nahid, A.A.; Alhumyani, H.A. Severity Classification of Diabetic Retinopathy Using an Ensemble Learning Algorithm through Analyzing Retinal Images. *Symmetry* **2021**, *13*, 670. [CrossRef]
9. Bakator, M.; Radosav, D. Deep learning and medical diagnosis: A review of literature. *Multimodal Technol. Interact.* **2018**, *2*, 47. [CrossRef]
10. Litjens, G.; Kooi, T.; Bejnordi, B.E.; Setio, A.A.A.; Ciompi, F.; Ghafoorian, M.; van der Laak, J.A.; van Ginneken, B.; Sánchez, C.I. A survey on deep learning in medical image analysis. *Med. Image Anal.* **2017**, *42*, 60–88. [CrossRef] [PubMed]
11. Lu, L.; Zheng, Y.; Carneiro, G.; Yang, L. *Deep Learning and Convolutional Neural Networks for Medical Image Computing*; Springer: Berlin/Heidelberg, Germany, 2017; [CrossRef]
12. Tan, M.; Le, Q.V. EfficientNet: Rethinking model scaling for convolutional neural networks. In Proceedings of the 36th International Conference on Machine Learning, ICML 2019, Beach, CA, USA, 10–15 June 2019; pp. 6105–6114.
13. Redmon, J.; Farhadi, A. YOLOv3: An Incremental Improvement. *arXiv* **2018**, arXiv:1804.02767.
14. Pal, P.; Kundu, S.; Dhara, A.K. Detection of red lesions in retinal fundus images using YOLO V3. *Curr. Indian Eye Res. J. Ophthalmic Res. Group* **2020**, *7*, 49.
15. Pires, R.; Avila, S.; Wainer, J.; Valle, E.; Abramoff, M.D.; Rocha, A. A data-driven approach to referable diabetic retinopathy detection. *Artif. Intell. Med.* **2019**, *96*, 93–106. [CrossRef]
16. Kaggle 2015 Dataset. Available online: https://kaggle.com/c/diabetic-retinopathy-detection (accessed on 1 April 2019).
17. Decenciere, E.; Zhang, X.; Cazuguel, G.; Lay, B.; Cochener, B.; Trone, C.; Gain, P.; Ordonez, R.; Massin, P.; Erginay, A.; et al. Feedback on a publicly distributed image database: The messidor database. *Image Anal. Stereol.* **2014**, *33*, 231–234. [CrossRef]
18. Jiang, H.; Yang, K.; Gao, M.; Zhang, D.; Ma, H.; Qian, W. An Interpretable Ensemble Deep Learning Model for Diabetic Retinopathy Disease Classification. In Proceedings of the 2019 41st Annual International Conference of the IEEE Engineering in Medicine and Biology Society (EMBC), Berlin, Germany, 23–27 July 2019; pp. 2045–2048. [CrossRef]
19. Szegedy, C.; Ioffe, S.; Vanhoucke, V.; Alemi, A.A. Inception-v4, inception-resnet and the impact of residual connections on learning. In Proceedings of the Thirty-First AAAI Conference on Artificial Intelligence, San Francisco, CA, USA, 4–9 February 2017; pp. 4278–4284.
20. Szegedy, C.; Vanhoucke, V.; Ioffe, S.; Shlens, J.; Wojna, Z. Rethinking the Inception Architecture for Computer Vision. In Proceedings of the IEEE Conference on Computer Vision and Pattern Recognition, Las Vegas, NV, USA, 26 June–1 July 2016; pp. 2818–2826. [CrossRef]

21. He, K.; Zhang, X.; Ren, S.; Sun, J. Deep Residual Learning for Image Recognition. In Proceedings of the IEEE Conference on Computer Vision and Pattern Recognition, Las Vegas, NV, USA, 26 June–1 July 2016; pp. 770–778. [CrossRef]
22. Liu, Y.P.; Li, Z.; Xu, C.; Li, J.; Liang, R. Referable diabetic retinopathy identification from eye fundus images with weighted path for convolutional neural network. *Artif. Intell. Med.* **2019**, *99*, 101694. [CrossRef] [PubMed]
23. Das, S.; Kharbanda, K.; Suchetha, M.; Raman, R.; Dhas, E. Deep learning architecture based on segmented fundus image features for classification of diabetic retinopathy. *Biomed. Signal Process. Control* **2021**, *68*, 102600. [CrossRef]
24. Wang, X.; Lu, Y.; Wang, Y.; Chen, W.B. Diabetic retinopathy stage classification using convolutional neural networks. In Proceedings of the International Conference on Information Reuse and Integration for Data Science, Salt Lake City, UT, USA, 6–9 July 2018; pp. 465–471. [CrossRef]
25. Wan, S.; Liang, Y.; Zhang, Y. Deep convolutional neural networks for diabetic retinopathy detection by image classification. *Comput. Electr. Eng.* **2018**, *72*, 274–282. [CrossRef]
26. Mobeen-Ur-Rehman.; Khan, S.H.; Abbas, Z.; Danish Rizvi, S.M. Classification of Diabetic Retinopathy Images Based on Customised CNN Architecture. In Proceedings of the 2019 Amity International Conference on Artificial Intelligence, AICAI 2019, Dubai, United Arab Emirates, 4–6 February 2019; pp. 244–248. [CrossRef]
27. Zhang, W.; Zhong, J.; Yang, S.; Gao, Z.; Hu, J.; Chen, Y.; Yi, Z. Automated identification and grading system of diabetic retinopathy using deep neural networks. *Knowl. Based Syst.* **2019**, *175*, 12–25. [CrossRef]
28. Harangi, B.; Toth, J.; Baran, A.; Hajdu, A. Automatic screening of fundus images using a combination of convolutional neural network and hand-crafted features. In Proceedings of the 2019 41st Annual International Conference of the IEEE Engineering in Medicine and Biology Society (EMBC), Berlin, Germany, 23–27 July 2019; pp. 2699–2702. [CrossRef]
29. Shanthi, T.; Sabeenian, R.S. Modified Alexnet architecture for classification of diabetic retinopathy images. *Comput. Electr. Eng.* **2019**, *76*, 56–64. [CrossRef]
30. Li, X.; Hu, X.; Yu, L.; Zhu, L.; Fu, C.W.; Heng, P.A. CANet: Cross-disease Attention Network for Joint Diabetic Retinopathy and Diabetic Macular Edema Grading. *IEEE Trans. Med Imaging* **2020**, *39*, 1483–1493. [CrossRef] [PubMed]
31. Dekhil, O.; Naglah, A.; Shaban, M.; Ghazal, M.; Taher, F.; Elbaz, A. Deep Learning Based Method for Computer Aided Diagnosis of Diabetic Retinopathy. In Proceedings of the IST 2019—IEEE International Conference on Imaging Systems and Techniques, Abu Dhabi, United Arab Emirates, 9–10 December 2019; pp. 1–4. [CrossRef]
32. He, A.; Li, T.; Li, N.; Wang, K.; Fu, H. CABNet: Category Attention Block for Imbalanced Diabetic Retinopathy Grading. *IEEE Trans. Med. Imaging* **2020**, *40*, 143–153. [CrossRef] [PubMed]
33. Kassani, S.H.; Kassani, P.H.; Khazaeinezhad, R.; Wesolowski, M.J.; Schneider, K.A.; Deters, R. Diabetic retinopathy classification using a modified xception architecture. In Proceedings of the 2019 IEEE International Symposium on Signal Processing and Information Technology (ISSPIT), Ajman, United Arab Emirates, 10–12 December 2019; pp. 1–6.
34. Bodapati, J.D.; Shaik, N.S.; Naralasetti, V. Composite deep neural network with gated-attention mechanism for diabetic retinopathy severity classification. *J. Ambient. Intell. Humaniz. Comput.* **2021**, 1–15. [CrossRef]
35. Hsieh, Y.T.; Chuang, L.M.; Jiang, Y.D.; Chang, T.J.; Yang, C.M.; Yang, C.H.; Chan, L.W.; Kao, T.Y.; Chen, T.C.; Lin, H.C.; et al. Application of deep learning image assessment software VeriSee™ for diabetic retinopathy screening. *J. Formos. Med Assoc.* **2021**, *120*, 165–171. [CrossRef]
36. Zago, G.T.; Andreão, R.V.; Dorizzi, B.; Teatini Salles, E.O. Diabetic retinopathy detection using red lesion localization and convolutional neural networks. *Comput. Biol. Med.* **2019**, *116*, 103537. [CrossRef] [PubMed]
37. Li, T.; Gao, Y.; Wang, K.; Guo, S.; Liu, H.; Kang, H. Diagnostic assessment of deep learning algorithms for diabetic retinopathy screening. *Inf. Sci.* **2019**, *501*, 511–522. [CrossRef]
38. Wang, J.; Luo, J.; Liu, B.; Feng, R.; Lu, L.; Zou, H. Automated diabetic retinopathy grading and lesion detection based on the modified R-FCN object-detection algorithm. *IET Comput. Vis.* **2020**, *14*, 1–8. [CrossRef]
39. Krizhevsky, A.; Sutskever, I.; Hinton, G.E. ImageNet Classification with Deep Convolutional Neural Networks. *Commun. ACM* **2017**, *60*, 84–90. [CrossRef]
40. Zisserman, K.S.; Zisserman, A. Very deep convolutional networks for large-scale image recognition. In Proceedings of the International Conference on Learning Representations, San Diego, CA, USA, 7–9 May 2015
41. Szegedy, C.; Liu, W.; Jia, Y.; Sermanet, P.; Reed, S.; Anguelov, D.; Erhan, D.; Vanhoucke, V.; Rabinovich, A. Going Deeper with Convolutions. In Proceedings of the IEEE Conference on Computer Vision and Pattern Recognition (CVPR), Boston, MA, USA, 7–12 June 2015; pp. 1–9. [CrossRef]
42. He, K.; Zhang, X.; Ren, S.; Sun, J. Spatial Pyramid Pooling in Deep Convolutional Networks for Visual Recognition. *IEEE Trans. Pattern Anal. Mach. Intell.* **2015**, *37*, 1904–1916. [CrossRef] [PubMed]
43. Chollet, F. Xception: Deep learning with depthwise separable convolutions. In Proceedings of the IEEE Conference on Computer Vision and Pattern Recognition (CVPR), Honolulu, HI, USA, 21–26 July 2017; pp. 1251–1258.
44. Huang, G.; Liu, Z.; van der Maaten, L.; Weinberger, K.Q. Densely Connected Convolutional Networks. In Proceedings of the IEEE Conference on Computer Vision and Pattern Recognition (CVPR), Honolulu, HI, USA, 21–26 July 2017; pp. 4700–4708.
45. Porwal, P.; Pachade, S.; Kamble, R.; Kokare, M.; Deshmukh, G.; Sahasrabuddhe, V.; Meriaudeau, F. Indian Diabetic Retinopathy Image Dataset (IDRiD): A Database for Diabetic Retinopathy Screening Research. *Data* **2018**, *3*, 25. [CrossRef]
46. APTOS 2019 Blindness Detection. Available online: https://www.kaggle.com/c/aptos2019-blindness-detection/overview/evaluation (accessed on 1 January 2020).

47. Alyoubi, W.L.; Shalash, W.M.; Abulkhair, M.F. Diabetic Retinopathy Detection through Deep Learning Technique: A Review. *Inform. Med. Unlocked* **2020**, *20*, 1–11. [CrossRef]
48. Hu, J.; Shen, L.; Sun;, G. Squeeze-and-excitation networks. In Proceedings of the IEEE Conference on Computer Vision and Pattern Recognition, Salt Lake City, UT, USA, 18–23 June 2018; pp. 7132–7141.
49. Ren, S.; He, K.; Girshick, R.; Sun, J. Faster R-CNN: Towards real-time object detection with region proposal networks. *IEEE Trans. Pattern Anal. Mach. Intell.* **2017**, *39*, 1137–1149. [CrossRef]
50. Dai, J.; Li, Y.; He, K.; Sun, J. R-FCN: Object detection via region-based fully convolutional networks. *arXiv* **2016**, arXiv:1605.06409.
51. Li, T.; Bo, W.; Hu, C.; Kang, H.; Liu, H.; Wang, K.; Fu, H. Applications of Deep Learning in Fundus Images: A Review. *Med. Image Anal.* **2021**, *69*, 101971. [CrossRef]
52. Esfahani, M.T.; Ghaderi, M.; Kafiyeh, R. Classification of diabetic and normal fundus images using new deep learning method. *Leonardo Electron. J. Pract. Technol.* **2018**, *17*, 233–248.
53. Dutta, S.; Manideep, B.C.; Basha, S.M.; Caytiles, R.D.; Iyengar, N.C.S.N. Classification of Diabetic Retinopathy Images by Using Deep Learning Models. *Int. J. Grid Distrib. Comput.* **2018**, *11*, 99–106. [CrossRef]
54. Zhou, M.; Jin, K.; Wang, S.; Ye, J.; Qian, D. Color Retinal Image Enhancement Based on Luminosity and Contrast Adjustment. *IEEE Trans. Biomed. Eng.* **2018**, *65*, 521–527. [CrossRef] [PubMed]
55. Pisano, E.D.; Zong, S.; Hemminger, B.M.; Deluca, M.; Johnston, R.E.; Muller, K.; Braeuning, M.P.; Pizer, S.M. Contrast Limited Adaptive Histogram Equalization Image Processing to Improve the Detection of Simulated Spiculations in Dense Mammograms. *J. Digit. Imaging* **1998**, *11*, 193–200. [CrossRef]
56. Zuiderveld, K. Contrast Limited Adaptive Histogram Equalization. *Graph. Gems IV* **1994**, 474–485. [CrossRef]
57. Sonali.; Sahu, S.; Singh, A.K.; Ghrera, S.; Elhoseny, M. An approach for de-noising and contrast enhancement of retinal fundus image using CLAHE. *Optics Laser Technol.* **2019**, *110*, 87–98. [CrossRef]
58. Pratt, H.; Coenen, F.; Broadbent, D.M.; Harding, S.P.; Zheng, Y. Convolutional Neural Networks for Diabetic Retinopathy. *Procedia Comput. Sci.* **2016**, *90*, 200–205. [CrossRef]
59. Ketkar, N. *Deep Learning with Python*; Springer: Berlin/Heidelberg, Germany, 2017; pp. 1–235. [CrossRef]
60. Shalash, W.M. Driver Fatigue Detection with Single EEG Channel Using Transfer Learning. In Proceedings of the 2019 IEEE International Conference on Imaging Systems and Techniques (IST), Abu Dhabi, United Arab Emirates, 9–10 December 2019.
61. COVER, T.; HART, P.. Nearest Neighbor Pattern Classfication. *IEEE Trans. Inf. Theory* **1967**, *13*, 21–27. [CrossRef]
62. Keras. Available online: https://keras.io/ (accessed on 1 January 2019).
63. Lee, W.Y.; Park, S.M.; Sim, K.B. Optimal hyperparameter tuning of convolutional neural networks based on the parameter-setting-free harmony search algorithm. *Optik* **2018**, *172*, 359–367. [CrossRef]
64. Bergstra, J.; Bengio, Y. Random search for hyper-parameter optimization. *J. Mach. Learn. Res.* **2012**, *13*, 281–305
65. Huang, Q.; Mao, J.; Liu, Y. An improved grid search algorithm of SVR parameters optimization. In Proceedings of the 2012 IEEE 14th International Conference on Communication Technology, Chengdu, China, 9–11 November 2012; pp. 1022–1026.
66. Maclaurin, D.; Duvenaud, D.; Adams, R. Gradient-based hyperparameter optimization through reversible learning. In Proceedings of the International Conference on Machine Learning, PMLR, Lille, France, 7–9 July 2015; pp. 2113–2122.
67. Smith, L.N. Cyclical learning rates for training neural networks. In Proceedings of the IEEE Winter Conference on Applications of Computer Vision, WACV 2017, Santa Rosa, CA, USA, 24–31 March 2017; pp. 464–472. [CrossRef]
68. Ahn, S.; Pham, Q.; Shin, J.; Song, S.J. Future Image Synthesis for Diabetic Retinopathy Based on the Lesion Occurrence Probability. *Electronics* **2021**, *10*, 726. [CrossRef]
69. Anton, N.; Dragoi, E.N.; Tarcoveanu, F.; Ciuntu, R.E.; Lisa, C.; Curteanu, S.; Doroftei, B.; Ciuntu, B.M.; Chiseliţă, D.; Bogdănici, C.M. Assessing Changes in Diabetic Retinopathy Caused by Diabetes Mellitus and Glaucoma Using Support Vector Machines in Combination with Differential Evolution Algorithm. *Appl. Sci.* **2021**, *11*, 3944. [CrossRef]
70. Aziz Computer. Available online: http://hpc.kau.edu.sa (accessed on 1 January 2019).

sensors

MDPI

Article

Novel MRI-Based CAD System for Early Detection of Thyroid Cancer Using Multi-Input CNN

Ahmed Naglah [1], Fahmi Khalifa [1], Reem Khaled [2], Ahmed Abdel Khalek Abdel Razek [2], Mohammad Ghazal [3], Guruprasad Giridharan [1] and Ayman El-Baz [1,*]

[1] Department of Bioengineering, University of Louisville, Louisville, KY 40292, USA; ahmed.naglah@louisville.edu (A.N.); fakhal01@louisville.edu (F.K.); guruprasad.giridharan@louisville.edu (G.G.)
[2] Faculty of Medicine, Mansoura University, Mansoura 35516, Egypt; reemkhaled@mans.edu.eg (R.K.); arazek@mans.edu.eg (A.A.K.A.R.)
[3] Electrical and Computer Engineering Department, Abu Dhabi University, Abu Dhabi 59911, United Arab Emirates; mohammed.ghazal@adu.ac.ae
* Correspondence: ayman.elbaz@louisville.edu

Abstract: Early detection of thyroid nodules can greatly contribute to the prediction of cancer burdening and the steering of personalized management. We propose a novel multimodal MRI-based computer-aided diagnosis (CAD) system that differentiates malignant from benign thyroid nodules. The proposed CAD is based on a novel convolutional neural network (CNN)-based texture learning architecture. The main contribution of our system is three-fold. Firstly, our system is the first of its kind to combine T2-weighted MRI and apparent diffusion coefficient (ADC) maps using a CNN to model thyroid cancer. Secondly, it learns independent texture features for each input, giving it more advanced capabilities to simultaneously extract complex texture patterns from both modalities. Finally, the proposed system uses multiple channels for each input to combine multiple scans collected into the deep learning process using different values of the configurable diffusion gradient coefficient. Accordingly, the proposed system would enable the learning of more advanced radiomics with an additional advantage of visualizing the texture patterns after learning. We evaluated the proposed system using data collected from a cohort of 49 patients with pathologically proven thyroid nodules. The accuracy of the proposed system has also been compared against recent CNN models as well as multiple machine learning (ML) frameworks that use hand-crafted features. Our system achieved the highest performance among all compared methods with a diagnostic accuracy of 0.87, specificity of 0.97, and sensitivity of 0.69. The results suggest that texture features extracted using deep learning can contribute to the protocols of cancer diagnosis and treatment and can lead to the advancement of precision medicine.

Keywords: thyroid; cancer; CNN; MRI; DWI; radiomics

Citation: Naglah, A.; Khalifa, F.; Khaled, R.; Abdel Razek, A.A.K.; Ghazal, M.; Giridharan, G.; El-Baz, A. Novel MRI-Based CAD System for Early Detection of Thyroid Cancer Using Multi-Input CNN. *Sensors* **2021**, *21*, 3878. https://doi.org/10.3390/s21113878

Academic Editor: Loris Nanni

Received: 3 May 2021
Accepted: 2 June 2021
Published: 4 June 2021

Publisher's Note: MDPI stays neutral with regard to jurisdictional claims in published maps and institutional affiliations.

1. Introduction

In the United States, approximately 52,890 new cases of thyroid cancer and about 2180 deaths were estimated in 2020 according to the American Cancer Society's most recent statistics [1]. The prevalence of thyroid nodules is approximately 5% in women and 1% in men [2]. Among the cases of thyroid nodules, 7–15% evolve into malignant tumors (cancerous tissue), and this rate depends on age, sex, radiation exposure history, family history, and other factors [2]. Malignant tumors can be classified into three major categories: Differentiated thyroid cancer (DTC), medullary thyroid cancer, and anaplastic thyroid cancer. DTC has the biggest share of thyroid cancer, with a share of more than 90%. DTC includes two main subcategories: papillary thyroid carcinoma (PTC) and follicular thyroid carcinoma (FTC). PTC accounts for more than 80% of all thyroid cancers [2].

The diagnostic criteria of thyroid nodules involve different procedures that include physical examination, blood test, ultrasound (US) imaging, magnetic resonance imaging (MRI), and a biopsy procedure. The detection of smaller nodules becomes easier over time due to the current advances in US and MRI. However, cancer diagnosis and early stratification of nodules is still challenging and mainly performed using biopsy [2]. Although biopsy, either fine-needle aspiration or surgical excision of the nodule, is still the definitive way of clinical evaluation, this invasive procedure is costly and may introduce a false negative error depending on the biopsy technique and the size of the nodule being aspirated [3–6].

Non-invasive-based approaches have been proposed by several researchers to provide accurate detection and stratification of thyroid cancer [7–10]. These methods utilize different types of medical images. The type of imaging technology used as an input to artificial intelligence (AI) algorithms can affects the accuracy of the desired computer-aided diagnosis (CAD) system. US imaging is currently used as a first-line evaluation of suspected thyroid nodules [2], and specific features of thyroid nodules in US imaging can be associated with higher risk of malignancy. However, the appearance of those features in US images is operator-dependent, and also multiple features need to be considered simultaneously during the evaluation in order to provide sufficient malignancy diagnostic power [2]. These factors cause various limitations in AI-based systems that use US images for thyroid nodule classification [7–9]. Compared to US, MR imaging modalities have also been used in the literature recently. For instance, T1-weighted MRI and T2-weighted MRI were used in a recent study to perform thyroid nodule classification [10]. Some MRI modalities can help distinguish between different substances in the tissue. For example, fats appear bright in T1-weighted MRI images [11], while fluids appear bright in T2-weighted MRI images. Studying T2-weighted MRI images can help in the modeling of fluid patterns in the tissue [12]. Over and above that, diffusion-weighted MRI (DWI) can model the diffusivity of fluids in the tissue by measuring constraints of fluid diffusion in different directions [13,14]. Therefore, DWI can model the dynamics of fluids in the tissue, and these dynamics can be presented by computing the apparent diffusion coefficient (ADC).

The cell proliferation process associated with malignant thyroid nodules can have a significant effect on the patterns and the dynamics of the extracellular matrix (ECM) in the thyroid tissue. Studies suggest that statistical analysis between ADC value and T2-weighted images, and therefore can differentiate between malignant and benign nodules [15–17]. Thus, in the preliminary analysis of our work, we examined if the intensity variations between malignant and benign groups are significantly different or not, see Figure 1. To achieve this, we employed a statistical analysis test to determine the differences between the two groups as observed in each of the T2-weighted images and the ADC maps (three different gradient coefficients were used to generate the ADC maps). Our analysis showed significant heterogeneity in intensity variance between T2-weighted images and ADC maps, which suggests that feeding the T2-weighted images and the ADC maps each to a separate input branch of the CNN would enables learning of independent textures in each branch and therefore this would enhance the accuracy of our system.

Inspired by our preliminary statistical analysis results, our initial exploratory work [18], and other studies [15–17], we propose a novel CNN-based CAD system that integrate T2-weighted images and ADC maps using a multi-input CNN network for thyroid nodules detection and classification, see Figure 2. Our work is in contrast to one recent study that proposed a CNN-based system using multimodel MRI but does not include ADC maps [10]. ADC maps can be considered as an indication of cell density in tissues [19] and therefore can be used to search for cancer biomarkers, which usually involve high rates of cell proliferation. Similar to a recent study [20] that uses multiparametric MRI radiomics for prediction, we use a CNN-based structure instead of hand-crafted features—namely, we utilize a process of independent convolutions for ADC and DWI before fusing them using the dense fully connected layer. This process increases the possibility to detect deep texture patterns from each modality without loosing the capability for automatic searching for visual features, provided by the CNN. Our system integrates multiple ADC maps obtained from different gradient coefficients (a configurable parameter in the MRI scanner) for each sample. Then, the combination of all inputs is fed to our CNN model as a multichannel 3D input in order to achieve enhanced learning of texture features, thus providing a more accurate diagnosis.

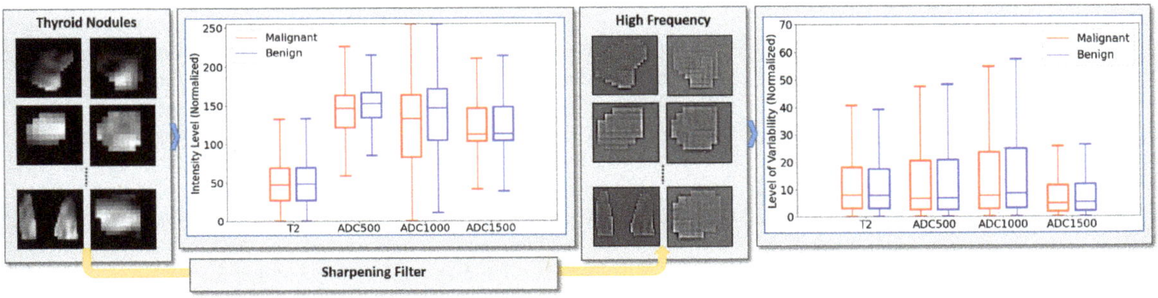

Figure 1. Illustrative diagram of the preliminary statistical study performed on our dataset. A high-pass Laplacian spacial filter was applied to the images to estimate intensity variation at the pixel level. Following that, statistical analysis was performed to calculate the mean difference between malignant and benign nodules.

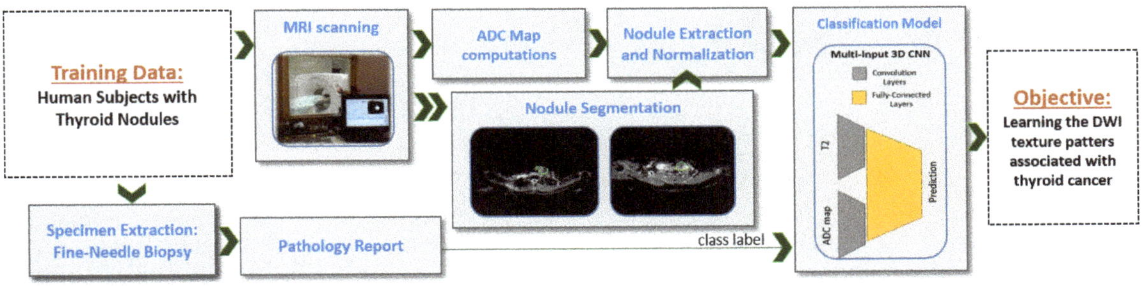

Figure 2. Schematic diagram that represents the training pipeline for the proposed system. MRI data were collected from human subject cohort. ADC maps were computed in order to prepare the two inputs for the CNN. The objective of the proposed system was to learn the texture patterns in DWI images and correlate them with pathological finding.

2. Materials and Methods

2.1. Study Participants and Data Collection

Data were collected in this study from 49 patients with pathologically proven thyroid nodules. The age range is 25 to 70 years. Imaging of the thyroid gland was performed at Mansoura University, Egypt with a 1.5 T Ingenia MR scanner (Philips Medical Systems, Best, Netherlands) using a head/neck circular polarization surface coil. All participants were fully informed about the aims of the study and provided their informed consent. The inclusion criteria for the study were untreated patients with thyroid nodules whose malignancy status was unclear from ultrasound examination. Patients underwent thyroid core biopsy or surgery after MR imaging. Histopathologic diagnoses were provided by an experienced cytologist or pathologist. In total, there are 17 malignant nodules in 17 patients and 40 benign nodules in 32 patients included in our study.

DWI volumes that employ a multislice, single-shot, spin-echo, echo-planar imaging sequence with TR = 10,000 ms, TE = 108 ms, and 125 kHz bandwidth were extracted. Axial diffusion-weighted slices over the region of interest were 5 mm thick with an inter-slice gap of 1 mm, 25 cm or 30 cm FOV, and 256 $\times$ 256 acquisition matrix. For DWI, a diffusion gradient was applied during scanning with *b*-values of $b = 500$ s/mm^2, $b = 1000$ s/mm^2, and $b = 1500$ s/mm^2. T2-weighted images are extracted using b-value of $b = 0$ s/mm^2.

2.2. ADC Map Calculation and Nodule Segmentation

Multiple steps were applied to the collected MR images in order to prepare the dataset to be used by the training model, see Figure 2. Nodule segmentation was performed manually in our study. An experienced radiologist segmented each nodule as it appeared in each T2-weighted slice ($b = 0$ s/mm^2) and in each DWI slice. Diffusion-weighted MRI scans were taken in the same session and using the same resolution, number of slices, and inter-slice gap. Therefore, no registration was applied to align the different b-values. We have future plans to implement an automated segmentation algorithm for nodule extraction. The produced manual segmentation was stored in the form of binary images. The binary image produced from DWI slice with $b = 0$ s/mm^2 was re-used during processing phases on the corresponding slice at all other b-values, and also was re-used for the corresponding slice at ADC500, ADC1000, and ADC1500. We extracted each nodule in both T2-weighted images and ADC maps using a square-bounding box. We regularized the spatial domain by resizing extracted box into unified $48 \times 48 \times 20$ volumes by adding zero-padding channels. We then normalized the voxel-intensity in that volume to be in 0–1 range. Each segmented nodule was provided for the network model on a black background and padding. Apparent diffusion coefficients (ADC maps) were calculated at each non-zero b-value (500, 1000, and 1500) by combining the diffusion images at the corresponding b-value with the image at $b = 0$ s/mm^2, and then we substituted, at the voxel level, this into the Stejskal–Tanner equation [21]. The generated images of this process are referred to as ADC500, ADC1000, and ADC1500. Since diffusion-weighted MRI (DW-MRI) as an absolute value usually does not reflect direct biological activity, the relative differences between DW-MRI at different b-values were used instead (i.e., ADC) to model the diffusivity in the tissue. Usually, a b-value of 0 is taken as reference, and which is why we computed three ADC values that correspond to 3 b-values of 500, 1000, and 1500 referenced to a b-value of 0.

2.3. Proposed Learning Model: Multi-Input CNN

To build our diagnostic system, we propose a novel multi-input deep-learning network. Our architecture follows the feed-forward convolutional neural network (CNN) structure. Our implementation uses the Keras package in Python, and the parameters used in our training model are summarized in Table 1. The proposed architecture, shown in Figure 3, consists of two identical branches in the structure. The advantages of our network compared with others is that the generated kernels are governed by the fusion of T2-weighted images and ADC maps of the training samples during the forward propagation and backward propagation of our neural network. Additionally, a $1 \times 1 \times 1$ *3Dconv* layer was added to the proposed design in order to perform compression for the features maps. The advantage of this addition is that the number of weights that needs to be learned during the training phase is extremely minmized, thus ensuring fast learning and diagnosis. For the analysis, each of the base images and the ADC maps was fed to the respective branch. The convolution layers were constructed from $3 \times 3 \times 3$ *3Dconv* (with 32 filters and $3 \times 3 \times 3$ kernel size), $1 \times 1 \times 1$ *3Dconv* (with 16 filters and $1 \times 1 \times 1$ kernel size), pooling block ($2 \times 2 \times 1$ pool size, maximum value pooling). Each branch had two convolution blocks before being concatenated into the dense fully connected layers (2 layers). Those layers were one hidden layer of 10 neurons with ReLU activation function [22] and one output layer of 1 neuron with sigmoid activation function [23]. The total number of parameters in our proposed network is 127,829 parameters.

The condition of unbalanced classes during the training phase was handled by configuring the weights in the mean-square error (MSE) loss function we used in the back propagation of the network. The ratio of the weight of malignant class to the weight of benign class was set to 16/32 when leaving out one malignant sample for testing, and the same ratio was set to 17/31 when leaving-out one benign sample for testing. The loss function used is given in Equation (1), where N is the number of training samples, y is the output of the neural network observed during forward propagation, y_i is the label of the sample, and w_i is the weight of each training sample.

$$Loss = \frac{1}{N} \sum_{i=0}^{N} w_i (y - y_i)^2 \tag{1}$$

We used Adam stochastic to update the parameters of the network during learning [24]. The learning rate and other parameters of the optimizer were tuned and kept constant during our evaluation. Additionally, we used the ratio of 1 to 3 of the samples as validation data during the learning phase.

Table 1. Summary of the network parameters used during model training.

Parameter	Value
Kernel Size	$3 \times 3 \times 3$
Number of Convolution Kernels	32
Number of 1×1 Kernels	16
Fully Connected Layers	2
Convolutional Layers	2
Activation	ReLU
Pooling Size	$2 \times 2 \times 2$
Pooling	MaxPooling
Number of Epochs	100
Input Shape	$48 \times 48 \times 20$

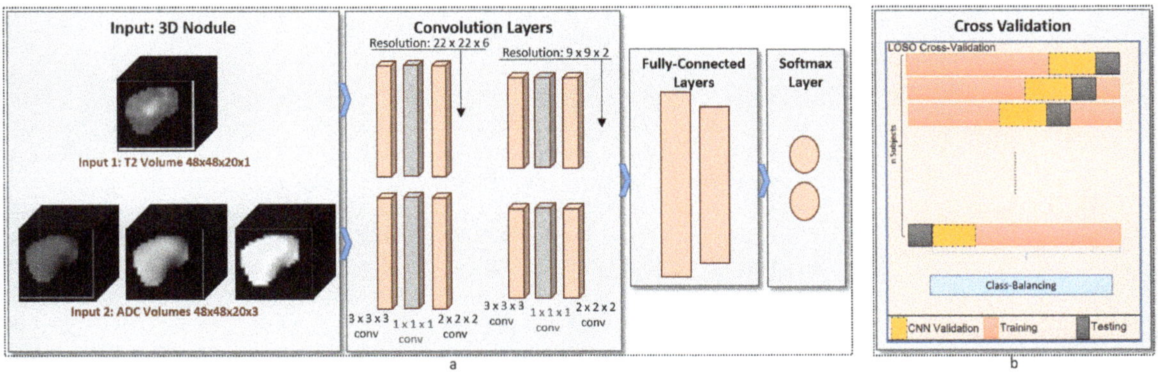

Figure 3. (**a**) Schematic diagram of the proposed CAD system that shows the design and the layers of the multi-input 3D CNN deep-learning framework. (**b**) Illustrative diagram that shows the cross-validation criteria used in our processing.

2.4. Other Learning Models

In order to perform bench-marking for our system, we compared its performance with other methods. We first compared the results with ML methods that use hand-crafted features, and then we compared the results with two state-of-the-art CNN models. Regarding the first comparison, the used hand-crafted features can be classified into three groups: shape features, statistical features, and hand-crafted texture patterns features. Starting with the shape features, we used nodule size (in voxels), convex hull ratio (defined as the ratio between the nodule size and the convex hull size), bounding rectangle ratio (defined as the ratio between the nodule size and the bounding rectangle size), and spherical harmonics of 3D contour encapsulating the nodules. We estimated the spherical harmonics inspired by [25] by the use of infinite set of harmonic functions defined on a spherical representation. They arise from solving the angular portion of Laplace's equation in spherical coordinates using separation of variables. The degree of the spherical harmonics can define the level of non-homogeneity of the surface, and we can map this to the ability to differentiate between malignant and benign nodules.

For the statistical features, we calculated the histogram of each image, and then in each histogram we summarized their statistical profile using 5 features (mean, standard deviation, entropy, skewness, kurtosis). This type of features is designed to summarize the whole image by presenting it using certain values. The overall appearance of thyroid nodule can reflect the first impression by experienced radiologists while examining the MRI scan. Finally, for the hand-crafted texture patterns we built a filter-bank of 9 filters to evaluate intensity variations between neighbor voxels. The used filter-bank is designed to capture edges in 4 orientations, lines in 4 orientations, and the point response (all-directions variability). The four orientations are horizontal, vertical and 2 diagonal orientations.

All features from the three hand-crafted features groups were evaluated for malignancy detection capability using four different classifiers: decision tree (DT) [26], random forest (RF) [27], Naive Bayes (NB) [28] and support vector machine (SVM) [29]. The classification models used in the benchmark were optimized to ensure appropriate comparison. In DT, min sample split was examined. In RF, number of estimators and maximum depth were examined. In SVM, C parameter is examined to tune the soft margin.

In addition to traditional ML methods, we compared our methods accuracy against other CNN-based methods. For bench marking purpose, we used two state-of-the-art CNN models for detection; AlexNet [30] and ResNet18 [31]. AlexNet is chosen as it is the first deep learning computer vision to be recognized as a classification-winner of ILSVRC [32] back in 2012. ResNet is chosen because it is the first ILSVRC winner that overachieve human accuracy in classification under different appearance conditions [33]. For both methods, we used Keras implementations in Python with the default configuration. AlexNet and ResNet were applied to the combined T2-ADC input in the form of multiple input channels.

2.5. Evaluation Criteria

The evaluation criteria of our system use a leave-one-out cross-validation. We kept the common network configuration fixed for our reported results, including the ablation study, as well as when compared with other techniques. The proposed system evaluation is based on four classification metrics: accuracy, precision, recall, and dice coefficient.

Additionally, further evaluation of the system robustness has been conducted using the the receiver operating characteristics (ROC) analysis curve. The ROC curve is a plot between the false positive rate and the true positive rate when we adjust the decision threshold. Figure 4c shows ROCs of the proposed multi-input CNN framework compared to the other frameworks discussed in this section. The area under the curve (AUC) of the voting between two CNNs gives slightly higher value, but our system achieved the best AUC compared with all other methods.

For the purpose of this analysis, the slice at which each thyroid nodule appears with biggest size was extracted and processed as a 2D image for each of T2-weighted image and ADC maps. Local intensity variations were modeled by high-pass filtering using a 3×3 Laplacian filter invariant to 45° rotations [34]. Tumor pixels were grouped into benign and malignant groups (35,625 and 15,764 pixels, respectively). Supported by the high number of samples, a Welch two-sample t-test was applied to determine difference the mean between groups. A statistical package in R was used to generate the results.

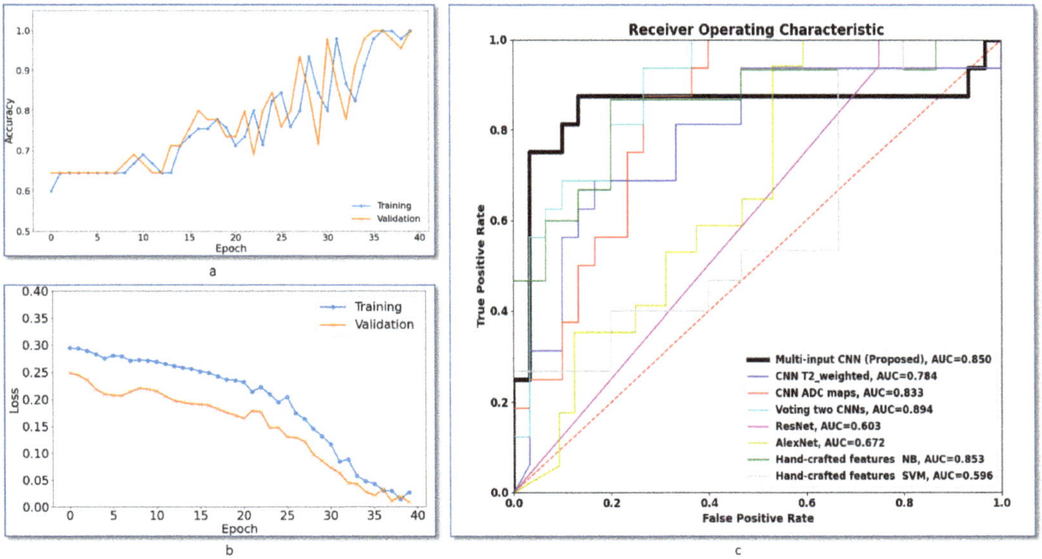

Figure 4. (**a**) Training versus validation accuracy curves with the number of epochs during network training. (**b**) Training versus validation loss curves with the number of epochs during network training. (**c**) Receiver operating characteristic curves (ROCs) of the proposed multi-input CNN framework compared to other methods. AUC is the area under the curve."DT"—Decision Tree. "RF"—random forest; "NB"—Naive Bayes; "SVM"—support vector machine.

2.6. Nodule Texture Visualization

Achieved kernels applied to each of the T2-weighted images and the ADC maps were extracted from CNN network after the last epoch of training cycles. The extracted kernels are converted from the 3D to 2D form by averaging the 3 depth channels. The kernels were then clustered using hierarchical agglomerative clustering [35,36]. Silhouette score was used for evaluating the fit of the estimated clusters [37]. The Sklearn package in Python was used for both clustering processing and evaluation.

3. Experimental Results

The overall proposed framework is depicted in Figure 3. In this section, we present our results, which include: (1) preliminary statistical analysis, (2) the performance of the proposed CAD system compared to other machine learning models that use hand-crafted features, (3) the performance of the proposed CAD system compared to state-of-the-art CNN models, and (4) the results obtained of analyzing the texture patterns after learning.

3.1. Significant Differences in T2 and ADC Local Intensity Variations between Malignant and Benign Groups

The results of analyzing local intensity variations in each of the T2-weighted images and the ADC maps show that there is a significant difference in the mean of those variations between benign and malignant groups. Table 2 presents the results obtained from the Welch two-sample t-test that shows a significant difference with $p < 0.05$. Table 2 also presents the achieved t value and the 95% confidence interval (CI). The CI values are normalized with respect to the standard deviation (SD) of the benign group. By observing the sign of CI, the malignant group has higher mean observed in T2-weighted images while the benign group has a higher mean in ADC maps. This result suggests that having convolution filters of T2-weighted images that are independent from those of ADC maps enables conducting enhanced texture-learning process. Convolution filters map the conv kernels in our proposed CNN architecture.

Table 2. Statistical analysis results for the Welch *t*-test on the pixel-level intensity variations between the malignant and benign groups.

	Welch Two-Sample *t*-Test		
MRI Parameter	**CI Δmean**	*t*	*p*
T2	−4% to −1%	−2.28	0.023
ADC500	5% to 9%	7.87	<0.001
ADC1000	26% to 34%	14.87	<0.001
ADC1500	4% to 8%	6.12	<0.001

3.2. Comparison with ML Methods That Use Hand-Crafted Features

The results are summarized in Table 3. As can be seen, the proposed multi-input CNN system outperform all compared classifiers. Our proposed CAD system achieved the best performance when compared to machine learning models that are based on hand-crafted features. Our system achieved an AUC of 0.85 compared to 0.59 when using linear support vector machine (SVM) classifier, see Figure 4c. Additionally, it achieved an accuracy, sensitivity, and specificity of 0.87, 0.69, and 0.97, respectively, compared to an 0.77, 0.67 and 0.77 when using random forest (RF) classifier, which achieved the best accuracy among the pool of classifiers used with hand-crafted features. The results in Table 3 show that using automatic feature selection by the aid of CNN helps in achieving better diagnostic accuracy.

Table 3. Comparative performance for the proposed multi-input CNN system and machine learning methods that use hand-crafted features. "DT"—Decision Tree. "RF"—Random Forest; "NB"—Naive Bayes; "SVM"—Support Vector Machine.

	Evaluation Metrics			
Method	**Accuracy**	**Sensitivity**	**Specificity**	**Dice Coefficient**
DT classifier	0.70	0.66	0.70	0.57
NB classifier	0.76	0.73	0.77	0.63
RF classifier	0.77	0.67	0.77	0.53
SVM classifier	0.56	0.40	0.73	0.48
Proposed Multi-Input CNN	0.87	0.69	0.97	0.79

3.3. Comparison with State-of-the-Art CNNs

In addition to the comparison with the handcrafted-based ML approaches, comparison against other state of the arts CNN models have been conducted. The comparative results, shown in Table 4 also showed that the proposed CAD system achieved the best diagnostic performance. It is worth mentioning that our system has relatively low number of layers compared to the compared models. It achieved an AUC of 0.85 compared to 0.67 and 0.60 obtained using AlexNet and ResNet 18, respectively. Additionally, it achieved an accuracy of 0.87, sensitivity of 0.69 and specificity of 0.97. The accuracy, sensitivity and specificity using AlexNet were 0.61, 0.53, and 0.66, respectively, and those obtained using ResNet18 are 0.49, 1.00 and 0.22, respectively. Results document that using lower number of CNN layers can achieve better diagnostic accuracy, which is considered an advantage of the proposed method compare with other CNN-based techniques.

3.4. Texture Features of T2-Weighted Images Are Visually Different Compared to ADC Maps

The convolution kernels (filters) extracted from the CNN after learning were clustered, see Figure 5a, and the clustering process was repeated for multiple runs each with different number of target clusters $k = 2, 4, 5, ..., 9$. Figure 5b shows the evaluation of the generated clusters using the Silhouette score. The clusters generated from the T2-weighted kernels (green curve) achieved better clusters compared to ADC kernels (blue curve). Additionally, $k = 3$ achieved the highest score in both T2-weighted and ADC images. Figure 5c,d show the visualization of the generated clusters of T2-weighted and ADC kernels, respectively.

The runs (with the corresponding number of clusters, or k) are represented on the y-axis. Each row includes the generated clusters of the corresponding run, and the cluster index inside each run is presented on the x-axis. Each cluster is illustrated by the mean of its member kernels, and then each mean is normalized from 0 to 1. A gray-scale visualization of each normalized mean is presented (at each row-column position) using a 3×3 board image in a way that 0–1 is mapped to a white–black gradient.

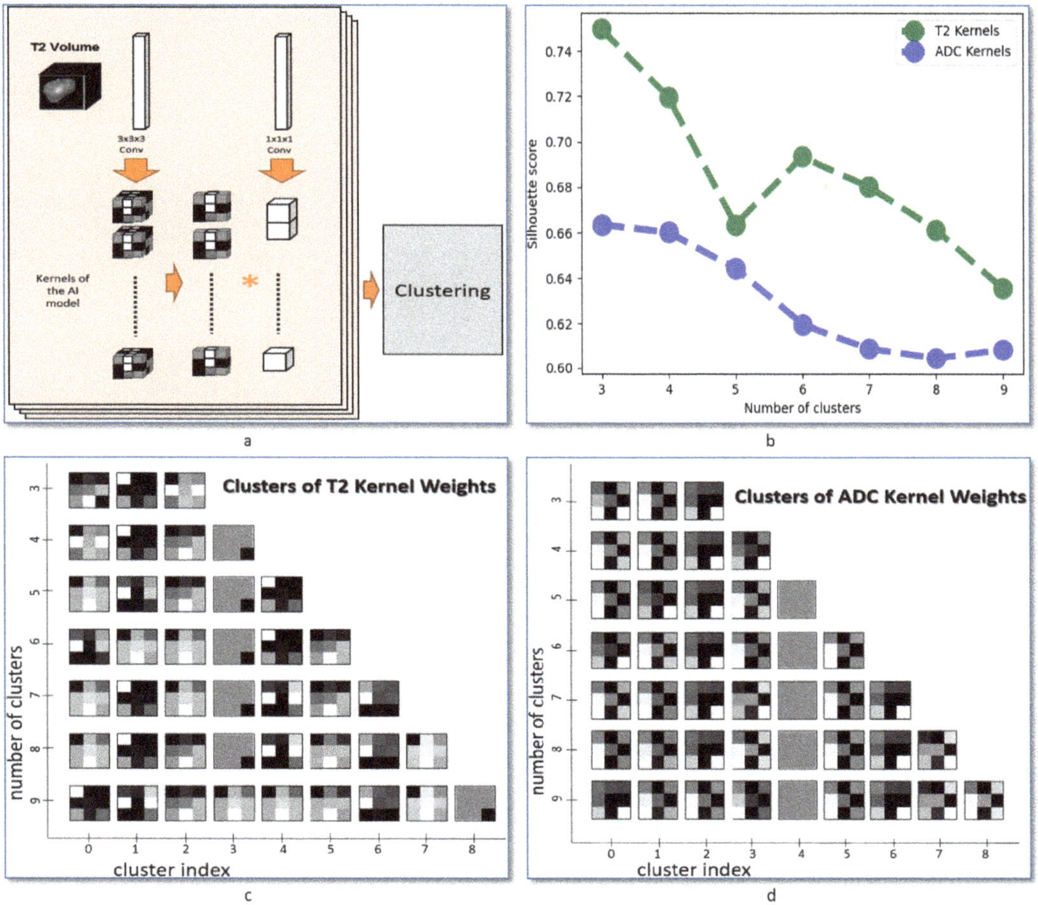

Figure 5. Analysis of the patterns extracted from the CNN after training phase. (**a**) Illustrative diagram of the process of extracting the kernels from the weights of each layer, and the processing of those kernels using a clustering technique (hierarchical agglomerative clustering) in order to analyze the patterns found in T2-weighted MRI images and ADC maps. (**b**) Evaluation metric of the clustering algorithm by computing Silhouette score while varying the number of clusters in the clustering algorithm. (**c**) Visualization of the results of our analysis on the features extracted from T2-weighted images. (**d**) Visualization of the results of our analysis on the features extracted from ADC maps. We can notice that the texture patterns that distinguish between malignant and benign thyroid nodules are having a degree of heterogeneity according to this visualization.

Table 4. Comparative performance of the proposed multi-input CNN system with state-of-the-art CNN-based classification.

	Evaluation Metrics			
Method	**Accuracy**	**Sensitivity**	**Specificity**	**Dice Coefficient**
AlexNet	0.61	0.53	0.66	0.49
ResNet18	0.49	1.00	0.22	0.58
Proposed Multi-Input CNN	0.87	0.69	0.97	0.79

4. Discussion and Conclusions

We proposed a new CAD system to distinguish between malignant and benign thyroid nodules. The main contributions of the proposed pipeline is the use of multi-input CNN that can detect texture patterns from each input independently. The first branch of our CNN models the fluids patterns in the thyroid tissue by learning the texture patterns in T2-weighted MRI images. The second branch of our CNN models the dynamics of tissue fluids by learning the texture patterns in ADC maps. We validated our method by applying leave-one-out cross-validation on multimodal data collected from 49 patients with pathologically confirmed nodules. We compared the classification accuracy obtained from our system with other ML and deep learning approaches. Experimental results from our system surpass results obtained from other models.

To assess the advantage of integrating multiple MRI modalities as separate inputs of the proposed network, we conducted a preliminary study that shows heterogeneity in the intensity variation between malignant and benign samples. In this experiment, a Welch two-sample *t*-test was used to assess the significant difference in mean variation between the two groups (Table 2) across all modalities. The difference in mean between the two groups in T2-weighted images has an opposite sign when compared to the corresponding difference in ADC maps (Table 2). This also suggests that using independent features in each input can enable finding more optimal features.

To assess the performance of our system, we compared it to other ML methods that use hand-crafted features. In the comparison, we used three categories of hand-crafted features. The first category is based on the statistical profile of image intensity. We evaluated that statistical profile using five features (mean, standard deviation, entropy, skewness, kurtosis). This category is designed to summarize the whole image by presenting it using the profile of each features. The overall appearance of the tumor can reflect the first impression by the physician while examining the MRI scan. The linear SVM classifier exhibited the worst performance, which suggests a lack of a linear border between classes. Results of the NB classifier showed the possibility of having a fairly distinguished statistical distribution of the hand-crafted features extracted from benign and malignant nodules. In order to benchmark our system, Figure 4c shows ROCs of the proposed multi-input CNN framework compared to the other systems under comparison. As demonstrated, the area under the curve (AUC) of our system is higher compared with all compared methods, which highlights the higher accuracy of our method. Figure 4a,b show the training versus validation accuracy and loss curves during the model training. Overall, the results showed that handcrafted features failed to provide a good modeling of our classification problem, and this suggests having multi-input CNNs that learn from paired features can enhance diagnostic accuracy of the CAD system.

To further support our method, an ablation study has been conducted to assess the accuracy of the proposed method. The study shows that the proposed fusion using multi-input CNN outperformed single-input frameworks. In that study, a single input CNN with the same structure was built and evaluated. Four scenarios were evaluated. Scenarios 1 and 2 use T2-weighted images and ADC maps, respectively. Scenario 3 uses a probability voting scheme between the prediction of scenarios 1 and 2. We used the following equation to acquire the resultant probability after voting: $P_v = \frac{1}{2}(P_{T2_{Weighted}} + P_{ADC})$. Scenario 4 uses a single input that combines T2-weighted images and ADC maps in the input channels.

Results obtained from the four scenarios are shown in Table 5. Using a multi-input CNN enhances the classification accuracy. The two-CNN voting scenario showed high specificity, but a low accuracy, sensitivity and dice coefficient compared to the proposed method. This ablation study suggests that having independent features for each input can enhance the detection performance of the CAD system.

Table 5. Ablation study results for the proposed system.

	Evaluation Metrics			
Method	**Accuracy**	**Sensitivity**	**Specificity**	**Dice Coefficient**
Single-Input CNN (T2-Weighted only)	0.76	0.56	0.87	0.62
Single-Input CNN (ADC only)	0.72	0.63	0.77	0.61
Two-CNN voting (base-images + ADC)	0.83	0.63	0.93	0.71
Multi-Input CNN (Proposed Method)	0.87	0.69	0.97	0.79

The main focus of this study is to investigate the ability to extract the texture features associated with thyroid cancer by combining the texture in two input CNN with two independent branches. The network was designed to minimize the number of layers in order to extract the texture patterns that can be linked to the anatomical structure in the nodules. This optimized architecture also supports fast processing, which can enable further integration with MRI scanner devices to present the visual features automatically extracted from MRI images. As a follow-up step in our study to evaluate the heterogeneity of texture features between MRI modalities, we applied a method to extract and cluster the learned features for each modality. An illustration is presented in Figure 5a and the obtained feature visualization in each input is presented in Figure 5c,d. That visualization suggests a heterogeneity in texture patterns between MRI modalities and supports the use of our method for thyroid nodule classification.

Our system yielded promising results. However, there are some limitations that need to be addressed in order to go forward with further clinical trials. The number of samples is limited under the scope of our study, and the results can reflect the pattern that exists in this cohort. Our model needs to be applied to another cohort with a higher number of subjects in order to assess the homogeneity of texture across cohorts. More samples can be collected to sufficiently cover the full spectrum of thyroid cancer.

In total, this paper shows that extracting texture patterns using deep learning can improve the diagnostic performance and can help in performing accurate diagnosis of thyroid cancer. For future work, our experiments can be applied to bigger cohort. Additionally, our model can be adapted to perform classification of the types of thyroid cancer. It can be also adapted to perform staging of thyroid cancer. Other modalities can be added to the model to study the heterogeneity of MRI texture patterns in a more advanced way. Our model can also be adapted to study the texture patterns of thyroid tissues while using other imaging techniques such as US. Although, US can provide a limited capability of modeling thyroid cancer compared to MRI, having a model that combines US and MRI can contribute to establishing more accurate models to ensure precise and personalized medicine.

Data collection can be also expanded to collect multiple scan from each subject in a different time points. By doing this, we can study the correlation between DWI patterns and the patterns of the cell proliferation process, which is associated with thyroid nodules at different stages of thyroid cancer.

Author Contributions: Conceptualization and formal analysis: A.N., F.K., R.K., A.A.K.A.R., M.G., G.G. and A.E.-B.; methodology: A.N., F.K., M.G., G.G. and A.E.-B.; software development: A.N.; validation and visualization: A.A.K.A.R., F.K. and A.E.-B.; initial draft: A.N., F.K. and R.K.; resources, data collection, and data curation: A.A.K.A.R. and R.K.; review and editing: M.G., G.G., A.A.K.A.R. and A.E.-B.; project administration: A.E.-B.; project directors: A.E.-B. and A.A.K.A.R. All authors have read and agreed to the published version of the manuscript.

Funding: This research received no external funding.

Institutional Review Board Statement: The study was conducted according to the guidelines of the Declaration of Helsinki and approved by the Institutional Review Board of Mansoura University (protocol code 18.12.389 and date of approval 15 December 2018).

Informed Consent Statement: Informed consent was obtained from all subjects involved in the study.

Data Availability Statement: Requests made to the corresponding author will be addressed and the available data can be provided.

Conflicts of Interest: The authors declare no conflict of interest.

References

1. Society, A.C. *Cancer Facts and Figures 2020*; American Cancer Society: Atlanta, GA, USA, 2020.
2. Haugen, B.R.; Alexander, E.K.; Bible, K.C.; Doherty, G.M.; Mandel, S.J.; Nikiforov, Y.E.; Pacini, F.; Randolph, G.W.; Sawka, A.M.; Schlumberger, M.; et al. 2015 American Thyroid Association management guidelines for adult patients with thyroid nodules and differentiated thyroid cancer: The American Thyroid Association guidelines task force on thyroid nodules and differentiated thyroid cancer. *Thyroid* **2016**, *26*, 1–133. [CrossRef]
3. Rojo, I.L.; Valdazo, A.G.; Ramirez, J.G. Current Use of Molecular Profiling for Indeterminate Thyroid Nodules. *Cirugía Española (Engl. Ed.)* **2018**, *96*, 395–400. [CrossRef]
4. Pescatori, L.C.; Torcia, P.; Nicosia, L.; Mauri, G.; Rossi, U.G.; Cariati, M. Which needle in the treatment of thyroid nodules? *Gland. Surg.* **2018**, *7*, 111. [CrossRef] [PubMed]
5. Alexander, L.F.; Patel, N.J.; Caserta, M.P.; Robbin, M.L. Thyroid Ultrasound: Diffuse and Nodular Disease. *Radiol. Clin.* **2020**, *58*, 1041–1057. [CrossRef]
6. Mistry, R.; Hillyar, C.; Nibber, A.; Sooriyamoorthy, T.; Kumar, N. Ultrasound Classification of Thyroid Nodules: A Systematic Review. *Cureus* **2020**, *12*, e7239. [CrossRef] [PubMed]
7. Ardakani, A.A.; Gharbali, A.; Mohammadi, A. Classification of benign and malignant thyroid nodules using wavelet texture analysis of sonograms. *J. Ultrasound Med.* **2015**, *34*, 1983–1989. [CrossRef]
8. Verburg, F.; Reiners, C. Sonographic diagnosis of thyroid cancer with support of AI. *Nat. Rev. Endocrinol.* **2019**, *15*, 319–321. [CrossRef]
9. Ouyang, F.S.; Guo, B.L.; Ouyang, L.Z.; Liu, Z.W.; Lin, S.J.; Meng, W.; Huang, X.Y.; Chen, H.X.; Qiu-Gen, H.; Yang, S.M. Comparison between linear and nonlinear machine-learning algorithms for the classification of thyroid nodules. *Eur. J. Radiol.* **2019**, *113*, 251–257. [CrossRef] [PubMed]
10. Zhang, R.; Liu, Q.; Cui, H.; Wang, X.; Song, S.; Huang, G.; Feng, D. Thyroid classification via new multi-channel feature association and learning from multi-modality MRI images. In Proceedings of the 2018 IEEE 15th International Symposium on Biomedical Imaging (ISBI 2018), Washington, DC, USA, 4–7 April 2018; IEEE: Piscataway, NJ, USA, 2018; pp. 277–280.
11. Wokke, B.H.; Bos, C.; Reijnierse, M.; van Rijswijk, C.S.; Eggers, H.; Webb, A.; Verschuuren, J.J.; Kan, H.E. Comparison of dixon and T1-weighted MR methods to assess the degree of fat infiltration in duchenne muscular dystrophy patients. *J. Magn. Reson. Imaging* **2013**, *38*, 619–624. [CrossRef]
12. Gupta, S.; Soellinger, M.; Boesiger, P.; Poulikakos, D.; Kurtcuoglu, V. Three-dimensional computational modeling of subject-specific cerebrospinal fluid flow in the subarachnoid space. *J. Biomech. Eng.* **2009**, *131*, 021010. [CrossRef]
13. Seo, H.; Choi, J.; Oh, C.; Han, Y.; Park, H. Isotropic diffusion weighting for measurement of a high-resolution apparent diffusion coefficient map using a single radial scan in MRI. *Phys. Med. Biol.* **2014**, *59*, 6289. [CrossRef] [PubMed]
14. Koh, D.M.; Collins, D.J. Diffusion-weighted MRI in the body: Applications and challenges in oncology. *Am. J. Roentgenol.* **2007**, *188*, 1622–1635. [CrossRef]
15. Hao, Y.; Pan, C.; Chen, W.; Li, T.; Zhu, W.; Qi, J. Differentiation between malignant and benign thyroid nodules and stratification of papillary thyroid cancer with aggressive histological features: Whole-lesion diffusion-weighted imaging histogram analysis. *J. Magn. Reson. Imaging* **2016**, *44*, 1546–1555. [CrossRef]
16. Brown, A.M.; Nagala, S.; McLean, M.A.; Lu, Y.; Scoffings, D.; Apte, A.; Gonen, M.; Stambuk, H.E.; Shaha, A.R.; Tuttle, R.M.; et al. Multi-institutional validation of a novel textural analysis tool for preoperative stratification of suspected thyroid tumors on diffusion-weighted MRI. *Magn. Reson. Med.* **2016**, *75*, 1708–1716. [CrossRef]
17. Schob, S.; Meyer, H.J.; Dieckow, J.; Pervinder, B.; Pazaitis, N.; Höhn, A.K.; Garnov, N.; Horvath-Rizea, D.; Hoffmann, K.T.; Surov, A. Histogram analysis of diffusion weighted imaging at 3T is useful for prediction of lymphatic metastatic spread, proliferative activity, and cellularity in thyroid cancer. *Int. J. Mol. Sci.* **2017**, *18*, 821. [CrossRef] [PubMed]
18. Naglah, A.; Khalifa, F.; Khaled, R.; El-Baz, A.; Abdel Khalek Abdel Razek, A. Thyroid cancer computer-aided diagnosis system using MRI-based multi-input CNN model. In Proceedings of the 2021 IEEE 18th International Symposium on Biomedical Imaging (ISBI 2021), Nice, France, 13–16 April 2021; IEEE: Piscataway, NJ, USA, 2021; pp. 1691–1694.
19. Surov, A.; Garnov, N. Proving of a mathematical model of cell calculation based on apparent diffusion coefficient. *Transl. Oncol.* **2017**, *10*, 828–830. [CrossRef]

20. Wang, H.; Song, B.; Ye, N.; Ren, J.; Sun, X.; Dai, Z.; Zhang, Y.; Chen, B.T. Machine learning-based multiparametric MRI radiomics for predicting the aggressiveness of papillary thyroid carcinoma. *Eur. J. Radiol.* **2020**, *122*, 108755. [CrossRef]
21. Stejskal, E.O.; Tanner, J.E. Spin diffusion measurements: Spin echoes in the presence of a time-dependent field gradient. *J. Chem. Phys.* **1965**, *42*, 288–292. [CrossRef]
22. Agarap, A.F. Deep learning using rectified linear units (relu). *arXiv* **2018**, arXiv:1803.08375.
23. Finney, D.J. *Probit Analysis: A Statistical Treatment of the Sigmoid Response Curve*; Cambridge University Press: Cambridge, UK, 1952.
24. Kingma, D.P.; Ba, J. Adam: A method for stochastic optimization. *arXiv* **2014**, arXiv:1412.6980.
25. Müller, C. *Spherical Harmonics*; Springer: Berlin/Heidelberg, Germany, 2006; Volume 17.
26. Friedl, M.A.; Brodley, C.E. Decision tree classification of land cover from remotely sensed data. *Remote Sens. Environ.* **1997**, *61*, 399–409. [CrossRef]
27. Liaw, A.; Wiener, M. Classification and regression by randomForest. *R News* **2002**, *2*, 18–22.
28. McCallum, A.; Nigam, K. A comparison of event models for naive bayes text classification. In *AAAI-98 Workshop on Learning for Text Categorization*; Association for the Advancement of Artificial Intelligence (AAAI): Palo Alto, CA, USA, 1998 ; Volume 752, pp. 41–48.
29. Suykens, J.A.; Vandewalle, J. Least squares support vector machine classifiers. *Neural Process. Lett.* **1999**, *9*, 293–300. [CrossRef]
30. Krizhevsky, A.; Sutskever, I.; Hinton, G.E. Imagenet classification with deep convolutional neural networks. *Commun. ACM* **2017**, *60*, 84–90. [CrossRef]
31. He, K.; Zhang, X.; Ren, S.; Sun, J. Deep residual learning for image recognition. In Proceedings of the IEEE Conference on Computer Vision and Pattern Recognition, Las Vegas, NV, USA, 27–30 June 2016; pp. 770–778.
32. Russakovsky, O.; Deng, J.; Su, H.; Krause, J.; Satheesh, S.; Ma, S.; Huang, Z.; Karpathy, A.; Khosla, A.; Bernstein, M.; et al. ImageNet Large Scale Visual Recognition Challenge. *Int. J. Comput. Vis. (IJCV)* **2015**, *115*, 211–252. [CrossRef]
33. Dodge, S.; Karam, L. A study and comparison of human and deep learning recognition performance under visual distortions. In Proceedings of the 2017 26th International Conference on Computer Communication and Networks (ICCCN), Vancouver, BC, Canada, 31 July–3 August 2017; IEEE: Piscataway, NJ, USA, 2017; pp. 1–7.
34. Negi, S.S.; Bhandari, Y.S. A hybrid approach to image enhancement using contrast stretching on image sharpening and the analysis of various cases arising using histogram. In Proceedings of the International Conference on Recent Advances and Innovations in Engineering (ICRAIE-2014), Jaipur, India, 9–11 May 2014; IEEE: Piscataway, NJ, USA, 2014; pp. 1–6.
35. Murtagh, F.; Legendre, P. Ward's hierarchical agglomerative clustering method: Which algorithms implement Ward's criterion? *J. Classif.* **2014**, *31*, 274–295. [CrossRef]
36. Murtagh, F.; Legendre, P. The clustering validity with silhouette and sum of squared errors? *Learning* **2015**, *3*, 274–295.
37. Thinsungnoena, T.; Kaoungkub, N.; Durongdumronchaib, P.; Kerdprasopb, K.; Kerdprasopb, N. The clustering validity with silhouette and sum of squared errors. In Proceedings of the 3rd International Conference on Industrial Application Engineering 2015, Kitakyushu, Japan, 28–31 March 2015; Volume 3. Available online : https://pdfs.semanticscholar.org/8785/b45c92622ebbbffee055aec198190c621b00.pdf (accessed on 1 May 2021).

sensors

MDPI

Article

Validation of a Low-Cost Electrocardiography (ECG) System for Psychophysiological Research

Ruth Erna Wagner [1], Hugo Plácido da Silva [2] and Klaus Gramann [1,*]

[1] Chair Biological Psychology and Neuroergonomics, TU Berlin, 10623 Berlin, Germany; ruth@wagner2web.eu
[2] IT-Instituto de Telecomunicações, 1049-001 Lisbon, Portugal; hsilva@lx.it.pt
* Correspondence: klaus.gramann@tu-berlin.de; Tel.: +49-(0)30-314-79-508

Abstract: Background and Objective: The reliability of low-cost mobile systems for recording Electrocardiographic (ECG) data is mostly unknown, posing questions regarding the quality of the recorded data and the validity of the extracted physiological parameters. The present study compared the BITalino toolkit with an established medical-grade ECG system (BrainAmp-ExG). Methods: Participants underwent simultaneous ECG recordings with the two instruments while watching pleasant and unpleasant pictures of the "International Affective Picture System" (IAPS). Common ECG parameters were extracted and compared between the two systems. The Intraclass Correlation Coefficients (ICCs) and the Bland–Altman Limits of Agreement (LoA) method served as criteria for measurement agreement. Results: All but one parameter showed an excellent agreement (>80%) between both devices in the ICC analysis. No criteria for Bland–Altman LoA and bias were found in the literature regarding ECG parameters. Conclusion: The results of the ICC and Bland–Altman methods demonstrate that the BITalino system can be considered as an equivalent recording device for stationary ECG recordings in psychophysiological experiments.

Keywords: BITalino; BrainAmp; ICC; intraclass correlation coefficient; Bland–Altman method

Citation: Wagner, R.E.; Plácido da Silva, H.; Gramann, K. Validation of a Low-Cost Electrocardiography (ECG) System for Psychophysiological Research. *Sensors* **2021**, *21*, 4485. https://doi.org/10.3390/s21134485

Academic Editors: Guruprasad A. Giridharan, Ali H. Mahmoud, Ahmed Shalaby, Ayman El-baz and Mohammed Ghazal

Received: 6 April 2021
Accepted: 28 June 2021
Published: 30 June 2021

1. Introduction

In psychophysiological research, Electromyography (EMG), Electrocardiography (ECG), Electrodermal Activity (EDA) and Electroencephalography (EEG) are common electrophysiological methods to investigate the relationship between human behavior and its physiological basis [1,2]. Current instruments are usually stationary, and hence the transmission of the collected data is done by wire, restricting the movement of participants. This is especially detrimental when using such systems in conditions that usually would require movement of participants (e.g., during naturalistic behavior or in virtual reality). Nowadays, there are multiple wearable recording devices on the market. These wearables are mobile and most of them can transmit ECG data wirelessly. However, not all wearables provide access to the data while recording, and they are relatively expensive. Often, proprietary software is necessary for data recording and export for subsequent analyses, adding additional costs and restrictions for the measurement device. Recently, the BITalino has been introduced as an inexpensive hardware and software toolkit specifically designed to deal with the requirements of electrophysiological signal acquisition [3]. The BITalino device transmits data wirelessly and provides the opportunity to access the data while recording.

To ensure that the data recorded with new wearables devices is of sufficient quality to be used in a research context or for non-scientific applications, new devices have to be verified before using them in psychophysiological experiments. Regarding the BITalino, only one study by Carreiras et al. [4] exists in which the BITalino was compared with an established ECG system. However, the main focus of that study was to analyze the morphological similarities between individual heartbeat waveforms and the general similarity between the synchronized time series. Further, the authors used dry electrodes and the electrodes were applied to the hand palms or fingers and thus do not represent standard ECG electrode placement. In addition, Carreiras et al. [4] did not use time or frequency domain measures to compare the two devices. While time domain parameters such as heart rate (HR) and heart rate variability (HRV) are established features that can be computed effectively from the ECG, the use of frequency domain parameters provides additional insights into the function of the cardiovascular system [5]. Specifically, the power spectrum of HRV allows for conclusions regarding the involvement of the parasympathetic and sympathetic system in cardiovascular responses. The computation of these features, however, critically depends on the data quality and data processing pipelines, as missing or artifactual beats impact the frequency domain significantly [6–8]. The present study thus used both time and frequency domain parameters to compare the two recording systems and to provide a systematic analyses of ECG parameters.

While the test for concordance of ECG features recorded with two different recording devices could be done based on non-specific ECG signals, the present study used an established psychophysiological protocol to evoke specific ECG activity. We used the "International Affective Picture System" (IAPS) [9] to provoke pronounced differences in ECG features in different test blocks to increase variability in the recordings for a later, more conservative, test for similarity. The IAPS allows for presenting different categories of emotional stimuli (positive, negative and neutral) that are matched regarding their arousal and dominance and that have been used in a large number of psychophysiological studies to evoke different affective responses while controlling for the arousal and dominance associated with a specific affective state [10].

Therefore, the aim of this study was to compare a medical-grade electrocardiography (ECG) system with an ECG sensor of the low-cost DiY (Do-it-Yourself) hardware toolkit BITalino. To evoke clear variation in ECG activity, an experimental protocol inducing different affective states and associated cardiovascular changes was implemented. Several established ECG parameters were extracted from both recordings and tested for similarity between the parameters. Since a statistical test for differences of two or more measures only provides information about differences between conditions, or, as in our case, between two measurement devices, the absence of significance in such tests does not provide evidence for similarity in performance. Correlational measures derived from two different system, in contrast, explain the strength of the relation between two measures but do not indicate their agreement [11]. Testing the agreement or similarity between two measures has to be done using specific statistical approaches that test for the concordance between the measures. There are several methods to test for the concordance of two or more measure with the Intraclass Correlation Coefficients (ICCs) and the Bland–Altman Limits of Agreement (LoA) method representing the most established and tested methods for continuous data with two or more groups [12].

The present study demonstrates that it is possible to reliably record research-grade ECG data with a wearable low-cost device. Reliable data acquisition with a system that does not require proprietary software and can access the recorded data in real time while providing wireless data transmission provides new opportunities for future mobile ECG investigations that do not require expensive laboratory equipment and that allow movement of participants.

The remainder of the work is organized as follows. Section 2 describes the material and methods. Section 3 provides an overview of the ICC and LoA statistical methods. Section 4 summarizes the reliability assessment results. Section 5 presents a discussion and main limitation of the work. Finally, Section 6 outlines the main conclusions and future work perspectives.

2. Methods

2.1. Participants

Twenty-four participants were recruited through advertisement at the Technical University of Berlin. Only healthy participants without any history of heart disease or pharmacological treatment of heart conditions were accepted. After the recordings, one participant reported to take medication that influenced cardiovascular parameters, leading to the exclusion of this participant. Thus, the final sample consisted of 23 participants (12 women, 11 men) with an age range from 22 to 57 (M = 28.3 years, SD = 8.8 years). Participation was voluntary and participants received course credit. They were told not to consume any form of caffeine for 2 h before the experiment and not to drink alcohol on the day of the experiment. They also got a picture with all electrode positions indicated, so that they could choose appropriate clothing. All subjects gave their consent before being enrolled in the study. The study was approved by the Ethical Commission of IT—Instituto de Telecomunicações with the matriculation number TUB-1234567. Participants provided written informed consent, and the study was conducted in accordance with the Declaration of Helsinki.

2.1.1. Hardware

The medical-grade ECG module ExG from BrainProducts was used as the standard ECG system, hereinafter referred to as the BrainAmp-ExG. The BrainAmp-ExG amplifier is an extension available for simultaneous measurement of EEG and other psychophysiological signals such as ECG, EMG and EDA, but it can also be used separately. The BrainAmp-ExG amplifier has a bandwidth from 0 to 1000 Hz. The BrainAmp system is separated from the power grid by the use of a power pack. Electrodes from the BrainAmp-ExG are connected via cables to the amplifier, which is connected to a PC.

As a DiY system, the BITalino version "Plugged BT Kit" was used in the experiment. It contains a control block and sensors for ECG, EMG and EDA, as well as a photo resistor (LUX) and an accelerometer (ACC). The BITalino ECG sensor has a bandwidth between 0.5 and 40 Hz. The electrodes of the BITalino are connected to the BITalino ECG module, which is connected by cable to the BITalino control block. The data can be sent via standard Bluetooth to a recording device. The recording device can be an Android tablet or smartphone, as well as a PC.

2.1.2. Software

To allow for a direct comparison of both ECG recordings, the data of the two different amplifier systems were synchronized using the Lab Streaming Layer (LSL) (Christian Kothe, https://github.com/sccn/labstreaminglayer). In Figure 1, the general data acquisition approach is presented. LSL catches data streams in the network, which can be recorded time synchronously by the Lab Recorder software (a part of the LSL package). For providing the data streams to the network, applets were used. The ECG signal from the BrainAmp system is usually recorded with the BrainAmp-Recorder software. An applet for redirecting the data stream from the BrainAmp-Recorder to the network already exists and is part of the LSL package. The applet for the BITalino had to be programmed for this study. The BITalino team provided the BITalino Matlab API, which was added as an official Matlab toolbox [13]. Using that API, the BITalino stream was forwarded to LSL based on the applet for Matlab (9.2.0.538062 (R2017a)).

When different streams are available in the local network, the Lab Recorder detects them and records all selected streams. The Lab Recorder saves the data streams to one file in the open source "extensible data format" (.xdf). XDF is "a general purpose container format for multi-channel time series data with extensive associated meta information. XDF is tailored towards biosignal data such as EEG, EMG, EOG, ECG, GSR, MEG ... " [14].

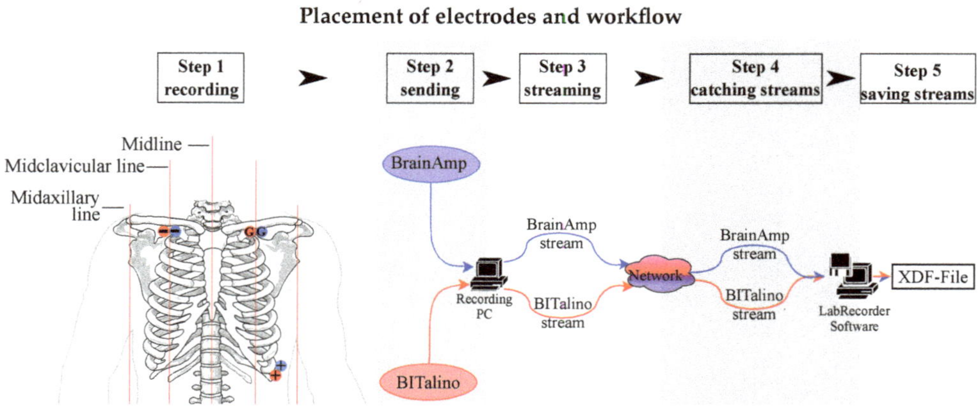

Figure 1. The left side of the image shows the adopted placement of electrodes. The BITalino leads are depicted in red and the BrainAmp leads in blue: −, below right clavicular; +, left side of chest midclavicular line beneath last rib; G, below left clavicular. The right side of the image shows the data acquisition workflow used for recording.

2.1.3. ECG Electrode Placement and Recording

A variation of Einthoven lead II was selected for the experiment, referred to as "alternative leads". To allow recordings of the ECG signal concurrently with two devices, electrodes were placed according to the schema presented in Figure 1.

Because ECG is a fast changing signal, a high sampling rate was used. While for the BrainAmp system it is possible to variably set different filters, the filters on the BITalino system are fixed. The BITalino allows data acquisition at sampling rates of 10, 100 and 1000 Hz, and, consequently, a sampling rate of 1000 Hz was selected for both ECG systems, resulting in one sample per millisecond. In addition, to reduce artifacts in the recordings, high- and low-pass filters were used according to the options available in the two amplifier systems. All settings are listed in Table 1.

Table 1. Hardware filtering specifications and settings used in the experiment. * Note that 0.016 Hz = time constant of 10 s ($f = \frac{1}{2\pi c}$, with f the frequency and c a time constant).

	BrainAmp	BITalino
high-pass filter	0.016 Hz *	0.5 Hz
low-pass filter	250 Hz	40 Hz
sampling rate	1000 Hz	1000 Hz

2.2. *Materials*

Stimuli (IAPS)

The result of this study aimed at establishing whether ECG data recorded with the BITalino system are comparable to an established medical-grade ECG system used in psychophysiological research. To this end, an established psychophysiological paradigm to evoke affective responses that are associated with changes in heart rate was used. Brouwer et al. [15] (p. 3) noted in their study that "most perception studies show valence rather than arousal effects, where pleasant stimuli correlate with higher heart rate acceleration than unpleasant stimuli [16–22]".

We used IAPS pictures to induce two emotional states, pleasant and unpleasant. For the pleasant conditions, pictures with medium arousal ratings were selected, while, for the unpleasant condition, pictures with medium to high arousal ratings were chosen. If the data quality of both the BrainAmp-ExG and the BITalino ECG is comparable, changes in HR dependent on the emotional picture condition should reveal similar values for both systems.

2.3. Procedure

Participants were seated in front of a monitor with a distance of approximately 50 cm to the screen. They were instructed to sit still for the time of the experimental task, which took 35 min on average. Stimuli were presented in four blocks (two blocks with pictures of the unpleasant and 2 blocks with pictures of the pleasant condition), consisting of 60 pictures each (Figure 2A). The order of blocks was counterbalanced across participants.

Each picture was presented for 4 s and stimulus presentations was separated by a fixation cross with 1 s duration (Figure 2B). After a block of 60 pictures, participants were asked to rate valence and arousal of the entire block on a 10-point scale from 0 to 9, with 9 indicating the highest arousal or valence, respectively. Before and after two blocks, a 5 min baseline block consisting of a gray fixation cross on black background was added. To control the potential impact of the picture order, pictures were randomly selected from the pool of pictures for each condition and blocks with pleasant and unpleasant pictures were counterbalanced across participants.

After participants were prepared and electrodes were attached, a first baseline block was used for acclimatization. The second baseline block was introduced in the middle of the experiment to recover to the resting heart rate before the last two experimental blocks were presented. After all blocks with picture presentations, a third and final baseline block followed.

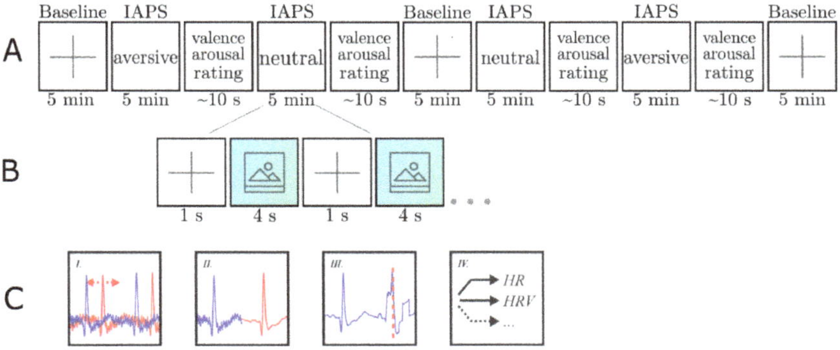

Figure 2. Block diagram of the experimental protocol and analyses pipeline, depicting the stimuli blocks (**A**), the fixation cross and picture presentation (**B**), and the overall processing pipeline (**C**).

2.4. Data Analysis

2.4.1. Data Processing

Data processing was done in Matlab version 9.2.0.538062 (R2017a) with the use of ECG tool, Matlab-based software developed in-house. The ECG tool offers the option to load .xdf-files. As a result of LSL, both signals were combined with markers in an .xdf-file. Streaming the BITalino data to LSL, after receiving them via Bluetooth from the BITalino devices, had never been tested before. Therefore, visual inspection was done by plotting both signals of one participant in one graph. The overall processing pipeline is depicted in Figure 2C. Due to temporal incongruity of both graphs, alignment was done before data processing. To this end, R-peaks were identified and exported with the corresponding timestamp for each participant. A window of 201 ms (100 before the R-peak and 100 after the R-peak) was searched to find the timestamp of the corresponding R-peak of the other system. This comparison resulted in differences with a mean difference per participant varying from 19 to 28 ms. The signals were re-synchronized using the mean difference for each participant.

After alignment, the signals from both devices were filtered with a third-order high-pass Butterworth filter at 1 Hz and a third-order low-pass filter at 40 Hz. Then, artifacts were manually identified and subsequently interpolated. For automated R-peak detection and to avoid false positives as far as possible, the allowed number of beats per minute (bpm) was set to range between 40 and 125 bpm. After automated R-peak detection, false R-peaks were marked and rejected and, in the case of missing peaks, the data were interpolated based on the mean peak interval 5 periods before the missing R-peak.

2.4.2. Dependent Variables

According to the Task Force of the European Society of Cardiology and others [23], we computed selected heart rate variability measurements that can be used for short-term analysis. The aim of the study was to determine whether the BITalino can be used in psychophysiological experiments and, as such, measures were selected which were used in previous experiments. According to Gramann and Schandry [24], the number of heartbeats per minute (designated as heart rate (HR)) is still the most common indicator in psychophysiology to measure cardiovascular events. Heart rate changes accompany almost every change of physical and mental load.

In addition to heart rate measures, measures of heart rate variability were used. For short-term HRV time domain measures, the ref. [23] recommends using RMSSD as an estimate of the short-term components of HRV, which is often used in psychophysiological research. Brouwer et al. [15] also used RMSSD as an estimate for HRV in their study.

In the frequency domain, the ref. [23] recommends three main spectral components for short-term analyses: the very low-frequency (VLF), the low-frequency (LF) and the high-frequency (HF) components. According to the [23] "the distribution of the power and the central frequency of LF and HF are not fixed but may vary in relation to changes in automatic modulations of the heart period ... ". The LF component reflects parasympathetic innervation, whereas HF reflects sympathetic and parasympathetic innervation. In addition to this, the ratio between LF and HF (LF/HF) is an indicator of ANS balance. We did not analyze the VLF component as it is not as well defined as the other parameters according to the [23]. In this study, LF, HF and LF/HF ratio were used to investigate whether both systems recorded comparable signals in the experiment.

We expected to see increased HR in blocks with pleasant stimuli as compared to unpleasant stimuli while no directed hypothesis were put forward regarding HRV due to inconsistent results in the literature [16–22,25–28]. While these results would confirm the general validity of our experimental manipulation, the main research question concerned the comparability of the features as measured with the two different ECG systems.

A summary of all measures used in this study can be seen in Table 2.

Table 2. Dependent variables.

HR Measures		**HR**	**Heart Rate**	**[bpm]**
HRV measures	time domain	RMSSD	root mean square of successive differences	[ms]
	frequency domain	LF	low frequency	$[ms^2]$
		HF	high frequency	
		LF/HF	ratio between LF and HF	

3. Statistical Methods

To investigate whether the BITalino system allows for recordings of comparable quality as the established ECG recordings with the BrainAmp system, two methods were used: the Intraclass Correlation Coefficient (ICC) and Bland–Altman Limits of Agreement (LoA) method.

3.1. *Intraclass Correlation Coefficient (ICC)*

According to Müller and Büttner [29] (p. 2465), ICCs are used in medicine to "assess agreement of quantitative measurements in the sense of consistency and conformity". The

ICC ranges, similar to other correlation coefficients, from 0.00 to 1.00 and is presented in this work as a percentage.

ICCs above 80% are usually regarded as indicating good to excellent reliability, whereas an ICC between 0.6 and 0.8 (60% and 80%) may be taken to represent substantial reliability [30]. Portney and Watkins [31] indicated that clinical measurements should show reliability of at least 90%. In addition to the ICC, the lower 95% confidence interval (lower CI) of the ICC can be calculated. Lee et al. [32] reported that an agreement sufficient for the interchangeable use of two methods is suggested only when a lower CI value of >75% is observed.

In this study, the ICC form for two-way mixed-effects using single measurements was used to investigate the absolute agreement defined by McGraw and Wong [33]. This approach is mathematically identical to ICC (2,1), as defined by Shrout and Fleiss [34].

3.2. Bland–Altman Limits of Agreement (Loa) Method

"The limits of agreement (LoA) method (Altman and Bland [35]; Bland and Altman [11]) for assessing the agreement between two methods of medical measurement is widely used (Bland and Altman [36], Ryan and Woodall [37])" [38] (p. 571).The Bland–Altman method obtains "the differences between measurements by the two methods for each individual" [38] (p. 571) and calculates "the mean and standard deviation" [38] (p. 571). In [38], the authors proposed methods for analyzing repeated data. The LoA were calculated according to the formulas presented in [38].

4. Results

4.1. Descriptive Results

The HR and HRV parameters in the time and frequency domain revealed only minimal differences in all selected parameters between the two recording devices (Table 3). Moreover, the extracted parameters from both systems during the baseline and the IPAS conditions showed only small differences overall. During blocks with unpleasant stimuli, the heart was lowest for unpleasant followed by pleasant and lastly the baseline blocks. For the RMSSD measures, the lowest HRV was observed during pleasant blocks, followed by unpleasant and baseline blocks. A similar pattern was observed for the ratio LF/HF.

Table 3. Descriptive results.

	BITalino Mean	BrainAmp Mean	BITalino SD	BrainAmp SD
HR				
Fixation Cross	73.065	73.025	10.190	10.205
Pleasant	72.624	72.625	10.274	10.276
Unpleasant	71.515	71.504	9.379	9.381
RMSSD				
Fixation Cross	0.045	0.045	0.025	0.025
Pleasant	0.043	0.043	0.025	0.025
Unpleasant	0.044	0.044	0.023	0.022
ratio LF/HF				
Fixation Cross	3.109	2.973	3.970	3.797
Pleasant	2.993	2.988	4.220	4.204
Unpleasant	3.081	3.078	4.889	4.875

4.2. ANOVA

A 2 × 3 analysis of variance with two levels of the factor "device" (BrainAmp, BITalino) and three levels of the factor "condition" (Baseline (Fixation Cross), pleasant IAPS, unpleasant IAPS) was calculated for all dependent variables. For this analysis, the first fixation block was excluded as it was for acclimatization. Thus, the mean for the factor condition was built of two blocks each. There was a significant main effect of the factor "condition" for HR (F (1.486, 32.685) = 4.694, $p = 0.025$), as shown in Table 4. For RMSSD, LF, HF and LF/HF ratio, the main effect of condition was not significant and there was no interaction effect for "condition × device" for any dependent variable.

Table 4. Results of 2 × 3 ANOVA for the factor "condition" all dependent variables.

Dependent Variable	Main Factor "Condition"	
HR	$F(1.486, 32.685) = 4.694$ *	$p = 0.025$ *
RMSSD	$F(2, 44) = 0.567$	$p = 0.571$
HRV LF	$F(1.200, 26.408) = 6.204$ *	$p = 0.15$ *
HRV HF	$F(1, 44) = 0.127$	$p = 0.881$
HRV LF/HF	$F(1.454, 31.997) = 0.910$ *	$p = 0.384$ *

* Greenhouse–Geisser corrected.

A post hoc pairwise comparison with Bonferroni correction was done for heart rate with an alpha value of 0.05. None of the pairwise comparisons was significant.

4.3. *Intraclass Correlation Coefficient*

The ICCs and the lower CIs were calculated for all dependent variables over all blocks and, in addition, for each block separately. To gain good to excellent agreement of both devices, the ICC should be higher than 90% for clinical measurements [31] and the lower CI should be higher than 75% for the interchangeable use of two methods [32]. The ICC estimates over all blocks for all dependent variables were over 90% and the lower CIs were over 75% (Tables 5 and 6). Therefore, all dependent variables met the criterion for good to excellent agreement. For each block separately, the ICC estimates were over 90% and the lower CIs were over 75% for all blocks and dependent variables, except for the LF/HF ratio in the second fixation cross (Block 4) (Tables 5 and 6).

Table 5. ICC in percent for each block and dependent variable.

	Overall	B1 Fix 1	B2 P 1	B3 UP 1	B4 Fix 2	B5 P 2	B6 UP 2	B7 Fix 3
HR	100.0%	100.0%	100.0%	100.0%	99.9%	100.0%	100.0%	100.0%
RMSSD	99.6%	99.9%	100.0%	100.0%	97.4%	99.8%	100.0%	100.0%
HRV LF	100.0%	100.0%	100.0%	100.0%	99.9%	100.0%	100.0%	100.0%
HRV HF	99.6%	99.9%	99.8%	100.0%	97.3%	99.9%	100.0%	99.9%
HRV LF/HF	98.8%	100.0%	100.0%	100.0%	83.6%	100.0%	100.0%	99.8%

B1–B7, block number; Fix, fixation cross; P, pleasant IAPS; UP, unpleasant IAPS.

Table 6. Lower CI in percent for each block and dependent variable.

	Overall	B1 Fix 1	B2 P 1	B3 UP 1	B4 Fix 2	B5 P 2	B6 UP 2	B7 Fix 3
HR	100.0%	100.0%	100.0%	100.0%	99.8%	100.0%	100.0%	100.0%
RMSSD	99.4%	99.8%	100.0%	100.0%	94.0%	99.6%	100.0%	99.8%
HRV LF	99.9%	99.9%	100.0%	100.0%	99.8%	100.0%	100.0%	100.0%
HRV HF	99.4%	99.8%	100.0%	100.0%	93.8%	99.7%	100.0%	99.9%
HRV LF/HF	98.4%	99.9%	100.0%	100.0%	65.6%	100.0%	100.0%	99.6%

B1–B7, block number; Fix, fixation cross; P, pleasant IAPS; UP, unpleasant IAPS.

4.4. *Bland–Altman Method*

An assumption for calculating Bland–Altman bias and limits of agreement is that the difference between both devices are normally distributed. A Shapiro–Wilk test [39] revealed that the data were not normally distributed. Bland and Altman [40] recommended a logarithmic transformation of differences in that case, which also revealed non-normal distribution of the transformed data. Quantile-Quantile plots (Q-Q plots) of the difference between data of the two devices were made to detect the problem on normality tests. The Q-Q plot for the difference of low-frequency measures is shown in Figure 3.

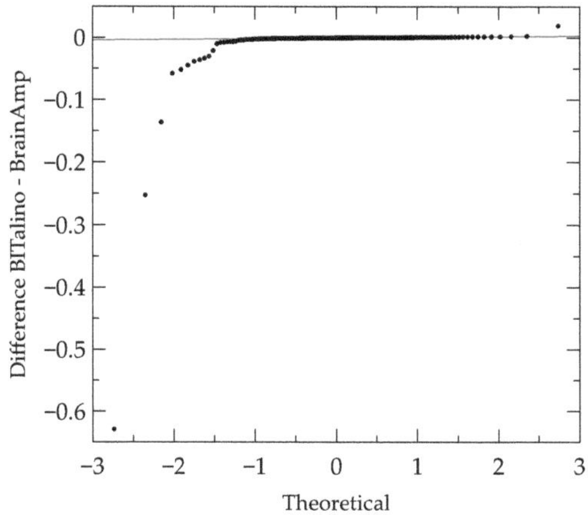

Figure 3. Q-Q plot of differences between the BrainAmp and the BITalino for LF.

In the Q-Q plot, it can be seen that there were several outliers, which may have negatively affected the results of the normality test. Therefore, outliers were excluded and tested again for normality. In some measurements, more than half of the data points had to be excluded to reach normal distribution. However, this heavy reduction of data points may distort the results. According to Bland and Altman [40] (p. 139), a non-normal distribution of the differences values may not be a comparably serious issue for the Bland–Altman method as compared to other statistical tests. Non-normal distributed differences will lead to more conservative results than normally distributed differences. For this reason, the non-normal distributed data were used for Bland–Altman analysis even though the normality assumption was violated. The results of the Bland–Altman analysis for non-normal distributed differences are presented in Table 7.

Table 7. Results of Bland–Altman absolute bias and absolute limits of agreement (LoA) for all dependent variables.

Measure	Bias	Lower LoA	LoA -	Upper LoA	Outlier (in %)
HR	−0.01990803	−0.33662671	-	0.29681066	4.83%
RMSSD	0.00003761	−0.00439510	-	0.00447032	3.22%
HRV LF	−0.00000880	−0.00011612	-	0.00009852	4.83%
HRV HF	0.00000290	−0.00019657	-	0.00020236	4.83%
HRV LF/HF	−0.06054003	−1.32977327	-	1.20869321	3.22%

The bias was close to 0 and limits of agreements were quite narrow for all dependent variables. Different results for low and high frequency were found, which may influence the result of the LF/HF ratio negatively. Next, percentages of differences lying outside the LoA were calculated for all dependent variables, as Weippert et al. [41] did in their analysis. The results are presented in Table 7. The percentage of outliers was lower than 5% for all measures. Therefore, more than 95% of differences between the two devices were observed within the limits of agreement. Although the results of Bland–Altmam bias and limits of agreement were quite different, they revealed the same percentage of differences lying outside the limits of agreement.

Visual Inspection of Bland–Altman Plots

Bland and Altman [40] suggested "to plot the difference between the measurements by the two methods for each subject against their mean" (p.140). This kind of plot allows for investigating possible relationships between the discrepancies and the true value. In contrast to R-peak analysis, the extracted parameters in the current study were mean values built over a period of time (here over one block). Thus, only seven measures by the two methods were available for each subject. Due to this small amount of measures per subject, Bland–Altman plots of all subjects were created [41]. Percentage of differences lying outside the LoA was under 5% for each measure, therefore the y-axes of the plots were restricted to the LoA.

The results for Heart Rate (HR) show a bias of −0.01991 bpm and LoA were at ±0.31672 bpm. Therefore, the BITalino yields on average 0.01991 bpm higher values than the BrainAmp-ExG, and the BITalino may yield between ±0.31672 bpm compared to the BrainAmp-ExG. The Bland–Altman plot for HR can be seen in Figure 4.

Due to some extreme data points below 0, the bias was probably shifted away from 0 to negative. The distribution of data points with the bias of −0.01991 bpm showed that the BrainAmp was consistently higher than the BITalino for most of the data points.

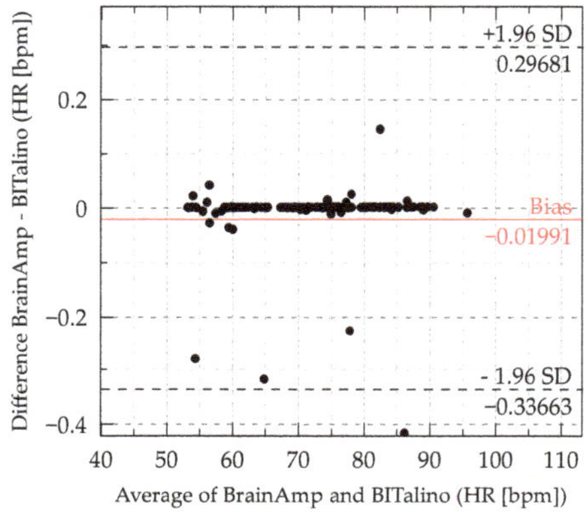

Figure 4. Bland–Altman plot of heart rate. (Some data points outside the LoA are cutoff to offer a more detailed view of the distribution inside the LoA.)

RMSSD. The bias for RMSSD of the complete dataset was at 0.00004 ms and limits of agreement were at ±0.00443 ms. Thus, the BITalino yielded on average 0.00004 ms lower values than the the BrainAmp-ExG, and the BITalino may yield ±0.00443 ms compared to the BrainAmp system. The Bland–Altman plot for RMSSD can be seen in Figure 5.

The distribution of the data showed that most of the data points were near the bias, but that there was a tendency for values of the BrainAmp-ExG to be slightly smaller than the values of the BITalino. Again, limits of agreement were quite narrow despite some extreme values (data points below −0.00075 ms and data points above 0.003 ms).

Low and high frequency. The bias for LF was at −0.0088 ms^2 and limits of agreement were at ±0.10732 ms^2. Thus, the BITalino yields on average 0.0088 ms^2 higher values than the BrainAmp, and the BITalino may yield ±0.10732 ms^2 compared to the BrainAmp.

The bias for HF was at 0.0029 ms^2 and limits of agreement were at ±0.19946 ms^2 . Thus, the BITalino yields on average 0.0029 ms^2 higher values than the BrainAmp, and the BITalino may yield ±0.199 ms^2 compared to the BrainAmp.

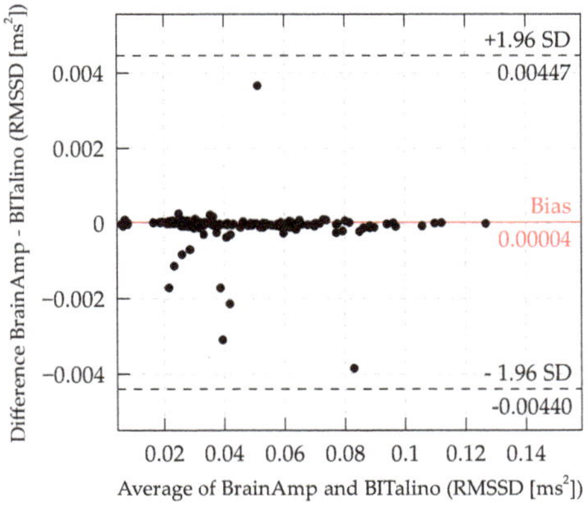

Figure 5. Bland–Altman plot of RMSSD. (Some data points outside the LoA are cutoff to offer a more detailed view of the distribution inside the LoA).

The Bland–Altman plot of high- and low-frequency components of HRV are shown in Figures 6 and 7. In the Bland–Altman plot of the low-frequency component (Figure 6), it can be seen that there were several data points above the bias and a few below the bias. The data points below may have influenced the results of bias and LoA negatively. They may result from interpolated artifacts, which occurred only in one of the systems.

A similar distribution of differences was found for the high-frequency component of HRV (Figure 7). For HF, the bias was positive and most of the data points were below the bias. For both frequency components, there was an increased variability of small values. This may indicate that there is less reliability at small values.

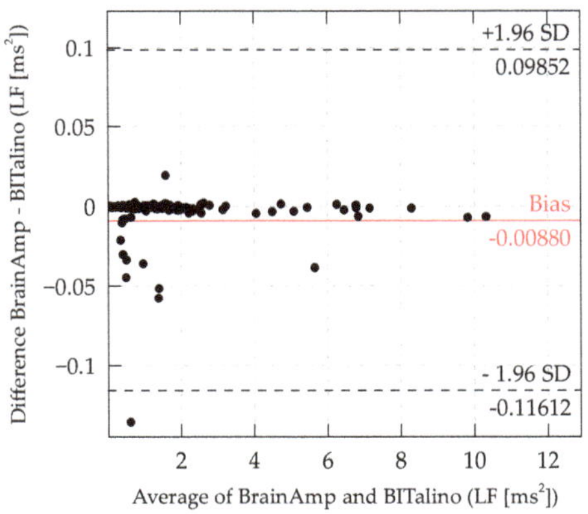

Figure 6. Bland–Altman plot of LF. (Some data points outside the LoA are cutoff to offer a more detailed view of the distribution inside the LoA.)

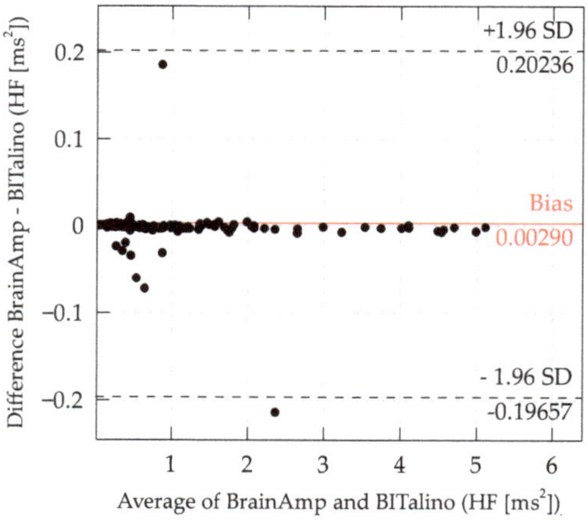

Figure 7. Bland–Altman plot of HF. (Some data points outside the LoA are cutoff to offer a more detailed view of the distribution inside the LoA.)

LF/HF ratio. The bias for LF/HF was at −0.06054 and limits of agreement were ±1.26923, which was the largest bias and widest LoA of all measures. Therefore, the Bland–Altman plot was inspected for LF/HF ratio too (Figure 8).

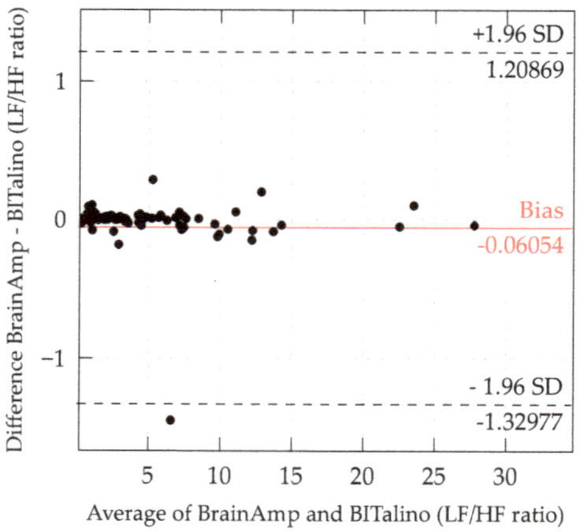

Figure 8. Bland–Altman plot of LF/HF ratio. (Some data points out- side the LoA are cutoff to offer a more detailed view of the distribution inside the LoA.)

Although all the parameters have different measurement scales, differences between measurement devices should always be close to 0. Therefore, a comparison of limits of agreement between measurements can be done. For the LF/HF ratio, the limits of agreement were 6 times larger than for the HF and 11 times larger than for the LF. Due to the fact that the ratio is built by both components, artifacts may influence the LF/HF ratio even more than both frequency components separately. One extreme difference of −8 (this point is not shown in the graph) may be the result of artifact interpolation in one of the measurements. Both frequency components showed agreement between the measurement devices. However, these different results may indicate that there is probably no or little agreement for the ratio of LF and HF.

5. Discussion

5.1. Overall ICC and Bland–Altman Method

All blocks were used in the overall ICC and Bland–Altman analysis. The results reveal that all measures show good to excellent agreement with the ICC method when using the criterion for clinical measurements (ICC > 90%). This result is consistent with the result of the study by Sandercock et al. [42], who found good to excellent agreement for all measures (LF, LF(nu), HF, HF(nu), LF:HF, RMSSD, SDNN and Mean R- R) when comparing different devices. They also used the Bland–Altman method in addition to the ICC.

In contrast to the ICC, Sandercock et al. [42] found no acceptable agreement between three instruments in the Bland–Altman analysis. They found one acceptable Bland–Altman result for the high frequency band of the HRV in one condition for two of the three instruments. They found a bias of -1 ms and a LoA of $\pm$264.6 ms. In contrast to Sandercock et al. [42], the present study analyzed high and low frequency measures of HRV in ms^2 and not in ms.

The results of the analyses demonstrate a bias for the high-frequency components of the HRV with 0.0029 ms^2 and LoA at $\pm$0.19946 ms^2 . Similar results were found for the low-frequency component of HRV with a bias of $-$0.0088 ms^2 and a LoA of $\pm$0.10732 ms^2. Based on the results and comparison with previous studies, it can be concluded that the low- and high-frequency components of HRV measured with the BITalino and the BrainAmpp-ExG showed a high level of agreement between the two systems.

In addition, the limits of agreement were more conservative for these non-normally distributed differences than for normally distributed differences.

5.2. ICC for Each Block

All measures showed a good to excellent agreement in all blocks except the ratio of LF/HF in the second baseline block (Block 4). The second unpleasant IAPS block (Block 3) and the second baseline block (Block 4) each contained more than 40 a of artifacts only in the BrainAmp recordings. However, the LF/HF showed 100% agreement in Block 3 but only 83.6% in Block 4. This might indicate that there was no evidence of artifact interpolation to influence the result of the ICC. The poor agreement of the LF/HF ratio in the second baseline block (Block 4) may be the result of movement, as participants had to sit still already for 15 min when beginning with the fourth block. Due to the fact that Bland–Altman uses all blocks as repeated measurements, the poor agreement for Block 4 may explain the wider limits of the LF/HF ratio in Bland–Altman analysis.

5.3. Conclusion of Method Comparison

As mentioned above, ICC and Bland–Altman analysis as clinical measurements are discussed controversially in the literature. Most of the researched studies investigating ECG comparisons [42,43] used both methods. In the case of Bland–Altman analyses, calculations depended on the design of the study. In the present study, measures of different blocks were used as repeated measurements. None of the referenced comparison studies described which Bland–Altman calculation was used. In addition, criteria for accepting both devices as interchangeable were not mentioned in these studies. For the ICC method, criteria were defined and therefore the interpretation of the results shows higher validity as compared to the Bland–Altman analysis.

Evaluating both methods and comparing their results, as well as inspecting Bland–Altman plots, allowed for an objective conclusion about the agreement of measures based on the two systems. Unfortunately, there are no guidelines for a Bland–Altman plot inspection. As demonstrated for the heart rate measure, scaling of the y-axis may mislead the interpretation of the distribution of differences. Furthermore, in the current study, the differences of all measures were not normally distributed, nor were the logarithmic transformed differences normally distributed. Nevertheless, Bland–Altman analysis was computed for the non logarithmic transformed and non-normal distributed data, violating the assumptions of distribution values bias and LoA.

ICC showed good to excellent agreement, Bland–Altman bias was small and LoA were narrow for almost all variables. The bigger bias and LoA for LF/HF may be explained by the influence of artifacts on one of the devices. If there is a big difference in LF and a small difference in HF, the ratio will be large and vice versa. However, taking all results, the data provide good evidence that both instruments showed very good agreement and can be used in further experiments interchangeably.

5.4. Limitation of Comparison Methods in the Current Study

The study was carried out with a sample composed of healthy participants, spanning an age range between 22 and 57 years old. To further encompass the variance that studies in psychophysiology require, future work should be developed focusing on replicating the current study for other sample profiles. Nevertheless, the critical comparison of the two systems was a within-subject design that should not be influenced by a restricted sample profile. The current study is in line with the state-of-the-art, in terms of sample size, and demonstrates the validity of the low-cost system under analysis for the sample enrolled in the study.

Integrating the BITalino stream via LSL required the use of an applet. In the current study, signals of both systems were not aligned. The validity of synchronously acquired data was already demonstrated by da Silva et al. [44]. This non-constant difference between R-peaks of both devices may arise from the working memory load of the Matlab-applet receiving data from the BITalino and forwarding it as a data stream over the network to LSL. The applet for receiving and forwarding the signal from the BITalino to LSL may be implemented in another programming language for future experiments to avoid this non-constant shift.

Furthermore, the BrainAmp ECG was used in comparison as the standard method. However, 93.52% of artifacts were found in the signals of the BrainAmp ECG. Different leads were used for the BrainAmp and the BITalino, because of the different connection of the leads to the specific system. The BrainAmp leads had been used very often before this experiment which might may have caused some material degradation and, as a consequence, worse signal quality as compared to the new BITalino sensors. Therefore, the BrainAmp-ExG leads had a higher sensitivity to movements and resulting movement artifacts. In the pretests before the experiments, both devices showed no artifacts and therefore the same leads were used in the experiment.

6. Conclusions and Future Work

Due to the comparison results of ICC and the Bland–Altman method, the BITalino can be considered as an equivalent recording device for stationary ECG recordings in psychophysiological experiments. The applet to stream the data will be implemented in another programming language and will be tested for future experiments. A new version of the BITalino called "(r)evolution" was introduced in the middle of 2017. Cable plugs were improved (from Molex Sherlock connectors to USB-like UC-E6 connectors); WiFi and BLE (Bluetooth Low Energy or Bluetooth 4.0) were added as technologies for data transmission; and new sensors were introduced. The first BITalino used Molex Sherlock connectors for the electrode leads, which was highly sensitive to cable movement. This may be fixed with the new UC-E6 plugs. The connectivity for data transmission was limited to Bluetooth 2.0. With the new version of BITalino, data can also be sent via BLE or WiFi, which can be advantageous in several use cases. This may fix some of the problems associated with receiving data from the BITalino in the current study. The improvements of the new BITalino (r)evolution and the sensors will be tested in further experiments, following the procedure of the current study. Overall, the results of the present study demonstrate good agreement between an inexpensive DiY system and an established medical grade ECG system. This provides a basis for the BITalino to be used for research in the lab and due to its portability, potentially mobile ECG system outside the lab.

Author Contributions: Conceptualization, R.E.W. and K.G.; methodology, R.E.W., H.P.d.S. and K.G.; formal analysis, R.E.W.; investigation, R.E.W.; and supervision, H.P.d.S. and K.G. All authors have read and agreed to the published version of the manuscript.

Funding: This work was supported in part by the Ministry of Economy and Competitiveness of the Spanish Government co-founded by the ERDF (PhysComp project) under Grant TIN2017-85409-P, and in part by the Instituto de Telecomunicaç oes (IT) in the scope of program under Grant UID/EEA/50008/2019.

Institutional Review Board Statement: The study was conducted according to the guidelines of the Declaration of Helsinki, and approved by the Ethics Committee of IT—Instituto de Telecomunicações (protocol code TUB-1234567, April 2021).

Informed Consent Statement: Informed consent was obtained from all subjects involved in the study.

Data Availability Statement: The data presented in this study are available upon reasonable request made to the corresponding author. The data are not publicly available due to privacy restrictions.

Acknowledgments: The authors would like to thank Ole Traupe from the department of Biological Psychology and Neuroergonomics at the Technical University of Berlin, for the developed Matlab-based software that supports part of the experimental component.

Conflicts of Interest: The funders had no role in the design of the study, in the collection, analyses, or interpretation of data, in the writing of the manuscript, or in the decision to publish the results. H.S. is one of the creators of the BITalino platform and one of the co-founders of the company currently commercializing it.

Abbreviations

The following abbreviations are used in this manuscript:

ACC	accelerometer
ANS	autonomic nervous system
API	application programming interface
BLE	Bluetooth Low Energy/Bluetooth 4.0
Bpm/bpm	beats per minute
CI	confidence interval
DiY	do-it-yourself
ECG	electrocardiography
EDA	electrodermal activity
EEG	electroencephalography
EMG	electromyography
EOG	electrooculography
GSR	galvanic skin response
HF	High Frequency
HF(nu)	High Frequency normalized unit
HR	Heart Rate
HRV	heart rate variability
Hz	Hertz
IAPS	International Affective Picture System
ICC	Intraclass Correlation Coefficient
LF	Low Frequency
LF(nu)	Low Frequency normalized unit
LF/HF	ratio between low frequency and high frequency
LoA	Limits of Agreement
LSL	Lab Streaming Layer
LUX	photo transistor

MEG	magnetoencephalography
Q-Q plot	quantile-quantile plot
RMSSD	Root Mean Square of Successive Differences
SDNN	Standard deviation of the NN (R-R) intervals
USB	Universal Serial Bus
VLF	very low frequency
XDF	extensible data format

References

1. Jimenez-Molina, A.; Retamal, C.; Lira, H. Using psychophysiological sensors to assess mental workload during web browsing. *Sensors* **2018**, *18*, 458. [CrossRef] [PubMed]
2. Manzey, D.; Luz, M.; Mueller, S.; Dietz, A.; Meixensberger, J.; Strauss, G. Automation in surgery: The impact of navigated-control assistance on performance, workload, situation awareness, and acquisition of surgical skills. *Hum. Factors* **2011**, *53*, 584–599. [CrossRef] [PubMed]
3. Da Silva, H.P.; Fred, A.; Martins, R. Biosignals for Everyone. *IEEE Pervasive Comput.* **2014**, *13*, 64–71. [CrossRef]
4. Carreiras, C.; Lourenço, A.; Silva, H.; Fred, A. Comparative Study of Medical-grade and Off-the-Person ECG Systems. In Proceedings of the International Congress on Cardiovascular Technologies—IWoPE (CARDIOTECHNIX), Vilamoura, Portugal, 20–21 September 2013; INSTICC, SciTePress: Setúbal, Portugal, 2013; pp. 115–120. [CrossRef]
5. Ishaque, S.; Khan, N.; Krishnan, S. Trends in Heart-Rate Variability Signal Analysis. *Front. Digit. Health* **2021**, *3*, 13. [CrossRef]
6. Baek, H.J.; Shin, J. Effect of missing inter-beat interval data on heart rate variability analysis using wrist-worn wearables. *J. Med. Syst.* **2017**, *41*, 1–9. [CrossRef] [PubMed]
7. Morelli, D.; Rossi, A.; Cairo, M.; Clifton, D.A. Analysis of the impact of interpolation methods of missing RR-intervals caused by motion artifacts on HRV features estimations. *Sensors* **2019**, *19*, 3163. [CrossRef] [PubMed]
8. Clifford, G.D.; Tarassenko, L. Quantifying errors in spectral estimates of HRV due to beat replacement and resampling. *IEEE Trans. Biomed. Eng.* **2005**, *52*, 630–638. [CrossRef]
9. Lang, P.J.; Bradley, M.M.; Cuthbert, B.N. *International Affective Picture System (IAPS): Affective Ratings of Pictures and Instruction Manual*; Technical Report A-8; Technical Report; The Center for the Study of Emotion and Attention (CSEA): Gainesville, FL, USA, 2008.
10. Bota, P.J.; Wang, C.; Fred, A.L.; Da Silva, H.P. A review, current challenges, and future possibilities on emotion recognition using machine learning and physiological signals. *IEEE Access* **2019**, *7*, 140990–141020. [CrossRef]
11. Bland, J.M.; Altman, D. Statistical methods for assessing agreement between two methods of clinical measurement. *Lancet* **1986**, *327*, 307–310. [CrossRef]
12. Ranganathan, P.; Pramesh, C.; Aggarwal, R. Common pitfalls in statistical analysis: Measures of agreement. *Perspect. Clin. Res.* **2017**, *8*, 187. [CrossRef]
13. Team, M.I.C.T. BITalino Toolbox-File Exchange-MATLAB Central. 2018. Available online: https://ww2.mathworks.cn/matlabcentral/fileexchange/53983-bitalino-toolbox?requestedDomain=zh (accessed on 2 June 2021).
14. Kothe, C.; Brunner, C. *Extensible Data Format (XDF)*; Swartz Center for Computational Neuroscience (SCCN), University of California: San Diego, CA, USA, 2018.
15. Brouwer, A.M.; van Wouwe, N.; Mühl, C.; van Erp, J.; Toet, A. Perceiving blocks of emotional pictures and sounds: Effects on physiological variables. *Front. Hum. Neurosci.* **2013**, *7*. [CrossRef]
16. Greenwald, M.K.; Cook, E.W.; Lang, P.J. Affective judgment and psychophysiological response: Dimensional covariation in the evaluation of pictorial stimuli. *J. Psychophysiol.* **1989**, *3*, 51–64.
17. Bradley, M.M.; Cuthbert, B.N.; Lang, P.J. Startle Reflex Modification: Emotion or Attention? *Psychophysiology* **1990**, *27*, 513–522. [CrossRef]
18. Lang, P.J.; Bradley, M.M.; Cuthbert, B.N. Emotion, motivation, and anxiety: Brain mechanisms and psychophysiology. *Biol. Psychiatry* **1998**, *44*, 1248–1263. [CrossRef]
19. Bradley, M.M.; Lang, P.J. Affective reactions to acoustic stimuli. *Psychophysiology* **2000**, *37*, 204–215. [CrossRef]
20. Anttonen, J.; Surakka, V. Emotions and heart rate while sitting on a chair. In *Proceedings of the SIGCHI Conference on Human Factors in Computing Systems*; ACM Press: Portland, OR, USA, 2005; pp. 491–499. [CrossRef]
21. Codispoti, M.; De Cesarei, A. Arousal and attention: Picture size and emotional reactions. *Psychophysiology* **2007**, *44*, 680–686. [CrossRef]
22. Sokhadze, E.M. Effects of Music on the Recovery of Autonomic and Electrocortical Activity After Stress Induced by Aversive Visual Stimuli. *Appl. Psychophysiol. Biofeedback* **2007**, *32*, 31–50. [CrossRef]
23. Task Force of the European Society of Cardiology and Others. Heart Rate Variability: Standards of Measurement, Physiological Interpretation, and Clinical Use. *Circulation* **1996**, *93*, 1043–1065. [CrossRef]
24. Gramann, K.; Schandry, R. *Psychophysiologie: Körperliche Indikatoren Psychischen Geschehens*, 4th ed.; vollst. überarb. aufl, Ed.; Beltz PVU: Weinheim, Germany, 2009.
25. Hare, R.; Wood, K.; Britain, S.; Shadman, J. Autonomic Responses to Affective Visual Stimulation. *Psychophysiology* **1970**, *7*, 408–417. [CrossRef]

26. Libby, W.L.; Lacey, B.C.; Lacey, J.I. Pupillary and Cardiac Activity During Visual Attention. *Psychophysiology* **1973**, *10*, 270–294. [CrossRef]
27. Winton, W.M.; Putnam, L.E.; Krauss, R.M. Facial and autonomic manifestations of the dimensional structure of emotion. *J. Exp. Soc. Psychol.* **1984**, *20*, 195–216. [CrossRef]
28. Lang, P.J.; Greenwald, M.K.; Bradley, M.M.; Hamm, A.O. Looking at pictures: Affective, facial, visceral, and behavioral reactions. *Psychophysiology* **1993**, *30*, 261–273. [CrossRef]
29. Müller, R.; Büttner, P. A critical discussion of intraclass correlation coefficients. *Stat. Med.* **1994**, *13*, 2465–2476. [CrossRef]
30. Pinna, G.; Maestri, R.; Torunski, A.; Danilowicz-Szymanowicz, L.; Szwoch, M.; La Rovere, M.; Raczak, G. Heart rate variability measures: A fresh look at reliability. *Clin. Sci.* **2007**, *113*, 131–140. [CrossRef] [PubMed]
31. Portney, L.G.; Watkins, M.P. *Foundations of Clinical Research: Applications to Practice*, 3rd ed.; Pearson/Prentice Hall: Upper Saddle River, NJ, USA, 2009.
32. Lee, J.; Koh, D.; Ong, C.N. Statistical evaluation of agreement between two methods for measuring a quantitative variable. *Comput. Biol. Med.* **1989**, *19*, 61–70. [CrossRef]
33. McGraw, K.O.; Wong, S.P. Forming inferences about some intraclass correlation coefficients. *Psychol. Methods* **1996**, *1*, 30–46. [CrossRef]
34. Shrout, P.E.; Fleiss, J.L. Intraclass correlations: Uses in assessing rater reliability. *Psychol. Bull.* **1979**, *86*, 420–428. [CrossRef] [PubMed]
35. Altman, D.G.; Bland, J.M. Measurement in Medicine: The Analysis of Method Comparison Studies. *Statistician* **1983**, *32*, 307. [CrossRef]
36. Bland, J.M.; Altman, D.G. Comparing Methods of Clinical Measurement-A Citation-Classic Commentary on Statistical-Methods for Assessing Agreement between 2 Methods of Clinical Measurment. *Curr. Contents* **1992**, *40*, 8.
37. Ryan, T.P.; Woodall, W.H. The most-cited statistical papers. *J. Appl. Stat.* **2005**, *32*, 461–474. [CrossRef]
38. Bland, J.M.; Altman, D.G. Agreement Between Methods of Measurement with Multiple Observations Per Individual. *J. Biopharm. Stat.* **2007**, *17*, 571–582. [CrossRef]
39. Shapiro, S.S.; Wilk, M.B. An Analysis of Variance Test for Normality (Complete Samples). *Biometrika* **1965**, *52*, 591. [CrossRef]
40. Bland, J.M.; Altman, D.G. Measuring agreement in method comparison studies. *Stat. Methods Med. Res.* **1999**, *8*, 135–160. [CrossRef]
41. Weippert, M.; Kumar, M.; Kreuzfeld, S.; Arndt, D.; Rieger, A.; Stoll, R. Comparison of three mobile devices for measuring R-R intervals and heart rate variability: Polar S810i, Suunto t6 and an ambulatory ECG system. *Eur. J. Appl. Physiol.* **2010**, *109*, 779–786. [CrossRef]
42. Sandercock, G.R.H.; Shelton, C.; Bromley, P.; Brodie, D.A. Agreement between three commercially available instruments for measuring short-term heart rate variability. *Physiol. Meas.* **2004**, *25*, 1115–1124. [CrossRef]
43. Nunan, D.; Donovan, G.; Jakovljevic, D.G.; Hodges, L.D.; Sandercock, G.R.H.; Brodie, D.A. Validity and Reliability of Short-Term Heart-Rate Variability from the Polar S810. *Med. Sci. Sport. Exerc.* **2009**, *41*, 243–250. [CrossRef]
44. Da Silva, H.P.; Carreiras, C.; Lourenço, A.; Fred, A.; das Neves, R.C.; Ferreira, R. Off-the-person electrocardiography: Performance assessment and clinical correlation. *Health Technol.* **2015**, *4*, 309–318. [CrossRef]

sensors

MDPI

Article

Ambient Healthcare Approach with Hybrid Whale Optimization Algorithm and Naïve Bayes Classifier

Majed Alwateer [1], Abdulqader M. Almars [1], Kareem N. Areed [2], Mostafa A. Elhosseini [1,2], Amira Y. Haikal [2] and Mahmoud Badawy [2,*]

1 College of Computer Science and Engineering, Taibah University, Yanbu 46421, Saudi Arabia; MWATEER@taibahu.edu.sa (M.A.); Amars@taibahu.edu.sa (A.M.A.); melhosseini@mans.edu.eg (M.A.E.)
2 Computers and Control Systems Engineering Department, Faculty of Engineering, Mansoura University, Mansoura 35516, Egypt; ek8819@gmail.com (K.N.A.); amirayh@mans.edu.eg (A.Y.H.)
* Correspondence: engbadawy@mans.edu.eg; Tel.: +20-1008008814

Abstract: There is a crucial need to process patient's data immediately to make a sound decision rapidly; this data has a very large size and excessive features. Recently, many cloud-based IoT healthcare systems are proposed in the literature. However, there are still several challenges associated with the processing time and overall system efficiency concerning big healthcare data. This paper introduces a novel approach for processing healthcare data and predicts useful information with the support of the use of minimum computational cost. The main objective is to accept several types of data and improve accuracy and reduce the processing time. The proposed approach uses a hybrid algorithm which will consist of two phases. The first phase aims to minimize the number of features for big data by using the Whale Optimization Algorithm as a feature selection technique. After that, the second phase performs real-time data classification by using Naïve Bayes Classifier. The proposed approach is based on fog Computing for better business agility, better security, deeper insights with privacy, and reduced operation cost. The experimental results demonstrate that the proposed approach can reduce the number of datasets features, improve the accuracy and reduce the processing time. Accuracy enhanced by average rate: 3.6% (3.34 for Diabetes, 2.94 for Heart disease, 3.77 for Heart attack prediction, and 4.15 for Sonar). Besides, it enhances the processing speed by reducing the processing time by an average rate: 8.7% (28.96 for Diabetes, 1.07 for Heart disease, 3.31 for Heart attack prediction, and 1.4 for Sonar).

Keywords: big healthcare data; classification; decision-making; feature selection; whale optimization; naive bayes

Citation: Alwateer, M.; Almars, A.M.; Areed, K.N.; Elhosseini, M.A.; Haikal, A.Y.; Badawy, M. Ambient Healthcare Approach with Hybrid Whale Optimization Algorithm and Naïve Bayes Classifier. *Sensors* **2021**, *21*, 4579. https://doi.org/10.3390/s21134579

Academic Editors: Ayman El-baz, Guruprasad A. Giridharan, Ahmed Shalaby, Ali H. Mahmoud and Mohammed Ghazal

Received: 3 June 2021
Accepted: 2 July 2021
Published: 4 July 2021

1. Introduction

Recently, many medical devices are equipped with sensors to collect, communicate, and integrate the massive generated medical data. Modern healthcare systems are based on emerging technology such as Wireless Sensor Networks (WSN) and the Internet of Things (IoT). Moreover, there is a widespread deployment for smart mobility initiatives that increase the development of intelligent healthcare systems. The objective is to maximize the use of real-time data streaming out of various medical, sensory services. The IoT generates diverse and complex big healthcare data. This data poses many challenges to the storage and analysis infrastructure. The convergence of IoT and several fundamental technologies such as cloud computing has become necessary to address the aforementioned challenges [1]. As shown in Figure 1, IoT-based healthcare systems may deploy a wide range of computing technologies such as cloud, edge, and fog computing, as a virtual resource utilization infrastructure.

Big data has become a slogan for many scientific and technological enterprises, researchers, data analysts, and technical practitioners. Big data can be defined as any large and complex data source (gold mine) combined with a combination of old and new data-management technologies and architecture. Organizations can gather, store, manage, and manipulate extremely large volumes and a wide variety of data from many sources at the required speed and the proper time to gain the right insights [2]. Big data offers the basic functionalities that enable different organizations to manage data rapidly, timely conducted, and obtain smart decisions to gain the value of big data [3]. Big data is characterized by three V's (Volume, Velocity, and Variety), according to industrial data analyst Doug Laney [4]. Three V's are increased by four more V's (Variability, Veracity, Validity, and Volatility) up to seven V's later, as shown in Figure 2. To cope, the big biomedical data is characterized by scale, diversity, and complexity. Biomedical data processing consists of phases that are collecting, processing, and managing data. The main objective is to produce new information for end-users [5]. There are four steps for big data analysis, defined as four A's: Acquisition, Assembly, Analyze, and Action.

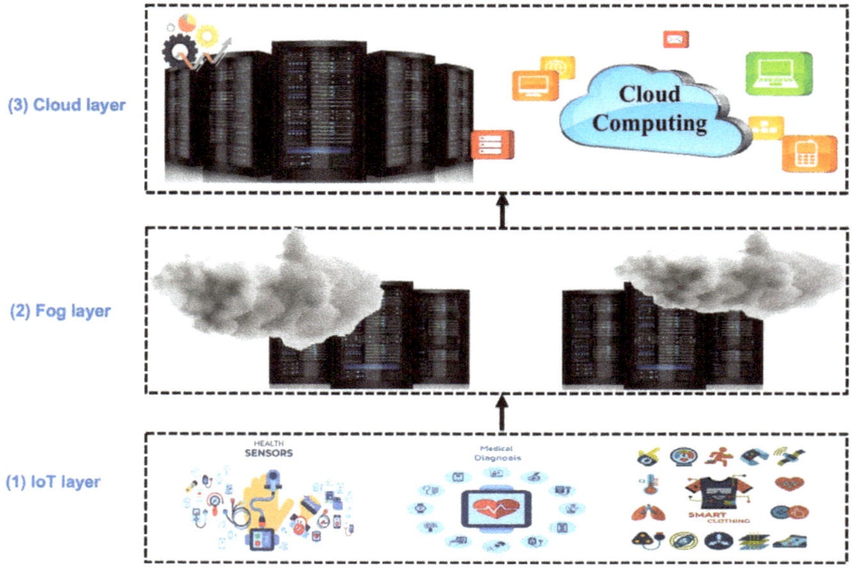

Figure 1. Modern healthcare systems' structure.

The main objective of big data architecture is to extract value from a wide range of data by collecting the raw generated data from various data sources (Acquisition) [2]. Data collection techniques are used to collect raw data from various data formats. Analyze means using analytical methods, algorithms, and tools to find new insights and extract value. Data mining simultaneously helps to generate insight and forecasting patterns and provides smart query functions, then decisions (Action) must be available [6].

The biomedical domain also joins the era of the development of big data. The big data contains patient information, essential signals, and others from a wide range of data sources. Big data technology stores, analyzes, and exploits patient information. However, a cloud-based IoT healthcare system suffers from challenging problems that are demanding prompt solutions. The following list surveys some barriers [7] such as:

- The massive collected data storage;
- Eliminate privacy and security leakage at a different platform level;
- Energy management with continuous monitoring leads to an increase in data volume and analytical demands;
- Deliver the information at the proper time and in a reliable manner;
- Heterogeneity: the diversity of the connected things;
- High dynamics: the dynamic global network infrastructure;

- Quality of Service (QoS) supports both QoS and functional properties concerning a Service-Level Agreement (SLA).

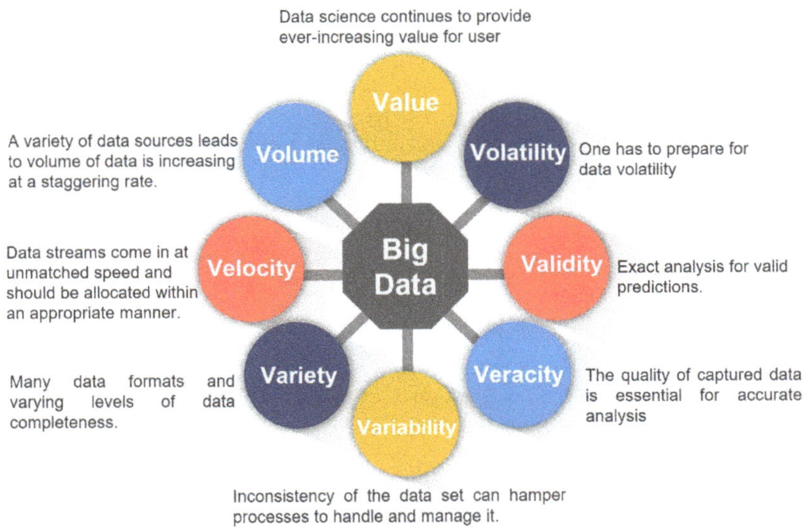

Figure 2. Big data multi-V's model.

Speed, efficiency, and high computational cost problems can be solved by saving time and reducing processing costs. We need to reduce the volume of data, and this can be implemented by reducing the feature of big data being processed. Data volume minimization can be achieved via the implementation of a Feature Selection (FS) technique. FS affects performance and offers faster decisions. FS determines the features that should be employed to improve performance [2].

The metaheuristic algorithms find the optimal settings of the application parameters and hyperparameters [8]. Metaheuristic algorithms can be categorized into three categories: evolutionary algorithms (EAs), trajectory-based algorithms, and swarm-based algorithms. Swarm-based algorithms are intuitive and inspired by nature, humans, and animals. While working with these algorithms, the researcher should make a compromise between exploration and exploitation. It turns out that the exploration process is searching far from the current candidate solution, while the exploitation is searching in the vicinity, near the current solution. The Whale Optimization Algorithm (WOA) has a low number of adjustable hyperparameters. The WOA mimics the humpback whale in searching for prey. The WOA consists of three operators to model the behavior of humpback whales. The WOA can accomplish data optimization missions by minimizing the number of features with high performance and making data ready to classify. The data are currently ready to be categorized, and several classification algorithms are included, including Decision Tree, Deep Learning (DL), K-Nearest Neighbor (KNN), and Naïve Bayes (NB). The NB classifier is a Bayes theorem-based model of probabilistic machine learning. NB can accomplish data classification as fast, simple to enforce, and real-time action support.

The main objective of this study is to propose a suitable approach for processing medical data rapidly in real-time and increasing its accuracy in a form that saves computational costs. This can be achieved by proposing an Ambient Healthcare approach with the Hybrid Whale Optimization Algorithm and Naïve Bayes Classifier (AHCA-WOANB) to perform feature selection on data and then classify it to reduce processing time while increasing performance.

The remaining of this paper will be as following: Section 2 will discuss related work and put a spotlight on the pros and cons of every discussed contribution; Section 3 will introduce the proposed AHCA-WOANB approach and the way of embedding the hybrid algorithm; Section 4 will introduce the experimental results that obtained; Finally, Section 5 will introduce the conclusion and future work.

2. Related Work

Medical services expect significant advancements through IoT and cloud computing integration. This integration introduces new forms of intelligent medical equipment and applications. The recently developed and introduced medical systems are targeted at the industry and academia to implement modern healthcare systems. IoT-based health architecture captures, processes, and analyzes medical data. In this vein, developing healthcare architectures, feature selection, and data classification has received significant attention in academia and the industry in the last few years [9]. In the next subsections, there will be a detailed description of the recent healthcare architecture. The WoA and NB classifier will also be surveyed.

2.1. Healthcare Architectures

Abawajy et al. [6] suggested a Cloud-based Patient monitoring architecture. There are three stages to their proposed architecture: collection station, data center, and monitoring station. Andriopoulou et al. [10] proposed a healthcare service framework based on fog computing that intermediates between clouds and loT devices and allows for new forms of computing and services. Their architecture comprises three main layers: data aggregation fog nodes, information storage, data processing and analysis fog servers, and data storage clouds. The same study introduced an IoT-based architecture for fog-based healthcare networks [10]. The design and implementation of the proposed architecture were in three layers. The first layer is IoT-based devices. The second layer consists of fog, while the third layer consists of the cloud layer. This architecture reduces cloud service traffic and provides low delays and immense permanent storage space. The integrated edge, fog, healthcare IoT-based cloud infrastructure was implemented by Dimosthenis et al. [11]. Their architecture consists of three layers for acquiring operation, data storage, and decision-making in real-time. The three layers are the edge layer that is close to the patients, the fog layer responsible for storing and processing data, and the cloud infrastructure that stores and analyzes data extracted from the fog and edge layers. Hassan et al. [9] have developed a 4-layer hybrid architecture named HAAL-NBFA, inspired by a growing interest in the use of AmI to develop care assistance systems for elderly patients. The HAAL-NBFA used both local monitoring and cloud-based architectures. The goal was to predict a patient's health status from contextual circumstances. They suggested a five-stage cloud classification model that can deal with broad imbalanced datasets. The Deep Learning Three-Layer Architecture called HealthFog was proposed by Shreshth Tuli et al. [12]. HealthFog shows its performance in energy usage, latency, and execution time. QoS attributes are not taken into account. The comparison of recent health system architectures in the literature is shown in Table 1.

Table 1. Recent healthcare system architecture.

Architecture	No. of Layers	Scalability	Flexibility	Real-Time Support	Energy-Efficiency	Computational Cost
PPHM [6]	Three Layer	Scalable	Flexible	N/A	Energy-efficient	High
HSDA [10]	Three Layers	Moderate	Moderate	support	Moderate	Moderate
EFCHioT [11]	Three Layers	Scalable	Limited	support	Energy-efficient	High
HAAL-NBFA [9]	Four Layers	Scalable	Limited	support	Moderate	High
HealthFog [12]	Three Layers	Limited	Moderate	support	Energy-efficient	Low

2.2. Whale Optimization Algorithm

One of the well-known metaheuristic optimization algorithms is the Whale Optimization Algorithm (WOA) [13,14]. WOA is considered a Wrapper-based Feature Selection technique, influenced by nature, proposed by Seyedali Mirjalili et al. [13,14]. The main inspiration for WOA is the actions of humpback whales. Whether by encircling or bubble-net approaches, they strike the prey. The current optimal location in the surrounding activity is treated as the prey, and according to Equations (1) and (2), the whale updates its position.

$$\vec{D} = \left| C.\vec{X}^*(t)) - X(t) \right| \tag{1}$$

$$\vec{X}(t+1) = \vec{X}^*(t) - \vec{A}.\vec{D} \tag{2}$$

where t refers to the current iteration, X^* is the vector that corresponds to the best solution, and X defines the position vector of the whale. The absolute value is $||$ and . is the element-wise multiplication. $\vec{A}$ and $\vec{C}$ are determined as follows in Equations (3) and (4).

$$\vec{A} = 2\vec{a}.\vec{r} - \vec{a} \tag{3}$$

$$\vec{C} = 2.\vec{r} \tag{4}$$

where a is linearly decreased from 2 to 0 throughout iterations, and r indicates a random number in $[0, 1]$.

There are only two ways to simulate bubble-net behavior. The first is to shrink the enclosing using Equation (3) with a reduced range of A by a. The search agent's new position can be defined anywhere between the best possible current position and the original position. Figure 3 depicts the feasible position from (X, Y) to (X^*, Y^*) that $\vec{A}$ can obtain in a 2D space, as given by Equation (3). The second one is the spiral updating positions; Equation (5) is used as a logarithmic spiral equation. The movement of humpback whales around the prey is helix-shaped, which is mimicked using Equation (5).

$$\vec{X}(t+1) = \vec{D'}.e^{bl}.cos(2\pi l) + \vec{X^*}(t) \tag{5}$$

Here, $\vec{D'} = \left| \vec{X^*}(t) - X(t) \right|$ is the distance from the ith whale to the victim, and B is a parameter for determining the form of the logarithmic spiral. l denotes a random number in $[-1, 1]$ that determines how close the next location of the whale is to the victim. $l = -1$ is the nearest location to the victim as shown in Figure 4.

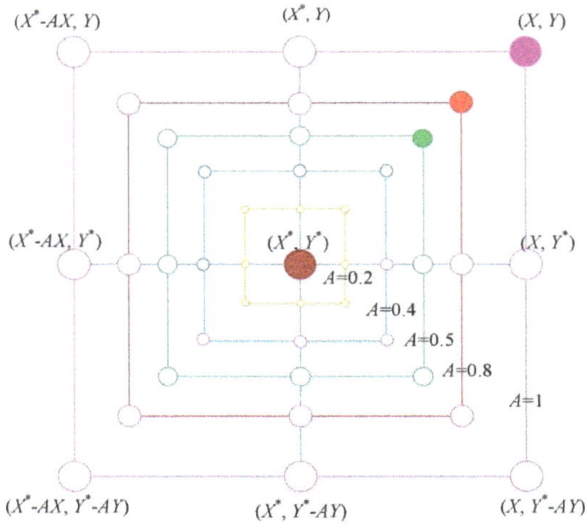

Figure 3. The WOA shrinking encircling mechanism.

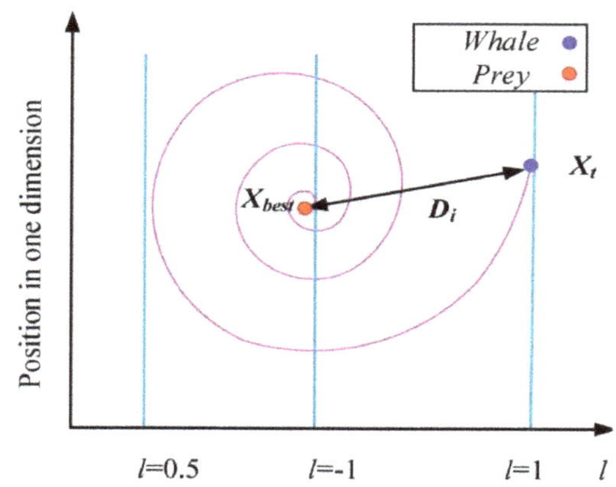

Figure 4. The spiral updating position.

It is worth remembering that humpback whales will simultaneously swim around the prey and along spiral-shaped tracks in a shrinking circle. To model this concurrent activity, the researchers believe that the processes of shrinking or the spiral model for adjusting the whale's location are equally probable. Equation (6) defines the mathematical model as follows.

$$\vec{x}(t+1) = \begin{cases} \vec{X}^*(t) - \vec{A}.\vec{D} & \text{if } p < 0.5 \\ X(t+1) = \vec{D}'.e^{bl}.cos(2\pi l) + \vec{X}^*(t) & \text{if } p \geq 0.5 \end{cases} \quad (6)$$

Here, p is a random number in $[0,1]$, which decides when to use the spiral model or the shrinking encircling method to change the whale position. In addition, humpback whales will search randomly, depending on the location of each other. The mechanism can be accomplished as follows:

$$\vec{D} = \left| \vec{C}.\vec{X_{rand}}(t) - \vec{x}(t) \right| \quad (7)$$

$$\vec{X}(t+1) = \vec{X_{rand}}(t) - \vec{A}.\vec{D} \quad (8)$$

where $\vec{X_{rand}}$ is a random whale (a random position vector) chosen from the current population. The WOA algorithm's pseudo-code is shown in Algorithm 1. The WOA algorithm randomly chooses X as the optimal way to enhance exploration.

The X^* value is chosen in the WOA algorithm for moving randomly selected whales rather than the best one to boost exploration. Besides Features Selection as a way to process data, there are other methods, including data classification. Data classification can be done in more than one form and by using many algorithms that differ in how they classify the big data.

Algorithm 1: The WOA

Initialize search agents.
Evaluate fitness function.
$it \leftarrow 0$
X^* = the best search agent.
while $t < MaxIteration$ **do**
    foreach $SearchAgent$ **do**
        Update A, C, l, p, and a.
        if $p \geq 0.5$ **then**
            $X(t+1)$ = Updating the search agent's position using the spiral method (Equation (5)).
        else
            if $|A| < 1$ **then**
                $X(t+1)$ = Updating the position of the current search agent using the encircling mechanism (Equation (1)).
            else if $|A| \geq 1$ **then**
                Random search agent is selected.
                $X(t+1)$ = Updating the position of the current search agent by using the prey searching method (Equation (8)).
            end
        end
    end
    If there is better solution, update $X^* = X(t+1)$.
    $t = t + 1$
end
return X^*

2.3. *Naïve Bayes Algorithm*

The Naïve Bayes Algorithm (NB) is a Bayes Theorem-based classification technique with an assumption of independence among predictors. It can be used for spam filters, text analysis, and medical diagnosis [15]. Naïve Bayes is considered one of the best algorithms with several advantages, such as easy implementation, high speed, and efficiency. NB requires less training data, is scalable, handles both continuous and discrete data, and is best suited for text data and fog computing support. The Naïve Bayes model is simple to construct and especially effective for very large datasets. Naïve Bayes also provides highly advanced classification methods as well as simplicity. The theorem of Bayes provides a way of calculating posterior probability $P(c \mid x)$ from $P(c)$, $P(x)$, and $P(x \mid c)$. The equation will be:

$$P(c \mid x) = \frac{P(x \mid c).P(c)}{P(x)} \tag{9}$$

The equation parameters are:

- $P(c \mid x)$: the posterior probability of class (c, target) given predictor (x, attributes).
- $P(c)$: the prior probability of class.
- $P(x \mid c)$: the likelihood which is the probability of the predictor given class.
- $P(x)$: the prior probability of the predictor.

The classification process can easily be described in three simple steps: (i) create the frequency table from the dataset, (ii) establish a Likelihood table by specifying the probabilities, and (iii) use the Bayesian equation to measure the post-class probability. The prediction result is the class with the highest posterior probability. In practice, it is nearly impossible to obtain a set of completely independent predictors. Assume the categorical variable in the test data has a category but not in the train data; in this case, the probability of this category is set to zero, and prediction is impossible.

To summarize, medical data has a very large size and has many features that can be decreased to make processing faster. There is a need to find a suitable method for processing medical data rapidly in real-time and increasing its accuracy in a form that saves computational cost. Many attempts were spotted on this point, and many solutions were introduced but with drawbacks in processing time and performance.

3. Methods

3.1. The Ambient Intelligent Healthcare Approach

Data evolves over time in most challenging data analysis applications and must be analyzed in near real-time. Patterns and relationships in such data frequently evolve over time, so models built to analyze such data quickly become obsolete. This phenomenon is known as concept drift in machine learning and data mining. In machine learning and data mining, concept drift refers to changes in the relationships between input and output data in the underlying problem over time. There are several approaches to dealing with concept drift; the most common is ignoring it and assuming that the data does not change. If you suspect that your dataset may be subject to concept drift, you can use a static model to detect Concept Drift Detection and a Baseline Performance. This should be your starting point and benchmark for comparing other methods. Solving the problem of increased processing time and high computational cost for medical big data systems is crucial. This can be achieved via (i) proposing an approach for processing various types of medical data, (ii) predicting useful information with minimum computational costs, and (iii) processing data in real-time. Therefore, a hybrid algorithm that consists of two phases is proposed. First, a feature selection technique is used to minimize the number of features. Thereafter, the second phase of the proposed hybridized algorithm is data classification.

As shown in Figure 5, the block structure of the proposed Ambient Healthcare approach with the Hybrid Whale Optimization Algorithm and the Naïve Bayes Classifier (AHCA-WOANB) consists of three main phases, which are the data collection phase, data processing phase, and services layer. Based on fog computing, the AHCA-WOANB gains most of its benefits, including enhanced business agility, improved security, deeper privacy knowledge, and reduced cost of operation.

The proposed approach phases are working according to specific steps. The first phase starts collecting data from various sources. Data diversity is concerned at this phase. For performing the data management process, data are transferred to the second phase. In the second phase, data are stored, then optimized and classified in a suitable way that facilitates the third phase to work correctly and introduce perfect services. In the next sections, there will be a detailed description of the phases of the AHCA-WOANB approach.

3.1.1. The Data Collection Phase

This phase consists of two steps: one for data perceptions and the second one responsible for transferring collected data to the next phase. The data comes from various sources such as hospitals, research institutes, wearable devices, and public organizations. After that, the collected data is transferred to the next phase via a networking medium.

3.1.2. The Data Management Phase

Fog technology is used to provide low latency and real-time communication between the data management phase and the other phases. To this end, this phase is applied using Hadoop [16,17], which is an open-source, Java-based software framework. The main objective of deploying Hadoop is to distribute data stores and applications processing on large clusters.

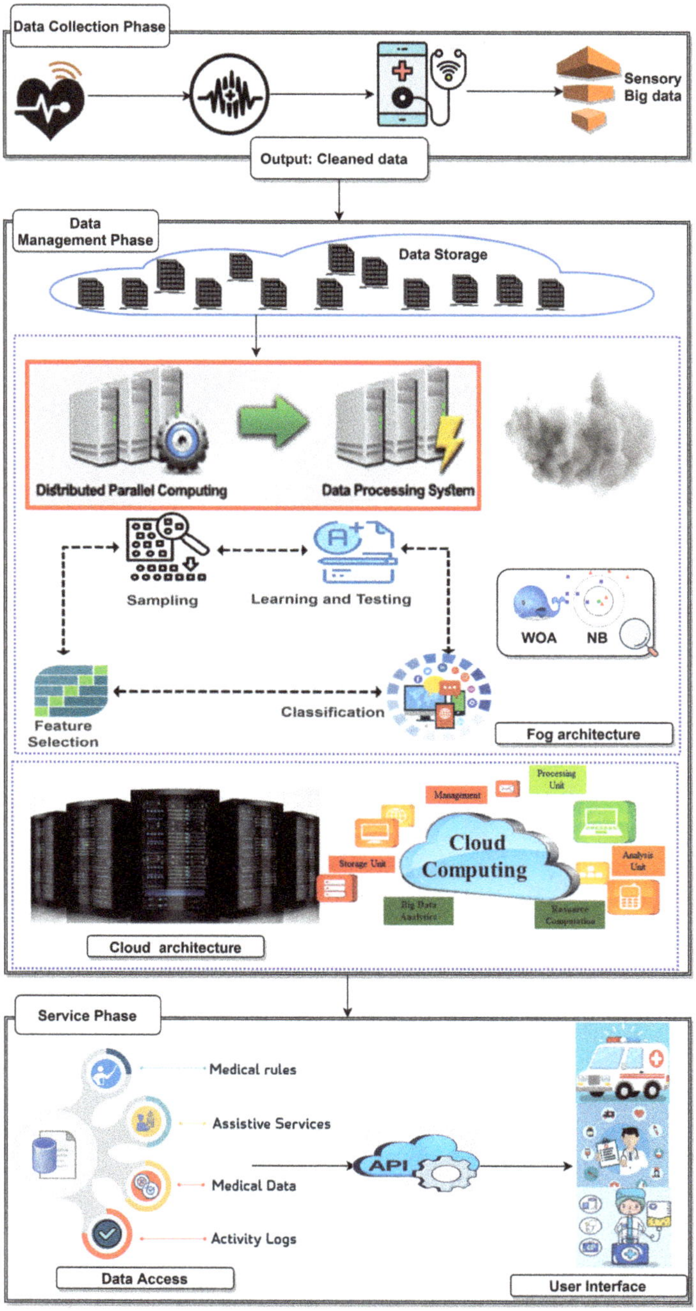

Figure 5. The proposed Ambient Intelligent Healthcare approach.

Hadoop provides massive storage for any kind of data, which is called the Hadoop Distributed File System (HDFS), and enormous processing power that is accomplished by Hadoop MapReduce programming, and this processing is easily made based on parallel computing. These support Hadoop with the ability to handle virtually limitless concurrent tasks or jobs and make it highly fault-tolerant and deployable on low-cost hardware. All of this makes it easy to depend on Hadoop as a backbone of any modern big data framework.

The data management phase consists of two modules that are responsible for data storage and processing. The first module is data storage, in which data are stored in the HDFS [16]. HDFS can store and spread massive datasets on hundreds of low-cost parallel servers. This supports the proposed approach with cost efficiency, flexibility, speed, and resilience to failure. The second module is data processing and classification, which uses Hadoop MapReduce [17] programming based on the proposed hybrid algorithm (WOA for feature selection then NB for classifying) and parallel computing to process many types of data.

The processing in this phase means optimizing data by using a hybrid algorithm. This algorithm performs a feature selection on big data that is stored in the HDFS using WOA, then classifies this optimized data using NB, and this processing is accomplished by MapReduce programming and parallel computing, as shown in Figure 6.

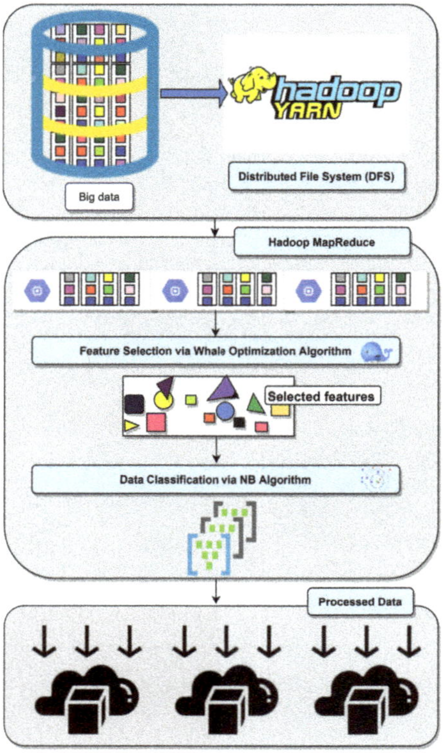

Figure 6. The proposed AHCA-WOANB approach data processing steps.

Data optimization and classification, as shown in Figure 7, are performed using MapReduce programming and parallel computing. This step is executed with the WOA for optimizing data by reducing the number of features of the currently processed dataset.

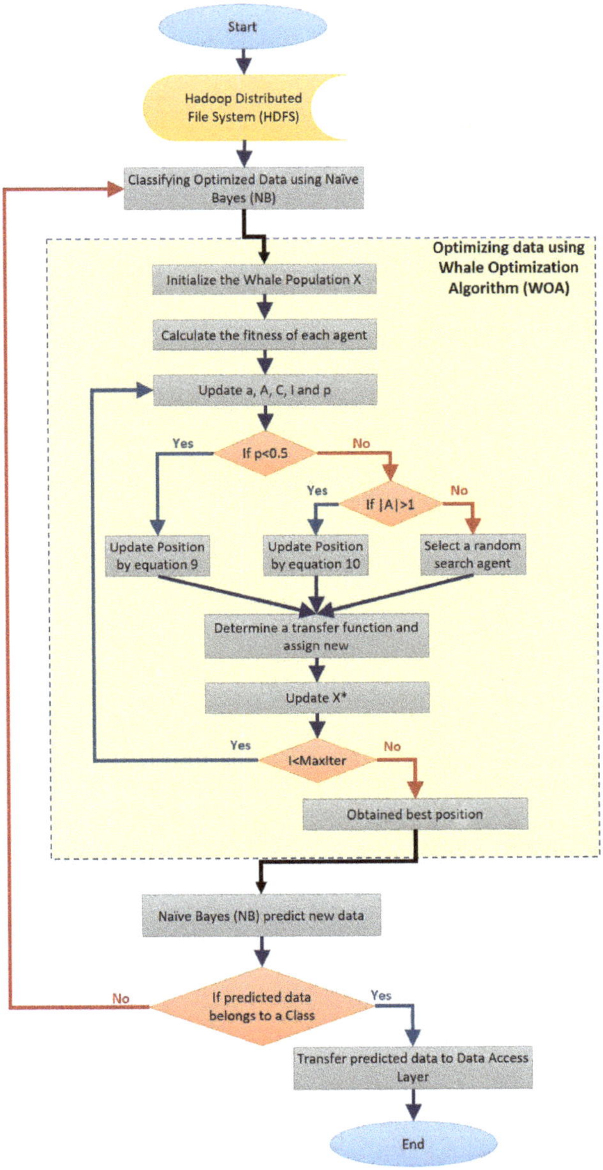

Figure 7. The proposed AHCA-WOANB approach flowchart.

Whales in the classical WOA move within the continuous search space to change their positions, referred to as continuous space. However, to solve Feature Selection problems, the solutions are limited to only 0 and 1 values. Therefore, continuous (free position) solutions must be converted to binary solutions to solve feature selection problems. As a result, a binary version of WOA is introduced to investigate the Feature Selection problem. The conversion is carried out by utilizing specific transfer functions, such as the S-shaped function. As a result, several studies have considered that the FS problem is an optimization problem; thus, the fitness function for the optimization algorithm has been changed to classifier accuracy, which the chosen features may maximize.

In this case, the proposed WOA algorithm is used to find the best features in an adaptive feature space search. This combination is obtained by achieving the highest classification accuracy while using the fewest features. The fitness function is depicted in Equation (10) below and the two proposed versions for evaluating individual whale positions.

$$F = \alpha\gamma_R(D) + \beta\frac{|C - R|}{|C|} \tag{10}$$

where:

- F denotes fitness function.
- R: the length of the selected feature subset.
- C: the total feature numbers.
- $\gamma_R(D)$: classification accuracy of the subset with length R.
- α: argument $\in [0, 1]$.
- β: argument $= 1 - \alpha$.

As a result, the fitness function with the highest classification accuracy will be produced. Based on the classification error rate and selected features, the equation above can be converted to a minimization problem. As a result, the obtained minimization problem can be solved, as shown in Equation (11).

$$F = \alpha E_R(D) + \beta\frac{|R|}{|C|} \tag{11}$$

where $E_R(D)$ is the classification error.

The method entails dividing a dataset into two subsets. The first subset, referred to as the training dataset 70%, is used to fit the model. The second subset is not used to train the model; rather, the model is fed the dataset's input element, and predictions are made based on the expected values. The second dataset is referred to as the test dataset 30%. The NB algorithm received the optimized datasets and started its mission to classify them and prepare for the predicting data stage. This means that while fewer features result in less computational complexity (both storage and execution), fewer features usually result in less accurate results due to the absence of useful information. The exception to this is when there are outliers and irrelevant features.

3.1.3. The Service Phase

The service phase consists of a set of modules: data access, Application Programming Interface (API), and User Interface (UI) modules. These modules interact with each other for performing the appropriate decision making. The data access module receives data and statistics from the processing and classification module then prepares the data to be used with the API and UI modules.

4. Simulation and Computer Results

This section evaluates the performance of the proposed AHCA-WOANB approach. The performance metrics that the system is seeking to improve are:

1. Accuracy: The validity of the predicted data by the system; improving this factor makes the decision making easier and more convenient.
2. Time: The time that the system will take to classify the data; eliminating this factor will minimize the cost.
3. Data Variety: The amount of accepted data by the system; this indicates how flexible the approach is by accepting more forms of data.

4.1. Used Datasets and Physical Meaning

This section explores the common datasets that were obtained from Kaggle [18]. These datasets will be used to test the approach and produce results. They are also various types, and the proposed approach will accept them easily, as mentioned in the first phase's description. Table 2 summarizes the characteristics of the used datasets.

Table 2. The characteristics of the used datasets.

Dataset	# Instances	# Features	Clasisfication Type	Availability
Heart disease UCI	303	14	Multiclass	The data set is publicly available on the Kaggle website https://www.kaggle.com/ronitf/heart-disease-uci (accessed on 2 July 2021)
Pima Indians Diabetes Database	768	9	Binary class	The data set is publicly available on the Kaggle website https://www.kaggle.com/uciml/pima-indians-diabetes-database (accessed on 2 July 2021)
Heart Attack Prediction	294	76	Multiclass	The data set is publicly available on the Kaggle website https://www.kaggle.com/imnikhilanand/heart-attack-prediction (accessed on 2 July 2021)
Sonar	1334	60	Binary class	The data set is publicly available on the Kaggle website https://www.kaggle.com/ypzhangsam/sonaralldata (accessed on 2 July 2021)

4.1.1. Diabetes

The dataset comes from the Diabetes and Digestive and Kidney Diseases National Institute. The dataset's purpose is to predict based on certain measures contained in the dataset whether a patient has diabetes or not. The collection of these instances from a large database has been limited by many constraints. All patients here are women of Pima's Indigenous Heritage who are at least 21 years old. The dataset contains multiple variables of the medical indicator and one variable objective, Outcome. Predictor variables (e.g., the number, BMI level, insulin level, age, and so on) of pregnancies that the patient has had.

4.1.2. Heart Disease Uci

There are 76 attributes in this database, but recent research refers to the use of a subset of 14. The only one used by ML researchers to date was the Cleveland database. The target area applies to the patient's involvement in heart disease. The integer value is between 0 (no presence) and 4. This set of data includes age, sex, type of chest pain (4 values), blood pressure, serum cholesterol in mg/dL, fasting blood sugar >120 mg/dL, electrocardiographic rest results (values, 1.2), achieved maximum heart rate, exercise inducing angina, exercise-induced ancient peak = ST exercise-induced depression, peak ST slopes, and the number of major vessels (0–3).

4.1.3. Heart Attack Prediction

The content of the cardiac disease directory is listed in this database. The data collection consists of various sources, including the Cleveland Clinical Foundation (Cleveland data) and the University Hospital, Zurich, Switzerland (SWID). Data are available from a wide variety of sources, including the VA Medical Center, Long Beach, CA (long-beach-va.data).

4.1.4. Sonar

This data collection includes 60 patterns derived from photos during pregnancy, which are used to assess fetal biometrics through ultrasound imagery. One such measurement is the circumference of the fetal head (HC). The HC can be used to estimate the pregnancy and to track fetal development. In a certain cross-section of the fetal head, called the default plane, HC is calculated. A total of 1334 2D images of the Standard Plane can be used to calculate the HC in the dataset for this challenge. In this challenge, algorithms built to calculate the fetal head circumference automatically can be compared in 2D ultrasound images.

4.2. Computer Results

This section presents the results that were achieved from testing the hybrid WOA-NB algorithm. First, we will introduce a comparison between the accuracy and speed of processing for every tested dataset using two ways. The first one is by executing classification only by using NB. The second one is by executing feature selection then classification by using WOA then NB, and this is the hybrid algorithm mentioned previously. The first-way results are introduced in Liangxiao et al. [19], which give NB results without other algorithms on multiple datasets. The second-way results will be calculated after executing the proposed hybrid algorithm. The comparison results will be shown in Table 3. Figures 8–11 depict the original and predicted data shapes for different datasets.

Table 3. Accuracy and speed comparison between NB and WOA-NB.

Classifier		Datasets			
Algorithm(s)	**Parameters**	**Diabetes**	**Heart-C**	**Heart-H**	**Sonar**
NB	No. of Features	8 of 8	13 of 13	13 of 13	60 of 60
	Accuracy (%)	77.24	83.04	83.91	85.4
	Time (s)	1.3151	0.81224	0.82374	0.87044
WOA and NB	No. of Features	4 of 8	12 of 13	12 of 13	52 of 60
	Accuracy (%)	79.82	85.48	87.07	88.94
	Time (s)	0.93421	0.80358	0.79651	0.85827

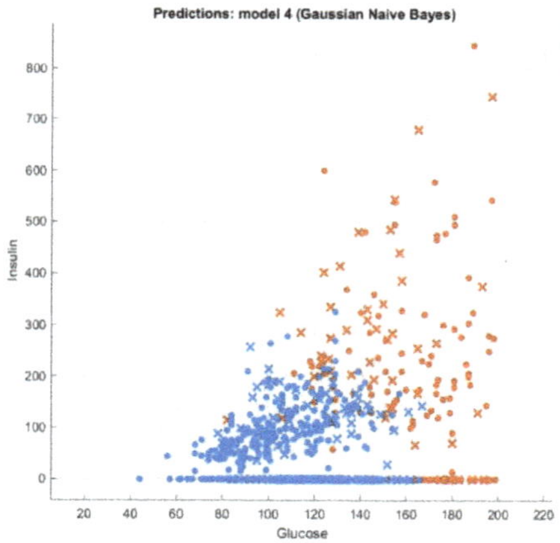

Figure 8. The Diabetes original and predicted data.

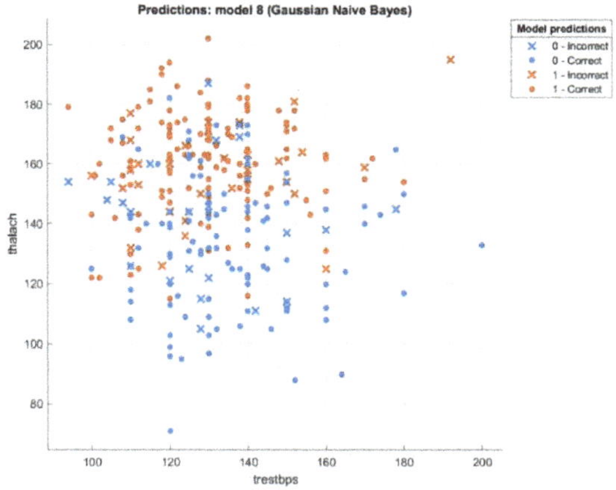

Figure 9. The Heart-C original and predicted data.

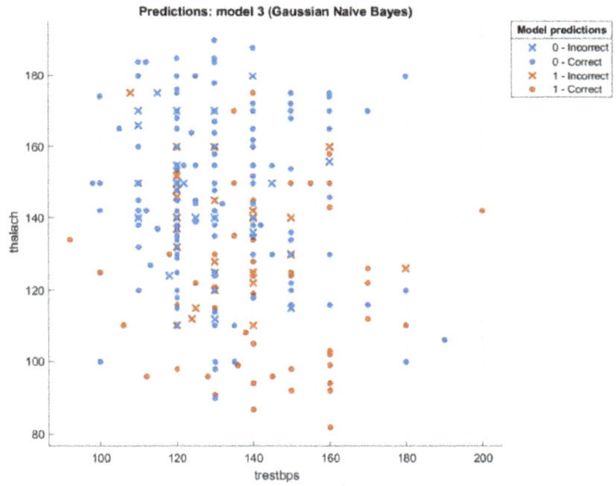

Figure 10. The Heart-H original and predicted data.

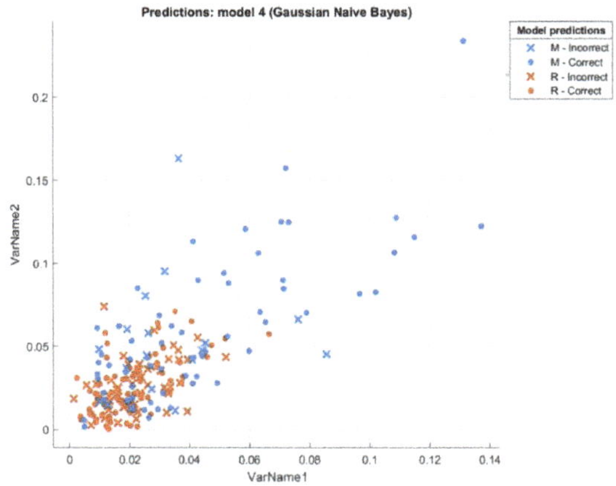

Figure 11. The Sonar original and predicted data.

The results show an enhancement in accuracy and time using the proposed approach over classification with only NB [19]. The enhancement is based on the number of reduced features after applying the WOA feature selection technique. In the Diabetes dataset, there are four of eight fewer features, and this enhanced the accuracy by 3.34% and reduced the computational time by 28.96%. In the Heart disease UCI dataset, there are 12 of 13 reduced features, and this enhanced the accuracy by 2.94% and reduced computational time by 1.07%. In the Heart attack prediction dataset, there are 12 of 13 reduced features, and this enhanced the accuracy by 3.77% and reduced the computational time by 3.31%. There are 52 of 60 fewer features in the Sonar dataset, which enhanced the accuracy by 4.15% and reduced the computational time by 1.4%. Figures 12 and 13 compare accuracy results and processing time results calculated from both Jiang [19] and the proposed approach.

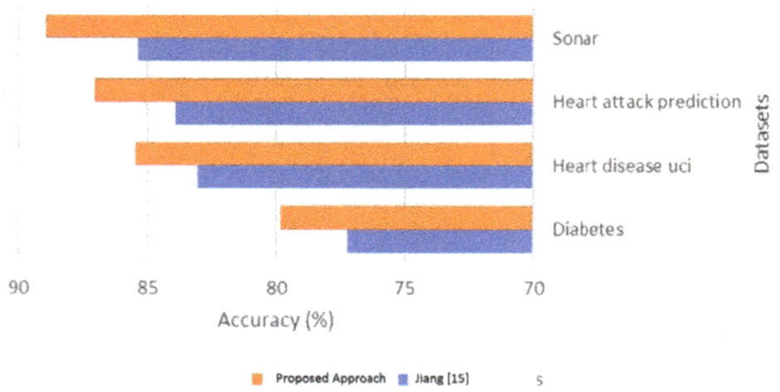

Figure 12. Accuracy comparison between NB and the proposed approach.

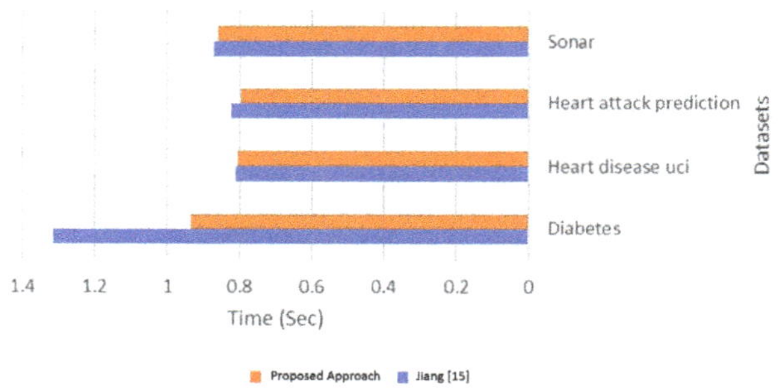

Figure 13. Time comparison between and the proposed approach.

The confusion matrix [20] is a performance calculation for a classification problem of learning machines that can measure the effectiveness of the proposed approach. The output can be two or more classes, as shown in Figure 14. It is a table of four different expected and true value combinations.

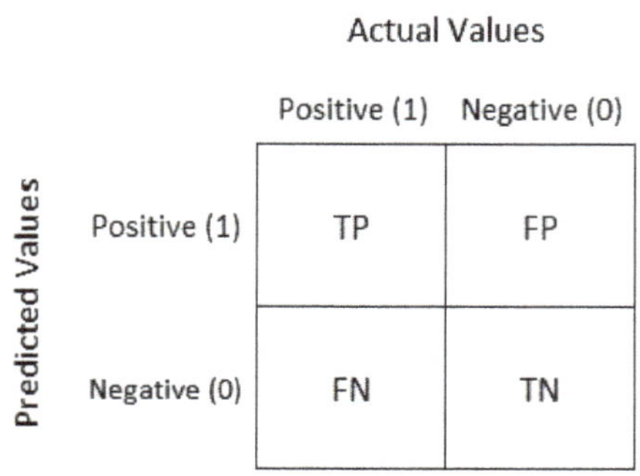

Figure 14. The confusion matrix.

There are two classes (Class 1: Positive and Class 2: Negative), and there are many terms as follows: Positive (P), Negative (N), True Positive (TP), False Negative (FN), True Negative (TN), and False Positive (FP) as follows:

- Positive (P): Observation is positive (for example: is an apple).
- Negative (N): Observation is not positive (for example: is not an apple).
- True Positive (TP): Observation is positive and is predicted to be positive.
- False Negative (FN): Observation is positive but is predicted negative.
- True Negative (TN): Observation is negative and is predicted to be negative.
- False Positive (FP): Observation is negative but is predicted positive.

The Classification Rate or Accuracy can be calculated from Equation (12). Now, the confusion matrix results of the proposed WOA-NP algorithm are depicted in Table 4. Precision, as in Equation (13), tells us how many samples were actual positive out of all positive predicted samples. Recall, Equation (14), tells us how many positive samples were detected out of all actual positive samples.

$$Accuracy = (TP + TN)/(TP + TN + FP + FN) \tag{12}$$

$$Precision = (TP)/(TP + FP) \tag{13}$$

$$Recall = (TP)/(TP + FN) \tag{14}$$

Sensitivity represents a positive data points proportion, which is correctly considered positive to all positive data points and calculated using Equation (15).

$$Sensitivity = \frac{TP}{TP + FN} \tag{15}$$

Specificity is a negative data point proportion that is incorrectly considered positive to all negative data points. It can be calculated using Equation (16).

$$Specificity = \frac{TN}{FP + TN} \tag{16}$$

The confusion matrix is useful to calculate the Recall, Precision, Specificity, and most significantly, the Receiver Operating Characteristic (ROC) curve (simply AUC) [21], and the confusion matrix is also useful for accuracy. The ROC curve is a graphical approach to demonstrate the difference between a classifier's true-positive and false-positive rates. This allows for an approach under the ROC curve (AUC) to determine which classifier is on average better.

Table 4. The confusion matrix results.

Datasets/Metrics	TP	FP	FN	TN	Precision	Recall	Specificity	Sensitivity
Diabetes	4730	410	1140	1400	92%	80.57%	77%	81%
Heart disease uci	1120	260	180	1470	81%	86.15%	85%	86%
Heart attack prediction	1660	250	130	900	82%	90%	78%	93%
Sonar	980	130	100	870	88%	91%	87%	91%

AUC is a threshold invariant of classification. It tests the accuracy of model's predictions regardless of the classification threshold selected. This implies the classifier is the greater the area under the curve more efficiently. Furthermore, there is a point on the curve that represents the optimal operating point of the classifier. Figures 15–18 show the ROC curves for every tested dataset while processing. From these curves, we notice that the area under every curve is excellent, proving that the AHCA-WOANB approach classification is efficient.

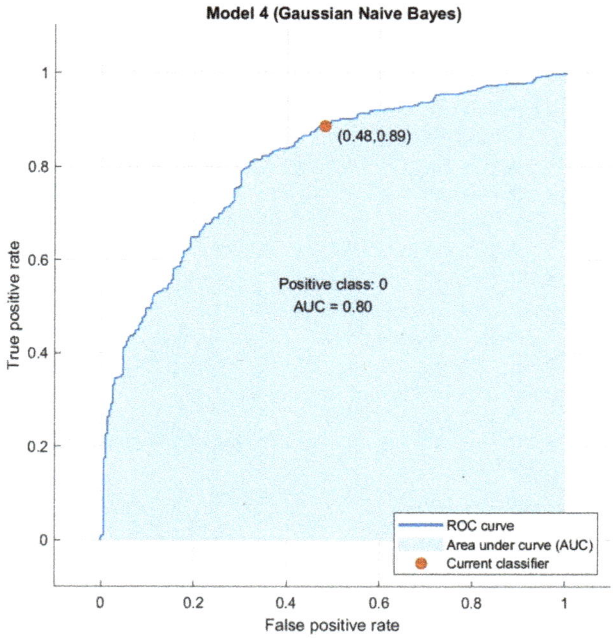

Figure 15. The ROC curve: Diabetes.

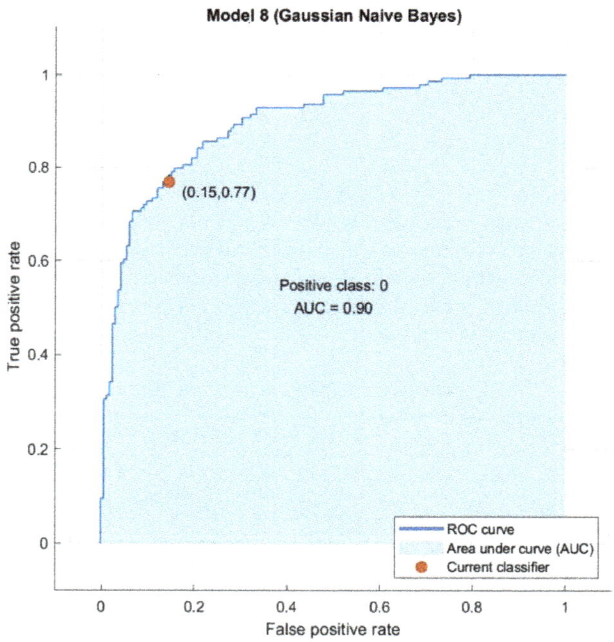

Figure 16. The ROC curve: Heart-C.

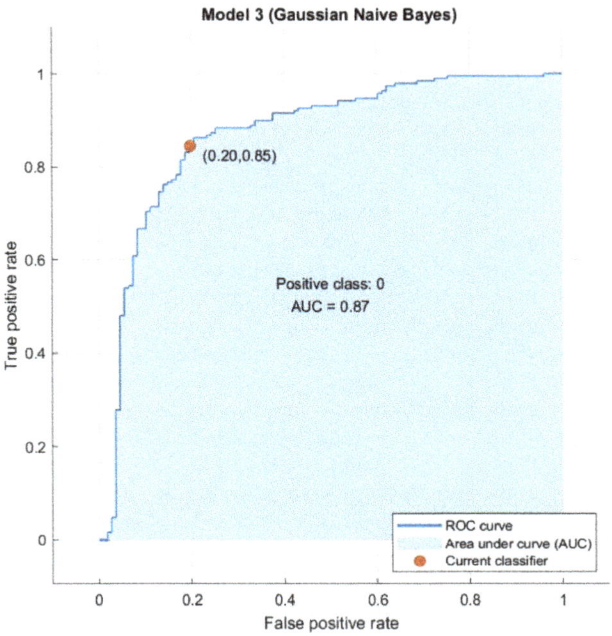

Figure 17. The ROC curve: Heart-H.

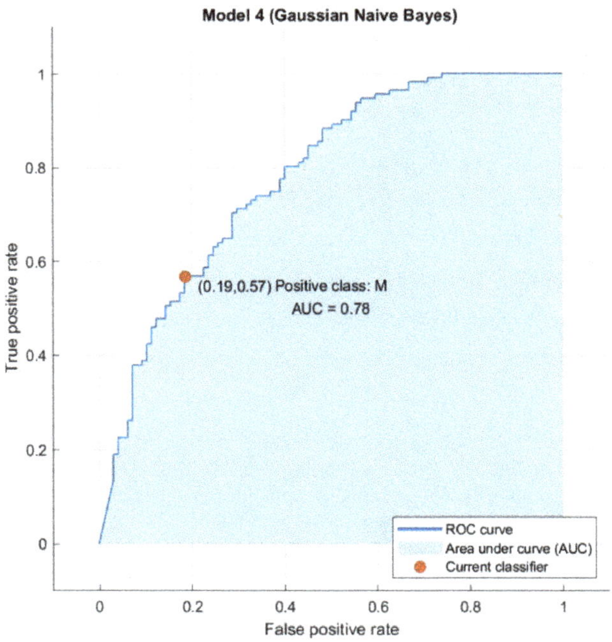

Figure 18. The ROC curve: Sonar.

Finally, all of these results lead us to clearly determine that the AHCA-WOANB hybrid algorithm (WOA for optimization and NB for classification) increases and enhances the accuracy by the average rate: 3.6% (3.34 for Diabetes, 2.94 for Heart disease UCI, 3.77 for Heart attack prediction, and 4.15 for Sonar) also can enhance the processing speed by reducing the processing time by the average rate: 8.7% (28.96 for Diabetes, 1.07 for Heart disease UCI, 3.31 for Heart attack prediction, and 1.4 for Sonar). The rate of these improved results, which are based on Datasets' Characteristics, should be aware that whenever the optimization step can reduce the number of dataset features, this will improve the accuracy and reduce the processing time even more than improving them for those datasets that have less few features.

5. Conclusions

Many healthcare big data needs too much effort to give humanity useful information that can help develop and enhance this field reasonably with the low computational cost. Therefore, the AHCA approach with a hybrid algorithm has been proposed to process various types of medical data. Then it can be easy for us to predict data and introduce useful information and statics to submit it to several parties that concerned this area. The AHCA-WOANB approach has two steps of processing. This is to optimize data to make the second one more efficient, while the second one is responsible for classifying the optimized data. The proposed algorithm increases and enhances the accuracy by approximately 4%. It can also enhance the processing speed by reducing the processing time by approximately 9%. (These results are the average of the results for all tested datasets that are based on characteristics of data and the number of features that have been reduced by the WOA.)

The future mission is to try to support the proposed algorithm by modifying the WOA parameters set automatically by using a conventional neural network algorithm to get better results because it optimizes the used data perfectly before it is processed with the NB algorithm. This will reduce human interactions, so it will reduce human mistakes, reduce the duration time of processing, and give better accuracy than before.

Author Contributions: Conceptualization, M.A., A.M.A., K.N.A., M.A.E., A.Y.H., and M.B.; Formal analysis, K.N.A., M.A.E., A.Y.H., and M.B.; Investigation, K.N.A., M.B., M.A.E.; Methodology, K.N.A., M.A.E., A.Y.H., and M.B.; Project administration, M.A., A.M.A., K.N.A., M.A.E., A.Y.H., and M.B.; Software, K.N.A., M.A.E., A.Y.H., and M.B.; Supervision, M.A., A.M.A., K.N.A., M.A.E., A.Y.H., and M.B.; Validation, M.A., A.M.A., K.N.A., M.A.E., A.Y.H., and M.B.; Visualization, M.A., A.M.A., K.N.A., M.A.E., A.Y.H., and M.B.; Writing—original draft, K.N.A., M.A.E., A.Y.H., and M.B.; Writing—review and editing, M.A., A.M.A., K.N.A., M.A.E., A.Y.H., and M.B. All authors have read and agreed to the published version of the manuscript.

Funding: This research received no external funding.

Institutional Review Board Statement: Not applicable.

Informed Consent Statement: Not applicable.

Data Availability Statement: Data available upon request.

Conflicts of Interest: The authors declare no conflict of interest.

References

1. Tariq, N.; Asim, M.; Al-Obeidat, F.; Zubair Farooqi, M.; Baker, T.; Hammoudeh, M.; Ghafir, I. The security of big data in fog-enabled IoT applications including blockchain: A survey. *Sensors* **2019**, *19*, 1788. [CrossRef]
2. Shehab, N.; Badawy, M.; Arafat, H. Big Data Analytics Concepts, Technologies Challenges, and Opportunities. In *Proceedings of the International Conference on Advanced Intelligent Systems and Informatics, Cairo, Egypt, 19–21 October*; Springer: Berlin, Germany, 2019; pp. 92–101.
3. Katal, A.; Wazid, M.; Goudar, R.H. Big data: Issues, challenges, tools and good practices. In Proceedings of the 2013 Sixth International Conference on Contemporary Computing (IC3), Noida, India, 8–10 August 2013; pp. 404–409.
4. Gantz, J.; Reinsel, D. Extracting value from chaos. *IDC Iview* **2011**, *1142*, 1–12.
5. Sin, K.; Muthu, L. Application of big data in education data mining and learning analytics–A literature review. *ICTACT J. Soft Comput.* **2015**, *5*, 1035–1049. [CrossRef]
6. Abawajy, J.H.; Hassan, M.M. Federated internet of things and cloud computing pervasive patient health monitoring system. *IEEE Commun. Mag.* **2017**, *55*, 48–53. [CrossRef]
7. Labrinidis, A.; Jagadish, H.V. Challenges and opportunities with big data. *Proc. VLDB Endow.* **2012**, *5*, 2032–2033. [CrossRef]
8. Reda, M.; Haikal, A.Y.; Elhosseini, M.A.; Badawy, M. An innovative damped cuckoo search algorithm with a comparative study against other adaptive variants. *IEEE Access* **2019**, *7*, 119272–119293. [CrossRef]

9. Hassan, M.K.; El Desouky, A.I.; Badawy, M.M.; Sarhan, A.M.; Elhoseny, M.; Gunasekaran, M. EoT-driven hybrid ambient assisted living framework with naïve Bayes–firefly algorithm. *Neural Comput. Appl.* **2019**, *31*, 1275–1300. [CrossRef]
10. Andriopoulou, F.; Dagiuklas, T.; Orphanoudakis, T. Integrating IoT and fog computing for healthcare service delivery. In *Components and Services for IoT Platforms*; Springer: Berlin, Germany, 2017; pp. 213–232.
11. Masouros, D.; Bakolas, I.; Tsoutsouras, V.; Siozios, K.; Soudris, D. From edge to cloud: Design and implementation of a healthcare Internet of Things infrastructure. In Proceedings of the 2017 27th International Symposium on Power and Timing Modeling, Optimization and Simulation (PATMOS), Thessaloniki, Greece, 25–27 September 2017; pp. 1–6.
12. Tuli, S.; Basumatary, N.; Gill, S.S.; Kahani, M.; Arya, R.C.; Wander, G.S.; Buyya, R. Healthfog: An ensemble deep learning based smart healthcare system for automatic diagnosis of heart diseases in integrated iot and fog computing environments. *Future Gener. Comput. Syst.* **2020**, *104*, 187–200. [CrossRef]
13. Mirjalili, S.; Lewis, A. The whale optimization algorithm. *Adv. Eng. Softw.* **2016**, *95*, 51–67. [CrossRef]
14. Cortés-Toro, E.M.; Crawford, B.; Gómez-Pulido, J.A.; Soto, R.; Lanza-Gutiérrez, J.M. A new metaheuristic inspired by the vapour-liquid equilibrium for continuous optimization. *Appl. Sci.* **2018**, *8*, 2080. [CrossRef]
15. Diab, D.M.; El Hindi, K.M. Using differential evolution for fine tuning naïve Bayesian classifiers and its application for text classification. *Appl. Soft Comput.* **2017**, *54*, 183–199. [CrossRef]
16. Shvachko, K.; Kuang, H.; Radia, S.; Chansler, R. The hadoop distributed file system. In Proceedings of the 2010 IEEE 26th Symposium on Mass Storage Systems and Technologies (MSST), Incline Village, NA, USA, 3–7 May 2010; pp. 1–10.
17. White, T. *Hadoop: The Definitive Guide*; O'Reilly Media, Inc.: Newton, MA, USA, 2012.
18. Learning, Kaggle Your Machine, Data Science Community. Available online: https://www.kaggle.com (accessed on 4 July 2021).
19. Jiang, L.; Zhang, L.; Yu, L.; Wang, D. Class-specific attribute weighted naive Bayes. *Pattern Recognit.* **2019**, *88*, 321–330. [CrossRef]
20. Fawcett, T. An introduction to ROC analysis. *Pattern Recognit. Lett.* **2006**, *27*, 861–874. [CrossRef]
21. Ling, C.X.; Huang, J.; Zhang, H. AUC: A statistically consistent and more discriminating measure than accuracy. *IJCAI* **2003**, *3*, 519–524.

sensors

MDPI

Article

A Comprehensive Computer-Assisted Diagnosis System for Early Assessment of Renal Cancer Tumors

Mohamed Shehata [1,†], Ahmed Alksas [1,†], Rasha T. Abouelkheir [2,†], Ahmed Elmahdy [2], Ahmed Shaffie [1], Ahmed Soliman [1], Mohammed Ghazal [3], Hadil Abu Khalifeh [3], Reem Salim [3], Ahmed Abdel Khalek Abdel Razek [4], Norah Saleh Alghamdi [5] and Ayman El-Baz [1,*]

1 BioImaging Lab, Bioengineering Department, University of Louisville, Louisville, KY 40292, USA; mnsheh01@louisville.edu (M.S.); ammost01@louisville.edu (A.A.); amshaf02@louisville.edu (A.S.); ahmed.soliman@louisville.edu (A.S.)
2 Department of Radiology, Urology and Nephrology Center, University of Mansoura, Mansoura 35516, Egypt; rashataha2020@gmail.com (R.T.A.); ahmed.elmahdy89@yahoo.com (A.E.)
3 College of Engineering, Abu Dhabi University, Abu Dhabi 59911, United Arab Emirates; mohammed.ghazal@adu.ac.ae (M.G.); hadil.abukhalifeh@adu.ac.ae (H.A.K.) ; reem.salim@adu.ac.ae (R.S.)
4 Department of Radiology, Faculty of Medicine, Mansoura University, Mansoura 35516, Egypt; arazek@mans.edu.eg
5 College of Computer and Information Science, Princess Nourah Bint Abdulrahman University, Riyadh 11564, Saudi Arabia; nosalghamdi@pnu.edu.sa
* Correspondence: aselba01@louisville.edu
† These authors contributed equally to this work.

Citation: Shehata, M.; Alksas, A.; Abouelkheir, R.T.; Elmahdy, A.; Shaffie, A.; Soliman, A.; Ghazal, M.; Abu Khalifeh, H.; Salim, R.; Abdel Razek, A.A.K.; et al. A Comprehensive Computer-Assisted Diagnosis System for Early Assessment of Renal Cancer Tumors. *Sensors* **2021**, *21*, 4928. https://doi.org/10.3390/s21144928

Academic Editor: Hyungsoon Im

Received: 8 June 2021
Accepted: 17 July 2021
Published: 20 July 2021

Abstract: Renal cell carcinoma (RCC) is the most common and a highly aggressive type of malignant renal tumor. In this manuscript, we aim to identify and integrate the optimal discriminating morphological, textural, and functional features that best describe the malignancy status of a given renal tumor. The integrated discriminating features may lead to the development of a novel comprehensive renal cancer computer-assisted diagnosis (RC-CAD) system with the ability to discriminate between benign and malignant renal tumors and specify the malignancy subtypes for optimal medical management. Informed consent was obtained from a total of 140 biopsy-proven patients to participate in the study (male = 72 and female = 68, age range = 15 to 87 years). There were 70 patients who had RCC (40 clear cell RCC (ccRCC), 30 nonclear cell RCC (nccRCC)), while the other 70 had benign angiomyolipoma tumors. Contrast-enhanced computed tomography (CE-CT) images were acquired, and renal tumors were segmented for all patients to allow the extraction of discriminating imaging features. The RC-CAD system incorporates the following major steps: (i) applying a new parametric spherical harmonic technique to estimate the morphological features, (ii) modeling a novel angular invariant gray-level co-occurrence matrix to estimate the textural features, and (iii) constructing wash-in/wash-out slopes to estimate the functional features by quantifying enhancement variations across different CE-CT phases. These features were subsequently combined and processed using a two-stage multilayer perceptron artificial neural network (MLP-ANN) classifier to classify the renal tumor as benign or malignant and identify the malignancy subtype as well. Using the combined features and a leave-one-subject-out cross-validation approach, the developed RC-CAD system achieved a sensitivity of 95.3% ± 2.0%, a specificity of 99.9% ± 0.4%, and Dice similarity coefficient of 0.98 ± 0.01 in differentiating malignant from benign tumors, as well as an overall accuracy of 89.6% ± 5.0% in discriminating ccRCC from nccRCC. The diagnostic abilities of the developed RC-CAD system were further validated using a randomly stratified 10-fold cross-validation approach. The obtained results using the proposed MLP-ANN classification model outperformed other machine learning classifiers (e.g., support vector machine, random forests, relational functional gradient boosting, etc.). Hence, integrating morphological, textural, and functional features enhances the diagnostic performance, making the proposal a reliable noninvasive diagnostic tool for renal tumors.

Keywords: renal cell carcinoma; CE-CT; morphology; texture; functionality; RC-CAD

1. Introduction

Renal cancer is one of the most common malignancies, being the sixth most prevalent type of cancer among men and the eighth most prevalent among women. For the past several decades, an increasing number of new patients have been diagnosed with renal cancer. The year 2020 saw approximately 74,000 diagnoses of renal cancer in the United States [1,2], and 15,000 patients are expected to have died from renal cancer in that same time period [1,2]. Roughly two thirds of the time, renal cancer is diagnosed before it has metastasized, in which case the 5 y survival rate is 93%. Once it has spread to the lymph nodes or the surrounding abdominal structures (i.e., other organs or tissues), the 5 y survival rate falls to 70%. In the worst case of metastasis to distant parts of the body, the 5 y survival rate is a mere 12% [1,2]. In addition, the National Cancer Institute had an approximated cost estimate of $5.1 billion for renal cancer care in the United States by the end of 2020 [3].

Renal cancer is a heterogeneous disease in which the renal cells become malignant (cancerous) and form tumors called renal masses. These renal masses, if not detected early and treated promptly, will lead to mortality. The most common, and also the most aggressive, renal cancer is renal cell carcinoma (RCC), accounting for 70% of all cases [4,5]. In turn, 70% of RCC are clear cell renal cell carcinoma (ccRCC), and of the remaining nonclear cell subtypes (nccRCC), the most prevalent are papillary (paRCC) and chromophobe (chrRCC) renal cell carcinomas, accounting for 15% and 5% of all RCC, respectively [6]. The World Health Organization (WHO) taxonomy of RCC [6] has clinical significance because the various subtypes can have very different prognoses [6–8]. Differential diagnosis of RCC must look out for the benign tumors angiomyolipoma (AML) and oncocytoma (ONC), which are easily confused with RCC using conventional diagnostic techniques [9–13]. AMLs with low fat content are particularly prone to misdiagnosis [14]. Diagnostic error leads to unnecessary surgical intervention for benign lesions, to the point where 15–20% of surgically resected "RCC" may actually be AML [15]. Therefore, accurate characterization of such renal masses at an early stage is crucial to the identification of appropriate intervention plans and/or treatment courses.

1.1. Current Diagnostic Techniques and Their Limitations

Evidence of renal cancer can be found in complete blood count (CBC) to check for the number of red blood cells; urine tests to look for blood, bacteria, or cancerous cells in urine; and blood chemistry tests to quantify renal function by checking the levels of certain chemicals in the blood. These signs are suggestive at best, and inadequate for diagnosis or typing of renal cancer. Only biopsy, performed using interventional radiology, can provide a definite diagnosis of renal cancer, and thus remains the gold standard [1,2]. However, it can only be used as the last resort due to its high invasiveness, cost, and turnaround and recovery times (approximately a week). Therefore, the investigation of noninvasive imaging modalities (e.g., computed tomography (CT), magnetic resonance imaging (MRI), and ultrasounds) to provide an early, reliable, accurate, cost-effective, and rapid diagnosis of renal tumors is underway [16–19].

1.2. Related Work

One of the most important diagnostic imaging modalities for the accurate diagnosis of renal tumors is contrast-enhanced CT (CE-CT) [20,21]. Besides specifying the location, shape, and size of a tumor, CE-CT can also distinguish RCC from benign lesions with 77–84% accuracy based on their different uptake of the contrast agent [18,22,23]. For this purpose, texture analysis (TA) is performed on the CE-CT images to extract quantitative features [24,25]. As a radiomic technique, TA has seen an array of applications in typing, staging, and grading tumors and even in predicting treatment response and survival rates [24]. A recent study by Deng et al. [26] utilized TA techniques along with CE-CT to discriminate malignant from benign renal tumors. Their study included 501 renal tumors of which 354 were RCCs and 147 were benign lesions. From the portal-venous phase, they manually placed a region of interest (ROI) in the largest CE-CT cross-section of the tumor volume. Then, they extracted four textural features, namely entropy, kurtosis, mean positive pixel density, and skewness. Utilizing logistic regression, they found that higher values of entropy were significantly associated with a greater likelihood of malignancy ($p = 0.022$). As a diagnostic indicator of RCC, the entropy feature had high specificity (85.5%), but quite low sensitivity (31.3%) [26].

Another study was conducted by Kunapuli et al. [27] to explore the potential of CE-CT along with TA to identify malignant renal tumors. Their dataset included images of 100 malignant (70 ccRCC, 20 paRCC, and 10 chrRCC) and 50 benign (20 AML and 30 ONC) tumors. After segmenting renal tumors manually using image-rendering software, 2D and 3D TAs were performed on tumor with the largest diameter and the entire tumor volume, respectively. Fifty-one 2D and 3D textural features were extracted from each of four different CT phases, yielding a total of two-hundred and four features per subject. These comprised 8 histogram features (i.e., first-order textural features), 40 s-order textural features (20 grey-level co-occurrence matrix (GLCM) and 20 grey-level difference matrix (GLDM)), and 3 spectral features derived from the 2D Fourier transform. Recursive feature elimination [28] was used to reduce the number of features to 10 per phase, or a total of 40. Their classification algorithm incorporating these features, using relational functional gradient boosting, had a reported 82% accuracy and an 0.83 area under the curve. The classifier was developed to discriminate between malignant and benign tumors only, and the authors did not investigate the subtype classification of malignant RCC [27].

Kocak et al. [29] conducted a study to classify ccRCC renal tumors from nccRCC ones using CE-CT along with TA. A total of 68 RCCs were included for internal validation (N = 48 ccRCC and N = 20 nccRCC). For external validation purposes, they included an additional 26 RCC from a public dataset (N = 13 and N = 13 nccRCC). Their study utilized MaZda image-rendering software [30] to manually segment renal tumors on the largest/middle cross-section. This was followed by an extraction of 275 textural-related features from each subject in both the enhanced CT phase and the unenhanced phase. In addition, a wrapper-based nested cross-validation approach was employed to select the reproducible features in both phases and to optimize their classification model. Artificial neural networks (ANNs) were used, and a classification accuracy of 86.7%, a sensitivity of 80%, and a specificity of 89.6% on internal data and an accuracy of 84.6%, a sensitivity of 69.2%, and a specificity of 100% on external data were reported in differentiating ccRCC from nccRCC. Although their study reported a good overall classification performance between ccRCC and nccRCC, they were limited by their low sensitivity. In addition, they reported a very poor diagnostic performance to differentiate chrRCC from paRCC and from ccRCC. They suggested that CE-CT is more powerful at providing useful textural features than the unenhanced CT.

A bigger study was performed by Sun et al. [31] to compare between the diagnostic performance of machine learning approaches and four expert radiologists in differentiating malignant from benign renal tumors, as well as ccRCC from nccRCC malignant tumors using CE-CT. Their study included 254 malignant tumors (ccRCC = 190, nccRCC = 64 (chrRCC = 38, paRCC = 26)), 26 AML benign tumors, and 10 ONCs. After performing manual delineation of the tumor lesions, they used open-source software packages to extract and analyze textural features and used another open-source software to complete their analysis. Then, they utilized a support vector machine (SVM) classifier with a radial basis function along with a 10-fold cross-validation approach to obtain the final diagnosis. They reported sensitivities of 90%, 86.3%, and 73.4% using SVM compared to 73.7–96.8%, 73.7–96.8%, and 28.1–60.9% obtained by the 4 expert radiologists in differentiating ccRCC from nccRCC, ccRCC from AML and ONC, and nccRCC from AML and ONC, respectively. Hence, they concluded that machine learning approaches along with textural features have potential power, as well as low-variance performance in diagnosing renal tumors.

Lee et al. [32] used TA and CE-CT in their study to differentiate between ccRCC malignant and AML benign renal tumors. Their study included 80 renal tumors (ccRCC = 41 and AML = 39). They combined several hand-crafted textural features extracted from a 2D manually annotated central image of the entire mass with automated deep features extracted by different ImageNet pretrained convolutional neural network (CNN) classification models, namely AlexNet [33], VGGNet [34], GoogleNet [35], and ResNet [36]. Then, they used the combined features to train and test a random forest (RF) classifier. Using a leave-one-out cross-validation approach, their combined model achieved a diagnostic accuracy of 76.6% $\pm$ 1.4%, outperforming the individual diagnostic results using either the hand-crafted features alone or the deep features alone.

Oberai et al. [37] investigated the potential power of CNN along with multiphasic CE-CT images to differentiate benign from malignant renal masses. Their study included 143 patients (malignant = 97 and benign = 46). After performing manual segmentation of the whole tumor volume, they selected the largest axial segmented tumor image from each CE-CT phase to input in the CNN for training and validation. Using an 8-fold cross-validation approach, they reported an accuracy of 78%, a sensitivity of 70%, and a specificity of 81%. However, their dataset had an approximately 2:1 class imbalance, which might contribute to the reduced diagnostic performance. Although their study included different types of malignant tumors, they did not investigate the subtyping of malignant class.

Zhou et al. [38] conducted a study to distinguish between malignant and benign renal tumors using CE-CT along with an ImageNet-pretrained InceptionV3 model. This model was then cross-trained using transfer learning on their own dataset of 192 renal tumors (malignant: ccRCC = 117 and nccRCC = 17, benign: renal cyst = 50 and AML = 8). Several image-level models were considered, using whole CT slices, ROIs, and rectangular subregions of the CT-CT data. Then, during the transfer learning, different number of layers were frozen, resulting in two-patient level models based on the optimal image-level models. Using a five-fold cross-validation approach, they reported a 69% accuracy using the slice dataset, a 97% accuracy using the ROI dataset, and a 93% accuracy using the RBR dataset. In spite of achieving a high accuracy in differentiating malignant from benign renal tumors, 50 out of 58 benign cases were renal cysts, which are much easier to distinguish from RCC compared to AML. In addition, they did not investigate discriminating ccRCC from nccRCC renal tumors.

Shehata et al. [39] published a recent study to differentiate malignant RCC from benign AML renal tumors, as well as to identify the malignant RCC subtype using CE-CT. Their data included 105 biopsy-confirmed cases (ccRCC = 40, nccRCC = 30, and AML = 35). After performing manual segmentation to delineate the renal tumor, they extracted 22 first- and second-order textural features, as well as two functional features represented by wash-in and wash-out slopes. These features were subdivided into four groups. To differentiate RCC from AML, they obtained four preliminary diagnoses using separate RF classifiers on each feature group, then used weighted-majority voting to produce the final diagnosis. They reported a 96% accuracy, a 100% sensitivity, and an 89% specificity. Subsequently, for cases diagnosed as RCC, they utilized SVM classifiers along with the weighted-majority voting technique to specify the subtype of malignancy as ccRCC or nccRCC, for which the reported accuracy was 71.4%. In spite of correctly identifying 70 of 70 RCC cases, their system was not specific enough. This could be a consequence of the imbalance between the RCC and AML group sizes. In addition, their technique did not achieve a sufficient diagnostic performance in malignancy subtyping.

Most of the studies referenced above were pure applications of TA to CE-CT imaging. That is to say, they did not integrate other features (e.g., morphological and functional) with two- or three-dimensional textural features to diagnose RCC. Only a few studies addressed typing of RCC, i.e., discrimination between ccRCC and nccRCC, which is vital information for deciding the course of treatment from the beginning. To overcome these limitations, we developed RC-CAD, a two-stage system for comprehensive computer-assisted diagnosis of renal cancer based on CE-CT imaging. RC-CAD (Figure 1) incorporates 3D morphological features, first- and second-order 3D textural features, and time-dependent metrics of renal function (wash-in/-out slopes) to provide a high diagnostic accuracy of cancerous renal tumors. The developed RC-CAD system has the ability to (i) discriminate malignant (RCC) from benign (AML) renal tumors and (ii) specify the subtype of malignant tumors as ccRCC vs. nccRCC. To the best of our knowledge, the developed CE-CT-based RC-CAD system is unique with the ability to integrate 3D morphological features with 3D textural features and functional features for early discrimination of RCC malignant tumors from AML benign tumors and determine the subtype of malignancy as ccRcc or nccRCC.

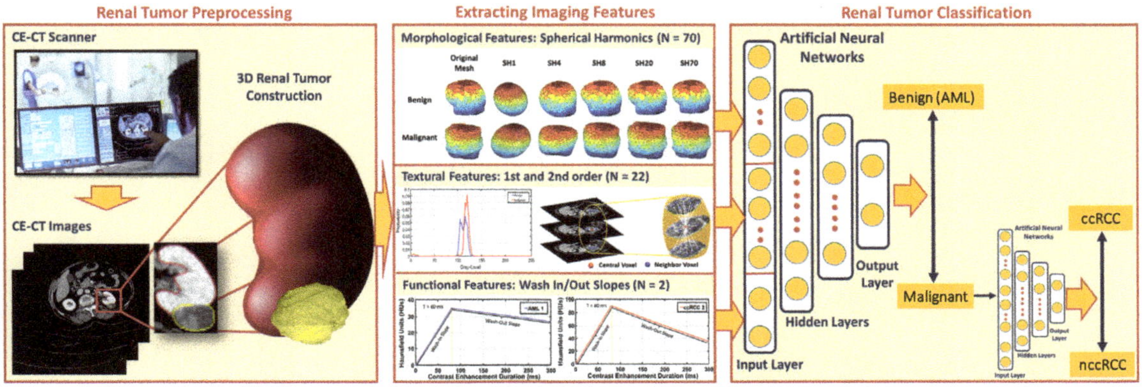

Figure 1. The proposed renal cancer computer-assisted diagnosis (RC-CAD) system.

It is worth noting that this paper extends our recent work [39] with the following substantial modifications: (i) increasing the sample size from 105 (70 RCC vs. 35 AML) to 140 renal tumors (70 RCC vs. 70 AML) to ensure data balancing and to avoid any possible classification bias towards the majority class, (ii) applying a new parametric spherical harmonic technique to estimate the morphological features from the segmented renal tumors to capture the surface complexity/irregularity between different types of renal tumors, (iii) integrating/concatenating the estimated morphological features with the first- and second-order textural features and functional features, and (iv) modeling a two-stage classification using a multilayer perceptron artificial neural network (MLP-ANN) whose inputs comprise all the aforementioned discriminant features. The first stage decides if the renal tumor is malignant (RCC) or benign (AML). In the former case, the second stage identifies the malignancy subtype as ccRCC or nccRCC.

2. Materials

Patients who had undergone renal biopsy for suspected cancer ($N = 140$) ranged from 15 to 87 years of age (mean = 50.5 years and standard deviation = 13.4 years). There were 72 patients who were males, while the remaining 68 were female. Informed consent was obtained from the patients themselves or their parents/legal guardians (age < 18 years) to participate in this study. Biopsy reports confirmed that 70 patients had RCC (40 ccRCC and 30 nccRCC, of which 17 were paRCC and 13 were chrRCC), while the other 70 had benign AML tumors. Study participants had undergone a multiphase CT examination prior to biopsy. Imaging was performed with a Brilliance CT 64 multislice scanner (Philips Medical Systems, Best, The Netherlands). A mechanical injector was used to administer contrast agent into an antecubital vein with a dose of 120 mL at a rate of 4.0 mL/s. The abdomen scanning included three main phases: a precontrast phase, a portal-venous phase, and a delayed-contrast phase acquired at $t = 0$, $t = 80$, and $t = 300$ s, respectively. All images were acquired using the following parameters: slice thickness = 2.5 mm; pitch = 0.984; rotation time = 0.75 s.

3. Methods

The proposed RC-CAD system pipeline (see Figure 1) performs the following steps to obtain the final diagnosis: (i) constructs 3D models of renal tumors from manually segmented 2D ROIs, (ii) applies a new parametric spherical harmonic technique to estimate the morphological features of the tumor boundary, (iii) constructs a rotation-invariant gray-level co-occurrence matrix (GLCM) to extract the textural features of the tumor volume, (iv) estimates the wash-in/wash-out slopes inside the 3D region, and (v) performs two-stage classification using an MLP-ANN whose inputs comprise all aforementioned discriminant features. The first stage decides if the renal tumor is malignant (RCC) or benign (AML). These steps are presented in detail next.

3.1. Renal Tumor Preprocessing

To provide a more accurate extraction of morphological, textural, and functional discriminating imaging features, for each subject, each CT slice intersecting the renal tumor was accurately and manually segmented by expert radiologists to define the 2D ROI. Then, all 2D ROIs were stacked together to construct the 3D renal tumor object (3D ROI), as shown in Figure 2.

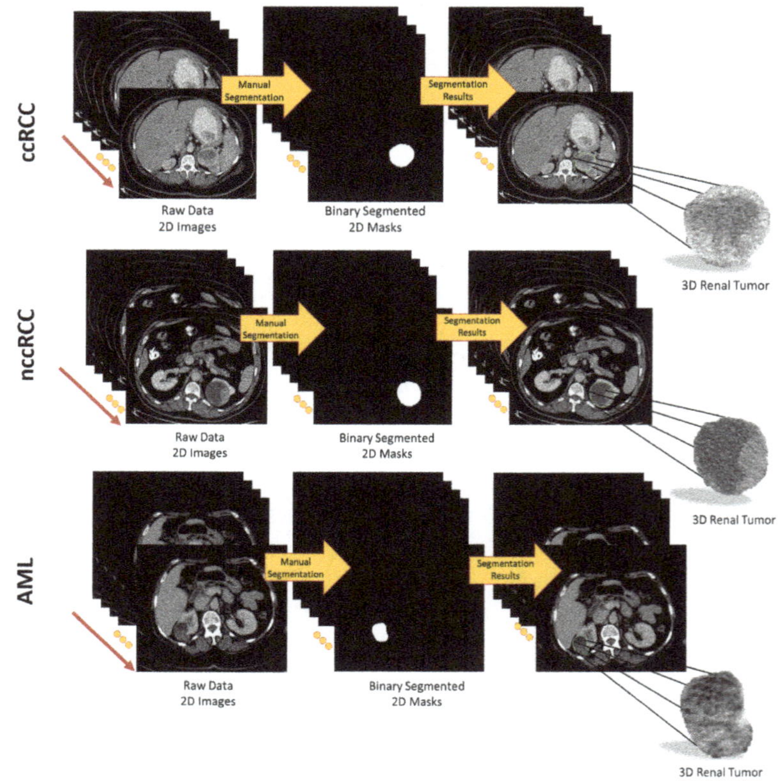

Figure 2. Visualization of the segmentation process to obtain 3D renal tumors.

3.2. Extracting Imaging Features

For accurate identification of malignant renal tumors and the associated subtype, all 3D segmented volumes were characterized by their morphological, textural, and functional features, as described below.

Morphological features: To enhance both the sensitivity and specificity of early renal cancer diagnosis, morphological features of the tumor are incorporated into the algorithm.

These features were designed to quantify the complex shape of the tumor boundary. This was motivated by the hypothesis that rapidly growing, malignant tumors develop more irregular/complex shapes relative to more slowly growing, benign tumors. Therefore, the utilization of such shape descriptors would enhance the performance of the automatic diagnosis. Examples of this phenomenon are illustrated in Figure 3.

Naturally, in order to measure the irregularity of the boundary, we must first construct an accurate shape model of the tumor. In this paper, we incorporated a state-of-the-art spectral decomposition in terms of spherical harmonics (SHs) [40] to construct this shape model. An arbitrary point in the interior of the tumor, or more specifically, the interior of its convex kernel, was selected as the origin $(0,0,0)$. In this coordinate system, the tumor's surface may be considered a function of the polar and azimuthal angle, $f(\theta,\varphi)$, which can be expressed as a linear combination of basis functions $Y_{\tau\beta}$ defined on the unit sphere. Starting with a discrete approximation of the surface, i.e., a triangular mesh, the proposed algorithm uses an attraction–repulsion technique [41] to map this mesh to the unit sphere. The mapping fixes the image of each mesh vertex at the unit distance from the origin, while preserving the mesh topology and maintaining the distance between adjacent vertices as much as possible.

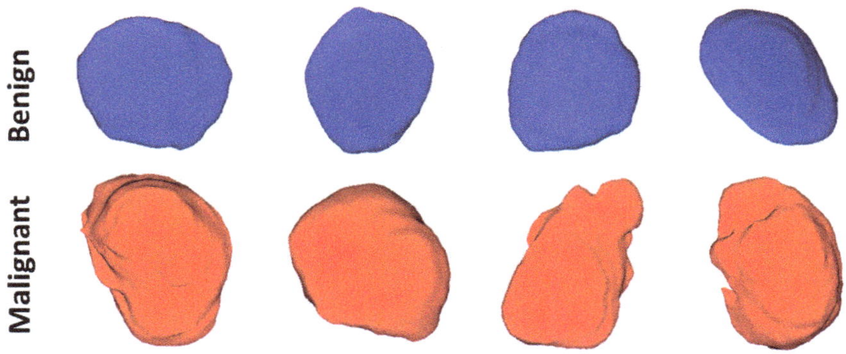

Figure 3. Visualizing 3D surface complexity differences between different renal tumors (benign are shown in blue, while malignant are shown in red).

Each iteration α of the attraction-repulsion works as follows. Let $\mathbf{C}_{\alpha,i}$ be the coordinates of the node on the unit sphere corresponding to mesh vertex i at the beginning of iteration α. Denote the vector from node i to node j by $\mathbf{d}_{\alpha,ji} = \mathbf{C}_{\alpha,j} - \mathbf{C}_{\alpha,i}$; then, the Euclidean distance between nodes i and j is $d_{\alpha,ji} = \left\|\mathbf{d}_{\alpha,ji}\right\|$. Finally, let J_i denote the index set of neighbors of vertex i in the triangulated mesh. Then, the attraction step updates the position of each node to keep it centered with respect to its neighbors:

$$\mathbf{C}'_{\alpha+1,i} = \mathbf{C}_{\alpha,i} + C_{A,1} \sum_{j \in J_i} \left(\mathbf{d}_{\alpha,ji} d^2_{\alpha,ji} + C_{A,2} \frac{\mathbf{d}_{\alpha,ji}}{d_{\alpha,ji}} \right), \tag{1}$$

The quantities $C_{A,1}$ and $C_{A,2}$ are implementation-defined parameters that determine the strength of the attractive force. The next step, repulsion, inflates the spherical mesh to prevent it from degenerating (the attraction step by itself would allow nodes to become arbitrarily close to one another).

$$\mathbf{C}''_{\alpha+1,i} = \mathbf{C}'_{\alpha+1,i} + \frac{C_R}{2I} \sum_{j=1; j \neq i}^{I} \frac{\mathbf{d}_{\alpha,ji}}{\mathbf{d}^2_{\alpha,ji}}, \tag{2}$$

Just as the attraction step, the repulsion step uses an implementation-defined parameter C_R to set the strength of the repulsive force. Subsequently, the nodes are projected back onto the sphere by giving them the unit norm, and these are their coordinates at the beginning of the next iteration, $\mathbf{C}_{\alpha+1,i} = \mathbf{C}''_{\alpha+1,i} / \|\mathbf{C}''_{\alpha+1,i}\|$.

At the terminal iteration α_f of the attraction–repulsion algorithm, the surface of the renal tumor is in a one-to-one correspondence with the unit sphere. Each node $\mathbf{C}_i = (x_i, y_i, z_i)$ of the original mesh is mapped to a corresponding point $\mathbf{C}_{\alpha_f,i} = (\sin\theta_i \cos\phi_i, \sin\theta_i \sin\phi_i, \cos\theta_i)$ with polar angle $\theta_i \in [0, \pi]$ and azimuthal angle $\phi_i \in [0, 2\pi)$. Considering these points as samples of a continuous function $f(\theta, \varphi)$ defining the boundary, the tumor shape may be estimated by fitting an SH series to the sample nodes, since the SHs form an orthogonal basis for functions on a sphere. The SH $Y_{\tau\beta}$ of degree τ and order β is defined as:

$$Y_{\tau\beta} = \begin{cases} c_{\tau\beta} G_\tau^{|\beta|} \cos\theta \sin(|\beta|\varphi) & -\tau \leq \beta \leq -1 \\ \frac{c_{\tau\beta}}{\sqrt{2}} G_\tau^{|\beta|} \cos\theta & \beta = 0 \\ c_{\tau\beta} G_\tau^{|\beta|} \cos\theta \cos(|\beta|\varphi) & 1 \leq \beta \leq \tau \end{cases} \quad (3)$$

where $c_{\tau\beta}$ is the SH factor and $G_\tau^{|\beta|}$ is the associated Legendre polynomial of degree τ and order β.

In practice, of course, the SH series is truncated by discarding harmonics above degree N, yielding an Nth order approximation. $N = 70$ suffices to accurately model the surface of renal tumors. Finally, the renal tumor object is reconstructed from the SHs of Equation (3). The first few harmonics describe the rough extent of the tumor, while higher degree harmonics provide the finer details of its surface. Therefore, benign tumors are accurately represented by a lower-order SH model, while malignant tumors, with their more complex morphology, require higher-order SH model to describe their shape.

Figure 4 shows the morphology approximation for three different renal tumors: malignant ccRCC, malignant nccRCC, and benign AML tumors. A summary of the attraction–repulsion algorithm is provided below.

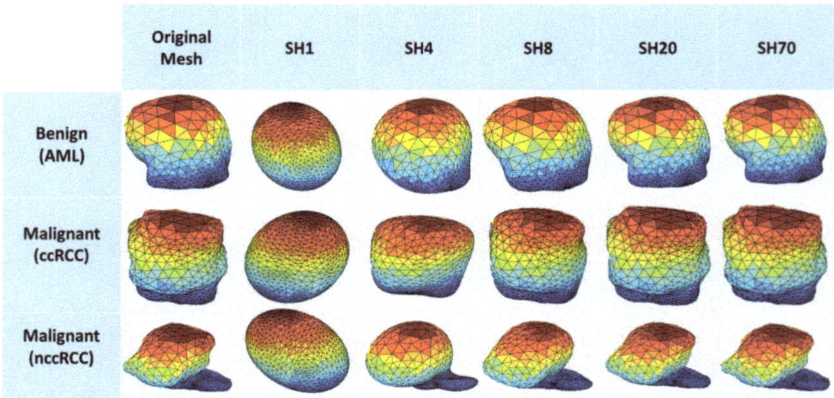

Figure 4. Renal tumors' reconstruction meshes showing the morphological differences among malignant ccRCC, malignant nccRCC, and benign AML tumors.

Initialization:
- Triangulate the surface of the tumor.
- Smooth the triangulated mesh with Laplacian filtering.
- Initialize the spherical parameterization with an arbitrary, topology-preserving map onto the unit sphere.
- Fix values of $C_{A,1}$, $C_{A,2}$, C_R, and threshold T.

Attraction–repulsion:
- **For** $\alpha = 0, 1, \ldots$
  - **For** $i = 1, \ldots, I$

- * Calculate $\mathbf{C}'_{\alpha+1,i}$ using Equation (1)
- **For** $i = 1, \ldots, I$
  - * Calculate $\mathbf{C}''_{\alpha+1,i}$ using Equation (2)
  - * Let $\mathbf{C}_{\alpha+1,i} = \mathbf{C}''_{\alpha+1,i} / \|\mathbf{C}''_{\alpha+1,i}\|$
- **If** $\max_i \|\mathbf{C}_{\alpha+1,i} - \mathbf{C}_{\alpha,i}\| \leq T$ **Then**, let $\alpha_f = \alpha + 1$, and **Stop**.

Textural features: Recently, TA has become a popular research topic, particularly in the field of medical imaging. New techniques of TA provide different quantitative patterns/descriptors by combining the grey values of each pixel/voxel in a tumor image/volume. As a result of these abilities, TA has been used in the diagnosis of several tumors and their related subtypes with encouraging classification abilities [24,25,42–48]. Therefore, in this manuscript, TA techniques were applied on the segmented 3D renal tumor volumes to precisely extract first- and second-order textural features that best describe the homogeneity/heterogeneity between renal tumors with different diagnoses. The use of such comprehensive textural features relies on the fact that malignant tumors mostly show high textural heterogeneity when compared to benign ones. The success of these findings would enhance the sensitivity and the specificity towards an early identification of renal cancer tumors. Figure 5 demonstrates the lesion texture differences of two malignant ccRCC subjects, two malignant nccRCC subjects, and two benign (AML) subjects.

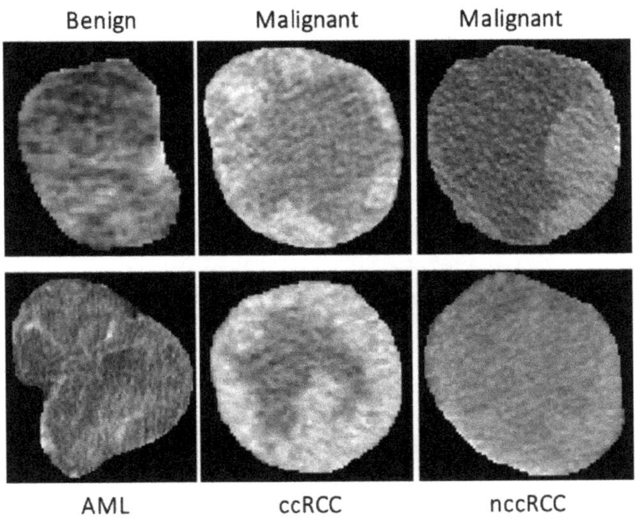

Figure 5. An illustrative example showing differences in texture between various renal tumor types.

First-order textural features: These textural features include any quantity that can be derived from the gray-level histogram of the tumor volume. In particular, mean, variance, standard deviation, entropy, skewness, kurtosis, cumulative distribution functions, and the grey-level percentiles [49] were extracted.

Figure 6 shows the average normalized histogram curves for all benign subjects (blue) vs. malignant (red). To construct these curves, the grey-level range was normalized first by dividing by the maximum grey-level value obtained from all subjects. Then, all histograms were constructed for all subjects within the new normalized grey-level range from 0 to 255. For each subject, the individual grey-level probability was obtained by dividing the histogram values by the corresponding number of voxels. Then, all normalized histograms from a particular group (malignant or benign) were averaged pointwise to obtain the final curve.

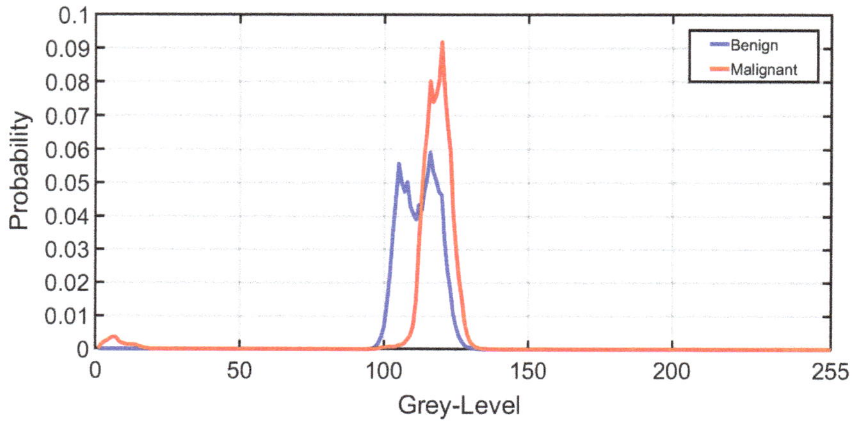

Figure 6. A visualization of the average normalized histogram curves for all benign subjects (blue) vs. malignant (red).

Second-order textural features: Since the first-order textural features might not be sufficient, with their range of values exhibiting significant overlap across classes, especially between subtypes of malignant tumor, second-order textural features were incorporated into the system. These features describe the joint distribution of gray values in multiple voxels that are considered to be neighbors of each other. In particular, the grey-level co-occurrence matrix (GLCM) [50] was used to capture the heterogeneous appearance of renal tumors.

To construct the GLCM, we must count the number of times an ordered pair of two grey values occurs in two neighboring voxels within the renal tumor object. This technique is continued until all conceivable occurrence frequencies within the grey-level range of the renal tumor item are found, which covers all possible pairs of neighbors. For this, we first contrast stretched the renal tumor object's original grey-level range to fit the desired span 0–255, yielding a GLCM matrix with a size of 256 × 256. Then, all feasible pair combinations were identified to construct the GLCM matrix (i.e., neighbors with gray levels i and j contribute to row i, column j of the GLCM). To define our neighborhoods, we used a distance criterion that voxels must be separated by $\leq\sqrt{2}$ mm, making the calculations rotation invariant (see Figure 7). The resultant GLCM was then normalized and used to extracting the following second-order texture features [49,50]: contrast, dissimilarity, homogeneity, angular second moment (ASM), energy, and correlation.

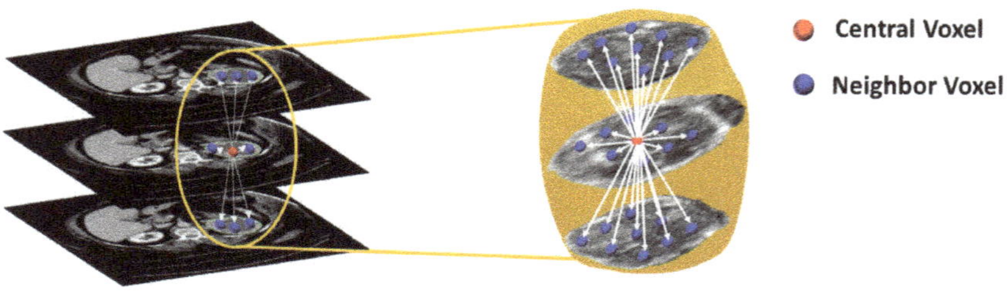

Figure 7. Visualization of the rotation-invariant neighborhood calculation system used to construct the grey-level co-occurrence matrix (GLCM). The GLCM can be constructed by counting the occurrence frequency of different grey-level pairs in-plane and in adjacent planes accounting for the 26-neighbor voxels (blue) of the central voxel (red).

The definitions of all first- and second-order textural features are provided in Tables 1 and A1 in Appendix A.

Table 1. Definition of first- and second-order textural features.

Textural Feature	Definition
	First-Order
Mean	The average grey value of voxels within the tumor.
Variance	Second central moment of gray values.
Standard deviation	Square root of variance.
Skewness (Skew)	Asymmetry of the distribution of gray values about the mean. If Skew < 0, that means the grey level spreads out more to the left of the mean than to the right, and if Skew > 0, that means the grey level spreads out more to the right of the mean than to the left. Skew will equal zero in the case of normal distributions.
Kurtosis (Kurt)	Measures the tail weight, or tendency to extreme values, of the object grey-level distribution. The normal distribution has Kurt = 3; distributions with heavier tails have Kurt > 3; distributions with less weight in the tails have Kurt < 3.
Entropy	A measure of randomness of grey values within an input image.
CDFs	A distribution function that accumulates voxel-wise grey values from the whole tumor object with minimum value = 0 and maximum value = 1.
Percentiles	Grey values percentiles corresponding to the CDFs (from 10% to 100%)
	Second-Order
Contrast	Measures the disparity in grey-level values between neighbors.
Dissimilarity	Finds to what extent voxels are different from their neighbors.
Homogeneity	Expresses the inverse difference moment among neighbors.
Angular second moment (ASM)	Determines the gray levels' local uniformity (orderliness).
Energy	The square root of the ASM.
Correlation	Determines the grey-level linear dependency in neighborhood blocks.

Functional features: Discriminating RCC from AML, as well as ccRCC from nccRCC might be achieved using time-dependent characteristics of CE-CT imaging. The most relevant CE-CT findings for this purpose are generally homogenous and prolonged enhancement patterns [51]. The time dependency can be expressed by the slopes of wash-in and wash-out. Wash-in is described as the rate of increasing attenuation (in HU) from the precontrast to portal-venous phase. Similarly, wash-out is the rate of decrease in attenuation between the portal-venous and delayed-contrast phase [52]. Higher slopes of wash-in and wash-out are typically associated with malignancy. Moreover, nccRCC demonstrates wash-in and wash-out slopes intermediate between those of AML and those of ccRCC [53]. Therefore, we constructed both wash-in and wash-out slopes for all renal tumor subjects for the classification of the renal tumor status. Examples of wash-in/-out slopes showing the differences across ccRCC, nccRCC, and AML are shown in Figure 8.

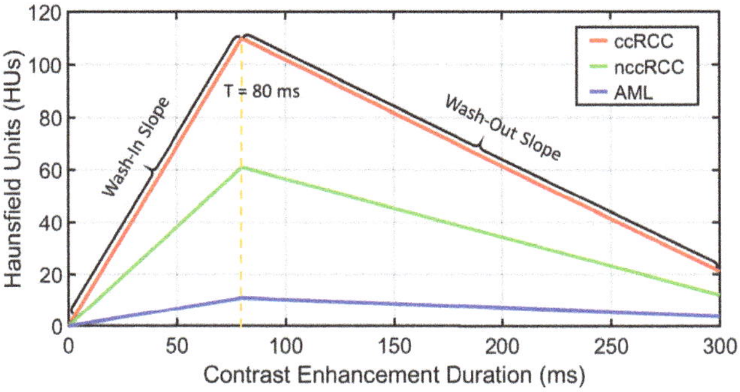

Figure 8. Example of the wash-in and wash-out slopes construction process for various types of renal tumors. When compared to nccRCC (green) and AML (blue), ccRCC tumors exhibit higher and faster wash-in/-out slopes (red).

3.3. Feature Integration and Renal Tumor Classification

Following the extraction of morphological, textural, and functional features from all given renal tumors, RC-CAD proceeds with two-stage diagnostic classification. The first stage aims to differentiate malignant (RCC) from benign (AML) tumors. In the case of malignancy, the second stage provides the classification of RCC tumors as ccRCC or nccRCC.

The multilayer perceptron (MLP) artificial neural network (ANN) consists of at least three layers: an input layer, one or more hidden layers, and an output layer, each with arbitrarily many activation/processing units, known as nodes/neurons. Each layer is fully connected to the next layer in sequence. Neurons use nonlinear activation functions to give the MLP-ANN the capability to divide the feature space into arbitrarily complex regions. The MLP-ANN mainly utilizes supervised backpropagation learning technique in the training phase, in which gradient descent methods are utilized to update the connection weights and additive biases in order to minimize the loss function. To achieve our goal, we utilized the MLP-ANN in both classification stages to obtain the final diagnosis. Classifier performance was assessed using five different feature sets (Table 2) as the ANN input in both stages. Feature Set 1 includes first-order histogram textural features ($N = 6$; mean, variance, standard deviation, skewness, kurtosis, and entropy); Feature Set 2 includes first-order percentile textural features ($N = 10$; from the 10th to the 100th percentile in 10% point steps); Feature Set 3 includes second-order GLCM textural features ($N = 6$; contrast, dissimilarity, homogeneity, ASM, energy, and correlation); Feature Set 4 includes SH reconstruction error (SHRE) morphological features ($N = 70$); and Feature Set 5 includes functional features ($N = 2$; wash-in slope and wash-out slope). At each classification stage, the individual feature sets were concatenated to obtain the combined features ($N = 94$) and were fed to a MLP-ANN to obtain the final diagnosis.

Table 2. Details of the extracted feature sets used in the two-stage renal tumor classification.

Texture Features	
Feature Set 1: First-order (histogram features)	6 features
Feature Set 2: First-order (percentiles)	10 features
Feature Set 3: Second-order (GLCM)	6 features
Shape Features	
Feature Set 4: Spherical harmonic reconstruction errors	70 features
Functional Features	
Feature Set 5: Wash-in/out slopes	2 features
Combined Features	
Feature Sets 1, 2, 3, 4, and 5	94 features

4. Results

The diagnostic performance of the RC-CAD system on our dataset of 140 renal tumors was assessed using leave-one-subject-out (LOSO) cross-validation. The system's diagnostic capabilities were assessed, evaluated, and compared in both classification stages using the individual feature sets, as well as the combined features. Each classification process was repeated 10 times, and the results were tabulated in terms of the mean $\pm$ the standard deviation to provide a more quantitative expression of the diagnostic performance.

The first stage classification (RCC vs. AML) performance for the RC-CAD system was first evaluated using individual Feature Sets 1, 2, 3, 4, and 5 (see Table 2) along with different MLP-ANN classification models. Then, the RC-CAD system was evaluated using the combined features, resulting in a noticeably enhanced diagnostic performance. A summary of the first stage performance in terms of the sensitivity, specificity, and Dice similarity coefficient (DSC) [54,55] is presented in Table 3.

Table 3. Diagnostic performance results of the first stage classification (RCC vs. AML) using different individual feature sets along with multilayer perceptron artificial neural network (MLP-ANN) classification models. The RC-CAD system diagnostic performance using the combined features outperformed the diagnostic abilities using individual feature sets. Sens: sensitivity, Spec: specificity, DSC: Dice coefficient of similarity, hl_n: size of hidden layer n.

	RCC vs. AML Classification Performance (Mean $\pm$ SD $\approx$)			
Feature Set	**Sens%**	**Spec%**	**DSC**	**MLP-ANN**
Set 1	94.1 ± 1.5	97.9 ± 1.5	0.96 ± 0.01	hl_1 = 10 nodes
Set 2	92.4 ± 2.9	95.1 ± 3.5	0.94 ± 0.02	hl_1 = 10 nodes
Set 3	94.9 ± 2.2	95.3 ± 2.5	0.95 ± 0.02	hl_1 = 10 nodes
Set 4	92.0 ± 2.4	96.6 ± 2.0	0.94 ± 0.02	hl_1 = 10 nodes, hl_2 = 5 nodes
Set 5	82.7 ± 4.1	91.7 ± 2.0	0.87 ± 0.02	hl_1 = 10 nodes
RC-CAD	**95.3 ± 2.0**	**99.9 ± 0.4**	**0.98 ± 0.01**	**hl_1 = 50 nodes, hl_2 = 25 nodes**

Hyperparameters: MLP-ANN (optimization function: trainlm, max epochs = 500, goal = 0, max validation failure = 6, min gradient = 10^{-7}, training gain (μ): initial μ = 0.001, μ decrease factor = 0.1, μ increase factor = 10, max μ = $1e^{10}$).

The diagnostic performance of the second stage classification (ccRCC vs. nccRCC) of the RC-CAD system was evaluated using the same LOSO cross-validation approach. As before, specially tailored MLP-ANN models were used with different feature sets. The best second stage classifier performance was obtained using the concatenated feature set (Table 4).

Table 4. Results from the second stage classification (ccRCC vs. nccRCC) using individual feature sets (1, 2, 3, 4, and 5) along with the multilayer perceptron artificial neural network (MLP-ANN) classification models. The RC-CAD system diagnostic performance using the combined features outperformed the diagnostic abilities using individual feature sets. Acc: accuracy, hl_n: size of hidden layer n.

	ccRCC vs. nccRCC Classification Performance (Mean $\pm$ SD $\approx$)	
Feature Set	**Acc%**	**MLP-ANN Architecture**
Set 1	76.8 ± 2.6	hl_1 = 10 nodes
Set 2	75.7 ± 3.8	hl_1 = 10 nodes
Set 3	83.3 ± 5.6	hl_1 = 10 nodes
Set 4	81.4 ± 5.1	hl_1 = 10 nodes, hl_2 = 5 nodes
Set 5	76.2 ± 2.33	hl_1 = 10 nodes
RC-CAD	**89.6 ± 5.0**	**hl_1 = 50 nodes, hl_2 = 25 nodes**

Hyperparameters: MLP-ANN (optimization function: trainlm, max epochs = 500, goal = 0, max validation failure = 6, min gradient = 10^{-7}, training gain (μ): initial μ = 0.001, μ decrease factor = 0.1, μ increase factor = 10, max μ = $1e^{10}$).

Figure 9 demonstrates a difficult case presentation for two ccRCC, two nccRCC, and two AML renal tumors. This figure visualizes the texture differences, wash-in and wash-out slope differences, and morphological differences between the different types of renal tumors, which emphasizes the potential power of the integration process of such features in providing a precise identification of a given renal tumor.

To ensure that our system is not prone to overfitting and to validate the reproducibility and robustness of RC-CAD, we performed a randomly stratified 10-fold cross-validation approach in both stages using the combined features. Likewise, the classification process was repeated 10 times using the same MLP-ANN classification model, and the results are tabulated in terms of the mean $\pm$ the standard deviation (Table 5).

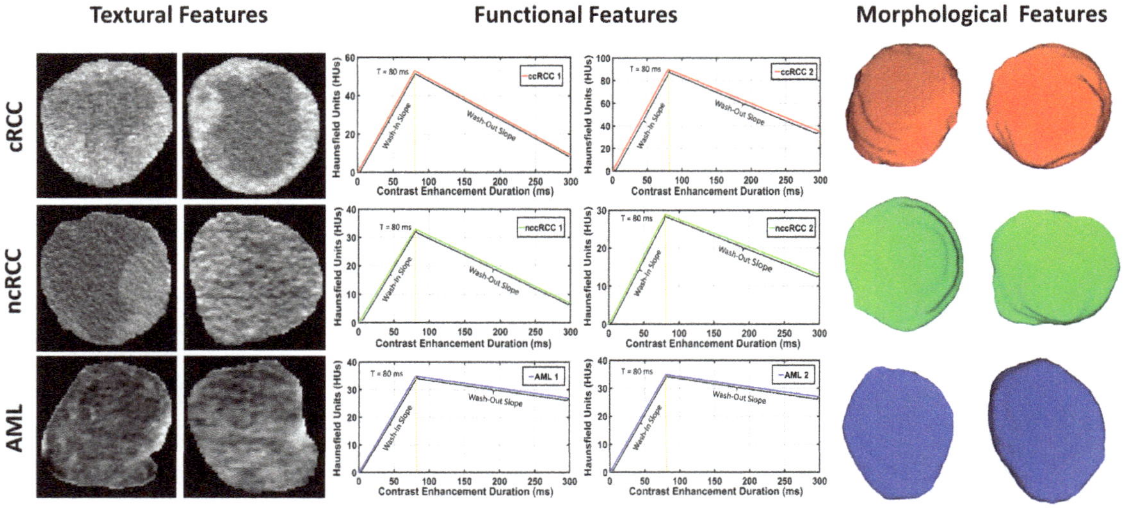

Figure 9. A difficult case presentation showing the textural differences, wash-in and wash-out slope differences, and shape differences between two ccRCC, two nccRCC, and two AML renal tumors.

Table 5. Diagnostic performance comparison for both classification stages between the developed RC-CAD system and other classification approaches (e.g., random forest (RF) and support vector machine (SVM)). Using leave-one-subject-out (LOSO) and a randomly stratified 10-fold cross-validation approach, the diagnostic abilities of the RC-CAD outperformed the others. Let Sens: sensitivity, Spec: Specificity, DSC: Dice similarity coefficient, and Acc: Accuracy.

First Stage Classification (RCC vs. AML) Performance (Mean $\pm$ SD $\approx$)				
Method	**Validation**	**Sens%**	**Spec%**	**DSC**
RC-CAD (Proposed)	**LOSO**	**95.3 $\pm$ 2.0**	**99.9 $\pm$ 0.4**	**0.98 $\pm$ 0.01**
	10-fold	**89.0 $\pm$ 3.4**	**91.0 $\pm$ 2.7**	**0.90 $\pm$ 0.02**
RFs	LOSO	89.0 $\pm$ 1.7	92.7 $\pm$ 2.7	0.91 $\pm$ 0.02
	10-fold	88.4 $\pm$ 1.0	90.7 $\pm$ 3.0	0.89 $\pm$ 0.01
SVM_{Quad}	LOSO	82.9 $\pm$ 0.0	88.6 $\pm$ 0.0	0.85 $\pm$ 0.00
	10-fold	81.9 $\pm$ 2.2	87.7 $\pm$ 2.5	0.84 $\pm$ 0.02

Second Stage Classification (ccRCC vs. nccRCC) Performance (Mean $\pm$ SD $\approx$)		
Method	**Validation**	**Acc%**
RC-CAD (Proposed)	**LOSO**	**89.6 $\pm$ 5.0**
	10-fold	**78.6 $\pm$ 5.7**
RFs	LOSO	53.7 $\pm$ 3.7
	10-fold	51.9 $\pm$ 2.6
SVM_{Quad}	LOSO	52.9 $\pm$ 0.0
	10-fold	54.3 $\pm$ 3.0

Hyperparameters: MLP-ANN (optimization function: trainlm, max epochs = 500, hidden layers: hl_1 = 50 nodes, hl_2 = 25 nodes, goal = 0, max validation failure = 6, min gradient = 10^{-7}, training gain (μ): initial μ = 0.001, μ decrease factor = 0.1, μ increase factor = 10, max μ = $1e^{10}$); RF (method: Bag, number of learning cycles = 30); SVM (kernel function: quadratic, box constraint = 1).

To highlight the advantages of using the MLP-ANN classifier, we compared RC-CAD with other, well-known machine learning classifiers (e.g., SVM_{Quad} and RF). As documented in Table 5, the diagnostic performance obtained by the developed RC-CAD system outperformed all other machine learning classifiers in both classification stages, which justifies the potential of such MLP-ANN classifiers being utilized for the developed RC-CAD system. It is worth mentioning that, in each classification stage, a grid search algorithm was employed to find the optimal set of hyperparameters, with the classification accuracy optimization criterion, for each of the classifier techniques being evaluated. The results of the hyperparameter optimization are appended to Table 5.

For the comparison with RC-CAD, we applied the existing state-of-the-art approach [27] using a total of 10 textural markers extracted from the portal-venous phase only along with the gradient boosting classification technique. In addition, we applied the state-of-the-art deep learning CNN approaches proposed by Lee et al. [32] and Oberai et al. [37] on our own datasets (first stage: N = 140; second stage: N = 70). To highlight the advantages of the RC-CAD system, all results are compared in Table 6. The diagnostic performance of RC-CAD exceeded that of other approaches in both classification stages.

Table 6. Diagnostic performance comparison for both classification stages between the developed RC-CAD system and the state-of-the-art approaches by [27,32,37]. The diagnostic abilities of the RC-CAD outperformed all other methods in both classification stages. Let Sens: sensitivity, Spec: Specificity, DSC: Dice similarity coefficient, and Acc: Accuracy.

First Stage Classification (RCC vs. AML) Performance (Mean $\pm$ SD $\approx$)				
Method		**Sens%**	**Spec%**	**DSC**
RC-CAD (Proposed)		**95.3 $\pm$ 2.0**	**99.9 $\pm$ 0.4**	**0.98 $\pm$ 0.01**
Kunapuli [27]		81.4 $\pm$ 0.0	95.7 $\pm$ 0.0	0.88 $\pm$ 0.00
Oberai [37]		88.9 $\pm$ 1.7	87.4 $\pm$ 1.4	0.91 $\pm$ 0.01
Lee [32]	AlexNet	84.0 $\pm$ 1.7	93.4 $\pm$ 1.9	0.88 $\pm$ 0.02
	GoogleNet	88.3 $\pm$ 1.7	95.1 $\pm$ 1.9	0.91 $\pm$ 0.01
	ResNet	88.0 $\pm$ 3.5	95.7 $\pm$ 0.9	0.91 $\pm$ 0.02
	VGGNet	86.9 $\pm$ 0.6	91.4 $\pm$ 2.4	0.89 $\pm$ 0.01
Second Stage Classification (ccRCC vs. nccRCC) Performance (Mean $\pm$ SD $\approx$)				
Method		**Acc%**	**ccRCC/40**	**nccRCC/30**
RC-CAD (Proposed)		**89.6 $\pm$ 5.0**	**35 $\pm$ 2**	**28 $\pm$ 3**
Kunapuli [27]		60.6 $\pm$ 2.7	28 $\pm$ 1	15 $\pm$ 1
Oberai [37]		84.3 $\pm$ 3.1	34 $\pm$ 1	25 $\pm$ 2
Lee [32]	AlexNet	71.7 $\pm$ 1.9	31 $\pm$ 2	19 $\pm$ 2
	GoogleNet	68.0 $\pm$ 1.5	32 $\pm$ 1	15 $\pm$ 1
	ResNet	70.3 $\pm$ 2.5	32 $\pm$ 0	17 $\pm$ 2
	VGGNet	72.6 $\pm$ 2.3	33 $\pm$ 1	18 $\pm$ 1

Hyperparameters: MLP-ANN (optimization function: trainlm, max epochs = 500, hidden layers: hl_1 = 50 nodes, hl_2 = 25 nodes, goal = 0, max validation failure = 6, min gradient = 10^{-7}, training gain (μ): initial μ = 0.001, μ decrease factor = 0.1, μ increase factor = 10, max μ = $1e^{10}$).

5. Discussion

The developed RC-CAD system demonstrated high diagnostic performance in terms of accuracy, sensitivity, specificity, and DSC in discrimination between benign (AML) and malignant (RCC) and in classification of the RCC subtype into ccRCC or nccRCC. This early and precise identification of the malignancy status of a given renal tumor and its associated subtype can enable clinicians to provide the appropriate early intervention/treatment plan and improve the outcomes. CE-CT was utilized as it is an imaging modality with the ability to provide different aspects of features, including but not limited to, morphological features, textural features, and functional features. The integration of these features is effective in determining the malignancy status of a given renal tumor when combined with a powerful machine learning classifier such as the MLP-ANN.

The grade of malignancy of a given renal tumor largely specifies the morphology of the tumor. Typically, malignant tumors demonstrate a more complex morphology than benign ones. Therefore, morphological features based on using spherical harmonics were utilized to capture possible surface complexity differences between malignant and benign renal tumors, as well as differences between different subtypes of malignancy.

First- and second-order textural features have been widely utilized to identify a given renal tumor status as malignant or benign, as well as to describe the malignancy subtype [26,27,29,31,32,38]. These features capture all possible textural homogeneity/heterogeneity across renal tumors with different diagnoses. In line with these studies, the extracted textural features provided high diagnostic performance in discriminating malignant ccRCC and nccRCC from benign (AML) renal tumors.

Additionally, functionality was utilized in identifying the malignancy status of a given renal tumor. The slopes of wash-in and wash-out can capture the existing differences in the enhancement characteristics [51,52]. In this study, the results obtained by the functionality metrics demonstrated the efficacy of such features in discriminating between benign (AML) and malignant (RCC) and identifying the malignancy subtype as ccRCC or nccRCC.

Although individual features have provided a reasonable diagnostic performance, they are not sufficient to rule out surgical intervention in (what may turn out to be) benign lesions. Therefore, the integration process of these features is critical to enhance the diagnostic accuracy to the point of clinical utility. The integration process produced a reliable and accurate RC-CAD system with an enhanced diagnostic performance in both classification stages as documented in Tables 3–5.

This study has some limitations: (i) benign tumors only included AMLs and did not include any ONCs; (ii) the datasets in this study were all collected from the same geographical area, and thus, we did not account for population diversity; (iii) demographics such as age and sex were not included in our analysis; (iv) differentiation between paRCC and chrRCC was not performed due to the limited number of subjects; and (v) the RC-CAD system in its current form still requires expert knowledge to segment the renal tumor manually before the handcrafted features are extracted. Despite these limitations, the RC-CAD system demonstrated the efficacy and feasibility of integrating various types of features to account for different aspects, making the developed RC-CAD a reliable noninvasive diagnostic tool.

6. Conclusions and Future Work

The developed RC-CAD system demonstrated a high classification sensitivity of 95.29% $\pm$ 2.03%, a specificity of 99.86% $\pm$ 0.43%, an ad DSC of 0.98 $\pm$ 0.01 in differentiating benign AML from malignant RCC renal tumors. In addition, the RC-CAD achieved an overall classification accuracy of 89.57% $\pm$ 5.03% in distinguishing ccRCC from nccRCC to provide the proper management plan. Integrating accurate morphological features with functional features and multiple first-order and second-order textural features was adequate to significantly enhance the diagnostic capabilities. Future work will obtain data from a larger cohort spanning different geographical areas to test the RC-CAD system's generalizability. In addition, new types of renal tumors including oncocytomas and malignant lymphomas will be included to expand the subclassification abilities of the RC-CAD system. This greater amount of data will necessitate a fully automated segmentation approach to be incorporated into the system, as manual segmentation will become too burdensome. Furthermore, fully automated extraction of diagnostic image features might be achieved using state-of-the-art deep learning approaches (e.g., convolutional neural networks and stacked auto-encoders).

Author Contributions: Conceptualization, M.S., A.A., R.T.A., M.G., A.A.K.A.R. and A.E.-B.; Data curation, R.T.A., A.E., M.G., A.A.K.A.R. and A.E.-B.; formal analysis, M.S., A.A., R.T.A., A.E., M.G., H.A.K., R.S., A.A.K.A.R., N.S.A. and A.E.-B.; methodology, M.S., A.A., R.T.A., A.E., A.S. (Ahmed Shaffie), A.S. (Ahmed Soliman), M.G., A.A.K.A.R. and A.E.-B.; project administration, A.E.-B.; resources, M.G., H.A.K., R.S., A.A.K.A.R., N.S.A. and A.E.-B.; software, M.S., A.A., A.S. (Ahmed Shaffie), A.S. (Ahmed Soliman) and A.E.-B.; supervision, A.A.K.A.R. and A.E.-B.; Validation, R.T.A., M.G., H.A.K., R.S., A.A.K.A.R., N.S.A. and A.E.-B.; visualization, M.S., A.A., A.A.K.A.R. and A.E.-B.; writing—original draft, M.S., A.A., R.T.A., A.S. (Ahmed Shaffie) and A.E.-B.; writing—review and editing, M.S., A.A., R.T.A., A.S. (Ahmed Soliman), M.G., H.A.K., R.S., A.A.K.A.R., N.S.A. and A.E.-B. All authors have read and agreed to the published version of the manuscript.

Funding: This research was funded by the Deanship of Scientific Research at Princess Nourah bint Abdulrahman University through the Fast-track Research Funding Program.

Institutional Review Board Statement: The study was conducted according to the guidelines of the Declaration of Helsinki and approved by the Institutional Review Board of Mansoura University (MS.19.02.481).

Informed Consent Statement: Informed consent was obtained from all subjects involved in the study.

Data Availability Statement: Data could be made available after acceptance upon a reasonable request to the corresponding author.

Conflicts of Interest: The authors declare no conflict of interest.

Appendix A

In this Appendix, we detail the mathematical formulas used to extract the textural features:

Basic notation:

- μ: mean;
- n: total number of voxels in the object;
- v_i: gray-level value of Voxel i;
- σ^2: variance;
- σ: standard deviation;
- N_g: the normalized grey levels;
- p: the normalized histogram counts;
- ϵ: an initial random small number;
- N_g: grey-levels (normalized 0–255);
- G_N: the GLCM (normalized 0–1);
- $\bar{x}, \sigma_x(i)$: the row margins (mean and standard deviation);
- $\bar{y}, \sigma_y(i)$: the column margins (mean and standard deviation).

Table A1. Texture features formulas.

Feature	Formula	
First-Order		
Mean (μ)	$\frac{1}{n}\sum_{i=1}^{n} v_i = \frac{v_1 + v_2 + \cdots + v_n}{n}$	(A1)
Variance (σ^2)	$\frac{\sum_{i=1}^{n}(v_i - \mu)^2}{n}$	(A2)
Entropy (Ent)	$-\sum_{i=1}^{N_g} p(i) \log_2 (p(i) + \epsilon)$	(A3)
Skewness (Skew)	$\frac{1}{n}\sum_{i=1}^{n}\left(\frac{v_i - \mu}{\sigma}\right)^3$	(A4)
Kurtosis (Kurt)	$\frac{1}{n}\sum_{i=1}^{n}\left(\frac{v_i - \mu}{\sigma}\right)^4$	(A5)

Table A1. *Cont.*

Feature	Formula	
	Second-Order	
Contrast	$\sum_{i=0}^{N_g}\sum_{j=0}^{N_g}(i-j)^2 G_N(i,j)$	(A6)
Dissimilarity	$\sum_{i=0}^{N_g}\sum_{j=0}^{N_g}\lvert i-j\rvert G_N(i,j)$	(A7)
Homogeneity	$\sum_{i=0}^{N_g}\sum_{j=0}^{N_g}\frac{G_N(i,j)}{1+(i-j)^2}$	(A8)
ASM	$\sum_{i=0}^{N_g}\sum_{j=0}^{N_g}\left(G_N(i,j)\right)^2$	(A9)
Energy	$\sqrt{ASM}$	(A10)
Correlation	$\frac{\sum_{i=0}^{N_g}\sum_{j=0}^{N_g} G_N(i,j)ij-\bar{x}\bar{y}}{\sigma_x(i)\sigma_y(j)}$	(A11)

References

1. ASCO. Kidney Cancer. Available online: https://www.cancer.net/cancer-types/kidney-cancer/ (accessed on 10 April 2020).
2. American Cancer Society. Key Statistics About Kidney Cancer. Available online: https://www.cancer.org/cancer/kidney-cancer/ (accessed on 10 April 2020).
3. National Cancer Institute. Cancer Prevalence and Cost of Care Projections. 2018. Available online: https://costprojections.cancer.gov/graph.php (accessed on 3 January 2018).
4. Siegel, R.L.; Miller, K.D.; Jemal, A. Cancer statistics, 2015. *CA Cancer J. Clin.* **2015**, *65*, 5–29. [CrossRef]
5. Chen, W.; Zheng, R.; Baade, P.D.; Zhang, S.; Zeng, H.; Bray, F.; Jemal, A.; Yu, X.Q.; He, J. Cancer statistics in China, 2015. *CA Cancer J. Clin.* **2016**, *66*, 115–132. [CrossRef]
6. Moch, H.; Cubilla, A.L.; Humphrey, P.A.; Reuter, V.E.; Ulbright, T.M. The 2016 WHO classification of tumours of the urinary system and male genital organs—Part A: Renal, penile, and testicular tumours. *Eur. Urol.* **2016**, *70*, 93–105. [CrossRef] [PubMed]
7. Delahunt, B.; Bethwaite, P.B.; Nacey, J.N. Outcome prediction for renal cell carcinoma: Evaluation of prognostic factors for tumours divided according to histological subtype. *Pathology* **2007**, *39*, 459–465. [CrossRef] [PubMed]
8. Cheville, J.C.; Lohse, C.M.; Zincke, H.; Weaver, A.L.; Blute, M.L. Comparisons of outcome and prognostic features among histologic subtypes of renal cell carcinoma. *Am. J. Surg. Pathol.* **2003**, *27*, 612–624. [CrossRef] [PubMed]
9. Rendon, R.A. Active surveillance as the preferred management option for small renal masses. *Can. Urol. Assoc. J.* **2010**, *4*, 136. [CrossRef] [PubMed]
10. Mues, A.C.; Landman, J. Small renal masses: Current concepts regarding the natural history and reflections on the American Urological Association guidelines. *Curr. Opin. Urol.* **2010**, *20*, 105–110. [CrossRef] [PubMed]
11. Heuer, R.; Gill, I.S.; Guazzoni, G.; Kirkali, Z.; Marberger, M.; Richie, J.P.; de la Rosette, J.J. A critical analysis of the actual role of minimally invasive surgery and active surveillance for kidney cancer. *Eur. Urol.* **2010**, *57*, 223–232. [CrossRef]
12. Xipell, J. The incidence of benign renal nodules (a clinicopathologic study). *J. Urol.* **1971**, *106*, 503–506. [CrossRef]
13. Gill, I.S.; Aron, M.; Gervais, D.A.; Jewett, M.A. Small renal mass. *N. Engl. J. Med.* **2010**, *362*, 624–634. [CrossRef] [PubMed]
14. Hodgdon, T.; McInnes, M.D.; Schieda, N.; Flood, T.A.; Lamb, L.; Thornhill, R.E. Can quantitative CT texture analysis be used to differentiate fat-poor renal angiomyolipoma from renal cell carcinoma on unenhanced CT images? *Radiology* **2015**, *276*, 787–796. [CrossRef]

15. Mindrup, S.R.; Pierre, J.S.; Dahmoush, L.; Konety, B.R. The prevalence of renal cell carcinoma diagnosed at autopsy. *BJU Int.* **2005**, *95*, 31–33. [CrossRef] [PubMed]
16. American Cancer Society. Test for Kidney Cancer. Available onilne: https://www.cancer.org/cancer/kidney-cancer/detection-diagnosis-staging/how-diagnosed.html (accessed on 10 April 2020).
17. Lim, R.S.; Flood, T.A.; McInnes, M.D.F.; Lavallee, L.T.; Schieda, N. Renal angiomyolipoma without visible fat: Can we make the diagnosis using CT and MRI? *Eur. Radiol.* **2018**, *28*, 542–553. [CrossRef]
18. Chandarana, H.; Rosenkrantz, A.B.; Mussi, T.C.; Kim, S.; Ahmad, A.A.; Raj, S.D.; McMenamy, J.; Melamed, J.; Babb, J.S.; Kiefer, B.; et al. Histogram analysis of whole-lesion enhancement in differentiating clear cell from papillary subtype of renal cell cancer. *Radiology* **2012**, *265*, 790–798. [CrossRef]
19. Zhou, X.; Yan, F.; Luo, Y.; Peng, Y.-L.; Parajuly, S.S.; Wen, X.-R.; Cai, D.-M.; Li, Y.-Z. Characterization and diagnostic confidence of contrast-enhanced ultrasound for solid renal tumors. *Ultrasound Med. Biol.* **2011**, *37*, 845–853. [CrossRef]
20. Dyer, R.; DiSantis, D.J.; McClennan, B.L. Simplified imaging approach for evaluation of the solid renal mass in adults. *Radiology* **2008**, *247*, 331–343. [CrossRef]
21. Zhang, J.; Lefkowitz, R.A.; Ishill, N.M.; Wang, L.; Moskowitz, C.S.; Russo, P.; Eisenberg, H.; Hricak, H. Solid renal cortical tumors: Differentiation with CT. *Radiology* **2007**, *244*, 494–504. [CrossRef] [PubMed]
22. Young, J.R.; Margolis, D.; Sauk, S.; Pantuck, A.J.; Sayre, J.; Raman, S.S. Clear cell renal cell carcinoma: Discrimination from other renal cell carcinoma subtypes and oncocytoma at multiphasic multidetector CT. *Radiology* **2013**, *267*, 444–453. [CrossRef] [PubMed]
23. Kim, J.K.; Kim, T.K.; Ahn, H.J.; Kim, C.S.; Kim, K.R.; Cho, K.S. Differentiation of subtypes of renal cell carcinoma on helical CT scans. *Am. J. Roentgenol.* **2002**, *178*, 1499–1506. [CrossRef]
24. Lubner, M.G.; Smith, A.D.; Sandrasegaran, K.; Sahani, D.V.; Pickhardt, P.J. CT texture analysis: definitions, applications, biologic correlates, and challenges. *Radiographics* **2017**, *37*, 1483–1503. [CrossRef]
25. Gillies, R.J.; Kinahan, P.E.; Hricak, H. Radiomics: images are more than pictures, they are data. *Radiology* **2016**, *278*, 563–577. [CrossRef]
26. Deng, Y.; Soule, E.; Cui, E.; Samuel, A.; Shah, S.; Lall, C.; Sundaram, C.; Sandrasegaran, K. Usefulness of CT texture analysis in differentiating benign and malignant renal tumours. *Clin. Radiol.* **2020**, *75*, 108–115. [CrossRef] [PubMed]
27. Kunapuli, G.; Varghese, B.A.; Ganapathy, P.; Desai, B.; Cen, S.; Aron, M.; Gill, I.; Duddalwar, V. A decision-support tool for renal mass classification. *J. Digit. Imaging* **2018**, *31*, 929–939. [CrossRef] [PubMed]
28. Guyon, I.; Weston, J.; Barnhill, S.; Vapnik, V. Gene selection for cancer classification using support vector machines. *Mach. Learn.* **2002**, *46*, 389–422. [CrossRef]
29. Kocak, B.; Yardimci, A.H.; Bektas, C.T.; Turkcanoglu, M.H.; Erdim, C.; Yucetas, U.; Koca, S.B.; Kilickesmez, O. Textural differences between renal cell carcinoma subtypes: Machine learning-based quantitative computed tomography texture analysis with independent external validation. *Eur. J. Radiol.* **2018**, *107*, 149–157. [CrossRef] [PubMed]
30. Szczypiński, P.M.; Strzelecki, M.; Materka, A.; Klepaczko, A. MaZda—A software package for image texture analysis. *Comput. Methods Programs Biomed.* **2009**, *94*, 66–76. [CrossRef]
31. Sun, X.Y.; Feng, Q.X.; Xu, X.; Zhang, J.; Zhu, F.P.; Yang, Y.H.; Zhang, Y.D. Radiologic-Radiomic Machine Learning Models for Differentiation of Benign and Malignant Solid Renal Masses: Comparison With Expert-Level Radiologists. *Am. J. Roentgenol.* **2020**, *214*, W44–W54. [CrossRef]
32. Lee, H.; Hong, H.; Kim, J.; Jung, D.C. Deep feature classification of angiomyolipoma without visible fat and renal cell carcinoma in abdominal contrast-enhanced CT images with texture image patches and hand-crafted feature concatenation. *Med. Phys.* **2018**, *45*, 1550–1561. [CrossRef]
33. Krizhevsky, A.; Sutskever, I.; Hinton, G.E. Imagenet classification with deep convolutional neural networks. In *Advances in Neural Information Processing Systems*; Neural Information Processing Systems Foundation, Inc. (NIPS): Lake Tahoe, NV, USA, 2012; pp. 1097–1105.
34. Simonyan, K.; Zisserman, A. Very deep convolutional networks for large-scale image recognition. *arXiv* **2014**, arXiv:1409.1556.
35. Szegedy, C.; Liu, W.; Jia, Y.; Sermanet, P.; Reed, S.; Anguelov, D.; Erhan, D.; Vanhoucke, V.; Rabinovich, A. Going deeper with convolutions. In Proceedings of the IEEE Conference on Computer Vision and Pattern Recognition, Boston, MA, USA, 7–12 June 2015; pp. 1–9.
36. He, K.; Zhang, X.; Ren, S.; Sun, J. Deep residual learning for image recognition. In Proceedings of the IEEE Conference on Computer Vision and Pattern Recognition, Las Vegas, NV, USA, 27–30 June 2016; pp. 770–778.
37. Oberai, A.; Varghese, B.; Cen, S.; Angelini, T.; Hwang, D.; Gill, I.; Aron, M.; Lau, C.; Duddalwar, V. Deep learning based classification of solid lipid-poor contrast enhancing renal masses using contrast enhanced CT. *Br. J. Radiol.* **2020**, *93*, 20200002. [CrossRef]
38. Zhou, L.; Zhang, Z.; Chen, Y.C.; Zhao, Z.Y.; Yin, X.D.; Jiang, H.B. A deep learning-based radiomics model for differentiating benign and malignant renal tumors. *Transl. Oncol.* **2019**, *12*, 292–300. [CrossRef] [PubMed]
39. Shehata, M.; Alksas, A.; Abouelkheir, R.T.; Elmahdy, A.; Shaffie, A.; Soliman, A.; Ghazal, M.; Khalifeh, H.A.; Razek, A.A.; El-Baz, A. A New Computer-Aided Diagnostic (CAD) System For Precise Identification Of Renal Tumors. In Proceedings of the 2021 IEEE 18th International Symposium on Biomedical Imaging (ISBI), Nice, France, 13–16 April 2021; pp. 1378–1381.

40. Shaffie, A.; Soliman, A.; Ghazal, M.; Taher, F.; Dunlap, N.; Wang, B.; Elmaghraby, A.; Gimel'Farb, G.; El-Baz, A. A new framework for incorporating appearance and shape features of lung nodules for precise diagnosis of lung cancer. In Proceedings of the IEEE International Conference on Image Processing (ICIP'17), Beijing, China, 17–20 September 2017; pp. 1372–1376. [CrossRef]
41. Nitzken, M.J. Shape Analysis of the Human Brain. Ph.D. Thesis, University of Louisville, Louisville, KY, USA, 2015.
42. Moya, L.; Zakeri, H.; Yamazaki, F.; Liu, W.; Mas, E.; Koshimura, S. 3D gray level co-occurrence matrix and its application to identifying collapsed buildings. *ISPRS J. Photogramm. Remote Sens.* **2019**, *149*, 14–28. [CrossRef]
43. Gonzales, R.C.; Woods, R.E. *Digital Image Processing*; Prentice Hall: Upper Saddle River, NJ, USA, 2002.
44. Kurani, A.S.; Xu, D.H.; Furst, J.; Raicu, D.S. Co-occurrence matrices for volumetric data. *Heart* **2004**, *27*, 25.
45. Tustison, N.; Gee, J. Run-Length Matrices For Texture Analysis. *Insight J.* **2008**, *1*, 1–6.
46. Barry, B.; Buch, K.; Soto, J.A.; Jara, H.; Nakhmani, A.; Anderson, S.W. Quantifying liver fibrosis through the application of texture analysis to diffusion weighted imaging. *Magn. Reson. Imaging* **2014**, *32*, 84–90. [CrossRef] [PubMed]
47. Castellano, G.; Bonilha, L.; Li, L.; Cendes, F. Texture analysis of medical images. *Clin. Radiol.* **2004**, *59*, 1061–1069. [CrossRef]
48. Anderson, S.W.; Jara, H.; Ozonoff, A.; O'Brien, M.; Hamilton, J.A.; Soto, J.A. Effect of disease progression on liver apparent diffusion coefficient and T2 values in a murine model of hepatic fibrosis at 11.7 Tesla MRI. *J. Magn. Reson. Imaging* **2012**, *35*, 140–146. [CrossRef]
49. Van Griethuysen, J.J.; Fedorov, A.; Parmar, C.; Hosny, A.; Aucoin, N.; Narayan, V.; Beets-Tan, R.G.; Fillion-Robin, J.C.; Pieper, S.; Aerts, H.J. Computational radiomics system to decode the radiographic phenotype. *Cancer Res.* **2017**, *77*, e104–e107. [CrossRef]
50. Haralick, R.M. Statistical and structural approaches to texture. *Proc. IEEE* **1979**, *67*, 786–804. [CrossRef]
51. Kim, J.K.; Park, S.Y.; Shon, J.H.; Cho, K.S. Angiomyolipoma with minimal fat: Differentiation from renal cell carcinoma at biphasic helical CT. *Radiology* **2004**, *230*, 677–684. [CrossRef]
52. Ye, X.D.; Ye, J.D.; Yuan, Z.; Dong, S.; Xiao, X.S. Characterization of solitary pulmonary nodules: Use of washout characteristics at contrast-enhanced computed tomography. *Oncol. Lett.* **2012**, *3*, 672–676. [CrossRef] [PubMed]
53. Xie, P.; Yang, Z.; Yuan, Z. Lipid-poor renal angiomyolipoma: Differentiation from clear cell renal cell carcinoma using wash-in and washout characteristics on contrast-enhanced computed tomography. *Oncol. Lett.* **2016**, *11*, 2327–2331. [CrossRef]
54. Dice, L.R. Measures of the amount of ecologic association between species. *Ecology* **1945**, *26*, 297–302. [CrossRef]
55. Carass, A.; Roy, S.; Gherman, A.; Reinhold, J.C.; Jesson, A.; Arbel, T.; Maier, O.; Handels, H.; Ghafoorian, M.; Platel, B.; et al. Evaluating White Matter Lesion Segmentations with Refined Sørensen-Dice Analysis. *Sci. Rep.* **2020**, *10*, 8242. [CrossRef] [PubMed]

sensors

MDPI

Review

Electrocardiogram-Based Emotion Recognition Systems and Their Applications in Healthcare—A Review

Muhammad Anas Hasnul [1], Nor Azlina Ab. Aziz [1,*], Salem Alelyani [2,3], Mohamed Mohana [2] and Azlan Abd. Aziz [1]

1 Faculty of Engineering and Technology, Multimedia University, Melaka 75450, Malaysia; 1141126389@student.mmu.edu.my (M.A.H.); azlan.abdaziz@mmu.edu.my (A.A.A.)
2 Center for Artificial Intelligence (CAI), King Khalid University, Abha 61421, Saudi Arabia; s.alelyani@kku.edu.sa (S.A.); mmuhanna@kku.edu.sa (M.M.)
3 College of Computer Science, King Khalid University, Abha 61421, Saudi Arabia
* Correspondence: azlina.aziz@mmu.edu.my

Abstract: Affective computing is a field of study that integrates human affects and emotions with artificial intelligence into systems or devices. A system or device with affective computing is beneficial for the mental health and wellbeing of individuals that are stressed, anguished, or depressed. Emotion recognition systems are an important technology that enables affective computing. Currently, there are a lot of ways to build an emotion recognition system using various techniques and algorithms. This review paper focuses on emotion recognition research that adopted electrocardiograms (ECGs) as a unimodal approach as well as part of a multimodal approach for emotion recognition systems. Critical observations of data collection, pre-processing, feature extraction, feature selection and dimensionality reduction, classification, and validation are conducted. This paper also highlights the architectures with accuracy of above 90%. The available ECG-inclusive affective databases are also reviewed, and a popularity analysis is presented. Additionally, the benefit of emotion recognition systems towards healthcare systems is also reviewed here. Based on the literature reviewed, a thorough discussion on the subject matter and future works is suggested and concluded. The findings presented here are beneficial for prospective researchers to look into the summary of previous works conducted in the field of ECG-based emotion recognition systems, and for identifying gaps in the area, as well as in developing and designing future applications of emotion recognition systems, especially in improving healthcare.

Keywords: electrocardiogram (ECG); affective computing; emotion recognition system; healthcare

Citation: Hasnul, M.A.; Aziz, N.A.H.; Alelyani, S.; Mohana, M.; Aziz, A.A. Electrocardiogram-Based Emotion Recognition Systems and Their Applications in Healthcare—A Review. *Sensors* **2021**, *21*, 5015. https://doi.org/10.3390/s21155015

Academic Editors: Ayman El-baz, Guruprasad A. Giridharan, Ahmed Shalaby, Ali H. Mahmoud and Mohammed Ghazal

Received: 17 June 2021
Accepted: 19 July 2021
Published: 23 July 2021

1. Introduction

Research interest in affective computing via physiological modalities has been popularized by the accelerated development of technological solutions, particularly within the healthcare industry. The field of affective computing originated from a paper written by Rosalind Picard in 1995, discussing neurological studies of human emotions and the possibility for computers to mimic them by expression recognition [1]. Affective computing is a multidisciplinary study that revolves around computer science, psychology, cognition, and physiology [2].

The significance of emotions in natural human interaction was demonstrated by Ekman et al. [3] from the premise "If B perceives A's facial expression of emotion, B's behavior toward A may change, and A's noticing this may influence or determine A's experience of emotion". Meanwhile, in a book by Reeves et al. [4], the authors claimed that humans treated computers as if they are just another living being too. From both arguments, it can be deduced that if computer systems are capable of discerning and responding to human affects, then the interactional gap between people and machines will be as naturalistic as talking to a friend and improve the human–computer interaction.

Adopting emotion recognition systems should be considered as a footstep towards instilling empathy, sympathy, and compassion into artificially intelligent machinery.

Emotion recognition systems have a lot of prospective applications, spanning healthcare, entertainment, e-learning, marketing, human monitoring, and security. According to [5], there were three major applications of emotion recognition systems specifically using ECG signals:

- Firstly, monitoring human emotions during certain tasks and assessing the behavioral response in critical situations. For example, in [6], the emotion recognition system focuses on studying a driver's performance during a race.
- Next, clinical application in monitoring patients' psychological condition for relevant drug prescriptions or treatment. In [7], emotion recognition is implemented in healthcare settings to promote relaxation and reduce stress. Three emotional services are provided in the design framework, which are relaxation, amusement, and excitement services.
- Finally, emotion recognition can be used for marketing. Emotion recognition can be utilized for website optimization [8], where the system can be designed to collect information on which adverts attract the most attention, which can allow catering appropriate contents according to audience demography.

The physiological approach towards emotion recognition has become a better alternative to facial expressions, gestures, and vocal traits. Machine vision-based emotion recognition systems are prone to fake emotions and can be manipulated easily [9–11]. This is why many studies focused on physiological signals, including the multimodal approach, by combining different physiological signals from biosensors such as an ECG, an electroencephalogram (EEG), an electromyogram (EMG), electrodermal activity (EDA) or galvanic skin response (GSR), a photoplethysmogram (PPG) or blood volume pressure (BVP), or a respiratory inductive plethysmograph (RIP). Although the multimodal emotion recognition approach commonly performed better, the unimodal approach has the advantages of a lower processing time and simpler data collection [12].

The brain and heart are connected via the autonomic nervous system (ANS), in which both indirectly influence each other's behavior [13]. The connection of the sympathetic nervous system (SNS) and parasympathetic nervous system (PNS) is part of the ANS. Thus, emotional experience does cause some changes in the heart rhythm, and this can be detected through ECG readings. The purpose of this review is to sum up the literature to date that has reported the adoption of ECG as an input of emotion recognition systems. This paper also discusses ECG features such as the heart rate (HR), as well as heart rate variability (HRV), and their relationship with the autonomic innervation of the heart.

The next sections discuss the review methodology, followed by the theoretical background of the autonomic innervation of the heart, electrocardiograms, various emotional models, and emotion elicitation and emotion evaluation techniques. ECG-inclusive datasets are reviewed and analyzed in Section 4. Section 5 discusses the methodology of developing an emotion recognition system from the pre-processing of ECG signals, feature extraction, feature selection and dimensionality reduction, classification, and validation. Section 6 focuses on the discussion of the summarized literature. The applications of emotion recognition systems in healthcare are reviewed in Section 7, and the discussion of the reviews is presented in Section 8. The last section concludes the work.

2. Review Methodology

The journals and articles reviewed in this work underwent a thorough selection process. Initially, keywords for the search criteria were identified. Studies associated with *"emotion recognition"*, *"ECG"*, and *"healthcare"* were searched throughout different academic databases. Table 1 shows the publisher database and number of studies reviewed for ECG-based emotion recognition, and healthcare applications of emotion recognition systems. Here, IEEE Xplore was the database with the most papers reviewed.

Table 1. Number of papers reviewed from the respective databases.

Publisher Database	ECG and Emotion Recognition	Healthcare Application
IEEE Xplore	26	9
Science Direct: Elsevier	4	1
Nature: Scientific Reports/Data	4	0
ACM DL	3	1
Springer Link	3	2
MDPI	2	0
IOP Science	2	1
J-Stage	1	0
Springer Nature	1	0
IOS Press	1	0
Wiley Online Library	1	0
Fuji Technology Press Ltd.	1	0
IJEECS	1	0
Frontiers	1	0
Total	**51**	**14**

The exclusion criteria after the first reading included the removal of duplicated publications, contextual irrelevancies, and non-English papers. The challenge in collecting the articles for review was the status of the article, that is, whether it is open access or included in our institutions' subscription or not.

In total, for ECG-based emotion recognition, 51 papers were reviewed, and the distribution according to the year the papers were published is shown in Figure 1. The trend shows that the number of works increases by year, and this reflects the growing interest of researchers in this field. The overview also shows the number of ECG-based emotion recognition studies conducted with unimodal and multimodal approaches.

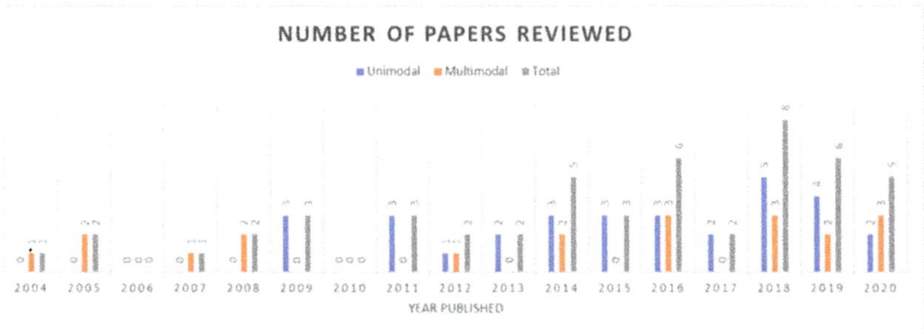

Figure 1. Overview of the years selected studies were published.

3. Theoretical Background

The contents covered here were cited from textbooks, academic journals, conference papers, and other sources with contextual benefits.

3.1. Autonomic Innervation of The Heart

The centers of the ANS's control over the heart rhythm are located at the medulla oblongata [14]. Without any external factor, both centers provide an infinitesimal amount of stimulation to the cardiac muscle and cause it to have an autonomic tune. However, upon excitation, the cardioaccelerator releases the neurotransmitter norepinephrine and causes the HR to increase drastically. This process occurs throughout the SNS, as well as at the sinoatrial (SA) node, and is commonly known as the "fight or flight" response [15]. As for the decrease in the HR, the cardioinhibitory centers release the neurotransmitter acetylcholine (Ach) to the PNS. Metaphorically, this activation can be referred to as the "rest and digest" operation [15]. SNS and PNS stimulation flows through the cardiac plexus, cervical ganglia, and superior thoracic ganglia to the SA and atrioventricular (AV) nodes, with the nerves' fibers reaching the atria and ventricles. Figure 2 shows the connection of the vagus nerve (PNS) and sympathetic cardiac nerves (SNS) in a simple model.

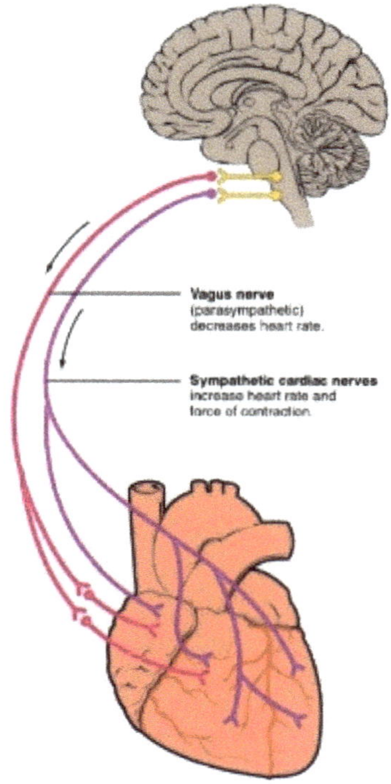

Figure 2. The ANS connection between the brain and heart [16].

The physiological interrelation between the heart and brain communication influences certain characteristic changes when it comes to emotion. The ANS's influence on emotional changes regulates various other body parameters [17]. According to the HeartMath Institute, the dynamic, continuous, and bidirectional communication of both organs affects one's perception, emotion, intuition, and general health [13]. Hence, detecting the cardiac rhythm for emotion recognition purposes based on autonomic innervation is necessary in healthcare as a preventive measure towards negative emotions such as stress [18].

3.2. Electrocardiogram (ECG)

An ECG measures the electrical activity of the heart in different phases and perspectives based on the situation and configuration [19]. The signal acquired provides a graphical depiction of the deflection and wave series produced by each cardiac cycle, as shown in Figure 3. The main purpose of an ECG in clinics is to detect pathological cardiac conditions such as arrhythmia, heart disease, and epilepsy [20].

A normal ECG signal should have three segmented waves in a single cycle [19]. The first wave materializes from the atrial depolarization, and it is called the P wave.

The second wave is the QRS complex, where it contains the highest amplitude caused by ventricular depolarization. The interval distance between R peaks is where the inter-beat interval (IBI) is usually calculated for HR detection [21]. Additionally, to extract HRV features from ECG signals, QRS detection is essential to sort out the RR intervals [22]. After a few milliseconds of plateau, a T wave appears because of ventricular repolarization [23], and the cycle repeats.

According to Rattanyu [24], and Bexton et al. [25], ECGs are one of the most widely used biosensors in emotion recognition because of their quality, and the information on human emotions contained in the signals. Various studies have used ECGs as a single modality for emotion recognition. Theekshana et al. [26] stated that there are four prime reasons that ECGs alone are sufficient for an emotion recognition system. Firstly, ECG signals capture the heart activity, and ANS stimulation towards each emotion causes rhythmic changes in the heart [25]. Secondly, an ECG can be extracted using a less intrusive, mobile, and wearable device [27]. Thirdly, an ECG is a versatile biosensor that can collect data from different parts of the body: the chest or the limbs, as shown in Figure 4. Lastly, ECG signals have a higher amplitude among other biosignals [24].

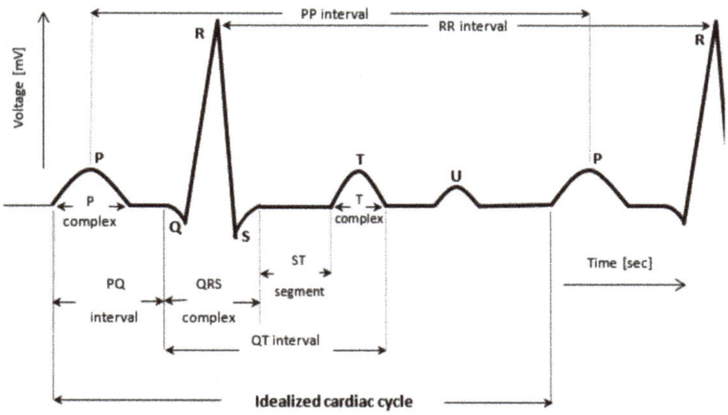

Figure 3. ECG cycle in a healthy and normal heart [28].

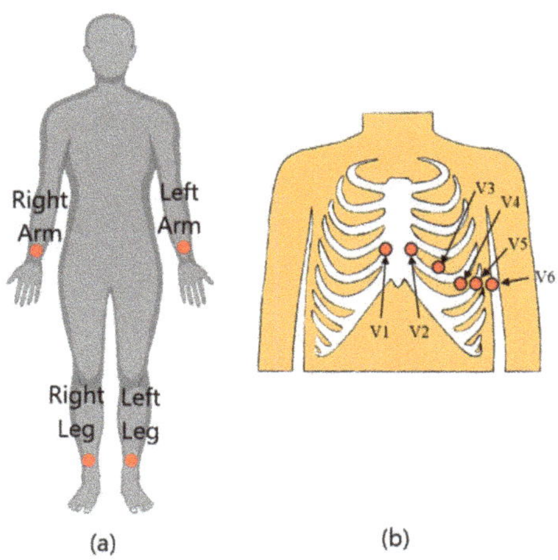

Figure 4. Possible electrode placements for ECG recordings [19]: (**a**) electrode placement for limbs lead configuration; (**b**) electrode placement for chest lead configuration [29].

3.3. Emotion Models

Emotion is a subjective and conscious mental experience accompanied by particular biological responses or changes [30]. Experts from different backgrounds have tried to uncover the universal definition of emotion; however, none of them have come to an agreement in establishing a single emotional model [15]. Despite this, the two most widely accepted and used emotional models are discrete categories and the affective dimension [1]. In addition, this paper also discusses another commonly used emotional model, the binary emotional model.

3.3.1. Discrete Emotional Model (DEM)

The DEM categorizes emotions into standard terms such as joy, fear, anger, disgust, sad, funny, and neutral [31]. This emotional model is standardized and shared across languages and cultures [32]. Cicero and Graver [33] named 4 basic categories, while Ekman [34] summarized 6, and Izard [35,36] suggested 10 basic emotions. Although the number of emotion classes in the DEM varies, there are similarities between them. Among the emotion labels, the most common are happiness, sadness, and anger [20,37–41]. The reason for the three of them being selected the most is because of the prominent arousal level that can be easily detected compared to more relaxed emotions [22].

3.3.2. Affective Dimensional Model (ADM)

The ADM, which is also known as the continuous dimension model, is a range of two-dimensional planes of valence and arousal. One researcher preferred to add another plane of dominance into the model [42]. The ADM was developed by Russell [43] and has been adopted widely by researchers from different backgrounds. Figure 5 shows the illustration of valence, arousal, and dominance on a positive and negative scale. Valence is the feeling of pleasantness, either being appetitive or aversive, while arousal is the intensity of the feeling being experienced [44]. The dominance scale represents the authority to be in control, ranging from submissive to feeling empowered.

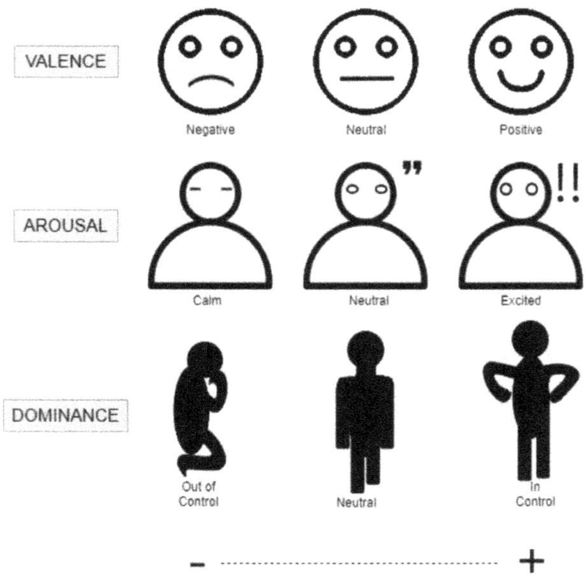

Figure 5. The graphical scheme provided to subjects to understand the ADM scales [45].

The versatility of the ADM compared to the DEM is demonstrated in Figure 6. Based on the valence and arousal scale, the categories of emotions can be segmented depending on the degree of intensity. High valence–high arousal (HVHA) is mapped to excitation, while high valence–low arousal (HVLA) is mapped to feeling calm, or relaxation. Low valence–high arousal (LVHA) is considered as anger and feeling distressed, while low valence–low arousal (LVLA) is related to sadness and feeling depressed. The middle of the scale is considered as a neutral state.

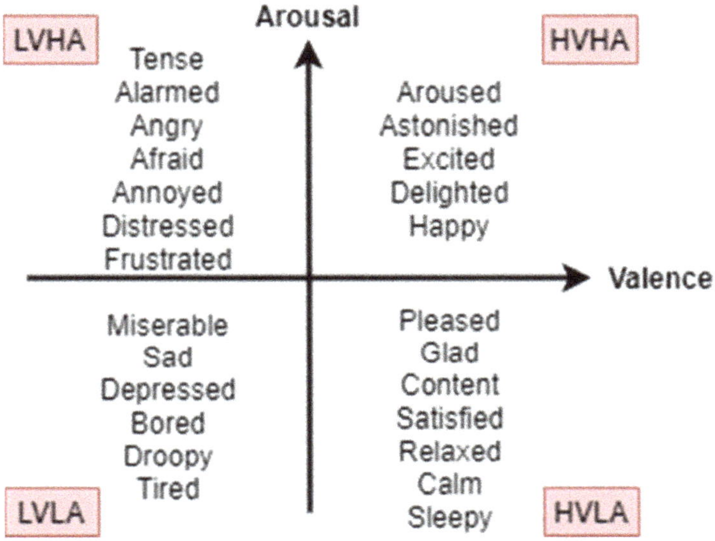

Figure 6. The mapping function between the ADM and DEM [46].

3.3.3. Binary Emotional Model

The binary emotional model consists of positive and negative emotional states (Pos/Neg) [47]. The purpose of this model is to simply generalize between which emotions are bad and which emotions are good. Negative emotions may cause mental stress to the bearer and the people around them. It is unhealthy to be exposed to prolonged negative emotions as it affects the physiological state of a person. Depression, anxiety, and bipolar disorder are known effects of emotional and mental stress [48,49]. Moreover, by simplifying the emotional model to two classes, a targeted application of an emotion recognition system can be built with less complexity. A higher accuracy of training and testing models can also be expected. Figure 7 shows the emotional stress model proposed by [39]. Instead of valence, the author used a pleasantness scale to describe the region of potential mental stressors. Any emotions categorized under negative valence such as sadness, anger, fear, and disgust are potential stress factors that may lead to complications. Thus, the binary emotional model is another important classification model for affective computing studies.

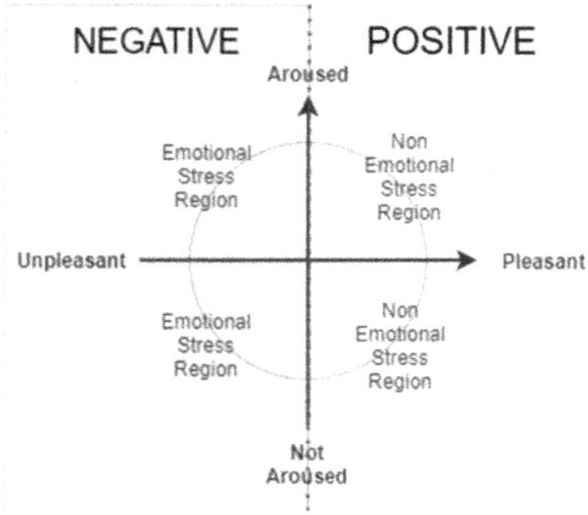

Figure 7. Pos/Neg as a model that identifies between good (no stress) and bad (stress) emotions.

3.4. Emotion Elicitation

Inducing basic emotions for data collection in an experiment requires certain guidelines and standard operating procedures. There are five common elicitation techniques which are audio visual, imagery, music, memory recall, and the situational procedure [50]. The less common approaches are naturalistic conversations or debates [51], driving [52], video games [53], and virtual reality [54].

Audio visual techniques can be segmented film clips for targeted emotions, or videos with the same purpose [31,45,55–59]. The length of the videos varies, as does the length of the recorded physiological signals. Imagery is the act of reading vignettes [50] and experiencing deep emotions through contemplation [60], but in addition to that, pictorial images such as the International Affective Picture System (IAPS) [61] have been used widely too. Music listening is another popular way to activate emotions through the lyrics, melody, and tempo variations [62]. The renowned dataset for affective audio stimulation is the International Affective Digitized Sounds system (IADS) [63]. Memory recall involves remembrance of personal experiences to reactivate the essence of emotions circa that moment [64]. The situational procedure necessitates fabricating a social environment that elicits the targeted emotion.

As it was described in [50], the most effective way to induce basic emotions is through audio visuals. Imagery is effective for happiness, surprise, fear, and anger. Music is only effective for happiness, sadness, and fear. Memory recall is recommended to induce happiness, anger, disgust, sadness, and fear, but not surprise. Finally, the situational procedure is a good approach for happiness, anger, fear, and surprise.

3.5. Emotion Evaluation

Emotion evaluation is an annotation perspective for emotion labeling on the data collected. The most common approach is through a first-person perspective or self-assessment. In this way, the subject personally labels their emotions on a Self-Assessment Manikin (SAM) [65]. The questionnaire varies depending on which emotional models are used. Usually, there will be a pictorial description of emotions and the intensity scale to ease the labeling process, as shown in Figure 5. The problem with internal annotation is that the subject might feel discomfort and insecure in sharing their true conscious and unconscious experiences towards the stimuli [15]. This indirectly reduces the reliability of the reported emotional experience.

Another perspective for emotion annotation is implicit assessment or external evaluation. This can be conducted through a second-person perspective and third-person perspective. The second-person perspective is someone who watches the subject experience the stimuli in real time and labels what they think the subject feels [51]. Meanwhile, third-person perspectives are external, conducted by watching the recordings of the subject's facial expression and body gestures, and then only annotating the guesses on what emotions the subject feels. Both methods have a disadvantage of bias, and they can easily be deceived [15]. Their perception often depends on personality, cultural bias, and environmental attributes.

4. ECG-Inclusive Affective Datasets

Affective datasets that have been collected using various physiological modalities are available in academic archives. Although they are not standardized, there are still commonalities between them. Since this review paper is only interested in ECG-based emotion recognition systems, the datasets enlisted are ECG-inclusive modalities. The focus is on the summary of the stimulation used, the data size, the modalities included, the ECG device used, the ECG configuration, emotional annotations, the model, and perspectives. Among the datasets with ECG signals are the following:

1. **AMIGOS** [55]: This stands for **A** dataset for **M**ultimodal research of affect, personality traits, and mood in **I**ndividuals and **G**r**O**up**S**. The data were collected from 40 subjects watching videos, with 16 samples each. Biosignals included are ECG, EEG, and GSR. The ECG device used was a Shimmer, at a 256 Hz sampling frequency. The ECG lead configurations used were right arm left leg (RA-LL), and left arm left leg (LA-LL). The emotion annotation labels were from a self-assessment, and third-person perspectives with a 3D ADM.
2. **ASCERTAIN** [56]: This stands for a multimodal datab**AS**e for impli**C**it p**ER**rsonali**T**y and **A**ffect recognit**I**o**N** using commercial physiological sensors. The data were collected from 58 subjects watching 36 video clips. The physiological signals used were ECG, EEG, and GSR. For ECG, the sampling rate was 256 Hz, with two unspecified lead configurations. The emotion annotation perspective was only from self-assessment, and the model used was the ADM on a scale of valence and arousal.
3. **AuBT** [66]: This stands for **Au**gsburg **B**iosignal **T**oolbox by the University of Augsburg. It contains a MATLAB GUI for emotion recognition purposes, together with a data corpus recorded from ECG, EMG, skin conductance (SC), and respiration (RSP). The data were from a single subject, with 100 samples collected within the span of 25 days while listening to music of the subject's choice. The ECG signal sampling rate was 256 Hz, with only one lead configuration. The emotions were labeled by self-assessment using the DEM. The four classes of emotions are joy, anger, sadness, and pleasure.
4. **CASE** [67]: This stands for the **C**ontinuously **A**nnotated **S**ignals of **E**motion. The data were collected from 30 subjects in real time while watching various videos. The physiological modalities included are ECG, BVP, EMG, and GSR (EDA). The ECG device used was from Thought Technology, and the configuration setup had three leads, 1 kHz. The annotation was by self-assessment using the ADM.
5. **CLAS** [68]: This stands for **C**ognitive **L**oad, **A**ffect and **S**tress Recognition. The data were collected from 62 subjects, with 32 samples each. The stimuli were separated equally between video clips and IAPS pictures. The biosignals included are ECG, PPG, and EDA. The ECG device used was the one-lead Shimmer3, with a right arm left arm configuration. The sampling rate was 256 Hz. Self-annotation of the valence and arousal ADM was performed by the subjects.
6. **DECAF** [57]: This stands for a multimodal dataset for **dec**oding user physiological responses to **af**fective multimedia content. The data were collected from 30 subjects with 76 samples. Here, 40 of the 76 samples were from music videos at a 1 min cap, while the others were from watching movie clips. The biosignals included are ECG, EMG, magnetoencephalogram (MEG), and electrooculogram (EOG). The sampling rate for the ECG was 1 kHz, and it was downsampled to 256 Hz. A one-lead configuration was used for this setup. The annotation was from a first-person perspective, and the ADM with a 3D scale was implemented.

7. **DREAMER** [58]: This dataset contains data collected from 23 participants, with 18 samples each. The stimuli used were video clips ranging from 1 to 3 min, with the focus on the ECG and EEG modalities. The ECG device used was a low-cost, wireless, portable, and wearable off-the-shelf device from Shimmer. The sampling rate was 256 Hz, with two-lead and three-lead configurations. Self-annotation of the subjects was conducted using a valence, arousal, and dominance ADM.
8. **DSDRWDT** [52]: This stands for **D**etecting **S**tress **D**uring **R**eal-**W**orld **D**riving **T**asks. The data were collected from 24 subjects while they were driving in a real-world condition. The biosignals included are ECG, EMG, SC, and RSP. The ECG device used was a FlexComp, with a 496 Hz sampling rate. The lead used was right arm left leg (RA-LL). The drivers labeled their stress levels through three stages: low, medium, and high. The emotional model considered was the Pos/Neg category model.
9. **EMDC** [69]: This **e**motion-specific **m**ultilevel **d**ichotomous **c**lassification dataset contains signals collected from 3 subjects, with 360 samples of music listening. The physiological modalities included are ECG, EMG, SC, and RSP. The ECG device used was a three-lead Procomp^2 Infiniti, at a 256 Hz sampling frequency. The affective annotations were from self-perspective with a 2D ADM.
10. **K-EmoCon** [51]: This dataset contains data collected from 32 subjects in real time from a naturalistic conversation (paired debates on social issues) to induce emotions. The physiological modalities included are ECG, EEG, BVP, EDA, and skin temperature (SKT). For the ECG signal, a Polar H7 was used, at a 1 Hz sampling rate. The only feature extracted was the HR. This paper claims to be the first publicly available dataset on emotion recognition that has a multi-perspective annotation from self-assessment, second person and third person. The ADM with valence and arousal scales was implemented.
11. **MANHOB-HCI** [59]: Data were collected from 27 subjects, with 20 samples, using ECG, EEG, GSR, EDA, RSP, and SKT. The ECG device used was a Biosemi Active II, with a three-lead configuration. The sampling rate was 1024 Hz and was downsampled to 256 Hz. Based on the emotional videos watched, the subjects self-reported their affective state with a 3D ADM.
12. **MPED** [31]: This stands for **M**ulti-Modal **P**hysiological **E**motion **D**atabase. The data were collected from 23 subjects, with 28 samples, watching video clips less than 5 min each. The biosgnals included are ECG, EEG, GSR, and RSP. The Biopac System with three-lead configurations and a 250 Hz sampling frequency was used for the ECG signal acquisition. The annotation perspective was from the first-person view using seven classes of the DEM: joy, funny, anger, fear, disgust, sad, and neutral.
13. **SWELL** [70]**:** This dataset is also known as SWELL knowledge work (SWELL-KW), and it is a new multimodal dataset for research on stress and user modeling. The data were collected from 25 subjects performing tasks such as writing, presenting, reading, and searching to elicit stress. The physiological signals recorded were ECG and SC. The ECG was recorded through a Mobi device (TMSi), with the electrodes placed in a triangular configuration on the chest. The sampling rate was 2048 Hz, with three leads attached. The assessment was conducted by the subjects through labeling two emotional models, which were the ADM and Pos/Neg.
14. **WESAD** [71]: This stands for **We**arable **S**tress and **A**ffect **D**etection. The data were collected from 15 subjects watching video clips and provided with public speaking and mental arithmetic tasks. The biosignals included are ECG, BVP, EDA, EMG, RSP, and temperature (TEMP). The ECG signal was acquired from a RespiBAN Professional using a three-lead configuration. The sampling rate was 700 Hz. The subject self-annotated their emotions using a three-class Pos/Neg model. Amusement, neutral, and stress were the classification categories implemented.

All of these ECG-inclusive datasets are summarized in Table 2. The stimulus used to induce the emotions during data collection, the data size, available modalities, details of the settings of ECG collection, the emotion annotations, the model, and perspectives are tabulated.

Dataset Popularity Analysis

Even though multiple datasets have been proposed and made available for others to use, not all datasets have been adopted by other researchers. Hence, based on the summarized literature from this review, the number of times a dataset has been adopted and cited in other studies (excluding self-citation) was calculated and is plotted in Figure 8. The most popular dataset being used for emotion recognition studies using ECG, as observed here, is AuBT, with six adoptions. Although the database was published in 2005, the citations observed here came from 2016 onwards. The popularity of the AuBT dataset is followed by AMIGOS, with four adoptions from 2018 to 2020. Third place goes to DREAMER, with two adoptions in 2020 and 2019. SWELL was published in 2014, but the adoption of the dataset is only found in two papers from 2020. The other three mentions are DECAF, MANHOB-HCI, and WESAD. All three have one adoption and citation in other research studies. Other datasets such as ASCERTAIN, CASE, and CLASS are not found in any other studies by far. Many of the works reviewed used their own collected data.

Table 2. Affective datasets available with the inclusion of the ECG modality.

Dataset	Stimuli	Data Size (Participants × Samples)	Physiological Modalities	ECG Device	ECG LEAD	Sampling Rate	Emotional Annotations	Emotional Model	Annotation Perspectives
AMIGOS [55]	51–150 s videos	40 × 16	ECG, EEG, GSR	Shimmer	RA-LL (Lead 2), LA-LL (Lead 3)	256 Hz	Valence, Arousal, and Dominance	ADM	Self and 3rd person
ASCERTAIN [56]	51–128 s videos	58 × 36	ECG, EEG, GSR	NA	2 Leads	256 Hz	Valence and Arousal	ADM	Self
AuBT [66]	2 min of music listening	1 × 100	ECG, EMG, RSP, SC	NA	1 Lead	256 Hz	Joy, Anger, Sadness, and Pleasure	DEM	Self
CASE [67]	<3 min videos	30 × 20 (real time)	ECG, BVP, EMG, GSR (EDA)	Thought Technology	RA-LA (Lead 1), RA-LL (Lead 2), LA-LL (Lead 3)	1000 Hz	Valence and Arousal	ADM	Self
CLAS [68]	16 video and 16 IAPS pictures	62 × 32	ECG, PPG, EDA	Shimmer3	RA-LA (Lead 1)	256 Hz	Valance and Arousal	ADM	Self
DECAF [57]	1 min music videos and ~ 80 s movie clips	30 × 76	ECG, EMG, EOG, MEG	NA	RA-LA (Lead 1)	1 KHz downsampled to 256 Hz	Valence, Arousal, and Dominance	ADM	Self
DREAMER [58]	65–393 s film clips	23 × 18	ECG, EEG	Shimmer ECG	RA-LL (Lead 2), LA-LL (Lead 3)	256 Hz	Valence, Arousal, and Dominance	ADM	Self
DSDRWDT [52]	50–90 min of driving	24	ECG, EMG, SC, RSP	FlexComp	RA-LL (Lead 2)	496 Hz	Low, Medium, and High Stress	Pos/Neg	Self
EMDC [69]	3–5 min of music listening	3 × 360	ECG, EMG, SC, RSP	Procomp2 Infiniti	3 Leads	256 Hz	Valance and Arousal	ADM	Self
K-EmoCon [51]	10 min naturalistic conversations	32 (real time)	ECG, EEG, BVP, EDA, SKT	Polar H7		1 Hz	Valence and Arousal	ADM	Self, 2nd and 3rd person
MANHOB-HCI [59]	35–117 s videos	27 × 20	ECG, EEG, GSR, EDA, RSP, SKT	Biosemi Active II	3 Leads	1024 Hz downsampled to 256 Hz	Valence, Arousal, and Dominance	ADM	Self
MPED [31]	<5 min videos	23 × 28	ECG, EEG, GSR, RSP	Biopac System	3 Leads	250 Hz	Joy, Funny, Anger, Fear, Disgust, Sad, and Neutral	DEM	Self
SWELL [70]	Writing, presenting, reading, and searching	25 × 3	ECG, SC	Mobi device (TMSi)	3 leads	2048 Hz	Valance, Arousal, and Stress	ADM and Pos/Neg	Self
WESAD [71]	Video clips, and public speaking and mental arithmetic tasks	15	ECG, BVP, EDA, EMG, RSP, TEMP	RespiBAN Professional	3 Leads	700 Hz	Neutral, Stress, and Amusement	Pos/Neg	Self

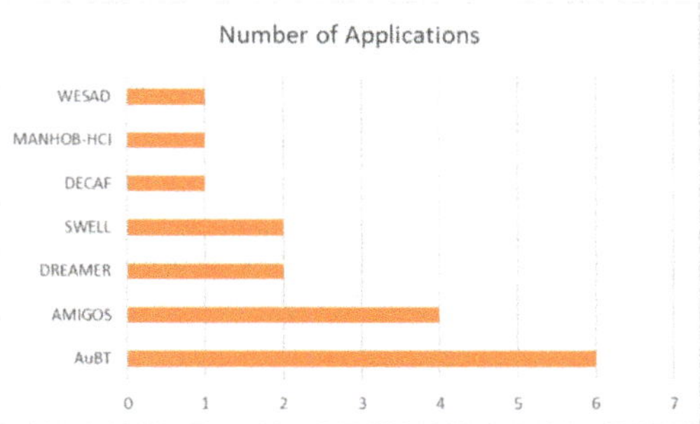

Figure 8. The number of times datasets were applied in different research studies found in the summarized literature.

5. Development of Emotion Recognition Systems

There are several steps in developing emotion recognition systems. This work focuses on the development of emotion recognition systems using machine learning techniques. The first step is pre-processing, which is to clean the signal from unwanted noises. Next is feature extraction using various techniques. The usage of feature selection as well as feature reduction to find the relevant emotion-related features is optional and can be included after feature extraction. The last step is classification and validation techniques using machine learning algorithms. The common adopted pipeline of emotion recognition models is presented in Figure 9.

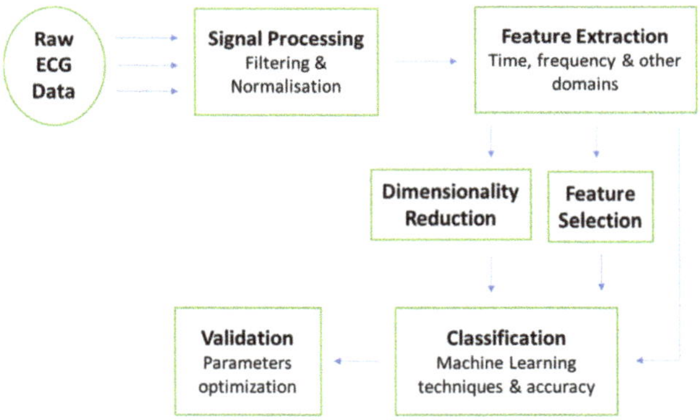

Figure 9. General methods for an ECG-based emotion recognition system using machine learning.

5.1. Pre-Processing

An ECG signal is considered as a high-sensitivity physiological signal with a low recording voltage between 0.5 and 5 mV [72]. Generally, the signal is susceptible to noise and corruption due to various internal and external factors depending on the method of application. The main sources of ECG noise are power line interference, muscle movements, electrode–skin contact, motion artifacts, baseline wander, electronic and electromagnetic device interference, external electrical system interference, internal high-frequency noise, and respiration or bowel sounds. The common frequency for muscle movements is 5–50 Hz, 0.12–0.5 Hz (at 8–30 beats per minute) for respiratory, 50/60 Hz on AC electrical systems, and >10 Hz on other electrical and electronic devices [73]. Although there is a wide variety of ECG filters, the applications depend on specific needs to denoise and reduce the amount of information complexity towards a desired level.

The multiple-configuration Butterworth filter is the most widely used filter based on the summarized papers. In [47,74], a low-pass Butterworth filter with a 60 Hz cut-off frequency was applied to remove a higher background noise of ECG signals. A 0.05–100 Hz Butterworth bandpass filter was used in [69] to remove noise, while a 49–51 Hz band-stop Butterworth filter was used in [75] for power line interference at 50 Hz. According to [72], although the bandpass filter may remove most of the stated noises, solely depending on it is discouraged as the result might not be the best. A fourth-order Butterworth filter with a 100 Hz cut-off frequency [76] and a sixth-order Butterworth filter with a 45 Hz cut-off frequency [40] were used to remove high-frequency noise and powerline interference. The lowest order of the Butterworth filter works best in the time domain, while in the frequency domain, a higher order is better.

In removing a high-frequency interference, [75] applied a 1–60 Hz bandpass filter, while [77] used a 5–15 Hz bandpass filter. In [24], an interpolation filter was utilized to remove signals of 30 Hz and below. A notch filter or a band-stop filter was applied in [20,78] at 50 Hz. A second-order infinite impulse response (IIR) notch filter was used to eliminate powerline noise and motion artifacts in [47]. A fourth-order notch filter at 50 Hz was used in [76] to eliminate power line interference, as suggested by [79].

The most common frequencies in ECG signals that should be preserved for further processing and feature extraction are 0.67–5 Hz (at 40–300 bpm) for detecting the HR and P wave. The QRS complex can be detected within 10 to 50 Hz, and the T wave at 1–7 Hz. A high-frequency potential may also be considered at 100–500 Hz [73]. To determine which filter is best to be used, the frequency setting and calibration pulse should always be informed first so that the ECG signal can be interpreted accurately.

5.2. Feature Extraction

ECG feature extraction has different approaches depending on the way raw signal calculations can be manipulated into meaningful information. This section begins with the most basic ECG signal processing through PQRST detection and the extraction of statistical features. Next, feature extraction for the HR and within beat (WIB) features is explained. The third part summarizes HRV and IBI as the most used features from ECG modalities to detect human emotions through ANS activity within the heart. The last part summarizes other feature extraction techniques used throughout the literature reviewed.

5.2.1. PQRST Detection and Statistical Features

The most basic features to be extracted from ECG signals are the PQRST points' allocations. Between the P wave, QRS complex and T wave, the QRS complex was considered important in defining the HR and HRV through IBI calculation [55,80]. The Pan–Tompkins QRS detection algorithm [81] is considered as the most common technique to find the R peak location [58,67,69]. In [39,40], the QRS complex was derived by applying a nonlinear transformation on the first derivative (Gaussian first-order differentiator) of the filtered ECG signal [82,83]. Continuous wavelet transforms (CWT) are applied to detect a precise R location and then the QS, P, and T waves [84]. Finally, in [83], a built-in R peak detection was embedded in Acknowkedge3.8.2 application software, and there is no need for the researcher to manually extract the features.

Based on PQRST detection, individual statistical features can also be extracted [58,66,85,86]. The statistical features extracted include mean, median (med), standard deviation (std) and quartile deviation, minimum (min), maximum (max), and range (max-min) of individual P, Q, R, S, and T. The authors of [84] extracted only the amplitude of P, R, and S, before proceeding to analyzing the other features.

5.2.2. HR and WIB Features

HR is measured in beats per minute (bpm). Considering that one cycle or one beat can be measured between two successive R peaks, the HR can be derived simply through averaging the overall signals collected through a period. The HR is proven to show distinct feature changes [87] and has been used in various ECG-based affective studies [6,24,39,51,53,55–57,67,71,75,78,85,88]. The benefits of HR over other features are the simplicity of the calculation and not requiring a highly accurate measurement. Even during an intensive exercise, the measurement of the HR is still reliable.

WIB features were proposed by [24], which calculate the statistical values of ECG intervals. Mean, med, max, min, and standard deviation are calculated from PR, ST, and QRS intervals [26]. Instead, in [58,66,85,86], PQ, QS, and ST intervals were used to calculate the statistical features stated, with an addition to the range. QRS morphologies were extracted in [89] based on clinical application. The morphology features are *qrsWBR* (width between R peaks and the next Q), *qrsWRE* (width between S and R peaks), *qrsABR* (difference between amplitude of R peaks and the next Q), *qrsARE* (difference between amplitude of R peaks and the consequential S), and *qrsMOR* (the shape of the QRS interval).

5.2.3. HRV and IBI Features

HRV measures specific changes between heart beats in the time domain. The time between beats is measured in milliseconds (ms) and is called an RR interval or IBI. The variation in IBI values contributes to the readings of HRV. HRV features are claimed to be one of the most used methods in ECG-based emotion recognition systems [69,90]. HRV is also known to have distinct changes in emotion variations [87] and used as an indication of stress and mental effort in healthy adults [69]. Moreover, HRV is the most precise non-invasive physiological technique in measuring the activity of the ANS throughout the body. The widely available and affordable consumer-grade ECG devices that can record a significantly good signal are sufficient for HRV feature extraction.

Out of the 51 studies summarized, 31 of them used HRV, with a slight common variation. However, in general, there are three domains of HRV feature analysis: time domain, frequency domain, and time–frequency domain. A detailed explanation of each domain is presented below:

- **Time domain** [26,91,92] (**Temporal** [15]): This measures the amount of variability in IBI, where the expression comes in the form of a natural logarithm (Ln) of original units, or the original units themselves, for a more normally distributed formation. There are short-term indices for recordings around minutes in length, and long-term indices which usually record over a period of 24 h. The first feature matrix is the standard deviation of the normal-to-normal interval (SDNN). This feature is represented in the unit of milliseconds (ms) for a standard short-term recording of 5 min [93], and 60 to 240 s for ultra-short term recordings [94,95]. SDNN changes also correlate with SNS and PNS activity in the heart. Next, the standard deviation of RR peaks (SDRR) is very similar to the previous case, but it includes false and abnormal beats measured at R peaks. NN50 and pNN50 are the number of adjacent normal-to-normal intervals and percentage of them that are more than 50 ms. These features are known to accommodate PNS activity in the heart [96]. Other variations are NN20 and pNN20, respectively. Next, the root mean square of successive differences (RMSSD) is an index of IBI variance in the HR. Finally, the HRV Triangular Index (TriInd) feature is usually combined with RMSSD to detect pathological cardiac complications, and triangular interpolation of a normal-to-normal interval histogram (TINN) is used as a histogram baseline for a normal-to-normal interval.
- **Frequency domain** [26,91,92] (**Spectral** [15]): This measures the amount of power at various frequencies using fast Fourier transformation (FFT). The amplitude of FFT can then be derived into a power spectral density (PSD). In spectrogram analysis, there is a range of feature levels available such as ultra-low frequency (ULF), very-low frequency (VLF), low frequency (LF) and high frequency (HF), as shown in Figure 10. However, in the emotion recognition system, ULF and VLF are not utilized as both need at least 24 h of ECG recording, which is not practical for emotion recognition. VLF, LF, and HF bands have a window range from 0.0033 to 0.04 Hz, 0.04 to 0.15 Hz, and 0.15 to 0.40 Hz. All three correlate with SNS and PNS activity changes. In fact, a low HF power reflects negative emotions such as anxiety, worrying, stress, and panic. Based on the bands, there are also variations of the normalized LF and HF, the LF/HF

ratio, and the total spectral power. Other statistical features that have been extracted from the frequency bands are spectral centroids, spread, kurtosis, skewness, slope, variation, decrease, roll-on/off, and total energy.

- **Nonlinear domain** [15,91] (**Geometrical** [15,26]): This measures the nonlinearity of time series of the unpredictability of the HRV complexity mechanism. The features are extracted from Poincare geometric plots and allow a refined pattern detection through a scatter plot. The parameters are the area of the total HRV eclipse (S), each point, the standard deviation from both axes (SD1), the standard deviation of each point from both axes plus the RR interval (SD2), and SD1/SD2. The feature variation includes SD12, Area0, Area1, Area2, Area3, and Area4.

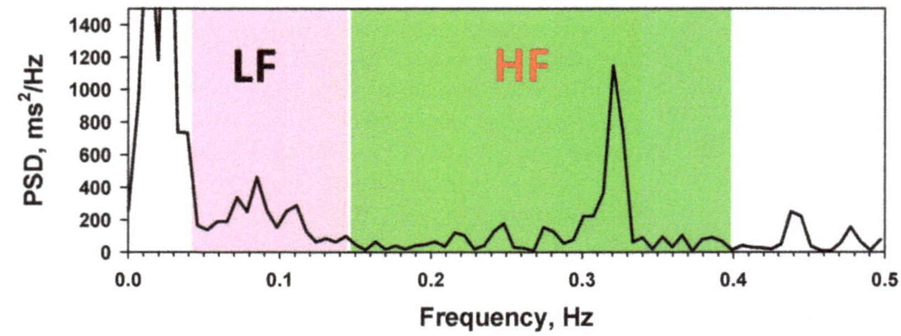

Figure 10. Power spectral density (PSD) features [97].

5.2.4. Empirical Mode Decomposition, Wavelet Transform, and Fourier Transform

Empirical mode decomposition (EMD), also known as the Hilbert–Huang transform (HHT), is a technique to transform signals into parts called intrinsic mode functions (IMF) [98]. This technique is suitable for nonlinear and nonstationary signals such as those from an ECG. With the IMF characteristic, the instantaneous frequency and amplitude of the signal can be defined. Moreover, the HHT also preserves the characteristic of frequency changes as the lengths of original signal and IMF are the same. The application of EMD for ECG feature extraction techniques to emotion recognition systems is seen in a few papers such as [21,26,54,76,99,100]. In [54], 35 features were extracted from IMF1 and IMF2. The features consist of statistical features such as mean, max, standard deviation, variance, skewness, kurtosis, and others.

The wavelet transform is a technique for multiresolution analysis [101] and divided into two forms. The continuous wavelet transform (CWT) has the capability of extracting features from the signal with the determination of extremum points and inflection points, while the discrete wavelet transform (DWT) can extract statistical and stochastic characteristics, and the energy spectrum. In general, the wavelet transform decomposes data into different frequency and time scales using a mathematical transformation function. The computing process involves dilation and translation of functions, or multiscale refinement of signals. The wavelet transform is also known to be able to solve difficult problems that Fourier transforms are not capable of [102]. In [84,101], the CWT is used to perform the feature extraction on ECG signals, while [89,103] applied the DWT in their framework process.

The Fourier transform is another technique for decomposing functions that are dependent on the time of space into functions that are dependent on the temporal or spatial frequency. The two common Fourier transforms in emotion recognition studies are the discrete Fourier transform (DFT) and the FFT. They are almost identical methods, with the FFT being a more efficient function, where the computation performs faster than the DFT. Again, in [76], the authors combined EMD and the DFT as IMF alone does not contain much information to provide any distinctive features. Another adoption of the DFT is also found in [26], where the application of feature extraction is paired with EMD and other methods. Finally, application of the FFT is only seen in one paper [69], where the features were derived from a partitioned coefficient within the frequency range into overlapping sub-bands with the same bandwidth. From that, the sub-band spectral entropy (SSE) is computed to identify the disorganization or uncertainty in a random variable. This helps the pattern recognition by scaling the intensity of a classifier's confidence.

5.2.5. Others

There are some independent feature extraction techniques based on ECG signals used for emotion recognition systems. Various novel approaches have been proposed to perform the task with the aim of extracting useful feature information that is relevant to the ANS activity of the heart. The prospective approach has been taken, from the mathematical process derivation function to pictorial plotting and statistical feature analysis.

Detrended fluctuation analysis (DFA) and detrended cross-correlation analysis (DCCA) were applied in [104]. Features from the multifractal spectra were also extracted in that paper. DFA is categorized under nonlinear feature analysis, and the work in [105] also applied this method along with Poincare plot feature extraction from HRV.

In [20], Coiflets wavelets (Coif5) at level 14, the discrete cosine transform (DCT), and Daubechies wavelet (db4) at level 8 were applied before using matching pursuit coefficients for feature extraction. The features extracted were statistical such as mean, variance, standard deviation, minimum, and maximum.

Instead of using the numerical values of ECG signals to extract the features, a graphical plot and image pattern recognition were applied in [47]. The methods used were the local binary pattern (LBP) and the local ternary pattern (LTP). The LBP is widely used in computer vision and image processing research, particularly in facial recognition. The LTP is the modification of the LBP by changing it from a binary operation of 1-0 to three operations of -1-0-1. The operation depends on the frame length and frame shift to extract the features.

Another method that has been reported is feature extraction through the Nonlinear Autoregressive Integrative (NARI) Point-Process Model [106]. The analysis of heartbeat dynamics started from detecting RR peaks, and following the Wiener–Voterra representation, a specific point process model was created for instantaneous identification up to the third order. The features are extracted from Lyapunov exponents as well as instantaneous spectra, and spectra. This evaluation is also known to be in the realm of high-order statistics (HOS).

A nonlinear approach based on Hurst was proposed in [40] by using rescaled statistics (RRS) and finite variance scaling (FVS). The new Hurst features are combined into HOS to be classified into six basic emotional states. The value of Hurst can also be obtained by EMD, the wavelet transform, and finite variance scaling. Before applying the feature extraction procedure, the QRS complex is extracted for further computation of RRS and FVS. In this process, six features are extracted from each sample in the study.

Other ECG feature extraction methods found in the reviewed works are the multivariant correlation method and spectrograms. In [107], the authors applied a linear multivariate approach for their feature function analysis. Meanwhile, in [108], the author extracted the features using deep learning by converting time series data to frequency domain-based images. Based on the images, only the 0–5 Hz range was converted into a spectrogram, and the data were fed into a VGG-16 network. Finally, 4096 features were extracted and studied.

5.3. Feature Selection and Dimensionality Reduction

Extracted features do not promise fully relevant correlations with physiological changes in emotion regulation. Feature selection is a method to optimize the classification architecture by only picking the best feature combinations and eliminating noninformative features. This can also reduce the computational cost of the classification in the later step. In [26], recursive feature elimination, the chi-square test, the P test, random forest feature selection (RF FS), extra tree feature selection, and random support vector machine feature selection were used. Moreover, swarm intelligence is also common in the feature selection process. The author of [74] applied the genetic algorithm, while ant colony optimization was used in [104]. Binary particle swarm optimization (BPSO) and hybrid particle swarm optimization (HPSO) have also been applied for feature selection [84]. The wrapper method and the Tabu search algorithm are found in [77] and [103]. In [109], the author used Kullback–Leibler divergence as a feature selection. Other common techniques are sequential forward selection (SFS) and sequential backward selection (SBS), which have been applied in [86,87,110].

Dimensionality reduction is a technique to reduce the number of features by transforming a higher dimension feature matrix into a lower dimension without losing the necessary information. The two most used techniques were principal component analysis (PCA) and linear discriminant analysis (LDA). The transformation of PCA is unsupervised, while LDA is supervised. The applications of PCA were viewed in [20,55,67,85,89,108,111]. LDA, also known as Fisher's linear discriminant analysis, was used in [20,24,53,87] as a dimension reduction procedure.

The applications of feature selection and dimensionality reduction techniques stated are reported to be beneficial in terms of improving the training and testing accuracy for emotion recognition systems. Moreover, the time taken to perform the classification is reduced significantly as less data need to be processed at a time. Finally, the chance to overfit the trained model is reduced, as the noisy data are eliminated from the final data fed to the classifier.

5.4. Classification

Classification techniques are divided into two main categories which are machine learning and deep learning. Commonly, if deep learning is adopted in physiological-based emotion recognition, there are no feature extraction and feature selection steps. If the deep learning architecture has a convolutional layer, it might somehow be considered as a dimensionality reduction stage.

Machine learning methods are divided into three learning categories which are supervised learning, unsupervised learning, and hybrid learning. In affective computing, the majority of the research adopted supervised learning through emotion labels such as ADM, DEM, and Pos/Neg through SAM. However, there is one work that used unsupervised learning, which is [112]. The ECG signals were unlabeled, and the convolutional neural networks (CNN) were trained to find any signal transformation for emotional patterns. Then, the weights were passed on to the labeled data for testing. The accuracy shows a significantly better result than most of the supervised learning techniques.

A classifier that has been frequently adopted and performed the best in emotion recognition systems is the support vector machine (SVM) [15]. From 24 out of the 51 studies summarized here (presented in the following section), SVM was adopted as either the only classifier or one of the machine learning algorithms to be compared. SVM kernels are simply the methods or behavior of making the hyperplane decision boundaries work in certain manners. In [89], SVM constantly performed better than random forest through every ratio of generated emotional data in the training set.

Although SVM is popular, it is not always the best classifier, as reported in several works. Other well-performing classifiers used are k-nearest neighbour (KNN) and naïve Bayes (NB). KNN was reported to perform better than SVM in [39,77]. Meanwhile, [56] showed that NB performed better than SVM in both valence and arousal classification using a single ECG modality. Classifiers that were also reviewed are decision tree (DT), random forest (RF), AdaBoost (AB), gradient boost (GB), quadratic classifier (QDA), and LDA. For less known classifiers such as extra tree, regression tree, and ensemble bag tree, their performance was reported to be considerably good in [26] when compared to RF and GB.

Neural network-based deep learning classifiers come in different forms and configurations. Based on the literature, there are a lot of neural network (NN) infrastructures such as 1-NN, deep convolution neural network (DCNN), probabilistic neural network (PNN), backpropagation neural network (BPNN), radial basis function neural network (RBFNN), multilayer perceptron (MLP), and extreme learning machine. Extreme learning machines alone were shown to improve the training accuracy of many databases [108]. DCNN also showed classification accuracy of the AMIGOS dataset in [113] for valence and arousal. The best accuracy was shown in [20] using PNN to classify five-class and three-class DEMs. However, the study was subjected to a credibility request as the result might be biased by overfitting.

5.5. Validation

Validation is a crucial step in building a machine learning model, especially when dealing with a subjective application such as emotion recognition. This step is designed to see the overall performance of the trained models when it comes to new data. The partitioning between training and testing datasets is to ensure the model can perform a validation step by imitating real-world scenarios outside of the experiment setup [15]. The generalization ability of validation allows the model to increase variability and reduce overfitting. The most common validation techniques are called cross-validation (CV) with different versions of approaches.

Non-exhaustive cross-validation of k-CV is a resampling procedure conducted with k number of folds to reshuffle and train the limited data sample, with 5 and 10 being the standard number of k when it comes to the number of folds in k-CV. When k is bigger than that, the subjected models are considered biased. The 5-fold CV was practiced in [54,74], while a rare 15-fold CV was only conducted in [54]. Moreover, 10-fold CV is the most widely practiced cross-validation technique, with 12 papers in total [6,26,39,47,53–55,88,99,112,114,115].

Exhaustive cross-validation techniques have two main variations. The first is leave-one-out cross-validation (LOOCV), where the models are tested and validated from end to end without leaving one participant or subject as a final validation. This method takes more time than leave-one-subject/participant-out cross-validation (LOSOCV/LpO CV). The main advantage of exhaustive CV over non-exhaustive CV is the lower bias as it trains the possible validation combination across all datasets. However, considering a large amount of computational work, the validation process takes a significantly longer time to complete. LOOCV was applied in [55,56,68,69,77,106,109,116], while LOSOCV was adopted in [71,105,110].

6. Review of ECG-Based Emotion Recognition Systems

The 51 reviewed works are summarized in Tables 3 and 4. Table 3 summarizes 31 studies on combinations of unimodal and multimodal ECG-based affective research that reported on ECG standalone results. Meanwhile, Table 4 summarizes 20 affective research studies that included ECG as one of their physiological modalities but did not mention the classification accuracy of using solely ECG as the input. In this section, the works that achieved more than 90% accuracy are highlighted.

Table 3. Research that only uses ECG as a unimodal approach or a multimodal physiological approach, with ECG standalone accuracy results included.

Source	Dataset	Modalities	ECG Pre-processing	ECG Extracted Features	Features Selection	Selected Features	Classifier	Validation	Accuracy
[20]	Own: 11 subjects, 56 music listening DEM (happiness, sadness, peacefulness, scary, neutral) and ADM (valence, arousal)	ECG, GSR	Digital notch filter at 50 Hz	Matching pursuit. Min, mean, max, var, std of Coif5 at level 14, db4 at level 8, DCT	LDA, PCA, Kernel-PCA	NA	PNN	NA	Subject-dependent and subject-independent using PCA: 100%
[21]	Own: 44 subjects, 5 images ADM (valence, active/passive arousal)	ECG	NA	EMD (bivariate extension of EMD), Hilbert–Huang Transform, local oscillation in every mode	NA	NA	LDA	NA	up to 89%
[24]	Own: 12 subjects, 60 samples each DEM (anger, fear, sadness, disgust, joy, neutral)	ECG	Interpolation filters remove 30 Hz and below	- IBI - WIB	Least Significant Difference—ANOVA	36 features: 11-feature approach and 3-feature approach	LDA, Adaptable KNN	NA	11-feature approach 37.23% 3-feature approach 61.44%
[26]	Own: 25 subjects, 488 samples DEM (anger, sadness, joy, pleasure)	ECG	Butterworth bandpass filter 0.05–100 Hz	- PQRST, HRV: sdnn, mn_nn, rmssd, m_nn, nn50, pnn50, hf, hfnu, lf_hf, lfnu, total_power, vlf, sd1, sd2 - WIB: PR, ST, QRS min, max, std, mean, med - EMD: spectral power of IMF in time and frequency domain, instantaneous frequency of IMF, spectral power of instantaneous frequency of IMF - TFB (ten-frequency band)	Recursive Feature Elimination, Chi-Square Test, P test, RF FS, Extra Tree FS, Random SVM FS	- EMD: spec_2, spec_4 - HRV: sdnn, mn_nn, m_nn - WIB: median_pr, max_pr, sd_pr, mean_qrs, max_qrs, min_qrs - TFB: band_2, band_3, band_5, band_7, band_10	RF, Extra Tree, Gradient Boost, AB SVM, AB DT, AB Naïve Bayes	10-fold CV	80% extra tree classifier and feature selection 79.23% RF classifier and extra tree feature selection 72.66% gradient boost classifier and RF FS
[39]	Own: 5 subjects, 15 video clips (Pos, Neg, Neutral)	ECG	Elliptic bandpass filter, DWT	Time domain: HR, MRAmp, MRRI	NA	NA	KNN, SVM	10-fold CV	Pos/Neg Neutral KNN: 66.49% 60:40 train/test, 66.22% 70:30 train/test, 67.54% 80:20 train/test Pos/Neg KNN: 74.67% 60:40 train/test, 77.69% 70:30 train/test, 77.42% 80:20 train/test Pos/Neg SVM: 64.98% 60:40 train/test, 65.52% 70:30 train/test, 66.04% 80:20 train/test
[40]	Own: 60 subjects, 60 samples DEM (happiness, sadness, fear, surprise, disgust, anger)	ECG	Baseline wander removed using wavelet-based algorithm, 6th-order Butterworth filter with 45 Hz cut-off	Nonlinear features "Hurst" using RRS and FVS from QRS. Combined HOS: Hurst, skewness based on Hurst, kurtosis based on Hurst	NA	NA	Bayesian classifier, Regression tree, KNN, Fuzzy KNN	Random validation, Subject-independent validation	Fuzzy KNN 6 Class: 92.87% RRS, 76.45% FVS
[47]	Own: 8 subjects DEM (joy, anger, sadness) + AuBT	ECG	2nd-order IIR notch filter, Butterworth low-pass filter with 60 Hz cut-off frequency	LBP, LTP: 3 s, 5 s, 10 s, 15 s frame length, and 1.5 s, 2.5 s, 5 s, 7.5 s frame shift	NA	NA	KNN	10-fold CV	LBP 84.17%, LTP 87.92%
[55]	AMIGOS	ECG, EEG, GSR	NA	Root mean square of IBI, mean IBI, 60 spectral power, LF, MF, HF of HRV spectral power, HR, HRV statistics: mean, std, skewness, kurtosis, % of time the future value above/below mean ± std	PCA	NA	Linear SVM	10-fold CV, LOOCV	Short video scenario: 53.5% V, 55.0% A Long video scenario: 55.0% V, 54.3% A Both: 54.5% V, 55.1% A

Table 3. *Cont.*

Source	Dataset	Modalities	ECG Pre-processing	ECG Extracted Features	Features Selection	Selected Features	Classifier	Validation	Accuracy
[56]	ASCERTAIN	ECG, EEG, GSR	NA	10 low-frequency PSD, 4 very slow response PSD, IBI, HR, HRV statistics: mean, std, skewness, kurtosis, % of time the future value above/below mean ± std	NA	NA	Linear SVM, NB	LOOCV	SVM: 56% V, 57% A NB: 60% V, 59% A
[58]	DREAMER	ECG, EEG	No pre-processing	- PQRST features: mean, med, std, min, max, range - HRV: RMMSD, PSD LF, PSD HF, LF/HF, total power	NA	NA	RBF SVM	NA	62.37% V, 62.37% A
[71]	WESAD	ECG, BVP, EDA, EMG, RSP, TEMP	NA	- HR, HRV: mean, std - HRV: NN50, pNN50, TINN, RMS, ULF, LF, HF, ULF, LF/HF, fULF-HF, relative power, normalized LF, normalized HF	NA	NA	DT, RF, AB, LDA, KNN	LOSO CV	3 Class: DT 57.81%, RF 60.36%, AB 61.71%, LDA 66.29%, KNN 54.76% Pos/Neg: DT 80.17%, RF 82.78%, AB 83.37%, LDA 85.44%, KNN 79.19%
[74]	Own: 16 subjects, 96 samples ADM (valence, arousal)	ECG	Butterworth low pass filter	HRV	Genetic Algorithm	NA	SVM	5-fold CV	ADM: 72.9% 89.6% V, 82.3% A
[75]	Own: 6 subjects, 36 film clips (Pos, Neg, Neutral)	ECG, EEG, RSP	Remove baseline drift, 1–60 Hz bandpass filter, 49–51 Hz band-stop Butterworth filter	HR, HR stability (HRstd), power (Hpow)	NA	NA	Linear SVM	NA	Pos/Neg, Neutral: HR 69.0%, HRstd 84.2%, Hpow 70.4%
[76]	Own: 30 subjects, 60 video clips DEM (happiness, sadness, fear, surprise, disgust, neutral)	ECG	4th-order notch filter at 50 Hz, 4th-order Butterworth filter 100 Hz cut-off, digital high-pass filters	EMD combined with Hilbert transform, EMD combined with DFT	NA	NA	LDA, KNN	NA	KNN: 52%
[77]	Own: 34 subjects, Pos/Neg (stress, no stress)	ECG, EDA, ST	5–15 Hz bandpass filter	HRV time and freq domains: mRR, medRR, mHR, SDRR, RMSSD, RR50, pRR50, LF, HF, LF/HF	Wrapper method	HRV: mRR, medRR, mHR, SDRR, RMSSD, RR50, LF, HF, LF/HF	LDA, QDA, SVM, KNN	LOOCV	KNN: 88.03%
[84]	Own: 391 subjects, 10 film clips (joy, sadness)	ECG	35 Hz low-pass filter and 50 Hz power source notch filter	CWT, 79 features: mean, std, med, min, max, range of intervals. P, R, S amp, HRV, and PSD	BPSO, HPSO	20, 16: Most selected: max R, range R, mean R, med R, range QS, std PQ, std S, mean QS, std QS, med P	Fisher classifier	Run 40 times	Joy: 84.45%, Sadness: 88.43%
[86]	AuBT DEM (only joy and pleasure data)	ECG	NA	81 features of HR and HRV	ANOVA: 44 features, SFS: 37 features, SBS: 3 features	R-range, Rampl-std, HRV-max, HRV-range, HRVDistr-range	SVM, LDA, Fisher's linear discriminant	NA	SVM + SFS-SBS-ANOVA: 92%
[89]	DECAF	ECG	Butterworth filter	HR, DWT, QRS morphology: qrsWBR, qrsWRE, qrsABR, qrsARE, qrsMOR	NA	NA	SVM, RF	NA	63.4% RF 64.5% SVM
[99]	AuBT	ECG, EMG, SC, RSP	Adaptive low-pass filter	HHT (EMD and Hilbert transform) fission and fusion	NA	4, 8, 12, 16 IMF features	SVM	10-fold CV	Fission 69%, Fusion 56%
[101]	AuBT	ECG, EMG, RSP, SC	NA	16 features of CWT Morlet wavelet coefficients	NA	NA	SVM	NA	75%
[102]	AuBT	ECG	NA	Wavelet transform: max and std of multiscale wavelet coefficients	NA	NA	BPNN, RBFNN	NA	BPNN: 87.5%, RBFNN 91.67%
[103]	Own: 391 subjects, 10 film clips DEM (joy, sadness)	ECG	NA	DWT, 79 features	Tabu Search Algorithm	23, 12: Most selected: std S, max R, std QS, range R, mean S, med R, med S, std R, min R, min S, PNN50 HRV, LF HRV	KNN, Fisher-KNN	Run 9 times	KNN: 75.85%, Fisher-KNN: 85.78%

Table 3. *Cont.*

Source	Dataset	Modalities	ECG Pre-processing	ECG Extracted Features	Features Selection	Selected Features	Classifier	Validation	Accuracy
[104]	Own: 20 subjects, 400 samples DEM (happy, sad, pleasant, angry)	ECG	NA	- Statistical features of time and frequency domain: max, min, mean, std, rmean, rrstd, energy, ratio - DFA: α, $\alpha 1$, $\alpha 2$ - Multifractal Features: $\alpha 0$, $\Delta\alpha$ - DCCA: ρDCCAh, ρDCCAm, ρDCCAl	Max–Min Ant System, Ant Colony Optimization	NA	KNN, SVM, DT	CV	Best Classifier: KNN 4 Class: 92% Happy 91% Sad 92% Pleasant 88% Angry 97%
[106]	Own: 30 subjects, 110 samples DEM (sadness, anger, happiness, relaxation) and ADM (valence, arousal)	ECG	Artifact removal and filtering	Instantaneous Spectrum and Bispectrum, Dominant Lyapunov Exponent	NA	NA	SVM	LOOCV	4 Class: 79.29% V/A: 79.15%, 83.55%
[108]	AMIGOS, DEAP, DREAMER, MANHOB-HCI	ECG, EEG, GSR, EDA, RSP, SKT, etc.	Moving average filter with 0.25 s window length	HRV: pNN50 Spectrogram: 4096 features	PCA	30 features	Extreme learning machine	NA	V/A (Individual): DEAP 70.86%, 71.09%; AMIGOS 81.89%, 82.74%; MANHOB-HCI 78.76%, 78.76%; DREAMER 80.43%, 80.68% (Combined): DEAP and AMIGOS 59.69%, 63.61%; DEAP, AMIGOS, and MANHOB-HCI 58.57%, 61.84% (Transfer Learning): Train (DEAP and AMIGOS) Test (MANHOB-HCI) 64.77%, 62.50%; Train (DEAP) Test MANHOB-HCI 63.59%, 61.46%
[111]	Own: 25 subjects, 50 samples each Pos/Neg and DEM (sad, angry, fear, happy, relax)	ECG	NA	- HRV: Time Domain (Mean RRI, CVRR, SDRR, SDSD) - Frequency Domain (LF, HF, LH ratio) - Statistic Analysis (Kurtosis coefficient, Skewness, Entropy) - Parameters of Poincare Plot (SD12, SD22, SD2SD1ratio)	PCA	Selected 5 from 13. CVRR, LF, HF, HF ratio, SD1	SVM	NA	Pos/Neg: 71.4% 5 Class: 56.9%
[112]	AMIGOS, DREAMER, WESAD, SWELL	ECG	High-pass IIR filter with bandpass of 0.8 Hz. Z-score normalization	High-level spatiotemporal features	NA	NA	Self-Supervised CNN	10-Fold CV	AMIGOS: 87.5% V, 88.9% A; DREAMER: 85.0% V, 85.9% A WESAD: 96.9% Pos/Neg; SWELL: 97.3% V, 96.7% A, 93.3% Stress
[114]	Own: 21 subjects, (Pos, Neg)	ECG, RIP	Tomkins's algorithm	9 features: heartbeat freq low, med, high, ratio low/high; QD, SD, 3.32QD	Correlation-based feature selection	HR power in Bands 1 and 3, mean, med, and 80th percentile of stretch	SVM	10-fold CV	~85%

Table 3. *Cont.*

Source	Dataset	Modalities	ECG Pre-processing	ECG Extracted Features	Features Selection	Selected Features	Classifier	Validation	Accuracy
[113]	AMIGOS	ECG, GSR	Pan–Tompkins QRS detection. 0.5–15 Hz cut-off frequency removal	- IBI time domain: meanNN, medNN, SDNN, rmSSD, pNN50, pNN20, coefVarSD, medADNN, coefVarNN, mCoeffVarNN, Shanon Entropy, HRV triangular, numArtifacts - Freq domain: peakHF, hTotalPowerRatio, normHF, peakLF, lfhfRatio, lfTotalPowerRatio, normLF, totalPower, ulfPeak, vhfPeak, vlfPeak - Nonlinear domain: correlation dimension, entropy, SVD, HF, LF, VLF, Shannon, fractal dimension Higushi and Petrosian, Fisher information	NA	NA	DCNN	NA	71% V, 81% A
[116]	Own: 25 subjects, 3 movies DEM (fear, disgust, neutral)	ECG	Quantization, Normalize Relative Compression Measure	NA	NA	NA	1-NN	Leave-one-out strategy	Fear: 77%, Disgust: 63%, Neutral: 74%
[117]	Own: 26 subjects Pos/Neg (stressed, not stressed)	ECG, RSP	Filtered and normalized	- HRV: var, quartile deviation, low freq energy, med freq energy, high freq energy, low/high freq energy ratio - Non-HRV: mean, med, 80th percentile, 20th percentile - HR	NA	NA	RBF SVM	Cross-subject validation	95% Not stressed, 89% Stressed

Table 4. Multimodal research that includes ECG model but did not perform an independent classification for the signal.

Source	Dataset	Physiological Modalities	ECG Pre-Processing	ECG Extracted Features	Features Selection	Selected Features	Classifier	Validation	Accuracy
[6]	Own: 10 subjects (Pos/Neg)	ECG, EMG, RSP, EDA	Low-pass filters at 100 and 500 Hz	HR, mean amp, mean abs first difference	NA	NA	SVM, adaptive neuro-fuzzy inference system (ANFIS)	10-fold CV	SVM 79.3%, ANFIS 76.7%
[51]	K-EmoCon	ECG, EEG, BVP, EDA, SKT	NA	HR	NA	NA	NA	NA	NA
[52]	Own: 24 subjects, 112 samples (Pos/Neg)	ECG, EMG, SC, RSP	NA	HRV: power spectrum, LF, HF, LF/HF, sympathovagal balance ratio, MF	ANOVA	NAs	Fisher projection matrix, linear discriminant	NA	97%
[53]	Own: 58 subjects DEM (anger, boredom, fear, frustration, happiness) and ADM (valance, arousal)	ECG, EDA, EMG, RSP	Baseline removal, filtering	- HRV/IBI, HR time domain: mean, med, max, min, range, var, std, ave derivative, abs deviation, kurtosis, skewness. - HR freq domain: 3 frequency bands, 4 energy bands	Fisher' linear discriminant	~ 8 selected ECG features out of 173 features	Linear SVM	10-fold CV	V/A: 58.5% 5 class: 63.4%
[54]	Own: 30 subjects, virtual reality DEM (disgust, fear happy, sad)	ECG, PPG	EMD	IMF1, IMF2; 35 features: mean, max, std, min, log energy, var, skewness, kurtosis, rms, crest factor, shape fac, impulse fac, margin fac, energy, med, mean freq, rom of square level, band power occupied bandwidth, change points, power bandwidth, Shannon energy, mad, third-order interception, interquartile range, spurious free dynamic range, peak to rms, snd, thd, total jitter, ave freq, entropy	NA	NA	Ensemble bagged trees	5-fold, 10-fold, 15-fold CV	85.7%
[57]	DECAF	ECG, EMG, EOG, MEG	NA	IBI, HR, HRV, PSD	NA	NA	Linear SVM	NA	60% V, 57% A

Table 4. *Cont.*

Source	Dataset	Physiological Modalities	ECG Pre-Processing	ECG Extracted Features	Features Selection	Selected Features	Classifier	Validation	Accuracy
[59]	MANHOB-HCI	ECG, EEG, GSR, EDA, RSP, SKT	NA	HRV, RMS of MSDFSB, SD, 56 spectral power, LF, MF, HF, HRV PS, Poincare analysis	NA	NA	RBF SVM	NA	(ECG + Peripherals): 45.5% V, 46.2% A
[67]	CASE	ECG, BVP, GSR, RSP, ST, EMG	NA	TEAP, Pan–Tompkins QRS detector: HR, IBI, SDNN	PCA	Mean HR	NA	MANOVA	NA
[68]	CLAS	ECG, PPG, EDA	NA	NA	NA	NA	Polynomial SVM	Leave one out	(ECG + PPG): V/A: ~70%
[69]	Own: 3 subjects, 120 samples ADM (valence, arousal)	ECG, EMG, SC, RSP	NA	FFT, SSE: meanEnergy_SubSpectra, meanHR_HRVtime, power-Low_HRVspec, mean_MSE, mean_SSE, etc.	NA	Valence 71, Arousal 45, 4 Class 77	SBS pLDA, EMDC	LOOCV	EMDC: Subject-dependent average: 95% Subject-independent: 70%
[78]	Own: 20 samples each ADM (valence, arousal)	ECG, EMG, EDA, ST, BVP, RSP	Low-pass filter with 90 Hz, sharp high-pass 0.5 Hz, notch filter 50 Hz	HR, HRV, IBI	NA	NA	NN	NA	89.93% V, 96.58% A
[107]	Own: 101 subjects, 4 video clips DEM (amusement, anger, grief, fear)	ECG, GSR, OXY	0.5 Hz high-pass filter, 35 Hz low-pass filter	Multi-variant correlation methods	NA	NA	RF	NA	74%
[85]	AuBT	ECG, EMG, SC, RSP	Low-pass filter, normalization	HR statistical values	ANOVA, SFS, SBS, PCA	NA	KNN, LDF, MLP	NA	4 Class: LDF-SFS 92.05% V/A: MLP-SFS-Fisher 88.64%, LDF-SFS 96.59%
[88]	Own: 22 subjects Pos/Neg (stress, stress-free)	ECG, EEG	NA	7 features: HR, HRV: VLF, LF, HF, LFnu, HFnu, LF/HF power ratio	Paired t-test, PCA		RBF and sigmoid SVM	10-fold CV	Sigmoid SVM 79.54%, RBF SVM 63.63%
[100]	AuBT	ECG, EMG, SC, RSP	NA	EEMD: Time Domain, Time Frequency Features, Nonlinear Features, IMF	NA	NA	C4.5 DT	NA	Joy 100%, Anger 100%, Sadness 88%, Pleasure 92%

Table 4. *Cont.*

Source	Dataset	Physiological Modalities	ECG Pre-Processing	ECG Extracted Features	Features Selection	Selected Features	Classifier	Validation	Accuracy
[105]	Own: 4 subjects, DEM (excited, happy, calm, tired, bored, sad, stressed, angry)	ECG, PPG, ST	NA	HRVAS Toolbox (HAR, PWTT): IBI, SDNN, RMSSD, pNN50, HRVi, TINN; PDS Welch, Lomb-Scargle periodogram, Autoregression: VLF, LF, HF, normLF, normHF, LF/HF; Nonlinear: sampen, DFA, Poincare plot SD1, SD2, SD1/SD2	NA	NA	KNN, DT, Bagged Ensembled (BE)-DT, Personalized-Baseline, BLD	LO-participant-OCV	Best classifier: BE-DT: Personalized 70.60%, Generalized BE-DT 62.14%
[109]	Own: 15 subjects Pos/Neg (Fear, Normal)	ECG, ST, EDA	NA	HRV time domain: mean, SDNN, RMSSD, NN50, pNN50	Kullback–Leibler Divergence	Mixed	NN, LDA, QDA	LOOCV	NN 92.5%, LDA 81.2%, QDA 85.6%
[110]	Own: 14 subjects, 10 samples DEM (sadness, disgust, fear, happiness, neutral)	ECG, SC, RPS, ST	NA	HRV: - Time domain (SDNN, RMSSD, SDSD, pNN50, pNN20, FF) - Frequency domain (LF, HF, normLF, normHF, LF/HF)	SFFS, SFFS-FP, mRMR, mRMR-FP, ReliefF, ReliefF-FP, IG, IG-FP, OneR, OneR-FP, Chi2, Chi2-FP	NA	KNN, SVM, RF, ML, RIPPER, C4.5 DT, NB	LOSOCV	MLP 60.3%
[115]	Own: 30 subjects DEM (amusement, fear, sad, joy, anger, disgust)	ECG, EEG	NA	HRV	NA	NA	MLP, SVM, Bayesian Network	10-fold CV	Bayesian Network 98.06%
[118]	Own: 47 subjects (Pos/Neg Neutral)	ECG, PPG	NA	- 11 statistical time domain: SDNN, NN50, pNN50, SDSD, RMSSD, SDRR, δx, Nδx, ϒx, Nϒx, STDDRRI, - HRV RRI using STFT (short-time Fourier transform): LF, HF, TP, LF/HF, HF/(LF + HF). - HRV Poincare plot: SD1, SD2, SD12, Area0, Area1, Area2, Area3, Area4	NA	NA	CNN	NA	75.4%

In Table 3, there are seven works that reported more than 90% accuracy in classifying emotions based on varying emotional models. Firstly, Sarkar and Etemad [112] performed a self-supervised emotion recognition study using four datasets which are AMIGOS, DREAMER, WESAD, and SWELL. Based on the raw ECG signals from each dataset, the neural network learned high-level abstract representations, and the weight was transferred to an emotion recognition network. The results show an improved performance compared to fully supervised learning. Although AMIGOS and DREAMER did not manage to pass 90% and above accuracy, WESAD and SWELL were claimed to be successfully classified, with accuracy above 90%. With 96.9% accuracy, the author managed to classify WESAD with the Pos/Neg Model. Moreover, with 97.3%, 96.7%, and 93.3%, the author managed to classify SWELL on a model based on a binary scale of valence, arousal, and stress.

In a study conducted by Zhang et al. [104], the data were labeled according to a DEM with four classes of emotions of happy, sad, pleasant, and angry. The overall accuracy based on the ECG unimodal approach was reported to be 92%. The individual accuracies were 97%, 92%, 91%, and 88% for angry, sad, happy, and pleasant. The best classification results among three classifiers were achieved using KNN from two sets of extracted features. The first feature set consisted of the time and frequency domains, with statistical characteristics of ECG signals, while the second set of features was correlation features. The correlation features were inclusive of the autocorrelation feature parameter, cross-correlation feature, and multifractal feature parameters. The feature selection used was the max–min ant system, which is a derivation of ant colony optimization.

Goshvarpour et al. [20] conducted an emotion recognition study based on ECG and GSR collected from 11 subjects that listen to music as an affective stimulation method. The result analysis was taken from the perspective of performance comparison between ECG and GSR unimodal approaches. Based on the matching pursuit method, three dictionaries were applied for feature extraction on the raw ECG signals, which were Coiflets wavelets (Coif5) at level 14, the discrete cosine transform (DCT), and Daubechies wavelet (db4) at level 8. Three feature selection methods were compared, and PCA was considered as the best one for the application of the study as the recognition rate was constantly 100% for subject-dependent and subject-independent scenarios across the ADM as well as the DEM. The classification was conducted using PNN with a 0.01 sigma value. By far, this paper reports the highest claimed accuracy for a unimodal ECG-based emotion recognition system.

The work by Hovsepian et al. [117], for ECG classification of binary stress and non-stress (Pos/Neg), reported 89% and 95% accuracy, respectively. The classifier used was SVM with RBF kernels trained using HR, HRV, and non-HRV features. The raw ECG signals were filtered and normalized before being extracted. Validation was also conducted between subjects as more than twenty subjects participated in the study.

In a study by Selvaraj et al. [40], six classes of emotions from the ECG unimodal approach were successfully classified with a maximum accuracy of 92.87%. The experiment was conducted on sixty subjects by inducing happiness, sadness, fear, disgust, surprise, and neutral emotions. The features that were extracted from ECG signals were nonlinear features or Hurst features. The features were derived from RRS and FVS. They also proposed a novel Hurst feature by merging RRS and FVS with HOS. The dataset was separated with a ratio of 70:30 for training and testing datasets. Four classifiers were considered: Bayesian classifier, regression tree, KNN, and fuzzy KNN, where the last classifier performed the best.

Xun and Zheng [86] also managed to obtain 92% accuracy in classifying joy and pleasure from the AuBT dataset. They only utilized the ECG signals from the database to perform the study. The ECG features were extracted using AuBT toolboxes, which provided a combination of HR and HRV features. A total of 81 features were extracted, but only 5 final features were selected using a combination of analysis of variance (ANOVA), SFS, and SBS. The final selected features were *R_range*, *ecgRampl-std*, *ecgHrv-max*, *ecgHrv-range*, and *ecgHrvDistr-range*. The classification was conducted using SVM, LDA, and Fisher's linear discriminant analysis with SVM as the best methods.

Guo [102] performed a comparison study between BPNN and RBFNN in classifying emotions using the AuBT dataset. The accuracy result for BPNN was 87.5%, while for RBFNN, it was 91.6%. The ECG features extracted were from the multiscale wavelet decomposition method for the extraction of the maximum value of wavelet coefficients and the standard deviation. The study highlighted that wavelet coefficients that are treated as eigenvectors are able to effectively characterize ECG signals.

Meanwhile, in Table 4, there are seven works that reported more than 90% accuracy in classifying emotions based on varying emotional models and multiple modalities inclusive of ECG. Lee and Yoo [109] collected multimodal physiological signals from ECG, EDA, and SKT from 15 subjects. The highest classification accuracy was found using NN at 92.5%, while 85.6% and 81.2% were found using QDA and LDA. The study also showed that a higher accuracy is expected by applying feature engineering through multimodal feature extraction and feature selection. The features extracted from ECG signals are time domain HRV features. The feature selection algorithm used was Kullback–Leibler divergence. EDA features were selected more frequently than the others, but as for ECG features, RMSSD, NN50, SDNN, and LF/HF were among the selected features in subject-dependent scenarios. The affective model used was Pos/Neg as the collected samples were based on fear as the negative label, and normal as neutral.

In [100], Gong et al. managed to classify joy and anger with 100% accuracy, while pleasure and sadness were classified at 92% and 88%. The study was conducted using the AuBT database and utilized a multimodal approach. The ECG, EMG, SC, and RSP were extracted using the ensemble empirical mode decomposition (EEMD) method, and the classifier used was C4.5 DT.

The authors of [115] focused on the combination of ECG and EEG for the application of an emotion recognition interface for interactive contents. The feature extracted from the ECG signals was HRV, and the classifiers tested were MLP, SVM, and a Bayesian network. By adopting 10-fold cross-validation, the best classifier reported was the Bayesian network, with 98.06% accuracy in recognizing six emotions from the DEM. Collected from 30 subjects, the emotions were amusement, fear, sadness, joy, anger, and disgust.

Kim and Andre [69] collected ECG, EMG, SC, and RSP signals from three subjects and performed a feature-based multiclass classification. The ECG features extracted were based on the HRV time, frequency, and nonlinear domains. Using a novel technique called emotion-specific multilevel dichotomous classification (EMDC), the authors managed to obtain a 95% average accuracy for subject-dependent and 70% for subject-independent scenarios. Among 110 combined extracted features, the best emotion-relevant feature from ECG was SD2 from the HRV Poincare plot for valence, arousal, and four classes of valence/arousal.

The study by Wagner et al. [85] adopted the AuBT multimodal physiological signal approach for emotion recognition. The ECG features extracted were HR statistical values. A few feature selection and classification techniques were tested to assess the recognition performance. With 92.05% accuracy, the four classes of emotion were classified using the linear discriminant function (LDF), and the features were selected using SFS. The same configuration obtained 96.59% accuracy on classifying arousal. However, for valence, the highest accuracy achieved was 88.64% using MLP and the combination of Fisher and SFS.

Healey and Picard [52] performed emotion recognition through detecting stress in a real-world driving scenario. A total of 24 drivers were tested through different traffic conditions in the greater Boston area while continuously providing feedback on their stress level. ECG, EMG, SC, and RSP sensors were attached to their body, and the data were recorded. The ECG features extracted were from the HRV power spectrum and sympathovagal balance ratio. The Fisher projection matrix and linear discriminant were used to determine the accuracy of the Pos/Neg emotional model. High, medium, and low stress recognition accuracies were 97.4%, 94.7%, and 100%, respectively.

Lastly, Haag et al. [78] took a multimodal approach towards emotion recognition by incorporating ECG, EMG, EDA, ST, RSP, and BVP. The ECG features extracted were HR, HRV, and IBI. Using NN, the study managed to classify arousal with 96.58% accuracy, and valence with 89.93% accuracy.

7. Application of Emotion Recognition System in Healthcare

A lot of treatments are available for physical illness, but it is not the same for psychological illness. Emotional health is important for the wellbeing of one's mental state. A negative emotional state may cause social and physical problems if left undiagnosed and untreated. For instance, prolonged exposure to stress or depression may lead someone to withdraw from a healthy relationship with the people around them and being aggressive, which could be dangerous for him/herself and the people around them. Moreover, negative emotions may also cause physical problems such as headaches, stomach upset, and muscle ache. An emotion recognition system can be utilized to improve the healthcare sector, especially in addressing metal health issues.

7.1. Emotion Recognition Application in Healthcare Utilizing ECG

The authors of [7,18] proposed a new healthcare system that focuses on emotional wellbeing. The system consists of physiological sensors (ECG and EEG) to measure and detect emotions. Based on that, the system provides necessary services such as relaxation, amusement, and excitement. These three emotional services are selected to balance out negative emotions detected from the subject with strong positive states. The relaxation service consists of a guided deep breathing exercise proven to benefit stress management. The exercise came with virtual objects in augmented reality and musical assistance for a calming effect. The system utilizes augmented reality as an output service channel, thus providing amusement and excitement services to the user interaction with the virtual objects. The interaction is enabled by Kinect's gesture detection.

A healthy workplace environment using a novel mood recognition solution that is able to identify eight different DEM emotions in every two-hour interval was proposed in [105]. The employees were provided with a wearable physiological device (ECG, PPG, and TEMP) along with a complimentary smartphone application called "HealthyOffice". The configuration setup was conducted to facilitate a periodical self-reporting towards the current emotional state in a structured manner. The objective of constantly monitoring employees' emotions in the workplace is to optimize the overall mental health of the organisation by eliminating anxiety, stress, and depression in the working environment. Thus, higher productivity is expected, and the output revenue can be significantly measured. A similar study of emotion healthcare application in the workplace environment was also conducted in [77], with a slightly different approach. This study used ECG, EDA, and TEMP as the physiological models. Rather than identifying the spectrum of basic emotions, the work only focused on stress and non-stress binary emotional classification.

A clinical application of emotion recognition systems was presented by [117]. The study utilized ECG and respiration sensors to detect stress symptoms in the patients. The targeted application of the work was towards patients who suffer migraine, addiction (substance or smoking), and stress-related disorders. The benefit of monitoring the patients' emotional stress condition is to ensure that a negative tendency is not triggered. Daily stress management can reduce severe addictive behavior and refrain from triggering migraine. The work also proposed a combination of physiological signals and other data such as visual exposure, social interactions, geoexposures, light and sound exposures, and digital trails to determine which parameters influence stress triggers. In [119], a home healthcare system using wearable physiological sensors that have an emotion recognition function was designed. The targeted groups for the application of the system were elderly and sub-healthy people. HR, TEMP, and SC were monitored at the wrist of the wearer in real time. The data were broadcast wirelessly to the family doctor or health practitioner who is responsible for the subject. An alert system was also embedded in the design to send a text message and notify the doctor, in case of a risky situation. The healthcare system can detect the states of joy, anger, and sadness.

The cardiac defense response (CDR) is a specific field of study that is closely related to psychophysiological reactivity towards an intense stimulation. CDR serves as a protective function of the fight or flight response in case of dangerous situations [120]. However, when exposed to it for a long period of time, anxiety, stress, depression, and other mental disorders might arise. The author of [121] proposed a novel integrated system using ECG signals to detect fear in real time. Since fear is the emotional response when a person is in danger, the system was designed to detect a prolonged CDR. In healthcare, this system is important for monitoring stress and early prevention of mental disorders.

7.2. General Healthcare Application of Emotion Recogntion Systems

The application of emotion recognition in military healthcare was studied in [122]. Since armed forces are constantly exposed to a highly stressful scenario and environment, many of them tend to develop psychiatric conditions such as depression, post-traumatic stress disorder (PTSD), and suicidal thoughts. To prevent dispatching emotionally unstable personnel into a risky mission, the work proposed the usage of emotion recognition screening to assess the mental health status of the subject. The system also analyzed the reaction towards stressful emotions of the subjects. However, further development is still needed for any practical application.

Next, an emotion recognition system was applied in [123] to improve the patient e-healthcare system in a so-called smart city. Medical doctors have difficulties in detecting and controlling the degree of pain experienced by their patients, especially for patients who cannot express it verbally such as babies. Thus, the study proposed a remote patient monitoring system that employs an automatic emotion detection architecture. The system is capable of achieving a more personalized pain detection index through emotion monitoring. With a proper analysis provided, the result of this system manages to obtain an accuracy of approximately 90% using SVM as the classifier.

Faiyaz et al. [124] proposed a novel e-healthcare support system with emotion recognition using fuzzy logic. The framework designed is suitable in the context of a real-life healthcare environment. Monitoring patients' emotions through the e-health system influences their satisfaction, wellbeing, and physical health. With the emotional feedback from their customers, healthcare providers can improve the quality of their services. The way of treating with empathy can be instilled in medical practitioners when they are aware of the affective state of their patients. This system is beneficial to both parties and improves the overall standards of the healthcare industry.

A fairly recent study was conducted in detecting the emotional state of patients during the spread of the virus SARS-COV-2, where face masks are mandatory [125]. A facial emotion recognition study was conducted with masked and unmasked versions of data. The unmasked faces in the database were modified digitally to add an artificial blue surgical mask over the face of the subjects. The system was designed to encourage pleasantness in doctor–patient interaction. However, with face masks being worn, inter-professional communication in healthcare is being upheld by the adoption of emotion recognition systems.

Another study that used computer vision to detect emotions in a healthcare center was presented in [126]. A multimodal visualization analysis was conducted on the facial expression of patients monitored using a monitoring camera at different intervals. The data were transmitted using the Internet of Things (IoT) and processed at the analysis center. If the system detected an abnormal expression, it would alert the physician in charge to check up on the patient.

Mental disorders and depression are serious illnesses that reduce the quality of life of individuals and the people around them. Early diagnosis of these psychiatric diseases can be conducted using an emotion recognition system, as proposed in [127]. The psychiatric patient-centric pervasive (P-cube) platform was designed to connect with the subject's smartphone or laptop to collect data for emotion recognition. Utilizing speech data recorded from the headset, the system can provide the therapist with deeper affective insights into a subject's mental state. Six basic emotions are detected using the system: anger, boredom, desperation, disgust, happiness, and pride.

Finally, ref. [128] proposed a speech signal-based emotion recognition system to analyze and detect compounded emotions. Prolonged anger, fear, and sadness are compounded with anxiety, where the person is prone to develop a more serious mental and physical health condition in the future. Compounded emotions might also drive a person to use substances, and, in the worst case, to commit suicide. The study designed a neural network-based autoencoder to extract suprasegmental features in voices and detect the early symptoms of anxiety disorder.

8. Discussion

8.1. Summary of the Review

The objective of this work was to perform a comprehensive review on emotion recognition systems that adopt ECG signals, and on their applications in healthcare. From the research reviewed, it is shown that with a combination of good pre-processing techniques, feature extraction and selection methods, and classification algorithms, human emotions can be recognized by machines with a medium to good accuracy. Even though the research on affective computing has been around for more than a decade, a standard universal emotional model has still not been achieved. Emotional models such as the ADM, DEM, and Pos/Neg are still ambiguous, particularly in the number of classes for the DEM. There are three-class, four-class, and even five-class labels for the DEM, which somehow raise the question of the purpose of recognizing each emotion. However, with the valence and arousal scale in the ADM, and the stress and non-stress binarization of Pos/Neg, the targeted application of emotion recognition systems is more focused and simpler.

The other angle reviewed here is how extracted ECG features are relevant to the ANS activity in the heart. Our eyes cannot visibly capture any characteristic changes in the raw ECG signal; however, the feature extraction techniques are sensitive enough to extract the informative features of ECG. Additionally, feature selection and dimensionality reduction allow only the most relevant features to be adopted to recognize the specific emotion, while features that are unnecessary are eliminated.

The classification and validation steps are the most important parts in emotion recognition systems. Different classifiers use different learning approaches towards the data being trained. Even though the most used machine learning algorithm for emotion recognition systems is SVM, it is not necessarily the best approach. As it was previously discussed, there are few studies that managed to outperform SVM's performance with other machine learning models. In addition, the reason most research on emotion recognition used machine learning instead of deep learning is because of the scarcity of the data available. As it was summarized, in the available databases, the number of subjects and samples are less compared to medical databases that deal with cardiac disease. Nonetheless, deep learning has been considered and has shown a promising performance. With more data, deep learning is a good direction for this area. However, collecting a large database to perform a subject-dependent and subject-independent analysis requires a lot of time and cost. Thus, it is important for researchers to properly decide the pipeline of their research and consider validation techniques in order to increase variability.

Finally, application of emotion recognition systems in healthcare focusing on mental health was reviewed in Section 6. Emotion recognition systems are able to help in assessing the mental state of an individual. The output of the system can then be used as an input for a system that responds to the emotion to provide comfort and regulate the emotion so that a positive emotion is experienced by the individual.

8.2. Research Challanges

Among the studies reviewed, the challenge for ECG-based emotion recognition systems is the lack of affective databases with a large number of samples taken from subjects with different backgrounds. Current affective databases are limited by an age group bias, where only university students participated in the data collection processes. Moreover, one of the regional experiments conducted caused the database used to have a homogenous locality sample from people with the same ethnic backgrounds.

The next challenge comes from the perspective of annotation, as well as unstandardized emotional models and scales. Since emotions are subjective experiences defined through different perspectives, the inexactness may cause classification fallacies. If the emotion experienced by a subject contradicts the perceived emotions by a second- or third-person perspective, this might cause a huge mess in the system. When dealing with insufficient datasets, researchers tend to combine datasets to increase the sample size. The unstandardized emotional models and scales cause a huge challenge in adopting different affective datasets in one study.

The last challenge is the applicability of emotion recognition systems designed for real-world situations, especially in healthcare. The majority of the studies summarized are not available for actual use because of the complexity of the design. The whole purpose of academic research is to promote intelligent solutions to issues or problems faced in real life. However, since the studies are not repeatable or are difficult to replicate, other researchers have difficulties in improving the steps taken from previous works. In order to make emotion recognition systems common in the healthcare industry, the models proposed have to be simple, efficient, and reliable, in addition to being tested vigorously.

8.3. Future Works

Further research should be conducted on emotion recognition systems based on ECG signals for healthcare purposes. Primarily, the relationship of different age groups, ethnicities, and personalities towards emotion stimuli and responses should be investigated. The bigger the sample size with a heterogenous background, the better the classification approach, and thus a universal system can be built. Next, the perspective of intercompatibility between one dataset and another should be reviewed if the same methodologies are to be applied to compensate the training and testing accuracy and promote the generalizability of the developed system. The research of emotion recognition should be closer to a real-life scenario, where the computer can learn to eliminate more outside noise, instead of working in a controlled environment. By applying this approach, the system should be robust and versatile for further application and commercialization. By deploying emotion recognition systems for healthcare usage, the architecture built must be reliable in dealing with different scenarios. Finally, various other possible real-world use cases of emotion recognition systems which allow personalization in real time should be explored.

9. Conclusions

This review has shown that emotion recognition systems are an essential subject in healthcare, and the application of them is possible via ECG as a unimodal or multimodal approach. The growing trend of research related to emotion recognition systems is a heathy step towards the maturity of this field. Future endeavours of incorporating emotional health in technological development will contribute to more responsible and sustainable innovations.

Author Contributions: Conceptualization, M.A.H. and N.A.A.A.; methodology, M.A.H. and N.A.A.A.; formal analysis, M.A.H. and N.A.A.A.; investigation, M.A.H.; resources, M.A.H. and S.A.; writing—original draft preparation, M.A.H.; writing—review and editing, N.A.A.A., A.A.A., S.A., and M.M.; visualization, M.A.H.; supervision, N.A.A.A. and A.A.A.; project administration, N.A.A.A. and M.M.; funding acquisition, N.A.A.A. and M.M. All authors have read and agreed to the published version of the manuscript.

Funding: This research was funded by the Ministry of Higher Education, Malaysia, under the Fundamental Research Grant Scheme, grant number FRGS/1/2019/ICT02/MMU/02/15, which is awarded to Multimedia University. The APC was co-funded by the Deanship of Scientific Research at King Khalid University under research grant number (R.G.P1/207/42).

Institutional Review Board Statement: Not applicable.

Informed Consent Statement: Not applicable.

Data Availability Statement: Not applicable.

Acknowledgments: We would like to acknowledge the input and assistance rendered to us by Chy Tawsif Khan, Sharifah Noor Masidayu Sayed Ismail, and Md Armanur Rahman from the Center for Engineering Computational Intelligence, and also the Multimedia University, Malaysia.

Conflicts of Interest: The authors declare no conflict of interest.

References

1. Picard, R.W. *Affective Computing*; Technical Report 321; MIT Media Laboratory Perceptual Computing Section: Cambridge, MA, USA, 1995.
2. Strauss, M.; Reynolds, C.; Hughes, S.; Park, K.; McDarby, G.; Picard, R.; Tao, J.; Tan, T. *Affective Computing: A Review*; Springer: Berlin/Heidelberg, Germany, 2005; pp. 699–706.
3. Ekman, P.; Friesen, W. Facial Sign Of Emotional Experience. *J. Personal. Soc. Psychol.* **1980**, *39*, 1125. [CrossRef]
4. Reeves, B. *The Media Equation: How People Treat Computers, Television, and New Media Like Real People and Places*; Cambridge University Press: Cambridge, UK, 1996.
5. Nikolova, D.; Georgieva, P.; Petkova, P.; Manolova, A. ECG-based emotion recognition: Overview of methods and applications. In Proceedings of the ANNA 2018—Advances in Neural Networks and Applications, St. Konstantin and Elena Resort, Bulgaria, 15–17 September 2018; pp. 118–122.
6. Katsis, C.D.; Katertsidis, N.; Ganiatsas, G.; Fotiadis, D.I. Toward emotion recognition in car-racing drivers: A biosignal processing approach. *IEEE Trans. Syst. Man Cybern. Part A Syst. Hum.* **2008**, *38*, 502–512. [CrossRef]
7. Tivatansakul, S.; Ohkura, M. Healthcare system focusing on emotional aspects using augmented reality: Implementation of breathing control application in relaxation service. In Proceedings of the 2013 International Conference on Biometrics and Kansei Engineering, Tokyo, Japan, 5–7 July 2013; pp. 218–222.
8. Kołakowska, A.; Landowska, A.; Szwoch, M.; Szwoch, W.; Wróbel, M.R. Emotion Recognition and Its Applications. In *Human-Computer Systems Interaction: Backgrounds and Applications 3*; Hippe, Z.S., Kulikowski, J.L., Mroczek, T., Wtorek, J., Eds.; Springer International Publishing: Cham, Switzerland, 2014; pp. 51–62. ISBN 978-3-319-08491-6.
9. Ghali, A.L.I.; Bassam Kurdy, M.H.D. Emotion Recognition Using Facial Expression Analysis. *J. Theor. Appl. Inf. Technol.* **2018**, *96*, 6117–6129.
10. Busso, C.; Deng, Z.; Yildirim, S.; Bulut, M.; Lee, C.M.; Kazemzadeh, A.; Lee, S.; Neumann, U.; Narayanan, S. Analysis of Emotion Recognition using Facial Expressions, Speech and Multimodal Information. In Proceedings of the 6th International Conference on Multimodal Interfaces, Sorrento, Italy, 25–29 November 2012; pp. 205–211.
11. Tarnowski, P.; Kołodziej, M.; Majkowski, A.; Rak, R.J. Emotion recognition using facial expressions. In Proceedings of the International Conference on Computational Science, Zurich, Switzerland, 12–14 June 2017; Volume 108, pp. 1175–1184.
12. Pantic, M.; Caridakis, G.; André, E.; Kim, J.; Karpouzis, K.; Kollias, S. Multimodal emotion recognition from low-level cues. *Cogn. Technol.* **2011**, 115–132.
13. McCraty, R. *Science of the Heart: Exploring the Role of the Heart in Human Performance*; HeartMath Institute: Boulder Creek, CA, USA, 2015; ISBN 1-879052-53-9.
14. Gordon Betts, J.; Young, K.A.; Wise, J.A.; Johnson, E.; Poe, B.; Kruse, D.H.; Korol, O.; Johnson, J.E.; Womble, M.; DeSaix, P. *Anatomy and Physiology II*; OpenStax: Houston, TX, USA, 2013.
15. Bota, P.J.; Wang, C.; Fred, A.L.N.; Placido Da Silva, H. A Review, Current Challenges, and Future Possibilities on Emotion Recognition Using Machine Learning and Physiological Signals. *IEEE Access* **2019**, *7*, 140990–141020. [CrossRef]
16. Betts, J.G.; Desaix, P.; Johnson, E.; Johnson, J.E.; Korol, O.; Kruse, D.; Poe, B.; Wise, J.A.; Womble, M.; Young, K.A. *Anatomy & Physiology-OpenStax*; Rice University: Houston, TX, USA, 2013.
17. Tecce, J.J. Psychophysiology: Human behavior and physiological response. *Int. J. Psychophysiol.* **1996**, *40*, 89–91. [CrossRef]
18. Tivatansakul, S.; Ohkura, M. Improvement of emotional healthcare system with stress detection from ECG signal. In Proceedings of the Annual International Conference of the IEEE Engineering in Medicine and Biology Society, EMBS, Milan, Italy, 25–29 August 2015.
19. Luthra, A. *ECG Made Easy*; Jaypee Brothers, Medical Publisher: Delhi, India, 2012.
20. Goshvarpour, A.; Abbasi, A.; Goshvarpour, A. An accurate emotion recognition system using ECG and GSR signals and matching pursuit method. *Biomed. J.* **2017**, *40*, 355–368. [CrossRef]

21. Agrafioti, F.; Hatzinakos, D.; Anderson, A.K. ECG pattern analysis for emotion detection. *IEEE Trans. Affect. Comput.* **2012**, *3*, 102–115. [CrossRef]
22. Bulagang, A.F.; Weng, N.G.; Mountstephens, J.; Teo, J. A review of recent approaches for emotion classification using electrocardiography and electrodermography signals. *Inform. Med. Unlocked* **2020**, *20*, 100363. [CrossRef]
23. Ali, M.; Mosa, A.H.; Al Machot, F.; Kyamakya, K. Emotion recognition involving physiological and speech signals: A comprehensive review. In *Studies in Systems, Decision and Control*; Springer International Publishing AG: Berlin/Heidelberg, Germany, 2018; Volume 109.
24. Rattanyu, K.; Mizukawa, M. Emotion recognition based on ecg signals for service robots in the intelligent space during daily life. *J. Adv. Comput. Intell. Intell. Inform.* **2011**, *15*, 582–591. [CrossRef]
25. Bexton, R.S.; Vallin, H.O.; Camm, A.J. Diurnal variation of the QT interval—Influence of the autonomic nervous system. *Br. Heart J.* **1986**, *55*, 253–258. [CrossRef]
26. Dissanayake, T.; Rajapaksha, Y.; Ragel, R.; Nawinne, I. An ensemble learning approach for electrocardiogram sensor based human emotion recognition. *Sensors* **2019**, *19*, 4495. [CrossRef]
27. Nemati, E.; Deen, M.J.; Mondal, T. A wireless wearable ECG sensor for long-term applications. *IEEE Commun. Mag.* **2012**, *50*, 36–43. [CrossRef]
28. Szczepański, A.; Saeed, K. A mobile device system for early warning of ECG anomalies. *Sensors* **2014**, *14*, 11031–11044. [CrossRef] [PubMed]
29. Tada, Y.; Amano, Y.; Sato, T.; Saito, S.; Inoue, M. A smart shirt made with conductive ink and conductive foam for the measurement of electrocardiogram signals with unipolar precordial leads. *Fibers* **2015**, *3*, 463–477. [CrossRef]
30. Merriam, W. Merriam-Webster Dictionary. 1828. Available online: http://webstersdictionary1828.com/ (accessed on 10 July 2021).
31. Song, T.; Zheng, W.; Lu, C.; Zong, Y.; Zhang, X.; Cui, Z. MPED: A multi-modal physiological emotion database for discrete emotion recognition. *IEEE Access* **2019**, *7*, 12177–12191. [CrossRef]
32. Ekman, P. An Argument for Basic Emotions. *Cogn. Emot.* **1992**, *6*, 169–200. [CrossRef]
33. Graver, M. *Cicero on the Emotions: Tusculan Disputations 3 and 4*; University of Chicago Press: Chicago, IL, USA, 2002; pp. 43–44.
34. Ekman, P. Basic Emotions. In *Handbook of Cognition and Emotion*; John Wiley & Sons: Hoboken, NJ, USA, 1999; pp. 45–60.
35. Izard, C.E. Basic Emotions, Natural Kinds, Emotion Schemas, and a New Paradigm. *Perspect. Psychol. Sci.* **2007**, *2*, 260–280. [CrossRef] [PubMed]
36. Izard, C.E. Emotion theory and research: Highlights, unanswered questions, and emerging issues. *Annu. Rev. Psychol.* **2009**, *60*, 1–25. [CrossRef]
37. Minhad, K.N.; Ali, S.H.M.D.; Reaz, M.B.I. A design framework for human emotion recognition using electrocardiogram and skin conductance response signals. *J. Eng. Sci. Technol.* **2017**, *12*, 3102–3119.
38. Kanagaraj, G.; Ponnambalam, S.G.; Jawahar, N. Trends in Intelligent Robotics, Automation, and Manufacturing. *Commun. Comput. Inf. Sci.* **2012**, *330*, 198–205.
39. Bong, S.Z.; Murugappan, M.; Yaacob, S. Analysis of electrocardiogram (ECG) signals for human emotional stress classification. In Proceedings of the Communications in Computer and Information Science, Kuala Lumpur, Malaysia, 20–22 February 2012; Volume 330, pp. 198–205.
40. Selvaraj, J.; Murugappan, M.; Wan, K.; Yaacob, S. Classification of emotional states from electrocardiogram signals: A non-linear approach based on hurst. *BioMed. Eng. Online* **2013**, *12*, 44. [CrossRef] [PubMed]
41. Wei, W.; Jia, Q.; Feng, Y.; Chen, G. Emotion Recognition Based on Weighted Fusion Strategy of Multichannel Physiological Signals. *Comput. Intell. Neurosci.* **2018**, *2018*, 5296523. [CrossRef]
42. Mehrabian, A. Comparison of the PAD and PANAS as models for describing emotions and for differentiating anxiety from depression. *J. Psychopathol. Behav. Assess.* **1997**, *19*, 331–357. [CrossRef]
43. Russell, J.A. A circumplex model of affect. *J. Personal. Soc. Psychol.* **1980**, *39*, 1161. [CrossRef]
44. Harmon-Jones, E.; Harmon-Jones, C.; Summerell, E. On the importance of both dimensional and discrete models of emotion. *Behav. Sci.* **2017**, *7*, 66. [CrossRef] [PubMed]
45. Koelstra, S.; Mühl, C.; Soleymani, M.; Lee, J.S.; Yazdani, A.; Ebrahimi, T.; Pun, T.; Nijholt, A.; Patras, I. DEAP: A database for emotion analysis; Using physiological signals. *IEEE Trans. Affect. Comput.* **2011**, *3*, 18–31. [CrossRef]
46. Alemi, O.; Li, W.; Pasquier, P. Affect-expressive movement generation with factored conditional Restricted Boltzmann Machines. In Proceedings of the 2015 International Conference on Affective Computing and Intelligent Interaction, ACII, Xi'an, China, 21–24 September 2015.
47. Tivatansakul, S.; Ohkura, M. Emotion Recognition using ECG Signals with Local Pattern Description Methods. *Int. J. Affect. Eng.* **2016**, *15*, 51–61. [CrossRef]
48. Yang, L.; Zhao, Y.; Wang, Y.; Liu, L.; Zhang, X.; Li, B.; Cui, R. The Effects of Psychological Stress on Depression. *Curr. Neuropharmacol.* **2015**, *13*, 494–504. [CrossRef]
49. Gershon, A.; Johnson, S.L.; Miller, I. Chronic stressors and trauma: Prospective influences on the course of bipolar disorder. *Psychol. Med.* **2013**, *43*, 2583–2592. [CrossRef] [PubMed]
50. Siedlecka, E.; Denson, T.F. Experimental Methods for Inducing Basic Emotions: A Qualitative Review. *Emot. Rev.* **2019**, *11*, 87–97. [CrossRef]

51. Park, C.Y.; Cha, N.; Kang, S.; Kim, A.; Khandoker, A.H.; Hadjileontiadis, L.; Oh, A.; Jeong, Y.; Lee, U. K-EmoCon, a multimodal sensor dataset for continuous emotion recognition in naturalistic conversations. *Sci. Data* **2020**, *7*, 293. [CrossRef] [PubMed]
52. Healey, J.A.; Picard, R.W. Detecting stress during real-world driving tasks using physiological sensors. *IEEE Trans. Intell. Transp. Syst.* **2005**, *6*, 156–166. [CrossRef]
53. Yang, W.; Rifqi, M.; Marsala, C.; Pinna, A. Physiological-Based Emotion Detection and Recognition in a Video Game Context. In Proceedings of the International Joint Conference on Neural Networks, Rio de Janeiro, Brazil, 8–13 July 2018.
54. Shahid, H.; Butt, A.; Aziz, S.; Khan, M.U.; Hassan Naqvi, S.Z. Emotion Recognition System featuring a fusion of Electrocardiogram and Photoplethysmogram Features. In Proceedings of the 2020 14th International Conference on Open Source Systems and Technologies (ICOSST), Lahore, Pakistan, 16–17 December 2020.
55. Miranda Correa, J.A.; Abadi, M.K.; Sebe, N.; Patras, I. AMIGOS: A Dataset for Affect, Personality and Mood Research on Individuals and Groups. *IEEE Trans. Affect. Comput.* **2018**, *12*, 479–493. [CrossRef]
56. Subramanian, R.; Wache, J.; Abadi, M.K.; Vieriu, R.L.; Winkler, S.; Sebe, N. Ascertain: Emotion and personality recognition using commercial sensors. *IEEE Trans. Affect. Comput.* **2018**, *9*, 147–160. [CrossRef]
57. Abadi, M.K.; Subramanian, R.; Kia, S.M.; Avesani, P.; Patras, I.; Sebe, N. DECAF: MEG-Based Multimodal Database for Decoding Affective Physiological Responses. *IEEE Trans. Affect. Comput.* **2015**, *6*, 209–222. [CrossRef]
58. Katsigiannis, S.; Ramzan, N. DREAMER: A Database for Emotion Recognition Through EEG and ECG Signals from Wireless Low-cost Off-the-Shelf Devices. *IEEE J. Biomed. Health Inform.* **2017**, *22*, 98–107. [CrossRef]
59. Soleymani, M.; Lichtenauer, J.; Pun, T.; Pantic, M. A multimodal database for affect recognition and implicit tagging. *IEEE Trans. Affect. Comput.* **2012**, *3*, 42–55. [CrossRef]
60. Mayer, J.; Allen, J.; Beauregard, K. Mood inductions for four specific moods: A procedure employing guided imagery vignettes with music. *J. Ment. Imag.* **1995**, *19*, 151–159.
61. Lang, P.J.; Bradley, M.M.; Cuthbert, B.N. *International Affective Picture System (IAPS): Instruction Manual and Affective Ratings*; University of Florida: Gainesville, FL, USA, 2005.
62. Krumhansl, C.L. Music: A link between cognition and emotion. *Curr. Dir. Psychol. Sci.* **2002**, *11*, 45–50. [CrossRef]
63. Bradley, M.M.; Lang, P.J. *The International Affective Digitized Sounds Affective Ratings of Sounds and Instruction Manual*; University of Florida: Gainesville, FL, USA, 2007.
64. Prkachin, K.M.; Williams-Avery, R.M.; Zwaal, C.; Mills, D.E. Cardiovascular changes during induced emotion: An application of Lang's theory of emotional imagery. *J. Psychosom. Res.* **1999**, *47*, 255–267. [CrossRef]
65. Bradley, M.M.; Lang, P.J. Measuring emotion: The self-assessment manikin and the semantic differential. *J. Behav. Ther. Exp. Psychiatry* **1994**, *25*, 49–59. [CrossRef]
66. Wagner, J. *Augsburg Biosignal Toolbox (Aubt)*; University of Augsburg: Augsburg, Germany, 2005.
67. Sharma, K.; Castellini, C.; van den Broek, E.L.; Albu-Schaeffer, A.; Schwenker, F. A dataset of continuous affect annotations and physiological signals for emotion analysis. *Sci. Data* **2019**, *6*, 1–3. [CrossRef] [PubMed]
68. Markova, V.; Ganchev, T.; Kalinkov, K. CLAS: A Database for Cognitive Load, Affect and Stress Recognition. In Proceedings of the International Conference on Biomedical Innovations and Applications, BIA, Varna, Bulgaria, 8–9 November 2019.
69. Kim, J.; André, E. Emotion recognition based on physiological changes in music listening. *IEEE Trans. Pattern Anal. Mach. Intell.* **2008**, *30*, 2067–2083. [CrossRef] [PubMed]
70. Koldijk, S.; Sappelli, M.; Verberne, S.; Neerincx, M.A.; Kraaij, W. The Swell knowledge work dataset for stress and user modeling research. In Proceedings of the ICMI 2014—International Conference on Multimodal Interaction, Istanbul, Turkey, 12–16 November 2014.
71. Schmidt, P.; Reiss, A.; Duerichen, R.; Van Laerhoven, K. Introducing WeSAD, a multimodal dataset for wearable stress and affect detection. In Proceedings of the ICMI 2018—International Conference on Multimodal Interaction, Boulder, CO, USA, 16–20 October 2018.
72. Nayak, S.; Soni, M.K.; Bansal, D. Filtering Techniques for Ecg Signal Processing. *Int. J. Res. Eng. Appl. Sci.* **2009**, *2*, 671–679.
73. Watford, C. Understanding Ecg Filtering. 2019. Available online: http://ems12lead.com/2014/03/10/understanding-ecg-filtering/#gref (accessed on 10 March 2014).
74. Xiefeng, C.; Wang, Y.; Dai, S.; Zhao, P.; Liu, Q. Heart sound signals can be used for emotion recognition. *Sci. Rep.* **2019**, *9*, 1–11. [CrossRef]
75. Liu, X.; Wang, Q.; Liu, D.; Wang, Y.; Zhang, Y.; Bai, O.; Sun, J. Human emotion classification based on multiple physiological signals by wearable system. *Technol. Health Care* **2018**, *26*, 459–469. [CrossRef]
76. Jerritta, S.; Murugappan, M.; Wan, K.; Yaacob, S. Electrocardiogram-based emotion recognition system using empirical mode decomposition and discrete Fourier transform. *Expert Syst.* **2014**, *31*, 110–120.
77. Anusha, A.S.; Jose, J.; Preejith, S.P.; Jayaraj, J.; Mohanasankar, S. Physiological signal based work stress detection using unobtrusive sensors. *BioMed. Phys. Eng. Express* **2018**, *4*, 6. [CrossRef]
78. Haag, A.; Goronzy, S.; Schaich, P.; Williams, J. Emotion recognition using bio-sensors: First steps towards an automatic system. In Proceedings of the Lecture Notes in Artificial Intelligence (Subseries of Lecture Notes in Computer Science), Mexico City, Mexico, 26–30 April 2004; Springer: Berlin/Heidelberg, Germany, 2004; Volume 3068.
79. Chavan, M.S.; Aggarwala, R.; Uplane, M. Suppression Of Baseline Wander And Power Line Interference in ECG Using Digital IIR Filter. *Int. J. Circuits Syst. Signal Process.* **2008**, *2*, 356–365.

80. Mahmoodabadi, S.Z.; Ahmadian, A.; Abolhasani, M.D.; Eslami, M.; Bidgoli, J.H. ECG feature extraction based on multiresolution wavelet transform. In Proceedings of the Annual International Conference of the IEEE Engineering in Medicine and Biology, Shanghai, China, 17–18 January 2006; pp. 3902–3905.
81. Pan, J.; Tompkins, W.J. A Real-Time QRS Detection Algorithm. *IEEE Trans. Biomed. Eng.* **1985**, *32*, 230–236. [CrossRef]
82. Wen, W.H.; Qiu, Y.H.; Liu, G.Y. Electrocardiography recording, feature extraction and classification for emotion recognition. In Proceedings of the 2009 WRI World Congress on Computer Science and Information Engineering, CSIE, Los Angeles, CA, USA, 31 March–2 April 2009; Volume 4, pp. 168–172.
83. Kathirvel, P.; Manikandan, M.S.; Prasanna, S.R.M.; Soman, K.P. An Efficient R-peak Detection Based on New Nonlinear Transformation and First-Order Gaussian Differentiator. *Cardiovasc. Eng. Technol.* **2011**, *2*, 408–425. [CrossRef]
84. Xu, Y.; Liu, G.Y. A method of emotion recognition based on ECG signal. In Proceedings of the 2009 International Conference on Computational Intelligence and Natural Computing, CINC 2009, Wuhan, China, 6–7 June 2009.
85. Wagner, J.; Kim, J.; André, E. From physiological signals to emotions: Implementing and comparing selected methods for feature extraction and classification. In Proceedings of the IEEE International Conference on Multimedia and Expo, Amsterdam, The Netherlands, 6 July 2005; Volume 2005.
86. Xun, L.; Zheng, G. ECG Signal Feature Selection for Emotion Recognition. *TELKOMNIKA Indones. J. Electr. Eng.* **2013**, *11*, 1363–1370. [CrossRef]
87. Rainville, P.; Bechara, A.; Naqvi, N.; Damasio, A.R. Basic emotions are associated with distinct patterns of cardiorespiratory activity. *Int. J. Psychophysiol.* **2006**, *61*, 5–18. [CrossRef]
88. Xia, L.; Malik, A.S.; Subhani, A.R. A physiological signal-based method for early mental-stress detection. *Biomed. Signal Process. Control* **2018**, *46*, 18–32. [CrossRef]
89. Chen, G.; Zhu, Y.; Yang, Z.; Hong, Z. Emotionalgan: Generating ECG to enhance emotion state classification. In Proceedings of the ACM International Conference Proceeding Series, Wuhan, China, 12 July 2019.
90. Ferdinando, H.; Seppanen, T.; Alasaarela, E. Comparing features from ECG pattern and HRV analysis for emotion recognition system. In Proceedings of the CIBCB 2016—Annual IEEE International Conference on Computational Intelligence in Bioinformatics and Computational Biology, Chiang Mai, Thailand, 5–7 October 2016.
91. Shaffer, F.; Ginsberg, J.P. An Overview of Heart Rate Variability Metrics and Norms. *Front. Public Health* **2017**, *5*, 258. [CrossRef] [PubMed]
92. Thayer, J.F. Heart Rate Variability: A Neurovisceral Integration Model. In *Encyclopedia of Neuroscience*; Elsevier: Amsterdam, The Netherlands, 2009.
93. Malik, M.; Camm, A.J.; Bigger, J.T.; Breithardt, G.; Cerutti, S.; Cohen, R.J.; Coumel, P.; Fallen, E.L.; Kennedy, H.L.; Kleiger, R.E.; et al. Heart rate variability. Standards of measurement, physiological interpretation, and clinical use. *Eur. Heart J.* **1996**, *17*, 1043–1065. [CrossRef]
94. Salahuddin, L.; Cho, J.; Jeong, M.G.; Kim, D. Ultra short term analysis of heart rate variability for monitoring mental stress in mobile settings. In Proceedings of the 2007 29th Annual International Conference of the IEEE Engineering in Medicine and Biology Society, Lyon, France, 23–26 August 2007; pp. 4656–4659.
95. Baek, H.J.; Cho, C.H.; Cho, J.; Woo, J.M. Reliability of ultra-short-term analysis as a surrogate of standard 5-min analysis of heart rate variability. *Telemed. E Health* **2015**, *21*, 404–414. [CrossRef]
96. Umetani, K.; Singer, D.H.; McCraty, R.; Atkinson, M. Twenty-four hour time domain heart rate variability and heart rate: Relations to age and gender over nine decades. *J. Am. Coll. Cardiol.* **1998**, *31*, 593–601. [CrossRef]
97. Hayano, J.; Kisohara, M.; Ueda, N.; Yuda, E. Impact of heart rate fragmentation on the assessment of heart rate variability. *Appl. Sci.* **2020**, *10*, 3314. [CrossRef]
98. Huang, N.E. Empirical Mode Decomposition and Hilbert Spectral Analysis. *Proc. R. Soc. A Math. Phys. Eng. Sci.* **1998**, *454*, 903–995. [CrossRef]
99. Zong, C.; Chetouani, M. Hilbert-Huang transform based physiological signals analysis for emotion recognition. In Proceedings of the 2009 IEEE International Symposium on Signal Processing and Information Technology (ISSPIT), Ajman, United Arab Emirates, 14–17 December 2009; IEEE: Ajman, United Arab Emirates, 2009; pp. 334–339.
100. Gong, P.; Ma, H.T.; Wang, Y. Emotion recognition based on the multiple physiological signals. In Proceedings of the 2016 IEEE International Conference on Real-Time Computing and Robotics, RCAR, Angkor Wat, Cambodia, 6–10 June 2016.
101. Guendil, Z.; Lachiri, Z.; Maaoui, C.; Pruski, A. Emotion recognition from physiological signals using fusion of wavelet based features. In Proceedings of the 2015 7th International Conference on Modelling, Identification and Control, ICMIC, Sousse, Tunisia, 18–20 December 2015.
102. Guo, X. Study of emotion recognition based on electrocardiogram and RBF neural network. *Procedia Eng.* **2011**, *15*, 2408–2412.
103. Cai, J.; Liu, G.; Hao, M. The research on emotion recognition from ECG signal. In Proceedings of the 2009 International Conference on Information Technology and Computer Science, Kiev, Ukraine, 25–26 July 2009; Volume 1.
104. Zhang, Z.; Wang, X.; Li, P.; Chen, X.; Shao, L. Research on emotion recognition based on ECG signal. *J. Phys. Conf. Ser.* **2020**, *1678*, 012091. [CrossRef]
105. Zenonos, A.; Khan, A.; Kalogridis, G.; Vatsikas, S.; Lewis, T.; Sooriyabandara, M. HealthyOffice: Mood recognition at work using smartphones and wearable sensors. In Proceedings of the 2016 IEEE International Conference on Pervasive Computing and Communication Workshops, PerCom Workshops, Sydney, NSW, Australia, 14–18 March 2016.

106. Valenza, G.; Citi, L.; Lanatá, A.; Scilingo, E.P.; Barbieri, R. Revealing Real-Time Emotional Responses: A Personalized Assessment based on Heartbeat Dynamics. *Sci. Rep.* **2014**, *4*, 4998. [CrossRef]
107. Wen, W.; Liu, G.; Cheng, N.; Wei, J.; Shangguan, P.; Huang, W. Emotion recognition based on multi-variant correlation of physiological signals. *IEEE Trans. Affect. Comput.* **2014**, *5*, 126–140. [CrossRef]
108. Siddharth, S.; Jung, T.-P.; Sejnowski, T. Utilizing Deep Learning Towards Multi-modal Bio-sensing and Vision-based Affective Computing. *IEEE Trans. Affect. Comput.* **2019**, *1*, 99. [CrossRef]
109. Lee, J.; Yoo, S.K. Design of user-customized negative emotion classifier based on feature selection using physiological signal sensors. *Sensors* **2018**, *18*, 4253. [CrossRef] [PubMed]
110. Kukolja, D.; Popović, S.; Horvat, M.; Kovač, B.; Ćosić, K. Comparative analysis of emotion estimation methods based on physiological measurements for real-time applications. *Int. J. Hum. Comput. Stud.* **2014**, *72*, 717–727. [CrossRef]
111. Guo, H.; Huang, Y.; Lin, C.; Chien, J.; Haraikawa, K.; Shieh, J. Heart Rate Variability Signal Features for Emotion Recognition by Using Principal Component Analysis and Support Vectors Machine. In Proceedings of the 2016 IEEE 16th International Conference on Bioinformatics and Bioengineering (BIBE), Taichung, Taiwan, 31 October–2 November 2016; pp. 274–277.
112. Sarkar, P.; Etemad, A. Self-supervised ECG Representation Learning for Emotion Recognition. *IEEE Trans. Affect. Comput.* **2020**. [CrossRef]
113. Santamaria-Granados, L.; Munoz-Organero, M.; Ramirez-Gonzalez, G.; Abdulhay, E.; Arunkumar, N. Using Deep Convolutional Neural Network for Emotion Detection on a Physiological Signals Dataset (AMIGOS). *IEEE Access* **2019**, *7*, 57–67. [CrossRef]
114. Plarre, K.; Raij, A.; Hossain, S.M.; Ali, A.A.; Nakajima, M.; Al'Absi, M.; Ertin, E.; Kamarck, T.; Kumar, S.; Scott, M.; et al. Continuous inference of psychological stress from sensory measurements collected in the natural environment. In Proceedings of the 10th ACM/IEEE International Conference on Information Processing in Sensor Networks, Chicago, IL, USA, 12–14 April 2011.
115. Shin, D.; Shin, D.; Shin, D. Development of emotion recognition interface using complex EEG/ECG bio-signal for interactive contents. *Multimed. Tools Appl.* **2017**, *76*, 11449–11470. [CrossRef]
116. Brás, S.; Ferreira, J.H.T.; Soares, S.C.; Pinho, A.J. Biometric and emotion identification: An ECG compression based method. *Front. Psychol.* **2018**, *9*, 467. [CrossRef]
117. Hovsepian, K.; Al'absi, M.; Ertin, E.; Kamarck, T.; Nakajima, M.; Kumar, S. CStress: Towards a gold standard for continuous stress assessment in the mobile environment. In Proceedings of the UbiComp 2015 ACM International Joint Conference on Pervasive and Ubiquitous Computing, Osaka, Japan, 7–11 September 2015.
118. Yang, C.J.; Fahier, N.; Li, W.C.; Fang, W.C. A Convolution Neural Network Based Emotion Recognition System using Multimodal Physiological Signals. In Proceedings of the 2020 IEEE International Conference on Consumer Electronics, Taoyuan, Taiwan, 28–30 September 2020.
119. Jiang, Z.; Lu, L.; Huang, X.; Tan, C. Design of wearable home health care system with emotion recognition function. In Proceedings of the 2011 International Conference on Electrical and Control Engineering, Yichang, China, 16–18 September 2011.
120. Vila, J.; Mata, J.L.; Guerra, P. Stress and Cardiac Response. In *International Encyclopedia of the Social & Behavioral Sciences*, 2nd ed.; Elsevier: Amsterdam, The Netherlands, 2015; pp. 539–545.
121. Covello, R.; Fortino, G.; Gravina, R.; Aguilar, A.; Breslin, J.G. Novel method and real-time system for detecting the Cardiac Defense Response based on the ECG. In Proceedings of the MeMeA 2013 IEEE International Symposium on Medical Measurements and Applications (MeMeA), Gatineau, QC, Canada, 4–5 May 2013.
122. Tokuno, S.; Tsumatori, G.; Shono, S.; Takei, E.; Yamamoto, T.; Suzuki, G.; Mituyoshi, S.; Shimura, M. Usage of emotion recognition in military health care. In Proceedings of the 2011 Defense Science Research Conference and Expo, DSR, Singapore, 3–5 August 2011.
123. Pujol, F.A.; Mora, H.; Martínez, A. Emotion recognition to improve e-healthcare systems in smart cities. In Proceedings of the Springer Proceedings in Complexity, Athens, Greece, 15–17 April 2019.
124. Doctor, F.; Karyotis, C.; Iqbal, R.; James, A. An intelligent framework for emotion aware e-healthcare support systems. In Proceedings of the 2016 IEEE Symposium Series on Computational Intelligence, SSCI, Athens, Greece, 6–9 December 2016.
125. Bani, M.; Russo, S.; Ardenghi, S.; Rampoldi, G.; Wickline, V.; Nowicki, S.; Strepparava, M.G. Behind the Mask: Emotion Recognition in Healthcare Students. *Med. Sci. Educ.* **2021**, 1–5. [CrossRef]
126. Altameem, T.; Altameem, A. Facial expression recognition using human machine interaction and multi-modal visualization analysis for healthcare applications. *Image Vis. Comput.* **2020**, *103*, 104044. [CrossRef]
127. Tacconi, D.; Mayora, O.; Lukowicz, P.; Arnrich, B.; Setz, C.; Tröster, G.; Haring, C. Activity and emotion recognition to support early diagnosis of psychiatric diseases. In Proceedings of the 2nd International Conference on Pervasive Computing Technologies for Healthcare 2008, PervasiveHealth, Tampere, Finland, 30 January–1 February 2008.
128. Rammohan, R.A.; Medikonda, J.; Pothiyil, D.I. Speech Signal-Based Modelling of Basic Emotions to Analyse Compound Emotion: Anxiety. In Proceedings of the 2020 IEEE International Conference on Distributed Computing, VLSI, Electrical Circuits and Robotics, DISCOVER, Udupi, India, 30–31 October 2020; pp. 218–223.

sensors

MDPI

Article

A Personalized Computer-Aided Diagnosis System for Mild Cognitive Impairment (MCI) Using Structural MRI (sMRI)

Fatma El-Zahraa A. El-Gamal [1,2], Mohammed Elmogy [2], Ali Mahmoud [1], Ahmed Shalaby [1], Andrew E. Switala [1], Mohammed Ghazal [3], Hassan Soliman [2], Ahmed Atwan [2], Norah Saleh Alghamdi [4,*], Gregory Neal Barnes [5,†] and Ayman El-Baz [1,†]

1 Bioengineering Department, University of Louisville, Louisville, KY 40292, USA; fatma_zahraa@mans.edu.eg (F.E.-Z.A.E.-G.); ahmahm01@louisville.edu (A.M.); ahmed.shalaby@louisville.edu (A.S.); andy.switala@louisville.edu (A.E.S.); aselba01@louisville.edu (A.E.-B.)
2 Information Technology Department, Faculty of Computers and Information, Mansoura University, Mansoura 35516, Egypt; melmogy@mans.edu.eg (M.E.); hsoliman@mans.edu.eg (H.S.); ahmed.atwan@nbu.edu.sa (A.A.)
3 Department of Electrical and Computer Engineering, Abu Dhabi University, Abu Dhabi 59911, United Arab Emirates; mohammed.ghazal@adu.ac.ae
4 College of Computer and Information Science, Princess Nourah Bint Abdulrahman University, Riyadh 11564, Saudi Arabia
5 Department of Neurology, University of Louisville, Louisville, KY 40292, USA; gregory.barnes@louisville.edu
* Correspondence: NOSAlghamdi@pnu.edu.sa
† Equivalent senior authors.

Citation: El-Gamal, F.E.-Z.A.; Elmogy, M.; Mahmoud, A.; Shalaby, A.; Switala, A.E.; Ghazal, M.; Soliman, H.; Atwan, A.; Alghamdi, N.S.; Barnes, G.N.; et al. A Personalized Computer-Aided Diagnosis System for Mild Cognitive Impairment (MCI) Using Structural MRI (sMRI). *Sensors* **2021**, *21*, 5416. https://doi.org/10.3390/s21165416

Academic Editors: James F. Rusling

Received: 21 June 2021
Accepted: 3 August 2021
Published: 11 August 2021

Abstract: Alzheimer's disease (AD) is a neurodegenerative disorder that targets the central nervous system (CNS). Statistics show that more than five million people in America face this disease. Several factors hinder diagnosis at an early stage, in particular, the divergence of 10–15 years between the onset of the underlying neuropathological changes and patients becoming symptomatic. This study surveyed patients with mild cognitive impairment (MCI), who were at risk of conversion to AD, with a local/regional-based computer-aided diagnosis system. The described system allowed for visualization of the disorder's effect on cerebral cortical regions individually. The CAD system consists of four steps: (1) preprocess the scans and extract the cortex, (2) reconstruct the cortex and extract shape-based features, (3) fuse the extracted features, and (4) perform two levels of diagnosis: cortical region-based followed by global. The experimental results showed an encouraging performance of the proposed system when compared with related work, with a maximum accuracy of 86.30%, specificity 88.33%, and sensitivity 84.88%. Behavioral and cognitive correlations identified brain regions involved in language, executive function/cognition, and memory in MCI subjects, which regions are also involved in the neuropathology of AD.

Keywords: Alzheimer's disease; personalized diagnosis; mild cognitive impairment; computer-aided diagnosis; sMRI

1. Introduction

Alzheimer's disease (AD) is considered the best-known neurodegenerative conditions targeting the central nervous system (CNS). Elderly people make up the preponderance of the sufferers of AD. However, younger people may be affected by early-onset AD [1]. Statistically speaking, disease risk increases with age among the elderly population, with 42% of those diagnosed with AD being 85 years or older, while only 6% of diagnosed cases are between 70 and 74 years old [2].

The characteristics of AD can be broadly grouped into clinical and anatomical features [3]. Features in either category vary from one patient to another. Clinically, AD patients show progressive deficits in cognition and memory in addition to disturbances in thought, perception, and behavior. Pathologically, patients incur a neuronal loss, granulovacuolar degeneration, and the formation of the two definitive diagnostic markers of AD: neurofibrillary tangles and neuritic plaques [4]. Up-regulated expression of the amyloid-β precursor protein (APP) is followed by a cascade of processing involving BACE1, PSEN1, PSEN2, and APH1, resulting in production of amyloid-β peptide, including its pathogenic species Aβ42. The Aβ42 conformations fuse into oligomers containing up to 100 units of Aβ42, and form neurotoxic protofibrils. Aβ42 oligomers itself leads to synaptic loss, neurotoxicity, and neuronal death. Aβ42 oligomers, under the influence of ApoE4, can undergo aggregation and formation of Aβ seniles plaques in affected brain regions [5].

As a neurodegenerative condition, AD is progressive. The severity of affliction is typically divided into three phases, beginning with a mild phase, then proceeding to moderate phase, and ending with severe phase [6]. The emergence of the disease's pathological features 10–15 years before being clinically discovered hinders the early diagnosis of the disease. Furthermore, the subject-dependent influence of AD between its sufferers adds another obstacle to diagnosing the disease in its early stage [4].

Various tests of a patient's mental and physical state can assist in AD diagnosis, including urinalysis, blood panels, and neurological, neuropsychological, psychiatric examinations. The patient's medical history, as well as brain imaging in various modalities, can also inform the diagnosis [1]. Regarding brain imaging, these technologies play a notable role in identifying the disease, specifically speaking in the pre-clinical and MCI phases [7]. Further information about the impact of brain imaging in this research area can be found in the study presented by Johnson et al. [8]. Additionally, a scientific work presented by Jack et al. [9] aimed to illustrate the function of each of the brain biomarkers along the cascade of AD. Relying on the study findings, for the earliest signs of the disease, positron emission tomography (PET) amyloid imaging, as well as cerebrospinal fluid (CSF) levels of amyloid beta (Aβ_{42}), reveal evidence of the underlying Aβ pathology. CSF levels of tau protein, structural magnetic resonance imaging (sMRI), 2-[18F] fluoro-2-deoxy-d-glucose (FDG-PET), and the cognitive and clinical symptoms can help follow patients as pathology accumulates with disease progression. sMRI discloses the structural abnormalities while FDG-PET or CSF-tau reveal neuronal injury and dysfunction.

Previous scientific research has attempted, through several methodologies, to different groups defined by cognitive status (normal control (NC), MCI, or AD) using neuroimaging data. For instance, a computer-assisted diagnostic (CAD) system was presented in [10] to diagnose AD at its earliest phase using independent component analysis (ICA) as well as support vector machines (SVM) for the feature extraction and the classification purposes, respectively. Additionally, a CAD system using Gaussian discriminant analysis was presented in [11] to screen the disease's phases where the features of the entorhinal cortex showed significant discriminatory power between both the normal group (NC) and abnormal group (MCI + AD). Additionally, the study could achieve an improvement regarding the classification performance through defining two separate spaces of the decision, for both hemispheres of the brain (left and right hemispheres), following by combining their obtained result. Beheshti et al. [12] used feature ranking in addition to genetic algorithms (GA) to propose a CAD system that addressed differentiating between NC, stable MCI (sMCI), progressive MCI (pMCI), as well as AD groups. The pMCI group comprises subjects who progressed clinically to the overt AD where their neuropsychological tests have a poorer performance than the NC group.

On the other hand, the sMCI, who either remains in the stable stage or may improve, shows no or marginal neuropsychological changes [13,14]. Zhang et al. [15] addressed the three-way classification problem between the NC, MCI, and AD groups. In this system, the principle analysis is used for feature detection, while the kernel support vector machine decision tree (kSVM-DT) was used for the classification purpose. Then, Zhang et al. [16] used the idea behind the eigenbrains along with the machine learning for building their CAD system. Therefore, Welch's t-test was used to find significant eigenbrain while the prediction task was accomplished using SVM with the implementation of different kernels.

Tong et al. [17] exploited the multiple instance learning (MIL) method to present a system aimed to diagnose both AD and MCI phases. In this system, the extracted features were in the form of local intensity patches. The MIL method was applied to address the case when some patches may not characterize the morphological association with AD because of the variable influence of the disease on these patches. Finally, Westman et al. [18] used orthogonal partial least squares to latent structures (OPLS) analysis to discriminate between the groups of AD through combining local and global volumetric measures obtained from MRI scans.

Despite the achievements mentioned above, there are several notes regarding these achievements that led to making the door still open in front of this research topic, and specifically speaking this AD-related research point (i.e., differentiating between NC and MCI groups). First, the previously mentioned studies addressed either a diagnosis of whole-brain findings consistent with impairment or else considered local, brain region-specific diagnosis while excluding the MCI group. Despite the importance of those researchers' findings in the diagnosis task, targeting the brain-based regional diagnosis might add more advantages due to the disease's subject-dependent influence that could impede the early diagnosis. Furthermore, the local/regional diagnosis can aid in revealing the disease-related ambiguity. Secondly, in general, the diagnosis performance when using sMRI in the AD early stage is fair and still needs more improvements. Due to the literature, the sMRI scans can be used to follow patients as pathology accumulates with disease progression. In contrast, at the early stages, the scan might look normal [9,19]. The aim of this paper is primarily to introduce a system for the local/regional diagnosis, using sMRI technology, for serving the goal of personalized diagnosis of MCI. Therefore, the proposed system studies the impact of MCI locally (i.e., in the term of the local brain regions), specifically speaking its impact on the brain cortical regions. Targeting the cortical regions is due to the essential role of the medical imaging-based measurement of the cerebral cortex's shape, composition, as well as function in the diagnosis of the neurodegenerative conditions and explicitly speaking in diagnosing AD [20–22]. To support the performed cortical regions diagnosis, further analysis of the obtained results has been performed to confirm the fitness of the results with the neurocircuits defined by the National Institute of Mental Health Research Domain Criteria (RDoC). In addition, the paper offers a global diagnosis where the results are promising, as evaluated, in addressing the challenging task of differentiating between the NC and MCI groups primarily through brain structuring features at the early stage of the disease. This paper is organized as follows. Section 2 explains the used material as well as the applied methods. Section 3 presents the evaluation results of the proposed CAD system. Section 4 discusses the obtained findings. In the end, a conclusion of the proposed study is shown in Section 5.

2. Materials and Methods

2.1. Materials

Data from the Alzheimer's Disease Neuroimaging Initiative (ADNI) database (adni.loni.usc.edu, (Last accessed on 1 July 2021)) was used to build the proposed system. ADNI is considered to be a standard database, which was established in 2003 as a public-private partnership under the lead of Michael W. Weiner, MD as a Principal Investigator. The aim behind the ADNI was to evaluate the role of combining serial MRI, PET, or other markers, along with the clinical and neuropsychological assessments, in measuring the evolution of MCI as well as AD. All the data on ADNI are provided for both the informational as well as the review purposes where according to ADNI, the IRB in approved for research use only. In the proposed work, we used 146 baseline sMRI scans of 60 normal plus 86 mildly cognitively impaired subjects, classified in ADNI as being either sMCI or pMCI. Table 1 shows the demographic distribution of the used dataset. As reported by ADNI, the NC participants represent the control subjects who do not show any depression, MCI, or dementia signs. On the other hand, the MCI subjects are the subjects with subjective memory concern that is reported by an informant, a clinician, or oneself. Despite this reported concern, the daily living activities of the MCI participants are basically preserved. The subjects neither show any significant impairment levels in other cognitive domains nor show dementia signs [23]. Please note here that in our paper, we did not focus on differentiating between the sMCI and the pMCI groups. This is due to our ultimate goal of presenting a personalized CAD system of either belonging to the NC or the MCI group without addressing whether the subject will proceed to AD, as in the pMCI group, or will remain stable, as in the sMCI group.

Table 1. Demographic data relating to baseline sMRI scans selected from ADNI. Note: MMSE is the Mini Mental State Examination, and CDR is the Clinical Dementia Rating.

	60 Normal Subject	86 MCI
Age (Mean ± std)	75.49 ± 4.78	73.98 ± 7.72
Gender		
Women	38	33
Men	22	54
MMSE scores	24–30	24–30
CDR	0	0.5

2.2. Methods

This paper aims to present a cortical region-based CAD system to perform the personalized diagnosis of MCI through the framework illustrated in Figure 1. The system begins with preprocessing the scans as well as segmenting the cerebral cortex and parcellating by hemisphere. Second, a triangular mesh reconstruction of the cortical surface is performed using the marching cubes (MC) algorithm. This is followed by the extraction of shape-based features at each node of the cortical mesh. The cortical region-based features are then defined through applying the Automated Anatomical Labeling (AAL) atlas to the reconstructed cortex. Third, a fusion of the obtained features is performed using canonical correlation analysis (CCA) to produce more representative features. Fourth, a two-stage diagnostic classifier is constructed, producing cortical region-specific diagnoses that are combined into a final diagnosis, of the subject's cognitive status.

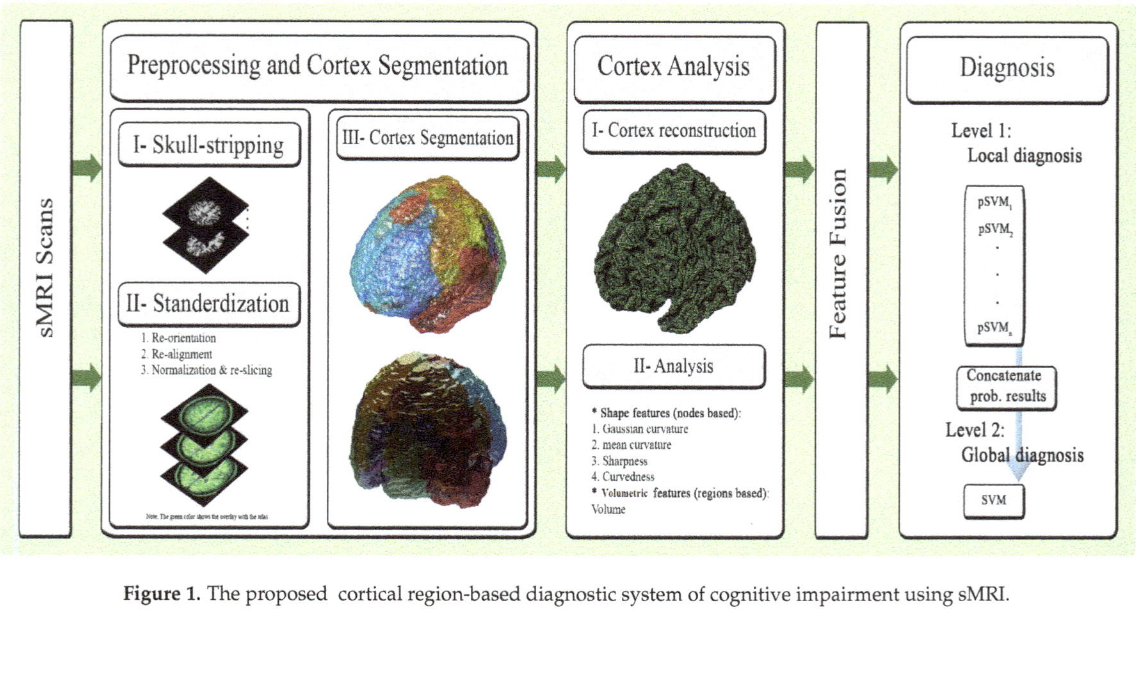

Figure 1. The proposed cortical region-based diagnostic system of cognitive impairment using sMRI.

2.2.1. Preprocessing and Brain Cortex Segmentation

This step serves the cortical regions-based diagnosis goal through standardizing them to the parcellation atlas space. Using the SPM toolbox, images are resampled and re-oriented (if necessary), skull-stripped, aligned, and spatially normalized. Skull stripping in this case had already been performed, so we convolved the sMRI scans with their corresponding brain masks that in turn are provided as part of the ADNI dataset. Then, the orientation of the atlas template's space, MNI space, had been matched with the scans through re-aligning re-orientating, spatial normalize as well as re-slicing the scans. The data were re-sliced and aligned with the MNI-152 standard template. One scan, selected as a reference, was rotated and shifted to align as near as possible to the template, with the line between the anterior and posterior commissures (AC-PC line) of the template and reference aligning exactly. The rest of the scans in the dataset were registered to the chosen reference with a rigid body transformation calculated to optimize the mutual information criterion. The particular choice of reference image is not significant, since all MRI in the ADNI database have roughly the same spatial orientation. Subsequently, the algorithm of Ashburner and Friston [24] was used to register each pre-aligned image precisely with the MNI-152 template using a combination of affine and nonlinear deformations. Figure 2 shows examples of preprocessed scans overlaid on the atlas template [25]. Following this step, segmentation of the cerebral cortex was performed using the xjview MATLAB toolbox.

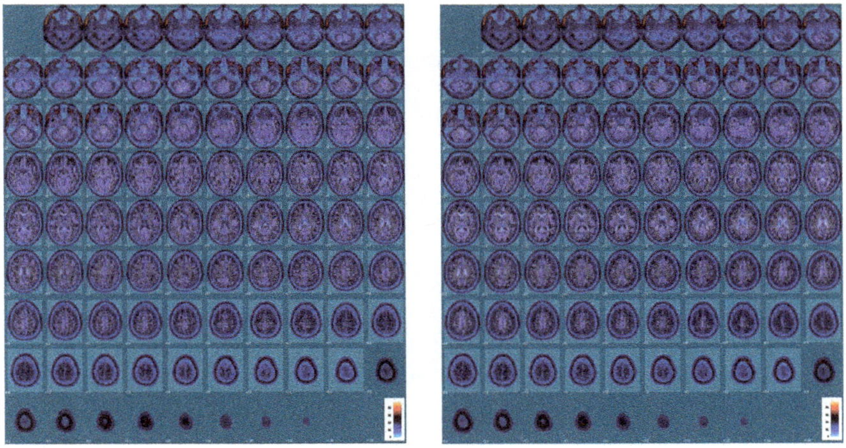

(a) (b)

Figure 2. Example of preprocessed and overlaid subjects' scans with the AAL atlas template from each studied group where (**a**) is for a normal subject, while (**b**) is for a mildly cognitive impairment subject).

2.2.2. Brain Cortex Reconstruction and Analysis

The shape descriptors to be used later by the algorithm depend upon the accurate representation of the cortical surface. Therefore, the MC algorithm is initially used for cortex reconstruction since it is best-known isosurface extraction method and produces high-resolution results [26,27]. Then, having obtained the triangulated mesh representation of the cortical surface, several shape features are calculated at each node individually through Equations (1)–(4) after calculating the principal curvature directions and values. Algorithm 1 summarizes the steps of the MC algorithm as well as the calculation of the principal curvature directions and values while Figure 3 illustrates results of cortical surface reconstruction for both NC and MCI subjects.

Algorithm 1 The MC algorithm and the calculation of the principal curvature directions and values.

Input: The dataset of the scalar volumetric
Output: The directions and values of the principle curvature
Steps:

1. Use the volume lattice for defining the cubes (C_l) in which the corner vertices are defined through the points ($P(x_i, y_j, s_k)$) of the lattice for the column $x_i(\forall_i), y_i(\forall_j)$ and the slice $S_k(\forall_n)$ where n represent the number of the volume slices.
2. Construct, in a sequential form of cube-by-cube manner throughout the rows of the dataset, a fecetized isosurface. In this procedure and when the value of the $V_i \geqslant$ isovalue (α), mark V_i and keep the remaining ones as unmarked. Consequently, the "active" edges are defined as an edge (E_j) ended with a marked vertex ($V_j m$) and an unmarked vertex ($V_j u$). Note: the value of α was calculated through applying the histogram to the labeled volume, remove the large first max value, and obtain the value of a middle bar of non-small values as the α value.
3. Use a look-up table to factorize the interacted isosurface of the intersection topologies in which the linear interpolation is applied for the location estimation of the intersection between the isosurface-edge through:
$$I(x, y, s) = V_{m(x,y,s)} + \rho(V_{u(x,y,s)} - V_{m(x,y,s)})$$
where: $\rho = \frac{\alpha - L_m}{L_u - L_m}$, L_m and L_u are the scalars values V_m as well as V_u, respectively.
4. Through the face and vertex lists of the resulting triangulated mesh and to calculate the principal curvature directions and values, describe the input by XY rather than XYZ through rotating the input so the current vertex's normal becomes [−1 0 0].
5. Fit a patch of the least-squares quadratic to the local neighborhood of a vertex "$f(x, y) = ax^2 + by^2 + cxy + dx + ey + f$".
6. Use the hessian-based eigenvectors and eigenvalues to calculate the principal curvature.

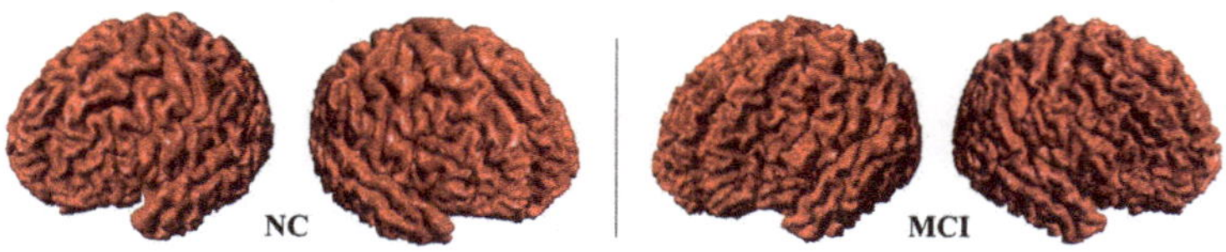

Figure 3. Examples of the marching cubes reconstruction output for normal and mildly cognitively impaired subjects. As shown, although it is not that obvious since it is still the early stage of the disorder, the brain atrophy starts to take place in the MCI case, where this atrophy defines the beginning of losing the neurons and the connections that exist between them.

Please note that the sharpness and curvedness features were used as in [28]. Next, labeling of each of the mesh nodes to its corresponding cortical regions is performed using the AAL atlas, which defines a total of 76 cortical regions. It is important to note here that alternative brain parcellation schemes could be used, as in [15,29,30]. In the proposed system, the AAL atlas was chosen because of its relatively fine granularity. Here, to make sure of the matching between the labels and the surface, the preprocessing steps of the proposed framework were first applied to standardize the scans to the geometry of the atlas template's space, MNI space. Then, converts MNI coordinate to a description of brain structure in AAL atlas using a standard list of the MNI space of the parcellation atlas to label the required brain cortical regions.

$$C_{\text{Gaussian}} = \lambda_1 \lambda_2 \tag{1}$$

$$C_{\text{mean}} = \frac{1}{2}(\lambda_1 + \lambda_2) \tag{2}$$

$$\text{Sharpness} = (\lambda_1 - \lambda_2)^2 \tag{3}$$

$$\text{Curvedness} = \sqrt{(\lambda_1^2 + \lambda_2^2)/2} \tag{4}$$

where λ_1 and λ_2 denote the principal curvatures. Quantities are estimated at the locus of each node of the triangulated surface.

Although grey matter volume has a significant impact in the AD research area, where it is considered to be the most popular cross-sectional quantitative metric [31], the demographic variability between the subjects can bias results. For this reason, the volume is used here in conjunction with the previously obtained features to increase the precision of the results while avoiding this biasing possibility. To calculate the volume: (1) apply the AAL atlas to the to the preprocessed scans to define the cortical regions of the brain, (2) the MC algorithm is applied to reconstruct each region separately, (3) calculate the volume for each of the reconstructed regions separately. By the end of this step, there are a total of five features calculated for each of the 76 brain cortical regions, and they are now ready for the next step of fusion.

2.2.3. Shape Feature Fusion

This step aims to fuse the previously extracted features to produce more informative discriminative features between the tested groups. For this purpose, the CCA-based technique of feature fusion is used due to its role in finding the associations between two sets of variables [32]. Obtaining the linear combinations helps in discovering this association that consequently enlarge the correlation between the two variable sets in the way that presented in Algorithm 2. Here and due to the number of studied features, five features, the CCA technique is implemented sequentially working with two features at a time until ending up with the final fusion-based feature vector for each labeled region. Note, due to the different scales of the extracted features, before fuse the features using the CCA technique, each of the features are normalized to be between 0 and 1 using Equation (5).

$$normFeat = (oldFeat - oldFeat_{min})/(oldFeat_{max} - oldFeat_{min}) \tag{5}$$

Algorithm 2 The algorithm for feature fusion based on CCA technique.

Input: Two matrices of the features, $X \in R^{p \times n}$ and $Y \in R^{q \times n}$, of the extracted $(p+q)$ features for the n samples.
Output: The fused features in the form of matrix.
Steps:

1. Compute the covariance matrix, S, for the two matrices X and Y using:

$$S = \begin{pmatrix} cov(x) & cov(x,y) \\ cov(y,x) & cov(y) \end{pmatrix} = \begin{pmatrix} S_{xx} & S_{xy} \\ S_{yx} & S_{yy} \end{pmatrix}$$

where the $S_{xx} \in R^{p \times p}$ and the $S_{yy} \in R^{q \times q}$ are within-sets matrices of the covariance of the X as well as the Y, respectively. The $S_{xy} \in R^{p \times q}$ is the matrix of the between-set covariance while $S_{yx} = S_{xy}^T$

2. Determine both of the linear combinations X^* and Y^* through using CCA to be able to enlarge the correlations among the matrices X and Y through:

$$corr(X^*, Y^*) = \frac{cov(X^*,Y^*)}{var(X^*).var(Y^*)}$$

where W_x and W_y represent the matrices of the transformation. $cov(X^*, Y^*) = W_x^T S_{xy} W_y$, $var(X^*) = W_x^T S_{xx} W_x$, and $var(Y^*) = W_y^T S_{yy} W_y$. The usage of Lagrange multipliers is to attain the maximization goal by maximizing $cov(X^*, Y^*)$ with a constrain of $var(X^*) = var(Y^*) = 1$.

Algorithm 2 *Cont.*

3. Determine W_x and W_y by:
   (a) Solve the equations of the eigenvalue:

$$S_{xx}^{-1} S_{xy} S_{yy}^{-1} S_{yx} \hat{W}_x = \Delta^2 \hat{W}_x$$

   where $\hat{W}_x$ and $\hat{W}_y$ are the eigenvectors while Δ^2 is the eigenvalues that corresponds to either the diagonal matrix or the canonical correlations square.
   (b) Determine d that represent the overall non-zero eigenvalues in every aforementioned equation, by $d = rank(S_{xy}(n, p, q))$.
   (c) Perform a decreasing order-based sorting operation of the previous step results $\delta_1 \geq \delta_2 \geq \ldots \geq \delta_d$.
   (d) Let the sorted eigenvectors be indicated by W_x and W_y where they consequently represent the non-zero eigenvalues in which X^* and $Y^* \in R^{dn}$ represent the canonical variates.
4. Calculate the sample covariance matrix of the transformed data, S^*, using:

$$S^* = \left[\begin{array}{cccc|cccc} 1 & 0 & \cdots & 0 & \delta_1 & 0 & \cdots & 0 \\ 0 & 1 & \cdots & 0 & 0 & \delta_2 & \cdots & 0 \\ \vdots & & \ddots & \vdots & \vdots & & \ddots & \vdots \\ 0 & 0 & \cdots & 1 & 0 & 0 & \cdots & \delta_d \\ \delta_1 & 0 & \cdots & 0 & 1 & 0 & \cdots & 0 \\ 0 & \delta_2 & \cdots & 0 & 0 & 1 & \cdots & 0 \\ \vdots & & \ddots & \vdots & \vdots & & \ddots & \vdots \\ 0 & 0 & \cdots & \delta_d & 0 & 0 & \cdots & 1 \end{array}\right]$$

Concatenate the features-based transformed vectors to obtain the feature fusion vector through:

$$Z = \begin{pmatrix} X^* \\ Y^* \end{pmatrix} = \begin{pmatrix} W_x^T X \\ W_y^T Y \end{pmatrix} = \begin{pmatrix} W_x & 0 \\ 0 & W_y \end{pmatrix}^T \begin{pmatrix} X \\ Y \end{pmatrix}$$

2.2.4. Diagnosis

The last step of the proposed system is to use the fused features to train the two diagnostic layers: regional and global. For this purpose, a probabilistic SVM (pSVM) support vector machine (pSVM) is used in the first diagnosis layer, where for each anatomical region a separate pSVM is trained to produce a probabilistic measure of association of that particular region's features with MCI. For this purpose, the fusion feature vector produced by the CCA technique was used as an input to the pSVM to produce the final probabilistic regional diagnosis result. Then, a standard SVM is used, in the second layer, where the probabilistic outputs of the first layer are input to it, and the output is the global diagnosis of NC or MCI.

3. Results

The system was trained and tested using the 146 baseline scans, previously mentioned, downloaded from ADNI. For the evaluation process, three types of experiments are performed: (1) evaluating the performance of different SVM kernels, (2) comparing the system's performance results with several some state-of-the-art methods, and (3) validating it with related work.

For testing classifier performance, k-fold cross-validation was applied to compare both the results of the SVM-related kernels, as shown in Figure 4, and our obtained results against some state-of-the-art methods, as shown in Figure 5. Regarding the k-fold cross-validation method, K = 4 and K = 10 were used to verify that the proposed system did not overfit while K = 10 was also used to evaluate the proposed linear-based CAD system with some state-of-the-art classifiers. As illustrated in Figure 4, the linear kernel could, in general, exceeds the overall performance of the other kernels (i.e., polynomial, and radial basis function (RBF) kernels) with the K = 4, and K = 10. For K = 4, the superior results of the linear kernel were around 86.3%, 85%, and 87.2% for the accuracy, specificity, and sensitivity, respectively. For K = 10, these superior results were around 86.3%, 88.33%, and 84.88% of accuracy, specificity, and sensitivity, respectively. Comparing the obtained results, at K = 10, with some other state-of-the-art classifiers (i.e., decision tree, ensemble classifier, and K nearest neighbors (KNN)), Figure 5, also showed that the linear-SVM generally could achieve better results.

Along with these quantitative performance results, an additional investigation has been performed to confirm the fitness of the obtained subjects' cortical regions-based diagnosis results with the neurocircuits defined by the National Institute of Mental Health RDoC. Therefore, Table 2 displays the modest correlations between the behavioral and cognitive data from ADNI and critical brain regions involved in memory and language. Finally, an illustration of different cortical region-based diagnoses is presented in Figure 6 where the disease's severity in each cortical region is represented in color.

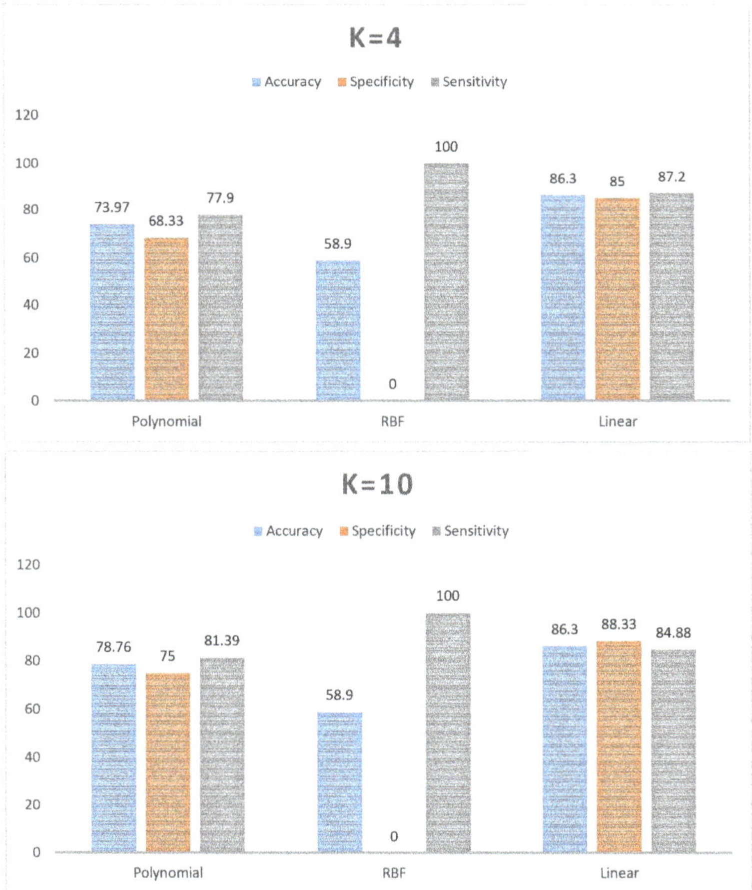

Figure 4. The results of the k-fold validation method in (%) for different SVM-based kernels

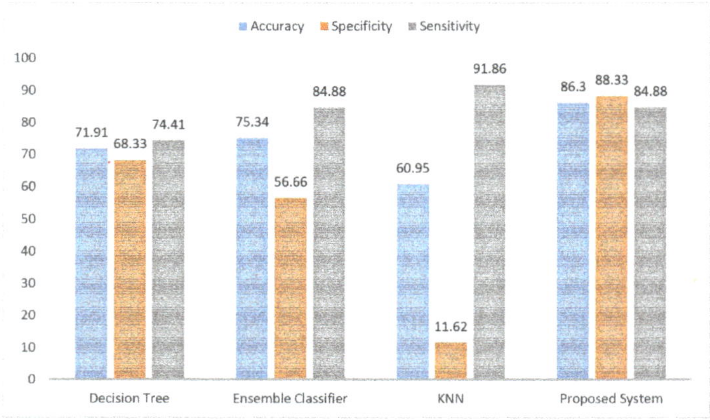

Figure 5. The comparison evaluation of our linear-based CAD system with some state-of-the-art classifiers with k-fold = 10.

Table 2. The person correlation for MRI parameters and distinct behavioral tasks in MCI subjects, where: BNTTOTAL: Total number correct on Boston Naming Test, BNTSPONT: number of spontaneously given correct responses, Partial Score of BNT, TOTAL11 (ADAS): total score on the 11 item cognitive subscale of the Alzheimer's Disease Assessment Scale (ADAS), FAQTOTAL: functional assessment questionnaire total score, CONMCXLA: number of targets hit on ADNI numbers cancellation task.

Brain Region	Behavioral Task	ADNI Category	r-Value	*p*-Value
Right Angular Gyrus	Language	BNTTOTAL	0.37	0.001
Right Angular Gyrus	Language	BNTSPONT	0.36	0.001
Left Angular Gyrus	Language	BNTTOTAL	−0.35	0.002
Left Angular Gyrus	Language	BNTSPONT	−0.37	0.001
Right Middle Cingulum	Language	BNTTOTAL	−0.29	0.010
Right Middle Cingulum	Language	BNTSPONT	−0.31	0.006
Right Inferior Frontal Opercularis	Cognitive	TOTAL11 (ADAS)	−0.32	0.004
Left Parahippocampal Gyrus	Adaptive	FAQTOTAL	−0.30	0.007
Left Parahippocampal Gyrus	Visual Spatial	CONMCXLA	0.30	0.008

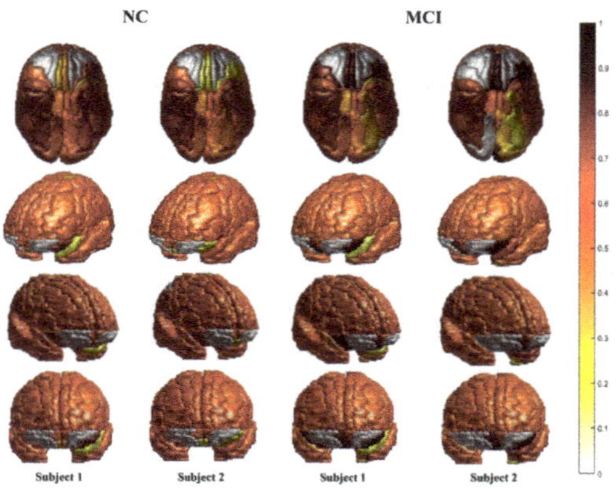

Figure 6. Different examples that show the cortical regions diagnosis for two different normal, and two different mildly cognitive subjects. Note: (1) the color-bar-based gradient colors represent the disease's severity in every studied region separately. (2) The blue arrows show examples of the cortical regions that show significant difference in the probabilistic diagnosis results between the NC and MCI subjects.

4. Discussion

Patients with mild cognitive impairment present with markedly reduced cognitive abilities when compared with unaffected people of the same age, and taking a level of education into account, but without meeting the criteria for dementia. One or more domains of cognition can be influenced by this impairment: memory, executive function, language, skills of the visuospatial domain, or attention. Regardless of the aforementioned impairments, the patients still can accomplish their daily tasks, such as occupational or social functions without confusion [33]. Therefore, MCI is considered to be an intermediate condition between typically seen age-related changes in cognition and dementia [33,34]. Although it is not guaranteed that all MCI cases proceed to AD, suffering from MCI increases the risk factor of ending up with AD [34,35].

To date, sMRI is one of the most developed modalities used for differential pathological diagnosis purposes due to its ability to detect the location and severity of atrophy through showing the detailed description of the soft tissues of the body [36,37]. sMRI can discriminate between tissue types through capturing proton density or magnetization properties (using spin-spin (T2) or spin-lattice (T1) relaxation times). Actually, T1-weighted, as well as T2-weighted images, are used for qualitative assessment that is designed to both differentiate between the tissues with a different relaxation time of T1/T2, and to evaluate the macroscopic lesions as well as tissues changes such as in sulci, cysts and ventricles [38].

Regarding AD, sMRI can, in general, reveals atrophy of the cerebral cortex during the progression of AD. Furthermore, the regions thought to distinguish AD from MCI and normal controls include MRI parameters of the putative earlier involved MCI regions (hippocampus, entorhinal cortex, supramarginal gyrus) vs. earlier involved AD regions (rate of hippocampal atrophy, cingulate cortex, and parietal cortex) [39]. Additionally, the analysis of sMRI helps in uncovering the relationship between both the elevated risks for MCI converting to AD and atrophy where this, in turn, assists in anticipating the future cognitive-based decline in the healthy adults. Additionally, the volumetric-based analysis using sMRI can aid in detecting crucial changes in the brain regions' size that in turn, effectively assist in the diagnosis procedure [40].

According to the literature, the shape, composition, and function of the cerebral cortex as measured by imaging modalities has a crucial role in diagnosing the neurodegenerative conditions, especially in AD [20–22]. Depending on imaging variability and due to the variability of AD effect among its sufferers, the ultimate goal of this paper is to introduce a cortical region-based diagnosis of MCI. Additionally, the paper aims to improve the overall performance of the discrimination between the NC and MCI Group, which is known to be a difficult task, as seen in the related literature.

We introduced a cortical region-based diagnostic system that serves the subject-dependent (i.e., personalized) diagnosis of MCI. Additionally, we target improving the diagnostic performance with respect to the related work. To achieve our goals, and because of the nature of the disease at this early stage, when underlying anatomical changes are subtle, it was necessary to choose high-resolution methods to accomplish this task. Therefore, in the proposed system, the MC algorithm was selected due to its role, as mentioned above in obtaining high-resolution extraction of isosurface results. Then, the shape-based features were addressed to serve the discrimination goal due to the nature of the disease's influence in the brain that could be detected through the sMRI scans. After obtaining these features and to present a more informative feature vector to the diagnosis step, as well as to overcome the biased results that can be obtained using the volume feature, a feature reduction/fusion process was applied. Finally, and based on its powerful role in addressing this type of problems as well as to serve the personalized diagnosis role, standard SVM and its variant, pSVM, was applied to provide two layers, regional followed by global diagnosis.

As previously mentioned, the system's performance has been evaluated from three different perspectives, which are evaluating the performance of different SVM kernels, comparing the obtained performance results with several state-of-the-art methods, and validating the system's performance with related work. Starting with the first evaluation,

Figure 4 shows a comparison of different SVM-related kernels' performance (i.e., polynomial, linear, and RBF) using k-fold cross-validation method, with K = 4, and K = 10 to exclude the possibility of overfitting, As shown in the figure, the linear kernel achieved superior results while the RBF kernel performed most poorly. The results of the linear-SVM reflect the power of the extracted features in providing linear separation between the tested groups. On the other hand, the low results of the nonlinear kernels can be justified as the result of the small dataset size that led to lower performance results of RBF-based SVM compared with the polynomial-based one. Additionally, the power of the extracted features that caused the superior results of the linear-SVM showed, as shown in the results that the RBF kernel failed to find a proper separating decision boundary between the studied groups.

Then, again through using the k-fold cross-validation method and specifically speaking K = 10, we compared the performance of the linear-SVM with some well-known methods (i.e., decision tree, ensemble classifier, and KNN), as presented in Figure 5. Broadly speaking, the linear-SVM showed better performance against the other methods. This indicates the proposed work's ability to deal with this research issue. In general, this better performance can be justified by several reasons. First, the discriminative power of the features that results in better classification performance ability of the linear-SVM to separate between the groups with linear hyperplanes. Second, the performance power of SVM, in general, to deal with high-dimensional space's dataset while this is not the case with other methods. Finally, the efficiency of SVM to deal with a small size of the datasets while other methods can suffer from under-performance results and/or overfitting.

Additionally, validating our system's performance against the literature showed the promise of the proposed work. For instance, in [15] a classification system was built, using the principal component analysis (PCA) kSVM-DT, and could reach a maximum accuracy result of 85%, specificity result of 80%, and sensitivity results of 87%. In [18], the OPLS analysis was used that led to a specificity result of 73% as well as a sensitivity result of 66%. Finally, in [41], an ICA/SVM system was proposed for the classification and could achieve accuracy, specificity, and sensitivity of 70.19%, 67.49%, and 72.89%, respectively. It is noteworthy that the results of the systems above have been obtained from those studies regardless of using different dataset as well as a different number of scans. The idea here is to validate our work against prior work focusing on the same research area.

The modest correlations between ADNI behavioral and cognitive data and brain regions (Table 2) critical to AD, involving memory and language, adds further validation to our approach. (Additional details about the ADNI categories can be found in [42–47].) Furthermore, a survey of statistically significant correlations between ADNI behavioral and cognitive data and brain regions suggest that regions linked to specific deficits in language (15 regions), executive function and cognition (10 regions), adaptive behavior (5 regions), and memory (3 regions) may point to early neuropathology in classic AD-involved regions in MCI subjects. Finally, Figure 6 illustrates some cortical regions-based diagnosis results of different normal as well as mildly cognitive impaired subjects. As shown in the figure, the system can visualize the disease's severity in the cortical regions separately. In turn, this illustration helps the experts to discover any local abnormality and its degree to consequently direct the treatment plans.

5. Conclusions

Among the neurodegenerative conditions, AD is considered one of the leading diseases that affect the CNS, where its main sufferers are elderly people. The principal goal of the presented work is to serve the subject-dependent (i.e., personalized) diagnosis of the MCI, the early phase of AD. This goal is achieved by demonstrating a cortical region-based CAD system that helps visualize the severity of the disease in different local brain regions. Because of the difficulty of addressing the classification task between the normal and the mildly cognitive impaired groups, our system aims to target a more promising performance than in the literature and some state-of-the-art methods. To achieve this purpose, the sMRI has been used where several shape-based features were extracted, and according to the obtained results, could provide powerful assistance in the targeted task. Comparing our system with some state-of-the-art methods and validating it with the related work shows promising results of ours in the studied research area. Therefore, the proposed system can be treated as an assistant tool that provides a highly performed diagnosis through focusing on the crucial related brain regions, cortical regions. Focusing on such areas is vital due to the variable effect of AD in its sufferers that in turn requires presenting different medical services to the sufferers according to the nature of the disease's influence and the degree of this influence in their cortical regions. Besides that, the proposed system can help analyze the disease and uncover the ambiguity surrounding it by providing a finely detailed computer-aided diagnosis system that targets the hardly discriminative early stage of the disease.

For future work, the authors plan to perform further evaluation of the presented diagnostic system with other datasets, improve the system's overall performance, and perform additional analysis processes involving multimodal imaging to enhance the goals in this research area. Additionally, the obtained promising results that in turn helped in proofing the targeted concept of this paper, encourages using the proposed system in addressing another AD-based discrimination task that is between the sMCI and pMCI groups, and evaluating the resulting diagnosis performance for further improvements. Additionally, regarding the surface reconstruction, the authors will try to implement some other reconstruction methods and compare their results with the MC algorithm.

Author Contributions: Conceptualization, F.E.-Z.A.E.-G., M.E., M.G., H.S., A.A., N.S.A., G.N.B. and A.E.-B.; Formal analysis, M.E., A.E.S., N.S.A. and A.E.-B.; Investigation, M.E., G.N.B. and A.E.-B.; Methodology, F.E-Z.E.-G., M.E., A.M., A.S., A.E.S., M.G., H.S., A.A., N.S.A. and A.E.-B.; Project administration, M.G., N.S.A. and A.E.-B.; Software, F.E.-Z.A.E.-G., A.E.S. and A.A.; Supervision, M.E., M.G., H.S., N.S.A., G.N.B. and A.E.-B.; Validation, M.E., M.G., H.S., N.S.A. and G.N.B.; Visualization, F.E.-Z.A.E.-G.; Writing—original draft, F.E.-Z.A.E.-G., M.E., M.G., H.S., A.A., N.S.A., G.N.B. and A.E.-B.; Writing—review and editing, F.E.-Z.A.E.-G., M.E., A.M., A.S., A.E.S., M.G., A.A., N.S.A., G.N.B. and A.E.-B. All authors have read and agreed to the published version of the manuscript.

Funding: This research was funded by the Deanship of Scientific Research at Princess Nourah bint Abdulrahman University through the Fast-track Research Funding Program.

Institutional Review Board Statement: A benchmark dataset, Alzheimer's Disease Neuroimaging Initiative (ADNI), was used to construct the proposed work where the terms of use are declared in the following link: http://adni.loni.usc.edu/terms-of-use/ (accessed on 1 July 2021).

Informed Consent Statement: A benchmark dataset, Alzheimer's Disease Neuroimaging Initiative (ADNI), was used to construct the proposed work where the informed consent has been obtained from the participants. More information can be found in the following link: http://adni.loni.usc.edu/study-design/ (accessed on 1 July 2021).

Data Availability Statement: The used data in this study was obtained from Alzheimer's Disease Neuroimaging Initiative (ADNI). More information regarding ADNI can be obtained from the following link: http://adni.loni.usc.edu/ (accessed on 1 July 2021).

Conflicts of Interest: The authors declare no conflict of interest.

Abbreviations

The following abbreviations are used in this manuscript:

AD	Alzheimer's disease
CNS	central nervous system
APP	amyloid-β precursor protein

BACE1	β secretase 1
PSEN1	presenilin 1
PSEN2	presenilin 2
APH1	anterior pharynxdefective 1
MCI	mild cognitive impairment
PET	positron emission tomography
CSF	cerebrospinal fluid
$A\beta_{42}$	amyloid beta
sMRI	structural magnetic resonance imaging
FDG-PET	2-[18F] fluoro-2-deoxy-d-glucose
NC	normal control
CAD	computer-assisted diagnostic
ICA	independent component analysis
SVM	support vector machines
GA	genetic algorithms
sMCI	stable MCI
pMCI	progressive MCI
kSVM-DT	kernel support vector machine decision tree
MIL	multiple instance learning
OPLS	orthogonal partial least squares to latent structures
RDoC	research domain criteria
ADNI	Alzheimer's disease neuroimaging initiative
MMSE	mini mental state examination
CDR	clinical dementia rating
MC	marching cubes
AAL	automated anatomical labeling
CCA	canonical correlation analysis
MNI	Montreal Neurological Institute
AC-PC	anterior and posterior commissures
pSVM	probabilistic support vector machines
BNTTOTAL	total number correct on Boston Naming Test
BNTSPONT	number of spontaneously given correct responses
ADAS	Alzheimer's Disease Assessment Scale-Cognitive Behavior
FAQTOTAL	functional assessment questionnaire total score
CONMCXLA	number of targets hit on ADNI numbers cancellation task
RBF	radial basis function
KNN	K nearest neighbors
PCA	principal component analysis

References

1. Disease and Dementia. What Is Alzheimer's? 2019. Available online: https://www.alz.org/alzheimers-dementia/what-is-alzheimers/ (accessed on 23 January 2019).
2. Brown, D. *Brain Diseases and Metalloproteins*; Pan Stanford: Singapore, 2013.
3. Jenner, P.; Goate, A.; Ashall, F. *Pathobiology of Alzheimer's Disease*; Elsevier Science: New York, NY, USA, 1995.
4. Gauthier, S. *Clinical Diagnosis and Management of Alzheimer's Disease*; CRC Press: Boca Raton, FL, USA, 2006.
5. Castellani, R.J.; Plascencia-Villa, G.; Perry, G. The amyloid cascade and Alzheimer's disease therapeutics: Theory versus observation. *Lab. Investig.* **2019**, *99*, 958–970. [CrossRef] [PubMed]
6. Kidd-Madison, N. *Alzheimer's Disease: Living with John, Caring for a Love One*; Xlibris US: Bloomington, IN, USA, 2014.
7. Osborn, A.G.; Salzman, K.L.; Jhaveri, M.D.; Barkovich, A.J. *Diagnostic Imaging: Brain E-Book*; Elsevier Health Sciences: Amsterdam, The Netherlands, 2015.
8. Johnson, K.A.; Fox, N.C.; Sperling, R.A.; Klunk, W.E. Brain imaging in Alzheimer disease. *Cold Spring Harb. Perspect. Med.* **2012**, *2*, a006213. [CrossRef]
9. Jack, C.R.; Knopman, D.S.; Jagust, W.J.; Shaw, L.M.; Aisen, P.S.; Weiner, M.W.; Petersen, R.C.; Trojanowski, J.Q. Hypothetical model of dynamic biomarkers of the Alzheimer's pathological cascade. *Lancet Neurol.* **2010**, *9*, 119–128. [CrossRef]
10. Khedher, L.; Illán, I.A.; Górriz, J.M.; Ramírez, J.; Brahim, A.; Meyer-Baese, A. Independent Component Analysis-Support Vector Machine-Based Computer-Aided Diagnosis System for Alzheimer's with Visual Support. *Int. J. Neural Syst.* **2017**, *27*, 1650050. [CrossRef]

11. Fang, C.; Li, C.; Cabrerizo, M.; Barreto, A.; Andrian, J.; Loewenstein, D.; Duara, R.; Adjouadi, M. A Novel Gaussian Discriminant Analysis-based Computer Aided Diagnosis System for Screening Different Stages of Alzheimer. In Proceedings of the 2017 IEEE 17th International Conference on Bioinformatics and Bioengineering (BIBE), Washington, DC, USA, 23–25 October 2017; pp. 279–284.
12. Beheshti, I.; Demirel, H.; Matsuda, H.; Alzheimer's Disease Neuroimaging Initiative. Classification of Alzheimer's disease and prediction of mild cognitive impairment-to-Alzheimer's conversion from structural magnetic resource imaging using feature ranking and a genetic algorithm. *Comput. Biol. Med.* **2017**, *83*, 109–119. [CrossRef]
13. Missonnier, P.; Deiber, M.P.; Gold, G.; Herrmann, F.; Millet, P.; Michon, A.; Fazio-Costa, L.; Ibanez, V.; Giannakopoulos, P. Working memory load-related electroencephalographic parameters can differentiate progressive from stable mild cognitive impairment. *Neuroscience* **2007**, *150*, 346–356. [CrossRef]
14. Wang, P.N.; Liu, H.C.; Lirng, J.F.; Lin, K.N.; Wu, Z.A. Accelerated hippocampal atrophy rates in stable and progressive amnestic mild cognitive impairment. *Psychiatry Res. Neuroimaging* **2009**, *171*, 221–231. [CrossRef]
15. Zhang, Y.; Wang, S.; Dong, Z. Classification of Alzheimer disease based on structural magnetic resonance imaging by kernel support vector machine decision tree. *Prog. Electromagn. Res.* **2014**, *144*, 171–184. [CrossRef]
16. Zhang, Y.; Dong, Z.; Phillips, P.; Wang, S.; Ji, G.; Yang, J.; Yuan, T.F. Detection of subjects and brain regions related to Alzheimer's disease using 3D MRI scans based on eigenbrain and machine learning. *Front. Comput. Neurosci.* **2015**, *9*, 66. [CrossRef]
17. Tong, T.; Wolz, R.; Gao, Q.; Guerrero, R.; Hajnal, J.V.; Rueckert, D. Multiple instance learning for classification of dementia in brain MRI. *Med. Image Anal.* **2014**, *18*, 808–818. [CrossRef] [PubMed]
18. Westman, E.; Simmons, A.; Zhang, Y.; Muehlboeck, J.S.; Tunnard, C.; Liu, Y.; Collins, L.; Evans, A.; Mecocci, P.; Vellas, B.; et al. Multivariate analysis of MRI data for Alzheimer's disease, mild cognitive impairment and healthy controls. *Neuroimage* **2011**, *54*, 1178–1187. [CrossRef]
19. American College of Radiology. Alzheimer's Disease. 2021. Available online: https://www.radiologyinfo.org/en/info/alzheimers (accessed on 19 June 2021).
20. Peters, A.; Morrison, J. *Cerebral Cortex: Neurodegenerative and Age-Related Changes in Structure and Function of Cerebral Cortex*; Springer: Berlin/Heidelberg, Germany, 1999.
21. Cechetto, D.; Weishaupt, N. *The Cerebral Cortex in Neurodegenerative and Neuropsychiatric Disorders: Experimental Approaches to Clinical Issues*; Elsevier Science: Amsterdam, The Netherlands, 2017.
22. Apostolova, L.G.; Thompson, P.M. Mapping progressive brain structural changes in early Alzheimer's disease and mild cognitive impairment. *Neuropsychologia* **2008**, *46*, 1597–1612. [CrossRef]
23. Alzheimer's Disease Neuroimaging Initiative. ADNI | Study Design. 2019. Available online: http://adni.loni.usc.edu/study-design/ (accessed on 22 May 2021).
24. Ashburner, J.; Friston, K.J. Unified segmentation. *Neuroimage* **2005**, *26*, 839–851. [CrossRef]
25. The Wellcome Centre for Human Neuroimaging. SPM12-Statistical Parametric Mapping. Filionuclacuk. 2017. Available online: https://www.fil.ion.ucl.ac.uk/spm/software/spm12/ (accessed on 28 January 201).
26. Hansen, C.; Johnson, C. *Visualization Handbook*; Elsevier Science: Amsterdam, The Netherlands, 2011.
27. Newman, T.S.; Yi, H. A survey of the marching cubes algorithm. *Comput. Graph.* **2006**, *30*, 854–879. [CrossRef]
28. Ismail, M.; Soliman, A.; ElTanboly, A.; Switala, A.; Mahmoud, M.; Khalifa, F.; Gimel'farb, G.; Casanova, M.F.; Keynton, R.; El-Baz, A. Detection of white matter abnormalities in MR brain images for diagnosis of autism in children. In Proceedings of the 2016 IEEE 13th International Symposium on Biomedical Imaging (ISBI), Prague, Czech Republic, 13–16 April 2016; pp. 6–9.
29. Su, S.S.; Chen, K.W.; Huang, Q. Discriminant analysis in the study of Alzheimer's disease using feature extractions and support vector machines in positron emission tomography with 18 F-FDG. *J. Shanghai Jiaotong Univ. (Sci.)* **2014**, *19*, 555–560. [CrossRef]
30. Salas-Gonzalez, D.; Segovia, F.; Martínez-Murcia, F.J.; Lang, E.W.; Gorriz, J.M.; Ramırez, J. An optimal approach for selecting discriminant regions for the diagnosis of Alzheimer's disease. *Curr. Alzheimer Res.* **2016**, *13*, 838–844. [CrossRef]
31. Vemuri, P.; Jack, C.R. Role of structural MRI in Alzheimer's disease. *Alzheimer's Res. Ther.* **2010**, *2*, 23. [CrossRef] [PubMed]
32. Haghighat, M.; Abdel-Mottaleb, M.; Alhalabi, W. Fully automatic face normalization and single sample face recognition in unconstrained environments. *Expert Syst. Appl.* **2016**, *47*, 23–34. [CrossRef]
33. Yaffe, K. *Chronic Medical Disease and Cognitive Aging: Toward a Healthy Body and Brain*; Oxford University Press: Oxford, UK, 2013.
34. Anderson, N.; Murphy, K.; Troyer, A. *Living with Mild Cognitive Impairment: A Guide to Maximizing Brain Health and Reducing Risk of Dementia*; Oxford University Press: Oxford, UK, 2012.
35. Lopez, O.L. Mild cognitive impairment. *Contin. Lifelong Learn. Neurol.* **2013**, *19*, 411–424. [CrossRef] [PubMed]
36. Haidekker, M.A. *Medical Imaging Technology*; Springer: Berlin/Heidelberg, Germany, 2013.
37. Smith, N.B.; Webb, A. *Introduction to Medical Imaging: Physics, Engineering and Clinical Applications*; Cambridge University Press: Cambridge, UK, 2010.
38. Ballabh, P.; Back, S.A. Advances in Neonatal Neurology. *Clin. Perinatol.* **2014**, *41*, xvii–xix. [CrossRef] [PubMed]
39. Leandrou, S.; Petroudi, S.; Kyriacou, P.A.; Reyes-Aldasoro, C.C.; Pattichis, C.S. Quantitative MRI brain studies in mild cognitive impairment and Alzheimer's disease: A methodological review. *IEEE Rev. Biomed. Eng.* **2018**, *11*, 97–111. [CrossRef]
40. Varghese, T.; Sheelakumari, R.; James, J.S.; Mathuranath, P.S. A review of neuroimaging biomarkers of Alzheimer's disease. *Neurol. Asia* **2013**, *18*, 239–248. [PubMed]

41. Khedher, L.; Ramírez, J.; Górriz, J.M.; Brahim, A. Automatic classification of segmented MRI data combining independent component analysis and support vector machines. *Innov. Med. Healthc.* **2015**, *207*, 271–279.
42. Nho, K.; Risacher, S.L.; Crane, P.K.; DeCarli, C.; Glymour, M.M.; Habeck, C.; Kim, S.; Lee, G.J.; Mormino, E.; Mukherjee, S.; et al. Voxel and surface-based topography of memory and executive deficits in mild cognitive impairment and Alzheimer's disease. *Brain Imaging Behav.* **2012**, *6*, 551–567. [CrossRef]
43. Gibbons, L.E.; Carle, A.C.; Mackin, R.S.; Harvey, D.; Mukherjee, S.; Insel, P.; Curtis, S.M.; Mungas, D.; Crane, P.K. A composite score for executive functioning, validated in Alzheimer's Disease Neuroimaging Initiative (ADNI) participants with baseline mild cognitive impairment. *Brain Imaging Behav.* **2012**, *6*, 517–527. [CrossRef] [PubMed]
44. Park, L.Q.; Gross, A.L.; McLaren, D.G.; Pa, J.; Johnson, J.K.; Mitchell, M.; Manly, J.J. Confirmatory factor analysis of the ADNI Neuropsychological Battery. *Brain Imaging Behav.* **2012**, *6*, 528–539. [CrossRef]
45. Ito, K.; Hutmacher, M.; Corrigan, B. Modeling of Functional Assessment Questionnaire (FAQ) as continuous bounded data from the ADNI database. *J. Pharmacokinet. Pharmacodyn.* **2012**, *39*, 601–618. [CrossRef] [PubMed]
46. Mohs, R.C.; Knopman, D.; Petersen, R.C.; Ferris, S.H.; Ernesto, C.; Grundman, M.; Sano, M.; Bieliauskas, L.; Geldmacher, D.; Clark, C.; et al. Development of cognitive instruments for use in clinical trials of antidementia drugs: Additions to the Alzheimer's Disease Assessment Scale that broaden its scope. *Alzheimer Dis. Assoc. Disord.* **1997**, *11*, 13–21. [CrossRef]
47. Battista, P.; Salvatore, C.; Castiglioni, I. Optimizing neuropsychological assessments for cognitive, behavioral, and functional impairment classification: A machine learning study. *Behav. Neurol.* **2017**, *2017*, 1850909. [CrossRef] [PubMed]

sensors

MDPI

Article

An Automated CAD System for Accurate Grading of Uveitis Using Optical Coherence Tomography Images

Sayed Haggag [1], Fahmi Khalifa [2], Hisham Abdeltawab [2], Ahmed Elnakib [2], Mohammed Ghazal [3], Mohamed A. Mohamed [1], Harpal Singh Sandhu [2], Norah Saleh Alghamdi [4] and Ayman El-Baz [2,*]

1 Electronics and Communications Engineering Department, Mansoura University, Mansoura 35516, Egypt; sshaggag@gmail.com (S.H.); mazim12@mans.edu.eg (M.A.M.)
2 Bioengineering Department, University of Louisville, Louisville, KY 40292, USA; fakhal01@louisville.edu (F.K.); hisham.abdeltawab@louisville.edu (H.A.); aaelna02@louisville.edu (A.E.); harpal.sandhu@gmail.com (H.S.S.)
3 Electrical and Computer Engineering Department, Abu Dhabi University, Abu Dhabi 59911, United Arab Emirates; mohammed.ghazal@adu.ac.ae
4 College of Computer and Information Science, Princess Nourah Bint Abdulrahman University, Riyadh 11564, Saudi Arabia; nosalghamdi@pnu.edu.sa
* Correspondence: aselba01@louisville.edu

Abstract: Uveitis is one of the leading causes of severe vision loss that can lead to blindness worldwide. Clinical records show that early and accurate detection of vitreous inflammation can potentially reduce the blindness rate. In this paper, a novel framework is proposed for automatic quantification of the vitreous on optical coherence tomography (OCT) with particular application for use in the grading of vitreous inflammation. The proposed pipeline consists of two stages, vitreous region segmentation followed by a neural network classifier. In the first stage, the vitreous region is automatically segmented using a U-net convolutional neural network (U-CNN). For the input of U-CNN, we utilized three novel image descriptors to account for the visual appearance similarity of the vitreous region and other tissues. Namely, we developed an adaptive appearance-based approach that utilizes a prior shape information, which consisted of a labeled dataset of the manually segmented images. This image descriptor is adaptively updated during segmentation and is integrated with the original greyscale image and a distance map image descriptor to construct an input fused image for the U-net segmentation stage. In the second stage, a fully connected neural network (FCNN) is proposed as a classifier to assess the vitreous inflammation severity. To achieve this task, a novel discriminatory feature of the segmented vitreous region is extracted. Namely, the signal intensities of the vitreous are represented by a cumulative distribution function (CDF). The constructed CDFs are then used to train and test the FCNN classifier for grading (grade from 0 to 3). The performance of the proposed pipeline is evaluated on a dataset of 200 OCT images. Our segmentation approach documented a higher performance than related methods, as evidenced by the Dice coefficient of 0.988 ± 0.01 and Hausdorff distance of 0.0003 mm ± 0.001 mm. On the other hand, the FCNN classification is evidenced by its average accuracy of 86%, which supports the benefits of the proposed pipeline as an aid for early and objective diagnosis of uvea inflammation.

Keywords: U-NET; deep learning; uveitis grading; OCT segmentation

Citation: Haggag, S.; Khalifa, F.; Abdeltawab, H.; Elnakib, A.; Ghazal, M.; Mohamed, M.A.; Sandhu, H.S.; Alghamdi, N.S.; El-Baz, A. An Automated CAD System for Accurate Grading of Uveitis Using Optical Coherence Tomography Images. *Sensors* **2021**, *21*, 5457. https://doi.org/10.3390/s21165457

Academic Editor: Ki H. Chon

Received: 6 July 2021
Accepted: 10 August 2021
Published: 13 August 2021

1. Introduction

In recent years, retinal imaging techniques have been greatly exploited by researchers to detect diseases that may cause vision loss. Particularly, optical coherence tomography (OCT) is a popular noninvasive technique that used for diagnosis and assessment of several retinal and corneal diseases [1,2]. Here, we are interested in vitreous inflammation diagnostic and grading [3]. Developing an accurate grading system for vitreous inflammation severity is clinically essential since the vitreous inflammation is considered an important medical diagnostic sign of uveitis. This paper proposes a fully automated computer aided diagnostic (CAD) system for grading of vitreous inflammation, based on extracting discriminatory features from the segmented vitreous regions of OCT images.

Uveitis [4–6] is generally a group of intraocular inflammatory diseases that may affect the uvea or destroy the eye tissues. It may affect all ages especially 20 to 60 years and it may last for short time (acute) or long time (chronic). It may be caused by diseases occurring in the eye or it can be part of an inflammatory diseases affecting other parts of the body. It may be infectious or autoimmune in origin. Uveitis may be classified more specifically according to the eye region that is affected by the inflammation into four types: (1) anterior uveitis, which refers to the inflammation affecting the anterior chamber of the eye; (2) intermediate uveitis, if the vitreous is affected; (3) posterior uveitis affecting the back of the eye, retina, and choroid; and (4) panuveitis when all eye major parts are affected: The vitreous inflammation grading is an important and critical target since its almost entirely subjective. Vitreal inflammation presents on examination as a haziness of the vitreous because protein and inflammatory cells leak into the vitreous. There are generally 6 grades of inflammation (0, 0.5, 1, 2, 3, 4) (but grade 4 cannot be assessed because it is not possible to get any clear OCT image from it).

In the literature, using deep learning in integration with neural networks can optimize solutions to several complex problems of classification [7]. machine and deep learning techniques show a potential to perform efficient segmentation of medical structures from OCT images and/or the classification and grading of OCT images [8–14]. For example, Pelosini et al. [8] developed a segmentation technique that based on a linear regression model, which has lower performance in pathological scans as compared to normal scans [15]. The computer aided diagnostic system of Eltanboly et al. [9] was designed to identify early signs of diabetic retinopathy; however, preprocessing and complicated computations are required for the segmentation of retina layers. Rossant et al. [13] succeeded to to segment the eight retina layers using a hybrid approach incorporating clustering, filtering, and both random field and active contour models. However, their proposed pipeline failed in segmentation of blurred images. Yazdanpanah et al. [14] used active contour energy minimization along with shape priors to segment retina layers. Of note, this was a very early study in the field of spectral-domain optical coherence tomography (SD-OCT), and worked on scans of rat retina obtained using custom hardware. Also, manual segmentation had to be initialized by the user. Haggag et al. [16] developed an automatic U-net convolutional neural network (U-CNN) for segmentation of the vitreous from OCT scans, where the input OCT images were directly applied to train the U-CNN. Their results showed the potential of using U-CNN to solve the problem of vitreous segmentation, but this technique has failed to segment most of severe inflammation images [16]. However, there are still many challenges to get perfect segmentation or classification in some cases of hardly separable images [8,9,15,16].

In trying to develop an automatic system for quantitative assessment of vitreous inflammation, Invernizzi et al. [17] described the inflammatory cells that appear in OCT scans as a hyper reflective dots. Vitreous haze, which may be indicative of inflammation, is also detectable by observing the variations in brightness of vitreous. Pearse et al. [18] developed an automatic technique to quantify the vitreous signal intensity from OCT scans. However, it has a significant limitation as an automatic system since it depends and needs manual segmentation. Schlegl et al. [19] utilized the U-CNN to develop a full automated pipeline to identify and then quantify the intra-retinal cystoid fluid and subretinal fluids.

Many studies used CNN and U-Net to improve OCT segmentation. Cecilia et al. [20] used a U-Net architecture for delineation of macular edema. This technique has achieved an acceptable accuracy which is evaluated by Dice metric of 0.91. He et al. [21] examined the performance of the U-Net architecture relative to a Random Forest-based approach. Finally, Leyuan et al. [22] identified the OCT layer boundaries by mixing the CNN with a graph based method.

To avoid the aforementioned limitations, the proposed CAD system is divided into two main stages (see Figure 1). The first stage segments the vitreous region using a U-net convolutional neural network aided with using the fused images as a training and testing dataset rather than using the original grayscale images directly in training and testing. The fused images are used as an auxiliary, pre-processing technique. This is followed by a grading stage that is conducted using a machine learning-based classifier into one of five grades (0, 0.5, 1, 2 and 3), where 0 refers to normal vitreous and 3 refers to the worst case of vitreous inflammation. The main contributions of this work are as follows:

- In contrast to [16], where the OCT images were directly applied to train the U-CNN, the first stage of the proposed CAD system trains the U-CNN model using a fused image (FI) dataset, which integrates the information of the original image with a proposed distance map, and a proposed adaptive appearance map (AAP), instead of the direct original images.
- Compared to previous work, the first stage of the proposed CAD system shows superior performance in vitreous segmentation from the OCT images in spite of the great similarity between the vitreous and the background.
- The second stage of the proposed CAD system shows great performance in classification accuracy in spite of the great overlap among the extracted features from the OCT vitreous images.

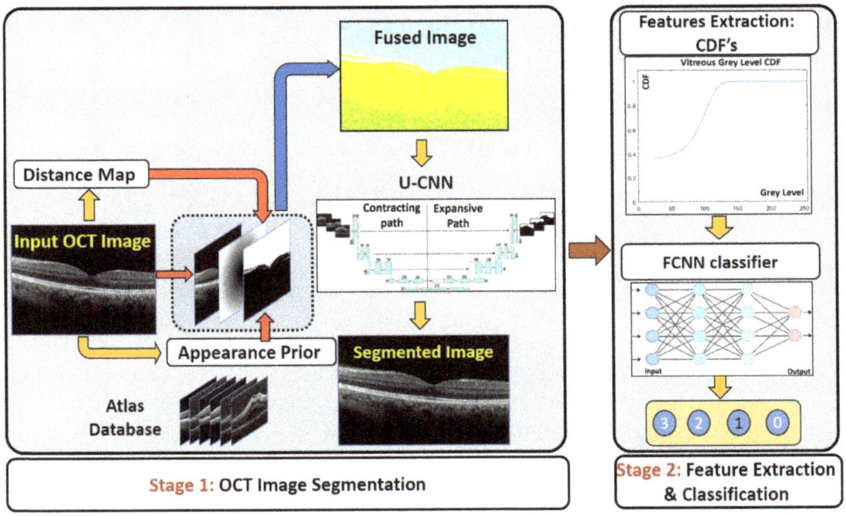

Figure 1. Illustration of the proposed CAD. The first stage is the segmentation stage depending on fused image and U-CNN. The second stage is the classifier to predict the grade of vitreous inflammation severity.

The rest of the paper is organized as follows. Section 2 details the methods used for the framework itself and for evaluating its accuracy in segmentation as well as classification. Section 3 discusses the experimental results and its details. Experimental results will show the potential of the U-CNN training using the proposed FI dataset to significantly improve the segmentation performance, evidenced by the obtained higher Dice similarity coefficient (DC) metric and the lower Hausdorff distance (HD). The results of vitreous inflammation grading using FCNN is also reported. Finally, Section 4 concludes the paper.

2. Materials and Methods

We developed a CAD system for accurate grading of vitreous inflammation from OCT images. The proposed pipeline is composed of two main stages. The first stage is to segment the vitreous region to simplify the processing in the next stage, i.e., grading of the inflammation severity. In our analysis, the total number of used images is 200 OCT of five different grades of severity (grades "0" through "3"). The details of each stage are described in the following subsections.

2.1. Segmentation Stage

The first stage of the CAD system is to extract the vitreous region from the images to be ready for accurate grading in the next stage. The segmentation stage is composed of two processes: the construction of a fused image and the application of the U-net CNN. The details of each are described as follows.

2.1.1. Construction of the Fused Image

Due to the similar visual appearance of the vitreous region and other tissues in the background, our pipeline extract different image descriptors from the OCT image to guide the U-CNN segmentation. The extracted image features are integrated with the original OCT intensity image to construct a three-layer image (called the fused image as shown in Figure 1) that is then used for CNN training and testing. The first layer of the fused image consists of the original grayscale OCT image. Since the vitreous region is typically located in the upper part of a given OCT image, we added in the second layer a distance-based image descriptor. Namely, the second layer is represented by a distance map for each image pixel with respect to the center of the image. It is measured from the center to encounter the possible rotation of incoming images.

In addition to the grayscale values and the distance-based image descriptor, we also incorporate a learned appearance prior. An adaptive probabilistic map is constructed for each input image to be segmented, using an atlas database. The atlas consists of grayscale OCT data sets (with their respective labels) from different subjects. The labeled data were obtained by manual delineation of the vitreous region by an OCT expert. During the testing phase, the specific appearance prior, $\mathbf{G}_i; i = 1, 2, \cdots N$, of an input grayscale image is constructed using the visual appearances of both the atlas grayscale images and their labeled images. A sliding window with a variable width (in our experiment below we start from 11×11 pixels) is centered at each pixel location in turn within the image to be segmented. The gray level g at each pixel location is noted, and an associated probability is computed from the atlas at the corresponding location. To effect this, the system first collects all grayscale values in the interval $[g - \Delta, g + \Delta]$ within the sliding window across all atlas OCT, along with their corresponding labels. Here Δ is a tunable threshold value that can be varied from 5 to 90. Then the probability assigned to the pixel location is $P = \frac{N_x}{N_t}$ where N_t is the total number of pixels within the given spatial and grayscale bounds, and N_x is the number of such pixels that are labeled as vitreous. This process is repeated for all pixel locations in a given image. The whole operation is repeated to compute the probability map for each test and training OCT image.

2.1.2. U-Net Segmentation

The second stage of our segmentation pipeline is the U-net CNN, shown in Figure 2. The input to the network is a fused image as constructed above. The U-CNN is composed of two consecutive paths, The first is a contracting path, similar in structure to image classification systems where the fused data are reduced in size and distilled into a set of feature information. The second path is an expansive and up-convolutional network to increase the spatial dimensions and adds context from the second path. Each consecutive block in U-CNN consists of a convolution layer followed by ReLU-activation functions and max pooling process.

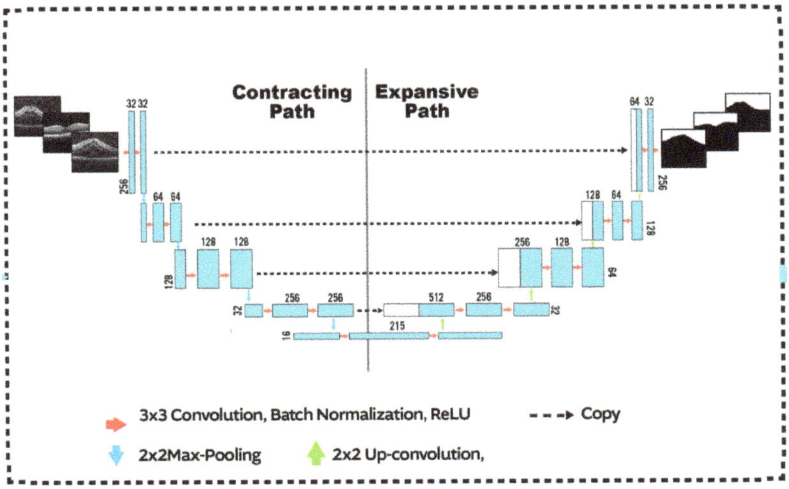

Figure 2. U-CNN structure: The input is a fused image of size 256 × 256 produced as shown in Figure 1. The segmented output has the same dimensions as the input. Convolution (with a 3 × 3 kernel), max-pooling, up-convolution operations are respectively indicted using the blue, red, and green arrows. The max-pooling (up-convolution) operation decreases (increases) the spatial dimensions by a factor of 2. The first path starts with 32 kernels and increases up to 512, where it decreases from 512 to 1 in the second. Zero-padding is employed at the boundaries. Copied contextual information afrom the contracting branch are concatenated to the expansive path (dashed arrows).

The architecture of the contracting or down-sampling section, which increases the number of feature maps, comprises several steps of convolution. Each convolutional block performs two steps of filtering with 3 × 3 kernels, having unit stride in x and y directions and ReLU activation functions. Finally, a 2 × 2 max-pooling is applied at the end of each block. The architecture of the up sampling section is similar to the down sampling section albeit in reversed order as shown.

A sigmoid layer is used at the network output to generate the probabilistic map. Finally, the bipolar cross entropy (BCE) loss function is applied to the network output through training mode, which is computed as

$$L_{BCE} = \sum_{i=1}^{M} -(T_{oi} \log(P_{oi}) + T_{bi} \log(P_{bi})) \quad (1)$$

where P_{oi}, and P_{bi}, are the predicted probabilities, computed from the U-net, that a given pixel i should be assigned to the vitreous or background segments, respectively. While, T_{oi} (T_{bi}) is the ground truth label, i.e., obtained from manual segmentation map, "1" for the object and "0" for the other tissues (vice versa for T_{bi}).

2.2. Grading Stage

Following the segmentation, the cumulative distribution function (CDF) of grayscale intensities within the segmented region is constructed for each image. These CDF's are used as the discriminatory features in our machine learning classifier.

For grading, we used a fully connected neural network to classify the vitreous region inflammation into one of five grades (0, 0.5, 1,2 and 3). '0' represents the normal eye '3' is the is most sever. The FCNN consists of an input layer, 5-nodes output layer, and two hidden layers. The input layer is chosen to be 50 nodes. Each CDF contains 256 points the last 70 points are truncated because all of them is ones and will not discriminate between the different severity degrees. The reminder points are 186 which are used as discriminatory features.

2.3. Performance Metrics

Among many different metrics of accuracy, we used the Dice Coefficient of similarity (DC) to measure the accuracy through out the stages of the proposed CAD. Also, we used the Hausdorff Distance (HD) metric to gauge the proximity of the boundary of segmented vitreous to its ground truth counterpart. Let **G** and **S** denote the sets of pixels labeled as vitreous in ground truth segmentation and machine segmentation, respectively. The DC metric is defined as follows [23]

$$DC = \frac{2 * TP}{2 * TP + FN + FP} \quad (2)$$

where TP is the cardinality of the intersection of **S** and **G**, $FP = |\mathbf{S} - \mathbf{G}|$, and $FN = |\mathbf{G} - \mathbf{S}|$. Another performance metric is the Hausdorff distance (HD) that measures the dissimilarity between the boundaries of ground truth and model segmentation. The HD from **G** to **S** is defined as the maximum Euclidean distance $d(g,s)$ between the points g from **G** and their closest points s in **S**:

$$HD_{\mathbf{G}\to\mathbf{S}} = \max_{g \epsilon G}\{\min_{s \epsilon S}\{d(g,s)\}\} \quad (3)$$

Note the asymmetry, in that $HD_{\mathbf{G}\to\mathbf{S}} \neq HD_{\mathbf{S}\to\mathbf{G}}$ in general. It is easy to define a symmetric version, bidirectional Hausdorff distance $BHD_{\mathbf{G}\to\mathbf{S}} = max\{HD_{\mathbf{G}\to\mathbf{S}}, HD_{\mathbf{S}\to\mathbf{G}}\}$. In order to reduce sensitivity to noise, a further modification is made, replacing the max operation in Equation (3) with taking the 95th percentile.

For the inflammation grading stage evaluation, we computed the average accuracy for all classified grades by the FCNN [24].

$$AverageAccuracy = \sum_{i=1}^{N} \frac{TP_i + TN_i}{TP_i + FN_i + FP_i} \quad (4)$$

3. Experimental Results and Discussions

3.1. Data Set

The proposed CAD system was applied and tested on 200 OCT images of eyes with different degrees of uveitis severity (0, 0.5, 1, 2, and 3). Sample of all applied inflammation grades and their corresponding segmentation are shown in Figure 3. Imaging was performed with a Spectralis spectral-domain optical coherence tomography (SD-OCT) machine (Heidelberg, Germany) having 4 micron axial resolution and 6 mm $\times$ 6 mm in-plane resolution. The rasters comprise thirty horizontal B-scans acquired in order from superior macula to the inferior macula. The entire field of view spans about 20° in both the nasal-temporal and inferior-superior directions, centered on the fovea. Imaging protocol ensured that at least 3 mm of posterior vitreous was visible. The scans that are used in the analysis are selected such that the central horizontal B scan passes through the fovea.

These images were identified using patient database from the uveitis service at the University of Louisville. After the uveitis specialist identified images of patients with uveitis, the images themselves were de-identified for the purpose of analysis. After that, two ophthalmologists graded every image, an attending ophthalmologist with subspecialty expertise and a uveitis fellow (i.e., a fully trained general ophthalmologist who was then undergoing additional subspecialty training in uveitis). They further set together to provide one diagnosis.

The dataset is organized such that 20 images were selected randomly to construct the atlas. The dimensions of the CNN input layer is 256 $\times$ 256, so the images are scaled from its original dimensions of 400 $\times$ 474 to 256 $\times$ 256 to fit the CNN input dimensions. For training and testing, the remainder of the OCT images were partitioned into four groups in order to perform fourfold cross-validation. The accuracy metrics reported are the the average of fourfold results.

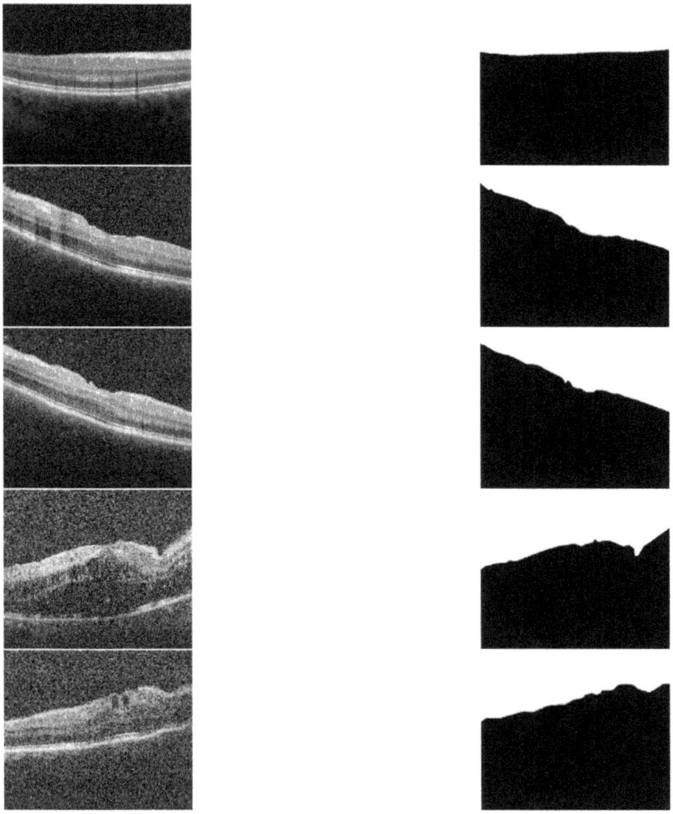

Figure 3. Sample of different grades and their segmentation results. First column (up–to–down) represents the grades 0, 0.5, 1, 2 and 3. The second column represents the corresponding segmentation results, respectively.

3.2. Fused Image Construction

Using original gray level images directly in training U-CNN as in [16] results in high accuracy in testing mode but for normal eyes or eyes with low or moderate vitreous haze. But in severe eyes, the vitreous region is very similar to other tissues and hence U-CNN performance is not acceptable. The results of segmentation have many artifacts in either vitreous (false positive) or in other tissues (false negative). To overcome this problem, we propose using the fused images in training and testing rather than the original gray level. The fused image, as explained in Section 2, consists of three layers, original gray level, distance map and appearance prior map (AP). To extract the AP map, an atlas is constructed from 20, randomly selected images that contains all grades of vitreous inflammation. Two parameters control the construction of the atlas which are sliding window width, and Δ. Sliding window is selected on average as 11×11 pixels.

The choice of the Δ value has greatly affected the segmentation results. To optimize the value of Δ, many experiments are carried out by different values of Δ. These values range from 5 up to 90. Each time, a complete dataset is produced, trained and tested on the proposed U-Net. Dice similarity and HD are computed for the testing set results. The results are summarized in Figure 4. As shown in the two graphs, it is clear that $\Delta = 25$ results in the optimal performance. Considering the average of DC or HD in each experiment, there is no perceptible difference. But considering all the testing set, the segmentation is performed with almost equal quality at this optimal value of Δ.

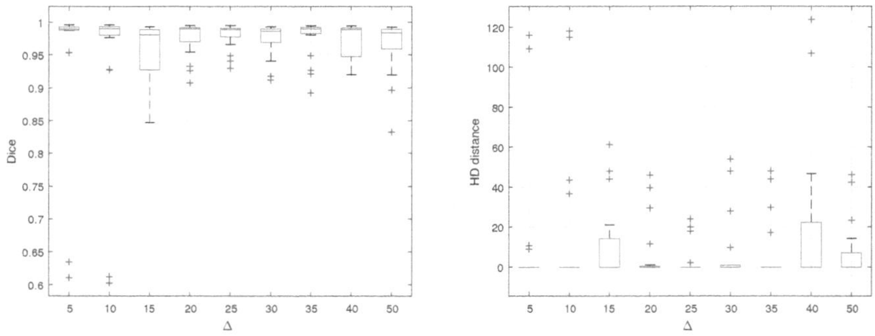

Figure 4. Effect of changing delta on segmentation accuracy evaluated by computing DC and HD distance for different empirically selected values.

3.3. Overall Segmentation Evaluation

To demonstrate the accuracy of our approach in the segmentation stage, some representative results are presented in Figures 5 and 6. As demonstrated in from Figure 5, it can be readily seen that the segmentation results have very high accuracy (DC = 0.99) despite the variations in vitreous inflammation degree, which is related to the contrast of the image. In the first row of Figure 5, the image is clear and the contrast between the object and non-object regions is easily spreadable. Although, in the second row, the image has low contrast, the accuracy of the segmentation is nearly the same as that of the first row.

Despite the fact that the selected images in Figure 6 (first row) have low contrast with high similarity between object and non-object regions, our approach has succeeded to segment the vitreous region with high accuracy. The DC for these images ranges from 0.961 to 0.978, which is acceptable but lower accuracy compared to the group of images in Figure 5. However, by visual inspection, the difference between the ground truth (yellow contour) and our system segmentation (green contour) in the first row of Figure 6 is not significant because the region in the middle of the retina is completely unclear. So, the difference between the two contours in the middle region is just a difference between the interpolation capability of two different techniques trying to predict the unclear region. The second row in Figure 6 contains the same images in the first row that with contours resulted from the previous technique. Also, we can confirm that, the high noise in the presented images proves the high efficiency of the proposed technique. Adaptive shape model has highly succeeded to reduce the effect of this noise by selecting proper values of Δ and/or the sliding window size.

To highlight the advantage of the proposed segmentation technique, we compare its performance with segmentation obtained from the previous technique that only utilizes OCT grayscale images [16]. Sample of the compared results are demonstrated in Figure 6 and the summary of the accuracy is given in Table 1. Statistical comparison between the current and previous segmentation methods was carried out using the two-sample Student's t-test. The obtained p-values (shown in Table 1) illustrate that there is a statistically significant difference (p-value ≤ 0.05) of the two methods.

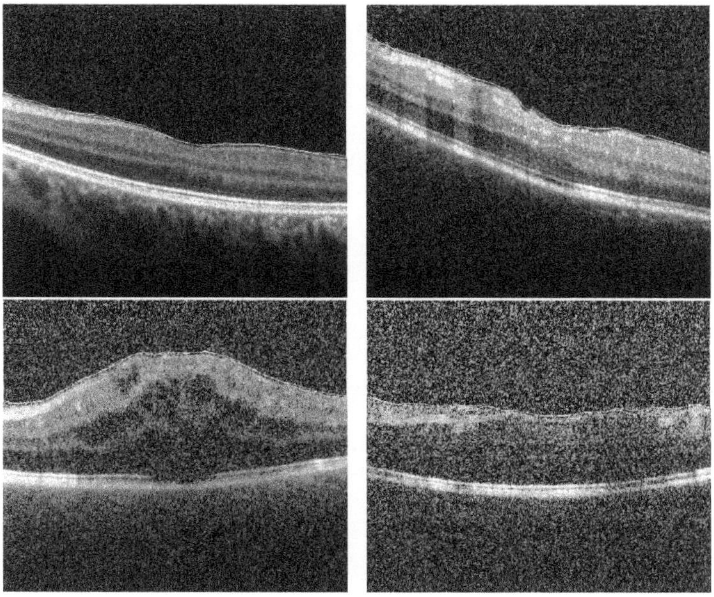

Figure 5. Sample of high accuracy segmentation. The first row represents grayscale images with high contrast, and the second row represents low contrast images with higher degree of vitreous inflammation. Green and yellow colors represents the ground truth and the CNN segmented respectively.

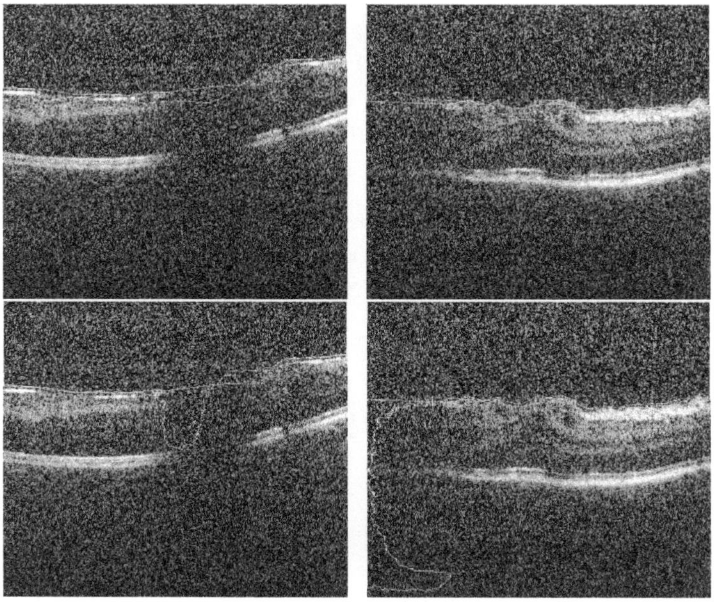

Figure 6. Sample of segmented images of our proposed approach (first row) compared with previous results using only U-Net [16] (second row). The green and yellow colors represents the ground truth and the CNN-segmented respectively.

3.4. Ablation Study

We added here an ablation study for the first stage, segmentation stage, to confirm the validation of our proposal. This study is divided into 2 sections. In the first one, the appearance prior map (AP) is replaced by the gray level in the fused images (FI). That is, the FI contains the distance map and 2 layers of gray level. A fixed number of epochs is maintained in all experiments to justify the results. However about 75% of images is segmented with acceptable accuracy, there are 25% of images still have errors. Sample of images for segmentation is added here to show this effect. In Figure 7 there are some artifacts in the background (FP) due to the similarity of this region in retina with vitreous region (left image). Also, in right image, there are some artifacts in vitreous (FN). These types of errors confirm the importance of the added AP layer to discriminate between the vitreous and the similar tissues in background.

The second section in the ablation study concerns the effect of removing the distance map from the FI images. The FI images contains the AP map in one layer and 2 layers contain the gray level. In this experiment, about 80% of testing images are segmented with acceptable accuracy. On the other hand, 20% have different types of errors. Sample of results are shown in Figure 8 and in Figure 9 to explain the importance of adding the distance map in our proposal. It is noted that, for limited number of training epochs (above 20 and less than 35) the results of segmentation are acceptable with average DC = 97 $\pm$ 2.1%, and the errors of segmentation are limited but still exists. Sample is shown in Figure 8. In trying to improve the accuracy by increasing the number of training epochs, greater errors appear as shown in Figure 9. It is clear that the AP map as well as the distance map increase the stability in training phase, which in turn results in ability to attain high accuracy even in those images of high level of haze.

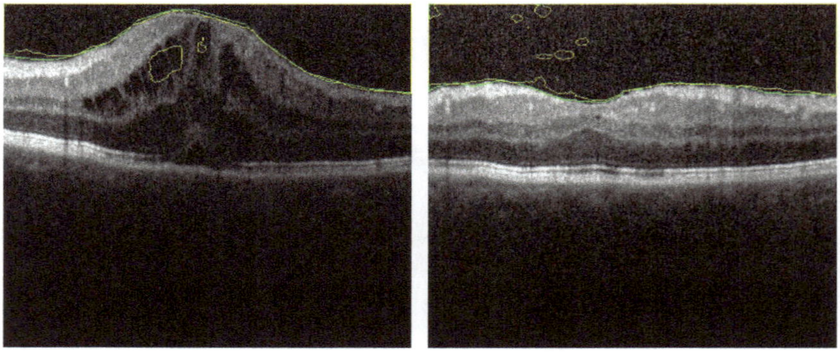

Figure 7. Segmentation sample when AP map is removed from fused images. There are artifacts in both retina layers (**left image**) and vitreous region (**right image**). These artifacts are removed when using the FI as described.

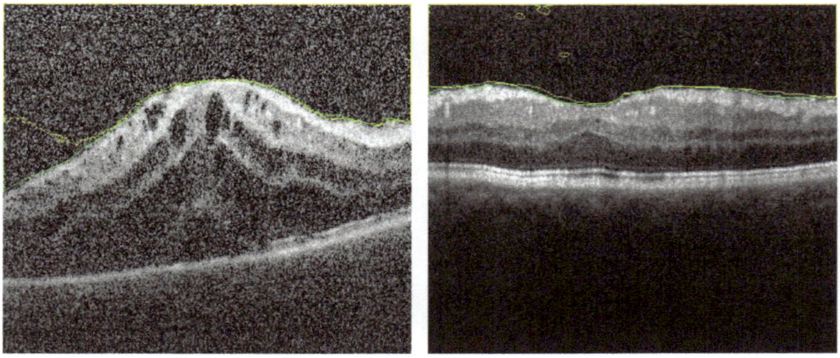

Figure 8. Segmentation sample when distance map is removed from fused images. Number of training epochs is limited. There are some artifacts which are removed when using the FI as described.

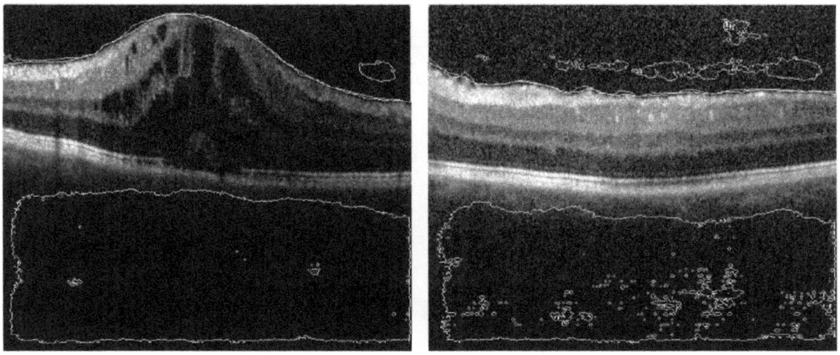

Figure 9. Segmentation sample when distance map is removed from fused images but with greater number of training epochs. There are large segmentation errors.

Table 1. Segmentation accuracy comparison of the proposed approach and the previous technique based on U-CNN only [16], using both area and distance-based metrics.

Metrics	This Paper	Haggag et al. [16]	p-Value
DC (%)	98.8 ± 1.03	94.0 ± 13.0	$\leq$0.0001
HD_{95} (mm)	0.0003 ± 0.001	0.0360 ± 0.086	$\leq$0.0001

3.5. Grading Stage

Following the segmentation stage, the cumulative distribution function (CDF) of gray scale intensity within the segmented region is constructed for each image of the dataset. The images are categorized into 5 classes according to the vitreous inflammation severity degree as (0, 0.5, 1, 2, 3) grades. Where '0' represents the normal eyes and '3' represents the most severe vitreous inflammation eyes as shown in Figure 3.

In classification process, we carried out many trials with different machine learning techniques to find the most suitable technique for this problem by computing the accuracy in each experiment. The most superior results were from, one hidden layer, fully connected neural networks (FCNN) and from support vector machine (SVM). The highest attained accuracy in SVM trials was 70.1%, and in FCNN trials was 73%. The other techniques results are limited to 53%. The best choice is to improve either SVM or FCNN.

The proposed improvement for SVM is to use two level classifier. In the first level, the image is classified as group I or group II: group I has 0 grade, while group II has grades 0.5, 1, 2, and 3. The second stage will discriminate group II into one of the other 4 grades. This technique has greatly improved the accuracy of grading up to 80%. For FCNN, the accuracy is greatly improved by using 2 hidden layers instead of one. Many experiments are carried out with different number of nodes in each layer and the final average accuracy of 86% is obtained.These results the are summarized in Table 2. Depending on the reported results, we selected to use the FCNN as the second stage of the proposed CAD system. A confusion matrix for the testing phase of FCNN results is shown in Figure 10 to clarify the performance of the FCNN in classification of vitreous inflammation grades.

Table 2. Grading accuracy comparison of the proposed approach compared with two-level classifier. Here, FCNN and SVM stand for fully connected neural network and support vector machine, respectively.

Metrics	FCNN	Two-Level SVM Classifier
Accuracy (%)	86.0 ± 1.0	80.0 ± 1.0

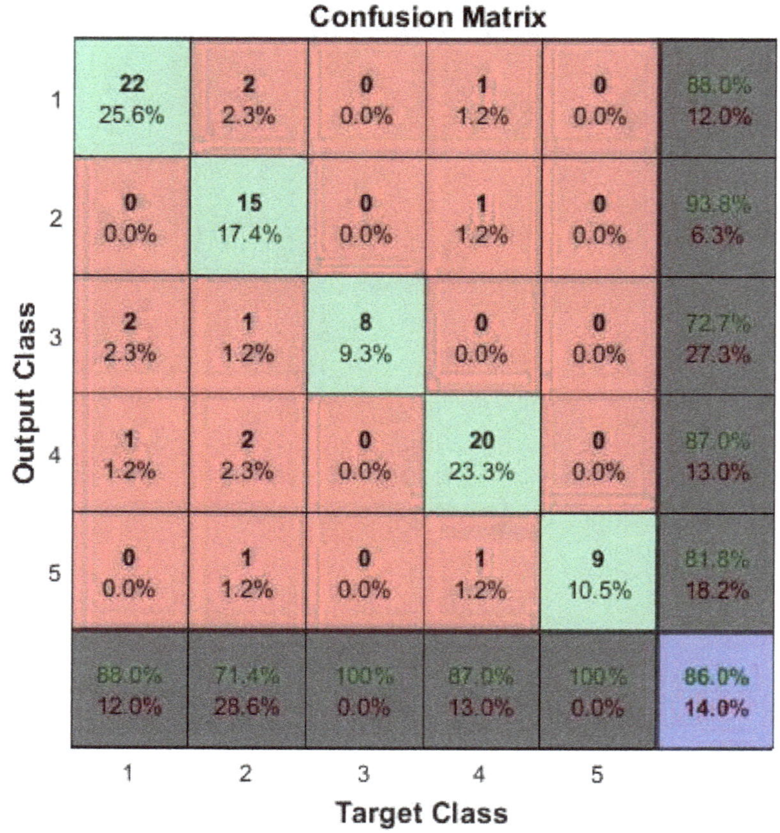

Figure 10. Confusion matrix for the grading details. The classes 1, 2, 3, 4 and 5 correspond to the grades 0, 0.5, 1, 2 and 3 respectively.

4. Conclusions

This paper has introduced a CAD system for vitreous inflammation automatic grading using OCT images. The proposed pipeline is based on a deep learning segmentation approach to extract the vitreous region. Vitreous inflammation severity is assessed by a Fully connected neural network classifier using the CDF of the uveitis intensity which computed from the segmented vitreous. The overall diagnostic accuracy of the proposed pipeline, evaluated using 200 OCT images, supports the benefits of our CAD system as an aid for early and objective diagnosis of uveitis. The proposed technique has proved very high accuracy in the segmentation section depending on the proposed fused images as an input to U-CNN rather than the traditional grey level images. This advantage can be attributed to the integration of appearance prior and distance map with the grey level image. By using this technique, the computational cost is greatly decreased in segmentation process as a result of the great reduction in the number of needed training epochs. One limitation in the grading stage is the very high similarity between the vitreous appearance in different inflammation degrees. This similarity has greatly limited the average accuracy of grading to 86%. In future work, we hope to use more features and to increase the number of images in the data set to improve this value of accuracy.

Author Contributions: Conceptualization, S.H., F.K., H.A., A.E., M.G., M.A.M., H.S.S., N.S.A. and A.E.-B.; Formal analysis, F.K., A.E., H.S.S., N.S.A. and A.E.-B.; Investigation, S.H., F.K., A.E., M.G., M.A.M. and H.S.S.; Methodology, S.H., F.K., H.A., A.E., M.G., N.S.A. and A.E.-B.; Project administration, A.E.-B.; Software, S.H., H.A. and M.A.M.; Supervision, F.K., A.E., M.G., N.S.A. and A.E.-B.; Validation, S.H., A.E. and H.S.S.; Visualization, S.H. and A.E.-B.; Writing—original draft, S.H., F.K., A.E., M.G., M.A.M., H.S.S., N.S.A. and A.E.-B.; Writing—review & editing, S.H., F.K., A.E., M.G., H.S.S., N.S.A. and A.E.-B. All authors have read and agreed to the published version of the manuscript.

Funding: This research was funded by the Deanship of Scientific Research at Princess Nourah bint Abdulrahman University through the Fast-track Research Funding Program.

Institutional Review Board Statement: The study was conducted according to the guidelines of the Declaration of Helsinki, and approved by the Institutional Review Board (protocol code 18.12.389 and date of approval 15 December 2018).

Informed Consent Statement: Informed consent was obtained from all subjects involved in the study.

Data Availability Statement: Data could be made available after acceptance upon a reasonable request to the corresponding author.

Conflicts of Interest: The authors declare no conflict of interest.

References

1. Park, J.; Lee, K.P.; Kim, H.; Park, S.; Wijesinghe, R.E.; Lee, J.; Han, S.; Lee, S.; Kim, P.; Cho, D.W.; et al. Biocompatibility evaluation of bioprinted decellularized collagen sheet implanted in vivo cornea using swept-source optical coherence tomography. *J. Biophotonics* **2019**, *12*, e201900098. [CrossRef] [PubMed]
2. Wijesinghe, R.E.; Park, K.; Kim, P.; Oh, J.; Kim, S.W.; Kim, K.; Kim, B.M.; Jeon, M.; Kim, J. Optically deviated focusing method based high-speed SD-OCT for in vivo retinal clinical applications. *Opt. Rev.* **2016**, *23*, 307–315. [CrossRef]
3. Huang, D.; Swanson, E.A.; Lin, C.P.; Schuman, J.S.; Stinson, W.G.; Chang, W.; Hee, M.R.; Flotte, T.; Gregory, K.; Puliafito, C.A.; et al. Optical coherence tomography. *Science* **1991**, *254*, 1178–1181. [CrossRef] [PubMed]
4. Barisani-Asenbauer, T.; Maca, S.M.; Mejdoubi, L.; Emminger, W.; Machold, K.; Auer, H. Uveitis-a rare disease often associated with systemic diseases and infections-a systematic review of 2619 patients. *Orphanet J. Rare Dis.* **2012**, *7*, 1–7. [CrossRef] [PubMed]
5. Miserocchi, E.; Fogliato, G.; Modorati, G.; Bandello, F. Review on the worldwide epidemiology of uveitis. *Eur. J. Ophthalmol.* **2013**, *23*, 705–717. [CrossRef] [PubMed]
6. Chang, J.H.M.; Wakefield, D. Uveitis: A global perspective. *Ocul. Immunol. Inflamm.* **2002**, *10*, 263–279. [CrossRef] [PubMed]
7. Khan, M.; Silva, B.N.; Han, K. Efficiently processing big data in real-time employing deep learning algorithms. In *Deep Learning and Neural Networks: Concepts, Methodologies, Tools, and Applications*; IGI Global: Hershey, PA, USA, 2020; pp. 1344–1357.
8. Pelosini, L.; Hull, C.C.; Boyce, J.F.; McHugh, D.; Stanford, M.R.; Marshall, J. Optical coherence tomography may be used to predict visual acuity in patients with macular edema. *Investig. Ophthalmol. Vis. Sci.* **2011**, *52*, 2741–2748. [CrossRef] [PubMed]
9. ElTanboly, A.; Ismail, M.; Shalaby, A.; Switala, A.; El-Baz, A.; Schaal, S.; Gimel'farb, G.; El-Azab, M. A computer-aided diagnostic system for detecting diabetic retinopathy in optical coherence tomography images. *Med. Phys.* **2017**, *44*, 914–923. [CrossRef] [PubMed]
10. Wang, Y.; Zhang, Y.; Yao, Z.; Zhao, R.; Zhou, F. Machine learning based detection of age-related macular degeneration (AMD) and diabetic macular edema (DME) from optical coherence tomography (OCT) images. *Biomed. Opt. Express* **2016**, *7*, 4928–4940. [CrossRef] [PubMed]
11. Murugeswari, S.; Sukanesh, R. Investigations of severity level measurements for diabetic macular oedema using machine learning algorithms. *Ir. J. Med. Sci.* **2017**, *186*, 929–938. [CrossRef] [PubMed]
12. Miri, M.S.; Abràmoff, M.D.; Kwon, Y.H.; Sonka, M.; Garvin, M.K. A machine-learning graph-based approach for 3D segmentation of Bruch's membrane opening from glaucomatous SD-OCT volumes. *Med. Image Anal.* **2017**, *39*, 206–217. [CrossRef] [PubMed]
13. Rossant, F.; Ghorbel, I.; Bloch, I.; Paques, M.; Tick, S. Automated segmentation of retinal layers in OCT imaging and derived ophthalmic measures. In Proceedings of the 2009 IEEE International Symposium on Biomedical Imaging: From Nano to Macro, Boston, MA, USA, 28 June–1 July 2009; pp. 1370–1373.
14. Yazdanpanah, A.; Hamarneh, G.; Smith, B.R.; Sarunic, M.V. Segmentation of intra-retinal layers from optical coherence tomography images using an active contour approach. *IEEE Trans. Med. Imaging* **2010**, *30*, 484–496. [CrossRef] [PubMed]
15. Wu, J.; Waldstein, S.M.; Montuoro, A.; Gerendas, B.S.; Langs, G.; Schmidt-Erfurth, U. Automated fovea detection in spectral domain optical coherence tomography scans of exudative macular disease. *Int. J. Biomed. Imaging* **2016**, *2016*, 7468953. [CrossRef] [PubMed]
16. Hagagg, S.; Khalifa, F.; Abdeltawab, H.; Elnakib, A.; Abdelazim, M.; Ghazal, M.; Sandhu, H.; El-Baz, A. A CNN-Based Framework for Automatic Vitreous Segemntation from OCT Images. In Proceedings of the 2019 IEEE International Conference on Imaging Systems and Techniques (IST), Abu Dhabi, United Arab Emirates, 8–10 Decemer 2019; pp. 1–5.

17. Invernizzi, A.; Cozzi, M.; Staurenghi, G. Optical coherence tomography and optical coherence tomography angiography in uveitis: A review. *Clin. Exp. Ophthalmol.* **2019**, *47*, 357–371. [CrossRef] [PubMed]
18. Keane, P.A.; Balaskas, K.; Sim, D.A.; Aman, K.; Denniston, A.K.; Aslam, T.; EQUATOR Study Group. Automated analysis of vitreous inflammation using spectral-domain optical coherence tomography. *Transl. Vis. Sci. Technol.* **2015**, *4*, 4. [CrossRef] [PubMed]
19. Schlegl, T.; Waldstein, S.M.; Bogunovic, H.; Endstraßer, F.; Sadeghipour, A.; Philip, A.M.; Podkowinski, D.; Gerendas, B.S.; Langs, G.; Schmidt-Erfurth, U. Fully automated detection and quantification of macular fluid in OCT using deep learning. *Ophthalmology* **2018**, *125*, 549–558. [CrossRef] [PubMed]
20. Lee, C.S.; Tyring, A.J.; Deruyter, N.P.; Wu, Y.; Rokem, A.; Lee, A.Y. Deep-learning based, automated segmentation of macular edema in optical coherence tomography. *Biomed. Opt. Express* **2017**, *8*, 3440–3448. [CrossRef] [PubMed]
21. He, Y.; Carass, A.; Yun, Y.; Zhao, C.; Jedynak, B.M.; Solomon, S.D.; Saidha, S.; Calabresi, P.A.; Prince, J.L. Towards topological correct segmentation of macular OCT from cascaded FCNs. In *Fetal, Infant and Ophthalmic Medical Image Analysis*; Springer: Berlin/Heidelberg, Germany, 2017; pp. 202–209
22. Fang, L.; Cunefare, D.; Wang, C.; Guymer, R.H.; Li, S.; Farsiu, S. Automatic segmentation of nine retinal layer boundaries in OCT images of non-exudative AMD patients using deep learning and graph search. *Biomed. Opt. Express* **2017**, *8*, 2732–2744. [CrossRef] [PubMed]
23. Babalola, K.O.; Patenaude, B.; Aljabar, P.; Schnabel, J.; Kennedy, D.; Crum, W.; Smith, S.; Cootes, T.; Jenkinson, M.; Rueckert, D. An evaluation of four automatic methods of segmenting the subcortical structures in the brain. *Neuroimage* **2009**, *47*, 1435–1447. [CrossRef] [PubMed]
24. Hossin, M.; Sulaiman, M. A review on evaluation metrics for data classification evaluations. *Int. J. Data Min. Knowl. Manag. Process* **2015**, *5*, 1.

sensors

MDPI

Article

Precise Segmentation of COVID-19 Infected Lung from CT Images Based on Adaptive First-Order Appearance Model with Morphological/Anatomical Constraints

Ahmed Sharafeldeen [1], Mohamed Elsharkawy [1], Norah Saleh Alghamdi [2,*], Ahmed Soliman [1] and Ayman El-Baz [1,*]

[1] BioImaging Laboratory, Department of Bioengineering, University of Louisville, Louisville, KY 40292, USA; a.sharafeldeen@louisville.edu (A.S.); mohamed.elsharkawy@louisville.edu (M.E.); ahmed.soliman@louisville.edu (A.S.)

[2] College of Computer and Information Science, Princess Nourah Bint Abdulrahman University, Riyadh 11564, Saudi Arabia

* Correspondence: nosalghamdi@pnu.edu.sa (N.S.A.); aselba01@louisville.edu (A.E.-B.)

Abstract: A new segmentation technique is introduced for delineating the lung region in 3D computed tomography (CT) images. To accurately model the distribution of Hounsfield scale values within both chest and lung regions, a new probabilistic model is developed that depends on a linear combination of Gaussian (LCG). Moreover, we modified the conventional expectation-maximization (EM) algorithm to be run in a sequential way to estimate both the dominant Gaussian components (one for the lung region and one for the chest region) and the subdominant Gaussian components, which are used to refine the final estimated joint density. To estimate the marginal density from the mixed density, a modified k-means clustering approach is employed to classify the Gaussian subdominant components to determine which components belong properly to a lung and which components belong to a chest. The initial segmentation, based on the LCG-model, is then refined by the imposition of 3D morphological constraints based on a 3D Markov–Gibbs random field (MGRF) with analytically estimated potentials. The proposed approach was tested on CT data from 32 coronavirus disease 2019 (COVID-19) patients. Segmentation quality was quantitatively evaluated using four metrics: *Dice similarity coefficient (DSC)*, *overlap coefficient*, *95th-percentile bidirectional Hausdorff distance (BHD)*, and *absolute lung volume difference (ALVD)*, and it achieved $95.67_{\pm 1.83}\%$, $91.76_{\pm 3.29}\%$, $4.86_{\pm 5.01}$, and $2.93_{\pm 2.39}$, respectively. The reported results showed the capability of the proposed approach to accurately segment healthy lung tissues in addition to pathological lung tissues caused by COVID-19, outperforming four current, state-of-the-art deep learning-based lung segmentation approaches.

Keywords: computed tomography (CT); lung; chest; segmentation; COVID-19

Citation: Sharafeldeen, A.; Elsharkawy, M.; Alghamdi, N.S.; Soliman, A.; El-Baz, A. Precise Segmentation of COVID-19 Infected Lung from CT Images Based on Adaptive First-Order Appearance Model with Morphological/Anatomical Constraints. *Sensors* **2021**, *21*, 5482. https://doi.org/10.3390/s21165482

Academic Editor: Yu-Dong Zhang

Received: 11 June 2021
Accepted: 10 August 2021
Published: 14 August 2021

1. Introduction

Pulmonary diseases are serious public heath threats that may happen after having inflammation or fluid accumulation in the lung, causing a respiratory failure, such as coronavirus disease 2019 (COVID-19). The primary reason for COVID-19 death is acute respiratory distress syndrome (ARDS) [1]. According to Gupta et al. [2], 83.9% of the COVID-19 patients in their study needed a mechanical ventilation support, of whom 87.95% had ARDS. Therefore, detection and diagnosis of COVID-19 grades is vital to prioritize patient's need for ventilator support. The accuracy attainable by computer-aided diagnostic (CAD) system using lung imaging data for COVID-19 depends on how accurate the segmentation is. Accurate lung segmentation is a challenging task as different pathologies affect the appearance of the lung, and if the infected regions are missed during the segmentation, it will affect the entire task. Therefore, this paper focuses on developing an automatic system to detect and segment the lungs in chest computed tomography (CT), which is one of the popular noninvasive clinical modalities used by physicians to diagnose lung pathologies.

In the last few years, many preliminary studies have been conducted to detect and segment lung as well as pathological lesions. Some of these studies [3–9] proposed threshold-based approaches for lung segmentation, which performed well on normal CT scans but failed in pathological cases, especially severe cases, whereas lungs in the normal CT scan can be discriminated easily from background due to huge differences in attenuation [10]. Therefore, to overcome this problem, more recent studies employed texture, shapes, deep learning, or hybrid techniques to accurately segment normal and different lung pathologies. These studies are briefly discussed below.

In [11–14], authors considered texture analysis, shape analysis, or both of them in their system to discriminate between objects. A recent study by Oulefki et al. [15] proposed a system to automatically segment COVID-19 lung infected region by applying a multi-level entropy-based threshold approach, namely a modified Kapur method. Their system achieved a sensitivity, specificity, Dice similarity coefficient (DSC), and precision of 73.3%, 99.4%, 71.4%, and 73.9%, respectively. Another study by Korfiatis et al. [16] employed k-means clustering to partition CT voxels into four classes: lung, muscle, fat, and bone based on intensity values. After that, the initial lung region was extracted by applying a filling operation. Finally, a support vector machine (SVM) was used to determine the final border of the lung based on intensity and wavelet-based descriptors. In [17], authors proposed a segmentation system by eliminating unwanted regions and segmenting lung initially using a threshold approach. Moreover, a 3D gray-level co-occurrence matrix (GLCM) was constructed for a window of size $15 \times 15 \times 15$ centered on each voxel. Then, predefined features were extracted from the GLCM, and a new image was constructed, being the product of the entropy and the inverse difference moment of the GLCM. Subsequently, the abnormal regions were identified from the constructed image using a threshold approach. Finally, the later and initial segmentation were merged together to determine the final segmentation. Dehmeshki et al. [18] used a genetic algorithm (GA) to construct a system to identify spherical nodules within CT images. First, the lung was segmented using adaptive thresholding. Then, the authors utilized a geometric feature, namely, volumetric shape index (VSI), for the segmented lung as a weighted factor in the fitness function of GA. VSI of a spherical object is 1, while that of a cylindrical object is 0.75, so the values of fitness function for nodules were higher than for blood vessels. Convergence criteria of GA to select the shape as a nodule was a threshold-based. The detection rate of their system was approximately 90% with a 14.6 false positive per scan. Moreover, Nakagomi [19] presented a min-cut graph segmentation algorithm based on multiple shapes and prior information of neighbors structure to detect and segment lung infected by pleural effusion. In [20], authors presented a lung segmentation system for different lung pathologies. Their system first determined two seed points within both lungs using a thresholding approach, then a fuzzy connectedness (FC) algorithm was used to extract the lung. Furthermore, multiple refinement stages based on machine learning classification and neighboring anatomy-guided learning mechanisms were included in their system to detect pathological regions during FC segmentation. A recent study by Houssein et al. [21] developed a segmentation system that employed a heuristic method, called manta ray foraging optimization (MRFO), based on an opposition-based learning (OBL), using Otsu's method as a fitness function, to get the best threshold values using COVID-19 CT images. More information about texture- and shape-based lung segmentation can be found in [22].

Recently, deep learning approaches have been employed to segment normal as well as pathological lung caused by COVID-19. For example, Saood et al. [23] investigated two deep learning approaches to semantically segment infected/non-infected lung using CT images. These included SegNet [24] and U-Net [25] networks. The author employed these networks for binary and multi-class classification. They conducted multiple experiments with different hyperparameters. The best reported results for the binary (multi-class) classification gave accuracy of $95.4_{\pm 2.9}$% ($90.7_{\pm 6}$%) and $94.9_{\pm 4.3}$% ($90.8_{\pm 6.5}$%) using SegNet and U-Net, respectively. A similar study [26] proposed a segmentation system using a convolution neural network (CNN). Their network employed feature variation block to enhance the efficiency of feature representation as well as progressive atrous spatial pyramid pooling to deal with appearance and shape differences caused by sophisticated infection. The DSC (sensitivity, specificity) of their system was 72.6% (75.1%, 72.6%) and 98.7% (98.6%, 99%) for COVID-19 infections and normal lung CT images, respectively. A multi-task deep learning-based system was implemented by Amyar et al. [27]. This study included reconstruction for better feature representation; segmentation to extract lesion regions; and classification to categorize the scan into normal, COVID-19, and other diseases. Their system employed encoder-decoder architecture based on U-Net network which used a common encoder for the three tasks. The best reported DSC of their segmentation task was 88%. Recent study by Fan et al. [28] developed a binary and multi-class segmentation system using CT chest images, called Inf-Net. This system was mainly based on a deep learning. Moreover, to compensate the limited number of labeled images, they included a random sampling-based semi-supervised learning, namely, Semi-Inf-Net. Their system employed edge attention as well as reverse attention to improve the feature representation by modeling lung boundaries. In addition, high-level features were exploited by their network and combined by a parallel partial decoder. The performance of their infection segmentation system achieved a DSC of 68.2% and 73.9%, sensitivity of 69.2% and 72.5%, and specificity of 94.3% and 96% using Inf-Net and Semi-Inf-Net, respectively. A similar study [29] proposed an automatic deep learning-based multi-class segmentation system of COVID-19 using CT chest images. The latter exploited aggregated residual transformations in addition to soft attention mechanism to better represent the features and to increase the system's ability to distinguish between different COVID-19 lesions. The reported DSC (accuracy, precision) of their system was 94% (89%, 95%) and 83% (79%, 82%) with and without data augmentation, respectively. Another study [30] proposed a semi-supervised deep learning-based segmentation system, called FSS-2019-nCov, to detect lesion infection in COVID-19 patients. The latter was based on encoder–decoder architecture with Res2Net [31] encoder backbone. In the proposed encoder–decoder architecture, the authors used a context enrichment module, namely, smoothed atrous convolution block and the multi-scale pyramid pooling block, to overcome any debilitation occurred in the represented knowledge generated in the encoder phase. This system was consisted of three modules: conditioner path, adaptive interaction module, and segmentation path. Conditioner path was responsible to learn feature maps from support sets which contain CT slice and its ground-truth. Subsequently, these feature maps were transmitted to the segmentation path using adaptive interaction module which was responsible for detecting lesion in the CT slice. The performance of their system achieved a DSC of 79.8%, sensitivity of 80.3%, and specificity of 98.6%. In [32], the authors employed V-Net [33] to segment lung in COVID-19 CT images that was refined by a shape deformation module. A similar study by Li et al. [34] employed U-Net to segment lung on CT images. Then, they proposed a deep learning network, called COVNet, with a ResNet-50 [35] backbone to detect COVID-19 lesions. A recent study [36] developed a deep learning-based segmentation system, called LungINFseg, to detect COVID-19 lesions in CT images. This system was built on the basis of encoder–decoder architecture. The authors employed a 2D discrete wavelet transform (DWT) with four Haar filters and a receptive field aware (RFA) module in the encoder phase, which were able to change the size of receptive field, to capture more relevant features related to infected regions. Their system achieved a DSC and intersection over union (IoU) score of 80.34% and 68.77%, respectively. Other studies have also employed deep learning as a segmentation system with varying accuracy as reported in [36–43].

Segmentation techniques for CT data using deep learning method consider the current, state-of-the-art approaches. However, they have some drawbacks in practical applications, such as the need for huge databases to learn the different pathology of the lung regions which makes the training of such network is very high computational [44]. Moreover, segmentation approaches based on deformable models, which optimize a trade-off between smoothness of the deformable boundary and homogeneity of the region inside the boundary, suffer from high computational complexity and limited capabilities when the desired boundary has concavities or encompasses a region that is naturally inhomogeneous, such as infected lung regions. To overcome the aforementioned limitations, we are proposing an unsupervised lung segmentation approach that is based on modeling the first-order appearance model of CT data by using a probabilistic model based on a linear combination of Gaussian (LCG) that estimates dominant components, corresponding to lung and chest regions, as well as subdominant components. Subsequently, these subdominant components are clustered to one of the dominant components for marginal density estimation. This model can capture the variability in the Hounsfield distributions that may come from changing the screening protocols and severity of lung infections. Finally, we refine the lung segmentation by applying 3D morphological constraints based on the Markov–Gibbs random field (MGRF) model with analytical parameter estimations.

2. Methods

A fully automated segmentation framework is presented to extract both healthy lung tissues as well as pathological lung tissues that may be caused by COVID-19. The major steps of the framework, depicted in Figure 1, are as follows: (i) preprocessing 3D chest CT scans to identify background voxels; (ii) modeling the gray-level distribution of the CT data as a Gaussian mixture model with parameters estimated using a novel, sequential, expectation-maximization (EM)-based approach; (iii) preliminary segmentation of the lung region based on the use of a Bayes classifier; and (iv) refining the segmentation using a three-dimensional, rotation- and translation-invariant MGRF to impose morphological constraint. Below, we will describe the details of each step.

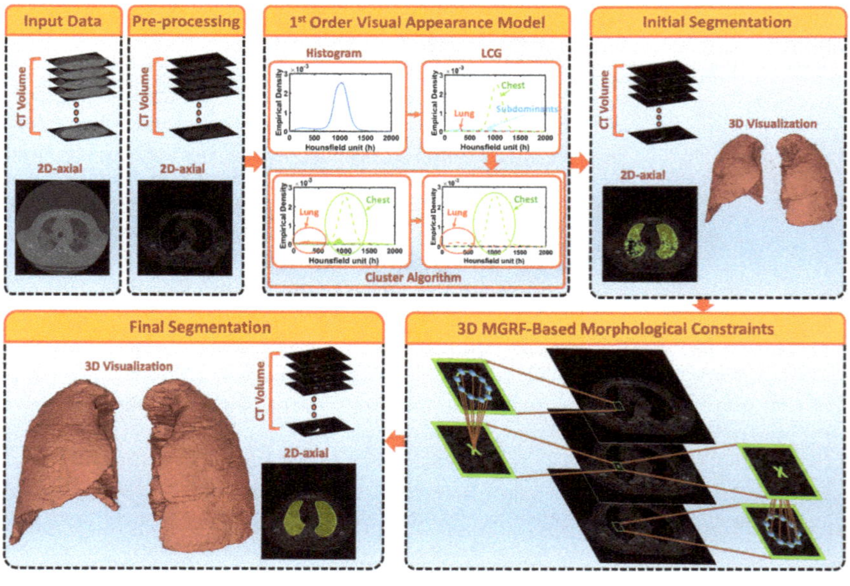

Figure 1. Schematic illustration of the pipeline of the proposed segmentation system using CT images.

2.1. First-Order Visual Appearance Model

The ultimate goal is accurate labeling of voxels as belonging to lung tissue or background, where accuracy is defined as close agreement with "ground-truth" lung region delineated by a radiologist. The main challenge in modeling the distribution of the radiodensities (in Hounsfield units) of lung and chest tissues, i.e., the relative frequency histogram of CT voxel values, is dependent upon slice thickness and the severity of lung infection as shown in Figure 2.

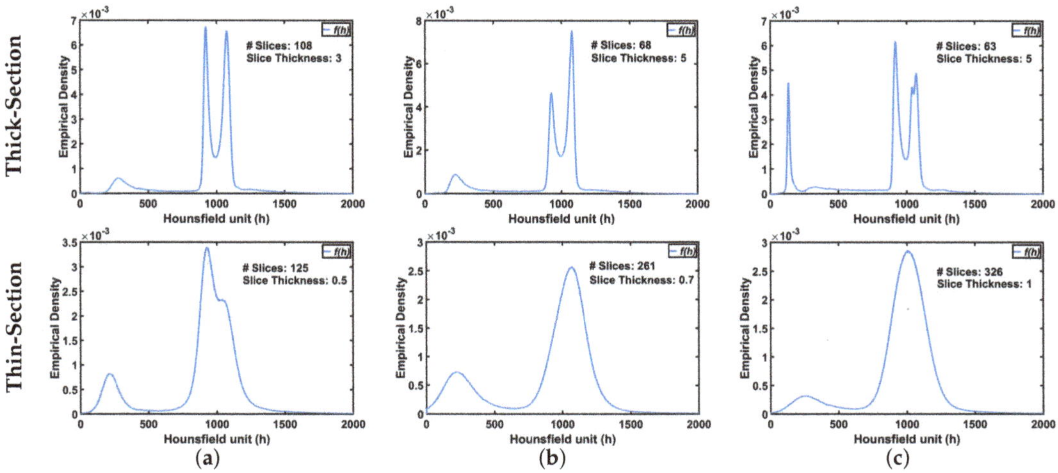

Figure 2. An illustrative example of variability of CT appearance (distribution of radiodensities) for (**a**) healthy/mild, (**b**) moderate, and (**c**) severe COVID-19 infections.

To address this challenge, we will assume that the first-order visual appearance model of the CT data (**H**) can be modeled with linear combination of Gaussian distributions with $K \geq 2$ components [45]. The first two components, called the dominant modes, corresponding to the lung region ($k = 1$) and the chest region exterior to the lungs ($k = 2$). The remaining Gaussian components $k = 3, \ldots, K$ are called subdominant modes. Thus, the proposed probabilistic model is

$$p(h) = w_1\varphi(h;\theta_1) + w_2\varphi(h;\theta_2) + \sum_{k=3}^{K} w_k\varphi(h;\theta_k), \tag{1}$$

where the $w_k > 0$ are mixing weights, and φ is a Gaussian density with parameters $\theta_k = (\mu_k, \sigma_k)$. In order for $p(h)$ to be a density function, the weights must satisfy the constraint

$$\sum_{k=1}^{K} w_k = 1. \tag{2}$$

Given the number K of Gaussian components, the $3K$ parameters of Equation (1), including mixing weights $\mathbf{W}$ and means and variances $\boldsymbol{\Theta}$, are estimated by maximizing the log-likelihood of the empirical data

$$L(\mathbf{W}, \boldsymbol{\Theta}) = \sum_{h=0}^{H} n(h) \log p(h; \mathbf{W}, \boldsymbol{\Theta}), \tag{3}$$

where $n(h)$ is the histogram of the CT data, whose voxel values range from 0 to H. The corresponding relative frequency histogram is denoted $f(h) = n(h)/N$, N being the total number of voxels. To maximize the likelihood in Equation (3), we employ an iterative block relaxation process as follows.

Let τ indicate an iteration such that $(\mathbf{W}^{[\tau]}, \boldsymbol{\Theta}^{[\tau]})$ are the parameter estimates on that iteration, and

$$p^{[\tau]}(h) = p(h; \mathbf{W}^{[\tau]}, \boldsymbol{\Theta}^{[\tau]}) = \sum_{k=1}^{K} w_k^{[\tau]}\varphi(h; \theta_k^{[\tau]}) \tag{4}$$

is the proposed probabilistic model for the CT data. The conditional weights are estimated as follows:

$$\pi^{[\tau]}(k|h) = \frac{w_k^{[\tau]}\varphi(h;\theta_k^{[\tau]})}{p^{[\tau]}(h)}; \quad (5)$$

This conditional probability specifies the relative contributions of voxel value h to each component at step τ. Using these variables, Equation (3) can be written in the equivalent form:

$$L(\mathbf{W}^{[\tau]}, \mathbf{\Theta}^{[\tau]}) = \sum_{h=0}^{H} n(h) \log\left[\sum_{k=1}^{K} \pi^{[\tau]}(k|h)\varphi(h;\theta_k^{[\tau]})\right] \quad (6)$$

From given starting values at $\tau = 0$, the block relaxation scheme converges to a local maximum of the likelihood function in Equation (6) through iteration of the following two steps:

1. E-step $[\tau+1]$: estimate $\mathbf{W}^{[\tau+1]}$, $\mathbf{\Theta}^{[\tau+1]}$, which maximize $L(\mathbf{W}, \mathbf{\Theta})$ under the fixed conditional weights of Equation (5) at step τ.
2. M-step $[\tau+1]$: recalculate weights, which maximize L holding parameters $\mathbf{W}^{[\tau+1]}$ and $\mathbf{\Theta}^{[\tau+1]}$ fixed.

The process is repeated until the changes of all the parameters become small.

The E-step maximizes the likelihood function of Equation (6) subject to the constraints Equation (2). The solution for the weights is

$$w_k^{[\tau+1]} = \sum_{h=0}^{H} f(h)\pi^{[\tau]}(k|h) \quad (7)$$

Then, parameters of each Gaussian component are found using the ordinary (unconstrained) maximum likelihood estimates:

$$\begin{aligned} \mu_k^{[\tau+1]} &= \frac{1}{w_k^{[\tau+1]}} \sum_{h=0}^{H} h \cdot f(h)\pi^{[\tau]}(k|h) \\ (\sigma_k^{[\tau+1]})^2 &= \frac{1}{w_k^{[\tau+1]}} \sum_{h=0}^{H} \left(h - \mu_k^{[\tau+1]}\right)^2 \cdot f(h)\pi^{[\tau]}(k|h) \end{aligned} \quad (8)$$

We will follow Algorithm 1 to illustrate the steps for estimating the parameters of the proposed probabilistic model. The final estimated density will consist of the two dominant Gaussian components and $K-2$ subdominant Gaussian components. Jensen–Shannon divergence (JSD) [46] is employed in this algorithm to measure the similarity between empirical density and mixed density for use as convergence criteria to determine the number of Gaussian components. The latter is a symmetric version of a Kullback–Leibler divergence [47].

Algorithm 1: Estimation of the proposed probabilistic model parameters

---

input : A test 3D CT image.
output: Estimated mixed density model $p(h)$ (Equation 1).
1. Use the block relaxation algorithm to estimate mixing weights, means, and variances for the two-component Gaussian mixture model representing the lung and chest regions.

2. **for** $K \leftarrow 3, 4, \ldots, K_{max}$ **do**

   1. Add one subdominant component to the model.
   2. Holding μ_k fixed only for dominant modes, update the other model parameters by block relaxation.
   3. Calculate the Jensen–Shannon divergence [46], $\text{JSD}(\text{f(h)}||\text{p(h)}) = \frac{KL(f(h)||M)+KL(p(h)||M)}{2}$. Here, $M = \frac{f(h)+p(h)}{2}$ and $KL(p(h)||M) = \sum_{h} p(h) \times \log_2 \frac{p(h)}{M}$ is the Kullback–Leibler divergence [47].

end
3. Select the K yielding the lowest value of JSD.

Estimation of the marginal density: The $K - 2$ subdominant components of the final estimated model $p(h)$ need to be partitioned among the two dominant modes. Each subordinate component is associated with one dominant component in order to minimize the expected misclassification rate. This is accomplished using the proposed Algorithm 2.

Algorithm 2: The proposed clustering algorithm

---

input : Estimated mixed density model $p(h)$ (Equation 1).
output: Marginal density function for lung $p_l(h)$ and for chest $p_c(h)$.

$p_l(h) = w_1 \varphi(h; \theta_1)$;
$(\mu_l, \sigma_l) = (\mu_1, \sigma_1)$;
$(\mu_{gl}, \sigma_{gl}) = (\mu_1, \sigma_1)$;
$p_c(h) = w_2 \varphi(h; \theta_2)$;
$(\mu_c, \sigma_c) = (\mu_2, \sigma_2)$;
$(\mu_{gc}, \sigma_{gc}) = (\mu_2, \sigma_2)$;
$M = \{\mu_3, \ldots, \mu_K\}$;
while *M is not empty* **do**
  $d_l = \min_{k \in M} \frac{|\mu_k - \mu_l|}{\sigma_l}$;
  $d_c = \min_{k \in M} \frac{|\mu_k - \mu_c|}{\sigma_c}$;
  if $d_l < d_c$ **then**
    $\hat{k} = \operatorname{argmin}_{k \in M} \frac{|\mu_k - \mu_l|}{\sigma_l}$;
    $p_l(h) = p_l(h) + w_{\hat{k}} \varphi(h; \theta_{\hat{k}})$;
    $\mu_{gl} = \mu_{gl} \cup \mu_{\hat{k}}$;
    $\mu_l = \text{mean}(\mu_{gl})$;
  else
    $\hat{k} = \operatorname{argmin}_{k \in M} \frac{|\mu_k - \mu_c|}{\sigma_c}$;
    $p_c(h) = p_c(h) + w_{\hat{k}} \varphi(h; \theta_{\hat{k}})$;
    $\mu_{gc} = \mu_{gc} \cup \mu_{\hat{k}}$;
    $\mu_c = \text{mean}(\mu_{gc})$;
  end
  $M = M - \{\mu_{\hat{k}}\}$
end

2.2. MGRF-Based Morphological Constraints

To get a consistent segmentation of the lung region, we applied rotation invariant spatial constraints by using a generic Markov–Gibbs model of region maps [45]. The model, which incorporates voxel–voxel interaction effects as shown in Figure 3, has, in general, an arbitrary interaction structure and corresponding Gibbs potentials. For simplicity, we restrict the interaction neighborhood system (**N**) to the nearest 9 neighbors in the above CT slice and 9 neighbors in the below CT-slice.

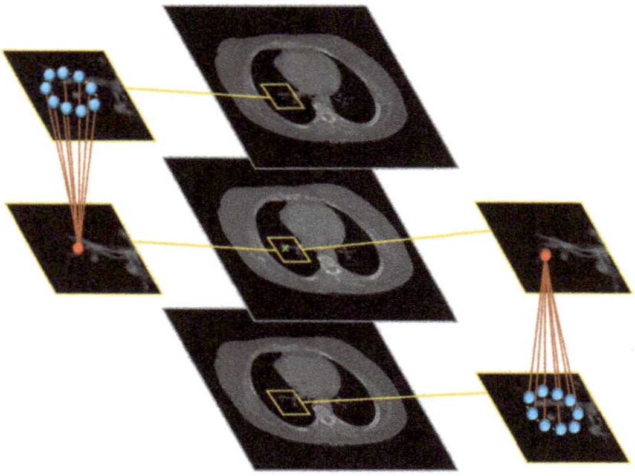

Figure 3. Illustration of the 3D MGRF-Based morphological constraints on the anatomical segmentation. The middle column shows the selected slice, and its upper and lower slices; the left column shows the selected pixel and its neighbors at the upper slice while the right column shows the selected pixel and its neighbors at the lower slice.

To model the interactions between the CT voxels, we will assume all the interactions as the same within each region. To estimate this interaction in analytical way, let $V : \mathbf{X} \times \mathbf{X} \rightarrow \{V_{\text{eq}}, V_{\text{ne}}\}$ denote a bi-valued Gibbs potential describing pairwise interactions, where

$$V(x, \chi) = \begin{cases} V_{\text{eq}} & x = \chi \\ V_{\text{ne}} & x \neq \chi \end{cases} \tag{9}$$

Then, the Gibbs probability distribution (GPD) of region maps on the 3D lattice **R** is as follows [45]:

$$P(\mathbf{m}) \propto \exp\left(\sum_{(i,j,z)\in\mathbf{R}} \sum_{(\xi,\eta,\zeta)\in\mathbf{N}} V(m_{i,j,z}, m_{i+\xi,j+\eta,z+\zeta}) \right) \tag{10}$$

By modifying the derivation scheme in [45] to fit our model, the following first approximation of the maximum likelihood estimator (MLE) of the potential values for a given map **m** is obtained:

$$\begin{aligned} V_{\text{eq}} &= \frac{X^2}{X-1}\left(f'(\mathbf{m}) - \frac{1}{X}\right) \\ V_{\text{ne}} &= \frac{X^2}{X-1}\left(f''(\mathbf{m}) - 1 + \frac{1}{X}\right) \end{aligned} \tag{11}$$

where $f'(\mathbf{m})$ and $f''(\mathbf{m})$ denote the relative frequency of the equal and non-equal pairs of the labels in all the equivalent voxels pairs $\{((i,j,z),(i+\xi,j+\eta,z+\zeta)) : (i,j,z) \in \mathbf{R};$ $(i+\xi,j+\eta,z+\zeta) \in \mathbf{R};$ $(\xi,\eta,\zeta) \in \mathbf{N}\}$, respectively.

2.3. *Joint MGRF Model and Lung Segmentation Algorithm*

In order to integrate the first-order appearance model with the spatial probabilistic model that describes the morphological/anatomical constrains, we will assume that the CT data ($\mathbf{g}$) consisting of visual appearance model and its spatial map ($\mathbf{m}$, data labels) follow the following two-level MGRF model:

$$P(\mathbf{g}, \mathbf{m}) = P(\mathbf{m})P(\mathbf{g}|\mathbf{m}) \tag{12}$$

Here, $P(\mathbf{m})$ is an unconditional distribution of maps that is modeled by MGRF probabilistic model that is demonstrated in Equation (10). $P(\mathbf{g}|\mathbf{m})$ is a conditional distribution of gray levels for a given labeling. The Bayesian maximum a posteriori estimation (MAP) of the labeling, given the image $\mathbf{g}$, $\mathbf{m}^* = \underset{\mathbf{m}}{\operatorname{argmax}} L(\mathbf{g}, \mathbf{m})$ maximizes the log-likelihood,

$$L(\mathbf{g}, \mathbf{m}) = \log P(\mathbf{g}|\mathbf{m}) + \log P(\mathbf{m}). \tag{13}$$

In order to summarize the proposed segmentation system, the basic steps are demonstrated in Algorithm 3.

Algorithm 3: Lung Extraction Algorithm

input : A test 3D CT image.
output: Final 3D lung segmentation.

1. **1st Order Density Estimation:** Estimate the marginal density function for lung ($p_l(h)$) and marginal density function for chest ($p_c(h)$).
2. **Initial Segmentation/Labeling:** Use Bayes classifier to delineate the initial lung region by using the marginal estimated densities.
3. **Estimation of Gibbs Potentials:** Applying Equation (11) on the initial segmentation to estimate the Gibbs potentials.
4. **Refine Segmentation:** Use iterative conditional mode (ICM) algorithm [45] to find the map that maximize the likelihood of joint MGRF model shown in Equation (13).

3. Evaluation Metrics

This section describes the metrics used to gauge the performance of our proposed system: *Dice similarity coefficient (DSC)*, *overlap coefficient*, and *absolute lung volume difference (ALVD)*. Each of these quantifies in some way either the agreement or dissimilarity between the segmentation algorithm result and the corresponding ground-truth segmentation. More detailed explanation is presented in Sections 3.1–3.3, respectively. Furthermore, a fourth metric, the *95th-percentile bidirectional Hausdorff distance (BHD)* (Section 3.4), is employed to quantify the accuracy of the boundary of the segmented region relative to ground-truth.

3.1. *Dice Similarity Coefficient (DSC)*

Dice similarity coefficient (DSC) is one of the most common similarity metric to measure the similarity between two different areas. This metric is used to evaluate the result of the proposed system by estimating the similarity between the black-white segmented lung (L) and the ground-truth (G), i.e., the percentage of common region (i.e., the green part) in both images as shown in Figure 4a. The range of this metric is between 0 and 1, as 0 and 1 mean dissimilar and similar, respectively. It is computed as follows:

$$DSC = \frac{2 \times n(L \bigcap G)}{n(L) + n(G)} \tag{14}$$

where $n(L \bigcap G)$ is the cardinality of white pixels in the intersection between the segmented lung (L) and the ground-truth (G), while $n(L)$ and $n(G)$ are the cardinality of the white pixels in the segmentation (L) and the ground-truth (G), respectively.

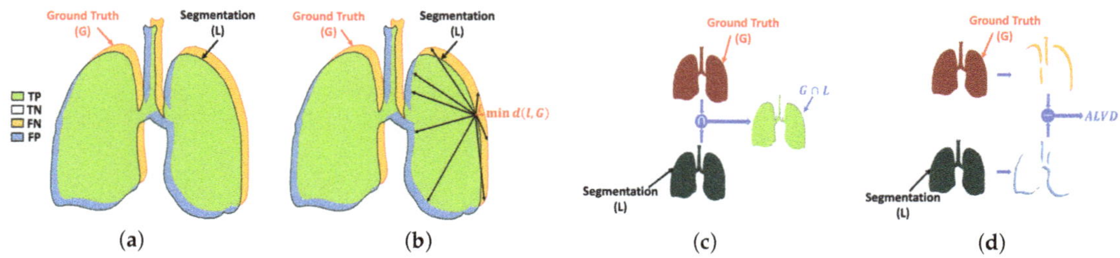

Figure 4. Illustration of the evaluation metrics: (**a**) DSC, (**b**) HD, (**c**) overlap coefficient, and (**d**) ALVD. Note that TP, TN, FP, and FN are true positive (correct lung pixel), true negative (correct background pixel), false positive (incorrect lung pixel), and false negative (incorrect background pixel).

3.2. Overlap Coefficient

Overlap coefficient is used in our assessment pipeline to measure the similarity between the predicted object and its ground-truth by computing the overlap percentage between them, see Figure 4c. The overlap coefficient of identical objects gives 1, while it gives 0 for heterogeneous one. The latter is estimated as follows:

$$overlap = \frac{n(L \bigcap G)}{n(L \bigcup G)} \tag{15}$$

where $n(L \bigcup G)$ is the cardinality of white pixels in the union between the segmented lung (L) and the ground-truth (G).

3.3. Absolute Lung Volume Difference (ALVD)

Another metric used to assess our work is absolute lung volume difference (ALVD). ALVD computes the similarity between two images by measuring the differences between the ground-truth (G) and the black-white segmented lung (L) (Figure 4d). The ALVD of similar objects gives 0. This metric is defined as

$$ALVD = \frac{|n(G) - n(L)|}{n(G)} \tag{16}$$

where $|n(G) - n(L)|$ is the absolute difference between the cardinality of white pixels in the ground-truth (G) and segmentation (L).

3.4. Bidirectional Hausdorff Distance (BHD)

This section describes the last metric called bidirectional Hausdorff distance (BHD), which is used to evaluate our proposed system in addition to the previous three metrics. BHD is the bidirectional estimation of Hausdorff distance (HD) between the black-white segmented lung (L) and the ground-truth (G), and vice versa. HD is the maximum Euclidean distance between the points in the border of the black-white segmented lung (L) and its closest point in the border of the ground-truth (G), as visualized in Figure 4b, which is computed as follows [48,49]:

$$HD(L, G) = \max_{l \in \mathbf{L}}\{\min_{g \in \mathbf{G}}\{d(l, g)\}\} \tag{17}$$

where l and g are sets of the points border in the L and G, respectively, and $d(g, l)$ is the Euclidean distance between the two points.

As, $BHD(L, G)$ is estimated as

$$BHD(L, G) = max\{\text{HD}(\mathbf{L}, \mathbf{G}), \text{HD}(\mathbf{G}, \mathbf{L})\} \tag{18}$$

In this paper, the 95th-percentile BHD is used to evaluate our proposed system. Instead of getting the maximum Euclidean distance between L and G, 95th-percentile of all computed distances is selected to overcome the outliers.

4. Experimental Results

The segmentation framework described above was applied to the problem of segmenting lung with pathological tissue in COVID-19 patients. The proposed segmentation system is evaluated and tested on 32 CT chest volume with different severity of COVID-19 infections, selected from 249 CT volume in COVID-19 [50]. Four of them had healthy/mild COVID-19 infections whose image size ranges from $512 \times 512 \times 51$ to $512 \times 512 \times 125$, while 17 patients of size $512 \times 512 \times$ 36–607 who had moderate infections as well as 11 CT chest volume of size $512 \times 512 \times$ 44–577 had severe COVID-19 infections. To compare our framework with other approaches that depend on a training dataset, we select another 34 3D CT chest volume (i.e., 3713 images in total) from the same dataset to use them as a training. Table 1 summarized the dataset characteristics used in our experimental results. The data are graded according to the radiology protocol in [51]. To obtain more accurate segmentation, we included morphological/anatomical constraints based on the use of a rotation invariant MGRF model.

Table 1. Dataset characteristics.

	Class	Resolution	#Slices	#Patients	Total
Training	Healthy/Mild	512×512	43–54	2	34
	Moderate		35–397	20	
	Severe		46–321	12	
Testing	Healthy/Mild		51–125	4	32
	Moderate		36–607	17	
	Severe		44–577	11	

To demonstrate step by step how our proposed approach works, Figure 5b shows empirical density for the 3D CT chest volume (Figure 5a), and the two Gaussian mixtures approximating its dominant modes are presented in Figure 5c. Furthermore, Figure 5c demonstrates the JSD between the empirical density and the two estimated dominant Gaussian components. Figure 5d shows the changes of JSD and the best-estimated number of Gaussian components that are demonstrated in Figure 5e. Figure 5f demonstrated the classification of the subdominant Gaussian components based on the use of the proposed clustering algorithm (Algorithm 2). Figure 5g,h demonstrates the final marginal densities for lung and chest as well as the final estimated mixed density. Figures 6 and 7 demonstrate the ability of the proposed probabilistic model to handle the variability in the empirical density that it may occur due to the severity of infections or the variability of the scanning protocol.

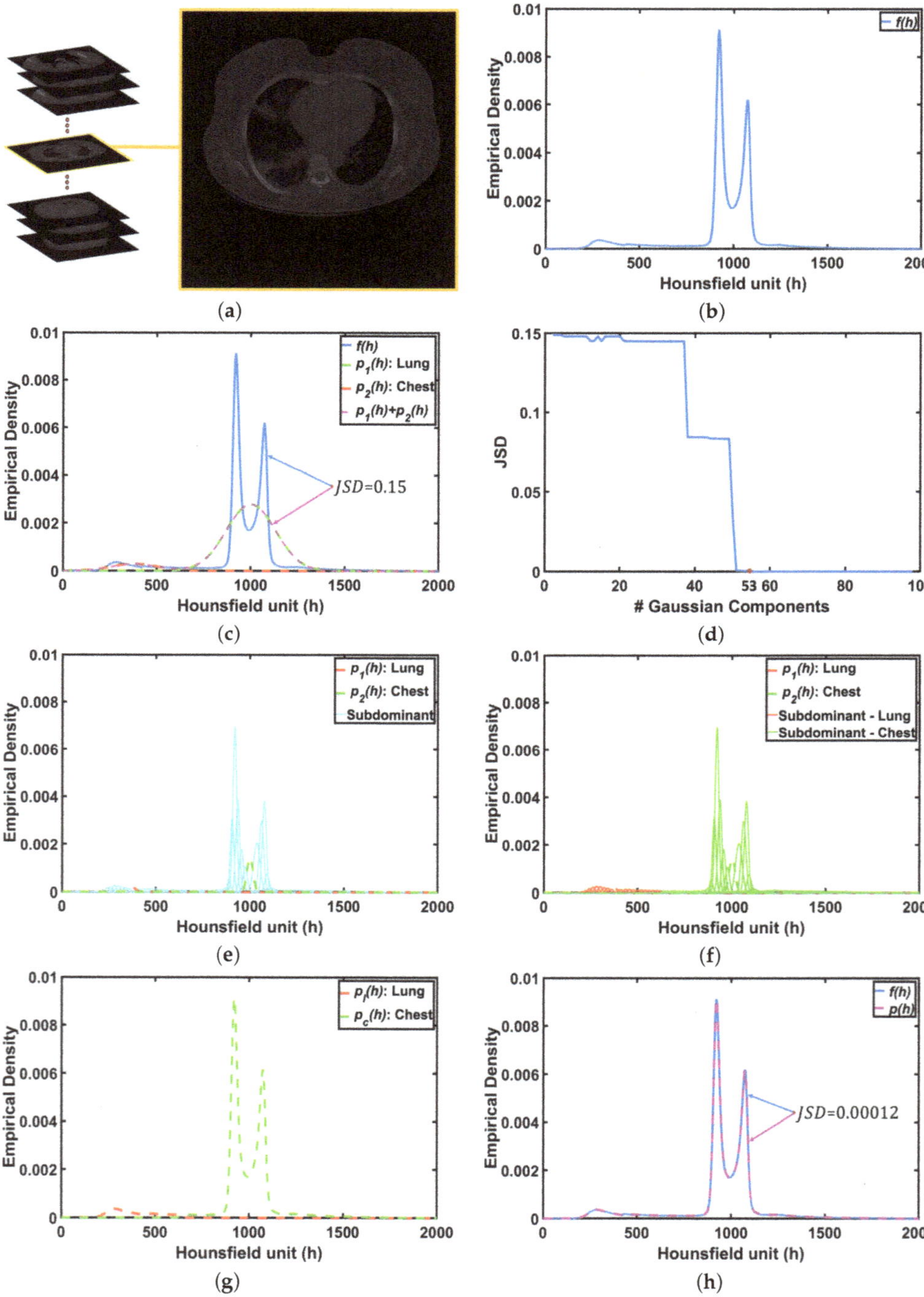

Figure 5. An illustrative example of the proposed system: (**a**) CT chest volume, (**b**) empirical density, (**c**) two dominants Gaussian components, (**d**) JSD between empirical density and mixed density, (**e**) two dominant and $K-2$ subdominant Gaussian components, (**f**) proposed cluster algorithm, (**g**) marginal density for lung and chest, and (**h**) final mixed density for all components. Note that JSD stands for Jensen–Shannon divergence.

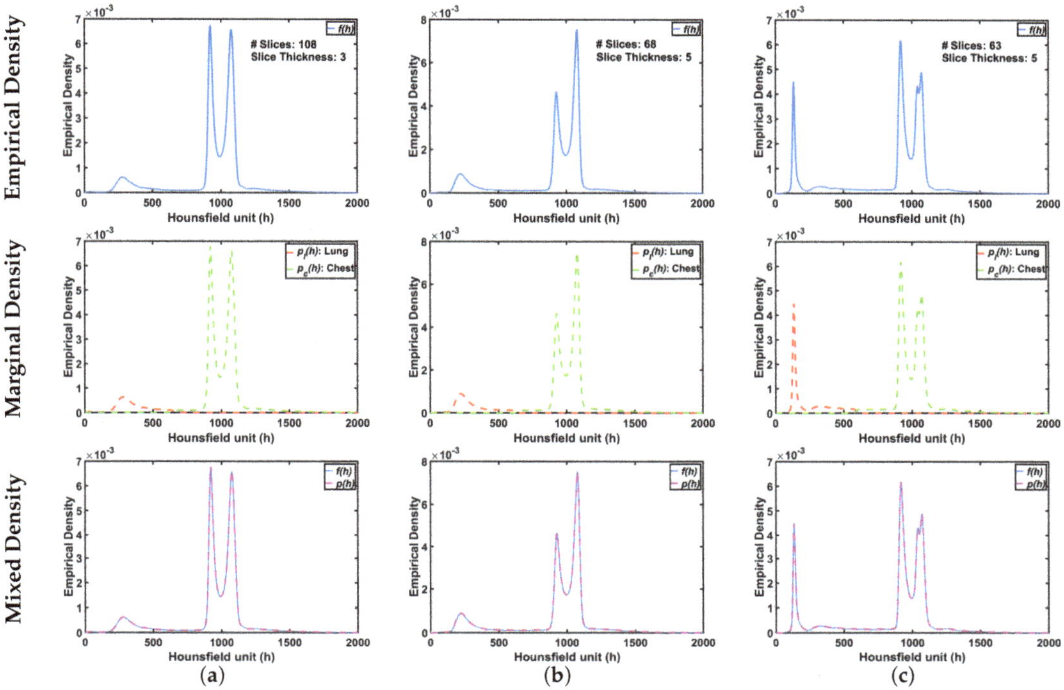

Figure 6. An illustrative example of the proposed appearance model estimated from Thick-Section CT appearance model for (**a**) healthy/mild, (**b**) moderate, and (**c**) severe COVID-19 infected lung. Note that first, second, and third rows represent empirical, marginal, and mixed densities, respectively.

To highlight the promise of including the rotation invariant MGRF-based morphological/anatomical constraints with the adaptive first-order appearance model, the system's performance is evaluated before and after inclusion, as demonstrated in Table 2. As shown in the table, the proposed segmentation is enhanced after including MGRF-based morphological/anatomical constraints, particularly in severe cases where the DSC is significantly increased from $82.51_{\pm 13.13}$% to $95.15_{\pm 1.91}$%. To more prove the attainable enhancement of the system, Figure 8 presents three examples of the proposed system before and after the inclusion for healthy/mild, moderate, and severe COVID-19 infected lung. As shown in the figure, the developed system outperforms the proposed appearance model alone (i.e., LCG) for three examples, whereas the proposed system shows its ability to segment a severe COVID-19 infection with 94.55% DSC compared to the proposed appearance model which gives 76.49% DSC. Moreover, Figure 9 presents the proposed segmentation for a severe lung COVID-19 infection at different cross-sections (i.e., 2D axial, coronal, and saggital) to visually show the efficiency of the proposed system. Overall, the proposed system achieves a DSC, overlap, BHD, and ALVD of $95.67_{\pm 1.83}$%, $91.76_{\pm 3.29}$%, $4.86_{\pm 5.01}$, and $2.93_{\pm 2.39}$, respectively. Finally, to prove the robustness of the proposed segmentation approach, deep learning approaches are adopted as a comparison: DeepLabv3+ [52] using ResNet-50 network as a backbone, Inf-Net [28] with backbone ResNet-50 network, U-Net [25], and 3D U-Net [53]. The results are reported in Table 3. As demonstrated in the table, the 3D U-Net approach gives a worst performance of $66.08_{\pm 35.99}$% DSC, $58.30_{\pm 34.81}$% overlap, $44.44_{\pm 48.60}$ BHD, and $66.77_{\pm 133.01}$ ALVD, while the proposed segmentation approach gives the best performance compared to these deep learning approaches. Moreover, to visually demonstrate the capability of the proposed system, three different examples of healthy/mild, moderate, and severe lung COVID-19 infections are segmented using these approaches, as presented in Figure 10. As demonstrated in the figure, the proposed approach segments the three examples better than the other four approaches. Moreover, the U-Net approach has a DSC close to the proposed approach. However, there are some parts that segment incorrectly as demonstrated in the figures, e.g., classifying part of trachea or chest as lung. Therefore, the proposed system is much better due to its segmentation being closer to the ground-truth. Therefore, it is highly recommended to use our approach to segment the lung infected by COVID-19 as it shows better performance than the state-of-the-art deep learning approaches. In addition, it is unsupervised technique, thus it will not suffer from the underfitting and overfitting problems.

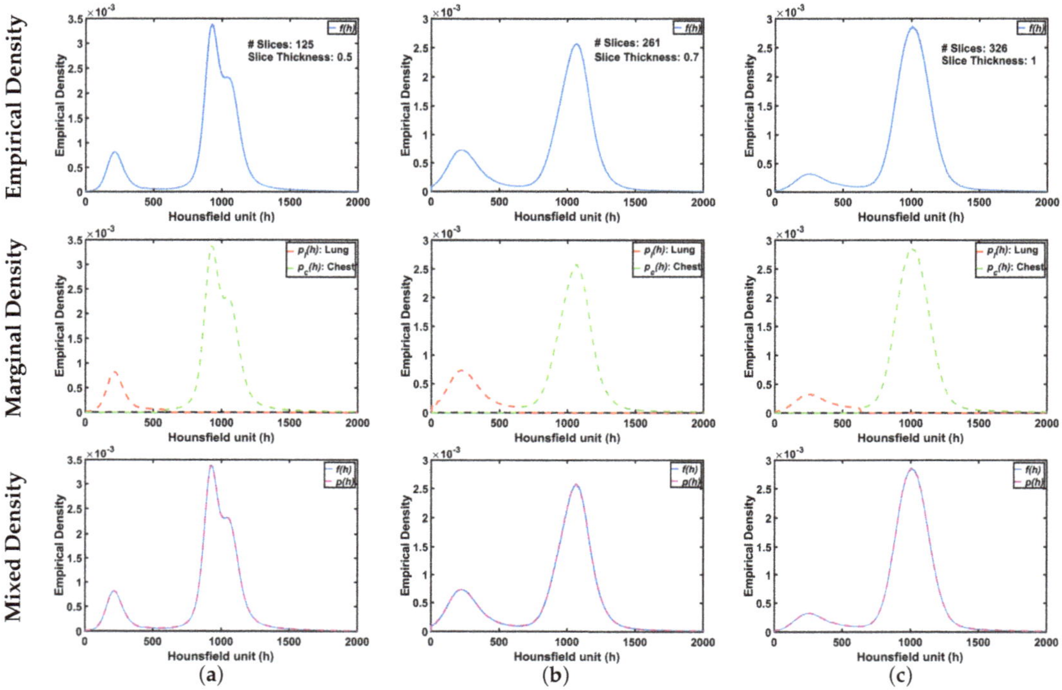

Figure 7. An illustrative example of the proposed appearance model estimated from Thin-Section CT appearance model for (**a**) healthy/mild, (**b**) moderate, and (**c**) severe COVID-19 infected lung. Note that first, second, and third rows represent empirical, marginal, and mixed densities, respectively.

Table 2. Quantitative evaluation of the proposed segmentation system before and after applying rotation invariant Markov–Gibbs random field (MGRF). Note that LCG, DSC, BHD, and ALVD stand for linear combination of Gaussian, Dice similarity coefficient, 95th-percentile bidirectional Hausdorff distance, and absolute lung volume difference, respectively.

		DSC	**Overlap**	**BHD**	**ALVD**
LCG-model	*Healthy/Mild*	$96.37_{\pm 0.47}$%	$92.99_{\pm 0.88}$%	$11.32_{\pm 4.59}$	$3.58_{\pm 2.06}$
	Moderate	$92.57_{\pm 4.64}$%	$86.47_{\pm 7.61}$%	$9.59_{\pm 5.30}$	$7.31_{\pm 7.39}$
	Severe	$82.51_{\pm 13.13}$%	$71.98_{\pm 17.26}$%	$13.77_{\pm 7.20}$	$23.16_{\pm 19.29}$
	Overall	$89.59_{\pm 9.76}$%	$82.31_{\pm 13.72}$%	$11.24_{\pm 6.08}$	$12.29_{\pm 14.63}$
Final System	*Healthy/Mild*	$\mathbf{97.53}_{\pm \mathbf{0.56}}$%	$\mathbf{95.18}_{\pm \mathbf{1.06}}$%	$\mathbf{2.41}_{\pm \mathbf{1.12}}$	$\mathbf{1.72}_{\pm \mathbf{1.09}}$
	Moderate	$\mathbf{95.54}_{\pm \mathbf{1.91}}$%	$\mathbf{91.53}_{\pm \mathbf{3.41}}$%	$\mathbf{4.25}_{\pm \mathbf{3.73}}$	$\mathbf{3.48}_{\pm \mathbf{2.59}}$
	Severe	$\mathbf{95.19}_{\pm \mathbf{1.66}}$%	$\mathbf{90.87}_{\pm \mathbf{3.01}}$%	$\mathbf{6.70}_{\pm \mathbf{6.97}}$	$\mathbf{2.52}_{\pm \mathbf{2.32}}$
	Overall	$\mathbf{95.67}_{\pm \mathbf{1.83}}$%	$\mathbf{91.76}_{\pm \mathbf{3.29}}$%	$\mathbf{4.86}_{\pm \mathbf{5.01}}$	$\mathbf{2.93}_{\pm \mathbf{2.39}}$

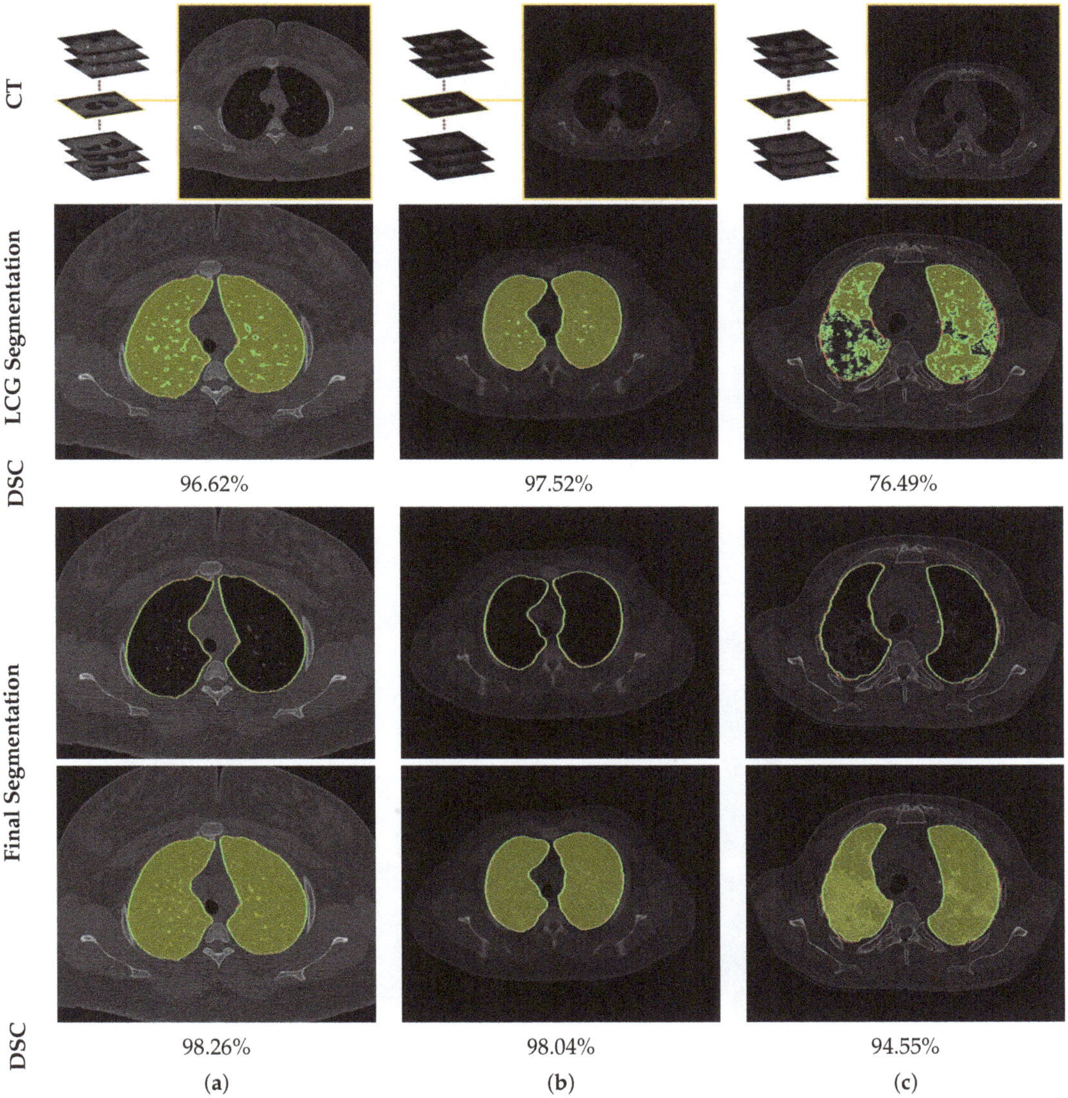

Figure 8. An illustrative example of the proposed segmentation for (**a**) healthy/mild, (**b**) moderate, and (**c**) severe COVID-19 infected lung. Note that red border (green border or yellow region) refers to ground-truth (segmentation).

Table 3. Quantitative evaluation of the proposed segmentation system compared with other deep learning approaches. Note that DSC, BHD, and ALVD stand for Dice similarity coefficient, 95th-percentile bidirectional Hausdorff distance, and absolute lung volume difference, respectively.

		DSC	Overlap	BHD	ALVD
DeepLabv3+ [52]	*Healthy/Mild*	80.32$_{\pm 32.97}$%	74.93$_{\pm 37.81}$%	23.58$_{\pm 40.93}$	116.36$_{\pm 220.88}$
	Moderate	95.15$_{\pm 1.52}$%	90.79$_{\pm 2.75}$%	8.85$_{\pm 21.37}$	7.32$_{\pm 3.68}$
	Severe	93.80$_{\pm 2.47}$%	88.41$_{\pm 4.29}$%	27.01$_{\pm 46.72}$	8.78$_{\pm 4.24}$
	Overall	92.88$_{\pm 11.49}$%	88.07$_{\pm 13.22}$%	16.79$_{\pm 34.17}$	21.41$_{\pm 77.87}$

Table 3. *Cont.*

		DSC	Overlap	BHD	ALVD
U-Net [25]	*Healthy/Mild*	$93.47_{\pm 7.46}$%	$88.39_{\pm 12.36}$%	$25.68_{\pm 15.60}$	$5.46_{\pm 6.00}$
	Moderate	$95.09_{\pm 2.02}$%	$90.71_{\pm 3.62}$%	$19.04_{\pm 35.58}$	$3.61_{\pm 3.36}$
	Severe	$91.68_{\pm 5.07}$%	$84.99_{\pm 8.30}$%	$44.81_{\pm 73.04}$	$9.41_{\pm 7.24}$
	Overall	$93.77_{\pm 4.30}$%	$88.56_{\pm 7.16}$%	$28.49_{\pm 50.08}$	$5.76_{\pm 5.80}$
Inf-Net [28]	*Healthy/Mild*	$89.77_{\pm 10.41}$%	$82.56_{\pm 15.81}$%	$17.41_{\pm 27.32}$	$14.41_{\pm 9.32}$
	Moderate	$92.73_{\pm 1.64}$%	$86.49_{\pm 2.85}$%	$13.40_{\pm 25.32}$	$13.43_{\pm 3.29}$
	Severe	$90.20_{\pm 4.56}$%	$82.42_{\pm 7.06}$%	$36.03_{\pm 38.77}$	$14.91_{\pm 5.65}$
	Overall	$91.54_{\pm 4.52}$%	$84.67_{\pm 6.99}$%	$21.44_{\pm 31.40}$	$14.00_{\pm 4.96}$
3D U-Net [53]	*Healthy/Mild*	$78.11_{\pm 35.98}$%	$72.80_{\pm 39.39}$%	$29.41_{\pm 41.91}$	$140.67_{\pm 276.19}$
	Moderate	$68.46_{\pm 35.82}$%	$60.58_{\pm 33.85}$%	$42.04_{\pm 51.53}$	$33.91_{\pm 35.35}$
	Severe	$55.72_{\pm 37.95}$%	$46.95_{\pm 35.31}$%	$55.25_{\pm 50.43}$	$93.15_{\pm 158.26}$
	Overall	$66.08_{\pm 35.99}$%	$58.30_{\pm 34.81}$%	$44.44_{\pm 48.60}$	$66.77_{\pm 133.01}$
Our System	*Healthy/Mild*	$\mathbf{97.53_{\pm 0.56}}$%	$\mathbf{95.18_{\pm 1.06}}$%	$\mathbf{2.41_{\pm 1.12}}$	$\mathbf{1.72_{\pm 1.09}}$
	Moderate	$\mathbf{95.54_{\pm 1.91}}$%	$\mathbf{91.53_{\pm 3.41}}$%	$\mathbf{4.25_{\pm 3.73}}$	$\mathbf{3.48_{\pm 2.59}}$
	Severe	$\mathbf{95.19_{\pm 1.66}}$%	$\mathbf{90.87_{\pm 3.01}}$%	$\mathbf{6.70_{\pm 6.97}}$	$\mathbf{2.52_{\pm 2.32}}$
	Overall	$\mathbf{95.67_{\pm 1.83}}$%	$\mathbf{91.76_{\pm 3.29}}$%	$\mathbf{4.86_{\pm 5.01}}$	$\mathbf{2.93_{\pm 2.39}}$

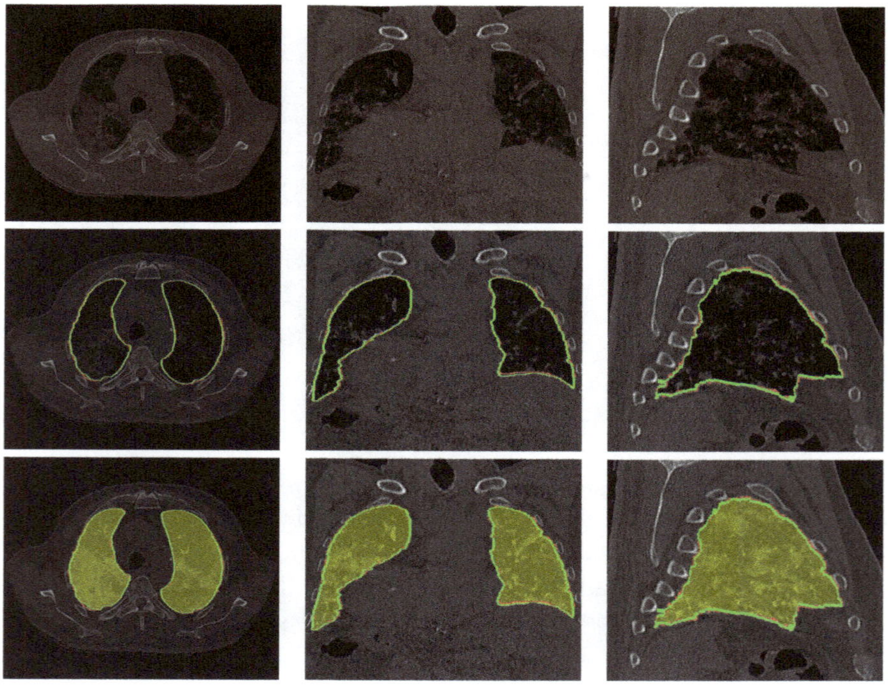

(**a**) (**b**) (**c**)

Figure 9. An illustrative example of the proposed segmentation (second and third rows) for a severe COVID-19 infected lung at (**a**) 2D axial, (**b**) coronal, and (**c**) sagittal cross sections of an original image (first row). Note that red border (green border or yellow region) refers to ground-truth (segmentation).

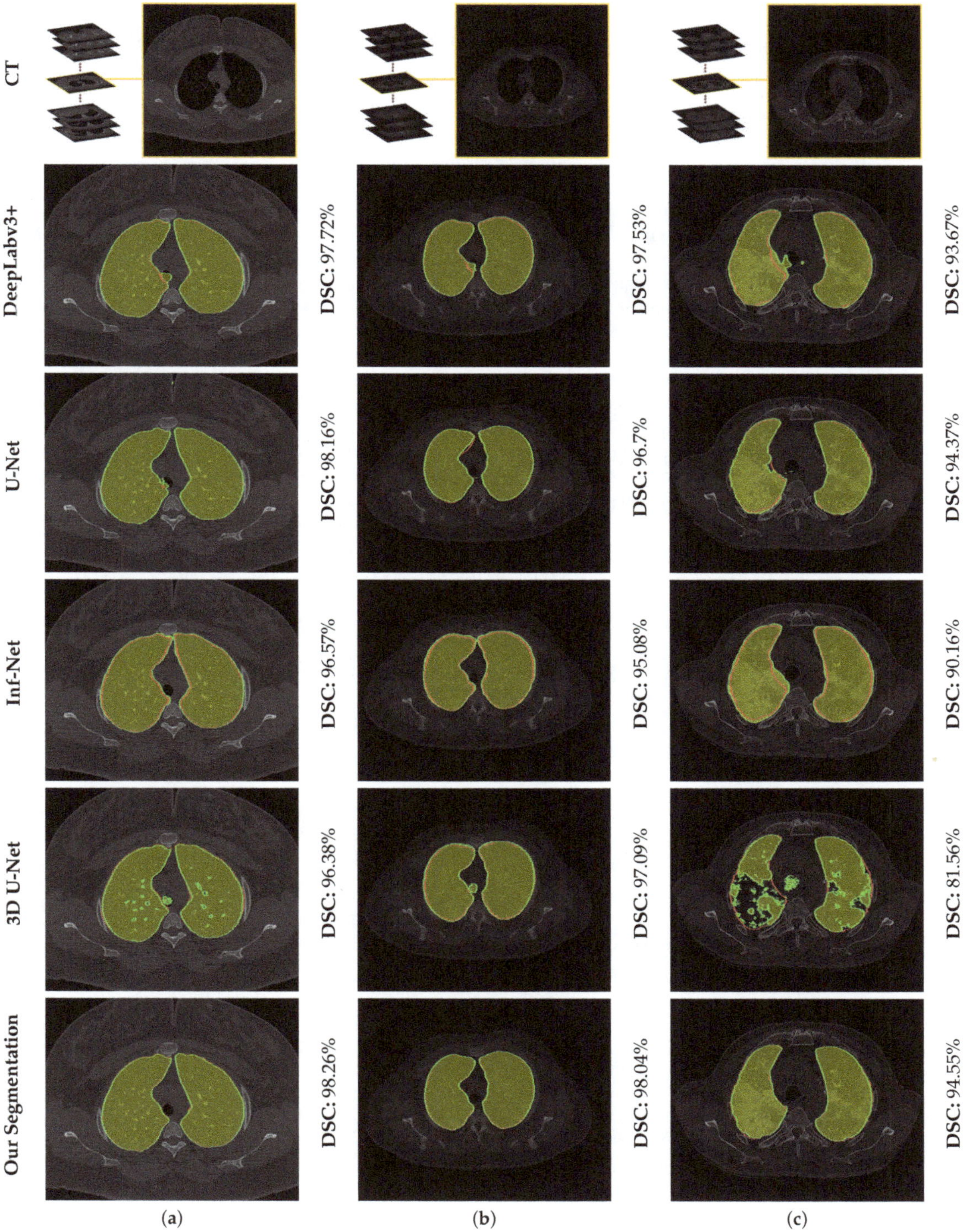

Figure 10. An illustrative example of the proposed segmentation compared to other deep learning approaches for (**a**) healthy/mild, (**b**) moderate, and (**c**) severe COVID-19 infected lung. Note that red border (green border or yellow region) refers to ground-truth (segmentation).

5. Discussion and Conclusions

Experiments demonstrate that the proposed framework is promising and achieved high accuracy, with identification of the first-order appearance model followed by 3D morphological constraints based on analytical estimation MGRF parameters producing good results when segmenting the COVID-19 infected lung region from CT images. Quantitative metrics of accuracy including the DSC, overlap coefficient, 95th-percentile BHD, and the ALVD metrics all show consistent performance on our sample data set of 32 subjects, outperforming current, state-of-the-art deep learning-based lung segmentation approaches. The results herein demonstrate the ability of the developed system to segment lung on a CT image, whose DSC is improved from $89.59_{\pm 9.76}\%$ to $95.67_{\pm 1.83}\%$ when 3D morphological MGRF-based constraints are included in the system pipeline. However, the accuracy of the proposed segmentation system will get affected if the lung is significantly damaged or filled with water, or the appearance of the lung is closed to the chest. Thus, separation based on appearance model will be very challenging task. Therefore, we plan to add some shape model approach in our system to overcome these problems. Moreover, a future extension of this work would integrate the proposed segmentation approach into a computer-aided diagnostic system to assess pulmonary function and risk of mortality in COVID-19 patients, which is the ultimate goal of our research group. Furthermore, the morphological constraints could be made to support large-scale inhomogeneity of the kind seen in severe lung infection. This will be accomplished by expanding the neighborhood system to include larger cliques so that the MGRF model incorporates higher order interaction effects.

Author Contributions: Methodology, A.S. (Ahmed Sharafeldeen), M.E., N.S.A., A.S. (Ahmed Soliman), and A.E.-B.; Software, A.S. (Ahmed Sharafeldeen) and A.E.-B.; Validation, A.S. (Ahmed Sharafeldeen) and A.E.-B.; Formal analysis, A.S. (Ahmed Sharafeldeen), M.E., N.S.A., A.S. (Ahmed Soliman), and A.E.-B.; investigation, A.E.-B.; Writing—original draft preparation, A.S. (Ahmed Sharafeldeen), M.E., N.S.A., A.S. (Ahmed Soliman), and A.E.-B.; Writing—review and editing, A.S. (Ahmed Sharafeldeen), M.E., N.S.A., A.S. (Ahmed Soliman), and A.E.-B.; Visualization, A.S. (Ahmed Sharafeldeen) and A.E.-B.; Supervision, A.E.-B.; Project administration, N.S.A. and A.E.-B. All authors have read and agreed to the published version of the manuscript.

Funding: The authors extend their appreciation to the Deputyship for Research & Innovation, Ministry of Education in Saudi Arabia for funding this research work through the project number (PNU-DRI-Targeted-20-001).

Institutional Review Board Statement: We used public data.

Informed Consent Statement: We used public data.

Data Availability Statement: The data presented in this study are openly available in The Cancer Imaging Archive (TCIA) at https://doi.org/10.7937/TCIA.2020.GQRY-NC81 accessed date 5 June 2021, reference number [50].

Conflicts of Interest: The authors declare no conflict of interest.

References

1. Machhi, J.; Herskovitz, J.; Senan, A.M.; Dutta, D.; Nath, B.; Oleynikov, M.D.; Blomberg, W.R.; Meigs, D.D.; Hasan, M.; Patel, M.; et al. The Natural History, Pathobiology, and Clinical Manifestations of SARS-CoV-2 Infections. *J. Neuroimmune Pharmacol.* **2020**, *15*, 359–386. [CrossRef] [PubMed]
2. Gupta, S.; Hayek, S.S.; Wang, W.; Chan, L.; Mathews, K.S.; Melamed, M.L.; Brenner, S.K.; Leonberg-Yoo, A.; Schenck, E.J.; Radbel, J.; et al. Factors Associated With Death in Critically Ill Patients With Coronavirus Disease 2019 in the US. *JAMA Intern. Med.* **2020**, *180*, 1436. [CrossRef]
3. Vijayaraj, J. Various Segmentation Techniques for Lung Cancer Detection using CT Images: A Review. *Turk. J. Comput. Math. Educ.* **2021**, *12*, 918–928. [CrossRef]
4. Silveira, M.; Nascimento, J.; Marques, J. Automatic segmentation of the lungs using robust level sets. In Proceedings of the 2007 29th Annual International Conference of the IEEE Engineering in Medicine and Biology Society, Lyon, France, 22–26 August 2007. [CrossRef]
5. Sun, X.; Zhang, H.; Duan, H. 3D Computerized Segmentation of Lung Volume With Computed Tomography. *Acad. Radiol.* **2006**, *13*, 670–677. [CrossRef] [PubMed]

6. Leader, J.K.; Zheng, B.; Rogers, R.M.; Sciurba, F.C.; Perez, A.; Chapman, B.E.; Patel, S.; Fuhrman, C.R.; Gur, D. Automated lung segmentation in X-ray computed tomography. *Acad. Radiol.* **2003**, *10*, 1224–1236. [CrossRef]
7. Hu, S.; Hoffman, E.; Reinhardt, J. Automatic lung segmentation for accurate quantitation of volumetric X-ray CT images. *IEEE Trans. Med. Imaging* **2001**, *20*, 490–498. [CrossRef]
8. Brown, M.S.; Goldin, J.G.; McNitt-Gray, M.F.; Greaser, L.E.; Sapra, A.; Li, K.T.; Sayre, J.W.; Martin, K.; Aberle, D.R. Knowledge-based segmentation of thoracic computed tomography images for assessment of split lung function. *Med. Phys.* **2000**, *27*, 592–598. [CrossRef]
9. Brown, M.; McNitt-Gray, M.; Mankovich, N.; Goldin, J.; Hiller, J.; Wilson, L.; Aberie, D. Method for segmenting chest CT image data using an anatomical model: Preliminary results. *IEEE Trans. Med. Imaging* **1997**, *16*, 828–839. [CrossRef]
10. Van Rikxoort, E.M.; de Hoop, B.; Viergever, M.A.; Prokop, M.; van Ginneken, B. Automatic lung segmentation from thoracic computed tomography scans using a hybrid approach with error detection. *Med. Phys.* **2009**, *36*, 2934–2947. [CrossRef]
11. Tan, J.H.; Acharya, U.R. Active spline model: A shape based model—Interactive segmentation. *Digit. Signal Process.* **2014**, *35*, 64–74. [CrossRef]
12. Gill, G.; Toews, M.; Beichel, R.R. Robust Initialization of Active Shape Models for Lung Segmentation in CT Scans: A Feature-Based Atlas Approach. *Int. J. Biomed. Imaging* **2014**, *2014*, 1–7. [CrossRef]
13. Lassen, B.; van Rikxoort, E.M.; Schmidt, M.; Kerkstra, S.; van Ginneken, B.; Kuhnigk, J.M. Automatic Segmentation of the Pulmonary Lobes From Chest CT Scans Based on Fissures, Vessels, and Bronchi. *IEEE Trans. Med Imaging* **2013**, *32*, 210–222. [CrossRef]
14. Birkbeck, N.; Kohlberger, T.; Zhang, J.; Sofka, M.; Kaftan, J.; Comaniciu, D.; Zhou, S.K. Lung Segmentation from CT with Severe Pathologies Using Anatomical Constraints. In *Medical Image Computing and Computer-Assisted Intervention–MICCAI 2014*; Springer International Publishing: Berlin/Heidelberg, Germany, 2014; pp. 804–811. [CrossRef]
15. Oulefki, A.; Agaian, S.; Trongtirakul, T.; Laouar, A.K. Automatic COVID-19 lung infected region segmentation and measurement using CT-scans images. *Pattern Recognit.* **2021**, *114*, 107747. [CrossRef]
16. Korfiatis, P.; Kalogeropoulou, C.; Karahaliou, A.; Kazantzi, A.; Skiadopoulos, S.; Costaridou, L. Texture classification-based segmentation of lung affected by interstitial pneumonia in high-resolution CT. *Med. Phys.* **2008**, *35*, 5290–5302. [CrossRef] [PubMed]
17. Wang, J.; Li, F.; Li, Q. Automated segmentation of lungs with severe interstitial lung disease in CT. *Med. Phys.* **2009**, *36*, 4592–4599. [CrossRef]
18. Dehmeshki, J.; Ye, X.; Lin, X.; Valdivieso, M.; Amin, H. Automated detection of lung nodules in CT images using shape-based genetic algorithm. *Comput. Med Imaging Graph.* **2007**, *31*, 408–417. [CrossRef] [PubMed]
19. Nakagomi, K.; Shimizu, A.; Kobatake, H.; Yakami, M.; Fujimoto, K.; Togashi, K. Multi-shape graph cuts with neighbor prior constraints and its application to lung segmentation from a chest CT volume. *Med. Image Anal.* **2013**, *17*, 62–77. [CrossRef] [PubMed]
20. Mansoor, A.; Bagci, U.; Xu, Z.; Foster, B.; Olivier, K.N.; Elinoff, J.M.; Suffredini, A.F.; Udupa, J.K.; Mollura, D.J. A Generic Approach to Pathological Lung Segmentation. *IEEE Trans. Med. Imaging* **2014**, *33*, 2293–2310. [CrossRef]
21. Houssein, E.H.; Emam, M.M.; Ali, A.A. Improved manta ray foraging optimization for multi-level thresholding using COVID-19 CT images. *Neural Comput. Appl.* **2021**. [CrossRef]
22. El-Baz, A.; Beache, G.M.; Gimel'farb, G.; Suzuki, K.; Okada, K.; Elnakib, A.; Soliman, A.; Abdollahi, B. Computer-Aided Diagnosis Systems for Lung Cancer: Challenges and Methodologies. *Int. J. Biomed. Imaging* **2013**, *2013*, 942353. [CrossRef]
23. Saood, A.; Hatem, I. COVID-19 lung CT image segmentation using deep learning methods: U-Net versus SegNet. *BMC Med. Imaging* **2021**, *21*. [CrossRef]
24. Badrinarayanan, V.; Kendall, A.; Cipolla, R. SegNet: A Deep Convolutional Encoder-Decoder Architecture for Image Segmentation. *IEEE Trans. Pattern Anal. Mach. Intell.* **2017**, *39*, 2481–2495. [CrossRef]
25. Ronneberger, O.; Fischer, P.; Brox, T. U-Net: Convolutional Networks for Biomedical Image Segmentation. In *Lecture Notes in Computer Science*; Springer International Publishing: Berlin/Heidelberg, Germany, 2015; pp. 234–241. [CrossRef]
26. Yan, Q.; Wang, B.; Gong, D.; Luo, C.; Zhao, W.; Shen, J.; Shi, Q.; Jin, S.; Zhang, L.; You, Z. COVID-19 Chest CT Image Segmentation—A Deep Convolutional Neural Network Solution. *arXiv* **2020**, arXiv:2004.10987.
27. Amyar, A.; Modzelewski, R.; Li, H.; Ruan, S. Multi-task deep learning based CT imaging analysis for COVID-19 pneumonia: Classification and segmentation. *Comput. Biol. Med.* **2020**, *126*, 104037. [CrossRef]
28. Fan, D.P.; Zhou, T.; Ji, G.P.; Zhou, Y.; Chen, G.; Fu, H.; Shen, J.; Shao, L. Inf-Net: Automatic COVID-19 Lung Infection Segmentation From CT Images. *IEEE Trans. Med Imaging* **2020**, *39*, 2626–2637. [CrossRef]
29. Chen, X.; Yao, L.; Zhang, Y. Residual Attention U-Net for Automated Multi-Class Segmentation of COVID-19 Chest CT Images. *arXiv* **2020**, arXiv:2004.05645.
30. Abdel-Basset, M.; Chang, V.; Hawash, H.; Chakrabortty, R.K.; Ryan, M. FSS-2019-nCov: A deep learning architecture for semi-supervised few-shot segmentation of COVID-19 infection. *Knowl. Based Syst.* **2021**, *212*, 106647. [CrossRef] [PubMed]
31. Gao, S.H.; Cheng, M.M.; Zhao, K.; Zhang, X.Y.; Yang, M.H.; Torr, P. Res2Net: A New Multi-Scale Backbone Architecture. *IEEE Trans. Pattern Anal. Mach. Intell.* **2021**, *43*, 652–662. [CrossRef] [PubMed]
32. Zhao, C.; Xu, Y.; He, Z.; Tang, J.; Zhang, Y.; Han, J.; Shi, Y.; Zhou, W. Lung segmentation and automatic detection of COVID-19 using radiomic features from chest CT images. *Pattern Recognit.* **2021**, *119*, 108071. [CrossRef]

33. Milletari, F.; Navab, N.; Ahmadi, S.A. V-Net: Fully Convolutional Neural Networks for Volumetric Medical Image Segmentation. In Proceedings of the 2016 Fourth International Conference on 3D Vision (3DV), Stanford, CA, USA, 25–28 October 2016. [CrossRef]
34. Li, L.; Qin, L.; Xu, Z.; Yin, Y.; Wang, X.; Kong, B.; Bai, J.; Lu, Y.; Fang, Z.; Song, Q.; et al. Using Artificial Intelligence to Detect COVID-19 and Community-acquired Pneumonia Based on Pulmonary CT: Evaluation of the Diagnostic Accuracy. *Radiology* **2020**, *296*, E65–E71. [CrossRef]
35. He, K.; Zhang, X.; Ren, S.; Sun, J. Deep Residual Learning for Image Recognition. In Proceedings of the 2016 IEEE Conference on Computer Vision and Pattern Recognition (CVPR), Las Vegas, NV, USA, 27–30 June 2016. [CrossRef]
36. Singh, V.K.; Abdel-Nasser, M.; Pandey, N.; Puig, D. LungINFseg: Segmenting COVID-19 Infected Regions in Lung CT Images Based on a Receptive-Field-Aware Deep Learning Framework. *Diagnostics* **2021**, *11*, 158. [CrossRef] [PubMed]
37. Shan, F.; Gao, Y.; Wang, J.; Shi, W.; Shi, N.; Han, M.; Xue, Z.; Shen, D.; Shi, Y. Abnormal lung quantification in chest CT images of COVID-19 patients with deep learning and its application to severity prediction. *Med. Phys.* **2021**, *48*, 1633–1645. [CrossRef] [PubMed]
38. Gerard, S.E.; Herrmann, J.; Xin, Y.; Martin, K.T.; Rezoagli, E.; Ippolito, D.; Bellani, G.; Cereda, M.; Guo, J.; Hoffman, E.A.; et al. CT image segmentation for inflamed and fibrotic lungs using a multi-resolution convolutional neural network. *Sci. Rep.* **2021**, *11*. [CrossRef]
39. Pan, F.; Li, L.; Liu, B.; Ye, T.; Li, L.; Liu, D.; Ding, Z.; Chen, G.; Liang, B.; Yang, L.; et al. A novel deep learning-based quantification of serial chest computed tomography in Coronavirus Disease 2019 (COVID-19). *Sci. Rep.* **2021**, *11*, 1–11. [CrossRef]
40. Ma, J.; Wang, Y.; An, X.; Ge, C.; Yu, Z.; Chen, J.; Zhu, Q.; Dong, G.; He, J.; He, Z.; et al. Toward data-efficient learning: A benchmark for COVID-19 CT lung and infection segmentation. *Med. Phys.* **2021**, *48*, 1197–1210. [CrossRef]
41. Elharrouss, O.; Subramanian, N.; Al-Maadeed, S. An encoder-decoder-based method for COVID-19 lung infection segmentation. *arXiv* **2020**, arXiv:2007.00861.
42. Müller, D.; Rey, I.S.; Kramer, F. Automated Chest CT Image Segmentation of COVID-19 Lung Infection based on 3D U-Net. *arXiv* **2020**, arXiv:2007.04774.
43. Tilborghs, S.; Dirks, I.; Fidon, L.; Willems, S.; Eelbode, T.; Bertels, J.; Ilsen, B.; Brys, A.; Dubbeldam, A.; Buls, N.; et al. Comparative study of deep learning methods for the automatic segmentation of lung, lesion and lesion type in CT scans of COVID-19 patients. *arXiv* **2020**, arXiv:2007.15546.
44. Tajbakhsh, N.; Jeyaseelan, L.; Li, Q.; Chiang, J.N.; Wu, Z.; Ding, X. Embracing imperfect datasets: A review of deep learning solutions for medical image segmentation. *Med. Image Anal.* **2020**, *63*, 101693. [CrossRef] [PubMed]
45. El-Baz, A.S.; Gimel'farb, G.L.; Suri, J.S. *Stochastic Modeling for Medical Image Analysis*; OCLC: 1086143882; CRC Press: Boca Raton, FL, USA, 2016.
46. Fuglede, B.; Topsoe, F. Jensen-Shannon divergence and Hilbert space embedding. In Proceedings of the International Symposium onInformation Theory 2004, Chicago, IL, USA, 27 June–2 July 2004. [CrossRef]
47. MacKay, D.J.C. *Information Theory, Inference, and Learning Algorithms*; Cambridge University Press: New York, NY, USA, 2003; p. 34
48. Gerig, G.; Jomier, M.; Chakos, M. Valmet: A New Validation Tool for Assessing and Improving 3D Object Segmentation. In *Medical Image Computing and Computer-Assisted Intervention–MICCAI 2001*; Springer: Berlin/Heidelberg, Germany, 2001; pp. 516–523. [CrossRef]
49. Soliman, A.; Khalifa, F.; Alansary, A.; Gimel'farb, G.; El-Baz, A. *Performance Evaluation of an Automatic MGRF-Based Lung Segmentation Approach*; AIP: College Park, MA, USA, 2013. [CrossRef]
50. An, P.; Xu, S.; Harmon, S.A.; Turkbey, E.B.; Sanford, T.H.; Amalou, A.; Kassin, M.; Varble, N.; Blain, M.; Anderson, V.; et al. CT Images in COVID-19. Available online: https://wiki.cancerimagingarchive.net/display/Public/CT+Images+in+COVID-19 (accessed on 5 June 2021).
51. Kasper, J.; Decker, J.; Wiesenreiter, K.; Römmele, C.; Ebigbo, A.; Braun, G.; Häckel, T.; Schwarz, F.; Wehler, M.; Messmann, H.; et al. Typical Imaging Patterns in COVID-19 Infections of the Lung on Plain Chest Radiographs to Aid Early Triage. In *RöFo-Fortschritte auf dem Gebiet der RöNtgenstrahlen und der Bildgebenden Verfahren*; Georg Thieme Verlag KG: New York, NY, USA, 2021. [CrossRef]
52. Chen, L.C.; Zhu, Y.; Papandreou, G.; Schroff, F.; Adam, H. Encoder-Decoder with Atrous Separable Convolution for Semantic Image Segmentation. In Proceedings of the European Conference on Computer Vision (ECCV), Munich, Germany, 8–4 September 2018.
53. Özgün Çiçek.; Abdulkadir, A.; Lienkamp, S.S.; Brox, T.; Ronneberger, O. 3D U-Net: Learning Dense Volumetric Segmentation from Sparse Annotation. In *Medical Image Computing and Computer-Assisted Intervention–MICCAI 2016*; Springer International Publishing: Berlin/Heidelberg, Germany, 2016; pp. 424–432. [CrossRef]

sensors

MDPI

Article

A CNN Deep Local and Global ASD Classification Approach with Continuous Wavelet Transform Using Task-Based FMRI

Reem Haweel [1,2], Noha Seada [1], Said Ghoniemy [1], Norah Saleh Alghamdi [3] and Ayman El-Baz [2,*]

[1] Faculty of Computer and Information Sciences, University of Ain Shams, Cairo 11566, Egypt; reem.t.haweel@cis.asu.edu.eg (R.H.); noha.seada@cis.asu.edu.eg (N.S.); said.Ghoniemy@cis.asu.edu.eg (S.G.)

[2] Bioengineering Department, University of Louisville, Louisville, KY 40208, USA

[3] College of Computer and Information Science, Princess Nourah Bint Abdulrahman University, Riyadh 11671, Saudi Arabia; nosalghamdi@pnu.edu.sa

* Correspondence: ayman.elbaz@louisville.edu

Abstract: Autism spectrum disorder (ASD) is a neurodegenerative disorder characterized by lingual and social disabilities. The autism diagnostic observation schedule is the current gold standard for ASD diagnosis. Developing objective computer aided technologies for ASD diagnosis with the utilization of brain imaging modalities and machine learning is one of main tracks in current studies to understand autism. Task-based fMRI demonstrates the functional activation in the brain by measuring blood oxygen level-dependent (BOLD) variations in response to certain tasks. It is believed to hold discriminant features for autism. A novel computer aided diagnosis (CAD) framework is proposed to classify 50 ASD and 50 typically developed toddlers with the adoption of CNN deep networks. The CAD system includes both local and global diagnosis in a response to speech task. Spatial dimensionality reduction with region of interest selection and clustering has been utilized. In addition, the proposed framework performs discriminant feature extraction with continuous wavelet transform. Local diagnosis on cingulate gyri, superior temporal gyrus, primary auditory cortex and angular gyrus achieves accuracies ranging between 71% and 80% with a four-fold cross validation technique. The fused global diagnosis achieves an accuracy of 86% with 82% sensitivity, 92% specificity. A brain map indicating ASD severity level for each brain area is created, which contributes to personalized diagnosis and treatment plans.

Keywords: autism; ASD; computer-aided diagnosis; deep learning; CNN; CWT

Citation: Haweel, R.; Seada, N.; Ghoniemy, S.; Alghamdi, N.S.; El-Baz, A. A CNN Deep Local and Global ASD Classification Approach with Continuous Wavelet Transform Using Task-Based FMRI. *Sensors* **2021**, *21*, 5822. https://doi.org/10.3390/s21175822

Academic Editors: Yu-Dong Zhang and Steve Ling

Received: 22 June 2021
Accepted: 25 August 2021
Published: 29 August 2021

1. Introduction

Autism spectrum disorder (ASD) is a neurodevelopmental disorder that affects social communication ability. ASD also causes language impairment and repetitive behaviors [1]. Individuals with ASD show different severity levels associated with each symptom [2]. The common ASD diagnostic standard utilizes history and expert clinical judgment together with behavioral modules of the autism diagnostic observation schedule (ADOS) [3,4]. Autism is diagnosed with the arising noticeable symptoms which start at the age of three to five years [5]. It is crucial to intervene and diagnose ASD early to allow for better assessment and treatment.

ASD can be diagnosed at the age of 12 months old, especially with the emergence of imaging diagnostic tools that employ brain imaging modalities such as structural (sMRI), functional (fMRI), and diffusion (DTI) magnetic resonance imaging [6]. Combining these scans to view the structure of the brain together with the brain functional activity during rest and performance of certain tasks constitute an early biomarker for ASD [7].

Resting state and task-based fMRI are types of fMRI scans that are adopted to manifest functional activity. Task-based fMRI measures evoked blood oxygen level-dependent (BOLD) signals during the performance of different tasks [8] such as auditory tasks, language tasks, visual processing tasks, motor tasks, and social tasks [9].

To investigate autistic brain abnormal functional response to speech compared to typically developed (TD) peers, several studies were performed [10]. Studies in [11–13] played an audio of a simple bedtime story and examined the sleep fMRI response. These studies included 40 autistic toddlers and 40 TD toddlers with ages that range from 12 to 48 months. Autistic toddlers showed abnormal laterality and hypoactivation in the left anterior portion of the superior temporal cortex (aSTG). On the other hand, TD toddlers exhibited the normal dominant activation of the left hemisphere aSTG. They also suggested early intervention and treatment as they demonstrated that as the age increases, lateralization abnormality increases.

Several studies up to 2013 that were reviewed in [14] concluded the involvement of atypical lateralization with language impairment. Individuals with ASD exhibited attenuation in the left hemisphere activation. Also, anomalous lateralization in the functional areas responsible for prelinguistics and language, specifically the fronto-temporal regions, were present. One of the reviewed studies [15] revealed atypical lateralization starts at an early age. Lower lateralization was present in high risk ASD infants, while higher lateralization was present in low risk peers. A review in [16] concluded similar results.

A meta-analysis of fMRI studies until 2013 was presented in [10]. Increased activation in the right precentral gyrus and decreased left activation were revealed in ASD individuals who performed language and auditory tasks, which contradicts the normal activation in TD individuals. Moreover, fMRI scans in TD individuals showed higher activation in the bilateral superior temporal gyri (STG) and left cingulate gyrus than ASD peers.

Literature on task-based fMRI analysis for ASD concludes fundamental differences in activation in ASD compared to TD individuals. These findings support the employment of task-based fMRI for early ASD diagnosis [17]. Machine learning (ML) has made it possible to develop intelligent and automated systems for several pattern recognition applications. The emergence of noninvasive or minimally invasive medical screening devices created massive informative data structures that allowed for the exploitation of ML for automated diagnosis. A research in [18] proposed a pipeline based on task fMRI scans for predicting treatment of social responsiveness scale outcome. They applied the general linear model (GLM) for brain feature extraction. Feature selection techniques were performed following feature extraction. For classification, they employed the random forest (RF) classifier. Twenty ASD children (5.90 ± 1.07 years) were included in the study. A recent study in [19] performed both local and global diagnosis for ASD toddlers. Brain areas parcellated with the Brainnetome atlas (BNT) were analyzed with a stacked nonnegativity constraint auto-encoder. The study included 30 ASD against 30 TD and classified between two groups with an accuracy of 75.8%. Another recent study graded the severity of autism into three groups [20,21]. GLM analysis for low individual level analysis, to extract features, and high group level analysis, to infer statistical differences between groups and validation, were applied. They utilized different approaches to extract features from GLM analyzed whole brain areas. Among the several classifier architectures they tested, Random Forest performed best with 78% accuracy. In [22], they enhanced their framework by performing a two stage classifier, included more data (92 mild, 32 moderate, and 33 severely autistic) and performed more validation techniques. Accuracies ranged between 70% and 83%.

ML and deep learning, which is a subset of ML that involves deep networks, have played a very important rule in many neuroscience applications. Convolutional neural network (CNN) is one of the most powerful DL network architectures. CNNs are deeply adopted in Brain-Computer Interfaces (BCI) as well as classification of EEG signals [23–25].

Recently, CNNs have been widely utilized for ASD diagnosis and analysis with fMRI [26]. Jinlong Hu et al. [27] adopted a multi-channel 2D CNN model to classify FMRI dataset of 995 subjects in a motor experiment. They proved that CNNs achieve good performance with high dimensional data, in comparison with other classifiers, mostly when the dataset is large as in their case. A study in [28] investigated the employment of spatial and temporal features of task-based fMRI. To capture the spatial information, they developed a 3D convolutional neural networks on two-channel images of mean and standard deviation that were created by the sliding window, which captures the temporal statistics. This framework achieved an 8.5% increase in the mean F-scores.

FMRI scans constitute 4D data of a brain 3D volume consisting of 1D time-dependent BOLD signals. Several signal processing techniques can be optimized to analyze these BOLD signals. Wavelet transform are considered one of the efficient time signal processing techniques for resolving time-series. Applications of the wavelet transform include compression, high resolution time, and frequency analysis and denoising [29]. It has also been utilized for fMRI analysis as an alternative to conventional GLMs. PS Lessa et al. [30] concluded that Wavelet correlation analysis achieves higher statistical power in comparison to GLMs. Moreover, wavelet transforms contribute to the achievement of efficient brain disorder diagnosis, such as ADHD, autism and Alzheimer diagnosis, when applied on fMRI feature processing. In an approach to diagnose ADHD, García et al. [31] performed continuous wavelet transform (CWT) to create scalograms of BOLD signals.

Most previous fMRI experiments were applied on adults [32,33], however, our proposed study includes toddlers/infants from 12 to 40 months old. The aim of our study is to develop an early autism computer aided local and global detection tool. Spatial dimensionality reduction with region of interest (ROI) selection and clustering have been performed to reduce the 4D fMRI data to a reduced number of BOLD signals. In order to provide a detailed frequency and scale representation, we have applied CWT on selected BOLD signals. CWT creates scalogram images that are used as input images to multi-channel 2D-CNNs for each area. Finally, brain maps that indicate level of ASD severity for each ROI is provided for each subject. The proposed framework works towards determining the neuro-circuits with abnormalities as well as creating personalized diagnosis and treatment plans that handles the specific case of each individual. Moreover, CWT achieved better results compared to other feature extraction and generation techniques.

2. Materials

2.1. *fMRI Data Collection*

This study includes subjects from "Biomarkers of Autism at 12 Months: From Brain Overgrowth to Genes" dataset. This dataset was collected between August 2007 and June 2014 and is provided by the national database for autism research (NDAR: http://ndar.nih.gov (accessed on 22 May 2019)) [11,34,35]. The dataset included 639 subjects that were tracked every 12 months roughly starting at 12 months and until they are 40 months old.

We have chosen some substantial criteria in selecting subjects for our study such that included subjects must have ADOS toddler module, sMRI (T1) and (T2), and response to speech task fMRI (T2*). Intensive validation on each report and scan has been conducted. Visual validation is performed for all sMRI scans to exclude inaccurate or corrupted ones. FMRI scans have been validated to have 154 volumes and visually validated to have no clear artifacts. One hundred subjects (50 ASD 50 TD) with ages ranging between 12–40 months old, are included in this study. Information about each subject , such as IDs and final diagnosis, as well as the extracted BOLD signals of this dataset are available in Supplementary Materials 1 and 2, respectively.

2.2. *Response to Speech Experiment*

The experiment that was used while task-based fMRI scans were acquired is a response to speech experiment. An audio record of a narrator telling a story was played during natural sleep. The audio consists of three different types of records, simple forward speech, complex forward speech, and backward speech. Such records alternate with silence periods and are repeated during a 6 min and 20 s span.

3. Methods

In this study, local and global ASD diagnosis have been developed. Figure 1 demonstrates the adopted framework. First, fMRI scans are preprocessed using FMRI expert analysis tool (FEAT) [36] developed in fMRI's software library (FSL) [37]. Brain parcellation is based on Harvard-Oxford probabilistic atlas https://identifiers.org/neurovault.collection:262. (accessed on 11 April 2019) The Detailed explanation of preprocessing steps is provided in [20].

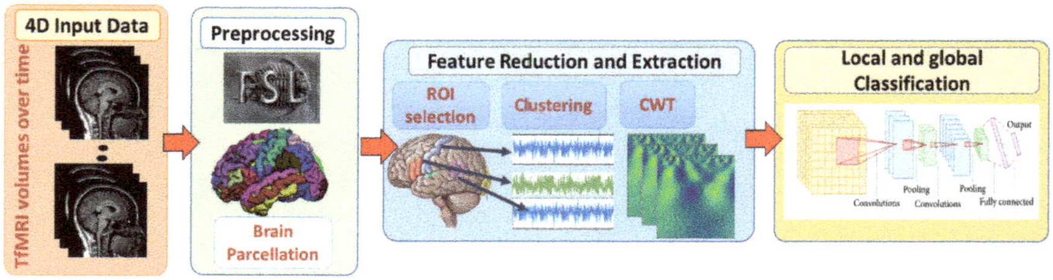

Figure 1. The proposed framework for local and global classification. First, 4D fMRI data are preprocessed with FSL. Brain extraction and parcellation to Harvard-Oxford probabilistic atlas are also performed. Second, spacial and temporal feature reduction and extraction techniques are performed. Finally, local classification models on each ROI are developed to provide a global classification decision.

3.1. Spatial Dimensionality Reduction

Applying neural networks on raw data without feature engineering is feasible when the raw data are easily separable. However, identifying autism biomarkers in task fMRI is a complex problem as autism follows a wide spectrum and is not easily separable. Moreover, fMRI raw data is a high dimensional data of 4D. CNN performance decreases when data dimensionality is high and input data size is small as in medical applications. Hence, it is crucial to reduce dimensionality. A comparison of fMRI feature extraction and reduction approaches have been presented in [38], proving higher ASD classification results. The following steps have been proposed for feature reduction:

- ROI selection: Based on literature of the response to speech experiment for toddlers, specific brain areas related to language circuits are activated. These areas include cingulate gyri (CG), superior temporal gyrus (STG), primary auditory cortex (PAC) and angular gyrus (AG) for both hemispheres. In this study, the most significantly activated brain areas are selected.
- Clustering: Each brain includes several commonly activated voxels, which are considered redundant data. Therefore, grouping similar BOLD signals in each area and extracting a single value for each group is efficient and can extensively enhance classification performance. Hence, each brain area's BOLD signals have been clustered with kmeans. Different number of clusters have been tested to achieve higher validation accuracies.Two methods to represent the signals of each cluster have been tested: averaging BOLD signals, or extracting the BOLD signal closest to the center of that cluster.

The advantage of the previous reduction approaches is that the brain structure is maintained. Each brain area is represented by a number of features. This technique allows for local analysis and obtaining brain maps.

3.2. Continuous Wavelet Transform

CWT is a technique used to represent a signal by convolving wavelets, that vary continuously in transition and scale, with the original signal. The result presents a power spectrum of the signal as in Figure 2. The CWT of a signal $x(t)$ at scale a ($a > 0$) and translation b is calculated by:

$$X_w(a,b) = \frac{1}{|a|^{1/2}} \int_{-\infty}^{\infty} x(t)\psi^*\left(\frac{t-b}{a}\right)dt \quad (1)$$

where ψ is the mother wavelet which is a continuous function in both the time domain and the frequency domain and the $*$ represents operation of complex conjugate. The mother wavelet is the source that generates daughter wavelets which are the translated and scaled versions of the mother wavelet. After extracting BOLD signals from clusters, the CWT is applied to produce scalograms that provide a detailed representation on these BOLD signals. The scalogram images are then rescaled to 64×64 and fed to multichannel 2D-CNNs for each area. In task-based fMRI experiments, quantifying the change in the BOLD signal across time is significantly important. As mentioned before, CWT scalograms hold information about both frequency and time in an image, and therefore, satisfy this requirement. Applying 2D CNN filters can extract trainable numerical weighted values from these images, during the training phase. During testing phase, these values are compared to classify each entry.

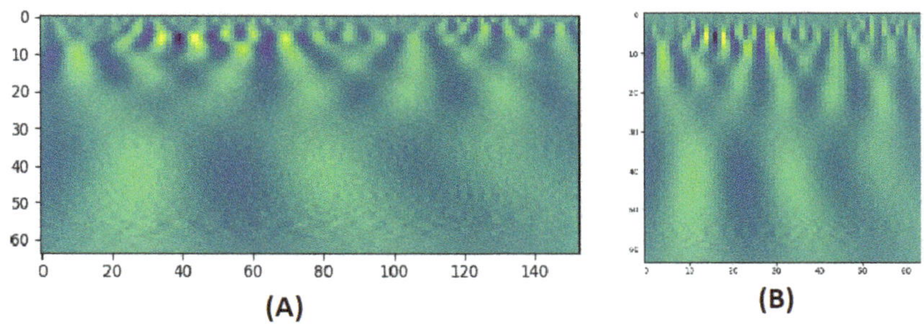

Figure 2. (**A**) A CWT scalogram example with 64 scales of a BOLD signal of 153 time points. (**B**) The resized version of size: 64×64.

3.3. 2D CNN Classification

CNN is a deep learning architecture gaining prominence in the analysis of images, including medical image data. CNN may be characterized by the dimensionality of their convolutional kernels, which in practice is typically between one and four, inclusive. Higher kernel dimensions incur a computational bottleneck, especially when paired with large input sizes, e.g., a 4D CNN that processes fMRI volumetric time series. We have developed a more tractable 2D CNN model four our framework. As a deep neural network, the CNN comprises a number of layers, including convolutional layers based on the aforementioned kernels, pooling layers for reducing the size of the activation map, and fully connected (FC) layers for higher order feature representations.

We have extensively tested several model hyper-parameters, as explained in detail in the experimental results. Our CNN model performs three successive passes of convolution and size reduction as shown in Table 1 (which is developed by the model summary method provided by Keras library). These are followed by FC layers (Dense), the final (output) layer having a softmax activation function for purposes of classification. As explained earlier, each brain area is represented with CWT power spectrum images. A separate CNN classifier is developed and tuned for better performance for each brain area. Global classification is obtained with majority voting by all areas, as shown in Figure 3.

Table 1. CNN network summary.

Layer	Output Shape	Param #
2Dconv	(None, 62, 62, 15)	1635
Max_pooling2D	(None, 31, 31, 15)	0
2Dconv_1	(None, 29, 29, 15)	2040
Max_pooling2D_1	(None, 14, 14, 15)	0
2Dconv_2	(None, 12, 12, 15)	2040
max_pooling2D_2	(None, 6, 6, 15)	0
Flatten	(None, 540)	0
Dense	(None, 10)	5410
Dense_1	(None, 2)	22
Total parameters: 11,147	Trainable parameters: 11,147	

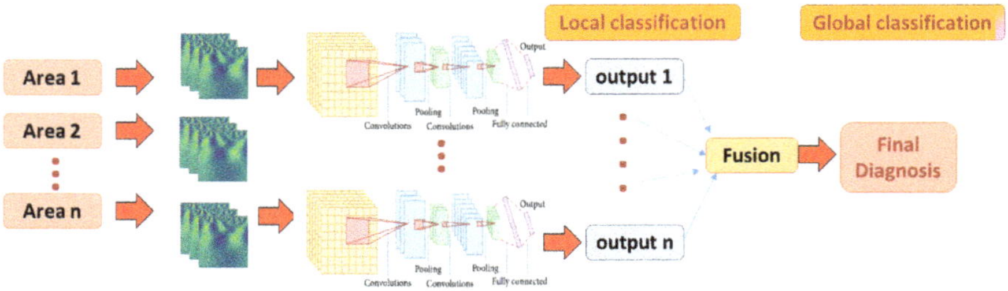

Figure 3. The local and global classification pipeline. A multi-channel 2D CNN local model is developed for each area, fed with corresponding CWT scalograms. The final global classification decision is fused using majority voting approach.

4. Experimental Results

The incorporated dataset includes 100 subjects (50 ASD and 50 TD). Performance evaluation has been conducted for local CNN model. The whole framework integration is performed using python. The CNN classification model is implemented with Keras library. Several parameters at each step on the proposed spatial dimensionality reduction and classification pipeline are evaluated. The 4-fold average classification accuracy with random shuffling is the score to be optimized. For clustering, 3 clusters provide discriminant average BOLD signals for each area. In the CWT stage, 32, 64 and 128 number of scales have been evaluated. best performance is obtained by 64 scales. Some wavelets have been tested such as: Mexican Hat, Gaussian Derivative and Morlets. Best results are obtained with Morlets.

A grid search method to determine classification parameters has been applied: number of filter (5, 10, 15), CNN kernal sizes (3, 5, 7), epchs (5:70 in order of 5), batch sizes (1, 32, 64, 100) learning rates (0.1, 0.001, 0.0001), optimizers ('SGD', 'Adagrad', 'RMSprop', 'Adadelta', 'Adamax', 'Adam', 'Nadam'), network activations ('softplus', 'softmax', 'softsign', 'tanh', 'relu', 'sigmoid', 'linear', 'hard_sigmoid'), and finally, kernal weight initializers ('uniform', 'normal', 'lecun_uniform', 'zero', 'glorot_uniform', 'glorot_normal', 'he_uniform', 'he_normal'). The parameters that achieved best results are represented in Table 2. 15 kernels, each with the size of 3×3, achieve better results. According to these parameters, the output shape and parameter columns in Table 1 are determined. The number of parameters is the number of trainable network weights at each stage. Only the convolutional and Dense layers contain trainable weights. The maxpooling layers (with size 2×2) only calculate the maximum without including a bias parameter. More explanation about how the model layer sizes are determined is provided in [39].

Table 2. CNN and CWT parameters.

Kernels	Kernel Size	Learning Rate	Batch Size	Optimizer	Network Activation	Kernel Initializer	Wavelet	Scales	Time Course Normalization
15	3	0.01	32	Adamax	Relu	Lecun_uniform	Morlet	64	Percent signal change

4.1. Local Classification

Each local CNN classifier is fed with CWT scalogram images extracted from both hemisphere and the inferior and posterior division, if present. Hence, each classifier has different number of extracted signals for it's input. Table 3 demonstrates the classification accuracy, sensitivity, specificity, and area under the curve (AUC) for the STG, CG, AG, and PAC areas. The AUC is an effective measure of sensitivity and specificity for assessing inherent validity of the proposed system. Higher AUC means that the proposed system is accurate in differentiating ASD with TD subjects. This implies both sensitivity and specificity are maximum and errors (false positive and false negative) are minimum.

The confusion matrix of each area is demonstrated in Figure 4. As can be noted, high percentages are concentrated in the diagonal of each matrix (True positive and True negative) and ranges around the corresponding total accuracy. Therefore, each matrix is balanced. Moreover, receiver operating characteristic (ROC) curves are plotted in Figure 5. After developing local 2D-CNN models, brain maps for each subject are created to represent the level of autism severity for each brain area.

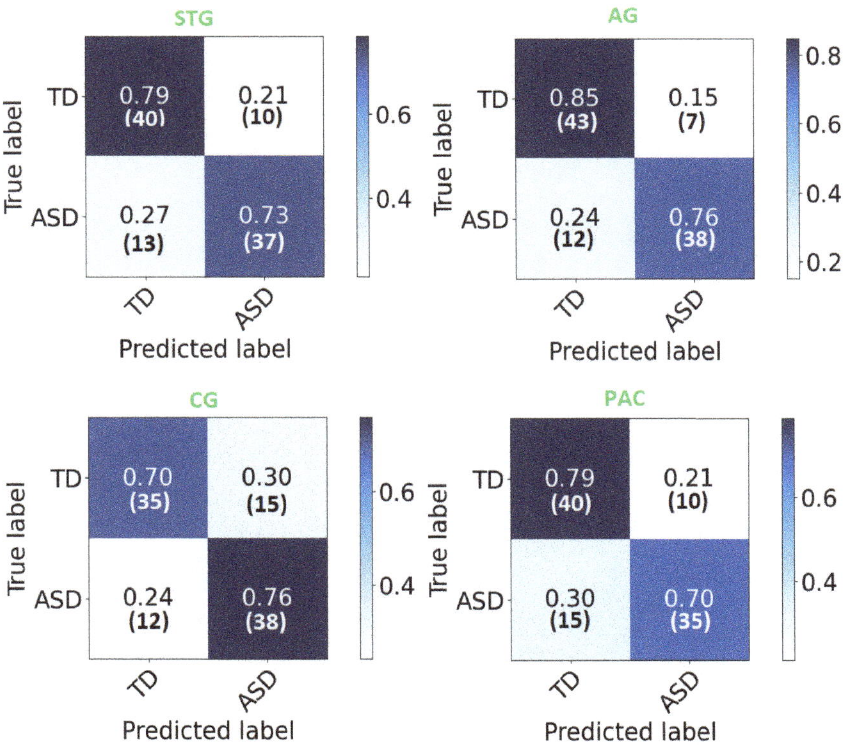

Figure 4. The confusion matrix for each ROI local classifier represented in percentage (number) for each row.

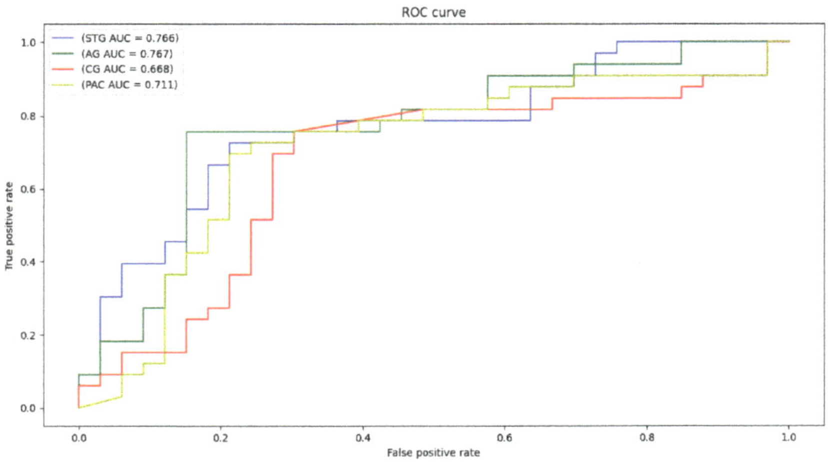

Figure 5. ROC curves and AUC for STG, CG, AG, and PAC selected areas.

Table 3. Accuracy, sensitivity, specificity, AUC of selected ROIs.

Classifier	Accuracy	Sensitivity	Specificity	AUC
STG	0.742	0.74	0.77	0.76
AG	0.80	0.78	0.83	0.77
CG	0.72	0.74	0.71	0.67
PAC	0.71	0.72	0.77	0.71

4.2. Global Classification

The global classification accuracy is obtained by fusing the decision from each local classifier with majority voting. The achieved accuracy is 86% (sensitivity 82%, specificity 92%). The confusion matrix is demonstrated in Figure 6. Same notes can be concluded from the confusion matrix. We have also tested a global 2D-CNN classifier that is trained with the scalogram images of all areas at once. This step is performed as a validation step and to highlight the advantage of classification that is based on local classifiers . The obtained accuracy is 82%. Figure 7 plots the ROC of the classifier.

The accuracy is close to the global accuracy of 86% which proves the stability of the system. The inferred reason for less accuracy can be related to the fact that higher number of input features (and hence higher number of parameters) introduced in the CNN network achieves lower accuracy. Therefore in this validation model, the increased number of channels increases the number of parameters and hence, leads to lower performance.

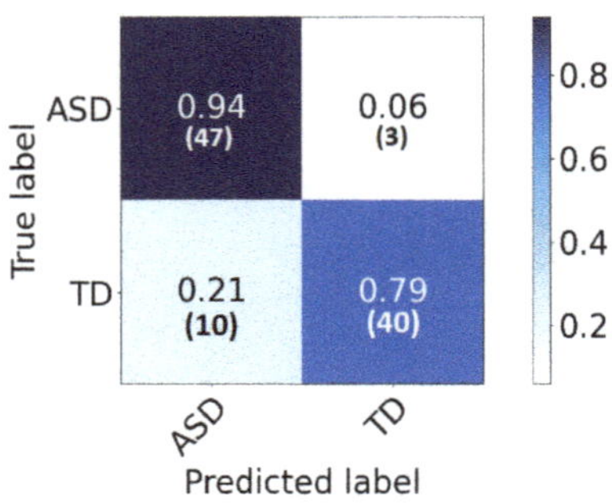

Figure 6. The confusion matrix for the global classifier represented in percentage (number) for each row.

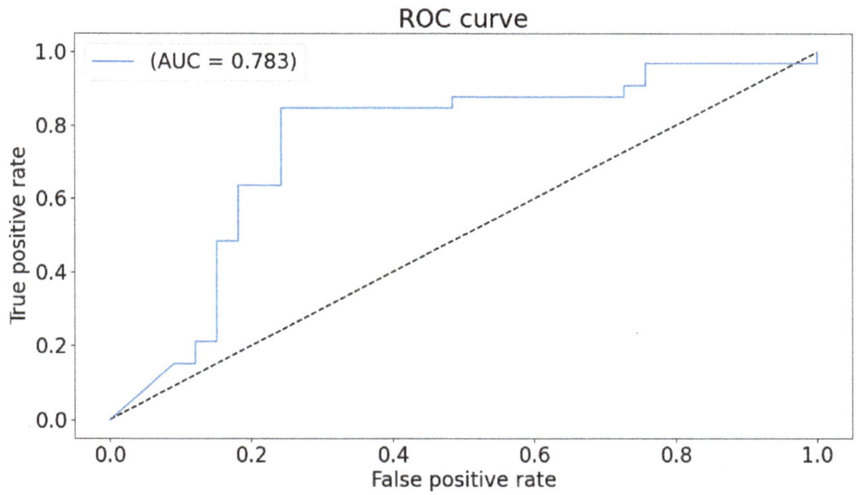

Figure 7. ROC curve and AUC for the global classifier.

The proposed framework achieves higher accuracies compared to other previous work performed on task-based fMRI scans of the same experiment, as presented in Table 4. A direct comparison between our research and other literature of other tasks would not be objective as other researches incorporate different data sets and task-based fMRI experiments. As a comparison with our previous approaches in [19,20,38], we can note that the accuracy of the proposed classification that is based on local classifiers is higher. The reason is believed to be the better learning of CNN local networks that have lower number of parameters. Majority voting reflects the advantage of building the decision based on the most affected brain areas, rather than all included areas.

Table 4. A comparison of the proposed CAD system with other GLM-based methods.

Method	Data Source	No. of Subjects	Modeling of BOLD	Classifier	Validation	Accuracy
[38]	NDAR	100 (50 ASD, 50 TD)	DWT	2D CNN	4-fold	78%
[19]	NDAR	60 (30 ASD, 30 TD)	GLM	SNCAE	4-fold	76%
[20]	NDAR	39 (13 Mild, 13 Moderate, 13 Severe)	GLM	RF	10-fold	72%
proposed	NDAR	100 (50 ASD, 50 TD)	CWT	multi-channel 2D CNN	4-fold	86%

4.3. Brain Maps

According to literature, not every brain area is affected by the same degree for each individual. Therefore, we obtain individual brain maps that explain the level of autism for each area. After the implementation and training of local classifiers, each subject's local brain area data is tested for each corresponding trained network. The resulted probabilities are represented in a brain map as demonstrated in Figure 8. As an example, the probabilities obtained for the first individual are: (STG: 0.037, AG: 0.36, CG: 0.31, PAC: 0.072). According to majority voting, the four areas has high probabilities for autism ($p > 0.5$), hence, this individual is TD. For the other individual, the obtained probabilities are: (STG: 0.77, AG: 0.97, CG: 0.61, PAC: 0.99). According to majority voting, the four areas has low probabilities for autism ($p <= 0.5$), hence, this individual is TD. Some individuals might have autistic areas and non autistic ones, as mentioned before. An example for the probability distribution (STG: 0.43, AG: 0.8, CG: 0.61, PAC: 0.99). Three areas are autistic ($p > 0.5$) and one area is non autistic ($p < 0.5$). Therefore, this subject is classified as autistic.

Figure 8 also demonstrates a 3D view. The viewing tool is FSLeyes through FSL. As can be noted, the grade of autism are higher (red colors) of ASD subjects, with variable grade on each area. The grade of autism for TD subjects is lower (yellow colors) with different grades.

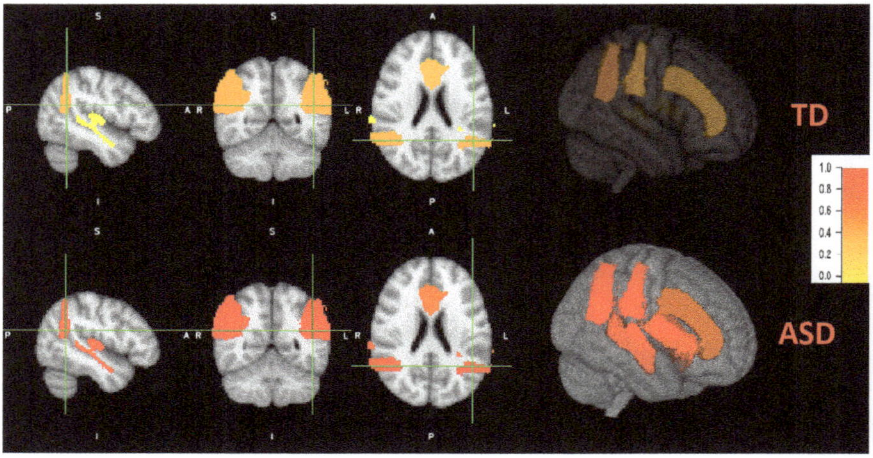

Figure 8. Coronal, sagital and axial 2D views and a 3D view of both ASD and TD example. Brain areas for the ASD individual are more severely distributed (red highlights) than TD peer (more yellow highlight distribution).

5. Conclusions and Future Work

In this paper, a novel CNN Deep learning based ASD local and global diagnosis system is introduced. The proposed system utilized task-based fMRI to achieve this goal. According to the response to speech experiment, hypoactivation of the bilateral superior temporal gyrus, bilateral primary auditory cortex, cingulate gyrus and angular gyrus are exhibited in ASD toddlers. Whereas, TD peers exhibited typical lateralized activation. Based on these results, local spatial and temporal features are extracted from each ROI separately. CWT is performed to extract scalogram images, from the extracted BOLD signals from spatially reduced clusters, that hold frequency specifications. A local CNN classifier is utilized for each area. Experimental results are reported for all activated brain areas. Accuracies range between 71% and 80%. Global classification is obtained from local results. Achieved accuracy is 86% (with 82% sensitivity and 92% specificity). Finally, local individual brain maps are created for each subject that indicate level of ASD severity.

Future work will include the application of the same approaches on rest-state fMRI of same dataset. Hence, a detailed report for each subject will be obtained for connected brain networks during rest and activated brain areas during task activities. Global decision will be more accurate and will consider all functional aspects of the brain. Researchers are encouraged to collect more data from different geographical sites. A protocol for generic experimental design is recommended to enable researchers to validate their work with other datasets. More validation steps will be performed, leading to a robust ASD diagnosis system. In addition, our future work will include genomic data (which is available in the collected data set used in this paper) to correlate affected brain areas with specific genome sequences to help in early ASD detection. Finally, local classification results will be investigated to identify malfunctioned neuro-circuits involved with ASD.

Supplementary Materials: The following are available online at: https://www.mdpi.com/article/10.3390/s21175822/s1 and https://cisasuedu-my.sharepoint.com/:u:/g/personal/reem_t_haweel_cis_asu_edu_eg/EYfDlDjzwEJDh3Sw_U8Cf7MBiW31QmgDaKpXLnupL77LGA?e=4%3aNDAvwR&at=9.

Author Contributions: Conceptualization, S.G.; Data curation, R.H.; Funding acquisition, N.S.A.; Investigation, N.S.; Methodology, S.G. and A.E.-B.; Project administration, N.S.A. and A.E.-B.;

Resources, A.E.-B.; Software, R.H.; Supervision, N.S., S.G. and A.E.-B.; Writing—original draft, R.H. All authors have read and agreed to the published version of the manuscript.

Funding: The Deanship of Scientific Research at PrincessNourah bint Abdulrahman University.

Institutional Review Board Statement: No IRB Required. It is a public dataset.

Informed Consent Statement: Written informed consent has been obtained from the patient(s) to use this dataset for research purposes and publishing this paper.

Data Availability Statement: The dataset adopted in this research is provided by the national database for autism research NDAR: http://ndar.nih.gov (accessed on 22 June 2021).

Acknowledgments: This research was funded by the Deanship of Scientific Research at Princess Nourah bint Abdulrahman University through the Fast-track Research Funding Program.

Conflicts of Interest: The authors declare no conflict of interest.

References

1. Amaral, D.G.; Schumann, C.M.; Nordahl, C.W. Neuroanatomy of autism. *Trends Neurosci.* **2008**, *31*, 137–145. [CrossRef]
2. Gotham, K.; Pickles, A.; Lord, C. Trajectories of autism severity in children using standardized ADOS scores. *Pediatrics* **2012**, *130*, e1278–e1284. [CrossRef]
3. Gotham, K.; Pickles, A.; Lord, C. Standardizing ADOS scores for a measure of severity in autism spectrum disorders. *J. Autism Dev. Disord.* **2009**, *39*, 693–705. [CrossRef] [PubMed]
4. Manning-Courtney, P.; Murray, D.; Currans, K.; Johnson, H.; Bing, N.; Kroeger-Geoppinger, K.; Sorensen, R.; Bass, J.; Reinhold, J.; Johnson, A.; et al. Autism spectrum disorders. *Curr. Probl. Pediatr. Adolesc. Health Care* **2013**, *43*, 2–11. [CrossRef] [PubMed]
5. Zwaigenbaum, L.; Bryson, S.; Rogers, T.; Roberts, W.; Brian, J.; Szatmari, P. Behavioral manifestations of autism in the first year of life. *Int. J. Dev. Neurosci.* **2005**, *23*, 143–152. [CrossRef] [PubMed]
6. Casanova, M.F.; El-Baz, A.; Suri, J.S. *Autism Imaging and Devices*; CRC Press: Boca Raton, MA, USA, 2017.
7. Ismail, M.M.T. A CAD System for Early Diagnosis of Autism Using Different Imaging Modalities. Ph.D. Thesis, University of Louisville, Louisville, KY, USA, 2016.
8. Van Horn, J.D.; Grethe, J.S.; Kostelec, P.; Woodward, J.B.; Aslam, J.A.; Rus, D.; Rockmore, D.; Gazzaniga, M.S. The Functional Magnetic Resonance Imaging Data Center (fMRIDC): The challenges and rewards of large–scale databasing of neuroimaging studies. *Philos. Trans. R. Soc. Lond. B Biol. Sci.* **2001**, *356*, 1323–1339. [CrossRef] [PubMed]
9. Casanova, M.F.; El-Baz, A.S.; Suri, J.S. *Imaging the Brain in Autism*; Springer: New York, NY, USA, 2013.
10. Philip, R.C.; Dauvermann, M.R.; Whalley, H.C.; Baynham, K.; Lawrie, S.M.; Stanfield, A.C. A systematic review and meta-analysis of the fMRI investigation of autism spectrum disorders. *Neurosci. Biobehav. Rev.* **2012**, *36*, 901–942. [CrossRef]
11. Eyler, L.T.; Pierce, K.; Courchesne, E. A failure of left temporal cortex to specialize for language is an early emerging and fundamental property of autism. *Brain* **2012**, *135*, 949–960. [CrossRef]
12. Lombardo, M.V.; Pramparo, T.; Gazestani, V.; Warrier, V.; Bethlehem, R.A.; Barnes, C.C.; Lopez, L.; Lewis, N.E.; Eyler, L.; Pierce, K.; et al. Large-scale associations between the leukocyte transcriptome and BOLD responses to speech differ in autism early language outcome subtypes. *Nat. Neurosci.* **2018**, *21*, 1680. [CrossRef]
13. Lombardo, M.V.; Pierce, K.; Eyler, L.T.; Barnes, C.C.; Ahrens-Barbeau, C.; Solso, S.; Campbell, K.; Courchesne, E. Different functional neural substrates for good and poor language outcome in autism. *Neuron* **2015**, *86*, 567–577. [CrossRef]
14. Lindell, A.K.; Hudry, K. Atypicalities in cortical structure, handedness, and functional lateralization for language in autism spectrum disorders. *Neuropsychol. Rev.* **2013**, *23*, 257–270. [CrossRef] [PubMed]
15. Seery, A.M.; Vogel-Farley, V.; Tager-Flusberg, H.; Nelson, C.A. Atypical lateralization of ERP response to native and non-native speech in infants at risk for autism spectrum disorder. *Dev. Cogn. Neurosci.* **2013**, *5*, 10–24. [CrossRef]
16. Mody, M.; Manoach, D.S.; Guenther, F.H.; Kenet, T.; Bruno, K.A.; McDougle, C.J.; Stigler, K.A. Speech and language in autism spectrum disorder: A view through the lens of behavior and brain imaging. *Neuropsychiatry* **2013**, *3*, 223. [CrossRef]
17. Haweel, R.; AbdElSabour Seada, N.; Ghoniemy, S.; ElBaz, A. A review on autism spectrum disorder diagnosis using task-based functional mri. *Int. J. Intell. Comput. Inf. Sci.* **2021**, *21*, 23–40.
18. Zhuang, J.; Dvornek, N.C.; Li, X.; Yang, D.; Ventola, P.; Duncan, J.S. Prediction of pivotal response treatment outcome with task fMRI using random forest and variable selection. In Proceedings of the 2018 IEEE 15th International Symposium on Biomedical Imaging (ISBI 2018), Washington, DC, USA, 4–7 April 2018; pp. 97–100.
19. Haweel, R.; Dekhil, O.; Shalaby, A.; Mahmoud, A.; Ghazal, M.; Khalil, A.; Ghoniemy, S.; Keynton, R.; Elmaghraby, A.; Barnes, G.; et al. Functional magnetic resonance imaging based framework for autism diagnosis. In Proceedings of the 2019 Fifth International Conference on Advances in Biomedical Engineering (ICABME), Tripoli, Lebanon, 17–19 October 2019; pp. 1–4.
20. Haweel, R.; Dekhil, O.; Shalaby, A.; Mahmoud, A.; Ghazal, M.; Khalil, A.; Keynton, R.; Barnes, G.; El-Baz, A. A Novel Framework for Grading Autism Severity Using Task-Based FMRI. In Proceedings of the 2020 IEEE 17th International Symposium on Biomedical Imaging (ISBI), Iowa City, IA, USA, 3–7 April 2020; pp. 1404–1407.

21. Haweel, R.; Dekhil, O.; Shalaby, A.; Mahmoud, A.; Ghazal, M.; Keynton, R.; Barnes, G.; El-Baz, A. A Machine Learning Approach for Grading Autism Severity Levels Using Task-based Functional MRI. In Proceedings of the International Conference on Imaging Systems and Techniques (IST'19), Abu Dhabi, United Arab Emirates, 9–10 December 2019.
22. Haweel, R.; Shalaby, A.; Mahmoud, A.; Ghazal, M.; Seada, N.; Ghoniemy, S.; Casanova, M.; Barnes, G.; El-Baz, A. A Novel Grading System for Autism Severity Level Using Task-based Functional MRI: A Response to Speech Study. *IEEE Access* **2021**, *9*, 100570–100582. [CrossRef]
23. Zhang, R.; Xu, P.; Guo, L.; Zhang, Y.; Li, P.; Yao, D. Z-score linear discriminant analysis for EEG based brain-computer interfaces. *PLoS ONE* **2013**, *8*, e74433. [CrossRef]
24. Bai, J.; Ding, B.; Xiao, Z.; Jiao, L.; Chen, H.; Regan, A.C. Hyperspectral Image Classification Based on Deep Attention Graph Convolutional Network. *IEEE Trans. Geosci. Remote Sens.* **2021**, 1–16. [CrossRef]
25. Subasi, A.; Ercelebi, E. Classification of EEG signals using neural network and logistic regression. *Comput. Methods Programs Biomed.* **2005**, *78*, 87–99. [CrossRef]
26. Wen, D.; Wei, Z.; Zhou, Y.; Li, G.; Zhang, X.; Han, W. Deep learning methods to process fMRI data and their application in the diagnosis of cognitive impairment: A brief overview and our opinion. *Front. Neuroinform.* **2018**, *12*, 23. [CrossRef] [PubMed]
27. Hu, J.; Kuang, Y.; Liao, B.; Cao, L.; Dong, S.; Li, P. A Multichannel 2D Convolutional Neural Network Model for Task-Evoked fMRI Data Classification. *Comput. Intell. Neurosci.* **2019**, *2019*, 5065214. [CrossRef] [PubMed]
28. Li, X.; Dvornek, N.C.; Papademetris, X.; Zhuang, J.; Staib, L.H.; Ventola, P.; Duncan, J.S. 2-channel convolutional 3D deep neural network (2CC3D) for fMRI analysis: ASD classification and feature learning. In Proceedings of the 2018 IEEE 15th International Symposium on Biomedical Imaging (ISBI 2018), Washington, DC, USA, 4–7 April 2018; pp. 1252–1255.
29. Amin, A.E. Automatic machine fault diagnosis based on wavelet transform and probabilistic neural networks. *Int. J. Intell. Comput. Inf. Sci.* **2014**, *14*, 63–79. [CrossRef]
30. Lessa, P.S.; Sato, J.R.; Cardoso, E.F.; Neto, C.G.; Valadares, A.P.; Amaro, E., Jr. Wavelet correlation between subjects: A time-scale data driven analysis for brain mapping using fMRI. *J. Neurosci. Methods* **2011**, *194*, 350–357. [CrossRef] [PubMed]
31. García, J.G.S.; López, J.M.H.; Barbosa, E.M.; Méndez, J.R.; Alonso, B.d.C. Diagnosis of ADHD children by wavelet analysis. *AIP Conf. Proc.* **2016**, *1747*, 030003.
32. Chanel, G.; Pichon, S.; Conty, L.; Berthoz, S.; Chevallier, C.; Grèzes, J. Classification of autistic individuals and controls using cross-task characterization of fMRI activity. *NeuroImage Clin.* **2016**, *10*, 78–88. [CrossRef] [PubMed]
33. Dvornek, N.C.; Yang, D.; Ventola, P.; Duncan, J.S. Learning Generalizable Recurrent Neural Networks from Small Task-fMRI Datasets. In Proceedings of the International Conference on Medical Image Computing and Computer-Assisted Intervention, Granada, Spain, 16–20 September 2018; Springer: New York, NY, USA, 2018; pp. 329–337.
34. Westfall, J.M.; Mold, J.; Fagnan, L. Practice-based research—"Blue Highways" on the NIH roadmap. *JAMA* **2007**, *297*, 403–406. [CrossRef]
35. Hall, D.; Huerta, M.F.; McAuliffe, M.J.; Farber, G.K. Sharing heterogeneous data: The national database for autism research. *Neuroinformatics* **2012**, *10*, 331–339. [CrossRef]
36. Woolrich, M.W.; Ripley, B.D.; Brady, M.; Smith, S.M. Temporal autocorrelation in univariate linear modeling of FMRI data. *Neuroimage* **2001**, *14*, 1370–1386. [CrossRef]
37. Jenkinson, M.; Beckmann, C.F.; Behrens, T.E.; Woolrich, M.W.; Smith, S.M. Fsl. *Neuroimage* **2012**, *62*, 782–790. [CrossRef]
38. Haweel, R.; Shalaby, A.; Mahmoud, A.; Seada, N.; Ghoniemy, S.; Ghazal, M.; Casanova, M.F.; Barnes, G.N.; El-Baz, A. A robust DWT–CNN-based CAD system for early diagnosis of autism using task-based fMRI. *Med. Phys.* **2020**, *48*, 2315–2326. [CrossRef]
39. LeCun, Y.; Bengio, Y.; Hinton, G. Deep learning. *Nature* **2015**, *521*, 436–444. [CrossRef]

sensors

MDPI

Article

Electrical Detection of Innate Immune Cells

Mahmoud Al Ahmad [1,*], Rasha A. Nasser [2], Lillian J. A. Olule [1] and Bassam R. Ali [2]

1 Department of Electrical Engineering, College of Engineering, UAE University, Al Ain 15551, United Arab Emirates; lolule@uaeu.ac.ae
2 Department of Genetics and Genomics, College of Medicine and Health Sciences (CMHS), UAE University, Al Ain 15551, United Arab Emirates; 201670412@uaeu.ac.ae (R.A.N.); bassam.ali@uaeu.ac.ae (B.R.A.)
* Correspondence: m.alahmad@uaeu.ac.ae

Abstract: Accurately classifying the innate immune players is essential to comprehensively and quantitatively evaluate the interactions between the innate and the adaptive immune systems. In addition, accurate classification enables the development of models to predict behavior and to improve prospects for therapeutic manipulation of inflammatory diseases and cancer. Rapid development in technologies that provide an accurate definition of the type of cell in action, allows the field of innate immunity to the lead in therapy developments. This article presents a novel immunophenotyping technique using electrical characterization to differentiate between the two most important cell types of the innate immune system: dendritic cells (DCs) and macrophages (MACs). The electrical characterization is based on capacitance measurements, which is a reliable marker for cell surface area and hence cell size. We differentiated THP-1 cells into DCs and MACs in vitro and conducted electrical measurements on the three cell types. The results showed average capacitance readings of 0.83 μF, 0.93 μF, and 1.01 μF for THP-1, DCs, and MACs, respectively. This corresponds to increasing cell size since capacitance is directly proportional to area. The results were verified with image processing. Image processing was used for verification because unlike conventional techniques, especially flow cytometry, it avoids cross referencing and by-passes the limitation of a lack of specificity of markers used to detect the different cell types.

Keywords: dendritic cells; electrical characterization; image processing; immune system; macrophages

Citation: Al Ahmad, M.; Nasser, R.A.; Olule, L.J.A.; Ali, B.R. Electrical Detection of Innate Immune Cells. *Sensors* **2021**, *21*, 5886. https://doi.org/10.3390/s21175886

Academic Editors: Ayman El-baz, Guruprasad A. Giridharan, Ahmed Shalaby, Ali H. Mahmoud and Mohammed Ghazal

Received: 26 July 2021
Accepted: 29 August 2021
Published: 1 September 2021

1. Introduction

Dendritic cells (DCs) and macrophages (MACs) are members of the mononuclear phagocyte system that perform multiple functions during an immune response [1]. Although both DCs and MACs are antigen-presenting cells, they differ in their functions. DCs are specialized in surveillance and the detection of pathogens and, as their name suggests, have elongated structures arising from their body called dendrites [2]. These dendrites increase the surface area of the DCs compared to the cell's volume [1,3,4]. On the other hand, MACs are mainly involved in the phagocytosis of microbial substances, pathogens, and even cancer cells [5]. MACs also play a significant role in regulating the immune system by releasing cytokines for anti-inflammation [6]. DCs and MACs have been regarded as clearly distinct in terms of cellular function although they occupy overlapping anatomical structures in many body tissues and systems [4]. DCs are stronger in processing antigens and presenting them to the adaptive immune system [7], while MACs are strong in migration to the site at which the pathogen resides and in phagocytosis [8]. DCs and MACs are the key players of the innate immune system as they are the link between the innate and adaptive immune systems [9]. The antigen is captured and processed by these cells and presented to the cells of the adaptive immune system, specifically, the T cells, at specific immunological locations.

In practice, the process of differentiating between DCs and MACs in vitro is not straightforward [10]. It has heavily relied on cell-surface markers thought to be solely present on one cell type and not on the other [1]. However, growing evidence suggests that many cell surface markers previously used to differentiate between these two cell types overlap [4]. This further complicates our understanding of the mononuclear phagocyte system and confirms the need for a more reliable system to distinguish between these two key immune cell types. Scientists have been using conventional techniques like western blot [11], flow cytometry (FACs) [12], immunohistochemistry [13], and PCR [14] to differentiate between DCs and MACs. Although these techniques are efficient, they are time and money-consuming and also require highly trained technicians. Flow cytometry, the most common technique used in classifying immune cells, depends on detecting cell surface markers present in one cell type and not the other. However, growing evidence suggests that when it is used to compare between DCs and MACs, the markers overlap and display a lack of specificity in comparing the cells, as presented in Figure 1.

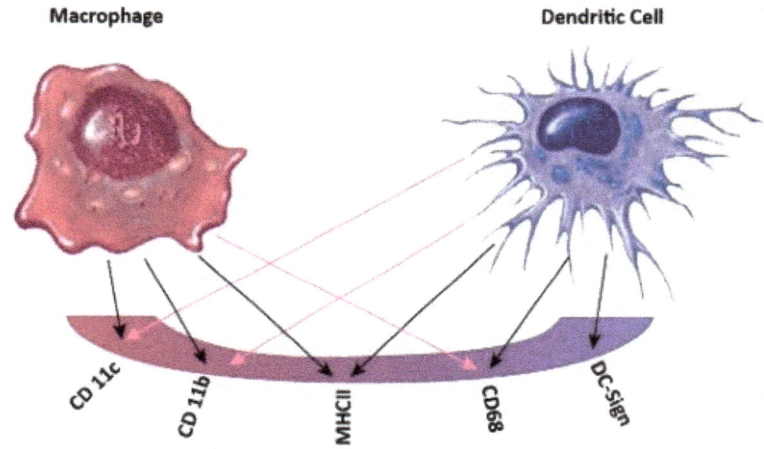

Figure 1. Overlapping of cell surface markers between MACs and DCs. DCs and MACs share the same surface markers CD11c, CD11b, MHCII, CD68.

Electrical characterization is widely used for the detection and accurate characterization of biological samples [15–17]. The last few years have witnessed a substantial growth in new electrical techniques that allow for the detailed study of cells, their characteristics, and functions [15,18,19]. Scientists have focused on studying the cells' electrical properties due to their relevance in cell activity [17]. These electrical properties are very important because they give insights into the changing biochemical and biophysical properties of the cell that control their interaction with other cells and their interaction with the environment [15].

Over the years, many studies have been conducted to extract biological data from electrical measurements [20]. Useful examples are the resting and membrane potential from the nervous system and the ECG of the heart. Electrical characterization has even expanded to study single cells, viruses, DNA, and even blood samples [18].

Electrical and electrochemical methods have been used widely in several biological applications. Electrical measurements have been used in three different important biological areas: (1) Detection of a disease: measuring the changes in dielectric properties to detect blood in urine samples (hematuria) without the use of inaccurate conventional techniques [21]; (2) characterizing healthy and cancerous cells in different tissue types [22]; and (3) using a label-free tracking method to study the development and progress of living cells in real-time. An example where this was used was to detect the life cycle of budding yeast. The capacitance–voltage dependency was exploited to detect changes in the cell cycle progression [23].

Coupled with electrical characterization is image processing. This has become a vital tool in biological applications for quantifying the phenotypic differences between various cell populations [24]. Screening biological samples has given scientists a deeper insight into the biological systems and their diverse processes such as gene expression, protein modification or interaction, signal transduction, and irregular RNA interference and mutations.

Traditionally, visual analysis is used for image processing. Cells are classified by measurements of cell shape, movement, and protein expression performed manually. This is conducted by suspending cells in a suitable medium, staining them with dye, then analyzing them under a microscope [25]. The manual approach is, however, time-consuming, subjective, and may require a large number of technicians working on the data. Nowadays, image processing is done almost automatically by large processing machines that can deal with high volumes of images, making it faster, more accurate, reliable, and less subjective [26]. Images are visualized as still images, videos, and more recently, 3D and 4D volumetric images. The acquired images can be enhanced by using different fluorescent technologies. The most basic type of analysis is morphological analysis, which does not only refer to metrics of the phenotypical shapes, but also the intensities, the spatial relationships, the staining patterns, and even migration and movement [27].

Automated imaging starts with the principle of extracting the physical parameters of the sample such as the area, density, and morphological properties [28]. Consequently, the data obtained from these images allow the mathematical modeling of biological kinetics and the studying of biochemical signaling networks [29]. The main imaging techniques used for cellular studies are fluorescent microscopy, multiphoton microscopy, atomic and electron microscopy [28]. The fluorescent microscope is mainly used for the visualization of sub-cellular structures and their compartmentalization [30]. It works by capturing the emissions of the excited biological samples using fluorophores. Multiphoton microscopy follows the same principle, but is mainly used for living samples and can image at a deeper scale in comparison to fluorescent microscopy [31]. These techniques have the advantage of high specific identification, but the limitation of photo-bleaching. On the other hand, atomic force microscopy uses Hooke's law (principle in physics that explains that the force used to compress or extend a spring is proportional to the same distance [32] to acquire the image from the sample [33]). The image is a representation of the forces between the sample and the tip of the probe that scans its surface, and the forces measured vary between chemical, magnetic, electrostatic, and mechanical contact forces. The advantage of this technique is that the sample does not require any special treatment, however, mechanical forces can damage the sample. The last technique, electron microscopy, uses an electron beam to image the object and magnifies it using electromagnetic fields [34]. It provides high resolution but sample preparation takes a long time and cannot be done on living samples.

The data obtained from the image acquisition techniques are processed in software to provide quantitative results [24]. The analysis of the results depends on the advances of the algorithms and processing of the software used. In general, the applications of these software include analyzing the stained tissues, gels, and obtaining the physical and morphological data of the sample [35]. After capturing the sample with the microscope, the software initiates the segmentation process, where the object is located and the boundaries are drawn along the object [36]. The main goal of this process is to simplify the image for quantification. Phenotype quantification is the critical step that follows, the software manages to quantify the image and obtain data such as sample size, distances between the objects, spatial distributions, and in the case of live imaging, tracking the sample movement [2,4]. Phenotypes and data collected from experiments conducted by scientists have also been collected and categorized in shared databases [27]. These databases provide an avenue for users to browse and inquire about experiments and for other scientists to develop more efficient analysis software. Additional experiments like western bot, FACs, and PCR along with the imaging data provide scientists with a better understanding of the biological data.

In this paper, we propose a new, easy, and efficient method to classify immune cells using electrical characterization techniques. The method allows for full differentiation between DCs and MACs. We believe that distinguishing between these cells using electrical characterization supported by image processing will ensure better classification of the innate immune cells during their steady state and inflammatory conditions in different tissues while playing different roles.

2. Methods

Two classification approaches are used to distinguish between the different innate immune cells: image processing and electrical characterization. The two approaches are illustrated in Figure 2. Cell differentiation by electrochemical characterization is based on the capacitance values, which are derived from current and voltage readings of cell samples. On the other hand, cell differentiation using image processing is based on analyzing the area, cell count, and morphology of visual data to distinguish the innate immune cells based on their size and morphological differences.

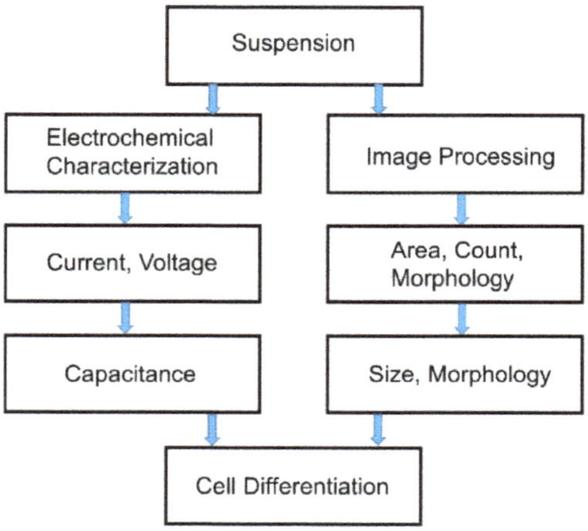

Figure 2. The two approaches for innate immune cell differentiation.

It should be noted that the markers used to specify each type of immune cell are not specific for one type of cell and this leads to the huge drawback of cross-referencing.

Table 1 summarizes the markers used and the specificity for each marker [31,37–40].

Table 1. Markers used for immune cells and their specifications.

Marker	Specificity	Ref.
CD83	Marker for mature DCs and very weak for THP-1	[31]
CD197	Receptor for T-cells, B cells, Natural killer cells and DCs	[37]
HLA-DR	Recognizes T cells, DCs, MACs, and B cells	[38]
CD1c	Subset of B cells and DCs	[39]
CD11c	For monocytes, MACs, DCs, Natural killer cells, T and B cells	[40]

Both experiments began with biological differentiation of cells and their preparation in suspensions. THP-1 was first cultured in RPMI-1640 media, then differentiated into DCs and MACs. Human monocytic THP-1 cell line (ATCC, Manassas, VA, USA) [41] were cultured in RPMI-1640 media supplemented with 10% fetal bovine serum (FBS), 1% sodium pyruvate, 0.01% of mercaptoethanol, and 1% penicillin/streptomycin at 37 °C, 5% CO_2, and 95% humidity.

Next, cell differentiation was carried out based on the protocol by Berges et al., using the activators specified [42]. For the DCs, THP-1 cells were harvested by centrifugation, then resuspended in culture medium supplemented with 10% FBS at a concentration of 2×10^5 cells/mL and transferred to a final volume of 20 mL into 200-mL tissue culture flasks. To induce differentiation, rhIL-4 (200 ng = 3000 IU/mL), rhGM-CSF (100 ng/mL = 1500 IU/mL), rhTNF-α (20 ng/mL = 2000 IU/mL), and 200 ng/mL ionomycin were added to the FBS- free media.

For the macrophages, the differentiating and activation protocols of THP-1-derived MACs were adapted and modified from Genin et al. [43]. THP-1 cells were terminally differentiated into uncommitted MACs (MPMA) with 300 nM phorbol 12-myristate 13-acetate (PMA; Sigma-Aldrich, Darmstadt, Germany) in RPMI 1640 media without the FBS supplement. After six hours, differentiating media were removed. The cells were then washed with phosphate-buffered saline (PBS) and rested for 24 h in RPMI 1640 without FBS supplement and PMA. Afterward, cells were activated for 48 h into pro-inflammatory MACs ($M_{LPS/IFN\gamma}$) by adding 10 pg/mL lipopolysaccharide (LPS; Sigma, St. Louis, MO, USA) and 20 ng/mL IFNγ (Biolegend, San Diego, CA, USA), or into anti-inflammatory MACs ($_{MIL\text{-}4/IL\text{-}13}$) with 20 ng/mL interleukin 4 (IL-4; Biolegend, USA) and 20 ng/mL interleukin 13 (IL-13; Biolegend, USA).

2.1. Flow Cytometry

To validate the differentiation of monocytes, fluorescent surface markers were evaluated using flow cytometry, based on their surface self-antigens. Cultured cells were washed, suspended at 3×10^4 in 200 µL cold FACS solution (DPBS; Gibco-Invitrogen, San Diego, CA, USA) and incubated with FITC- or PE-conjugated monoclonal antibodies or appropriate isotypic controls for 30 min. Cells were then washed twice and resuspended in 300 µL of cold FACS solution. Stained cells were analyzed with (BD Accuri C6 plus). Cell debris was excluded from the analysis by setting a gate on forward and side scatter that included only cells that were viable. Results were processed using FlowJo Software (version 7).

2.2. Image Acquisition and Processing

The image processing method consists of analyzing the cells based on visual data supported by their morphological and structural differences. Images were captured using an Olympus Fluorescent Microscope and quantified using ImageJ software (National Institute of Health, Gaithersburg, MD, USA) [44]. The software was used to obtain the ratio of THP-1 to DCs, THP-1 to MACs, and the average area of the three types of cells. ImageJ software segments the images, recognizes the cells, differentiates between the different types of cells, and automatically calculates the area.

2.3. Electrochemical Measurement

For the electrochemical approach, measurements were performed using the µSTAT 400 potentiostat (Metrohm DropSens, Oviedo, Spain) [45]. This was a portable BiPotentiostat/Galvanostat with maximum measurable current and potential of ±40 mA and ±4 V, respectively. It can be used for voltammetric, amperometric, or potentiometric measurements. It has connectors that allow for connection to screen printed or coaxial electrodes and can be used with a one- or two-working electrode configuration. It connects to a PC via USB or Bluetooth.

All measurements were carried out at room temperature. The electrochemical measurements were controlled using Dropview software. Prior to the experiments, two optimizations were performed: (1) identify the optimum step potential (Estep) and scan rate (S_{rate}); and (2) determine the best electrode option between the chip and coaxial cable.

2.3.1. System Optimization for E_{step} and S_{rate}

To find the optimum of S_{rate}, the voltage was swept from −0.9 V to 0.9 V while E_{step} was kept constant at 0.002 V and the S_{rate} was varied from 0.004 V/s to 2 V/s. An optimum S_{rate} of 0.004 V/s was selected, which allowed for accurate data (this value of S_{rate} limits the non-Faradic current and therefore background noise, which affects the sensitivity of the voltammetry system [46]), sufficient current flow, and absence of time-dependent charging and discharging effects. This value gave the highest capacitance resolution, which can aid with distinguishing between cells.

Second, both E_{step} and S_{rate} values were varied simultaneously from 0.009 V to 0.01 V and from 0.009 V/s to 2 V/s, respectively. It was found that corresponding low values did not allow for proper current flow and high values of S_{rate} did not allow for sufficient charge of the sample. Additionally, equal values of E_{step} and S_{rate} did not provide the correct shape for the cyclic voltammogram. Hence, from the experiments, the optimum values of E_{step} and S_{rate} were selected as 0.002 V and 0.04 V/s, respectively.

2.3.2. System Optimization for Electrode Selection

The screen printed electrode was tested for its performance. It comprised three electrodes: a working electrode, reference electrode and counter electrode. The sample was applied to all electrodes and then the electrode was connected to the DropSens machine via a port with silver contacts. It was found that although the screen printed electrode is low cost, disposable, and can give results for low volumes, current flow in the samples experienced interference, and as a result, not all cells were charged. Instead, a coaxial cable was used. The coaxial cable is easy to clean between trials and most importantly, guarantees equal current flow throughout the sample.

Using the coaxial cable, the DropSens machine was configured for two electrode measurements with one electrode used as the working electrode and the other electrode used as the reference/counter electrode. The cable is an open ended coaxial adaptor with inner and outer conductor electrode dimensions of 2 mm and 5 mm, respectively, and a length of 7 mm, which allows for a sample volume of 500 μL. Both electrodes are made from Nickel. The coaxial cable was secured to ensure stability during measurements. The electrolyte used was the RPMI full media supplemented with 10% FBS.

2.3.3. Measurement Procedure

Once optimization was completed, cyclic voltammetry measurements were performed between 0.9 V to −0.9 V, E_{step} of 0.002 V and S_{rate} of 0.04 s per step using the coaxial cable. Cells were prepared using RPMI full media supplemented with 10% FBS. After the activation process, cells were centrifuged and prepared at different dilutions from 10 to 10^5 per 500 μL. This was carried out by first counting the cells using a hemocytometer, then diluting them to the necessary concentrations. Data were extracted directly from drop view using the cyclic voltammetry technique. The results exported were current vs. voltage.

After extracting the current vs. voltage data, the capacitance of the biological cells was determined using MATLAB code based on the fact that the capacitive current is proportional to the rate of change of the potential with the constant of proportionality equal to the capacitance, as shown in Equation (1).

$$i(t) = C\frac{dv(t)}{dt} \tag{1}$$

where $Q(t)$ is the time-dependent charge; C is the capacitance in farads; and $V(t)$ is the time dependent voltage in volts.

2.4. Statistical Analysis

All measurements were performed at least three times, and the results represent the mean ± standard deviation. A two-tailed Student's t-test with a significance level of 0.05 was also performed.

3. Results and Discussion

The main goal of this work was to find a way to identify immune cells without the drawback of cross-referencing. For flow cytometry, cells were selected by a gating process. Debris were excluded and only stained cells were selected. The results are plotted in the histogram shown in Figure 3. Cell surface markers for CD83, CD197, HLA-DR, CD1c, and CD11c expression on THP-1 cells and the differentiated DCs and MACs were analyzed. Two sample t tests were performed with a p-value of 0.05. The p-values are tabulated in the Appendix A in Table A1.

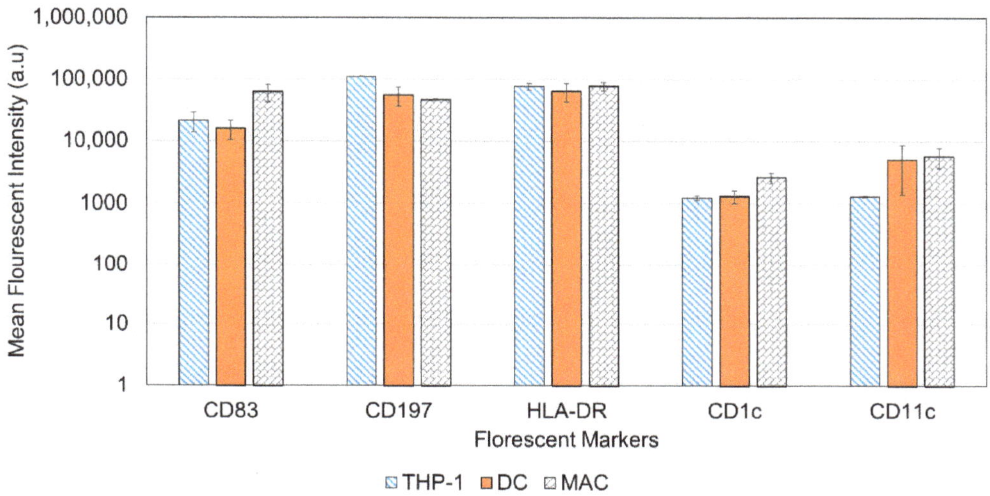

Figure 3. Average mean fluorescent intensity of different cell markers for THP-1, DCs, and MACs with S.E.M bars obtained for three measurements. Cultured cells were washed, suspended at 3×10^4 in 200 µL cold FACS solution (DPBS; Gibco-Invitrogen) and incubated with FITC- or PE-conjugated monoclonal antibodies or appropriate isotypic controls for 30 min. Cells were then washed twice and resuspended in 300 µL of cold FACS solution. Stained cells were analyzed with BD Accuri C6 plus. Cell debris was excluded from the analysis by setting a gate on forward and side scatter that included only cells that are viable.

To begin with, CD83 represents an important marker that is specific for DCs. However, our results showed that there is no significant difference between DCs and THP-1 or MACs, and this is supported by a study undertaken by D. Ferenbach and J. Hughes and others [4,47]. On the other hand, CD197 expression only showed differences between MACs against THP-1 and DCs against THP-1. This can be attributed to CD197 being a marker for antigen presenting cells, however, it cannot classify between the different types of antigen presenting cells. Regarding HLA-DR marker expression, it presented on all the three types of immune cells [37,38], hence, we could see no difference with the flow cytometry results. CD1c is a marker for DCs, this is supported by our results as they can classify DCs from MACs, but not from THP-1 cells. However, CD11c is a marker for all three cells [39] and as per our results, there were no differences between these cells, using this marker. Hence flow cytometry analyzes the data by giving statistical significance to values but fails to interpret it into biological significance, thus failing to give an identity to the immune cells [31].

The morphology and structure of the three types of immune cells identified using the image segmentation approach for electrical characterization are demonstrated in Figure 4. The THP-1 cells can be easily distinguished from DC by their round structure without elongations. Once activated, the non-adherent THP-1 cells differentiate to adherent cells that are morphologically different from their inactive forms. On the other hand, MACs and

DCs take more space to spread out due to the larger size of the former and the presence of dendrites in the latter, as shown in Figure 4.

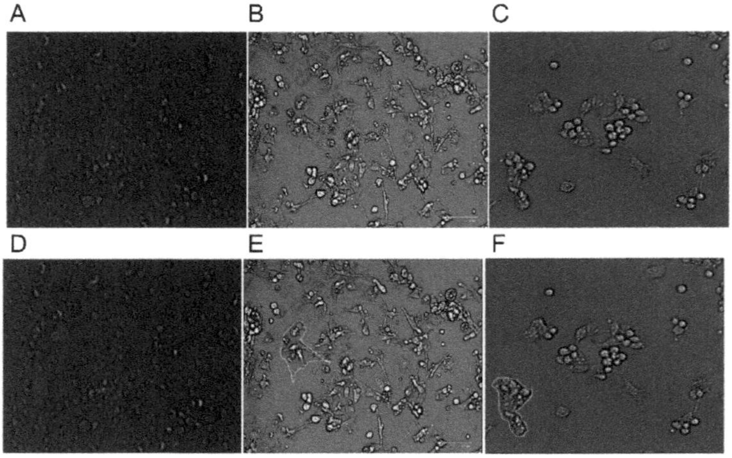

Figure 4. (**A**) THP-1 Immune cells before differentiation. THP-1 was first cultured in RPMI-1640 media, then differentiated into DCs and MACs. Human monocytic THP-1 cell line (ATCC, Manassas, VA, USA)35 were cultured in RPMI-1640 media supplemented with 10% fetal bovine serum (FBS), 1% sodium pyruvate, 0.01% of mercaptoethanol, and 1% penicillin/streptomycin at 37 °C, 5% CO_2, and 95% humidity. (**B**) DCs and (**C**) MACs after differentiation, respectively. DCs were differentiated based on the Berges et al. protocol. To induce differentiation rhIL-4 (200 ng = 3000 IU/mL) and rhGM-CSF (100 ng/mL = 1500 IU/mL), rhTNF-α (20 ng/mL = 2000 IU/mL), and 200 ng/mL ionomycin were added to the FBS-free media. For the macrophages, the differentiating and activation protocols of THP-1-derived macrophages were adapted and modified from Genin et al. [37]. THP-1 cells were terminally differentiated into uncommitted macrophages (MPMA) with 300 nM phor-bol 12-myristate 13-acetate (PMA; Sigma-Aldrich, Germany) in RPMI 1640 media without FBS supplement. Afterward, cells were activated for 48 h into pro-inflammatory macrophages (MLPS/IFNγ) by adding 10 pg/mL lipopolysaccharide (LPS; Sigma, USA) and 20 ng/mL IFNγ (Biolegend, San Diego, CA, USA), or into anti-inflammatory macrophages (MIL-4/IL-13) with 20 ng/mL interleukin 4 (IL-4; Bio-legend, USA) and 20 ng/mL interleukin 13 (IL-13; Biolegend, USA). THP-1 cells have a round shape and are suspended in the media, DCs are attached and spread their dendrites in the flask. MACs are also adherent, but without the elongations of the DCs. (**D**–**F**) show the selection undertaken in ImageJ software for the calculation of the area of the THP-1, DCs, and MACs, respectively.

Figure 4D–F shows the detailed selection of immune cells using the software. The software highlights the morphological differences (it marks the outside border of the cell yellow). After the selection of each cell, the software automatically calculates the area of the cell. Results were obtained from three different images to statistically compare the area of each cell. Figure 5 shows a summary of the results. The averages were obtained for measurements conducted on 200 cells of each type. The MACs were found to have the largest area and the THP-1s were the smallest due to their rounded shape. These results are supported by findings in the literature [48,49].

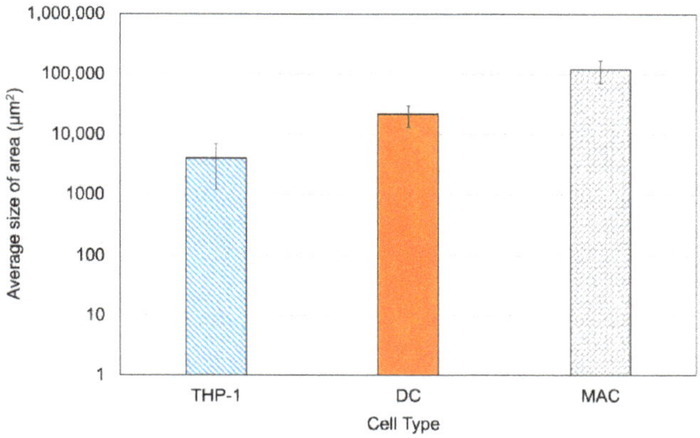

Figure 5. The calculated average area of each cell with S.E.M bars. MACs have the largest area, followed by DCs, and finally THP1 cells.

For electrochemical characterization, the DropSens technology was used to obtain the I–V curves for the three immune cells. The results are shown in Figure 6 for different cell concentrations. The current versus time and voltage versus time results are shown in Figure 7. When the positive voltage is applied, the cell suspensions begin to oxidize near the working electrode, this results in an increase in anodic current. This occurs until a peak potential of 0.9 V, wherein a peak anodic current is recorded. After this, a reductive scan is applied, that is, the applied potential is reduced, causing a re-reduction of the oxidized suspension. In other words, the reducing potential now results in a cathodic current (increasingly negative current). At a maximum negative potential of −0.9 V, the maximum cathodic current is recorded (maximum negative current). Although reduction peaks at −0.2 V were observed for all experiments, the regions of maximum and minimum potential were of more interest because the peaks corresponded to the sample concentrations [46]. The peak anodic and cathodic currents had equal magnitude and opposite sign. As the potential is increased positively again, the oxidation and increasing flow of anodic current repeats.

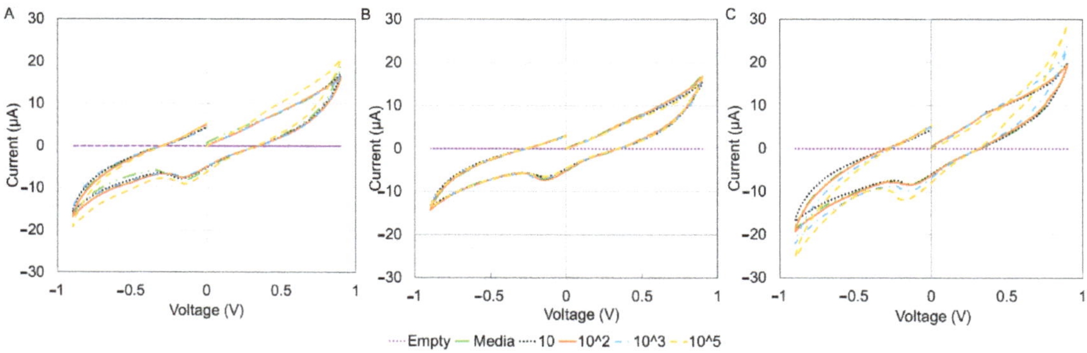

Figure 6. I–V curve for the three types of cells using drop sense technology. (**A**) THP1, (**B**) DCs, (**C**) MACs. There were no clear differences between the three graphs. RPMI full media supplemented with 10% FBS was used to dilute the cells. It was also used as the media. Measurements were conducted using a two nickel electrode configuration, scan range of −0.9 V to 0.9 V and a scan rate of 0.04 V/s.

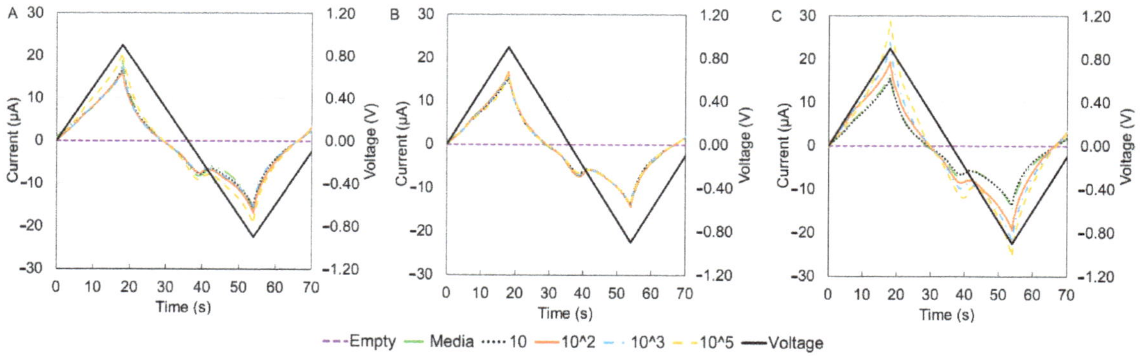

Figure 7. Current versus time and voltage versus time curves for the three types of cells from the drop sense technology. (**A**) THP-1, (**B**) DCs, (**C**) MACs. RPMI full media supplemented with 10% FBS used to dilute the cells. It was also used as the media. Measurements were conducted using a two nickel electrode configuration, scan range of −0.9 V to 0.9 V and a scan rate of 0.04 V/s.

However, since the voltammogram results showed no significant difference within the three types of cells hence, the capacitance was pursued as a means of identification and differentiation. Capacitance measurements have been shown to be a reliable marker for tracking cell surface area and therefore cell size [50]. The graphs of the extracted capacitance are shown in Figure 8.

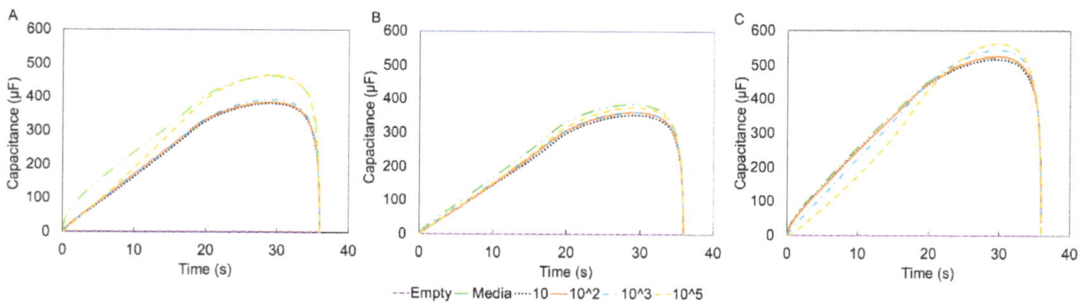

Figure 8. Capacitance–time curve for the three types of cells before media de-embedding (removing the value of media from the rest of the samples) (**A**) THP-1, (**B**) DCs, (**C**) MACs. Capacitance values were extracted using MATLAB, based on the fact that the capacitive current measured is proportional to the rate of change of the applied potential with the constant of proportionality equal to the capacitance. There is no consistent trend between the concentration and capacitance.

Comparing the three plots, it was noticed that only THP-1 cells displayed the expected trend of increased capacitance with increasing concentration. Electrochemical sensors react with the analyte under test to produce an electrical signal proportional to the analyte concentration [51]. The inconsistency with DCs and MACs was likely due to the lack of a homogenous suspension as cells might not have fully differentiated. Therefore, to obtain a better picture of the capacitance data, the value of the media was de-embedded from the other samples, that is, each concentration value was divided by the corresponding media value. Additionally, because electronic measurements of conductive solutions are often affected by ionic effects like electrode polarization that occurs within the Debye screening length of the solution, de-embedding can mitigate this effect since the electrode polarization is localized and remains constant for a particular ion concentration and device geometry [52]. Figure 9 displays the data for the three immune cells after the de-embedding process.

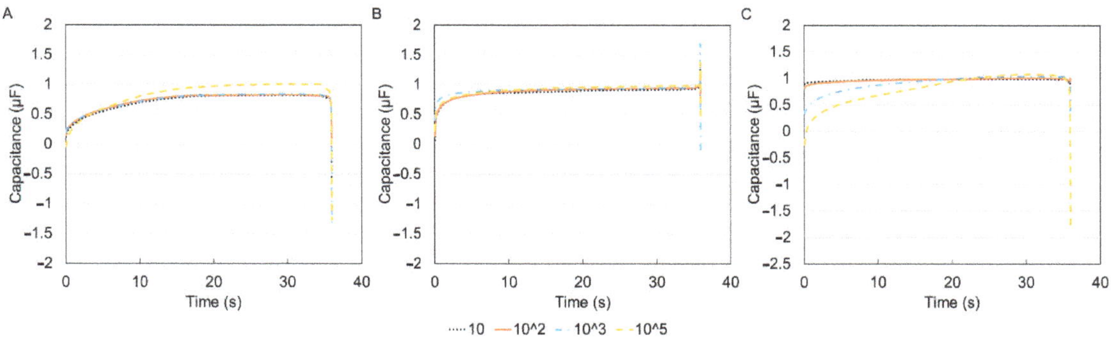

Figure 9. Capacitance–time curve for the three types of cells after media de-embedding (**A**) THP-1, (**B**) DCs, (**C**) MACs. De-embedding was performed by diving each of the concentration values in Figure 8 by their corresponding media value.

From the initial capacitance plot (Figure 8), it was seen that the capacitance peaked at about 29.2 s for all experiments. Therefore, the values of the capacitance for this time measurement were extracted from the de-embedded data and compared as shown in Figure 10. As expected for each cell type, there was a general increase in capacitance with concentration. This is illustrated in Figure 10A. This is attributed to the fact that an increase in the number of cells results in an increase in total surface area and since the area is directly proportional to capacitance, an increase in capacitance is observed. Although a clear distinction between the MACs and DCs can be seen (the MACs have a larger capacitance and therefore are larger and the DCs have a lower capacitance and therefore are smaller) to more clearly differentiate between all three cell types and by-pass the inconsistency at the 10^5 concentration, the average capacitance for three concentrations was plotted as shown in Figure 10B. It should be noted that the reason for the discrepancy at 10^5 was attributed to errors in pipetting or sample preparation. It is therefore recommended that several concentrations be used for proper validation. Additionally, more accurate results can be obtained by using polished, well cleaned electrodes and smaller sample volumes for greater sensitivity.

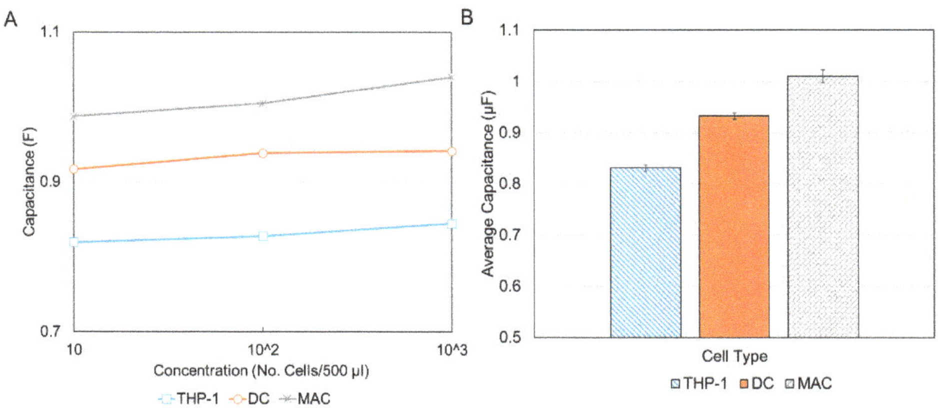

Figure 10. Capacitance vs. concentration for the three types of cells after the de-embedding process. (**A**) Capacitance versus concentration at 29.2 s where maximum capacitance occurs for each of the cell types. (**B**) Average capacitance for the three concentrations with S.E.M error bars. MACs had the highest values and DCs had the lowest values, consistent with the literature.

The results showed that the lowest average value of capacitance was for THP-1 (0.83 µF), followed by DCs (0.93 µF), and finally, the largest capacitance was reported for the MACs (1.01 μF). This corresponds to an increasing cell size from THP-1 to DCs to MACs, consistent with the results reported in Figure 6 and in the literature. Although from the results the distinction is possible with only the lowest concentration, the authors recommend the use of the three lowest concentrations used in this paper at a minimum. These concentration ranges are comparable to those used for flow cytometry, for example, Bio-Rad recommends concentrations of 10^5–10^7 cells/mL [53].

The assay described in this study can be practically functionalized by creating a compact battery powered and/or directly powered sensing unit and a control unit. The sensing unit will comprise two electrodes separated by a gap into which the specimen can be loaded via pipette. When voltage is applied to the electrode, the corresponding resultant current can be measured by the electrodes. The sensing unit will connect to the control unit where voltage value and step size can be controlled or swept. Once cyclic voltammetry measurements are performed, software in the control unit can perform further processing on the extracted current and voltage data to calculate the capacitance of the sample under test. The results could then be displayed in the control unit graphical user interface or to a PC via USB/wirelessly for further processing.

Author Contributions: M.A.A. conceived the experiments; M.A.A. and R.A.N. conducted the experiments; and M.A.A., R.A.N. and L.J.A.O. analyzed the results. All authors wrote and reviewed the manuscript. M.A.A. and B.R.A. supervised the project. All authors have read and agreed to the published version of the manuscript.

Funding: This research received no external funding.

Institutional Review Board Statement: Not applicable.

Informed Consent Statement: Not applicable.

Data Availability Statement: Data is contained within the article.

Conflicts of Interest: The authors declare no conflict of interest.

Appendix A. Supplementary Description of Datasets

Appendix A.1. Supplementary Materials for Flow Cytometry Experiments

For the flow cytometry results, a two-tailed Student´s *t*-test with a significance level of 0.05 was also performed. The *p* values are reported in Table A1. Significance was determined for *p*-values $p < 0.05$.

Table A1. Statistical analysis of the flow cytometry results. *p* values for two sample *t*-tests using unequal variance were determined using a significance level of 0.05.

Marker	THP-1 to DC	THP-1 to MAC	DC to MAC
CD83	0.37	0.04	0.06
CD197	0.04	0.00	0.50
HLA-DR	0.42	0.92	0.40
CD1c	0.21	0.06	0.79
CD11c	0.72	0.04	0.03

Appendix A.2. Supplementary Materials for System Optimization for Estep and Srate

To prepare the system for electrochemical measurements, two optimization steps were conducted to determine the best values for S_{rate} and E_{step}. S_{rate} determines the rate of voltage ramping and E_{step} defines the difference in voltage between two points at different distances from the source of energy. First, to find the optimum of S_{rate}, the voltage was swept from −0.9 V to 0.9 V while E_{step} was kept constant at 0.002 V and the S_{rate} was varied from 0.004 V/s to 2 V/s. Results for specific values are shown in Figure A1.

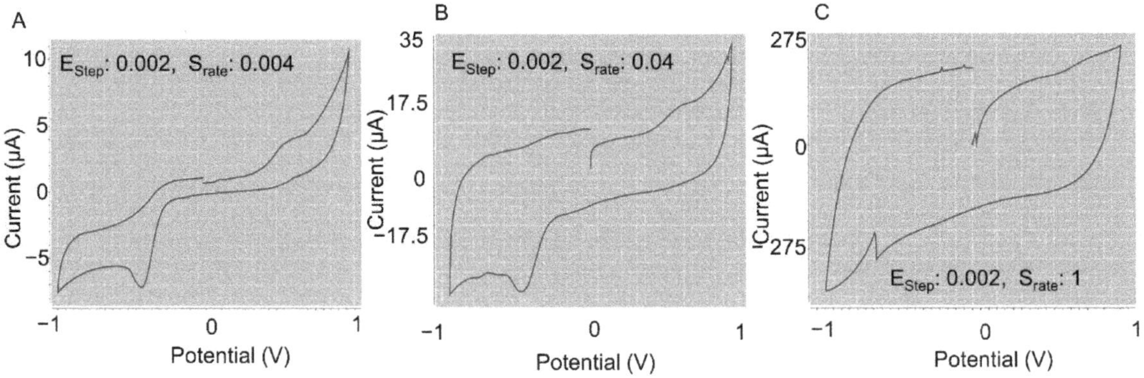

Figure A1. Electrochemical system optimization results for varying S_{rate}. (**A**) E_{step} = 0.002 and S_{rate} = 0.004, (**B**) E_{step} = 0.002 and S_{rate} = 0.04; (**C**) E_{step} = 0.002 and S_{rate} = 1.

Second, both E_{step} and S_{rate} values were varied simultaneously from 0.009 V to 0.01 V and from 0.009 V/s to 2 V/s, respectively. Results for specific values are shown in Figure A2.

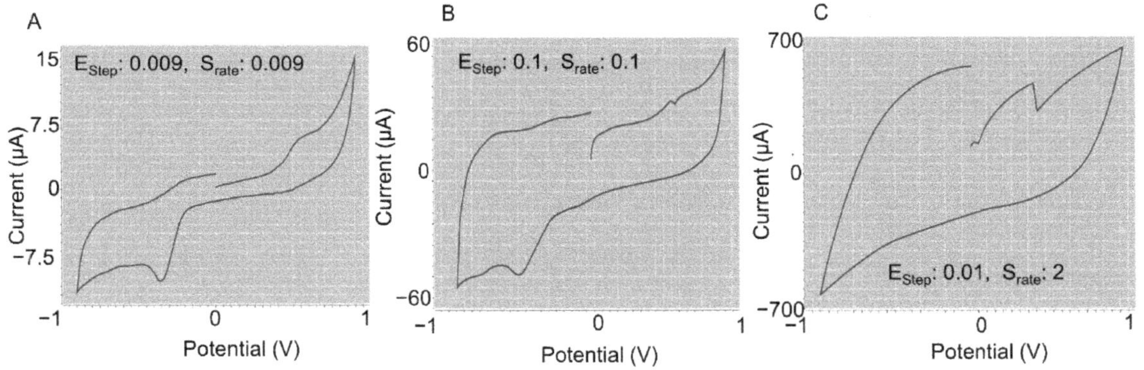

Figure A2. Electrochemical system optimization results for simultaneous varying of S_{rate} and E_{rate}. (**A**) E_{step} = 0.009 and S_{rate} = 0.009; (**B**) E_{step} = 0.1 and S_{rate} = 0.1; (**C**) E_{step} = 0.01 and S_{rate} = 2.

References

1. Guilliams, M.; Ginhoux, F.; Jakubzick, C.; Naik, S.H.; Onai, N.; Schraml, B.U.; Segura, E.; Tussiwand, R.; Yona, S. Dendritic cells, monocytes and macrophages: A unified nomenclature based on ontogeny. *Nat. Rev. Immunol.* **2014**, *14*, 571–578. [CrossRef]
2. Schraml, B.U.; Reis e Sousa, C. Defining dendritic cells. *Curr. Opin. Immunol.* **2015**, *32*, 13–20. [CrossRef] [PubMed]
3. Clark, G.; Angel, N.; Kato, M.; Lopez, J.A.; MacDonald, K.; Vuckovic, S.; Hart, D.N. The role of dendritic cells in the innate immune system. *Microbes Infect.* **2000**, *2*, 257–272. [CrossRef]
4. Ferenbach, D.; Hughes, J. Macrophages and dendritic cells: What is the difference? *Kidney Int.* **2008**, *74*, 5–7. [CrossRef]
5. Macrophage—An Overview. ScienceDirect Topics. Available online: https://www.sciencedirect.com/topics/materials-science/macrophage (accessed on 1 July 2020).
6. Cavaillon, J.M. Cytokines and macrophages. *Biomed. Pharmacother.* **1994**, *48*, 445–453. [CrossRef]
7. Hilligan, K.L.; Ronchese, F. Antigen presentation by dendritic cells and their instruction of CD4+ T helper cell responses. *Cell. Mol. Immunol.* **2020**, *17*, 587–599. [CrossRef] [PubMed]
8. Aderem, A.; Underhill, D. Mechanisms of phagocytosis in macrophages. *Annu. Rev. Immunol.* **1999**, *17*, 593–623. [CrossRef]
9. Hughes, C.E.; Benson, R.; Bedaj, M.; Maffia, P. Antigen-Presenting Cells and Antigen Presentation in Tertiary Lymphoid Organs. *Front. Immunol.* **2016**, *7*, 481. [CrossRef] [PubMed]
10. Hume, D.A. Macrophages as APC and the Dendritic Cell Myth. *J. Immunol.* **2008**, *181*, 5829–5835. [CrossRef]
11. Yang, P.-C.; Mahmood, T. Western blot: Technique, theory, and trouble shooting. *N. Am. J. Med Sci.* **2012**, *4*, 429–434. [CrossRef]
12. Cordier, G. Flow cytometry for immunology. *Biol. Cell* **1986**, *58*, 147–150. [CrossRef]

13. Haines, D.M.; West, K.H. Immunohistochemistry: Forging the links between immunology and pathology. *Veter-Immunol. Immunopathol.* **2005**, *108*, 151–156. [CrossRef] [PubMed]
14. Lew, A.; Brandon, R.B.; Panaccio, M.; Morrow, C.J. The polymerase chain reaction and other amplification techniques in immunological research and diagnosis. *Immunology* **1992**, *75*, 3–9. [PubMed]
15. Noble, D. Electrical properties of biological cells. *Nat. Cell Biol.* **1978**, *276*, 541. [CrossRef]
16. Woodward, A.M.; Kell, D. On the nonlinear dielectric properties of biological systems: Saccharomyces cerevisiae. *Bioelectrochem. Bioenerg.* **1990**, *24*, 83–100. [CrossRef]
17. Di Biasio, A.; Ambrosone, L.; Cametti, C. The Dielectric Behavior of Nonspherical Biological Cell Suspensions: An Analytic Approach. *Biophys. J.* **2010**, *99*, 163–174. [CrossRef]
18. Nasir, N.; Al Ahmad, M. Cells Electrical Characterization: Dielectric Properties, Mixture, and Modeling Theories. *J. Eng.* **2020**, *2020*, 9475490. [CrossRef]
19. Goldberger, J.J.; Subacius, H.; Sen-Gupta, I.; Johnson, D.; Kadish, A.H.; Ng, J. A new method to determine the electrical transfer function of the human thorax. *Am. J. Physiol. Circ. Physiol.* **2007**, *293*, H3440–H3447. [CrossRef] [PubMed]
20. Adams, K.L.; Puchades, M.; Ewing, A.G. In Vitro Electrochemistry of Biological Systems. *Annu. Rev. Anal. Chem.* **2008**, *1*, 329–355. [CrossRef]
21. Nasir, N.; Raji, S.; Mustafa, F.; Rizvi, T.A.; Al Natour, Z.; Hilal-Alnaqbi, A.; Al Ahmad, M. Electrical detection of blood cells in urine. *Heliyon* **2020**, *6*, e03102. [CrossRef]
22. Al Ahmad, M.; Al Natour, Z.; Mustafa, F.; Rizvi, T.A. Electrical Characterization of Normal and Cancer Cells. *IEEE Access* **2018**, *6*, 25979–25986. [CrossRef]
23. Al Ahmad, M.; Al Natour, Z.; Attoub, S.; Hassan, A.H. Monitoring of the Budding Yeast Cell Cycle Using Electrical Parameters. *IEEE Access* **2018**, *6*, 19231–19237. [CrossRef]
24. Chen, W.; Li, W.; Dong, X.; Pei, J. A Review of Biological Image Analysis. *Curr. Bioinform.* **2018**, *13*, 337–343. [CrossRef]
25. Von Bartheld, C.S.; Bahney, J.; Herculano-Houzel, S. The search for true numbers of neurons and glial cells in the human brain: A review of 150 years of cell counting. *J. Comp. Neurol.* **2016**, *524*, 3865–3895. [CrossRef] [PubMed]
26. Saraswat, M.; Arya, K. Automated microscopic image analysis for leukocytes identification: A survey. *Micron* **2014**, *65*, 20–33. [CrossRef]
27. Department of Engineering Science. Biological Image Processing. Available online: http://www.ibme.ox.ac.uk/research/biomedia/vicente-grau/biological-image-processing (accessed on 2 April 2020).
28. Kherlopian, A.R.; Song, T.; Duan, Q.; Neimark, M.A.; Po, M.J.; Gohagan, J.K.; Laine, A.F. A review of imaging techniques for systems biology. *BMC Syst. Biol.* **2008**, *2*, 74. [CrossRef]
29. Hornick, J.E.; Hinchcliffe, E.H. It's all about the pentiums: The use, manipulation, and storage of digital microscopy imaging data for the biological sciences. *Mol. Reprod. Dev.* **2015**, *82*, 508–517. [CrossRef]
30. MicroscopyU. Introduction for Fluorescence Microscopy. Available online: https://www.microscopyu.com/techniques/fluorescence/introduction-to-fluorescence-microscopy (accessed on 28 January 2021).
31. Basiji, D.A.; Ortyn, W.E.; Liang, L.; Venkatachalam, V.; Morrissey, P. Cellular Image Analysis and Imaging by Flow Cytometry. *Clin. Lab. Med.* **2007**, *27*, 653–670. [CrossRef]
32. Khan Academy. What Is Hooke's Law. Available online: https://www.khanacademy.org/science/physics/work-and-energy/hookes-law/a/what-is-hookes-law (accessed on 28 January 2021).
33. Binnig, G.; Quate, C.F.; Gerber, C. Atomic Force Microscope. *Phys. Rev. Lett.* **1986**, *56*, 930–933. [CrossRef]
34. Microbe Notes. Electron Microscope—Definition, Principle, Types, Uses, Images. Available online: https://microbenotes.com/electron-microscope-principle-types-components-applications-advantages-limitations (accessed on 28 January 2021).
35. Image Segmentation—An Overview. Available online: https://www.sciencedirect.com/topics/computer-science/image-segmentation (accessed on 28 March 2020).
36. NIST. Quantification of Cells with Specific Phenotypic Characteristics. Available online: https://www.nist.gov/programs-projects/quantification-cells-specific-phenotypic-characteristics (accessed on 28 March 2020).
37. HLA DR Antigen—An Overview. ScienceDirect Topics. Available online: https://www.sciencedirect.com/topics/medicine-and-dentistry/hla-dr-antigen (accessed on 1 July 2020).
38. Helm, O.; Held-Feindt, J.; Schäfer, H.; Sebens, S. M1 and M2: There is no "good" and "bad"—How macrophages promote malignancy-associated features in tumorigenesis. *Oncoimmunology* **2014**, *3*, e946818. [CrossRef]
39. Jacome-Galarza, C.E.; Lee, S.-K.; Lorenzo, J.A.; Aguila, H.L. Identification, characterization, and isolation of a common progenitor for osteoclasts, macrophages, and dendritic cells from murine bone marrow and periphery. *J. Bone Miner. Res.* **2012**, *28*, 1203–1213. [CrossRef] [PubMed]
40. Twigg, H.L. Macrophages in Innate and Acquired Immunity. *Semin. Respir. Crit. Care Med.* **2004**, *25*, 21–31. [CrossRef] [PubMed]
41. THP-1 TIB-202TM. ATCC. Available online: https://www.atcc.org/products/tib-202 (accessed on 1 July 2020).
42. Berges, C.; Naujokat, C.; Tinapp, S.; Wieczorek, H.; Höh, A.; Sadeghi, M.; Opelz, G.; Daniel, V. A cell line model for the differentiation of human dendritic cells. *Biochem. Biophys. Res. Commun.* **2005**, *333*, 896–907. [CrossRef] [PubMed]
43. Genin, M.; Clement, F.; Fattaccioli, A.; Raes, M.; Michiels, C. M1 and M2 macrophages derived from THP-1 cells differentially modulate the response of cancer cells to etoposide. *BMC Cancer* **2015**, *15*, 1–14. [CrossRef] [PubMed]

44. Schneider, C.A.; Rasband, W.S.; Eliceiri, K.W. NIH Image to ImageJ: 25 years of image analysis. *Nat. Methods* **2012**, *9*, 671–675. [CrossRef]
45. Metrohm DropSens. Potentiostats. Available online: http://www.dropsens.com/en/potentiostats_pag.html (accessed on 1 July 2020).
46. Wang, H.-W.; Bringans, C.; Hickey, A.; Windsor, J.; Kilmartin, P.; Phillips, A. Cyclic Voltammetry in Biological Samples: A Systematic Review of Methods and Techniques Applicable to Clinical Settings. *Signals* **2021**, *2*, 138–158. [CrossRef]
47. Li, Z.; Ju, X.; Silveira, P.A.; Abadir, E.; Hsu, W.-H.; Hart, D.N.J.; Clark, G. CD83: Activation Marker for Antigen Presenting Cells and Its Therapeutic Potential. *Front. Immunol.* **2019**, *10*, 1312. [CrossRef]
48. Krombach, F. Cell size of alveolar macrophages: An interspecies comparison. *Environ. Health Perspect.* **1997**, *105*, 1261–1263.
49. Dumortier, H.; Van Mierlo, G.J.D.; Egan, D.; Van Ewijk, W.; Toes, R.E.M.; Offringa, R.; Melief, C.J.M. Antigen Presentation by an Immature Myeloid Dendritic Cell Line Does Not Cause CTL Deletion In Vivo, but Generates CD8+ Central Memory-Like T Cells That Can Be Rescued for Full Effector Function. *J. Immunol.* **2005**, *175*, 855–863. [CrossRef] [PubMed]
50. Thomas, P.; Lee, A.K.; Wong, J.G.; Almers, W. A triggered mechanism retrieves membrane in seconds after Ca^{2+}-stimulated exocytosis in single pituitary cells. *J. Cell Biol.* **1994**, *124*, 667–675. [CrossRef] [PubMed]
51. Nikbakht, G.; Pakbin, B.; Brujeni, G.N. Evaluation of a new lymphocyte proliferation assay based on cyclic voltammetry; an alternative method. *Sci. Rep.* **2019**, *9*, 1–7. [CrossRef] [PubMed]
52. Sohn, L.L.; Saleh, O.A.; Facer, G.R.; Beavis, A.J.; Allan, R.S.; Notterman, D.A. Capacitance cytometry: Measuring biological cells one by one. *Proc. Natl. Acad. Sci. USA* **2000**, *97*, 10687–10690. [CrossRef] [PubMed]
53. Bio-Rad. Preparation of Tissue Culture Cells for Flow Cytometry. Available online: https://www.bio-rad-antibodies.com/preparation-of-cells-for-flow-cytometry.html (accessed on 8 August 2021).

sensors

MDPI

Article

Detection of COVID-19 from Chest X-ray Images Using Deep Convolutional Neural Networks

Natheer Khasawneh [1,*], Mohammad Fraiwan [2], Luay Fraiwan [3], Basheer Khassawneh [4] and Ali Ibnian [4]

1 Department of Software Engineering, Jordan University of Science and Technology, P.O. Box 3030, Irbid 22110, Jordan
2 Department of Computer Engineering, Jordan University of Science and Technology, P.O. Box 3030, Irbid 22110, Jordan; mafraiwan@just.edu.jo
3 Department of Biomedical Engineering, Jordan University of Science and Technology, P.O. Box 3030, Irbid 22110, Jordan; fraiwan@just.edu.jo
4 Department of Internal Medicine, Jordan University of Science and Technology, P.O. Box 3030, Irbid 22110, Jordan; basheerk@just.edu.jo (B.K.); amibnian@hotmail.com (A.I.)
* Correspondence: natheer@just.edu.jo; Tel.: +971-528310815

Abstract: The COVID-19 global pandemic has wreaked havoc on every aspect of our lives. More specifically, healthcare systems were greatly stretched to their limits and beyond. Advances in artificial intelligence have enabled the implementation of sophisticated applications that can meet clinical accuracy requirements. In this study, customized and pre-trained deep learning models based on convolutional neural networks were used to detect pneumonia caused by COVID-19 respiratory complications. Chest X-ray images from 368 confirmed COVID-19 patients were collected locally. In addition, data from three publicly available datasets were used. The performance was evaluated in four ways. First, the public dataset was used for training and testing. Second, data from the local and public sources were combined and used to train and test the models. Third, the public dataset was used to train the model and the local data were used for testing only. This approach adds greater credibility to the detection models and tests their ability to generalize to new data without overfitting the model to specific samples. Fourth, the combined data were used for training and the local dataset was used for testing. The results show a high detection accuracy of 98.7% with the combined dataset, and most models handled new data with an insignificant drop in accuracy.

Keywords: COVID-19; chest X-ray; deep learning; convolutional neural networks; diagnosis

Citation: Khasawneh, N.; Fraiwan, M.; Fraiwan, L.; Khassawneh, B.; Ibnian, A. Detection of COVID-19 from Chest X-ray Images Using Deep Convolutional Neural Networks. *Sensors* **2021**, *21*, 5940. https://doi.org/10.3390/s21175940

Academic Editor: Loris Nanni

Received: 29 July 2021
Accepted: 1 September 2021
Published: 3 September 2021

1. Introduction

Coronavirus disease 2019 (COVID-19), which is caused by the SARS-CoV-2 virus, has wreaked havoc on humanity, especially healthcare systems. For example, recently, the wave of infections in India has caused a great number of families to seek care at home due to a lack of intensive care units. Worldwide, millions have succumbed to this pandemic and many more have suffered long- and short-term health problems. The most common symptoms of this viral syndrome are fever, dry cough, fatigue, aches and pains, loss of taste/smell, and breathing problems [1]. Other less common symptoms are also possible (e.g., diarrhea, conjunctivitis) [2]. Infections are officially confirmed using real-time reverse transcription polymerase chain reaction (RT-PCR) [3]. However, chest radiographs using plain chest X-rays (CXRs) and computerized tomography (CT) play an important role confirming the infection and evaluating the extent of damage incurred to the lungs. CXR and CT scans are considered major evidence for clinical diagnosis of COVID-19 [4].

Chest X-ray images are one of the most common clinical diagnosis methods. However, reaching the correct judgement requires specialist knowledge and experience. The strain on medical staff worldwide incurred by the COVID-19 pandemic, in addition to the already inadequate number of radiologists per person worldwide [5], necessitates innovative accessible solutions. Advances in artificial intelligence have enabled the implementation of sophisticated applications that can meet clinical accuracy requirements and handle large volumes of data. Incorporating computer-aided diagnosis tools into the medical hierarchy has the potential to reduce errors, improve workload conditions, increase reliability, and replace by enhance the workflow and reduce diagnostic errors by providing radiologists with references for diagnostics.

The fight against COVID-19 has taken several forms and fronts. Computerized solutions offer contactless alternatives to many aspects of dealing with the pandemic [6]. Some examples include robotic solutions for physical sampling, vital sign monitoring, and disinfection. Moreover, image recognition and AI are being actively used to identify confirmed cases not adhering to quarantine protocols. In this work, we propose an automatic diagnosis artificial intelligence (AI) system that is able to identify COVID-19-related pneumonia from chest X-ray images with high accuracy. One customized convolutional neural networks model and two pre-trained models (i.e., MobileNets [7] and VGG16 [8]) were incorporated. Moreover, CXR images of confirmed COVID-19 subjects were collected from a large local hospital and inspected by board-accredited specialists over a period of 6 months. These images were used to enrich the limited number of existing public datasets and form a larger training/testing group of images in comparison to the related literature. Importantly, the reported results come from testing the models with this completely foreign set of images in addition to evaluating the models using the fused aggregate set. This approach exposed any overfitting of the model to a specific set of CXR images, especially as some datasets contain multiple images per subject.

2. Background and Related Work

COVID-19 patients who have clinical symptoms are more likely to show abnormal CXR [9]. The main findings of recent studies suggest that these lung images display patchy or diffuse reticular–nodular opacities and consolidation, with basal, peripheral, and bilateral predominance [10]. For example, Figure 1 shows the CXR of a mild case of lung tissue involvement with right infrahilar reticular–nodular opacity. Moreover, Figure 2 shows the CXR of a moderate to severe case of lung tissue involvement. This CXR shows right lower zone lung consolidation and diffuse bilateral airspace reticular–nodular opacities, which are more prominent on peripheral parts of lower zones. Similarly, Figure 3 shows the CXR of a severe case of lung tissue involvement. This is caused by diffuse bilateral airspace reticular–nodular opacities that are more prominent on peripheral parts of the lower zones, and ground glass opacity in both lungs predominant in mid-zones and lower zones. On the other hand, Figure 4 shows an unremarkable CXR with clear lungs and acute costophrenic angles (i.e., normal).

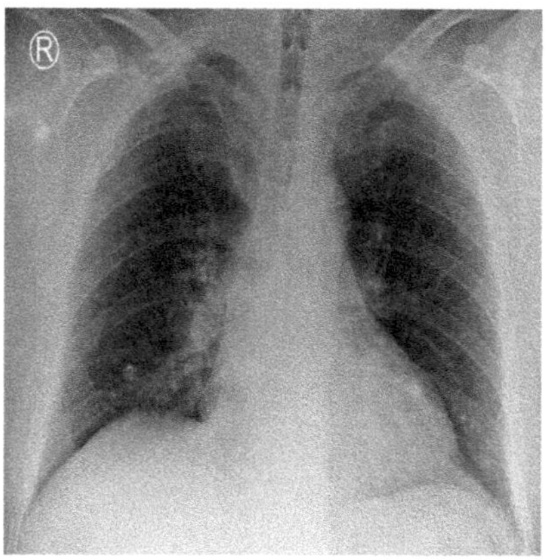

Figure 1. CXR of COVID-19 subject showing mild lung tissue involvement.

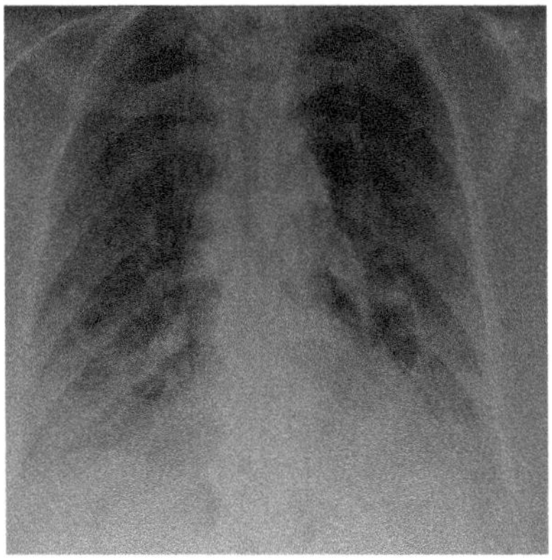

Figure 2. CXR of COVID-19 subject showing moderate to severe lung tissue involvement.

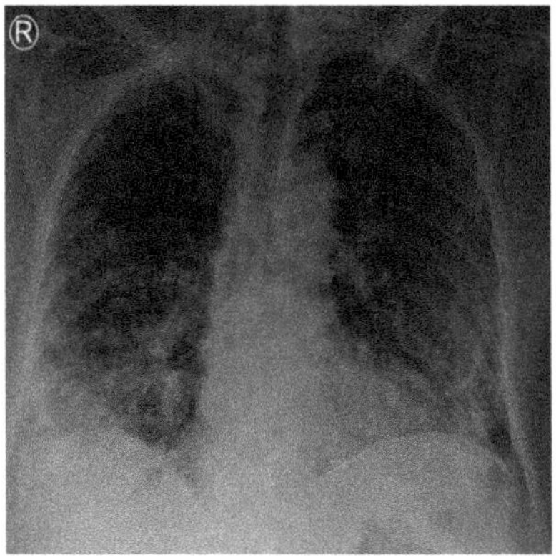

Figure 3. CXR of COVID-19 subject showing severe lung tissue involvement.

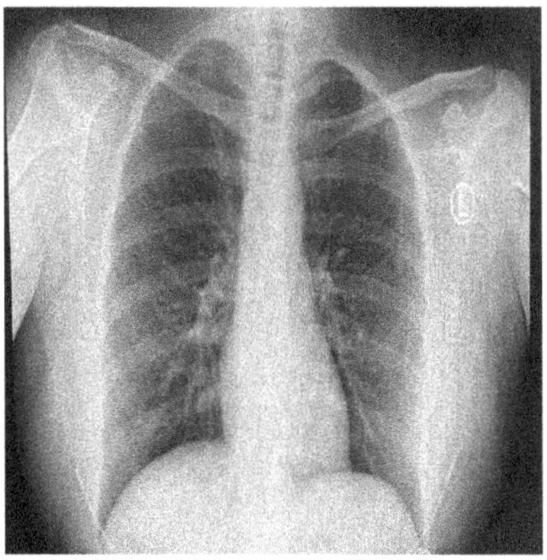

Figure 4. Normal CXR.

AI, with its machine learning (ML) foundation, has taken great strides toward deployment in many fields. For example, Vetology AI [11] is a paid service that provides AI-based radiograph reports. Similarly, the widespread research and usage of AI in medicine have been observed for many years now [12,13]. AI-based web or mobile applications for automated diagnosis can greatly aid clinicians in reducing errors, provide remote and cheap diagnosis in poor undermanned underequipped areas, and improve the speed and quality of healthcare [14]. In the context of COVID-19 radiographs, ML methods are feasible to evaluate CXR images to detect the aforementioned markers of COVID-19 infection and the adverse effects on the state of the patients' lungs. This is of special importance considering the fact that health services were stretched to their limits and sometimes to the brink of collapse by the pandemic.

Deep learning AI enables the development of end-to-end models that learn and discover classification patterns and features using multiple processing layers, rendering it unnecessary to explicitly extract features. The sudden spread of the COVID-19 pandemic has necessitated the development of innovative ways to cope with the rising healthcare demands of this outbreak. To this end, many recent models have been proposed for COVID-19 detection. These methods rely mainly on CXR and CT images as input to the diagnosis model [15,16]. Hemdan et al. [17] proposed the COVIDX-Net deep learning framework to classify CXR images as either positive or negative COVID-19 cases. Although they employed seven deep convolutional neural network models, the best results were 89% and 91% F1-scores for normal and positive COVID-19, respectively. However, their results were based on 50 CXR images only, which is a very small dataset to build a reliable deep learning system.

Several existing out-of-the-box deep learning convolutional neural network algorithms are available in the literature [18], and they have been widely used in the COVID-19 identification literature with and without modifications [15]. They provide track-proven image detection and identification capabilities in many disciplines and research problems. Some of the most commonly used models are: (1) GoogleNet, VGG-16, VGG-19, AlexNet, and LetNet, which are spatial exploitation-based CNNs. (2) MobileNet, ResNet, Inception-V3, and Inception-V4, which are depth based CNNs. (3) Other models include DenseNet, Xception, SqueezeNet, etc. These architectures can be used pre-trained with deep transfer learning (e.g., Sethy et al. [19]), or customized (e.g., CoroNet [20]).

Rajaraman et al. [21] used iteratively pruned deep learning ensembles to classify CXRs into normal, COVID-19, or bacterial pneumonia with a 99.01% accuracy. Several models were tested and the best results were combined using various ensemble strategies to improve the classification accuracy. However, such methods are mainly suitable for small numbers of COVID-19 images as the computational overhead of multiple model calculations is high, and there is no guarantee that they will retain their accuracy with large datasets [15,22]. Other works for three-class classification using deep learning were also proposed in this context. The studies by Ucar et al. [23], Rahimzadeh and Attar [24], Narin et al. [25], and Khobahi et al. [26] classify cases as COVID-19, normal, or pneumonia. Others replace pneumonia with a generic non-COVID-19 category [27,28], or severe acute respiratory syndrome (SARS) [29]. Less frequently, studies distinguish between viral and bacterial pneumonia in a four-class classification [18]. A significant number of studies conducted binary classification into COVID-19 or non-COVID-19 classes [19,30]. Although these methods achieved high accuracies (i.e., greater than 89%), the number of COVID-19 images from the total dataset is small. For example, Ucar et al. [23] used 45 COVID-19 images only. Moreover, subsequent testing of the models used a subset of the same dataset, which may give falsely improved results, especially as same subject may have multiple CXR images in the dataset.

3. Material and Methods

3.1. Subjects

The selected images were acquired from locally recorded chest X-rays of COVID-19 patients in addition to a publicly available dataset [31]. The combination of two datasets adds greater credibility to the developed identification models. This is because training/validation was performed on one set, and the testing was performed on a different dataset. In addition, it increased the size of the dataset, which is a problem with most of the related literature.

The first group of images was obtained locally at King Abdullah University Hospital, Jordan University of Science and Technology, Irbid, Jordan. The study was approved by the institutional review board (IRB 91/136/2020) at King Abdullah University Hospital (KAUH). Written informed consent was sought and obtained from all participants (or their parents in case of underage subjects) prior to any clinical examinations. The dataset included 368 subjects (215 male, 153 female) with a mean $\pm$ SD age of 63.15 $\pm$ 14.8. The minimum subject age was 31 months and maximum age was 96 years. All subjects had at least one positive RT-PCR test and were in need of hospital admittance as determined by the specialists at KAUH. The hospital stay ranged from 5 days to 6 weeks with some subjects passing away (exact number not available). The CXR images were taken after at least 3 days of hospital stay to ensure the existence of lung abnormalities, which were confirmed by the participating specialists. The CXR images were reviewed using the MicroDicom viewer version 3.8.1 (see https://www.microdicom.com/, accessed on: 28 May 2021), and exported as high-resolution images (i.e., 1850 $\times$ 1300 pixels).

The second group of images is publicly available [31], and was produced by the fusion of three separate datasets: (1) COVID-19 chest X-ray dataset [32]. (2) The Radiological Society of North America (RSNA) dataset [33]. (3) The U.S. National Library of Medicine (USNLM) Montgomery County X-ray set [34]. At the time of performing the experiments, the dataset contained 2295 CXR images (1583 normal and 712 COVID-19), which were used in this work. However, the dataset is continuously being updated [35].

3.2. Deep Learning Models

Deep learning is the current trend and most prolific AI technique used for classification problems [15]. It has been used widely and successfully in a range of applications, especially in the medical field. The next few paragraphs describe the models used in this work.

1. 2D sequential CN CNN models are one class in the deep learning literature. They are a special class of feedforward neural networks that have been found to be very useful in analyzing multidimensional data (e.g., images) [18]. However, CNNs conserve memory relative to multilayer perceptrons by sharing parameters and using sparse connections. The input images are transformed into a matrix to be processed by the various CNN elements. The model consists of several alternating layers of convolution and pooling (see Table 1), as follows:

   Convolutional layer

   The convolutional layer determines the features of the various patterns in the input. It consists of a set of dot products (i.e., convolutions) applied to the input matrix. This step creates an image processing kernel containing a number of filters, which outputs a feature map (i.e., motifs). The input is divided into small windows called receptive fields, which are convolved with the kernel using a specific set of weights. In this work, a 2D convolution layer was used (i.e., using the CONV2D class).

   Pooling layer

   This down-sampling layer reduces the spatial dimensions of the output volume by reducing the number of feature maps and network parameters. Moreover, pooling helps in improving the generalization of the model by reducing overfitting [36]. The output from this step is a combination of features invariant to translational shifts and distortions [37].

   Dropout

   Overfitting is a common problem in neural networks. Hence, dropout is used as a strategy to introduce regularization within the network, which eventually improves generalization. It works by randomly ignoring some hidden and visible units. This has the effect of training the network to handle multiple independent internal representations.

Fully connected layer

This layer accepts the feature map as input and outputs nonlinear transformed output via an activation function. This is a global operation that works on features from all stages to produce a nonlinear set of classification features. The rectified linear unit (ReLU) was used in this step as it helps in overcoming the vanishing gradient problem [38].

Table 1. Summary of the CNN models used in this work.

Layer	Output Shape	No. of Parameters
CONV2D-1	(None, 150, 150, 32)	2432
MaxPooling2D-1	(None, 75, 75, 32)	0
Dropout-1	(None, 75, 75, 32)	0
Conv2D-2	(None, 75, 75, 64)	51,264
MaxPooling2D-2	(None, 37, 37, 64)	0
Dropout-2	(None, 37, 37, 64)	0
Flatten	(None, 87,616)	0
Dense-1	(None, 256)	22,429,952
Dropout-3	(None, 256)	0
Dense-2	(None, 1)	257

2. Pre-trained models

MobileNets

The MobileNets model [7] is a resource-limited CNN architecture, which was chosen in this work with an eye on future mobile applications for disease diagnosis. It uses depth-wise separable convolutions, which significantly reduces the number of parameters. MobileNets was open-sourced by Google to enable the development of low-power, small, and low-latency applications for mobile environments.

VGG-16

VGG-16 [8] is a representative of the many models existing in the literature. It has gone through various refinements to improve its accuracy performance and resources consumption (e.g., VGG-19). The VGG model is a spatial exploitation CNN with 19 layers, 3×3 filters (computationally efficient), 1×1 convolution in between the convolution layers (for regularization), and max-pooling after the convolution layer. The model is known for its simplicity [18].

3.3. Model Implementation

The models were implemented and evaluated using the Keras [39] high-level application program interface (API) of TensorFlow 2 [40]. The experiments were run on a Dell Precision 5820 Tower (Dell Inc., Round Rock, TX, USA) with Intel Xeon W-2155, 64GB of RAM (Intel Inc., Santa Clara, CA, USA), and 16GB Nvidia Quadro RTX5000 GPU (Nvidia Inc., Santa Clara, CA, USA).

4. Results and Discussion

Four different approaches were used to evaluate the three deep learning models. First, only the public dataset was used to train and test the models. Second, the fused dataset was used to test and train the models (i.e., the sets were combined together and treated as one without any distinction). Third, the public dataset was used for training the model and the locally collected dataset was used for testing. This approach shows the ability of the model to generalize to new data and avoid overfitting to specific images/subjects. Fourth, the combined (i.e., fused) dataset was used for training and local dataset for testing. Table 2 shows the number of training and testing subjects used for each approach. Note that the local dataset did not include normal CXR images as those are abundantly available. The confusion matrices resulting from testing were analyzed to produce several standard performance measures. These include accuracy, specificity, sensitivity, F1-score, and precision as defined in Equations (1)–(5).

Table 2. The number of training and testing subjects used for each of the evaluation approaches.

Approach	Training		Testing	
	COVID-19	Normal	COVID-19	Normal
Public dataset	545	1266	167	317
Fused dataset	842	1266	238	317
Public dataset for training and local dataset for testing	545	1266	368	317
Fused dataset for training and local dataset for testing	842	1266	368	317

$$Accuracy = \frac{t_p + t_n}{t_p + f_n + f_p + t_n} \quad (1)$$

$$Sensitivity = \frac{t_p}{t_p + f_n} \quad (2)$$

$$Specificity = \frac{t_n}{t_n + f_p} \quad (3)$$

$$F1score = \frac{2 \times t_p}{2 \times t_p + f_p + f_n} \quad (4)$$

$$Precision = \frac{t_p}{t_p + f_p} \quad (5)$$

where t_p: true positive, represents the subjects correctly classified in predefined (positive) class. f_n: false negative, represents the subjects misclassified in the other (negative) class. f_p: false positive, represents the subjects misclassified in predefined (positive) class. t_n: true negative, represents the subjects correctly classified in the other (negative) class.

Figure 5 shows the training and validation loss for the two model training methods. The 2D CNN model required more epochs to reach the appropriate accuracy improvement, but the training was smooth with little oscillation. Moreover, the other two models required very few epochs (e.g., VGG-16 required one epoch with the fused dataset, hence the missing plot). Figure 6 shows the training and validation accuracy. The figures generally show that the models are able to properly fit training data and improve with experience. It is clear that the MobileNets and VGG-16 models achieve superior and high classification accuracy.

The testing dataset (i.e., the locally collected COVID-19 CXR images) is different from the training dataset.

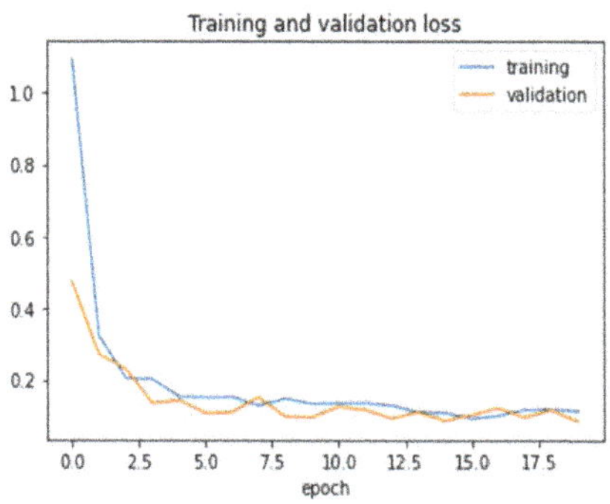

(**a**) CNN trained using the public dataset.

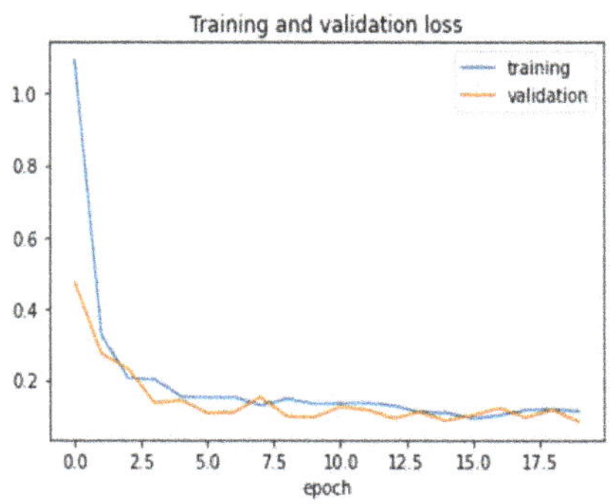

(**b**) CNN trained using the fused dataset.

Figure 5. *Cont.*

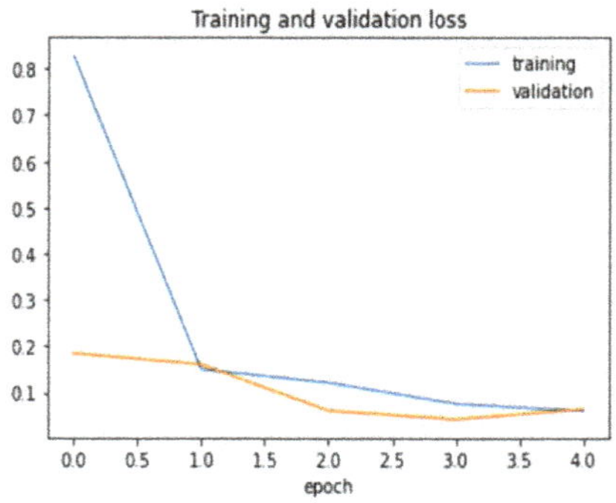

(**c**) MobileNets trained using the public dataset.

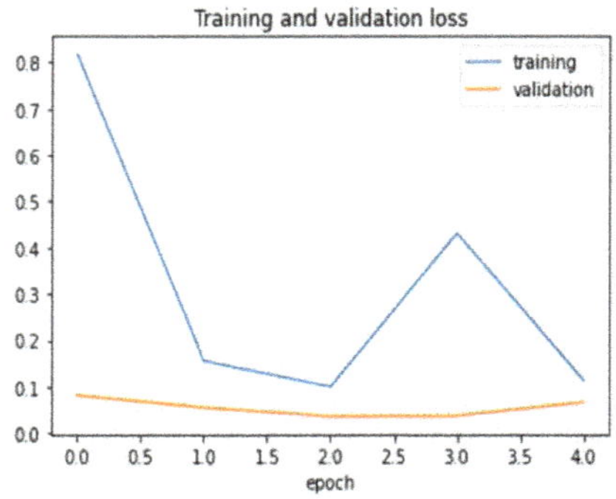

(**d**) MobileNets trained using the fused dataset.

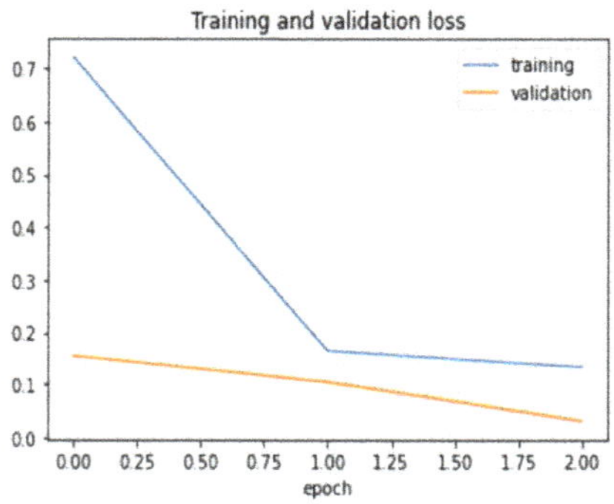

(**e**) VGG-16 trained using the public dataset.

Figure 5. Training and validation loss for the three architectures trained using the public and the fused datasets. Note that VGG-16 trained on the fused dataset ended after one epoch only, hence there is no corresponding figure. The models are able to properly fit training data and improve with experience (as seen in validation curves).

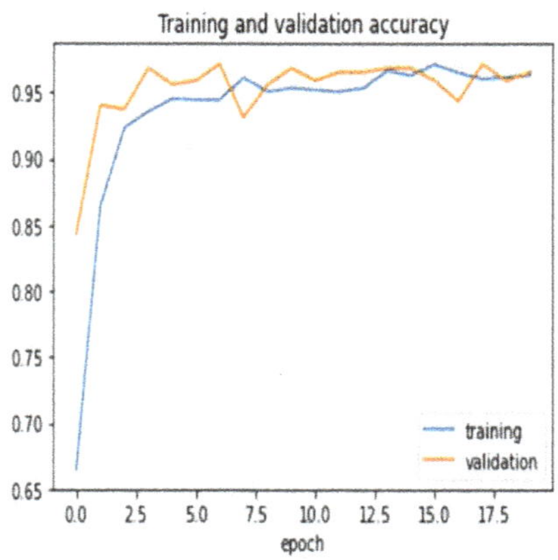

(**a**) CNN trained using the public dataset.

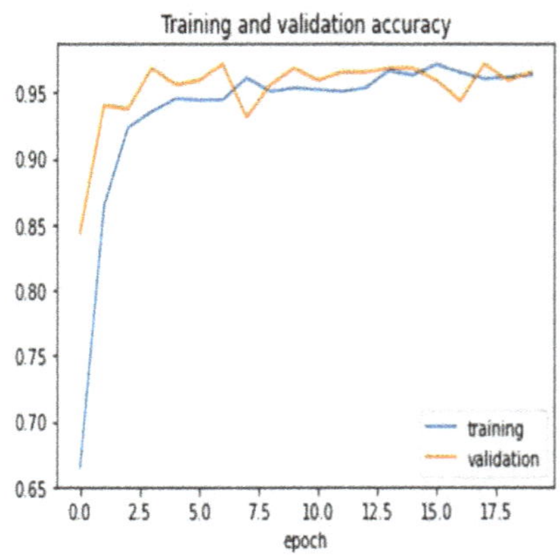

(**b**) CNN trained using the fused dataset.

Figure 6. *Cont.*

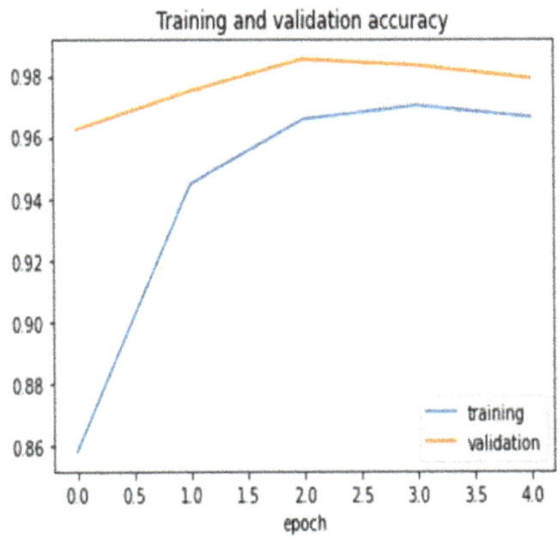

(**c**) MobileNets trained using the public dataset.

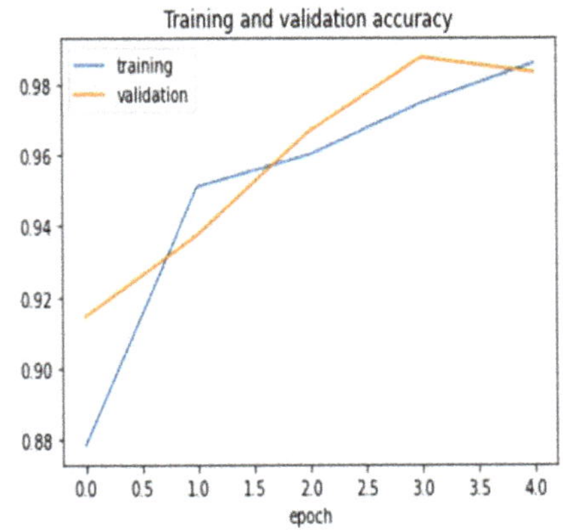

(**d**) MobileNets trained using the fused dataset.

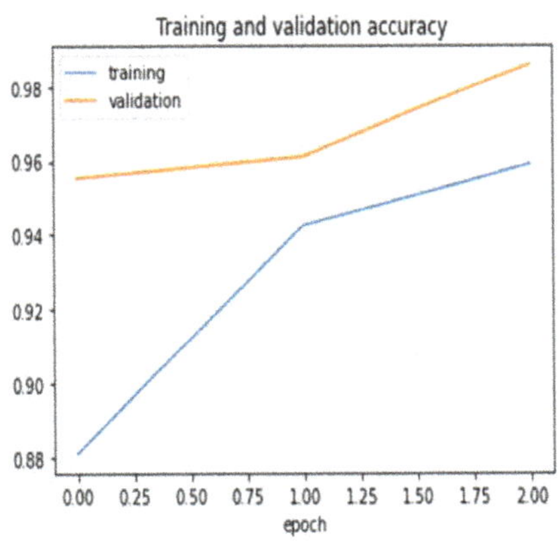

(**e**) VGG-16 trained using the public dataset.

Figure 6. Training and validation accuracy for the three architectures trained using the public and the fused datasets. Note that VGG-16 trained on the fused dataset ended after one epoch only, hence there is no corresponding figure. The models are able to properly fit training data and improve with experience (as seen in validation curves).

4.1. 2D Sequential CNN

Tables 3 and 4 show the values for the performance evaluation metrics and the corresponding confusion matrices for the 2D sequential CNN model. The architecture achieved the best accuracy of 96.1% over all training and testing methods. However, the accuracy drops sharply to 79% when the testing was carried out using a database (i.e., the locally collected COVID-19 CXR images) different from the training one (i.e., the public dataset). This indicates the failure of the model to generalize to new data, and that there may be subtle or obscure differences between the images from the two datasets. This is further confirmed by the fact that normal images (see Table 4c), which were taken from the public dataset, were mostly correctly classified. The source of errors came from false negative classifications (i.e., type II errors). However, the accuracy improved to 89.3%, when a separate part of the testing dataset was included in the training. Still, most of the errors were type II (see Table 4d). This is a model performance mismatch problem of the custom CNN, which is typically caused by unrepresentative data samples. However, since the other models were trained on the same data, then this reason could be discounted. The MobileNets and VGG-16 models were employed using transfer learning, which inherently reduces overfitting. Moreover, these models are larger and deeper than the custom CNN, which due to overparameterization can lead to better generalization performance [41].

Table 3. Performance evaluation metrics for the customized CNN model. Acc.: Accuracy, Sens.: Sensitivity, Spec.: Specificity, Prec.: Precision.

Dataset	Acc.	Sens.	Spec.	F1-Score	Prec.
Public dataset	96.1%	92.8%	97.8%	94.2%	95.7%
Fused dataset	93.7%	85.7%	99.7%	92.1%	99.5%
Public dataset for training and local dataset for testing	79%	62.8%	97.8%	76.2%	97.1%
Fused dataset for training and local dataset for testing	89.3%	80.4%	99.7%	89%	99.7%

Table 4. The confusion matrices resulting from the customized CNN model. Positive refers to confirmed COVID-19 case.

(a) Public Dataset

		Predicted diagnosis	
		Positive	Negative
Actual	Positive	155	12
	Negative	7	310

(b) Fused Public and Local Datsets

		Predicted diagnosis	
		Positive	Negative
Actual	Positive	204	34
	Negative	1	316

(c) Public Dataset for Training and Local Dataset for Testing

		Predicted diagnosis	
		Positive	Negative
Actual	Positive	231	137
	Negative	7	310

(d) Fused Dataset for Training and Local Dataset for Testing

		Predicted diagnosis	
		Positive	Negative
Actual	Positive	296	72
	Negative	1	316

4.2. MobileNets

Tables 5 and 6 show the values for the performance evaluation metrics and the corresponding confusion matrices for the MobileNets model. It achieved accuracy values between 97.1% and 98.7%, which shows stability when faced with new data, and the ability to generalize. Errors, although few, were caused by misclassifying COVID-19 CXR images as normal. However, the type I errors increased slightly (Table 6c).

Table 5. Performance evaluation metrics for the customized MobileNets model. Acc.: Accuracy, Sens.: Sensitivity, Spec.: Specificity, Prec.: Precision.

Dataset	Acc.	Sens.	Spec.	F1-Score	Prec.
Public dataset	98.3%	98.2%	98.4%	97.6%	97%
Fused dataset	97.1%	92.8%	99.4%	95.7%	98.7%
Public dataset for training and local dataset for testing	98%	97.6%	98.4%	98.1%	98.6%
Fused dataset for training and local dataset for testing	98.7%	98.1%	99.4%	98.8%	99.4%

Table 6. The confusion matrices resulting from the customized MobileNets model. Positive refers to confirmed COVID-19 case.

(a) Public Dataset			
		Predicted diagnosis	
		Positive	Negative
Actual	Positive	164	3
	Negative	5	312
(b) Fused Public and Local Datsets			
		Predicted diagnosis	
		Positive	Negative
Actual	Positive	155	12
	Negative	2	315
(c) Public Dataset for Training and Local Dataset for Testing			
		Predicted diagnosis	
		Positive	Negative
Actual	Positive	359	9
	Negative	5	312
(d) Fused Dataset for Training and Local Dataset for Testing			
		Predicted diagnosis	
		Positive	Negative
Actual	Positive	361	7
	Negative	2	315

4.3. VGG-16

Tables 7 and 8 show the values for the performance evaluation metrics and the corresponding confusion matrices for the VGG-16 model. The model achieved the best accuracy over all models (i.e., 99%) when the fused dataset was used for training and the local dataset was used for testing, which indicates its ability to capture various properties from different sets. However, it fell behind MobileNets slightly when the training dataset (i.e., the public dataset) was different from the testing dataset. Moreover, the model achieved the highest accuracy (98.7%) with the fused dataset for both training and testing. However, MobileNets achieved slightly higher accuracy when trained and tested with the public dataset alone. Such slight performance differences when the dataset is augmented with data from other sources may need further investigation. The confusion matrices show that, for VGG-16, the majority of errors are type I over all evaluation methods, which is different from the CNN or MobileNets errors (i.e., type II). Improving VGG-16's handling of normal images should cut the error rate significantly.

Table 7. Performance evaluation metrics for the customized VGG-16 model. Acc.: Accuracy, Sens.: Sensitivity, Spec.: Specificity, Prec.: Precision.

Dataset	Acc.	Sens.	Spec.	F1-Score	Prec.
Public dataset	97.1%	98.2%	96.5%	95.9%	93.7%
Fused dataset	98.7%	99.2%	98.4%	98.5%	97.9%
Public dataset for training and local dataset for testing	97.2%	97.8%	96.5%	97.4%	97%
Fused dataset for training and local dataset for testing	99%	99.5%	98.4%	99.1%	98.7%

Table 8. The confusion matrices resulting from the customized VGG-16 model. Positive refers to confirmed COVID-19 case.

(a) Public Dataset			
		Predicted diagnosis	
		Positive	Negative
Actual	Positive	164	3
	Negative	11	306
(b) Fused Public and Local Datsets			
		Predicted diagnosis	
		Positive	Negative
Actual	Positive	236	2
	Negative	5	312
(c) Public Dataset for Training and Local Dataset for Testing			
		Predicted diagnosis	
		Positive	Negative
Actual	Positive	360	8
	Negative	11	306
(d) Fused Dataset for Training and Local Dataset for Testing			
		Predicted diagnosis	
		Positive	Negative
Actual	Positive	366	2
	Negative	5	312

4.4. Comparison to Related Work

Table 9 shows a performance comparison of deep learning studies in binary classification using CXR images. Some studies did not report the accuracy as their datasets were largely imbalanced. Although most related studies reported high accuracy values, a common theme among them is the lack of a significant number of COVID-19 cases for this type of classification model. For example, Narin et al. [25] mention that the excess number of normal images resulted in higher accuracy in all of those models. This is useless considering the fact that very few differences exist among normal images of lungs across different subjects. Similarly, Hemdan et al. [17] stated the limited number of COVID-19 X-ray images as the main problem in their work. Moreover, the dataset that we included in this work contains only one image per subject, unlike other datasets which include more images than subjects. In addition, special consideration was paid to the type of cases included in the dataset, because the effect of COVID-19 on the lungs does not necessarily appear immediately with symptoms and it may take a few days.

The literature on deep learning for medical diagnosis in general and COVID-19 classification in particular is vast and expanding. However, large datasets are required to truly have reliable generalized models. We believe that development of mobile and easy access applications that capture and store data on the fly will enable better data collection and improved deep learning models.

Table 9. Performance comparison of deep learning studies in binary COVID-19 diagnosis (i.e., positive or negative) using CXR images. Some studies did not report the accuracy as their datasets were largely imbalanced. All websites were last accessed on 28 May 2021.

Study	No. of COVID-19 Images and Database	Method	Accuracy
Singh et al. [42]	50, https://github.com/ieee8023/covid-chestxray-dataset	MADE-based CNN	94.7%
Sahinbas et al. [43]	50, https://github.com/ieee8023/covid-chestxray-dataset	VGG16, VGG19, ResNet, DenseNet, InceptionV3	80%
Medhi et al. [44]	150, https://www.kaggle.com/bachrr/covid-chest-xray	Deep CNN	93%
Narin et al. [25]	341, https://github.com/ieee8023/covid-chestxray-dataset	InceptionV3, ResNet50, ResNet101	96.1%
Sethy et al. [19]	48, https://www.kaggle.com/andrewmvd/convid19-X-rays	most available models (e.g., DenseNet, ResNet)	95.3%
Minaee et al. [30]	71, https://github.com/ieee8023/covid-chestxray-dataset	ResNet18, ResNet50, SqueezeNet, DenseNet-121	–
Maguolo et al.[45]	144, https://github.com/ieee8023/covid-chestxray-dataset	AlexNet	–
Hemdan et al. [17]	25, https://github.com/ieee8023/covid-chestxray-dataset	VGG19, ResNet, DenseNet, Inception, Xception	90%
This work	712+368, doi.org/10.21227/x2r3-xk48+local	2D CNN, VGG16, MobileNets	up to 99%

5. Conclusions

Global disasters bring people together and spur innovations. The current pandemic and the worldwide negative consequences should present an opportunity to push forward technological solutions that facilitate everyday life. In this study, we have collected chest X-ray images from hospitalized COVID-19 patients. These data will enrich the current available public datasets and enable further refinements to the systems employing them. Moreover, deep learning artificial intelligence models were designed, trained, and tested using the locally collected dataset as well as public datasets, both separately and combined. The high accuracy results present an opportunity to develop mobile and easy access applications that improve the diagnosis accuracy, reduce the workload on strained health workers, and provide better healthcare access to undermanned/underequipped areas. Future work will focus on this avenue as well as development and evaluation of multiclass classification models.

Author Contributions: Conceptualization, N.K. and M.F.; methodology, N.K. and M.F.; software, N.K. and L.F.; validation, N.K., M.F. and B.K.; formal analysis, M.F. and L.F.; investigation, M.F., B.K. and A.I.; resources, N.K., M.F., A.I. and B.K.; data curation, N.K., M.F., A.I. and B.K.; writing—original draft preparation, N.K., M.F. and L.F.; writing—review and editing, N.K., M.F. and L.F.; funding acquisition, M.F. All authors have read and agreed to the published version of the manuscript.

Funding: This research is supported by the Deanship of Scientific Research at Jordan University of Science and Technology, Jordan, grants no. 20210027 and 20210047. The APC was not funded at the time of submission.

Institutional Review Board Statement: The current study was conducted according to the guidelines of the Declaration of Helsinki and approved by the Institutional Review Board (IRB) at King Abdullah University Hospital, Deanship of Scientific Research at Jordan University of Science and Technology in Jordan (Ref. 91/136/2020).

Informed Consent Statement: Informed consent was obtained from all subjects involved in the study.

Data Availability Statement: The dataset generated and/or analyzed during the current study is available from the corresponding author on reasonable request. The dataset will be made public in a separate data article.

Conflicts of Interest: The authors declare no conflict of interest.

Abbreviations

The following abbreviations are used in this manuscript:

AI	artificial intelligence
COVID-19	coronavirus disease 2019
CT	computerized tomography
CXR	chest X-rays
KAUH	King Abdullah University Hospital
RT-PCR	real-time reverse transcription polymerase chain reaction
SARS	severe acute respiratory syndrome

References

1. Huang, C.; Wang, Y.; Li, X.; Ren, L.; Zhao, J.; Hu, Y.; Zhang, L.; Fan, G.; Xu, J.; Gu, X.; et al. Clinical features of patients infected with 2019 novel coronavirus in Wuhan, China. *Lancet* **2020**, *395*, 497–506. [CrossRef]
2. CDC. Symptoms of COVID-19. 2021. Available online: https://www.cdc.gov/coronavirus/2019-ncov/symptoms-testing/symptoms.html (accessed on 25 May 2021).
3. Axell-House, D.B.; Lavingia, R.; Rafferty, M.; Clark, E.; Amirian, E.S.; Chiao, E.Y. The estimation of diagnostic accuracy of tests for COVID-19: A scoping review. *J. Infect.* **2020**, *81*, 681–697. [CrossRef]
4. Zu, Z.Y.; Jiang, M.D.; Xu, P.P.; Chen, W.; Ni, Q.Q.; Lu, G.M.; Zhang, L.J. Coronavirus Disease 2019 (COVID-19): A Perspective from China. *Radiology* **2020**, *296*, E15–E25. [CrossRef]
5. WHO. Medical Doctors (per 10 000 Population). 2021. Available online: https://www.who.int/data/gho/data/indicators/indicator-details/GHO/medical-doctors-(per-10-000-population) (accessed on 28 May 2021).
6. Khamis, A.; Meng, J.; Wang, J.; Azar, A.T.; Prestes, E.; Li, H.; Hameed, I.A.; Takács, Á.; Rudas, I.J.; Haidegger, T. Robotics and Intelligent Systems Against a Pandemic. *Acta Polytech. Hung.* **2021**, *18*, 13–35. [CrossRef]
7. Howard, A.G.; Zhu, M.; Chen, B.; Kalenichenko, D.; Wang, W.; Weyand, T.; Andreetto, M.; Adam, H. MobileNets: Efficient Convolutional Neural Networks for Mobile Vision Applications. *arXiv* **2017**, arXiv:1704.04861.
8. Simonyan, K.; Zisserman, A. Very Deep Convolutional Networks for Large-Scale Image Recognition. In Proceedings of the 3rd International Conference on Learning Representations, ICLR 2015, San Diego, CA, USA, 7–9 May 2015.
9. Samrah, S.M.; Al-Mistarehi, A.H.W.; Ibnian, A.M.; Raffee, L.A.; Momany, S.M.; Al-Ali, M.; Hayajneh, W.A.; Yusef, D.H.; Awad, S.M.; Khassawneh, B.Y. COVID-19 outbreak in Jordan: Epidemiological features, clinical characteristics, and laboratory findings. *Ann. Med. Surg.* **2020**, *57*, 103–108. [CrossRef] [PubMed]
10. Cozzi, D.; Albanesi, M.; Cavigli, E.; Moroni, C.; Bindi, A.; Luvarà, S.; Lucarini, S.; Busoni, S.; Mazzoni, L.N.; Miele, V. Chest X-ray in new Coronavirus Disease 2019 (COVID-19) infection: findings and correlation with clinical outcome. *La Radiol. Med.* **2020**, *125*, 730–737. [CrossRef] [PubMed]
11. AI Vetology. AI Vetology. 2021. Available online: https://vetology.ai/ (accessed on 25 May 2021).
12. Greenfield, D. Artificial Intelligence in Medicine: Applications, Implications, and Limitations. 2019. Available online: https://sitn.hms.harvard.edu/flash/2019/artificial-intelligence-in-medicine-applications-implications-and-limitations/ (accessed on 25 May 2021).
13. Amisha.; Malik, P.; Pathania, M.; Rathaur, V. Overview of artificial intelligence in medicine. *J. Fam. Med. Prim. Care* **2019**, *8*, 2328. [CrossRef]
14. Faust, O.; Hagiwara, Y.; Hong, T.J.; Lih, O.S.; Acharya, U.R. Deep learning for healthcare applications based on physiological signals: A review. *Comput. Methods Programs Biomed.* **2018**, *161*, 1–13. [CrossRef]
15. Islam, M.M.; Karray, F.; Alhajj, R.; Zeng, J. A Review on Deep Learning Techniques for the Diagnosis of Novel Coronavirus (COVID-19). *IEEE Access* **2021**, *9*, 30551–30572. [CrossRef]
16. Shi, F.; Wang, J.; Shi, J.; Wu, Z.; Wang, Q.; Tang, Z.; He, K.; Shi, Y.; Shen, D. Review of Artificial Intelligence Techniques in Imaging Data Acquisition, Segmentation, and Diagnosis for COVID-19. *IEEE Rev. Biomed. Eng.* **2021**, *14*, 4–15. [CrossRef] [PubMed]
17. Hemdan, E.E.D.; Shouman, M.A.; Karar, M.E. COVIDX-Net: A Framework of Deep Learning Classifiers to Diagnose COVID-19 in X-Ray Images. *arXiv* **2020**, arXiv:eess.IV/2003.11055.
18. Khan, A.; Sohail, A.; Zahoora, U.; Qureshi, A.S. A survey of the recent architectures of deep convolutional neural networks. *Artif. Intell. Rev.* **2020**, *53*, 5455–5516. [CrossRef]
19. Sethy, P.K.; Behera, S.K.; Ratha, P.K.; Biswas, P. Detection of coronavirus Disease (COVID-19) based on Deep Features and Support Vector Machine. *Int. J. Math. Eng. Manag. Sci.* **2020**, *5*, 643–651. [CrossRef]
20. Khan, A.I.; Shah, J.L.; Bhat, M.M. CoroNet: A deep neural network for detection and diagnosis of COVID-19 from chest x-ray images. *Comput. Methods Programs Biomed.* **2020**, *196*, 105581. [CrossRef] [PubMed]
21. Rajaraman, S.; Siegelman, J.; Alderson, P.O.; Folio, L.S.; Folio, L.R.; Antani, S.K. Iteratively Pruned Deep Learning Ensembles for COVID-19 Detection in Chest X-Rays. *IEEE Access* **2020**, *8*, 115041–115050. [CrossRef]
22. Chowdhury, M.E.H.; Rahman, T.; Khandakar, A.; Mazhar, R.; Kadir, M.A.; Mahbub, Z.B.; Islam, K.R.; Khan, M.S.; Iqbal, A.; Emadi, N.A.; et al. Can AI Help in Screening Viral and COVID-19 Pneumonia? *IEEE Access* **2020**, *8*, 132665–132676. [CrossRef]
23. Ucar, F.; Korkmaz, D. COVIDiagnosis-Net: Deep Bayes-SqueezeNet based diagnosis of the coronavirus disease 2019 (COVID-19) from X-ray images. *Med. Hypotheses* **2020**, *140*, 109761. [CrossRef]
24. Rahimzadeh, M.; Attar, A. A modified deep convolutional neural network for detecting COVID-19 and pneumonia from chest X-ray images based on the concatenation of Xception and ResNet50V2. *Inform. Med. Unlocked* **2020**, *19*, 100360. [CrossRef]
25. Narin, A.; Kaya, C.; Pamuk, Z. Automatic detection of coronavirus disease (COVID-19) using X-ray images and deep convolutional neural networks. *Pattern Anal. Appl.* **2021**, *24*, 1207–1220. [CrossRef]
26. Khobahi, S.; Agarwal, C.; Soltanalian, M. CoroNet: A Deep Network Architecture for Semi-Supervised Task-Based Identification of COVID-19 from Chest X-ray Images. Available online: https://www.medrxiv.org/content/early/2020/04/17/2020.04.14.20065722 (accessed on 25 May 2021).
27. Wang, L.; Lin, Z.Q.; Wong, A. COVID-Net: A tailored deep convolutional neural network design for detection of COVID-19 cases from chest X-ray images. *Sci. Rep.* **2020**, *10*, 19549. [CrossRef]

28. Afshar, P.; Heidarian, S.; Naderkhani, F.; Oikonomou, A.; Plataniotis, K.N.; Mohammadi, A. COVID-CAPS: A capsule network-based framework for identification of COVID-19 cases from X-ray images. *Pattern Recognit. Lett.* **2020**, *138*, 638–643. [CrossRef]
29. Abbas, A.; Abdelsamea, M.M.; Gaber, M.M. Classification of COVID-19 in chest X-ray images using DeTraC deep convolutional neural network. *Appl. Intell.* **2020**, *51*, 854–864. [CrossRef]
30. Minaee, S.; Kafieh, R.; Sonka, M.; Yazdani, S.; Soufi, G.J. Deep-COVID: Predicting COVID-19 from chest X-ray images using deep transfer learning. *Med. Image Anal.* **2020**, *65*, 101794. [CrossRef]
31. Punn, N.S.; Agarwal, S. COVID-19 Posteroanterior Chest X-Ray Fused (CPCXR) Dataset. Available online: https://ieee-dataport.org/documents/covid-19-posteroanterior-chest-x-ray-fused-cpcxr-dataset (accessed on 25 May 2021).
32. Cohen, J. COVID-19 Chest X-ray Dataset. Available online: https://github.com/ieee8023/covid-chestxray-dataset (accessed on 25 May 2021).
33. Radiological Society of North America. RSNA Pneumonia Detection Challenge. Available online: https://www.kaggle.com/c/rsna-pneumonia-detection-challenge (accessed on 25 May 2021).
34. Antani, S. Tuberculosis Chest X-ray Image Data Sets. - LHNCBC Abstract. Available online: https://lhncbc.nlm.nih.gov/LHC-publications/pubs/TuberculosisChestXrayImageDataSets.html (accessed on 25 May 2021).
35. Punn, N.S.; Agarwal, S. Automated diagnosis of COVID-19 with limited posteroanterior chest X-ray images using fine-tuned deep neural networks. *Appl. Intel.* **2020**, *51*, 2689–2702. [CrossRef]
36. Scherer, D.; Müller, A.; Behnke, S. Evaluation of Pooling Operations in Convolutional Architectures for Object Recognition. In *Artificial Neural Networks–ICANN 2010*; Springer: Berlin/Heidelberg, Germany, 2010; pp. 92–101._10. [CrossRef]
37. Ranzato, M.; Huang, F.J.; Boureau, Y.L.; LeCun, Y. Unsupervised Learning ofw Invariant Feature Hierarchies with Applications to Object Recognition. In Proceedings of the 2007 IEEE Conference on Computer Vision and Pattern Recognition, Minneapolis, MN, USA, 17–22 June 2007; pp. 1–8. [CrossRef]
38. Nwankpa, C.; Ijomah, W.; Gachagan, A.; Marshall, S. Activation Functions: Comparison of trends in Practice and Research for Deep Learning. *arXiv* **2018**, arXiv:1811.03378.
39. Keras. Keras Documentation: About Keras. Available online: https://keras.io/ (accessed on 25 May 2021).
40. TensorFlow. Available online: https://www.tensorflow.org/ (accessed on 25 May 2021).
41. Brutzkus, A.; Globerson, A. Why do Larger Models Generalize Better? A Theoretical Perspective via the XOR Problem. In Proceedings of the 36th International Conference on Machine Learning(ICML), Long Beach, CA, USA, 9–15 June 2019.
42. Singh, D.; Kumar, V.; Yadav, V.; Kaur, M. Deep Neural Network-Based Screening Model for COVID-19-Infected Patients Using Chest X-Ray Images. *Int. J. Pattern Recognit. Artif. Intell.* **2020**, *35*, 2151004. [CrossRef]
43. Sahinbas, K.; Catak, F.O. Transfer learning-based convolutional neural network for COVID-19 detection with X-ray images. In *Data Science for COVID-19*; Elsevier: Amsterdam, The Netherlands, 2021; pp. 451–466.
44. Medhi K.; Jamil, M.; Hussain, I. Automatic Detection of COVID-19 Infection from Chest X-ray Using Deep Learning. Available online: https://www.medrxiv.org/content/10.1101/2020.05.10.20097063v1 (accessed on 25 May 2021).
45. Maguolo, G.; Nanni, L. A Critic Evaluation of Methods for COVID-19 Automatic Detection from X-ray Images. *arXiv* **2020**, arXiv:eess.IV/2004.12823.

sensors

MDPI

Article

Portable Ultrasound Research System for Use in Automated Bladder Monitoring with Machine-Learning-Based Segmentation

Marc Fournelle [1,*], Tobias Grün [1], Daniel Speicher [1], Steffen Weber [1], Mehmet Yilmaz [2], Dominik Schoeb [2], Arkadiusz Miernik [2], Gerd Reis [3], Steffen Tretbar [1] and Holger Hewener [1]

1 Department of Ultrasound, Fraunhofer Institute for Biomedical Engineering, 66280 Sulzbach, Germany; tobias.gruen@ibmt.fraunhofer.de (T.G.); daniel.speicher@ibmt.fraunhofer.de (D.S.); steffen.weber@ibmt.fraunhofer.de (S.W.); steffen.tretbar@ibmt.fraunhofer.de (S.T.); holger.hewener@ibmt.fraunhofer.de (H.H.)
2 Department of Urology, Faculty of Medicine, Universitätsklinikum Freiburg University of Freiburg, Hugstetter Str. 55, 79106 Freiburg, Germany; mehmet.yilmaz@uniklinik-freiburg.de (M.Y.); dominik.stefan.schoeb@uniklinik-freiburg.de (D.S.); arkadiusz.miernik@uniklinik-freiburg.de (A.M.)
3 DFKI—German Research Center for Artificial Intelligence, Trippstadter Straße 122, 67663 Kaiserslautern, Germany; reis@dfki.de
* Correspondence: marc.fournelle@ibmt.fraunhofer.de

Abstract: We developed a new mobile ultrasound device for long-term and automated bladder monitoring without user interaction consisting of 32 transmit and receive electronics as well as a 32-element phased array 3 MHz transducer. The device architecture is based on data digitization and rapid transfer to a consumer electronics device (e.g., a tablet) for signal reconstruction (e.g., by means of plane wave compounding algorithms) and further image processing. All reconstruction algorithms are implemented in the GPU, allowing real-time reconstruction and imaging. The system and the beamforming algorithms were evaluated with respect to the imaging performance on standard sonographical phantoms (CIRS multipurpose ultrasound phantom) by analyzing the resolution, the SNR and the CNR. Furthermore, ML-based segmentation algorithms were developed and assessed with respect to their ability to reliably segment human bladders with different filling levels. A corresponding CNN was trained with 253 B-mode data sets and 20 B-mode images were evaluated. The quantitative and qualitative results of the bladder segmentation are presented and compared to the ground truth obtained by manual segmentation.

Keywords: POCUS; multichannel system; channel data; bladder monitoring; POUR; machine-learning; segmentation

Citation: Fournelle, M.; Grün, T.; Speicher, D.; Weber, S.; Yilmaz, M.; Schoeb, D.; Miernik, A.; Reis, G.; Tretbar, S.; Hewener, H. Portable Ultrasound Research System for Use in Automated Bladder Monitoring with Machine-Learning-Based Segmentation. *Sensors* **2021**, *21*, 6481. https://doi.org/10.3390/s21196481

Academic Editors: Ayman El-baz, Guruprasad A. Giridharan, Ahmed Shalaby, Ali H. Mahmoud and Mohammed Ghazal

Received: 24 June 2021
Accepted: 23 September 2021
Published: 28 September 2021

1. Introduction

Ultrasound imaging is a frequently used method for postoperative monitoring of the urinary bladder. Depending on the surgical context, different clinical conditions that need close monitoring can occur. Post-operative urinary retention (POUR) is a frequent problem for various reasons (e.g., intravesical blood clotting) that can lead to bladder overdistension and needs rapid detection and medical intervention. On the other hand, invasive procedures such as catheterization present significant discomfort for patients and can lead to infections or even trauma of the urinary tract. In contrast, ultrasound imaging is fully non-invasive and has already shown its potential for bladder monitoring [1–3]. Accurate bladder volumes can be extracted from 3D ultrasound data; however, reliable qualitative information about potential bladder overdistension can already be derived from 2D B-mode (brightness mode) ultrasound images.

In order to efficiently prevent POUR and directly initiate therapeutic measures if an increased amount of urine or blood is detected in the urinary bladder, the bladder should be monitored at frequent intervals, which is not possible in a clinical environment where ultrasound investigations are mostly performed using standard sonography equipment based on hand-held probes. Accordingly, when defining a tool for ideal postoperative follow-up and the prevention of related complications in the 24–48 h period after surgery, different challenges and requirements arise. First, the system must be portable, such that the mobility of the patient is ensured. Second, the probe must be self-adhesive or pad-like (in contrast to hand-held probes that require the presence of a sonographer). Third, (image or signal) data must be automatically analyzed to retrieve diagnostic features that are relevant for the identification of a potential complication (e.g., a bladder volume above a defined threshold in the context of POUR monitoring or specific scattering properties as a result of blood clots in the bladder). In a research context, where the optimal signal and image processing still needs to be defined, this results in a need for RF or even better pre-beamformed channel data access. In particular, the third requirement allows the use of analysis methods beyond pure image-based segmentation and classification. We recently showed in other applications that machine learning approaches can be applied to raw radio-frequent ultrasound data prior to image formation for classification tasks with a high accuracy [4]. Radio-frequent data with a high dynamic range (16-bit amplitude quantization) and ultrasonic wave phase information at high digitalization rates of up to 50 MHz contain a lot more informational content than scan-converted ultrasound images. During scan conversion, typically more than 90% of the raw ultrasound wave information is lost during image formation and cannot be used in image-based processing.

To the best of our knowledge, there are no systems available that fulfil the above defined requirements. The use of advanced classification approaches is not possible with classical clinical sonography systems, as they do not provide access to radio frequent ultrasound data. Ultrasound systems for research applications such as the Vantage Ultrasound System (Verasonics, Inc. Redmond, WA, USA), the ULA-OP [5], the systems from the Technical University of Denmark [6] or the DiPhAS by Fraunhofer IBMT (Sulzbach, Germany) [7] provide access to this type of data, but are mostly not certified for clinical use, and more importantly, they are complex, bulky and costly devices. The latest generation of point of care ultrasound (POCUS) devices, such as the Butterfly iQ or Vscan [8] by GE has decreased the costs by an order of magnitude when compared to high-end sonography machines, and can be used in bedside settings due to their miniaturization. However, the availability of care staff still represents a limiting factor when it comes to frequent monitoring postoperatively. Finally, dedicated devices for bladder monitoring such as DFree (Triple W, Tokyo, Japan) or SENS-U [9] (Novioscan, Nijmegen, The Netherlands) have a particular focus on incontinence management. These systems directly generate bladder filling level-related parameters and do not provide access to the underlying ultrasound signals. Other ultrasound systems optimized for urological applications such as BladderScan (Verathon, WA, USA) measure the bladder volume, but are based on hand-held probes, which limits their suitability for continuous monitoring.

In summary, all these devices optimized for the daily clinical routine (or for home-care settings in the case of DFree or SENS-U) are difficult to utilize in research applications, where customized signal and image processing algorithms need to be applied to the data. In particular, machine-learning based approaches have been shown to have tremendous potential for automated segmentation of ultrasound data [10], and have been reported in particular for breast imaging [11], coronary arteries [12], and thyroid [13] or different tumors [14]. In comparison to these applications, where the anatomy is more complex and the contrast difference is reduced, bladder segmentation represents an ideal use case for ML-based approaches due to the low echogenity and the resulting high contrast to surrounding tissue. Multiple ultrasound imaging devices, including mobile ones like Butterfly iQ+ (Butterfly Network Inc, Guilford, CT, USA), already include automated bladder segmentation and volume estimation, but the shape of the hand-held transducer does not allow long-time monitoring as a wearable.

In light of the somewhat contrary requirements of an ideal urinary bladder monitoring system that also provides full data access, and thereby can be flexibly used in research applications, we developed a new portable ultrasound system (mobile ultrasound equipment—MoUsE). Despite being validated in this first application in the context of bladder monitoring, the MoUsE can also be used as a general-purpose ultrasound research system since full access to the transmit and receive pipeline is provided.

2. Materials and Methods

2.1. Portable Multichannel Electronics with Research Interface

The MoUsE is a compact ultrasound system integrated into a 3D printed housing (Figure 1) with dimensions of 184 mm × 123 mm × 33 mm and a total weight of 610 g, thus ensuring its portability. It is driven by a 12V medical power supply which can be replaced by lithium-ion battery packs for future fully mobile applications. Detailed specifications are given in Table 1. All system functionalities, including generation of transmit signals, amplification and digitization of receive signals, storage and communication (via USB 3.0) to a PC/tablet controlling the device are implemented on the same main printed circuit board (PCB). Data management, communication and sequence control are handled in the integrated ZYNQ-7 FPGA. An on-board low voltage (LV) power supply generates the required power levels for the logic components.

Table 1. MoUsE system performance and features.

Dimensions	184 mm × 123 mm × 33 mm
Weight	610 g
Power consumption	12 W
Power supply	12 V DC, medical certified power supply, lithium-ion battery packs for future fully mobile applications
Transmitter	32 channels, Tri-state pulser, max voltage ± 100 V
Receiver	32 channels Bandwidth: 100 kHz–10 MHz Gain: up to 44.3 dB Up to 50 MHz sampling rate with a resolution of 12 Bit per sample
Interface	USB 3.0
RAM	8 GBit internal RAM
Imaging	Plane wave compounding, custom algorithms can be implemented
Software	Clinical type user interface USPilot, SDK for programming system from 3rd party applications in C#/C++/Matlab
Transducer specifications	32 elements Pitch = 500 µm Centre F\frequency = 3 MHz

A compact high voltage (HV) power supply that generates the ± 100 V of transmit voltage for each of the octal (8-channel) transmit receive ICs was implemented on a second PCB mounted on the main PCB. A frequency range of 100 kHz–10 MHz was defined as the transmit bandwidth.

In principle, transmit signals can be freely defined within the limits of the tri-state programmable ICs, for instance, using pulse width modulation (PWM); however, only rectangular bursts with adjustable length and frequency have been implemented in the software so far. The internal system clock of 160 MHz is used for the definition of the transmit signals. Receive signals are digitized with up to 50 MSa/s with a resolution of 12 bit and are transferred as pre-beamformed channel data via USB 3.0 to a PC/tablet for image reconstruction. The receive data can be amplified by up to 44.3 dB with different linear or customized TGC settings. No analog preprocessing is performed on-board beyond bandpass filtering and (optional) data accumulation (corresponding to averaging) for improvement of the signal to noise ratio (SNR). Interfaces for wireless (IEEE 802.11 b/g/n (1 × 1)) communication and the transfer of pre-beamformed channel data are foreseen in the hardware design but not yet implemented. The system uses a sleep mode to switch off the transceiver ICs for stand-by between long-term measurements to reduce power consumption.

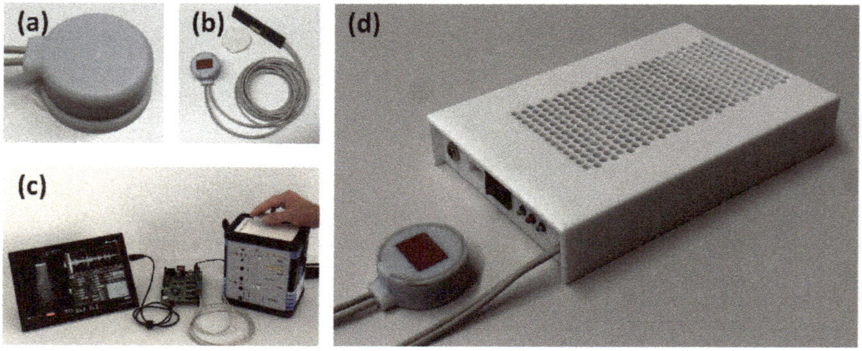

Figure 1. MoUsE system overview with close up of 32 element transducer housing (**a**), transducer with cable, custom connector PCB and disposable patch (**b**), MoUsE PCB tested on phantoms prior to integration (**c**), and the final system integrated with passive cooling in a 3D printed housing (**d**).

2.2. Transducer Design and Manufacturing

The MoUsE can be driven with all kinds of 32-element transducers using the given pinout or via transducer connection adapter. However, in the context of the first application being used for automated bladder monitoring, a 32-element phased array transducer was developed. The transducer properties were defined in a sound field simulation study using the in-house developed sound field simulation software tool SCALP based on point source synthesis (Figure 2). A pitch of 500 µm with a kerf of 50 µm and element sub-dicing were chosen as a compromise between sensitivity (profiting from larger element size) and beam steering capabilities (decreasing with larger element size). To improve the elevational resolution, a focusing silicon lens was applied to the element of elevational size of 11.5 mm. The array was manufactured from a soft PZT material (3203 HD), the center frequency was adjusted to 3 MHz and two matching layers were applied for improved bandwidth. Connection to the MoUsE electronics was achieved by two 16-core micro-coax cables directly soldered to the customized connector PCB, which was preferred over a solution involving a commercial connector for the sake of compactness. The acoustic block was finally integrated into a 3D printed cylindrical housing of 40 mm in diameter and a height of 17.5 mm. For long-term monitoring applications, a fixation concept involving an acoustically transparent adhesive tape could optionally be used.

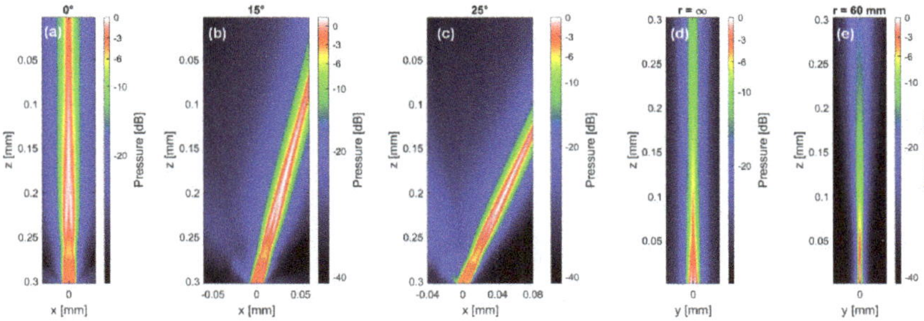

Figure 2. Acoustic pressure distribution simulation performed during specification phase of the MoUsE transducer. (**a**–**c**) Plane wave transmission under different angles to investigate the steering capabilities and the identify potential grating lobes, (**d**,**e**) single element elevational sound field without focusing (**d**) and with lens focusing to 60 mm (**e**).

2.3. Beamforming and Software

Image reconstruction is performed in real-time using a GPU (OpenCL, Khronos Group, Beaverton, OR, USA)-based implementation of plane wave compounding [15] approach in the in-house developed clinical style user interface USPilot (Figure 3). Other reconstruction methods can easily be implemented via an SDK. The number of plane wave angles, as well as the increment can be freely selected by the user. Other transmit parameters such as the frequency, the burst count or the voltage can be adjusted as well. On the receive side, the data sampling rate, averaging factor and TGC can be selected.

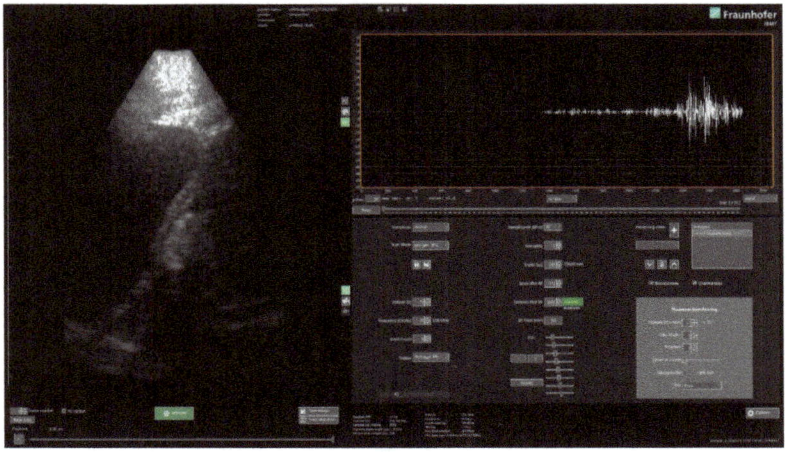

Figure 3. Clinical style user interface USPilot.

The reconstruction can be adjusted in terms of the size and resolution of the reconstruction grid (lateral and axial pixel/sample count), the speed of sound and apodization. Furthermore, customized algorithms (e.g., bandpass filtering or alternative beamforming approaches) can be inserted into the (real-time) reconstruction pipeline. The software allows the visualization of reconstructed (compounded) B-scan images as well as the pre-beamformed channel data (in time or frequency) domain, which makes it ideal not only for clinical research, but also for educational purposes or research on reconstruction algorithms. In addition to controlling the system via the USPilot, an open programming interface (C#/C++/Matlab with SDK) is made available, which provides access to the same transmit, receive and beamforming parameters as in the case of the UI. A custom but open binary data format (*.orb) is chosen for storage of the pre-beamformed and reconstructed ultrasound data. Meta-data such as transmit and receive parameters are stored with the actual ultrasound data by default and import tools for Matlab/Python/C/C++ are made available.

2.4. ML-Based Segmentation Algorithm

We trained a neural network to segment the bladder into abdominal ultrasound images and encountered two main challenges when implementing the network. On the one hand, the limited space and computational resources available at inference time and on the other hand, the quality of abdominal ultrasound images can be very challenging. Figure 4 shows an example: in the left sub-figure, a (partially filled) bladder appears mainly as a dark region in the image since little sound is reflected by the fluid. In addition, the bladder is only partially imaged and merges seamlessly into the black area outside the ultrasound fan. This situation is usually the case in corpulent patients. As can be seen in the upper part of the segment, weak echoes might occur in cases where the side lobes of the ultrasound beam intersect with the bladder tissue. A very different situation is shown in the middle sub-figure. Here, the (almost empty) bladder is located in the middle of the ultrasound fan. Lastly, the right sub-figure depicts a situation where other anatomical structures, e.g., the pubic bone or the colon, generate a large dark region that might fuse with the bladder. Please note that the appearance of different anatomical parts can be very similar in the images.

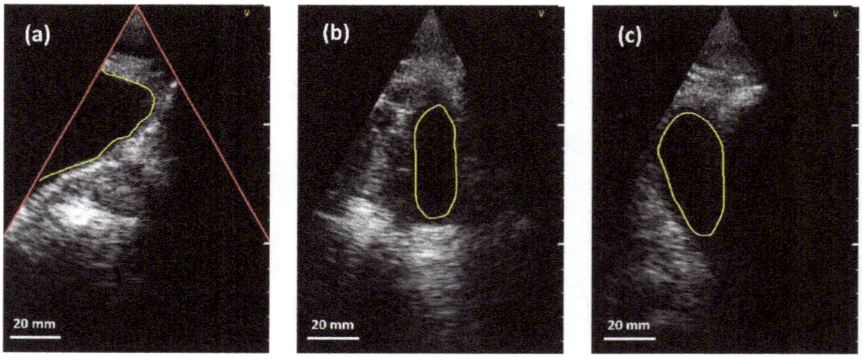

Figure 4. Examples of bladder segmentation (yellow). Red lines in the left sub-image indicate the borders of the ultrasound fan above which there is no valid information. (**a**) Partially visible bladder. (**b**) Almost empty bladder near the center of the US-fan. (**c**) Additional dark regions due to pubic bone shadow or colon.

We started development using a Mask-R-CNN architecture [16,17] to segment the bladder. However, we found that the model size of approximately 0.5 GByte was way too large for the intended purpose. A second drawback was that the network tended to overfit to the data, since only very few images (253) were available for training. We therefore decided to use a U-Net architecture [18] in a minimal configuration. We set the network up to compute a 2-class segmentation (bladder, non-bladder). The original ultrasound images (1056×720) were down-sampled to a resolution of 528×352 and reduced to a single color channel. In total, we acquired 253 data sets (each consisting of one B-mode image), which were acquired from 20 human volunteers as training data for the CNN. For both the contracting and expanding paths, we used 5 successive blocks. We started with 6 channels for the first layer and doubled the channel number with each successive layer, resulting in a total of 96 channels at the bottleneck. For expansion we used up-sampling followed by convolution. Training was performed using a batch size of 4 with a learning rate of 0.00002. Using these parameters, the network converged within 400 epochs. The resulting network was less prone to overfitting than the original attempt. We found however that the amount of data was still too low. More importantly, we found that the network had issues in detecting the virtual border of a scan in the image. In particular, if the ultrasound response for a partially imaged bladder was very weak, the resulting segment often extended into the illegal region of the image, i.e., outside the ultrasound fan. Additionally, we often found cases where other dark regions were segmented as bladder.

To this end, we extended the dataset by re-sampling the images so that one of the fan sides coincided with one of the image borders. Furthermore, we flipped images and ground truth on the vertical as well as the horizontal axis. This way we increased the number of images by a factor of 20. Training the network using the augmented data effectively prevented overfitting. Furthermore, and probably much more importantly, the network learned how artifacts and the bladder differ.

For the trained network, we computed an IoU above 0.75 but below 0.9 for all images. We checked segmentations and ground truth and found, interestingly, that the computed segmentations were consistently tighter (smaller) than the ground truth provided by medical experts. The ground truth segmentation was performed by one experienced urologist using the VIA annotation tool [19]. A second experienced urologist performed the validation of the ground truth. Consulting with the experts revealed that the network only segmented the interior of the bladder while the experts partially included the bladder tissue. This unintended result proved to be beneficial for the application at hand. Since we want to estimate the bladder volume, including the tissue would lead to a systematic error that, in particular, depends on the volume itself.

We are working on a further reduction in the network size. The original network size was 340 MBytes. We were able to reduce its size with various pruning strategies [20] to under 300 MBytes without significantly sacrificing the quality of the results. This size is still too large to be run efficiently on a mobile device. Additionally, the inference times need to be decreased significantly. Currently, the network does inference on the target device at approximately 6.4 s per frame. Although this would be more than sufficient for a regular check of the bladder volume, the system would not be able to perform any other tasks in the meanwhile. In the use-case of regular checks of the bladder volume and content, such an inference frame rate might still be acceptable for long-time monitoring. The integration of such a model in the processing pipeline will be implemented by supporting the ONNX model format with the C# runtime using Microsoft ML.NET in the future.

3. Results

3.1. Characterization of Electronics

The transmit and receive paths of the electronics were characterized with respect to the bandwidth. First, for the assessment of the transmit bandwidth, an 80 mVpp sinus signal of varying frequency from a signal generator was digitized by the electronics and the amplitude of the digitized signal was characterized (Figure 5a). As can be seen, the input bandwidths significantly decrease below 100 kHz and above 10 MHz. Furthermore, we evaluated the signal fidelity by generating rectangular bursts of 3 cycles at different frequencies (Figure 5b,c). The electrical signals were measured on the connector PCB with an oscilloscope and minor overshooting was observed.

3.2. Transducer Characterization

For the assessment of the transducer performance, echo signals from a steel reflector generated by excitation of individual transducer elements with a rectangular burst 1 were evaluated. Figure 6a shows a typical time domain echo signal of one of the transducer elements with the corresponding spectrum in Figure 6b. Each of the signals was analyzed with respect to the maximum signal amplitude in order to compare the transmit-receive sensitivity of the transducer elements. As can be seen in Figure 6c, the element sensitivity is very homogeneous with a relative standard deviation of only 5.6%.

For all elements, the maximum frequency is around 2.3 MHz with a standard deviation of 1% (Figure 6d). The center frequency and the −6 dB bandwidth seem to vary more strongly (Figure 6e,f); however, this is an artifact due to a frequency dip around 3 MHz just below the −6 dB line in the spectrum (red line in Figure 6b). If we neglect this minor dip, the average center frequency of the transducer is 2.9 MHz with a −6 dB bandwidth of approximately 60%.

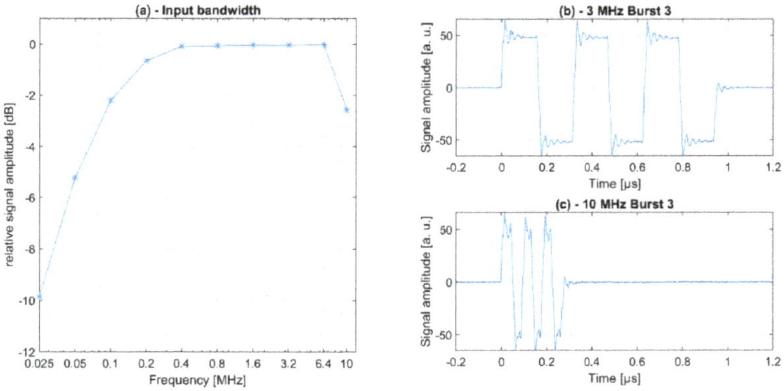

Figure 5. Assessment of MoUsE electronics input bandwidth (**a**) and signal fidelity (**b**,**c**) as a function of frequency.

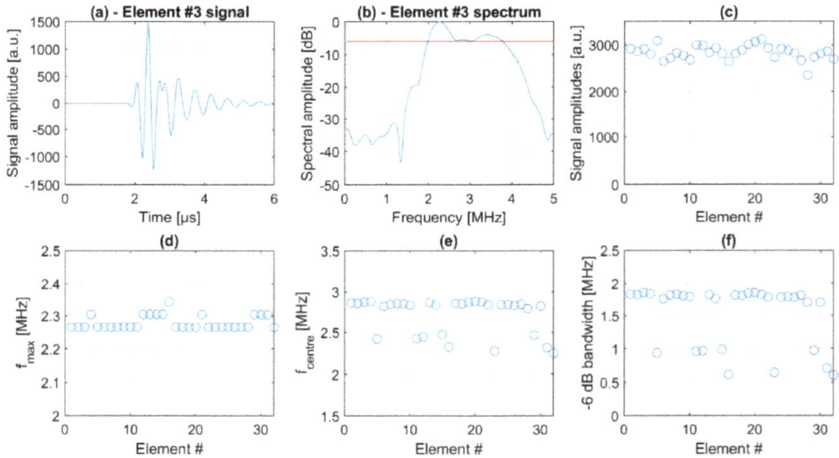

Figure 6. Analysis of transducer performance by charaterization of pulse-echo data from a steel reflector. Single element signals in time (**a**) and frequency (**b**) domain, where the red line depicts the −6 dB threshold. Element sensitivity statistics (**c**), maximum frequency, center frequency and bandwidth statistics (**d**–**f**).

3.3. System Characterization/Standards

In view of using the system on probands in the context of an exploratory clinical study, the system's compliance with respect to medical device standards was verified by certified laboratories. In particular, the acoustic output was characterized according to IEC 60601-2-37, where the maximum pressure, the mechanical and thermal index as well as the intensity were assessed. All parameters remain well below the threshold for diagnostic ultrasound (e.g., MI < 0.5 and I_{SPTA} < 5 mW/cm^2). Furthermore, the electrical safety was tested according to IEC 60601-1 and the electromagnetic compatibility (e.g., immunity and emission) was tested according to IEC 60601-1-2. The system complied with the standards in both tests.

3.4. Imaging Performance

3.4.1. Reconstruction Speed

When considering the achievable reconstruction speed and the system frame rate, the data transfer from the electronics to the PC/tablet, where the GPU-based reconstruction is implemented, represents a bottleneck, rather than the reconstruction itself. With the used setup (Surface Pro 7 with Intel Core i7-7660U, 16GB RAM, Intel Iris Plus Graphic 640, Microsoft, Redmond, WA, USA), up to 300 frames of pre-beamformed channel data could be transferred when a sampling rate of 40 MSa/s and an image depth of 8 cm were chosen. Both parameters have a direct impact on the number of transferred frames per second; however, this is not totally linear due to some communication overhead. Since less time is needed for GPU-reconstruction than for data transfer, plane wave imaging can be performed with 300 frames/s for the above-described parameters with 23 B-scans per second and using compounding with 13 angles.

3.4.2. Resolution

The image resolution was characterized using wires with a diameter of 150 μm in a water tank at different depths. Pre-beamformed channel data were acquired after transmitting 21 plane waves in an angle range of ± 16°. Reconstruction was performed offline in Matlab (The MathWorks, Inc., Natick, MA, USA) with the highest resolution to allow better assessment of the lateral extent of the point spread function (PSF).

The FWHM (Full Width Half Maximum) was characterized as a function of depth (wires in distances between 1 cm and 10 cm from the transducer aperture) and as a function of the number of compounding angles (from 1 to 21). Furthermore, different beamforming approaches were investigated from conventional delay and sum (DAS) to coherence beamforming (COH) [21,22] or non-linear filter approaches based on signal statistics (STD) [23].

The lateral FWHM ranges between 300–800 μm depending on the chosen algorithm for the targets closest to the aperture and between 1300–2800 μm for those that are 10 cm away. In all cases, the STD reconstruction significantly improves the lateral resolution when compared with simple DAS. Furthermore, Figure 7 shows that increasing the number of compounding angles does not always lead to an improved resolution. In fact, depending on the depth, an ideal resolution is achieved with 5–10 compounding angles. This can be explained by trailing wave artifacts, which are not taken into account in the DAS beamforming.

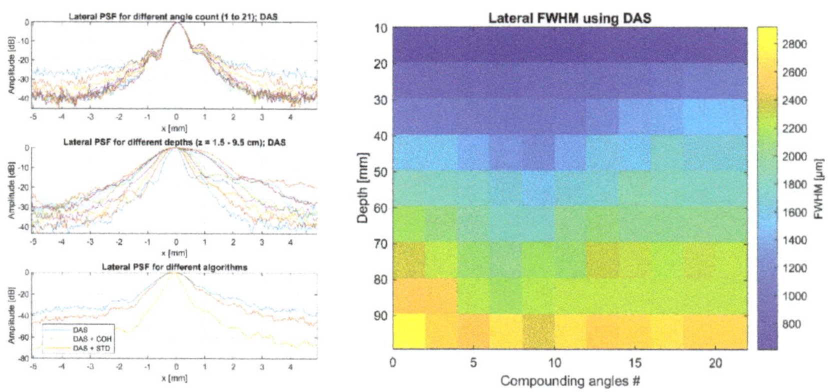

Figure 7. Lateral PSF of the MoUsE system equipped with our 32-element 3 MHz phased array probe. (**Left**) FWHM as a function of plane wave compounding angle count for a constant depth, as a function of depth for constant plane wave compounding angle count and FWHM obtained with different reconstruction approaches. (**Right**) 2D plot of FWHM as a function of angle count and depth for conventional DAS beamforming.

3.4.3. Signal to Noise Ratio

The depth-dependent system's *SNR* was characterized using data from a CIRS multipurpose phantom. One hundred consecutive image acquisitions were performed with the CIRS phantom in the same position and the reconstructed, compounded and enveloped filtered data were analyzed (prior to logarithmic compression). Each depth mean values μ and standard deviation values σ along a central image line in the yellow frame in Figure 8 were used to calculate the depth-dependent *SNR* as suggested in [24].

$$SNR(z) = 20 \cdot log_{10}(\mu(z)/\sigma(z)) \tag{1}$$

To achieve the ideal *SNR*, the data were acquired in a compounding mode with 21 angles in the range of $\pm$ 16°. Conventional delays-and-sum beamforming without additional contrast-enhancing filter was used to reconstruct the data.

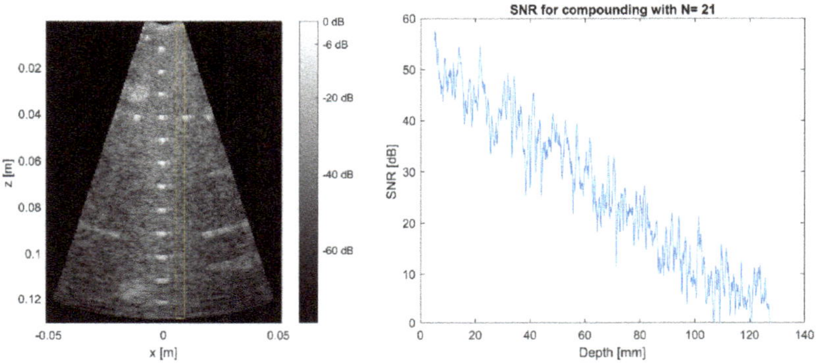

Figure 8. B-mode image acquired with 21 compounding angles used for calculation of the SNR (**left**). Depth-dependent SNR of compounded data (**right**).

3.4.4. Contrast

Assessment of the image contrast was performed by scanning lesions in a standard ultrasound imaging phantom (CIRS multipurpose phantom Model 040GSE, CIRS, Norfolk, VA, USA). The contrast ratio (*CR*) and the contrast to noise ratio (*CNR*) as defined in [25] were taken as metrics for quantification of the image contrast behavior:

$$CR = 20 \cdot log_{10}(\mu_{lesion}/\mu_{bck}) \tag{2}$$

$$CNR = \frac{|\mu_{bck} - \mu_{lesion}|}{\sqrt{\sigma_{bck}{}^2 - \sigma_{lesion}{}^2}} \tag{3}$$

Plane wave compounding data were acquired with a varying number of angles between 1 and 21. The metrics were then assessed as a function of the number of compounding angles. For this purpose, the mean values μ and the standard deviation σ inside defined image regions (red circle: lesion; yellow circle: background in Figure 9a) were calculated.

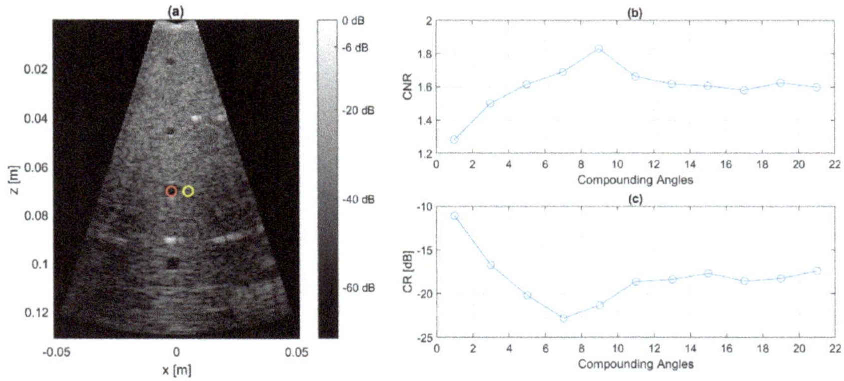

Figure 9. B-mode image of CIRS phantom (**a**) taken for assessment of CNR and CR by analysis of lesion (red ROI) and background (yellow ROI). The x-dimension is in the lateral dimension of the ultrasound array and the z-dimension is in the axial direction (ultrasound propagation direction). CNR and CR (**b**,**c**) are calculated as metrics based on the mean values and standard deviations inside the ROIs.

3.5. Segmentation

To validate the quality of the trained CNN, ultrasound B-mode images from human bladders with different filling levels were acquired from four male volunteers with the MoUsE system. In this first study, 20 data sets (each consisting of one reconstructed B-mode image) were collected. None of these data sets is included in the 253 data sets used for training of the CNN. For image acquisition, an ideal position for the probe on the abdomen was identified based on the real-time feedback of the MoUsE system. Images of the bladder at different filling levels were then acquired with the probe at this position. When it comes to the beamforming approach, plane wave compounding with 21 angles was chosen. Examples of different bladder images can be seen in Figure 10a–d. In a second step, the images were automatically segmented using the above-described CNN. Examples of the segmentation for four different data sets are given in Figure 10e–h, where different situations can be identified. In Figure 10e, the upper part of the bladder, which is closest to the probe, is not identified as part of the bladder by the CNN. This might be due to clutter signals in this part of the image. In Figure 10f, the bladder is correctly segmented; however, an additional surface, which does not correspond to the bladder, was identified as bladder tissue. Figure 10g represents an ideal case with a high correlation between the ground truth and the CNN-segmentation. Finally, Figure 10h shows a case where the bladder was not found by the algorithm due to the really low contrast between the (compressed and almost empty) bladder and the surrounding tissue, as can be seen in Figure 10d. Examples of the ground truth segmentation for the cases presented above are given in Figure 10i–l.

For a qualitative analysis of the segmentation quality, the percentage of the bladder surface that has not been identified as bladder by the CNN was assessed. Furthermore, the image fraction that was falsely identified as bladder tissue by the algorithm was assessed as well. Both parameters are expressed in relation to the bladder surface in the ground truth segmentation. The process of automated analysis is shown in Figure 11. First, the ground truth data were binarized for easy comparison with the CNN-segmentation, which provides binarized data by default. By comparing both images, missing bladder tissue and tissue falsely identified as bladder are identified. Finally, simple pixel counting was used to quantify the missing and false bladder surface. The analysis shows that only a very small tissue fraction (corresponding to 1.4% of the bladder surface) was falsely identified as bladder tissue. On the other side, significant parts of the bladder (median of 33%) were not recognized as such by the algorithm. As can be seen in Figure 10, this is mostly the case where clutter artifacts appear, leading to low contrast between bladder tissue and the background.

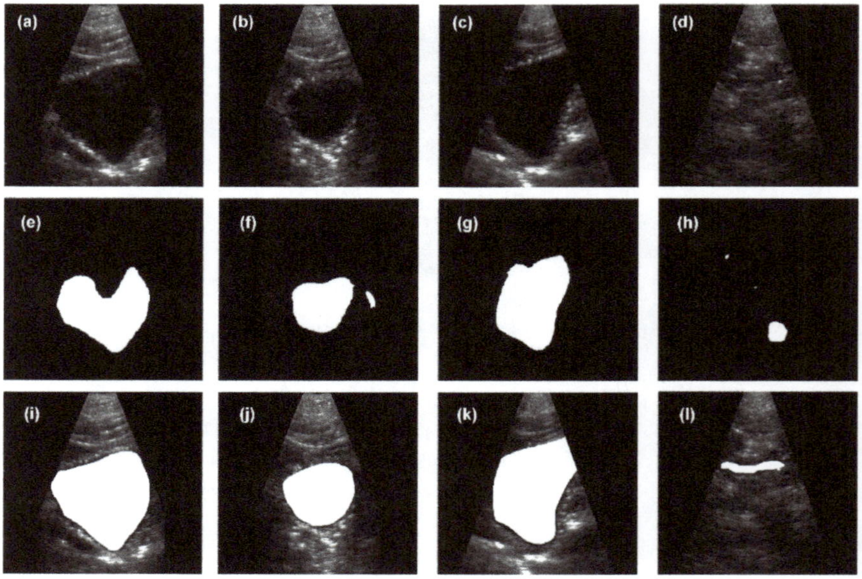

Figure 10. First investigation of the combination of ultrasound B-mode images acquired with the MoUsE system and the described CNN for automated segmentation of human bladder. (**a–d**) Ultrasound B-mode data (plane wave compounding, 21 angles), (**e–h**) segmentation results from the CNN, and (**i–l**) ground truth segmentation (performed manually by an experienced urologist).

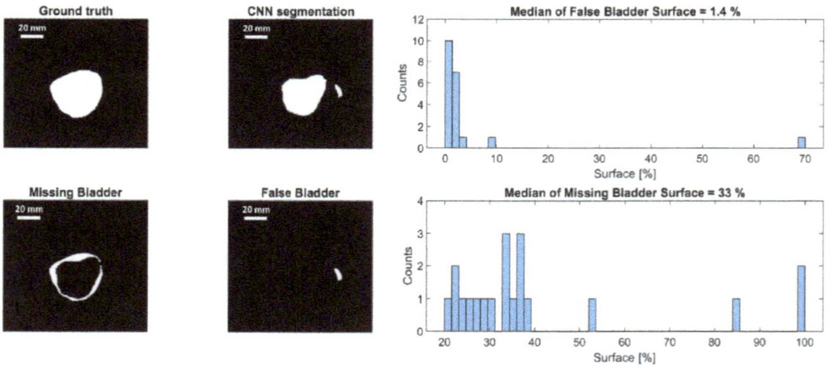

Figure 11. Statistical analysis of the accuracy of bladder segmentation and example of one segmentation highlighting the differences between the expert ground truth and the CNN segmentation. Areas not recognized as bladder by the CNN are marked as "missing bladder", areas erroneously segmented as bladder by the CNN are marked as "false bladder". The relative fractions of "missing" and "false" bladder in the different segmented data sets are shown as histogram in the right column.

4. Discussion

We developed a new portable low-cost ultrasound research system designed for continuous bladder imaging and characterized its (hard- and software) components in first phantom and proband experiments to assess its potential for later use in post-operative bladder monitoring. With dimensions of $18 \times 12 \times 3$ cm^3 and a weight of 610 g, the system is compact enough for applications where portability is required. The ultrasound probe was integrated into compact housing (diameter of 40 mm, height of 17.5 mm) and equipped with a self-adhesive foil, which allows long-term use without manual probe positioning. The system was designed, manufactured, assembled and tested in the ultrasound department of Fraunhofer IBMT. In the design process, the focus was set not only on the performance but also on cost efficiency and limiting the total material cost for the electronics to approximately €1000. The system was designed to be as flexible as possible, and therefore it provides full control to the transmit parameters and full access to the receive data pipeline, where receive and beamforming parameters can be selected and custom filters and reconstruction algorithms can be integrated into the real-time pipeline. Full data access to the receive pipeline and in particular real-time availability of the pre-beamformed channel data (up to 300 frames/s in our study) is not provided by clinical sonography systems and makes the system future-proof for other types of applications such as raw radio-frequent signal processing and ML modeling. On the other hand, most research systems are not certified for medical use. Accordingly, the combination of low-cost and the above-described flexibility makes the MoUsE system an ideal tool for research and educational purposes in ultrasound imaging. In order to ease the transfer of new ultrasound imaging approaches into clinics, the technical prerequisites such as data access must be provided and regulatory constraints must be respected as well. For this reason, we performed various tests according to safety standards for medical devices, such as electrical safety, electromagnetic compatibility and acoustic safety. Compliance to these standards was shown and the corresponding test protocols are available; this is of great value when seeking an ethics clearance for exploratory clinical studies.

In order to cover most of the clinical applications of diagnostic ultrasound, we chose a frequency range of 100 kHz–10 MHz as the target specification and validated the bandwidth in our study. The imaging performance of the MoUsE is mainly dependent on the transducer that is used. Our phased array probe with 32 elements represents a compromise between opening angle and sensitivity. A smaller pitch would have been preferred since a larger opening would have resulted, which is crucial for effective plane wave compounding. On the other hand, given the demonstrated image depth of more than 10 cm in the standard CIRS phantom and more than 15 cm in the human abdomen, imaging of the entire bladder would have been difficult to achieve with a smaller aperture size generating less acoustic energy output. The comparison of the image metrics obtained with different beamforming approaches underlines the potential of software-based reconstruction methods, and thereby, the need to have access to pre-beamformed channel data.

Having high-contrast image data is particularly needed when subsequent image processing steps are performed for automated analysis of the data, such as in our first application of bladder segmentation. We demonstrated the general functionality of our CNN for segmentation in abdominal ultrasound images. However, the analysis showed that a high contrast is crucial to prevent segmentation artifacts. This is underlined by the comparison with earlier work on the use of CNNs for bladder segmentation from ultrasound data [26,27], where a higher correlation between the automatically determined and the manually segmented bladder volumes was obtained. However, it should be mentioned, that the cited work was based on the use of high-end clinical ultrasound devices, which provide higher contrast, and two orthogonal B-mode images were acquired for obtaining quantitative values for the bladder volume [26]. The assessment of the actual bladder volume can hardly be achieved with high accuracy using single cross-sectional B-mode images, and therefore it is beyond the scope of the presented work. However, the impact of the lower SNR when compared to ultrasound data acquired with high-end clinical ultrasound machines needs to be closely investigated, particularly since the bladder cross-sectional surface was systematically underestimated. This was due to clutter signals occurring at the bladder border that were recognized as background tissue by the CNN. On the other hand, background tissue was very reliably identified with very few "false positive" areas (background tissue falsely identified as bladder).

Despite the first proof-of-concept, further investigation is needed to enhance the performance of the overall approach. In particular, the network size needs to be improved in order to allow better use on mobile devices with limited computing capabilities. Since the analysis has shown the importance of SNR for the accurate segmentation and the potential of more sophisticated beamforming approaches for contrast improvement, the optimization of image CR and CNR will be the focus of our future work. Furthermore, we will investigate if training the algorithm with more diverse data (different, and in particular, lower contrast levels) will yield higher accuracy. In summary, in applications such as the monitoring of POUR, where a significant or even dramatic and thereby potentially harmful increase in bladder volume can occur, the proposed approach provides sufficient sensitivity. However, for applications where a precise quantitative assessment of the bladder volume is needed, further enhancement of the performance is needed and will be investigated using refined beamforming approaches and improved training of the CNN.

Finally, beyond this first study on bladder monitoring, we will seek to use MoUsE and its unique combination of device mobility, flexibility and data access in other medical ultrasound applications. Although the number of transmit/receive channels is currently limited to 32, a synchronization scheme that combines several MoUsE systems for a higher total channel count is currently under development. A wireless interface is already available on the hardware, but is not implemented in software, which is also a work in progress and would allow easier use in future mobile ultrasound applications. A battery-powered version of MoUsE is in development as well. The possibility of transferring existing classification tasks using machine learning on radio-frequent data in addition to the image-based approach will also be investigated.

Author Contributions: Conceptualization, M.F., T.G., D.S. (Daniel Speicher), G.R., S.T. and H.H.; methodology, M.F., H.H. and G.R.; software, H.H. and S.W.; validation, M.F., T.G., D.S. (Daniel Speicher), A.M., M.Y. and D.S. (Dominik Schoeb); formal analysis, M.F. and A.M.; investigation, M.F., A.M. and G.R.; resources, M.F. and S.T.; data curation, M.F., A.M. and H.H.; writing—original draft preparation, M.F., H.H. and G.R.; writing—review and editing, M.F., H.H.; visualization, M.F., H.H., G.R. and S.W.; supervision, M.F. and H.H.; project administration, M.F.; funding acquisition, M.F., A.M. and G.R. All authors have read and agreed to the published version of the manuscript.

Funding: This research was funded by the German Federal Ministry for Education and Research BMBF under the project VISIMON (grant number 16SV7861K).

Institutional Review Board Statement: The study was conducted according to the guidelines of the Declaration of Helsinki, and approved by the Institutional Review Board (or Ethics Committee) of Albert-Ludwigs-Universität Freiburg (Antrag 9/18 EK-Freiburg, 7 July 2018).

Informed Consent Statement: Informed consent was obtained from all subjects involved in the study.

Conflicts of Interest: The authors declare no conflict of interest. The funders had no role in the design of the study; in the collection, analyses, or interpretation of data; in the writing of the manuscript, or in the decision to publish the results.

References

1. Brouwe, T.A.; van den Boogaard, C.; van Roon, E.N.; Kalkmann, C.J.; Veeger, N. Non-invasive bladder volume measurement for the prevention of postoperative urinary retention: Validation of two ultrasound devices in a clinical setting. *J. Clin. Monit. Comput.* **2018**, *32*, 1117–1126. [CrossRef] [PubMed]
2. Rosseland, L.A.; Stubhaug, A.; Breivik, H. Detecting postoperative urinary retention with an ultrasound scanner. *Acta Anaesthesiol. Scand.* **2002**, *46*, 279–282. [CrossRef] [PubMed]
3. Daurat, A.; Choquet, O.; Bringuier, S.; Charbit, J.; Egan, M.; Capdevilla, X. Diagnosis of postoperative urinary retention using a simplified ultrasound bladder measurement. *Anesth. Analg.* **2015**, *120*, 1033–1038. [CrossRef] [PubMed]
4. Brausch, L.; Hewener, H. Classifying muscle states with ultrasonic single element transducer data using machine learning strategies. *Proc. Meet. Acoust.* **2019**, *38*, 022001. [CrossRef]
5. Tortoli, P.; Bassi, L.; Boni, E.; Dallai, A.; Guidi, F.; Ricci, S. ULA-OP: An advanced open platform for ultrasound research. *IEEE Trans. Ultrason. Ferroelectr. Freq. Control* **2009**, *56*, 2207–2216. [CrossRef] [PubMed]
6. Jensen, J.A.; Holm, O.; Jerisen, L.J.; Bendsen, H.; Nikolov, S.I.; Tomov, B.G.; Munk, P.; Hansen, M.; Salomonsen, K.; Hansen, J. Ultrasound research scanner for real-time synthetic aperture data acquisition. *IEEE Trans. Ultrason. Ferroelectr. Freq. Control* **2005**, *52*, 881–891. [CrossRef] [PubMed]

7. Hewener, H.; Welsch, H.J.; Günther, C.; Fonfara, H.; Tretbar, S.; Lemor, R.M. A highly customizable ultrasound research platform for clinical use with a software architecture for 2d-/3d-reconstruction and processing including closed-loop control. In *World Congress on Medical Physics and Biomedical Engineering-IFMBE Proceedings*; Dössel, O., Schlegel, W.C., Eds.; Springer: Berlin/Heidelberg, Germany, 2009; Volume 25.
8. Prinz, C.; Voigt, J.U. Diagnostic Accuracy of a Hand-Held Ultrasound Scanner in Routine Patients Referred for Echocardiography. *J. Am. Soc. Echocardiogr.* **2011**, *24*, 111–116. [CrossRef] [PubMed]
9. Van Leuteren, P.G.; Nieuwhof-Leppink, A.J.; Dik, P. SENS-U: Clinical evaluation of a full-bladder notification—A pilot study. *J. Pediatric Urol.* **2019**, *15*, 381. [CrossRef]
10. Huang, Q.; Zhang, F.; Li, X. Machine Learning in ultrasound computer aided diagnostic systems: A survey. *Biomed Res. Int.* **2018**, *2018*, 5137904. [CrossRef]
11. Xu, Y.; Wang, Y.; Yuan, J.; Cheng, Q.; Wang, X.; Carson, P.L. Medical breast ultrasound imaging segmentation by machine learning. *Ultrasonics* **2019**, *91*, 1–9. [CrossRef]
12. Menchon-Lara, R.M.; Sancho-Gomez, J.L. Fully automatic segmentation of ultrasound common carotid artery images based on machine learning. *Neurocomputing* **2015**, *151*, 161–167. [CrossRef]
13. Poudel, P.; Illanes, A.; Ataide, E.J.G.; Esmaeili, N.; Balakrishnan, S.; Friebe, M. Thyroid ultrasound texture classification using autoregressive features in conjunction with machine learning approaches. *IEEE Access* **2019**, *7*, 79354–79365. [CrossRef]
14. Zhang, Z.; Han, Y. Detection of ovarian tumors in obstetric ultrasound imaging using logistic regression classifier with an advanced machine learning approach. *IEEE Access* **2020**, *8*, 44999–45008. [CrossRef]
15. Montaldo, G.; Tanter, M.; Bercoff, J.; Benech, N.; Fink, M. Coherent plane-wave compounding for very high frame rate ultrasonography and transient elastography. *IEEE Trans. Ultrason. Ferroelectr. Freq. Control* **2009**, *56*, 489–506. [CrossRef] [PubMed]
16. He, K.; Gkioxari, G.; Doll, P.; Girshick, R.B. Mask R-CNN. In Proceedings of the IEEE International Conference on Computer Vision (ICCV), Venice, Italy, 22–29 October 2017; pp. 2980–2988.
17. Wu, X.; Kirillov, A.; Massa, F.; Lo, W.-Y.; Girshick, R.B. Detectron2. Available online: https://github.com/facebookresearch/detectron2 (accessed on 27 March 2019).
18. Ronneberger, O.; Fischer, P.; Brox, T. U-Net: Convolutional Networks for Biomedical Image Segmentation. In *Medical Image Computing and Computer-Assisted Intervention—MICCAI*; Springer: Cham, Switzerland, 2015; Volume 2015, pp. 234–241.
19. Dutta, A.; Zisserman, A. The VIA Annotation Software for Images, Audio and Video. In Proceedings of the 27th ACM International Conference on Multimedia, New York, NY, USA, 21–25 October 2019.
20. Molchanov, P.; Mallya, A.; Tyree, S.; Frosia, I.; Kautz, J. Importance Estimation for Neural Network Pruning. In Proceedings of the IEEE Conference on Computer Vision and Pattern Recognition, Long Beach, CA, USA, 15–21 June 2019.
21. Li, P.C.; Li, M.L. Adaptive Imaging and the generalized coherence factor. *IEEE Trans. Ultrason. Ferroelectr. Freq. Control* **2003**, *50*, 128–141.
22. Matrone, G.; Ramalli, A.; D´hooge, J.; Tortoli, P.; Magenes, G. A comparison of coherence-based beamforming techniques in high frame rate ultrasound imaging with multi-line transmission. *IEEE Trans. Ultrason. Ferroelectr. Freq. Control* **2020**, *67*, 329–340. [CrossRef] [PubMed]
23. Fournelle, M.; Bost, W. Wave front analysis for enhanced time-domain beamforming of point-like targets in optoacoustic imaging using a linear array. *Photoacoustics* **2019**, *14*, 67–76. [CrossRef]
24. Hager, P.A.; Benini, L. LightProbe: A digital ultrasound probe for software defined ultrafast imaging. *IEEE Trans. Ultrason. Ferroelectr. Freq. Control* **2019**, *66*, 747–760. [CrossRef]
25. Matrone, G.; Savoia, A.S.; Caliano, G.; Magenes, G. The delay multiply and sum beamforming algorithm in ultrasound B-mode medical imaging. *IEEE Trans. Med. Imaging* **2015**, *34*, 940–946. [CrossRef]
26. Matsumoto, M.; Tsutaoka, T.; Yabunaka, K.; Handa, M.; Yoshida, M.; Nakagami, G.; Sanada, H. Development and evaluation of automated ultrasonographic detection of bladder diameter for estimation of bladder urine volume. *PLoS ONE* **2019**, *14*, e0219916. [CrossRef]
27. Akkus, Z.; Kim, B.H.; Nayak, R.; Gregory, A.; Alizad, A.; Fatemi, M. Fully automated segmentation of bladder sac and measurement of detrusor wall thickness from transabdominal ultrasound images. *Sensors* **2020**, *10*, 4175. [CrossRef] [PubMed]

sensors

MDPI

Article

Optical Detection of SARS-CoV-2 Utilizing Antigen-Antibody Binding Interactions

Mahmoud Al Ahmad [1,2,*], Farah Mustafa [2,3], Neena Panicker [3] and Tahir A. Rizvi [2,4]

1 Electrical Engineering Department, United Arab Emirates University, Al Ain 15551, United Arab Emirates
2 Zayed Center for Health Sciences, United Arab Emirates University, Al Ain 15551, United Arab Emirates; fmustafa@uaeu.ac.ae (F.M.); tarizvi@uaeu.ac.ae (T.A.R.)
3 Department of Biochemistry, College of Medicine & Health Sciences, Al Ain 20000, United Arab Emirates; ngpanicker@uaeu.ac.ae
4 Department of Microbiology and Immunology, College of Medicine & Health Sciences, Al Ain 20000, United Arab Emirates
* Correspondence: m.alahmad@uaeu.ac.ae; Tel.: +971-37135150

Abstract: Severe acute respiratory syndrome coronavirus 2 (SARS-CoV-2), the virus responsible for the coronavirus disease (COVID-19) pandemic, is sweeping the world today. This study investigates the optical detection of SARS-CoV-2, utilizing the antigen-antibody binding interactions utilizing a light source from a smart phone and a portable spectrophotometer. The proof-of-concept is shown by detecting soluble preparations of spike protein subunits from SARS-CoV-2, followed by detection of the actual binding potential of the SARS-CoV-2 proteins with their corresponding antigens. The measured binding interactions for RBD and NCP proteins with their corresponding antibodies under different conditions have been measured and analyzed. Based on these observations, a "hump or spike" in light intensity is observed when a specific molecular interaction takes place between two proteins. The optical responses could further be analyzed using the principle component analysis technique to enhance and allows precise detection of the specific target in a multi-protein mixture.

Keywords: COVID-19; NC protein; optical detection; protein–protein interactions; RBD; SARS-CoV-2

Citation: Ahmad, M.A.; Mustafa, F.; Panicker, N.; Rizvi, T.A. Optical Detection of SARS-CoV-2 Utilizing Antigen-Antibody Binding Interactions. *Sensors* **2021**, *21*, 6596. https://doi.org/10.3390/s21196596

Academic Editors: Ayman El-baz and Andrea Cusano

Received: 30 August 2021
Accepted: 28 September 2021
Published: 2 October 2021

1. Introduction

The world is currently facing the COVID-19 pandemic, caused by the appearance of a novel coronavirus in the human population at the end of 2019 [1]. Within a few months, this virus had spread to most countries across the world, infecting millions (>21 million as of 17 August 2020) and causing >770,000 deaths [2]. Rapid detection methods, independent of lab settings, have been identified as top priorities in promoting epidemic prevention and control. Currently, the molecular technique of quantitative real time polymerase chain reaction (qRT PCR) is the gold standard for SARS-CoV-2 detection using samples from respiratory secretions [3–7]. However, this time-consuming and cumbersome procedure involves long processing times (days) for results [8]. Several other molecular assays have been developed to detect SARS-CoV-2, such as enzyme-based assays, such as ELISAs, and rapid tests that aim to detect either antibodies against the virus or the viral antigen themselves [4]. Nevertheless, most of these antigen-antibody-based assays have failed quality control due to their rapid development without proper testing, resulting in either false negative or false positive detection, due to the long time it takes to develop serum responses to the viral infection (from days to weeks) [9]. Thus, most of the methods used so far require skilled manpower, are time consuming if accurate, or not reliable at all, if fast. On the other hand, biosensor technology provides excellent sensitivity, but it has its own caveats. For example, some biosensors require metal coating deposited on the device, thereby raising costs [10], while others suffer from temperature-dependence, which can be a hindrance for portable biosensors in outdoor conditions [11]. Some require expensive reagents and reaction times that are often longer [12]. Mavrikou et al. have used bioelectric recognition assays along with artificially engineered cells to demonstrate direct detection of SARS-CoV-2 surface antigens without prior sample processing [13]; however, they still have to show whether their systems will work in a real-world scenario. Optical, label-free biosensors have been utilized frequently in biomolecular detection due to their continuous monitoring abilities, and high sensitivity to local variations, including the refractive index change [14]. They are capable of detecting interactions between molecules and their surrounding media [15].

In terms of detection—the most prominent feature of the SARS-CoV-2 virus, like other coronaviruses, is the spike protein (S) that protrudes out of the virus particle, essentially like "spikes" as the name suggests. The spike protein forms a trimer that is used by the virus to enter susceptible cells using the angiotensin-converting enzyme 2 (ACE2) protein as the cellular receptor [16], the same protein used by the SARS-CoV-1 virus that caused the first SARS epidemic in 2003 (Figure 1a). The spike protein is cleaved by host proteases into two subunits: the surface subunit S1 and the transmembrane subunit S2 [17] (Figure 1b). The surface S1 subunit is used by the virus to interact with the ACE2 protein, using its receptor-binding domain (RBD) [18]. This allows the virus to attach to the susceptible cells, while the S2 protein is used for the actual fusion of the virus with the cell membrane, allowing the virus to be endocytosed and release its genomic RNA cargo, wrapped up in the nucleocapsid protein (NCP), into the cytoplasm [19,20]. The viral genomic RNA is immediately used to translate viral proteins that are used for successful virus replication in the susceptible cells [21]. The spike protein is also one of the most immunogenic proteins of the virus, towards which most of the neutralizing antibody responses against the virus are generated in infected individuals, making it an ideal candidate for a vaccine, as well as a target of drug development [22–24].

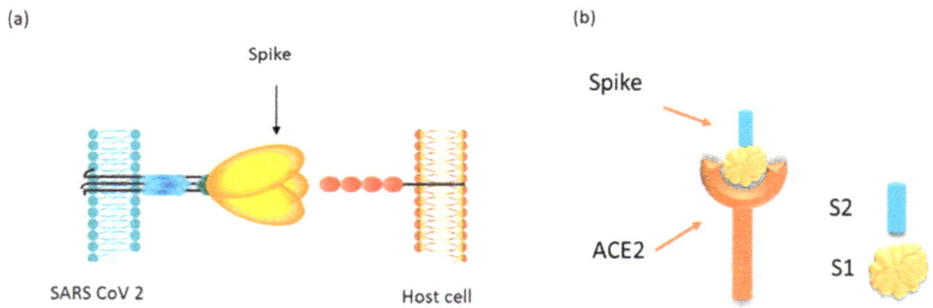

Figure 1. Schematic illustration of the SARS-CoV-2 spike protein and ACE2 receptor binding. (**a**) SARS-CoV-2 binding to the ACE2 receptor on the host cell surface. (**b**) Binding of ACE2 and the spike protein along with an illustration of the spike protein subunits, S1 and S2.

The receptor-binding domain of SARS-CoV-2 is the key region of the S protein that affects the virus spread. Xia et al. have confirmed these observations by showing that even the fusion capability of the SARS-CoV-2 S2 subunit is better than that of SARS-CoV-1, further explaining the increased infectivity of the virus compared with other coronaviruses [25,26]. They further show that lipopeptide inhibitors can be developed, which can disrupt such fusion capability to inhibit the ability of the virus to infect cells [27]. Similarly, Seydoux et al. have shown the utility of isolating S-specific antibody-producing B-cell clones from COVID-19 patients [28]. They further demonstrated that the most potent amongst these antibodies was targeted against the RBD of the S protein, which was able to block the interaction of the S protein with ACE2 successfully. Yang et al. tested several binding inhibitor peptides, targeting the virus early attachment stages [29]. Others have observed a strong correlation between levels of RBD-binding antibodies and SARS-CoV-2 neutralizing antibodies in patients [22,30–34]. Thus, study of spike protein interaction with the ACE2 receptor can be of importance, for not only virus entry into cells, but also as a means of inhibiting virus infection of susceptible cells, development of vaccines, and detection of virus infection.

In this work, an optical-based time detection method incorporating the smartphone light source and a portable mini spectrometer for SARS-CoV-2 detection was developed, based on the ability to measure antigen-antibody binding interactions.

2. Materials and Methods

2.1. Optical Mini-Spectrometers

C11708MA from Hamamatsu/Japan [35] was used to convert the variable attenuation of light waves as they passed from end-to-end or reflected off substances into signals with spectral responses, ranging from 640 to 1010 nm. The wavelength reproducibility ranged between −0.5 and 0.5 nm and had a maximum of 20 nm FWHM spectra, under constant light conditions. The measurements were conducted with the room lights on. The distances among the light source, the spectrometer, and the sample holder were adjusted to eliminate any possible interference and to stabilize the spectrometer performance. Furthermore, the spectrometer was aligned with the light source and the sample cuvette to achieve a straight path of light.

2.2. Smart Mobile Phone

The smartphone light source was used as the main light source [36]. The mobile light emits lights with the spectral range from 380 to 740 nm. The maximum optical power was emitted at a wavelength of 623 nm. In this work, iPhone 8 was employed, though any smart phone can be used.

2.3. Nucleocapsid Protein

The SARS-CoV-2 nucleocapsid protein (Sino Biologicals, Cat no. 40588-V08B) [37] and its corresponding nucleocapsid antibody (Sino Biologicals Cat no. 40588-T62) [37] were used for the binding affinity experiments. The lyophilized protein was resuspended at a stock concentration of 0.25 mg/mL, according to the manufacturer's instructions, in sterile water. The nucleocapsid rabbit polyclonal antibody was supplied at a stock concentration of 1 mg/mL.

2.4. The Receptor Binding Domain (RBD)

The receptor binding domain (RBD) of the SARS-CoV-2 spike protein (Sino Biologicals, Cat No 40592-V05H) [37] was expressed as a recombinant protein with the Fc region of mouse (mFc) at the C terminus end and its corresponding spike RBD antibody (Sino Biologicals, cat. no. 40592-T62) [37] was used for the binding affinity experiments. The RBD protein was prepared in sterile water at a stock concentration of 0.25 mg/mL, as per the manufacturer's instruction. The spike RBD rabbit polyclonal antibody was prepared at a stock concentration of 1 mg/mL and diluted further for analysis.

3. Results and Discussions

3.1. Experimental Design

The experimental setup utilized in this study is shown in Figure 2a, incorporating a mini spectrometer and a smart mobile phone that was employed as a light source with its power spectrum depicted in Figure 2b. The measured optical power of the beam exhibited maximum power at a wavelength of 623 nm [36]. The mini-spectrometer C11708MA (Hamamatsu/Japan) was used to measure the light intensity as it passed through test substances with spectral responses ranging from 640 to 1010 nm [35]. The wavelength reproducibility was between −0.5 and 0.5 nm and a maximum of 20 nm FWHM spectra, under constant light conditions. The sample under test was placed between the mobile light source and the mini-spectrometer, as shown in Figure 2a. The measurements were conducted with the room lights on. The distances among the light source, the spectrometer, and the sample holder were adjusted to eliminate any possible interference and to stabilize the spectrometer performance. Furthermore, the spectrometer was aligned with the light source and sample cuvette to achieve a straight path of light. Figure 2c illustrates the incident, reflected, and transmitted light intensities. The light intensities were linked through the Kirchhoff's Law of Radiation [38], which correlates the optical absorbance, transmittance, and reflection, along with the incident wave.

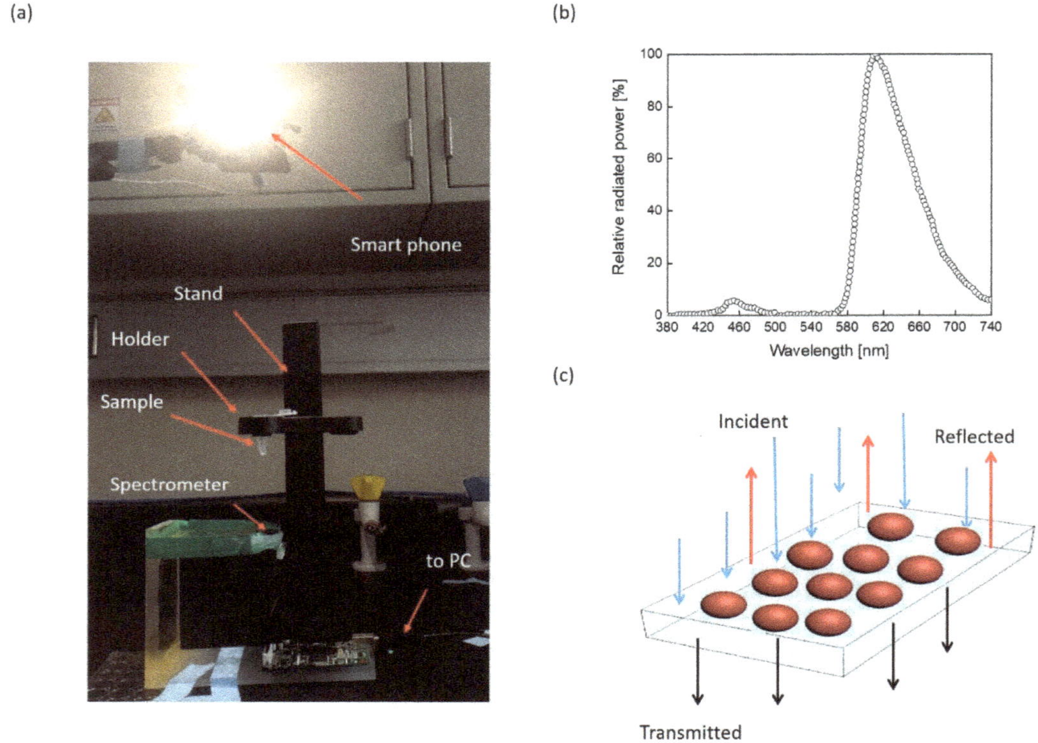

Figure 2. The proposed concept of optical detection and the experimental design: (**a**) the optical measurement setup is shown, consisting of a smart phone as a light source and the mini-spectrometer utilized to collect the light waves passing through the sample kept in the holder. (**b**) The smart phone power spectra vs. wavelength. (**c**) Illustration of the spectrometer detection principle.

This experimental setup was first used to characterize the two spike proteins subunits, S1 and S2, which are encoded by all coronaviruses and, as mentioned, allow virus entry into susceptible cells (Figure 1b). Figure 3a shows the optical responses for both proteins along with their corresponding blank samples. The measured optical intensity changed from 600 to 750 nm, within the light source spectrum measured earlier in Figure 2b. The response of the blank samples was performed first, followed by the two protein suspensions, the responses to which were recorded individually as shown in Figure 3a.

Figure 3a reveals that S2 exhibited a higher "back scattering" and/or absorbance than S1. The response of the two blank samples was quite comparable, showing the reproducibility of the results. Since the maximum difference between the blank and the two protein samples was observed at 623 nm, this wavelength was chosen for further experimentation, which is also the wavelength at which the optical power of the smart phone is at its maximum.

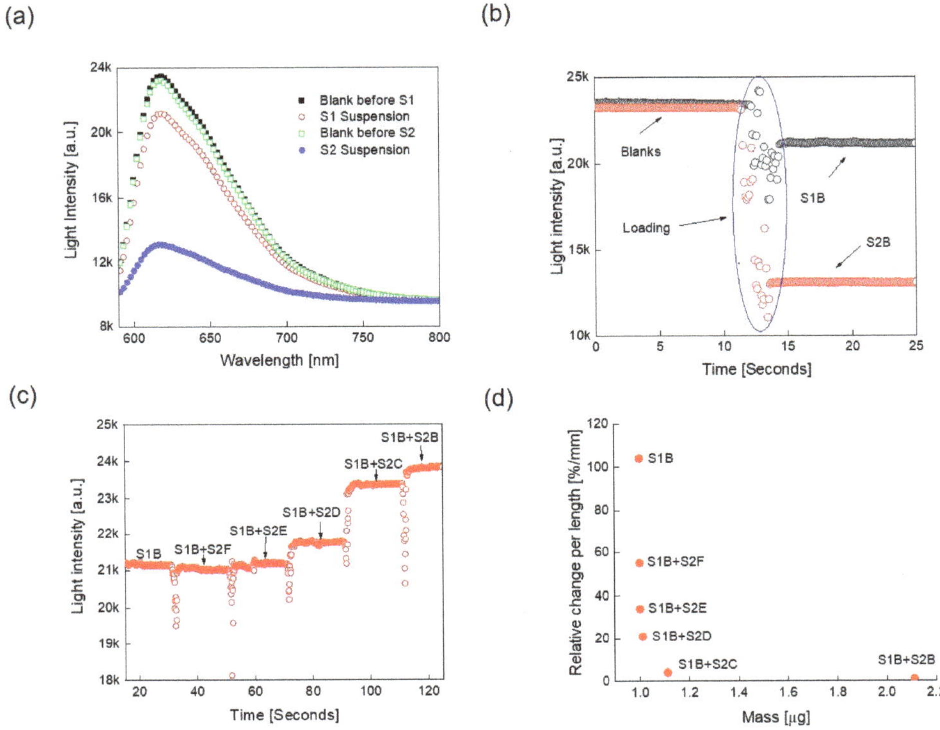

Figure 3. Optical measurements of the spike protein subunits S1 and S2: (**a**) measured responses for spikes proteins S1 and S2 at the highest concentration individually (S1B and S2B, respectively), along with their corresponding blanks. (**b**) Time domain measurements of the microcentrifuge tube, the blank (shown in gray circles) vs. water (red circles) at a wavelength of 623 nm. (**c**) Measured optical responses for the mixed protein samples vs. time. Samples S1B and S2B were at 5000 copies per ml, S2C, S2D, S2E, and S2F are the serial dilutions of S2B at 10-, 100-, 1000- and 10,000-fold, respectively. (**d**) Relative change in light intensity per light path vs. loaded mass. All optical responses were measured at 623 nm. Light intensity was measured as arbitrary units (a.u).

3.2. Optimization of the Sample Reading Conditions

An initial test of this experimental setup revealed that it had one major drawback; i.e., when samples were loaded into the holder, the angle and position of the microcentrifuge tube changed, which affected the results obtained. To ensure that the results were reproducible, the measurements for the same samples were conducted over different days, and on each day, the setup was standardized, since the position of the mobile phone, spectrometer, and samples could vary. To overcome this caveat and have more consistence measurements without constant standardization, advantage was made of the ability of the spectrometer to provide light intensity measurements over time. Hence, after placing the microcentrifuge tube into the holder, the measurement mode started and the corresponding "blank" recorded. Then the sample was added after ~100 ms, while keeping the measurement mode on. Figure 3b illustrates the corresponding measurement profile for S1B and S2B individual samples suspended in water over time. Initially, a fluctuation in the light intensity was observed with time, as each sample was added to the tube, but then it stabilized with time. As expected, the blank exhibited the maximum measured light intensity, while the suspended samples showed lower light intensity than the blank once stabilized.

3.3. *Test of the Spike Proteins Using the Proposed Experimental Set-Up*

To test the proof-of-principle, initially a mixing experiment was conducted at a light wavelength of 623 nm. Towards this end, 250 μL of S1B protein solution was tested at the same maximum concentration at 5000 copies/mL followed by addition of the same amount of S2B. Figure 3c shows the light intensity (as arbitrary units, a.u.) with time as the protein samples were added to the *transparent measurement container* in a sequential manner. This was followed by the addition of 250 μL of ten-fold serial dilutions of the S2 protein at equal time intervals to the S1B + S2B samples. As can be seen from Figure 3c, with the addition of the S2 protein, the light intensity increased. The biggest increase was observed with the concentrated S2B sample followed by its ten-fold dilution samples S2C, S2D, S2E, etc., until S2F addition as a 1:10,000 dilution had no extra effect on the increase in light intensity, revealing the limit of detection of the assay (5000 molecules per mL × 250 μL × 1/10,000 = 125 molecule per mL). These results reveal that the ratio between the S1 and S2 protein concentration plays an important role in the light intensity levels measured. The ratio of S1 and S2 in the virus is the same since both originate from the cleavage of the S protein. However, the S1 subunit is expressed on the cell surface, while the S2 subunit is embedded in the lipid bilayer of the cell membrane; therefore, S2 is less available at the cell surface, which should affect light intensity less than S1, despite equal ratios. Table 1 lists the extracted parameters at specific time points. The relative change in light intensity per light path length is a constructed parameter that should correlate with the loaded mass (concentration) of the protein in a suspension.

Table 1. List of measured and extracted parameters.

Sample Description	Light Intensity (a.u.)	Length of the Light Path (mm)	Mass of Protein Tested (μg)	ΔI_r Per Length (%/mm)
S1B	21,215	0.11111	1	104
S1B + S2F	21,080	0.22222	1.0001	55
S1B + S2E	21,265	0.33333	1.0011	34
S1B + S2D	21,785	0.44444	1.0111	21
S1B + S2C	23,440	0.55556	1.1111	4
S1B + S2B	23,875	0.66667	2.1111	0.8

Figure 3d shows the change in relative light intensity divided by the light path length vs. the total mass of the tested samples. As shown in Table 1, it reveals that, as the mass of the protein increased in our experimental system, the intensity of light also increased, revealing that length of the light path was directly proportional to the amount of protein in the sample.

Figure 4a,b illustrates the definition of the light intensities and light path length. The smart mobile integrated light source emits a light intensity (I_0) that is the maximum intensity that can be measured in this experimental setup. The blank intensity (I_b) is the measured intensity that goes through the empty container responsible for holding the sample, such as the microcentrifuge tube. The instantaneous measured intensity (I) is the recorded light when it passes through the sample. This amount of light intensity strongly depends on the buffer in which the sample is solubilized/dissolved in, its composition, the light path length, the kind of the suspended analytes, and its size in the buffer. The light path length depends on the loaded amount of suspension inside the container. The path length varies from zero up to the container length (L). For a sample with a specific volume (V), the corresponding path length is equal to the volume over the cross-sectional area of the container (A). Equation (1) expresses the relationship between the relative change in light intensity per light path length and loaded mass (m), as follows:

$$m = m_i + m_f e^{-\alpha(\Delta I/l)} \quad (1)$$

where m_i, m_f, and l are the initial mass of the buffer, the mass of the final suspension composite, and the light path length, respectively. α is the decay factor, unique for each control buffer. Its unit is in mm and could be correlated with the material absorptivity. ΔI is the relative change in light intensity expressed as follows:

$$\Delta I = (1 - I/I_b) \times 100\% \quad (2)$$

where I and I_b are the instantaneous measured light intensity of the suspension and the corresponding blank, respectively. Figure 4c shows the relationship between mass and the relative change per length after fitting the measured points with the exponential function. As can be seen, with more sample volume, the path length increases and light intensity decreases; hence, the relative change decreases dramatically.

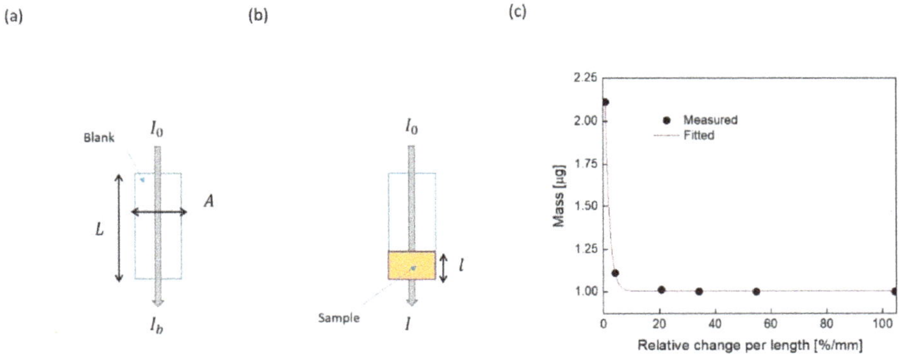

Figure 4. Illustration of light intensity and its path length: (**a**) the blank representation, and (**b**) light path length of the sample. L and A are the length and cross-sectional area of container, l is the light path length. I_0, I_b, and I are the incident, blank, and instantaneous sample intensities, respectively. (**c**) Loaded mass vs. relative change in light intensity per light-path length. The measured points were fitted with exponential function expressed by Equation (1) with the following parameters: m_i = 1.003µ ± 2.68n, m_f = 2.163µ ± 34.7n, and α-factor is 1.28435 ± 0.030. The other fitting model accuracy parameters are reduced Chi-Sqr, R-Square (COD), Adj. R-Square are 28.8 atto, 1 and 1, respectively, which indicates the best possible fit.

3.4. Test of Binding Interactions between Spike and ACE2 Using the Optical Assay

After successful demonstration that our set-up could detect spike proteins in solution using light, we asked if light intensity could be used to characterize the binding interactions of the spike protein with the viral receptor ACE2. Towards this end, two different variants of the S1 subunit of the spike protein, S1X and S1Y, were tested (one form that could bind ACE2 with a much stronger affinity than the other one), along with a non-specific control protein—bovine serum albumin (BSA)—that should not bind to ACE2. These proteins were selected to demonstrate the detection of the binding process with ACE2 over time. The measurement process started with the blank, and after 200 s, 250 µL of ACE2 protein suspension was tested (Figure 5a). This process was repeated for S1X, S1Y, and BSA, and their responses to light were measured individually in the same manner as ACE2. The corresponding individual profiles of ACE2, S1X, S1Y, and BSA are depicted in Figure 5a, which showed a straight constant line over time. Next, each protein was mixed with the ACE2 separately to detect any possible binding effect. The measurements started with first loading the ACE2 in the blank container, then after 200 ms, the test protein was added to the ACE2 in solution. The responses of the various protein mixtures were read over a period of 15 min and are shown in Figure 5b.

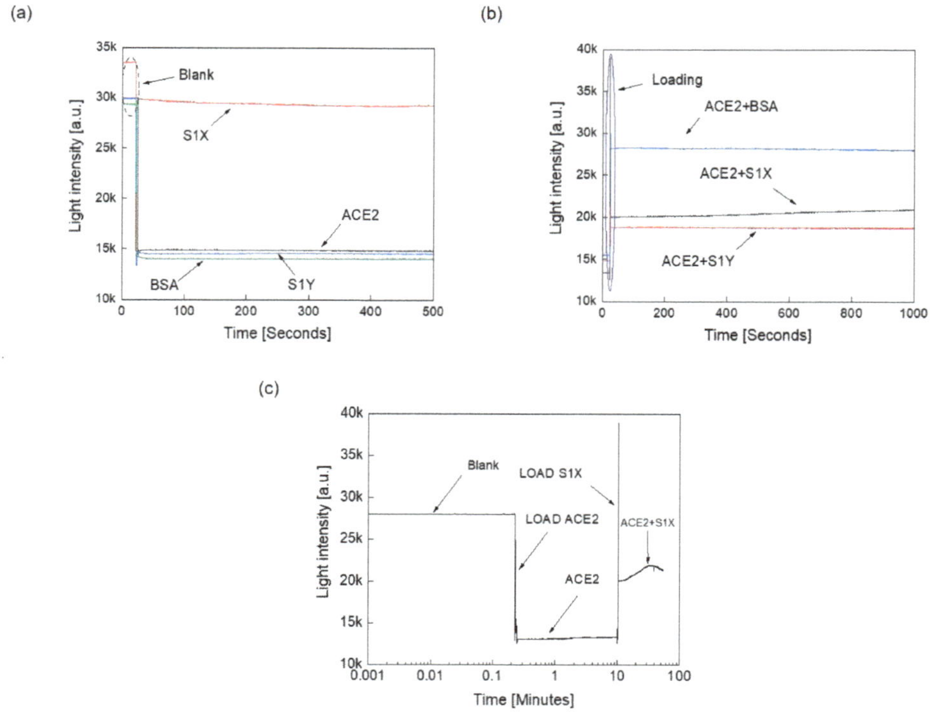

Figure 5. Optical detection of binding interactions between ACE2 and other proteins. (**a**) Measured light intensities over time for individual assessment of ACE2, S1X, S1Y, and BSA. (**b**) The measured mixed light intensities vs. time for ACE2 mixed with S1X, S1Y, or BSA. (**c**) The measured ACE2–S1X interaction profile for an extended time period.

Figure 5b shows the corresponding slopes that represent the change of the light intensities over time. The ACE2 + BSA and ACE2 + S1Y responses exhibited almost constant lines, suggesting highly reduced or lack of any interaction as observed when the proteins were tested individually Figure 5a. However, the ACE2 + S1X profile showed a linear straight line with the maximum-recorded slope. The corresponding light intensity line increased over time, suggesting an interaction between the SIX protein and the ACE2 receptor. We interpret this to mean that there was no protein–protein interaction if the slope of the line was zero; otherwise, protein–protein interaction occurred. Based on these observations, our results suggest that the S1X protein exhibits stronger interactions with ACE2, while BSA and S1Y had weaker interactions with ACE2. These observations are confirmed by the fact that S1X has a higher affinity for ACE2 (2 μg/mL S1X can bind 1.5–15 ng/mL ACE2), while S1Y reportedly has a much lower affinity (2 μg/mL S1B binds 0.5–8.7 ng/mL ACE2), as tested in enzyme-linked immunosorbent assays (ELISA) by the company that synthesized these proteins [39].

To explore the interaction and binding characteristics between ACE2 and S1X in more detail, the measurement time between the two proteins was extended over one hour, the results of which are plotted in Figure 5c. As can be seen, a nice "hump" was observed as an increase in arbitrary units (a.u.) with time that was not observed in the other protein mixtures tested, which we feel is indicative of the binding reaction between the two proteins.

3.5. Validation of the Optical Assay Using Known Antigen/Antibody Pairs

Next, we wanted to confirm our observations by using our optical system to detect protein–protein interactions using proteins that are well known to interact with each other.

This was addressed by testing the molecular interactions between an antigen and an antibody, which is similar to the interaction between the spike protein and its receptor. Towards this end, two proteins were tested along with their specific antibodies: the first protein was the receptor-binding domain (RBD) of SARS-CoV-2 spike protein and its antibody and the other was the nucleocapsid protein (NCP) of SARS-CoV-2 and its antibody. Similar to the procedure described earlier, the two proteins were tested individually in our optical assay followed by addition of their corresponding antibodies that were mixed and then tested for their interactions.

Figure 6a shows the binding between RBD and its antibody. Upon the addition of the antibody, as observed earlier, an "interaction peak" was recorded (circled in the blue color). Similarly, Figure 6b shows the binding between NCP and its antibody. However, in this case, we realized that the binding effect occurred at specific antibody concentrations; thus, when the antibody was added first, no interaction peak was observed. Therefore, we added more concentrated antibody and upon its addition, the interaction peak was observed. The addition of more antibody did not allow detection of further interaction peaks, revealing that the protein–protein interaction took place at a specific concentration, and once the interaction had taken place, no further interaction took place. For a virus-based suspension, it is therefore suggested to use a fixed antibody concentration and serially dilute the virus suspension to conduct the binding measurements. Certainly, at a specific virus concentration, binding effect will appear in the form of an optical response.

Figure 6c,d illustrates the corresponding optical responses for the NC protein and its corresponding antibody, when they were mixed inside (Figure 6c) or outside (Figure 6d) the microcentrifuge tube, respectively. Inside mixing means that the protein was added to the tube and the antibody was added after 10 s, while in the outside mixing scenario, both the protein and antibody were mixed prior to being loaded in the tube for optical measurements. As can be seen, the binding response could be detected in each case in the form of appearance of the hump. However, this "hump" was a lot more pronounced when the protein and the antibody were mixed prior to testing than when they were added sequentially. This is good news for the real-life scenario, where in a patient sample, the antibody should be already bound to the viral or bacterial antigen at the time of detection.

3.6. Test of the Optical Detection Assay Using a Solid Support

The nitrocellulose membrane is a popular matrix that is frequently used due to its high protein-binding affinity with a pore size of 0.25–0.45 μm in paper-based diagnostics. Protein molecules usually bind to the nitrocellulose membranes through hydrophobic interactions [40]. Due to the ease of their handling, cheap cost, and the presence of hydrophobic interactions between them and the suspended proteins, we tested whether the binding between the SARS-CoV-2 spike protein and antibody could be detected optically when both were added to each other on the nitrocellulose membrane. Using the experimental setup detailed in Figure 2a, the optical responses for nitrocellulose membrane, nitrocellulose membrane and spike protein alone, nitrocellulose membrane and antibody against spike protein alone, and nitrocellulose membrane spike protein–antibody were measured. Figure 7a shows that both the antibody alone and spike protein alone exhibited higher light intensity than the nitrocellulose membrane alone with almost a straight line with a constant slope over a time period of 10 s. The on-paper measured optical responses exhibited fluctuations as in the samples measured using microcentrifuge tubes. This implies that these fluctuations are not due to any interactions; rather, they are due to the spectrometer conversion process [41].

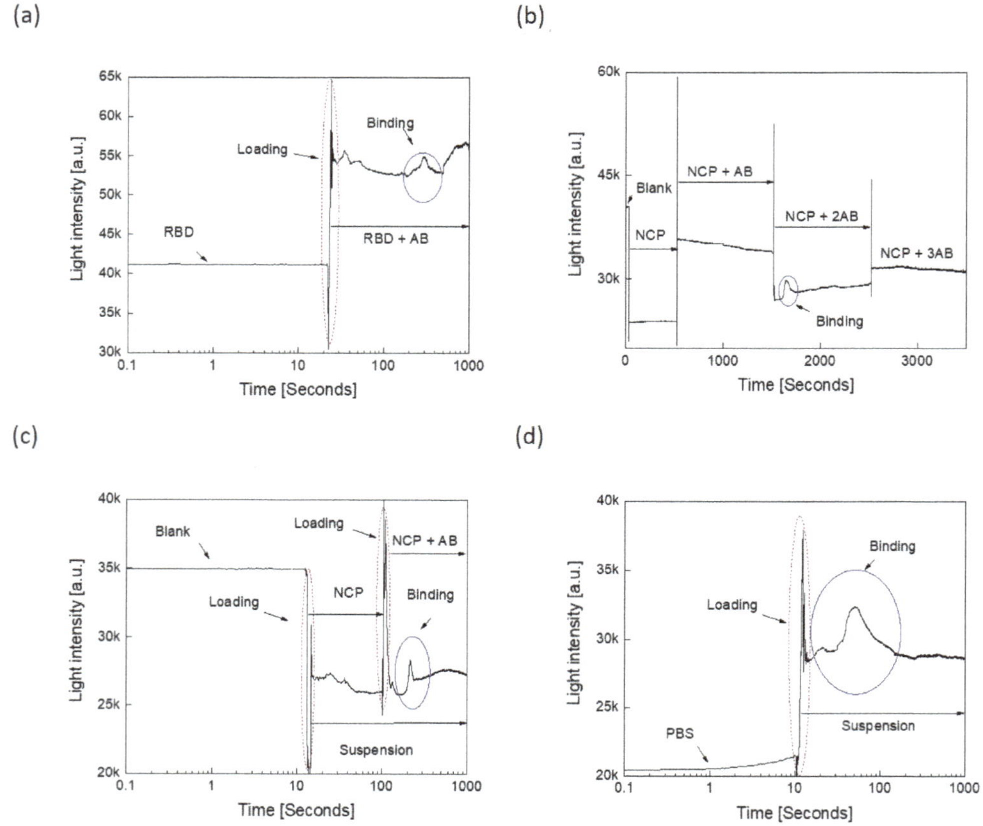

Figure 6. Optical detection of the binding affinities between: (**a**) the receptor-binding domain (RBD) of the spike protein with its antibody (AB), and (**b**) the nucleocapsid protein (NCP) and its antibody. The antibody was added again to NCP since no binding interaction was observed the first time. To confirm the result, the antibody was added a third time, but this time once again, the binding interaction was not apparent. (**c**) NCP binding with the antibody after mixing inside, and (**d**) NCP binding with the antibody after mixing outside. The interaction peak is circled.

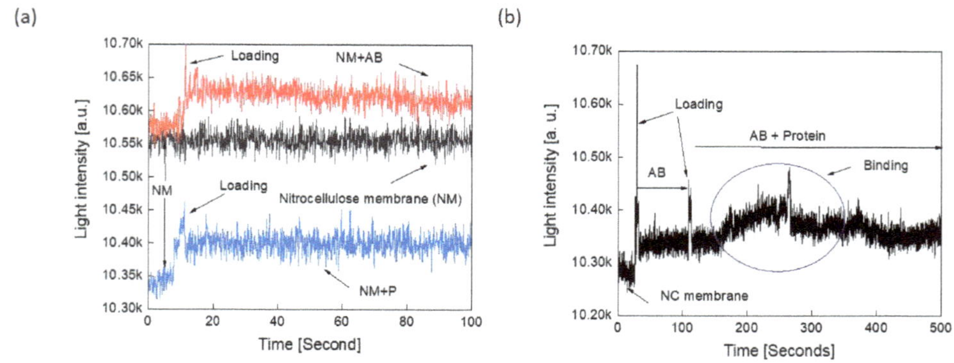

Figure 7. Test of protein–protein interaction measurements on solid support: (**a**) optical responses on nitrocellulose membrane (NM) alone, nitrocellulose membrane and spike protein (NM + P), and nitrocellulose membrane and antibody to spike protein (NM + AB) alone. (**b**) Optical responses to spike protein–antibody binding on the nitrocellulose membrane.

Figure 7b summaries the interaction measurements, which start with the membrane alone. After 20 s, the antibody suspension was loaded on the membrane and measurements were conducted up to 100 s. Next, the spike protein sample was loaded and measurements were continued up to 500 s. As revealed from Figure 7b, the interaction peak clearly appeared as circled in blue. It is worth noting that the membrane size, shape, and charge of biomolecules, pH, and viscosity of the control buffer, as well as the composition influences the corresponding optical response and binding interactions and must be carefully standardized [42].

3.7. Role of Electric Current in Disrupting Protein-Protein Interactions

Finally, we studied the effect of direct current (DC biasing) on the ability of two proteins to bind specifically. This was achieved by subjecting the NC protein solution to DC voltage bias, as depicted in Figure 8a. An applied bias should result in an induction of current across the suspension. If this current is high enough, it should have the potential to destroy the protein physiology and functionality, resulting in the loss of specific protein-protein interactions. To test this hypothesis, the NC protein solution was loaded in an electroporation cuvette (rather than a microcentrifuge tube) that incorporates two electrodes with a volume of 0.5 mL and a separation distance of 0.4 cm. This should result in a breakdown electric field of 7.5 V/cm. At this field onwards, the binding between the protein and the antibody should be affected. Above this field, the sample should be incapacitated for binding. Figure 8a reveals that the optical response decays slowly with the application of DC bias. At 3 volts DC bias, the optical response decays with a considerable step, and increasing the DC bias further should burn the suspension and destroy it.

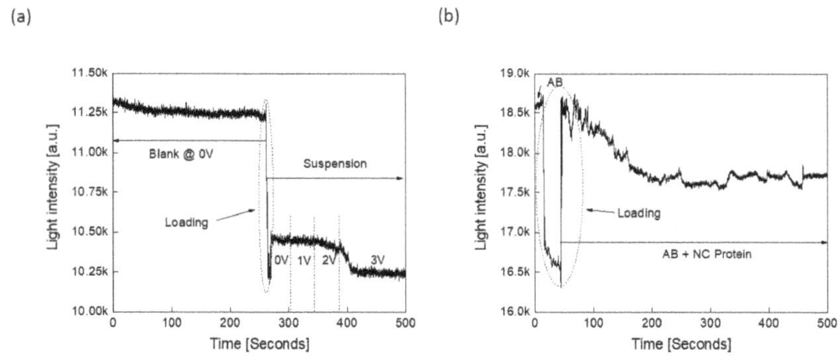

Figure 8. Opto-electrical measurements: (**a**) Measured NC protein optical response versus time at different DC bias voltages. (**b**) Binding measurements between NC protein and its corresponding antibody after subjected the solution to an electric field.

The breakdown field depends on the electrical characteristics of both the buffer and the analyte such as proteins, viruses, etc. To explore this further, the suspension of protein was subjected to 3 V for 1 min and then the antibody to NC was added to the NC protein solution. The corresponding measured response is shown in Figure 8b. The measured response was observed to be noisy and did not show a clear binding effect when compared with Figure 6c that reported the optical response for the same protein and antibody without the application of DC bias. It is worth mentioning that it may be possible to create a corresponding vaccine for a disease by subjecting the target viral protein to DC bias which will affect its function and destroy its physiology (denature it) and communicability (binding interactions). Furthermore, the proposed optical detection in time domain can also be used for monitoring and detecting the efficiency of vaccine process development.

4. Discussion

This study establishes the proof-of-principle that optical methods can be used to detect specific SARS-CoV-2 spike proteins or their subunits (S, S1, and S2) as well as their interactions with the ACE2 receptor in solution, whenever present (Figures 3 and 5). The principle was further validated by testing specific protein–protein interactions by testing two viral protein–antibody pairs (RBD and NC proteins with their specific antibodies) and testing them either in solution (Figure 6) or on a solid matrix (Figure 7). Finally, it was shown that application of a weak current into the system could lead to the disruption of NC protein–antibody interactions, which could be optically detected (Figure 8). In other words, our technique could be used not only to detect specific SARS-CoV-2 spike protein–receptor interactions, but also result in destruction of protein interactions important for virus replication; thus, inhibiting rate of infection. The proposed detection method can be performed within minutes, without the need to biochemically label the proteins. This system can be used to develop novel optical-based detection tests for any virus in a specific and sensitive manner, as long as one specific protein partner is available in the solution or on a solid support that can interact specifically with a specific viral protein. For instance, in the case of SARS-CoV-2, one could use either an antibody to the spike protein or the ACE2 protein to determine whether a particular patient sample may have the virus.

Figure 1c shows the spikes distribution suspended in a sample. As illustrated, the spike proteins are randomly distributed and exhibit Brownian motion by default [43]. The same scenario applies to the distribution of ACE2 as illustrated in Figure 1d [44]. If specific binding occurs between the spike proteins and ACE2, as represented by Figure 1e, their binding distribution should still exhibit random Brownian motion. Nevertheless, the SARS-CoV-2 spike protein binds with human ACE2 protein with a specific binding energy that has been measured and is estimated to be nearly -58.55 ± 8.75 $kmol^{-1}$ [45,46]. A conformational change occurs in the ACE2 receptor protein after binding with spike protein fragment [46]. Ov et al. showed that the refraction index changes due to the binding interactions after the virus-antibody incubation process [47]. To detect binding of living cells and viruses with potential drugs, they proposed a novel label-free real time approach, incorporating long-range surface waves on a one-dimensional photonic crystal surface along with microfluidic channel technology [48].

The photoelectric effect theory combines kinetic energy, binding energy, and photon energy all three of which are correlated through the theoretical physics fundamentals and principles [44]. Hence, if the generated photon energy due to the binding interactions is sufficient, it could give rise to light intensity at a specific wavelength. Wang et al. discussed the enhancement of receptor binding of SARS-CoV-2 through networks of hydrogen-bonding and hydrophobic interactions [46]. They provided explanations to better understand the structural and energetic details responsible for protein–protein interactions between the host receptor ACE2 and SARS-CoV-2. Their simulations reveal that both electrostatic complementarity and hydrophobic interactions are critical to enhance receptor binding and escape antibody recognition by the RBD of SARS-CoV-2. Ortega et al. conducted an in silico analysis to study the role of changes in SARS-CoV-2 spike protein during interaction with the ACE2 receptor. They concluded that the binding energy generated during the SARS-CoV-2 spike and ACE2 interactions can be reduced due to mutations in the sequence of the spike protein [18]. Dahal et al. demonstrated that binding probability increases with antibody concentration and the stability of protein [48].

Based on these observations, we believe that a "hump or spike" in light intensity is observed when a specific molecular interaction takes place between two proteins. This is mainly due to the physiochemical properties of the proteins that relate to binding affinity in the contact surface area, which incorporates the association/dissociation process [39].

As revealed from the corresponding binding measured light intensity profiles, they exhibit Gaussian-like peaks. Wang et al. demonstrated in their study that the molecular binding at the single molecule level displays such a peak [40]. Interestingly, Kozono et al. monitored the real-time Brownian motion and fitted it with Gaussian function [41]. The fitting parameters of the distributions can provide many features of the binding interactions [42]. This could provide a quantitative signature or characterization of a specific antigen binding to a specific antibody, such as intrinsic specificity and binding rate. It is also proven that the probability of the binding free energy to be Gaussian distributed near the mean and exponential-like distributed in the tail [43]. Figure 9 shows the binding interaction over the corresponding time intervals for RBD and NCP proteins with their corresponding antibodies under different conditions, as described in Figure 6. Similar interaction peaks were observed in each case, except they varied in the time of appearance and extent of light intensity. The time slot denoted by (i) represents the time just before the interaction occurs. As the interaction starts, the corresponding optical profile ascends incrementally as indicated by (ii) due to the increase in binding events, releasing more photons energy. The peak pointed by (iii) occurs at the maximum event of binding between antigens and their antibodies. The height of the peaks indicates stronger interactions and vice versa. The profile then descends until the end as the binding events become less, and no further interactions occur at the end, as illustrated by (iv). The distance in time to maximum peak reflects the speed of the binding interactions; thus, the earlier the peak appears, the faster the binding interaction takes place. As can be seen in Figure 9, the speed of NC protein binding to its antibody took place between 100 and 1000 s, irrespective of the dilution of the proteins.

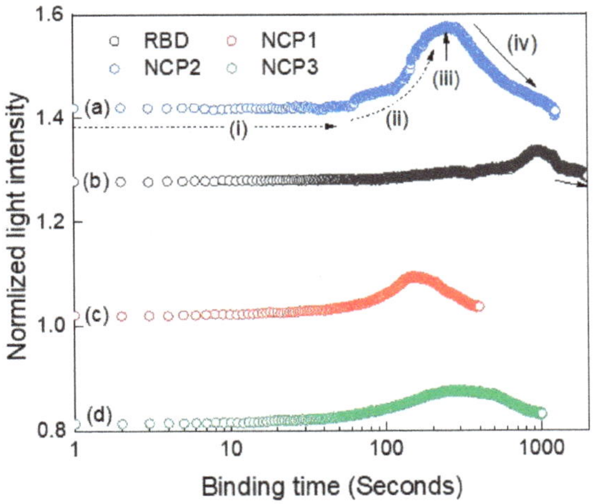

Figure 9. Optical profiles for normalized interactions vs. binding time under different conditions for RBD and NCP. (**a**) NCP with its antibody at the maximum concentration of 22 µg per mL; (**b**) RBD with its antibody; (**c**) NCP with its antibody at a 1:10 dilution; (**d**) NCP with its antibody at 1:10 with outside mixing.

Next, we analyzed the interaction profiles of these samples further by fitting them to Gaussian function. Table 2 lists their corresponding fitting parameters. The most important parameters are the width and the maximum peak amplitude. Base and center parameters represent the offset level and the maximum peak location, respectively. These two parameters provide minor information and could be set to fixed values, such as zero in all profiles. The multiplication of the maximum amplitude with its corresponding width can be utilized as an indicator to describe the speed of interaction. This "indicator" is listed in Table 2, last row. Accordingly, NCP2 exhibited the fastest binding, while NCP3 exhibited the slowest binding with the arrangement from fast to slow being as follows: NCP2, NCP1, RBD, and NCP3.

Table 2. Fitting parameters for interaction profiles depicted in Figure 9.

Fitting Parameters	NCP3	RBD	NCP2	NCP1
Base	1.43	1.29	1.03	0.83
Center	302	996	181	380
Width	130	252	68	194
Amplitude	0.13	0.04	0.06	0.05
Indicator	16.9	10.08	4.08	9.7

Practical Applications of the Proposed Technique

The optical approach presented in this study can be easily turned into a functional working system to detect SARS-CoV-2 or any other viral or bacterial pathogen against which an antibody is available that can detect it sensitively. Currently, there are several available handheld portable spectrophotometers, which are compact and lightweight, and equipped with wireless communication system for data transmission. The data can be received by the smart phone through Bluetooth or Wi-Fi technologies equipped with a mobile app designed to process the received optical profiles over time. The collected optical profiles vs. time can then be processed immediately using the smart phone processor and computational resources. The results can be displayed on the same smart phone immediately as well. The antibody could be coated on flexible strips and kept inside packs with medium. These strips can be used directly for loading the nasal swab in-position within a fabricated holder using 3D printing technology. The 3D printed holder can be designed to integrate the portable sensor and the smart phone as well. The concept of strips can be further used to detect different specimens taken from blood, breath, urine, nasal swabs, stool, etc. For example, the subject can breathe, exhale, or sniff into a device with a probe coated with antibodies. If binding occurs, the integrated device should be able to pick up the interaction, confirming that the patient is infected with the virus to which the antibodies are directed against.

The current methodology provides a rapid, reproducible, and accurate detection mechanism that can be used to create home-based COVID-19 detection tests that can be used by anyone. The authors envision that such tests would not require any laboratory setting, and could be performed using test strips coated with antibodies without prior sample processing. Interestingly, our approach does not require any electrode patterning, which makes it the best fit for massive production and high-volume use. It can be adapted as a point-of-care testing platform with high-throughput to be used in schools, airports, malls and public services places as well. The cost per test is expected to be less than one dollar, which will make it competitive with current market price. The detection platform can be easily equipped with standard electronic data transmission systems to transmit and process data in place and share it with family, doctors, and hospitals over wireless transmission. Furthermore, the platform can be deployed in high-risk areas with ease-of-use and clear steps to load the specimen and easy to understand instructions to operate.

Furthermore, when compared with other detection concepts and methodologies, the presented approach can distinguish between influenza and coronaviruses. ACE2 binds directly to the viral spike protein, while ACE2 plays an important role in acute lung injury induced by influenza viruses [49], which can be correlated with disease severity [50]. Hence, the proposed methodology can be used in reverse where the spike protein can be used for ACE2 detection.

5. Conclusions

In summary, this study provides proof-of-principle for an optical-based, quick, simple, and sensitive screening technology for the detection of SARS-CoV-2. It is based on the principle that when light passes through a sample, interactions between the photons and sample occurs within a specific range of *wavelengths*. The current approach utilizes a smartphone light source and a portable mini-spectrophotometer to convert the variations in light intensity into measured signal. The optical responses could further be analyzed using the principle component analysis technique to enhance and allow precise detection of the specific target in a multi-protein mixture. This approach can be further developed to accommodate mass screening that should provide fast and accurate positive or negative test results.

Author Contributions: M.A.A. conceived the study. M.A.A., F.M. and T.A.R. designed the experiments. M.A.A. and N.P. performed the experiments. M.A.A., F.M. and T.A.R. analyzed the data. All authors have read and agreed to the published version of the manuscript.

Funding: This work was supported by UAEU grant 31R129.

Institutional Review Board Statement: Not applicable.

Informed Consent Statement: Not applicable.

Data Availability Statement: Not Applicable.

Acknowledgments: We thank the research office at UAEU for their continuous help and support.

Conflicts of Interest: The authors declare no conflict of interest.

References

1. Wu, F.; Zhao, S.; Yu, B.; Chen, Y.-M.; Wang, W.; Song, Z.-G.; Hu, Y.; Tao, Z.-W.; Tian, J.-H.; Pei, Y.-Y.; et al. A New Coronavirus Associated with Human Respiratory Disease in China. *Nature* **2020**, *579*, 265–269. [CrossRef] [PubMed]
2. Center for Systems Science and Engineering. COVID-19 Dashboard by the Center for Systems Science and Engineering (CSSE) at Johns Hopkins University (JHU). Available online: https://coronavirus.jhu.edu/map.html (accessed on 7 July 2020).
3. Zou, L.; Ruan, F.; Huang, M.; Liang, L.; Huang, H.; Hong, Z.; Yu, J.; Kang, M.; Song, Y.; Xia, J.; et al. SARS-CoV-2 Viral Load in Upper Respiratory Specimens of Infected Patients. *N. Engl. J. Med.* **2020**, *382*, 1177–1179. [CrossRef] [PubMed]
4. Uddin, M.; Mustafa, F.; Rizvi, T.A.; Loney, T.; Al Suwaidi, H.; Al-Marzouqi, A.H.H.; Eldin, A.K.; Alsabeeha, N.; Adrian, T.E.; Stefanini, C.; et al. SARS-CoV-2/COVID-19: Viral Genomics, Epidemiology, Vaccines, and Therapeutic Interventions. *Viruses* **2020**, *12*, 526. [CrossRef] [PubMed]
5. Ghebreyesus, T.A. WHO Director-General's Opening Remarks at the Media Briefing on COVID-19. 3 March 2020. Available online: https://www.who.int/dg/speeches/detail/who-director-general-s-opening-remarks-at-the-media-briefing-on-covid-19---3-march-2020 (accessed on 1 October 2021).
6. Li, R.; Pei, S.; Chen, B.; Song, Y.; Zhang, T.; Yang, W.; Shaman, J. Substantial Undocumented Infection Facilitates the Rapid Dissemination of Novel Coronavirus (SARS-CoV-2). *Science* **2020**, *368*, 489–493. [CrossRef] [PubMed]
7. Liu, X.; Feng, J.; Zhang, Q.; Guo, D.; Zhang, L.; Suo, T.; Hu, W.; Guo, M.; Wang, X.; Huang, Z.; et al. Analytical Comparisons of SARS-COV-2 Detection by QRT-PCR and DdPCR with Multiple Primer/Probe Sets. *Emerg. Microbes Infect.* **2020**, *9*, 1175–1179. [CrossRef]
8. Tahamtan, A.; Ardebili, A. Real-Time RT-PCR in COVID-19 Detection: Issues Affecting the Results. *Expert Rev. Mol. Diagn.* **2020**, *20*, 453–454. [CrossRef]
9. Tang, Y.-W.; Schmitz, J.E.; Persing, D.H.; Stratton, C.W. Laboratory Diagnosis of COVID-19: Current Issues and Challenges. *J. Clin. Microbiol.* **2020**, *58*, e00512–e00520. [CrossRef]
10. Slaughter, G. Current Advances in Biosensor Design and Fabrication. In *Encyclopedia of Analytical Chemistry*; John Wiley & Sons, Ltd.: Chichester, UK, 2018; pp. 1–25. [CrossRef]
11. Srinivasan, B.; Tung, S. Development and Applications of Portable Biosensors. *J. Lab. Autom.* **2015**, *20*, 365–389. [CrossRef]
12. Bhalla, N.; Jolly, P.; Formisano, N.; Estrela, P. Introduction to Biosensors. *Essays Biochem.* **2016**, *60*, 1–8. [CrossRef]
13. Mavrikou, S.; Moschopoulou, G.; Tsekouras, V.; Kintzios, S. Development of a Portable, Ultra-Rapid and Ultra-Sensitive Cell-Based Biosensor for the Direct Detection of the SARS-CoV-2 S1 Spike Protein Antigen. *Sensors* **2020**, *20*, 3121. [CrossRef]
14. Helmerhorst, E.; Chandler, D.J.; Nussio, M.; Mamotte, C.D. Real-Time and Label-Free Bio-Sensing of Molecular Interactions by Surface Plasmon Resonance: A Laboratory Medicine Perspective. *Clin. Biochem. Rev.* **2012**, *33*, 161–173.
15. Heller, G.T.; Aprile, F.A.; Vendruscolo, M. Methods of Probing the Interactions between Small Molecules and Disordered Proteins. *Cell. Mol. Life Sci.* **2017**, *74*, 3225–3243. [CrossRef]
16. Hoffmann, M.; Kleine-Weber, H.; Schroeder, S.; Krüger, N.; Herrler, T.; Erichsen, S.; Schiergens, T.S.; Herrler, G.; Wu, N.-H.; Nitsche, A.; et al. SARS-CoV-2 Cell Entry Depends on ACE2 and TMPRSS2 and Is Blocked by a Clinically Proven Protease Inhibitor. *Cell* **2020**, *181*, 271–280.e8. [CrossRef]
17. Shang, J.; Wan, Y.; Luo, C.; Ye, G.; Geng, Q.; Auerbach, A.; Li, F. Cell Entry Mechanisms of SARS-CoV-2. *Proc. Natl. Acad. Sci. USA* **2020**, *117*, 11727–11734. [CrossRef] [PubMed]

18. Lan, J.; Ge, J.; Yu, J.; Shan, S.; Zhou, H.; Fan, S.; Zhang, Q.; Shi, X.; Wang, Q.; Zhang, L.; et al. Structure of the SARS-CoV-2 Spike Receptor-Binding Domain Bound to the ACE2 Receptor. *Nature* **2020**, *581*, 215–220. [CrossRef] [PubMed]
19. Yan, R.; Zhang, Y.; Li, Y.; Xia, L.; Guo, Y.; Zhou, Q. Structural Basis for the Recognition of SARS-CoV-2 by Full-Length Human ACE2. *Science* **2020**, *367*, 1444–1448. [CrossRef]
20. Ou, X.; Liu, Y.; Lei, X.; Li, P.; Mi, D.; Ren, L.; Guo, L.; Guo, R.; Chen, T.; Hu, J.; et al. Characterization of Spike Glycoprotein of SARS-CoV-2 on Virus Entry and Its Immune Cross-Reactivity with SARS-CoV. *Nat. Commun.* **2020**, *11*, 1620. [CrossRef] [PubMed]
21. Chen, Y.; Liu, Q.; Guo, D. Emerging Coronaviruses: Genome Structure, Replication, and Pathogenesis. *J. Med. Virol.* **2020**, *92*, 418–423. [CrossRef]
22. To, K.K.-W.; Tsang, O.T.-Y.; Leung, W.-S.; Tam, A.R.; Wu, T.-C.; Lung, D.C.; Yip, C.C.-Y.; Cai, J.-P.; Chan, J.M.-C.; Chik, T.S.-H.; et al. Temporal Profiles of Viral Load in Posterior Oropharyngeal Saliva Samples and Serum Antibody Responses during Infection by SARS-CoV-2: An Observational Cohort Study. *Lancet Infect. Dis.* **2020**, *20*, 565–574. [CrossRef]
23. Du, L.; He, Y.; Zhou, Y.; Liu, S.; Zheng, B.-J.; Jiang, S. The Spike Protein of SARS-CoV—A Target for Vaccine and Therapeutic Development. *Nat. Rev. Microbiol.* **2009**, *7*, 226–236. [CrossRef]
24. Du, L.; Tai, W.; Yang, Y.; Zhao, G.; Zhu, Q.; Sun, S.; Liu, C.; Tao, X.; Tseng, C.-T.K.; Perlman, S.; et al. Introduction of Neutralizing Immunogenicity Index to the Rational Design of MERS Coronavirus Subunit Vaccines. *Nat. Commun.* **2016**, *7*, 13473. [CrossRef] [PubMed]
25. Wrapp, D.; Wang, N.; Corbett, K.S.; Goldsmith, J.A.; Hsieh, C.-L.; Abiona, O.; Graham, B.S.; McLellan, J.S. Cryo-EM Structure of the 2019-NCoV Spike in the Prefusion Conformation. *Science* **2020**, *367*, 1260–1263. [CrossRef] [PubMed]
26. Xia, S.; Zhu, Y.; Liu, M.; Lan, Q.; Xu, W.; Wu, Y.; Ying, T.; Liu, S.; Shi, Z.; Jiang, S.; et al. Fusion Mechanism of 2019-NCoV and Fusion Inhibitors Targeting HR1 Domain in Spike Protein. *Cell. Mol. Immunol.* **2020**, *17*, 765–767. [CrossRef] [PubMed]
27. Xia, S.; Liu, M.; Wang, C.; Xu, W.; Lan, Q.; Feng, S.; Qi, F.; Bao, L.; Du, L.; Liu, S.; et al. Inhibition of SARS-CoV-2 (Previously 2019-NCoV) Infection by a Highly Potent Pan-Coronavirus Fusion Inhibitor Targeting Its Spike Protein That Harbors a High Capacity to Mediate Membrane Fusion. *Cell Res.* **2020**, *30*, 343–355. [CrossRef] [PubMed]
28. Seydoux, E.; Homad, L.J.; MacCamy, A.J.; Parks, K.R.; Hurlburt, N.K.; Jennewein, M.F.; Akins, N.R.; Stuart, A.B.; Wan, Y.H.; Feng, J.; et al. Analysis of a SARS-CoV-2-Infected Individual Reveals Development of Potent Neutralizing Antibodies with Limited Somatic Mutation. *Immunity* **2020**, *53*, 98–105.e5. [CrossRef] [PubMed]
29. Yang, J.; Petitjean, S.; Derclaye, S.; Koehler, M.; Zhang, Q.; Dumitru, A.; Soumillion, P.; Alsteens, D. Molecular Interaction and Inhibition of SARS-CoV-2 Binding to the ACE2 Receptor. *Nat. Commun.* **2020**, *11*, 1–21. [CrossRef]
30. Premkumar, L.; Segovia-Chumbez, B.; Jadi, R.; Martinez, D.R.; Raut, R.; Markmann, A.; Cornaby, C.; Bartelt, L.; Weiss, S.; Park, Y.; et al. The Receptor Binding Domain of the Viral Spike Protein Is an Immunodominant and Highly Specific Target of Antibodies in SARS-CoV-2 Patients. *Sci. Immunol.* **2020**, *5*, eabc8413. [CrossRef] [PubMed]
31. Alberts, B.; Johnson, A.; Lewis, J.; Raff, M.; Roberts, K.; Walter, P. Looking at the Structure of Cells in the Microscope. In *Molecular Biology of the Cell*; Garland Science: New York, NY, USA, 2002.
32. Hales, J.E.; Matmon, G.; Dalby, P.A.; Ward, J.M.; Aeppli, G. Virus Lasers for Biological Detection. *Nat. Commun.* **2019**, *10*, 3594. [CrossRef]
33. Liu, P.Y.; Chin, L.K.; Ser, W.; Chen, H.F.; Hsieh, C.-M.; Lee, C.-H.; Sung, K.-B.; Ayi, T.C.; Yap, P.H.; Liedberg, B.; et al. Cell Refractive Index for Cell Biology and Disease Diagnosis: Past, Present and Future. *Lab Chip* **2016**, *16*, 634–644. [CrossRef]
34. Li, Y.; Hua, N.; Li, J.; Zhong, Z.; Li, S.; Zhao, C.; Xue, X.; Zheng, X. Optical Spectrum Feature Analysis and Recognition for Optical Network Security with Machine Learning. *Opt. Express* **2019**, *27*, 24808. [CrossRef]
35. HAMAMATSU. Mini-Spectrometer MS Series C11708MA. Available online: https://www.hamamatsu.com/jp/en/product/type/C11708MA/index.html (accessed on 1 October 2021).
36. Kim, H.; Jung, Y.; Doh, I.-J.; Lozano-Mahecha, R.A.; Applegate, B.; Bae, E. Smartphone-Based Low Light Detection for Bioluminescence Application. *Sci. Rep.* **2017**, *7*, 40203. [CrossRef]
37. Sino Biological. Available online: https://www.sinobiological.com/ (accessed on 1 October 2021).
38. Al Ahmad, M.; Najar, A.; El Moutaouakil, A.; Nasir, N.; Hussein, M.; Raji, S.; Hilal-Alnaqbi, A. Label-Free Cancer Cells Detection Using Optical Sensors. *IEEE Access* **2018**, *6*, 55807–55814. [CrossRef]
39. Kastritis, P.L.; Bonvin, A.M.J.J. On the Binding Affinity of Macromolecular Interactions: Daring to Ask Why Proteins Interact. *J. R. Soc. Interface* **2013**, *10*, 20120835. [CrossRef]
40. Wang, H.; Tang, Z.; Wang, Y.; Ma, G.; Tao, N. Probing Single Molecule Binding and Free Energy Profile with Plasmonic Imaging of Nanoparticles. *J. Am. Chem. Soc.* **2019**, *141*, 16071–16078. [CrossRef] [PubMed]
41. Kozono, H.; Matsushita, Y.; Ogawa, N.; Kozono, Y.; Miyabe, T.; Sekiguchi, H.; Ichiyanagi, K.; Okimoto, N.; Taiji, M.; Kanagawa, O.; et al. Single-Molecule Motions of MHC Class II Rely on Bound Peptides. *Biophys. J.* **2015**, *108*, 350–359. [CrossRef] [PubMed]
42. Zheng, X.; Wang, J. The Universal Statistical Distributions of the Affinity, Equilibrium Constants, Kinetics and Specificity in Biomolecular Recognition. *PLoS Comput. Biol.* **2015**, *11*, e1004212. [CrossRef]
43. Zheng, X.; Wang, J. Universal Statistical Fluctuations in Thermodynamics and Kinetics of Single Molecular Recognition. *Phys. Chem. Chem. Phys.* **2016**, *18*, 8570–8578. [CrossRef] [PubMed]
44. Masters, B.R. Albert Einstein and the Nature of Light. *Opt. Photonics News* **2012**, *23*, 42. [CrossRef]
45. French, A.P.; Taylor, E.F. *An Introduction to Quantum Physics*, 1st ed.; M.I.T. Introductory Physics Series; CRC Press: Boca Raton, FL, USA, 1979.

46. Wang, Y.; Liu, M.; Gao, J. Enhanced Receptor Binding of SARS-CoV-2 through Networks of Hydrogen-Bonding and Hydrophobic Interactions. *Proc. Natl. Acad. Sci. USA* **2020**, *117*, 13967–13974. [CrossRef]
47. OV, M. Antiviral Properties and Toxicity of Ag-Cystine Complex. *J. Emerg. Dis. Virol.* **2016**, *2*. [CrossRef]
48. Dahal, N.; Nowitzke, J.; Eis, A.; Popa, I. Binding-Induced Stabilization Measured on the Same Molecular Protein Substrate Using Single-Molecule Magnetic Tweezers and Heterocovalent Attachments. *J. Phys. Chem. B* **2020**, *124*, 3283–3290. [CrossRef] [PubMed]
49. Chen, L.; Hao, G. The Role of Angiotensin-Converting Enzyme 2 in Coronaviruses/Influenza Viruses and Cardiovascular Disease. *Cardiovasc. Res.* 2020. [CrossRef]
50. Ni, W.; Yang, X.; Yang, D.; Bao, J.; Li, R.; Xiao, Y.; Hou, C.; Wang, H.; Liu, J.; Yang, D.; et al. Role of Angiotensin-Converting Enzyme 2 (ACE2) in COVID-19. *Crit. Care* **2020**, *24*, 422. [CrossRef] [PubMed]

sensors

MDPI

Article

A Deep Learning Pipeline for Grade Groups Classification Using Digitized Prostate Biopsy Specimens

Kamal Hammouda [1], Fahmi Khalifa [1], Moumen El-Melegy [2], Mohamed Ghazal [3], Hanan E. Darwish [4], Mohamed Abou El-Ghar [5] and Ayman El-Baz [1,*]

1 BioImaging Laboratory, Bioengineering Department, University of Louisville, Louisville, KY 40292, USA; kamal.hammouda@louisville.edu (K.H.); fahmi.khalifa@louisville.edu (F.K.)
2 Department of Electrical Engineering, Assiut University, Assiut 71515, Egypt; moumen@aun.edu.eg
3 Electrical and Computer Engineering Department, Abu Dhabi University, Abu Dhabi 59911, United Arab Emirates; mohammed.ghazal@adu.ac.ae
4 Mathematics Department, Faculty of Science, Mansoura University, Mansoura 35516, Egypt; Hedarwish@mans.edu.eg
5 Radiology Department, Urology and Nephrology Center, Mansoura University, Mansoura 35516, Egypt; maboelghar@mans.edu.eg
* Correspondence: aselba01@louisville.edu

Abstract: Prostate cancer is a significant cause of morbidity and mortality in the USA. In this paper, we develop a computer-aided diagnostic (CAD) system for automated grade groups (GG) classification using digitized prostate biopsy specimens (PBSs). Our CAD system aims to firstly classify the Gleason pattern (GP), and then identifies the Gleason score (GS) and GG. The GP classification pipeline is based on a pyramidal deep learning system that utilizes three convolution neural networks (CNN) to produce both patch- and pixel-wise classifications. The analysis starts with sequential preprocessing steps that include a histogram equalization step to adjust intensity values, followed by a PBSs' edge enhancement. The digitized PBSs are then divided into overlapping patches with the three sizes: 100 × 100 (CNN_S), 150 × 150 (CNN_M), and 200 × 200 (CNN_L), pixels, and 75% overlap. Those three sizes of patches represent the three pyramidal levels. This pyramidal technique allows us to extract rich information, such as that the larger patches give more global information, while the small patches provide local details. After that, the patch-wise technique assigns each overlapped patch a label as GP categories (1 to 5). Then, the majority voting is the core approach for getting the pixel-wise classification that is used to get a single label for each overlapped pixel. The results after applying those techniques are three images of the same size as the original, and each pixel has a single label. We utilized the majority voting technique again on those three images to obtain only one. The proposed framework is trained, validated, and tested on 608 whole slide images (WSIs) of the digitized PBSs. The overall diagnostic accuracy is evaluated using several metrics: precision, recall, F1-score, accuracy, macro-averaged, and weighted-averaged. The (CNN_L) has the best accuracy results for patch classification among the three CNNs, and its classification accuracy is 0.76. The macro-averaged and weighted-average metrics are found to be around 0.70–0.77. For GG, our CAD results are about 80% for precision, and between 60% to 80% for recall and F1-score, respectively. Also, it is around 94% for accuracy and NPV. To highlight our CAD systems' results, we used the standard ResNet50 and VGG-16 to compare our CNN's patch-wise classification results. As well, we compared the GG's results with that of the previous work.

Keywords: deep learning; classification; grade groups; CAD system; prostate cancer

Citation: Hammouda, K.; Khalifa, F.; El-Melegy, M.; Ghazal, M.; Darwish, H.E.; Abou El-Ghar, M.; El-Baz, A. A Deep Learning Pipeline for Grade Groups Classification Using Digitized Prostate Biopsy Specimens. *Sensors* **2021**, *21*, 6708. https://doi.org/10.3390/s21206708

Academic Editor: Yu-Dong Zhang

Received: 3 September 2021
Accepted: 4 October 2021
Published: 9 October 2021

1. Introduction

The most recent statistics from the American Cancer Society showed that prostate cancer (PC) is the most prevalent type of cancer with 248,530 (26%) cases, and it is also the second leading cause of cancer-related death with 34,130 (26%) [1] among men. Prostate tumors are like many other cancers in that the initial stage does not cause death or pain. By time the tumor is recognized, it has advanced to high grade with increase mortality [1]. The pathological evaluation of prostate biopsies determines the best treatment method of PC [2]. One of the methods used to characterize the heterogeneous tumor growth patterns is the Gleason grading system, which observes in a biopsy regarding their degree of discrimination or the Gleason pattern (GP).

The GP practically ranges from GP1 through GP5. The GP1 (stroma) and GP2 (benign) represent the nonepithelium tissue. While GP3, GP4, and GP5 represent the epithelium tissue. GP3 indicates moderately differentiated glands compared with that of GP5, which represents poorly differentiated cells [3,4]. Many factors contribute to determining the stage of PC, like the prostate-specific antigen (PSA) level. However, the primary factor is the Gleason score (GS). The GS is the grading system used to determine PC's aggressiveness depending on the two most frequent GP observed in the biopsy [5]. Typically, the GS ranges from 6 to 10, where 6 illustrates low-grade cancer, i.e., the cancer is likely to grow slowly, and 10 represents high-grade, i.e., the cancer is expected to spread more rapidly.

The GS grading system is often divided into only three categories, 6, 7, and 8–10 [5]. This classification is rather coarse. For example, GS7 could indicate that the most cells are GP3, followed by GP4, or that most cells are GP4, followed by GP3; however, the latter case has a much worse prognosis. Similarly, GS9 or GS10 has a worse prognosis than GS8 despite often being grouped together. Eventually, the 2014 International Society of Urological Pathology (ISUP) developed a simple grading system for PC: grade groups (GG) system, based on the visual assessment of cell differentiation and GP predominance [6], see Figure 1. The GG ranges from GG1 to GG5, with higher GG indicating greater clinical risk. Table 1 shows the relation between the Gleason grading (GP and GS) and the GG system, besides the shape of cell tissues for GP and the GG's risk level.

Table 1. Grading systems for a prostate biopsy specimen are the Gleason grading system, the Gleason pattern (GP) and Gleason score (GS), as well as the grade groups (GP) system.

Shape of Cell Tissues		GP	Risk Level	GS	GG
stroma (connective tissue, non-epithelium tissue)		GP1	-	-	-
healthy (benign) epithelium		GP2	-	-	-
moderately differentiated	Distinctly infiltration of cells form glands at margins	GP3	Low	GP3 + GP3 = GS6	GG1
			Favorable	GP3 + GP4 = GS7	GG2
moderately and Poorly differentiated	Irregular messes of neoplastic cells with few glands	GP4	Unfavorable	GP4 + GP3 = GS7	GG3
			High	GP4 + GP4 = GS8 GP3 + GP5 = GS8 GP5 + GP3 = GS8	GG4
Poorly differentiated	Lack of or occasional glands, sheets of cells	GP5	High	GP4 + GP5 = GS9 GP5 + GP4 = GS9 GP5 + GP5 = GS10	GG5

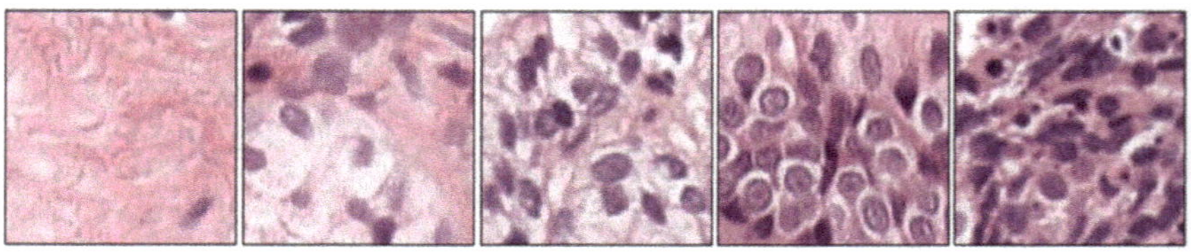

Figure 1. Examples of GP labels.

The discordance in GG diagnosis by different pathologists using the same biopsy is between 30–50% [3,7,8]. Agreement is greater among pathologists with urologic subspecialty training and high experience than among pathologists in general [9]. Accurate diagnosis of prostate biopsy specimens helps physicians to make essential treatment decisions [9,10]. Due to expert subspecialists' availability, the development of an automated system for assessing prostate biopsy specimens with expert-level performance could improve prostate biopsy's clinical utility.

In recent years, extensive research work was developed to diagnose the tumorous lesions for many organs, especially the prostate [11–14]. Deep learning (DL) combined with histopathology and radiology imaging, particularly magnetic resonance imaging (MRI), plays an essential role in grading the prostate's cancerous tissues [4,15–17]. For histopathology, Arvaniti et al. [18] developed a DL approach to identify automated Gleason grading of prostate cancer tissue microarrays with Hematoxylin and Eosin (H&E) staining. This model's advantages were that it was trained by a dataset of about 641 patients and tested on an independent cohort of 245 patients annotated by two pathologists. Cohen's quadratic kappa statistic was used to the interannotator agreements between the model and each pathologist. The authors reported the results for the GP and GS. However, they did not mention the final classification of the GG that is considered the simple grading system for PC. Also, Bulten et al. [19] introduced automated grading prostate biopsies using a DL system. They focus on classifying the GP for the prostate biopsies, and then identifying the GS depending on the GP predominance. Their DL approach was developed using 5834 biopsies from 1243 patients. The authors did not report the overall accuracy of the GP classification; they reported only the final results for the GG. Similarly, Nagpal et al. [4] used a DL approach to improve GS for whole-slide images of prostatectomies. The system was developed using 112 million pathologist-annotated image patches from 1226 slides and tested on an independent validation dataset of 331 slides. The author considered the GG4 with GG5 as one class and did not report the individual results for both of them. The view tissue for the GG5 is very similar to the GG4, and it is considered the big challenge to differentiate between them.

According to the previous studies, the general technique to classify the GG, (see e.g., the work in [19]) is that the DL systems are developed to segment digitized prostate biopsy specimens (PBSs) into regions according to GP, after which the GG is identified depending on the GS and GP grade and its predominance. However, no study reported the overall accuracy of the GP segmentation. They reported only the final results for the GG. Our work develops a DL-based computer-aided diagnostic (CAD) system for reading digitized PBSs sections and dealing with GP as a classification problem, not as a segmentation task using patch- and pixel-wise classification methodology. This is the first time this ideas was applied, to the best of our knowledge. Finally, GP labels are used to determine the GS and GG, and their performance is comparable to expert subspecialists.

The rest of the paper is structured as follows. Section 2 describes in details the proposed DL pipeline. The performance metrics used for evaluation and the details of experimental results are given in Section 3. The limitation and highlights for our pipeline are discussed in Section 4. Finally, Section 5 concludes the work.

2. Methods

This work's primary objective is to develop a CAD system for accurate GG diagnosis of PBSs. The proposed overall CAD system performs GP classification, as well as identifies the GS and GG. The GP classification pipeline consists of three stages: a DL system consisting of fusion three convolution neural networks (CNN); namely, a pyramidal CNN. Also, a patch and pixel-wise classification that divided the original image into patches and labeled them according to GP, the majority voting techniques is used in this step to merge the patches images into the original size, see Figure 2. Finally, identifying the GS and GG depends on the classification of the GP.

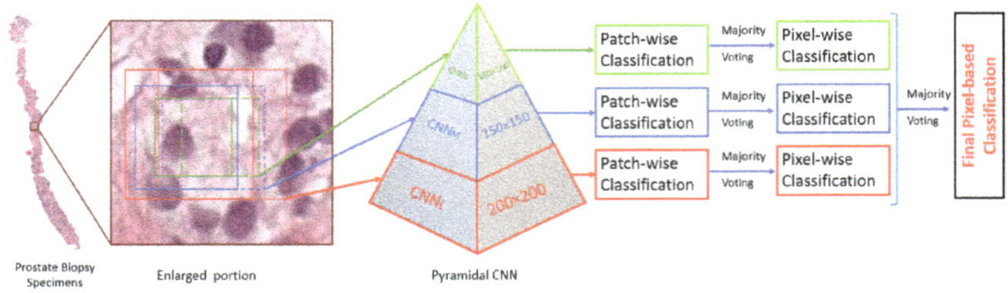

Figure 2. The proposed pipeline for our CAD system.

2.1. Deep Learning System

The CNN plays an essential role in many fields of medical image analysis, especially in the segmentation [12,20,21], and classification [22,23]. Our DL system has a pyramidal architecture containing three CNNs, see Figure 2. The overall framework for our DL system is depicted in Figure 3 , which shows the training and testing phases for for patch-wise classification. For the training model, the preprocessing step is applied to prepare the input data for the CNN. The preprocessing includes histogram equalization followed by edge enhancement [24,25]. The edge enhancement is applied to make the edges visible prominently by increasing the contrast of the pixels around the specific edges. The convolution matrix, namely, mask or kernel, is utilized to enhance the edges [24,25]. Figure 4 shows the effect of applying edge enhancement and histogram equalization on the original prostate patch. After that, the PBSs images are divided into overlapping patches with three different sizes: 100 × 100, 150 × 150, and 200 × 200 pixels, see Figure 2. The overlap between successive patches is 75%. The generation of overlapped patches provides different image viewpoints that enhance the DL framework's training and validation. We select for training those patches with no more than 30% of their area labeled as background in the ground truth. Each patch is assigned a single label, being the ground truth GP of most pixels in the patch. If the winning label matches the value of the center of the given patch, then this patch is selected for training. Otherwise, we remove it from the CNN training. Algorithm 1 presents all details about the preprocessing step.

The pyramidal CNN is composed of three CNNs, and each one has a different patch size, as shown in Figure 2. We designed the three CNNs such that they have the same architecture but with different sizes. The prominent architecture of any DL-CNN base consists of input layers, hidden layers, and an output layer [26]. Our CNN's input layer is fed with the patches from the first step (preprocessing) for our proposed framework. The small CNN (CNN_S) is fed with 100 × 100 patches, the medium CNN (CNN_M) is fed with 150 × 150 patches, and the large CNN (CNN_L) is provided with 200 × 200 patches. The core of CNN is the hidden layers that contain the number of CNN parameters and weights. The architecture of the hidden layers of our CNN is represented by a series of convolution layers (CLs) intervened by max-pooling layers (MPLs) and dropout layer, followed by two fully connected layers (FCls). Finally, there is a soft-max layer to give the probability for the five classes.

In the CL, the image is convolved with kernels (multiple kernels in each layer) to extract prominent features that describe the object of interest in the input patch; these features are called feature maps. Therefore, each CL results in a volume of feature maps. In our implementation, we use kernels of size 3 × 3. In MPLs, the spatial dimensions are reduced by a factor of two. Benefits are twofold: firstly, keeping only the most prominent features, discarding those less essential, and secondly, reducing computational cost and training time. In our implementation, the stride is equal to one for all layers.

Algorithm 1: Preprocessing step of developing input data for a convolution neural network (CNN). Value of N is 100, 150, or 200.

Input: Prostate biopsy specimens digitized.
Output: Classified selected patches into Gleason pattern labels .

1. Apply the histogram equalization and edge enhancement on the PBSs.
2. Divide the PBSs into overlapping patches, with size N × N pixels and 75% overlapping.
3. Selecting appropriate patches for training
    - Calculate the majority voting for the pathological patch, WL ← Winning Label.
    - Estimate two variables for corresponding label path, RB←ratio of Background and CV ←Center value.
    - If $(WL == CV)\&(RB \leq 0.3)$
        Select the patch
      Else
        Remove the patch

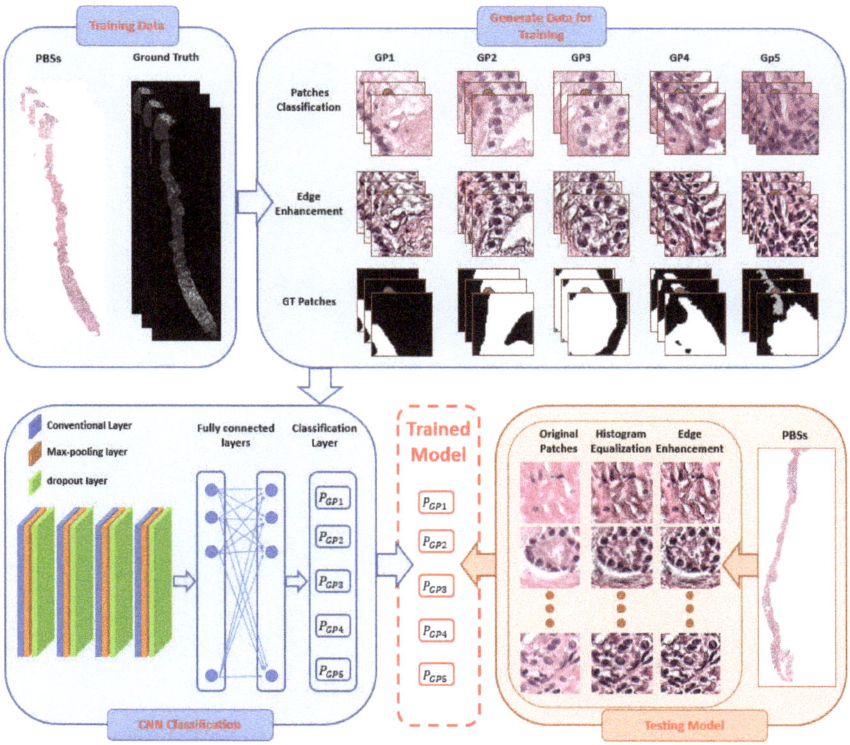

Figure 3. Proposed pipeline for patch-wise classification, while PBSs is prostate biopsy specimens and Gleason pattern labels (GP).

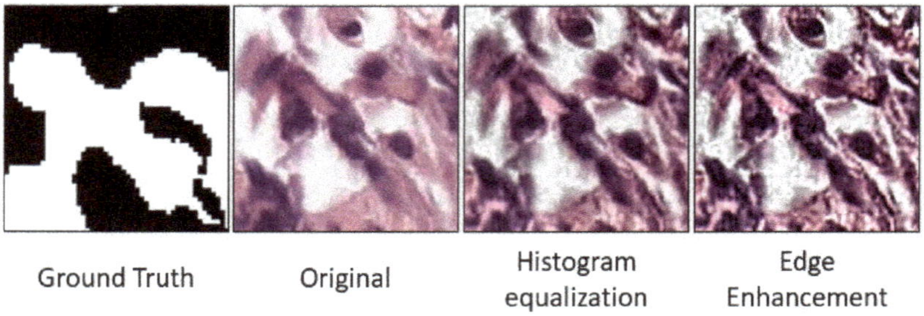

Figure 4. Example for applying prepossessing step on original patch: histogram equalization and edge enhancement.

The CNN contains four convolution layers, and the number of CLs filters is 16, 32, 64, and 128. The dropout layers weight 0.1, 0.1, 0.3, 0.3. The number of units for the FCLs is 64 and 512, respectively. The training seeks to minimize the cross-entropy loss between the predicted probabilities and the ground truth labels. The dropouts layers follow FCLs to minimize network overfitting, and the dropout rate is set to 0.15 for both layers. The total and trainable parameters for CNN_S, CNN_M, and CNN_L, are 264,421, 534,757, and 952,549, respectively, and there are no nontrainable parameters for all of them. The labeled patches are used to train the proposed CNN. During the training, the CNN uses iterative optimization to learn its weights to maximize the number of correctly classified samples during prediction.

Our DL model has numerous parameters. Therefore, we utilized a hyper-parameter tuning with a random search (RS) technique that helps to reduce overfitting and improves our model's performance. Our system's accuracy is assessed by performing training, validation, and testing for the patches. The curves for the accuracy and loss of training the CNN_L, the best accuracy among three CNN, are presented in Figure 5. Also, the validation (accuracy and loss) curves are shown in Figure 5. By increasing the number of epochs, the validation accuracy rises until it reaches around 0.78, and the validation loss decreases until it gets around 0.7.

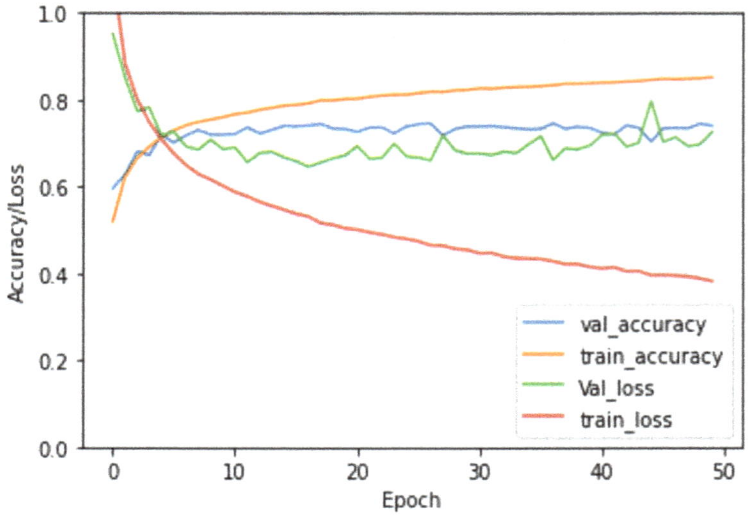

Figure 5. Training loss and accuracy as well as validation loss and accuracy in dataset for our proposed CNN_M.

2.2. Patch- and Pixel-Wise Classification

The goal for the patch-wise technique is to label all patches generated from the digitized PBS. We apply the patch-wise classification for all three CNNs individually during the test to assign each overlapped patch a label from one to five as GP categories. After that, a pixel-wise classification is applied to obtain three images of the same size as the original. The pixel-wise technique utilizes the output from the patch-wise classification, labeled patches generated from the three CNNs, to give all pixels that contain this patch the same label. Most of the pixels appear in several batches due to overlapped batches. Therefore, overlapped pixels have multiple labels depending on their position in the image. The majority voting is the core approach for the pixel-wise classification to get a single label for each overlapped pixel. The two techniques, patch- and pixel-wise, are used on the output of the three CNNs. The results after applying those techniques are three images of the same size as the original (each pixel has three labels); then, we applied majority voting again on those three images to obtain the final pixel-based classification.

2.3. Grade Groups System

The identification of the GG label is considered our goal in this work. Each digitized PBSs has labels between 1–5 according to its GP. We utilize Table 1 that demonstrates the relation between three measurements (GP, GS, and GG) to generate the GS from GP. Thus, identifying the GG from GS.

3. Results

The proposed framework is trained, validated, and tested on 416, 96, and 96, respectively, with whole slide images (WSIs) of the digitized PBSs from the Radboud University Medical Center, USA, and it was analyzed by the University of Louisville Hospital, USA [19,27]. A semiautomatic labeling technique was utilized to circumvent the need for full manual annotation by pathologists. Expert pathologists defined the GP, GS, and GG for all WSIs, and the digitized PBSs are divided into overlapping patches for patch and pixel-wise classification according to the GP ground truth. Our CAD software is primarily implemented in Python and Matlab programming environments. The experimental results were also performed on a Dell Precision workstation with an Intel Xeon eight-core CPU running at 3.31 GHz and 128 GB RAM.

The total number of patches for each CNN_S, CNN_M, and CNN_L are around 5.8, 3.6, and 1.7 million, respectively. Those patches belong to 608 (416, 96, and 96) of the WSIs of the digitized PBS. The WSIs, 608, are separated into training, validation, and testing before generating the patches that means the model doesn't see the validation or testing patches. We face a big challenge to train our model with a balanced dataset because the occurrence of the GP1 is very high with around 60% of the PBS, and the other four types (GP2, GP3, GP4, GP5) have almost 40%. Therefore, we utilized all batches generated from the four GP (GP2, GP3, GP4, GP5) during our training and randomly selected the number of patches from the GP1 that made the number of patches very close. The CNN_S, CNN_M, and CNN_L were trained with around 130, 45, and 25,000 patches, respectively, for each group.

Our goal for this automated system is to identify the GG. Therefore, there are many steps, and each one has its results before reaching our target. We show first the accuracy for each CNN, pyramidal CNN, especially the patch-wise classification, see Tables 2 and 3. After that, we demonstrate the system's accuracy for the GG. More details are presented in the following two subsections.

Table 2. Patch-wise classification accuracy for our proposed CNN_S and CNN_L using precision, recall, F1-score, accuracy, macro-averaged, and weighted-averaged.

	CNN_S			CNN_M			CNN_L		
	Precision	**Recall**	**F1-Score**	**Precision**	**Recall**	**F1-Score**	**Precision**	**Recall**	**F1-Score**
Class 1	0.86	0.97	0.91	0.92	0.97	0.94	0.96	0.94	0.95
Class2	0.74	0.79	0.76	0.77	0.80	0.78	0.81	0.82	0.81
Class3	0.66	0.63	0.76	0.68	0.62	0.65	0.75	0.68	0.71
Class4	0.66	0.44	0.52	0.63	0.55	0.59	0.64	0.66	0.65
Class5	0.53	0.66	0.59	0.46	0.63	0.53	0.42	0.53	0.47
Accuracy	0.70	0.70	0.70	0.73	0.73	0.73	0.76	0.76	0.76
Macro-averaged	0.68	0.70	0.69	0.69	0.71	0.70	0.72	0.73	0.72
Weighted-average	0.70	0.70	0.70	0.73	0.73	0.72	0.77	0.76	0.76

Table 3. Patch-wise classification accuracy for our proposed CNN_L and VGG-16 network using precision, recall, F1-score, accuracy, macro-averaged, and weighted-averaged.

	CNN_L			**VGG-16**			**ResNet50**		
	Precision	**Recall**	**F1-Score**	**Precision**	**Recall**	**F1-Score**	**Precision**	**Recall**	**F1-Score**
Class1	0.96	0.94	0.95	0.87	0.82	0.85	0.94	0.93	0.94
Class2	0.81	0.82	0.81	0.76	0.56	0.64	0.74	0.93	0.82
Class3	0.75	0.68	0.71	0.65	0.58	0.62	0.75	0.65	0.70
Class4	0.64	0.66	0.65	0.51	0.63	0.56	0.72	0.54	0.61
Class5	0.42	0.53	0.47	0.35	0.59	0.44	0.58	0.76	0.66
Accuracy	0.76	0.76	0.76	0.65	0.65	0.65	0.75	0.75	0.75
Macro-averaged	0.72	0.73	0.72	0.63	0.64	0.62	0.75	0.76	0.75
Weighted-average	0.77	0.76	0.76	0.68	0.65	0.65	0.77	0.76	0.76

3.1. Patch-Wise Classification for Each CNN

The overall diagnostic classification accuracy is evaluated using the accuracy metrics precision, recall, F1-score, accuracy, macro-averaged, and weighted-averaged [28,29]. The F1-score is computed by the formula:

$$F1\text{-}score = \frac{2 \times (precision \times recall)}{(precision + recall)} \tag{1}$$

The overall accuracy is the proportion of correctly classified samples out of all the samples; then, it must be equal for all metrics: precision, recall, F1-score. To summarize, the following always holds for the micro-F1.

$$micro\text{-}F1 = micro\text{-}precision = micro\text{-}recall = accuracy \tag{2}$$

since for the micro-averaging case, they are also equal to their harmonic mean; in other words, the micro-F1 case. The macro-average is also calculated for each metric and computed as simple arithmetic means of our per-class. The weighted average is the weighted of each class by the number of samples from that class.

The patch-wise classification results for our proposed pyramidal CNN are reported in Tables 2 and 3. For CNN_S, CNN_M, and CNN_L, the classification accuracy is in the range 0.70–0.76. The macro-averaged and weighted-average metrics are found to be around

0.68–0.77. To highlight the advantages of using our DL (CNN), the accuracy of our pipeline is compared against standard ResNet50, and VGG-16 [22,30]. The input patches are resized into 224 × 224 pixels to fit with the image input size of the ResNet50 and VGG-16. The F1-score of VGG-16 is in the range of 0.58–0.70. In addition, the macro-averaged and weighted-average metrics are both found to be 0.63. The accuracy of our CNN_L is high compared with that of the VGG-16 (0.65) and almost the same with that of ResNet50 (0.75), see Table 3. Besides the high accuracy for our CNN, there are two reasons for creating this CNN. Firstly, the computational cost for the RestNet50 and VGG-16 is high compared with that of our CNN. The number of parameters for ResNet50 and VGG-16 is almost 23 and 27 million, respectively, and our CNN is approximately one million. The second reason is that our pyramidal CNN needs a flexible size for the CNN, and a standard CNN like ResNet50 is a fixed-size that is 224 × 224.

3.2. Grade Group Results

After applying the patch- and pixel-wise classification for each CNN, we merge the CNN outputs to obtain the production of the digitized PBS as the exact size of the original one. The new digitized PBS defines the results for GP from our automated system. We identify the GS and GG, the goal of our pipeline, using the fundamental converting that presents in the Table 1. Figure 6 shows the GG examples for our automated system results, which compare the reference standard and the predicted GG from our system using the distribution of GG.

The overall GG diagnostic accuracy is summarized in Table 4, which presents the accuracy metrics precision, recall, F1-score, accuracy, and negative predictive value (NPV). Also, the confusion matrices for the grade groups results are shown in Figure 7. To validate our CAD system's results and demonstrate its value, we compared our results with the pathologists' estimated results, and previous work[19]. Firstly, the discordance for diagnosing the GG from the same biopsy is between 30% and 50% for various pathologists [3,7,8]. Therefore, our CAD system's accuracy compared with that of pathologists' estimated results is acceptable because our results are about 80% for precision, between 60–80% for recall and F1-score, and around 94% for accuracy and NPV. Secondly, the average accuracy and NPV for our automated CAD system to identify GG are 0.8767 and 0.9167, respectively, while the previous work [19] has 0.8500 and 0.9100, respectively. The obtained results show that our results compared with that of previous work are higher than two percent for an average of accuracy and almost the same for the NPV.

Table 4. Grade groups classification of our CAD system using precision, recall, F1-score, accuracy, and negative predictive value (NPV).

	Precision	Recall	F1-Score	Accuracy	NPV	Cases
Benign	0.75	0.75	0.76	0.92	0.95	8
GG1	0.71	0.71	0.71	0.92	0.95	7
GG2	0.75	0.50	0.60	0.92	0.93	6
GG3	0.71	0.45	0.56	0.84	0.86	11
GG4	0.23	0.50	0.32	0.80	0.92	6
GG5	0.73	0.67	0.70	0.86	0.89	12

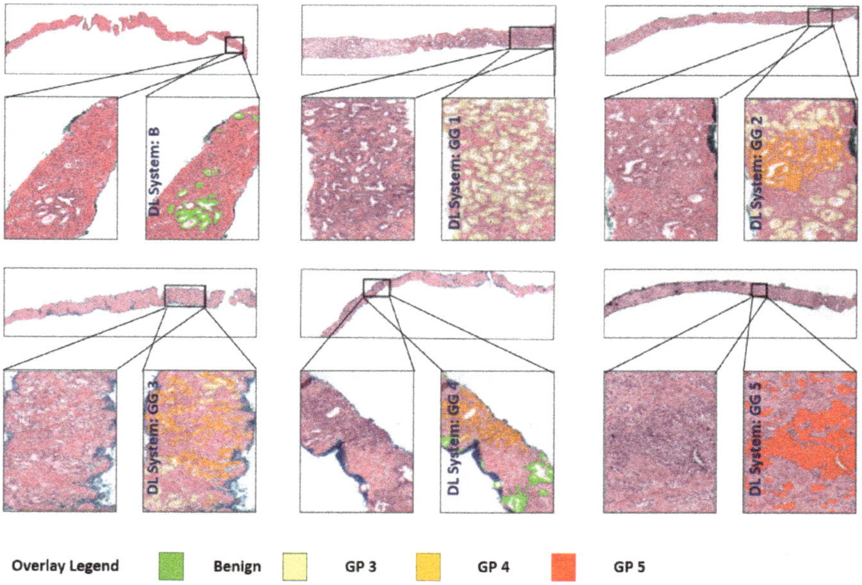

Figure 6. Examples of GG results from our system. In zoomed regions, system's GP prediction is shown as an overlay on tissue; B (benign).

Consensus \ Deep learning system	Benign	1	2	3	4	5
Benign	6	1	0	0	1	0
1	0	5	1	0	1	0
2	0	0	3	2	1	0
3	0	1	0	5	4	1
4	1	0	0	0	3	2
5	1	0	0	0	3	8

Figure 7. Confusion matrices on grade groups.

4. Discussion

The treatment for prostate cancer over the years improved for men with low-risk diseases. Notably, for patients with localized prostate cancer, active surveillance is safer compared with radical prostatectomy, as verified by many trials [31]. According to the American Society of Clinical Oncology, the GG and GP grading are considered the decision-maker according to the guideline of the American Society of Clinical Oncology [32]. The consults were recommended to enhance the consistency and quality of care due to the interobserver variability for the Gleason system [32,33]. Therefore, our automated CAD system could be a valuable decision support tool for patients' GG with localized disease and give significant downstream treatment implications.

For that purpose, we developed an automated DL architecture for classifying the GG of digitized PBS. The ground truth of our datasets was performed using many experienced urologic subspecialists. They have around 25 years of experience with diverse backgrounds, and accessed several histologic sections and immunohistochemically stained sections for every specimen. The overall accuracy for our CAD system showed a similar rate compared with that of general pathologists, which is 70%. According to [34,35], the DL system can be used to alert pathologists of what might be missed. Otherwise, defining small tissue regions depends on a pathologist's judgment that leads to overrule of false-positive categorizations. Therefore, our DL-CAD system has benefits for bolstering the selection of treatment modalities, especially for patients with localized disease.

Developing a framework with high accuracy is our ultimate goal in which DL, patch-, and pixel-wise classification were performed. The accuracy of the diagnostic results for the proposed framework using pyramidal CNN presents that CNN_L had higher accuracy than that of CNN_S and CNN_M, see Tables 2 and 3 and Figure 5 , which show the validation curves for the CNN_L. The comparison between the best CNN against the standard ResNet50 and VGG-16 [22,30], shown in Table 3, emphasizes the benefits of using the hyper-parameter tuning and the RS technique. Besides, using the new idea to identify the problem as classification one, not a segmentation, developed high accuracy.

The proposed CAD system can be helpful in healthcare systems in several ways, such as decreasing the consultation-associated costs, enhancing grading consistency, and reducing treatment-related morbidity for men with low-risk diseases. The performance metrics for GG estimation are higher for G1 and G2 grades compared with that of G3, G4, G5. Therefore, our automated system could be accurately classifying low-risk cases that are eligible for more conservative management.

The GG classification plays an essential role in prostate cancer treatment [31,36]. Still, it is not a straightforward task to the extent that there is no match the results between the subspecialists and the general pathologists' for the GG classification. The subspecialists' grading is more concordant than the general pathologists' grading [37]. However, due to the difficulty of GG and inherent subjectivity, there is discordance between subspecialists. Therefore, it is critical to enhance the risk stratification for prostate cancer by overcoming those disagreements. Developing a system with high precision that human graders and predict clinical risk is our priority. Machine learning, especially DL, models could distinguish novel histoprognostic signals that the human eye can not discover [38,39], as well as assistance in stratifying patient risk like existing molecular tests [40].

Despite the promising results, our automated DL system has some limitations. Firstly, our DL model was trained and tested from a single institution. Therefore, using an external test dataset for the different centers and WSI with various staining protocols should further enhance the robustness of our automated system. Secondly, our DL models, as well the pathologists who made the ground truth labeling, treated each biopsy as an independent sample. In clinical practice, multiple biopsies are sampled from various regions of the prostate. Therefore, an update to our model could take multiple biopsies into account and give a grade group prediction at the patient level. Finally, our study concentrated on the grading of acinar adenocarcinoma in prostate biopsies. However, prostate biopsies can contain other tumor types and foreign tissue, such as colon glands. The biopsies could also include additional prognostic information, such as the detection of intraductal carcinoma [41].

5. Conclusions

This paper introduced a Deep Learning-based CAD system to classify the grade groups (GG) system using digitized prostate biopsy specimens (PBSs) using pyramidal CNN, with patch- and pixel-wise classifications. The proposed pipeline results highlight our system's potential to classify all five GG of the PBSs in comparison with that of other standard CNNs. The agreement between our CAD system and pathologists is comparable to inter-rater reliability among pathologists. In future work, because the digitized PBSs do not have the same direction, adding a new preprocessing step to overcome this challenge will fit our results. This processing rotates the overlapped patches with angles 45 and 90, and flipping them will enhance our pyramidal CNN accuracy. In addition, to highlight our model, we will try to test our model with a dataset from another institution.

Author Contributions: K.H.: designed the algorithm and performed the CNN validation and testing. F.K. and K.H.: designed the algorithm and analysis methods and provided writing the initial manuscript draft. M.E.-M. and M.A.E.-G.: validated the results. A.E.-B. and M.E.-M. and M.A.E.-G.: secure funding. M.G. and H.E.D.: helped with the statistical analysis. K.H., F.K. and A.E.-B.: conceived the idea. All authors have read and agreed to the published version of the manuscript.

Funding: The authors like to acknowledge the support of the National Program for Research & Innovation in Health and Biomedical Sciences, Academy of Scientific Research and Technology in Egypt in this work.

Institutional Review Board Statement: This is a publicly available dataset.

Informed Consent Statement: Informed consent was obtained from all subjects involved in the study.

Data Availability Statement: The data used in this study is available from https://www.kaggle.com/c/prostate-cancer-grade-assessment, accessed on 3 October 2021.

Acknowledgments: The authors like to acknowledge the support of the National Program for Research & Innovation in Health and Biomedical Sciences, Academy of Scientific Research and Technology in Egypt in this work.

Conflicts of Interest: The authors declare no conflict of interest.

References

1. American Cancer Society. Cancer Facts and Figures. 2021. Available online: https://www.cancer.org/research/cancer-facts-statistics/all-cancer-facts-figures/cancer-facts-figures-2021.html (accessed on 3 October 2021).
2. Litwin, M.S.; Tan, H.J. The diagnosis and treatment of prostate cancer: A review. *JAMA* **2017**, *317*, 2532–2542. [CrossRef]
3. Veloso, S.G.; Lima, M.F.; Salles, P.G.; Berenstein, C.K.; Scalon, J.D.; Bambirra, E.A. Interobserver agreement of Gleason score and modified Gleason score in needle biopsy and in surgical specimen of prostate cancer. *Int. Braz. J. Urol.* **2007**, *33*, 639–651. [CrossRef]
4. Nagpal, K.; Foote, D.; Liu, Y.; Chen, P.H.C.; Wulczyn, E.; Tan, F.; Olson, N.; Smith, J.L.; Mohtashamian, A.; Wren, J.H.; et al. Development and validation of a deep learning algorithm for improving Gleason scoring of prostate cancer. *NPJ Digit. Med.* **2019**, *2*, 1–10. [CrossRef]
5. Matoso, A.; Epstein, J.I. Defining clinically significant prostate cancer on the basis of pathological findings. *Histopathology* **2019**, *74*, 135–145. [CrossRef]
6. Epstein, J.I.; Egevad, L.; Amin, M.B.; Delahunt, B.; Srigley, J.R.; Humphrey, P.A. The 2014 International Society of Urological Pathology (ISUP) consensus conference on Gleason grading of prostatic carcinoma. *Am. J. Surg. Pathol.* **2016**, *40*, 244–252. [CrossRef]
7. Melia, J.; Moseley, R.; Ball, R.; Griffiths, D.; Grigor, K.; Harnden, P.; Jarmulowicz, M.; McWilliam, L.; Montironi, R.; Waller, M.; et al. A UK-based investigation of inter-and intra-observer reproducibility of Gleason grading of prostatic biopsies. *Histopathology* **2006**, *48*, 644–654. [CrossRef]
8. Egevad, L.; Ahmad, A.S.; Algaba, F.; Berney, D.M.; Boccon-Gibod, L.; Compérat, E.; Evans, A.J.; Griffiths, D.; Grobholz, R.; Kristiansen, G.; et al. Standardization of Gleason grading among 337 European pathologists. *Histopathology* **2013**, *62*, 247–256. [CrossRef]
9. Kvåle, R.; Møller, B.; Wahlqvist, R.; Fosså, S.D.; Berner, A.; Busch, C.; Kyrdalen, A.E.; Svindland, A.; Viset, T.; Halvorsen, O.J. Concordance between Gleason scores of needle biopsies and radical prostatectomy specimens: A population-based study. *BJU Int.* **2009**, *103*, 1647–1654. [CrossRef]
10. Bottke, D.; Golz, R.; Störkel, S.; Hinke, A.; Siegmann, A.; Hertle, L.; Miller, K.; Hinkelbein, W.; Wiegel, T. Phase 3 study of adjuvant radiotherapy versus wait and see in pT3 prostate cancer: Impact of pathology review on analysis. *Eur. Urol.* **2013**, *64*, 193–198. [CrossRef]
11. Kasivisvanathan, V.; Rannikko, A.S.; Borghi, M.; Panebianco, V.; Mynderse, L.A.; Vaarala, M.H.; Briganti, A.; Budäus, L.; Hellawell, G.; Hindley, R.G.; et al. MRI-targeted or standard biopsy for prostate-cancer diagnosis. *N. Engl. J. Med.* **2018**, *378*, 1767–1777. [CrossRef]

12. Hammouda, K.; Khalifa, F.; Soliman, A.; Abdeltawab, H.; Ghazal, M.; Abou El-Ghar, M.; Haddad, A.; Darwish, H.E.; Keynton, R.; El-Baz, A. A 3D CNN with a Learnable Adaptive Shape Prior for Accurate Segmentation of Bladder Wall Using MR Images. In Proceedings of the 2020 IEEE 17th International Symposium on Biomedical Imaging (ISBI), Iowa City, IA, USA, 3–7 April 2020; pp. 935–938.
13. Wildeboer, R.R.; van Sloun, R.J.; Wijkstra, H.; Mischi, M. Artificial intelligence in multiparametric prostate cancer imaging with focus on deep-learning methods. *Comput. Methods Programs Biomed.* **2020**, *189*, 105316. [CrossRef] [PubMed]
14. Hammouda, K.; Khalifa, F.; Soliman, A.; Ghazal, M.; Abou El-Ghar, M.; Badawy, M.; Darwish, H.; Khelifi, A.; El-Baz, A. A multiparametric MRI-based CAD system for accurate diagnosis of bladder cancer staging. *Comput. Med. Imaging Graph.* **2021**, *90*, 101911. [CrossRef]
15. Reda, I.; Khalil, A.; Elmogy, M.; Abou El-Fetouh, A.; Shalaby, A.; Abou El-Ghar, M.; Elmaghraby, A.; Ghazal, M.; El-Baz, A. Deep learning role in early diagnosis of prostate cancer. *Technol. Cancer Res. Treat.* **2018**, *17*, 1533034618775530. [CrossRef]
16. Schelb, P.; Kohl, S.; Radtke, J.P.; Wiesenfarth, M.; Kickingereder, P.; Bickelhaupt, S.; Kuder, T.A.; Stenzinger, A.; Hohenfellner, M.; Schlemmer, H.P.; et al. Classification of cancer at prostate MRI: Deep learning versus clinical PI-RADS assessment. *Radiology* **2019**, *293*, 607–617. [CrossRef] [PubMed]
17. Mehrtash, A.; Sedghi, A.; Ghafoorian, M.; Taghipour, M.; Tempany, C.M.; Wells, W.M. III; Kapur, T.; Mousavi, P.; Abolmaesumi, P.; Fedorov, A. Classification of clinical significance of MRI prostate findings using 3D convolutional neural networks. In Proceedings of the Medical Imaging 2017: Computer-Aided Diagnosis, Orlando, FL, USA, 22 May 2017; International Society for Optics and Photonics: Bellingham, WA, USA, 2017; Volume 10134, p. 101342A.
18. Arvaniti, E.; Fricker, K.S.; Moret, M.; Rupp, N.; Hermanns, T.; Fankhauser, C.; Wey, N.; Wild, P.J.; Rueschoff, J.H.; Claassen, M. Automated Gleason grading of prostate cancer tissue microarrays via deep learning. *Sci. Rep.* **2018**, *8*, 1–11. [CrossRef]
19. Bulten, W.; Pinckaers, H.; van Boven, H.; Vink, R.; de Bel, T.; van Ginneken, B.; van der Laak, J.; de Kaa, C.H.v.; Litjens, G. Automated gleason grading of prostate biopsies using deep learning. *arXiv* **2019**, arXiv:1907.07980.
20. Hammouda, K.; Khalifa, F.; Abdeltawab, H.; Elnakib, A.; Giridharan, G.; Zhu, M.; Ng, C.; Dassanayaka, S.; Kong, M.; Darwish, H.; et al. A new framework for performing cardiac Strain Analysis from cine MRi imaging in Mice. *Sci. Rep.* **2020**, *10*, 1–15. [CrossRef] [PubMed]
21. Kamnitsas, K.; Ledig, C.; Newcombe, V.F.; Simpson, J.P.; Kane, A.D.; Menon, D.K.; Rueckert, D.; Glocker, B. Efficient multi-scale 3D CNN with fully connected CRF for accurate brain lesion segmentation. *Med Image Anal.* **2017**, *36*, 61–78. [CrossRef] [PubMed]
22. Russakovsky, O.; Deng, J.; Su, H.; Krause, J.; Satheesh, S.; Ma, S.; Huang, Z.; Karpathy, A.; Khosla, A.; Bernstein, M.; et al. Imagenet large scale visual recognition challenge. *Int. J. Comput. Vis.* **2015**, *115*, 211–252. [CrossRef]
23. Krizhevsky, A.; Sutskever, I.; Hinton, G.E. Imagenet classification with deep convolutional neural networks. *Adv. Neural Inf. Process. Syst.* **2012**, *25*, 1097–1105. [CrossRef]
24. Kaur, M.; Kaur, J.; Kaur, J. Survey of contrast enhancement techniques based on histogram equalization. *Int. J. Adv. Comput. Sci. Appl.* **2011**, *2*, 2011. [CrossRef]
25. Nnolim, U.A. Smoothing and enhancement algorithms for underwater images based on partial differential equations. *J. Electron. Imaging* **2017**, *26*, 023009. [CrossRef]
26. Shin, H.C.; Roth, H.R.; Gao, M.; Lu, L.; Xu, Z.; Nogues, I.; Yao, J.; Mollura, D.; Summers, R.M. Deep convolutional neural networks for computer-aided detection: CNN architectures, dataset characteristics and transfer learning. *IEEE Trans. Med Imaging* **2016**, *35*, 1285–1298. [CrossRef]
27. Website for the Dataset. 2021. Available online: https://www.kaggle.com/c/prostate-cancer-grade-assessment (accessed on 3 October 2021).
28. Hossin, M.; Sulaiman, M.N. A review on evaluation metrics for data classification evaluations. *Int. J. Data Min. Knowl. Manag. Process.* **2015**, *5*, 1.
29. McNee, S.M.; Riedl, J.; Konstan, J.A. Being accurate is not enough: How accuracy metrics have hurt recommender systems. In Proceedings of the CHI'06 Extended Abstracts on Human Factors in Computing Systems, New York, NY, USA, 22–27 April 2006; pp. 1097–1101.
30. He, K.; Zhang, X.; Ren, S.; Sun, J. Deep residual learning for image recognition. In Proceedings of the IEEE Conference on Computer Vision and Pattern Recognition, Las Vegas, NV, USA, 27–30 June 2016; pp. 770–778.
31. Lane, J.A.; Donovan, J.L.; Davis, M.; Walsh, E.; Dedman, D.; Down, L.; Turner, E.L.; Mason, M.D.; Metcalfe, C.; Peters, T.J.; et al. Active monitoring, radical prostatectomy, or radiotherapy for localised prostate cancer: Study design and diagnostic and baseline results of the ProtecT randomised phase 3 trial. *Lancet Oncol.* **2014**, *15*, 1109–1118. [CrossRef]
32. Chen, R.C.; Rumble, R.B.; Loblaw, D.A.; Finelli, A.; Ehdaie, B.; Cooperberg, M.R.; Morgan, S.C.; Tyldesley, S.; Haluschak, J.J.; Tan, W.; et al. Active surveillance for the management of localized prostate cancer (Cancer Care Ontario guideline): American Society of Clinical Oncology clinical practice guideline endorsement. *J. Clin. Oncol. Off. J. Am. Soc. Clin. Oncol.* **2016**, *34*, 2182–2190. [CrossRef] [PubMed]
33. Brimo, F.; Schultz, L.; Epstein, J.I. The value of mandatory second opinion pathology review of prostate needle biopsy interpretation before radical prostatectomy. *J. Urol.* **2010**, *184*, 126–130. [CrossRef]
34. Steiner, D.F.; MacDonald, R.; Liu, Y.; Truszkowski, P.; Hipp, J.D.; Gammage, C.; Thng, F.; Peng, L.; Stumpe, M.C. Impact of deep learning assistance on the histopathologic review of lymph nodes for metastatic breast cancer. *Am. J. Surg. Pathol.* **2018**, *42*, 1636. [CrossRef]

35. Liu, Y.; Kohlberger, T.; Norouzi, M.; Dahl, G.E.; Smith, J.L.; Mohtashamian, A.; Olson, N.; Peng, L.H.; Hipp, J.D.; Stumpe, M.C. Artificial intelligence–based breast cancer nodal metastasis detection: insights into the black box for pathologists. *Arch. Pathol. Lab. Med.* **2019**, *143*, 859–868. [CrossRef] [PubMed]
36. Gislén, A.; Dacke, M.; Kröger, R.H.; Abrahamsson, M.; Nilsson, D.E.; Warrant, E.J. Superior underwater vision in a human population of sea gypsies. *Curr. Biol.* **2003**, *13*, 833–836. [CrossRef]
37. Allsbrook, W.C., Jr.; Mangold, K.A.; Johnson, M.H.; Lane, R.B.; Lane, C.G.; Epstein, J.I. Interobserver reproducibility of Gleason grading of prostatic carcinoma: General pathologist. *Hum. Pathol.* **2001**, *32*, 81–88. [CrossRef] [PubMed]
38. Courtiol, P.; Maussion, C.; Moarii, M.; Pronier, E.; Pilcer, S.; Sefta, M.; Manceron, P.; Toldo, S.; Zaslavskiy, M.; Le Stang, N.; et al. Deep learning-based classification of mesothelioma improves prediction of patient outcome. *Nat. Med.* **2019**, *25*, 1519–1525. [CrossRef]
39. Wulczyn, E.; Steiner, D.F.; Xu, Z.; Sadhwani, A.; Wang, H.; Flament-Auvigne, I.; Mermel, C.H.; Chen, P.H.C.; Liu, Y.; Stumpe, M.C. Deep learning-based survival prediction for multiple cancer types using histopathology images. *PLoS ONE* **2020**, *15*, e0233678. [CrossRef] [PubMed]
40. Marrone, M.; Potosky, A.L.; Penson, D.; Freedman, A.N. A 22 gene-expression assay, Decipher®(GenomeDx Biosciences) to predict five-year risk of metastatic prostate cancer in men treated with radical prostatectomy. *PLoS Curr.* **2015**, *7*. [CrossRef]
41. Kweldam, C.F.; Kümmerlin, I.P.; Nieboer, D.; Verhoef, E.I.; Steyerberg, E.W.; Van der Kwast, T.H.; Roobol, M.J.; van Leenders, G.J. Disease-specific survival of patients with invasive cribriform and intraductal prostate cancer at diagnostic biopsy. *Mod. Pathol.* **2016**, *29*, 630–636. [CrossRef] [PubMed]

sensors

MDPI

Article

Determination of Chewing Count from Video Recordings Using Discrete Wavelet Decomposition and Low Pass Filtration

Sana Alshboul and Mohammad Fraiwan *

Department of Computer Engineering, Jordan University of Science and Technology, P.O. Box 3030, Irbid 22110, Jordan; smalshboul16@cit.just.edu.jo
* Correspondence: mafraiwan@just.edu.jo

Abstract: Several studies have shown the importance of proper chewing and the effect of chewing speed on the human health in terms of caloric intake and even cognitive functions. This study aims at designing algorithms for determining the chew count from video recordings of subjects consuming food items. A novel algorithm based on image and signal processing techniques has been developed to continuously capture the area of interest from the video clips, determine facial landmarks, generate the chewing signal, and process the signal with two methods: low pass filter, and discrete wavelet decomposition. Peak detection was used to determine the chew count from the output of the processed chewing signal. The system was tested using recordings from 100 subjects at three different chewing speeds (i.e., slow, normal, and fast) without any constraints on gender, skin color, facial hair, or ambience. The low pass filter algorithm achieved the best mean absolute percentage error of 6.48%, 7.76%, and 8.38% for the slow, normal, and fast chewing speeds, respectively. The performance was also evaluated using the Bland-Altman plot, which showed that most of the points lie within the lines of agreement. However, the algorithm needs improvement for faster chewing, but it surpasses the performance of the relevant literature. This research provides a reliable and accurate method for determining the chew count. The proposed methods facilitate the study of the chewing behavior in natural settings without any cumbersome hardware that may affect the results. This work can facilitate research into chewing behavior while using smart devices.

Keywords: chewing; smart devices; discrete wavelet decomposition; low pass filter; number of chews

Citation: Alshboul, S.; Fraiwan, M. Determination of Chewing Count from Video Recordings Using Discrete Wavelet Decomposition and Low Pass Filtration. *Sensors* **2021**, *21*, 6806. https://doi.org/10.3390/s21206806

Academic Editors: Ayman El-baz, Guruprasad A. Giridharan, Ahmed Shalaby, Ali H. Mahmoud and Mohammed Ghazal

Received: 5 September 2021
Accepted: 7 October 2021
Published: 13 October 2021

1. Introduction

Chewing (i.e., mastication) is the action of crushing and grounding food by the teeth. It is an important process that represents the first step of digestion by which the surface area of the food is increased to allow for easy swallowing and efficient breakdown by enzymes. Healthy nutrition is affected by several factors related to chewing, including; food intake, chewing behavior, chewing time, chewing speed and the bolus size.

Monitoring and study of the chewing process is important. Abnormal chewing behavior could be an indication of some ailments (e.g., anorexia, tooth decay, etc.), which may reduce the chewing speed or the bolus size. Moreover, people suffering from binge eating disorder tend to consume large amounts of food in a short time and are subject to greater risk of high blood pressure and cardiovascular diseases [1]. In addition, some researchers attempted to establish calibrated model for the caloric intake based on the number of bites and chew count [2]. Thus, there is a need to establish automated portable methods for the correct determination of the chew count [3]. Also, eating while using mobile handheld devices is becoming common with children. This phenomenon has a great effect on eating habits, which in turn influence the health of individuals (e.g., obesity and overweight). Recent research suggests that children who use electronics for longer hours or eat while using those devices have higher Body Mass Index (BMI) [4].

Manually counting chews by trained clinicians and the effort involved in studies enlisting even small number of subjects is large considering the number of chews per minute. The process is tedious, time consuming, and error prone. The objective of this paper is to automatically determine the chew count from video recordings of subject munching on food while using camera-equipped electronic devices. This research develops a method to automatically count the number of chews appearing in the video recording. The results from this work can facilitate greater research in chewing behavior and its relationship with human health. The contributions of this paper are as follows:

- We record chewing video data from 100 subjects at three speeds (slow, normal, and fast).
- We use image processing techniques to isolate and extract the videos of the subject's face away from artifacts.
- We extract signals corresponding to the various movements during the chewing action.
- We propose two algorithms to count the number of chews automatically based on Discrete Wavelet Decomposition and low pass filters.
- We achieve a low mean percentage error in automatically counting the number of chews.

The remainder of this paper is organized as follows: In Section 2 we provide a background into the chewing process and its health ramifications, and the related literature in automatic chew counting. Section 3 describes in detail the data collection process and the proposed methods for determining the chew count. Performance evaluation metrics and the corresponding results are reported in Section 4. This is followed by a discussion in Section 5 of the advantages and limitations of the reported work. The conclusion and future work are presented in Section 6.

2. Background and Related Work

Chewing is the process of grinding a large piece of food between the teeth to convert the food to small bolus that could be swallowed [5,6]. Recently, chewing behavior is considered one factor associated with increased risk of diseases such as obesity and diabetes, which may result from abnormal chewing behavior or from eating disorders [7]. Changes to chewing behavior may be attributed to social and economic factors that may affect food intake and food selection. For example, consuming food while driving or during the usage of smart devices may lead to fast food intake and a reduction in mealtime [7]. In the next subsection, we discuss the importance of investigating chewing behavior. Such literature signifies the importance and real-life applications of the automated count of chews. After that, we analyze the related works and their shortcomings.

2.1. Chewing and Health

The relationship between chewing behavior and various health aspects is continuously being investigated in the literature. [8] showed that eating slowly might reduce the risks of overweight and underweight in Japanese preschoolers. This was corroborated by the results of [9], wherein obese subjects had lower number of chews per gram of food in comparison to a subject having normal weight. In this regard, relevant literature has shown that increasing the chew count by 150–200% may reduce the food mass intake by up to 15% [10]. Similarly, other studies have shown that prolonged chewing before swallowing may lead to lower caloric intake [11,12].

Chewing has also been found to be beneficial to brain functions. Chen et al. [13] showed that chewing is an effective activity for maintaining the part of the nervous systems responsible for spatial memory and learning (i.e., the hippocampus). Preserving the hippocampus can reduce brain deterioration with age. Chuhuaicura et al. [14] supported the hypothesis of the correlation between mastication and cognitive protection, and they identified seven areas in the brain prefrontal cortex that could be affected by increasing the mastication [15]. In general, mastication plays as a protection factor from cognitive deterioration and neurodegenerative diseases [13,15,16].

2.2. Automatic Chew Counting

Traditional methods used for determining the chew count were either manual or automatic (i.e., using pervasive hardware) [17]. Manual methods are inherently tedious, prone to errors, and un-scalable to large number of subjects. They rely on inspecting visual recordings or direct viewing of subjects. For example, Moraru et al. [18] used visual observation to collect chewing count data from 34 subjects. Other studies [2,12] used similar approach.

Automated methods employ a range of devices that vary in sophistication and cost. Some studies used Electromyography (EMG) to record the chew count of a small number of subjects (i.e., less than 10), which is understood given that special electrodes, EMG device, and professional help are required to perform the recording [19–21]. In another study, piezoelectric and printed strain sensors were used in characterizing the chewing behavior of five subjects [22]. However, their approach relied on the subjects to report their own chewing behavior via a push button. Such an approach may be biased as the subjects positively influenced the quality of the input signal (i.e., the chewing behavior was unnatural). Nonetheless, the reported mean absolute error was 8% even with such input. Similarly, Fontana et al. [2] employed the same input method. They used the annotated data to train an artificial neural networks model (ANN) and their research achieved a mean absolute error of 15.01%. Amft et al. [23] proposed counting chews using sound analysis of audio recordings of the chewing process. However, such a method differs among subjects and may be prone to ambient and other types of noise especially if the subject is using an electronic device (e.g., playing multimedia) while eating. Nonetheless, noise-resilient algorithms for chewing detection were proposed by Bedri et al. [24] using a combination of acoustic, optical, and inertial sensors. They achieved an accuracy of 93% and an F1-score of 80.1% in unconstrained free living evaluation. Similarly, Papapanagiotou et al. [25] used convolutional neural networks to achieve a 98% accuracy and F1-score of 88.3%. Recently, Hossain et al. [26] used a similar approach to detect faces, which they followed by transfer learning using AlexNet to classify images as bite or not, and used affine optical flow to detection rotational movement in the detect faces. They reported a mean accuracy of $88.9 \pm 7.4\%$ for chew count. However, deep learning algorithms are known to be slow and consume significant resources.

In general, hardware-based methods may cause discomfort to child subjects and incur high cost in large-scale experiments. Additionally, remote or at a distance studies may not be possible if special procedures are required to fit the hardware. Cadavid et al. [27] used an active appearance model (AAM) to detect chewing events from captured images of the subject's face. They noticed that the AMM parameters displayed periodic variations in response to the chewing behavior, which were different from other facial activities (e.g., talking). Thus, spectral analysis was used to derive features for a support vector machine classification model. The dimensionality of the features was reduced using principle component analysis in order to reduce the system overhead. However, their approach requires extensive space and computational overhead [28]. They achieved an accuracy of 93%, but that was accomplished using leave one subject out validation, which is not recommended for their small dataset (i.e., 37 subjects) [29].

3. Material and Methods

3.1. Ethical Approvals

The current study was approved by the institutional review board (IRB No. 29/11/2018) at King Abdullah University Hospital (KAUH) and the Deanship of Scientific Research at Jordan University of Science and Technology in Jordan.

3.2. Procedure

Written informed consent was sought and provided prior to the study commencement. For underage subjects, their parents filled the consent form, which needed to be signed if they voluntarily accepted their child's participation. The research assistants received intensive training by the lead investigators on the data collection process, as well as the data entry. The information package included an information sheet describing the study purpose and procedure in details, the consent form (including consent to publication of images), and a parental/self-reporting questionnaire that contains demographics and other relevant information.

3.3. Participants

The current study enrolled 100 randomly selected subjects. A total of 375 information packages were randomly distributed prior to data collection. Of those, 275 (73.3%) recipients refused to participate. The subjects included a mix of children and adults, with an age range of 6–76 years (mean = 19.72, standard deviation = 11.03). Fifty-six of the subjects were children and 44 were adults, and 58 were males. There were no restrictions regarding skin color, facial hair, hairstyle, head cover, or wearing glasses (medical or otherwise).

3.4. Data Collection

A Huawei Y7 Prime 2018 smartphone main camera was used for video recording. It is a 13 MP camera with 1080p@30fps resolution. The subjects were asked to face the camera and eat a crunchy food sample (e.g., cucumber). Each subject recorded three one-minute clips corresponding to three speeds (i.e., slow, normal, and fast). There was no specific environment for the dataset collection, and no additional constrains were set during video recording. Videos were recorded in a variety of setups (i.e., outdoors, indoors in a room, and in public places) and with different light intensities.

Objective reference is required as a gold standard for performance evaluation. To this end, three annotators were trained by the principle investigators to count the number of chews in video recordings, and the training videos were not included in the dataset. Each annotator worked independently from all others and recorded the number of chews in each of the 300 video clips (i.e., 100 subjects with 3 recordings each). The annotators were allowed to pause and rewind the videos for accurate counting.

Upon completing the annotation, the reliability of the process was verified using Intra-class correlation coefficient (ICC) [30]. Table 1 shows the ICC values for all annotators as well as pair wise comparisons among them. The lowest value in the table is 0.83 between annotators 2 and 3, which is considered an excellent value [31].

Table 1. Annotator ICC values for the three chewing speeds.

Annotator\Chewing Speed	Fast	Medium	Slow
All	0.91	0.94	0.96
1 & 2	0.88	0.90	0.92
2 & 3	0.83	0.90	0.95
1 & 3	0.90	0.94	0.95

3.5. Determining the Chew Count

Figure 1 shows the general steps taken to count the number of chews. Given a video recording of the subject while eating, the algorithm works by first extracting individual frames as separate images. In each image, the face of the subject is identified using the Viola-Jones algorithm [32] (Section 3.5.1). However, not all of the face is of interest to chew counting, only a few landmarks, which are indicators of mastication, are important. Thus, the Kasemi and Sullivan landmark detector [33] was employed to detect facial landmarks (Section 3.5.2). The Euclidean distance between a reference point and each of the identified facial landmarks is measured and the average is calculated. Since chewing involves jaw motion, there is a need to treat successive Euclidean distance averages as time series data generated using the mean Euclidean distance from each video frame, which results in the chewing signal (Section 3.5.3). After that, filtering techniques employing LPF or DWD retrain the relevant frequencies (Section 3.5.4). Finally, a peak counting determines the number of chews excluding biting peaks (Section 3.5.5). In the next few subsections, we will go through each one of the steps in detail. These steps were implemented using Matlab 2020a software.

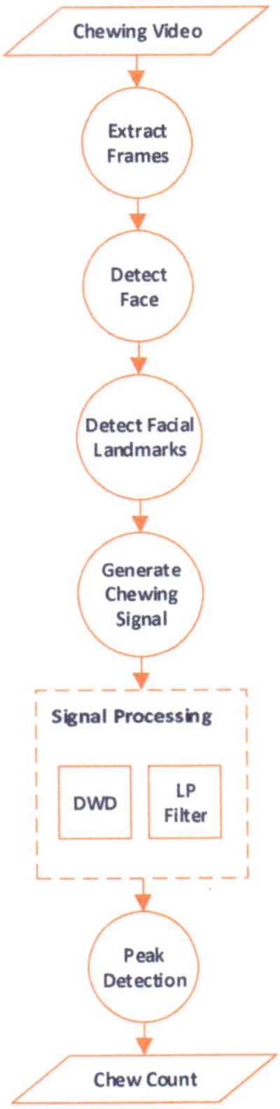

Figure 1. The general steps to count the number of chews from the input video clip.

3.5.1. Face Detection

The first step in the algorithm aims to detect the face of the subject. To this end, the Viola-Jones face detector was employed. The algorithm was chosen because it is fast and has high detection accuracy [32]. It works in the following steps:

1. The image is converted to gray scale, which reduces the overhead. However, once the face is detected, the location is marked in the colored image.
2. The image is scanned to search for intensity differences that may represent facial features. This is done using boxes called Haar rectangles [34].These boxes are moved so that every tile in the image is covered. Figure 2 shows a set of three Haar features (HFs); two-rectangle, three-rectangle, and four-rectangle. These features represent regions with different shades in an image. For example, the eyebrows will appear darker in comparison to the surrounding skin. Similarly, the top of the nose may seem brighter than the sides.
3. Each box is represented by a matrix of values corresponding to the pixel color intensities in that box. The darker the pixel the closer the corresponding value to 1. A Feature is generated by the difference between the sum of pixel values in the dark region and the sum of pixel values in the light region.
4. The previous calculations can cause high computational overhead because of the large number of pixels. Therefore, the process is adjusted to use an integral image (i.e.,

a summed-area table). Each value, $I(x,y)$, in the integral image is the summation of all pixel values that lie above and to the left of (x,y) in the original image inclusively, see Equation (1). Figure 3 shows an example matrix representing the original image and the corresponding integral image. Using the integral image, calculating the intensities of any rectangular area of any size in the original image requires four values only. Moreover, the integral image is calculated with a single pass over all pixels. This method greatly improves the efficiency of calculating the Haar feature rectangles.

5. Scanning the image using the rectangular boxes will generate a set of intensity values, which form the input to the classification process. The output of this step indicates whether or not a feature is likely to be part of the face. The Viola-Jones algorithm uses adaptive boosting (AdaBoost), which employs a weak learner constraint to select few features out of thousands of possible features. The algorithm training dataset contained 4960 annotated facial images as well as 9544 other images without faces [32].
6. Cascaded or ensemble classification. This step further refines the classification process by attempting to discard the background regions by increasing the complexity of classifiers in cascade. The collective effect of the weak classifiers selects the best combination of features and their associated weights.

$$I(x,y) = \sum_{x' \leq x, y' \leq y} v(x',y'), \tag{1}$$

where $v(x',y')$ is the value of the pixel at (x',y').

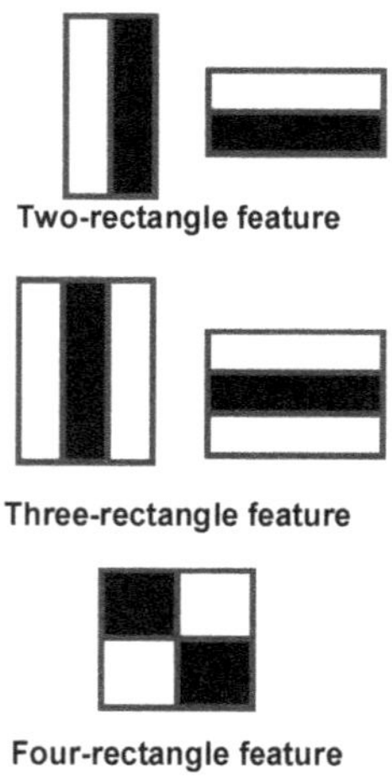

Figure 2. Haar rectangular features.

3.5.2. Facial Landmarks Detection

The Viola-Jones algorithm generates a bounding box around the face of the subject. However, the face as a whole is not useful by itself for chew counting. Thus, Kasemi and Sullivan landmark detector [33] was employed to identify key facial features and their location on the face. The facial landmark detector estimates the position of the facial landmarks using an ensemble of regression trees (ERT) based on sparse pixel set intensities, which are used as an input to the regressors. The pixel intensities are selected using a gradient boosting algorithm and a prior probability of the distance between pairs of input pixels. The face image is transformed into an initial shape and the features are extracted to update the current shape vector. This procedure is repeated several times until convergence is reached. After that, intensities of the sparse pixels are indexed on the initial shape. Each regressor estimates the current shape from an initial shape estimation to solve the problem of face alignment. The initial shape can be selected by the mean shape of the centered and scaled face image.

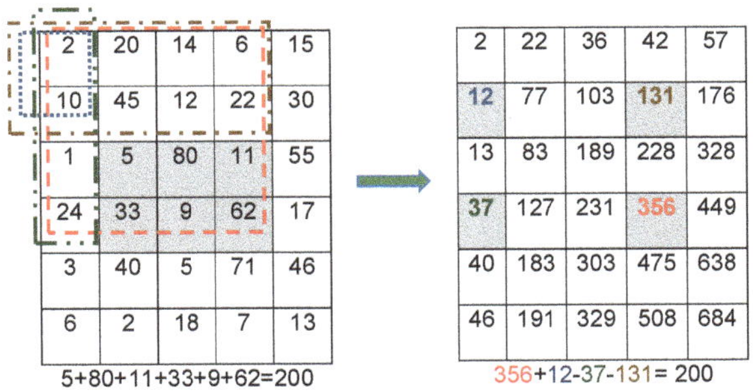

Figure 3. The intensities in the original image (**left**) and the corresponding integral image (**right**). Calculating the intensity of the shaded box requires only four indices in the integral image regardless of the number of pixels in the box.

This procedure results in a 192 × 2 vector representing the (x, y) coordinates of 192 points on the subject's face. However, such number of facial points is excessive, redundant, and consumes large space and processing power. The determination of the facial landmarks forms the basis for the identification of the chewing motion. Several useful observations were drawn from analyzing the chewing process, as follows:

1. The lower lip moves up and down during crushing the bolus in between the upper and lower jaws. Furthermore, the lower lip moves slightly to the left and right during the bolus motion in the mouth, but the motion of the lower lip decreases when the subject swallows. Moreover, the lower lip motion is undiscernible when the chewing speed is too slow and when the food texture is neither solid nor crispy. In addition, the separation between the two lips increases when the subject is taking a bite.
2. The upper lip motion is unbeneficial for counting chews as it is undiscernible across video frames. This mainly due to its connection to the immobile maxilla.
3. The corner points on the edge of the mouth move in an oval trajectory, which could be a result of smiling or other facial expressions. Thus, they were ignored.

Careful inspection of the chewing process revealed that most of the points responding to the chewing operation are located in the chin and jawline regions. Therefore, only 11 points in the chin and jawline were used, see Figure 4. They displayed consistency and a stable chewing pattern during chewing regardless of the speed. Moreover, the motion is immune to facial expressions (e.g., smiling). In addition, the points are visible during food intake. Thus, the motion of the jawline points was used for counting purposes. These points move in three ways, as follows:

1. Up and down during for crushing/chewing the food.
2. Sideways during bolus motion across the mouth sides.
3. A large downward movement for every food bite.

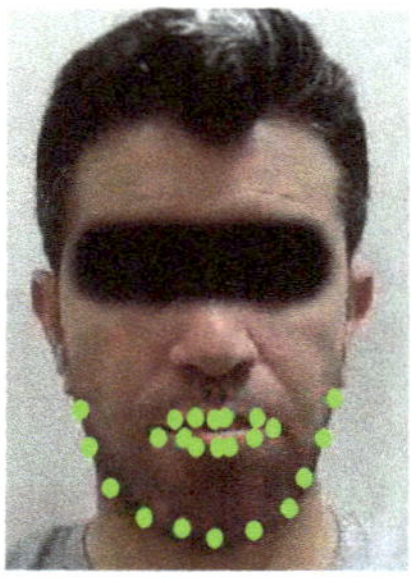

Figure 4. Facial landmark detection showing the 11 jaw and 15 mouth landmarks. Only the 11 jaw landmarks were used in counting chews.

3.5.3. Generation of the Chewing Signal

We define the up down mandible motion as one chew. To measure this motion, a reference point was required with the constraint that it is unaffected by the chewing motion, random movement, and may not be hidden during chewing. To this end, the upper left corner of the face bounding box was chosen as a reference for all movements. This box tracks the face throughout the recording and represents a fixed reference frame for the jawline points. The Euclidean distance (ED) was measured for each frame between every jawline point (x, y) and the reference point (u, v), and the average was taken for the 11 points, see Equation (2).

$$ED = \frac{1}{11}\sum_{p=1}^{p=11}\sqrt{(x-u)^2+(y-v)^2} \tag{2}$$

Figure 5 shows an example of the ED as measured between the reference point and the jawline points used for counting chews. The ED values measured throughout the duration of the chewing clip form a signal that represents the chewing pattern, see Figure 6. The labelled peaks in Figure 6 represent the subject taking a bite and they were discounted from the total chew count. Moreover, the signal inherently contains some noise due to the subject's movement and swallowing. For example, the sideways movement of the head. Therefore, signal processing techniques were required to correctly identify the patterns resulting from the actual chewing.

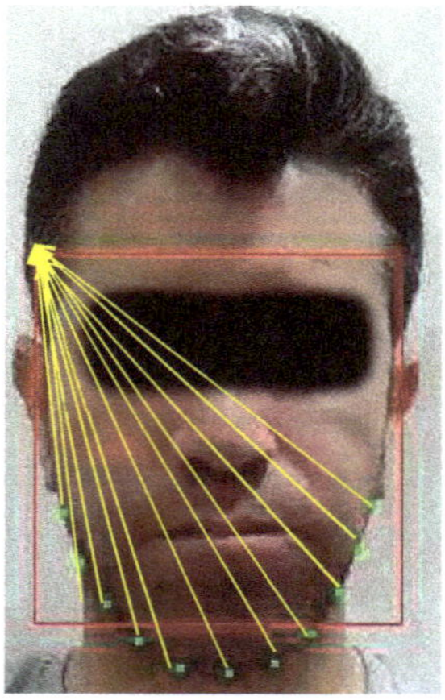

Figure 5. The Euclidean distance between chin/jaw landmarks and the upper left corner of the face rectangle.

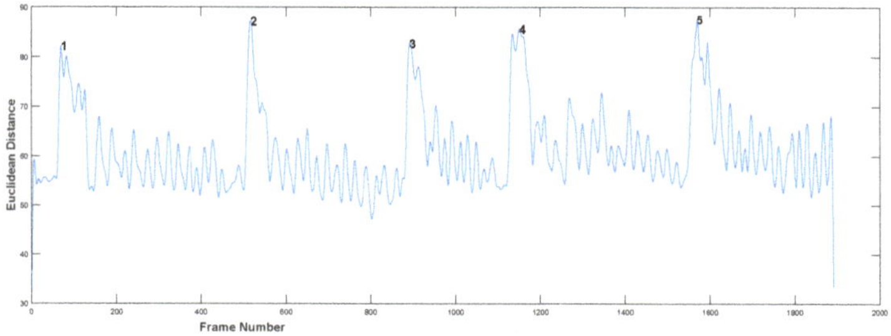

Figure 6. The chewing signal and five biting peaks.

3.5.4. Chewing Signal Processing

As previously stated, the chewing signal carries some noise due to the subject's movement, mandible motion, and other artefacts (e.g., variations in the head bounding box). We experiment with two signal processing methods to improve the signal usefulness, as follows:

- Low pass filter (LPF): a LPF was designed with a cut-off frequency of 1 Hz and a sampling rate of 30 Hz [35]. It is a linear phase minimum order finite impulse response filter. The measured frequencies in the collected dataset ranged between 0.4 and 2.3 Hz for all chewing speeds. However, some of these frequencies resulted from variations in the mandible motion before the completion of one chew. Thus, the frequencies that are not representing actual chewing were removed. This was accomplished by assigning a proper passband frequency. Several passband frequencies and sampling rates were tested, and a 1 Hz passband frequency and 50 Hz sampling rate achieved the best results. Figure 7 shows the original signal with many fake peaks caused by noise. Whereas Figure 8 shows the smoothing of the signal and the elimination of most of these peaks after LPF application.
- Discrete wavelet decomposition (DWD): DWD is a discrete version of the continuous wavelet transform [36]. It retains the important features and reduces the computational complexity in comparison to the continuous wavelet transform [37]. In DWD, the signal is decomposed using low and high pass filters into approximation (A) and detail (D) coefficients, respectively. Further reduction to the frequency was achieved by applying the same procedure to the resulting approximation coefficients. A Daubechies mother wavelet with tab equal 4 was used, which achieve the best smoothing effect while retaining the important features. The sampling rate in the chewing signal was 30 Hz and the chewing signal frequency was 0–16 Hz, because of the noise in the signal that comes from the unwanted movements and from the fast chewing speed videos. Thus, three levels of decomposition were required to reach the closest frequency of chewing (i.e., 1–2 Hz) for normal speed, see Figure 9. This corresponds to 1 to 2 chews per second. The frequency resolution can be increased/decreased to match the chewing speed and the associated chewing signal frequency, see Figure 10.

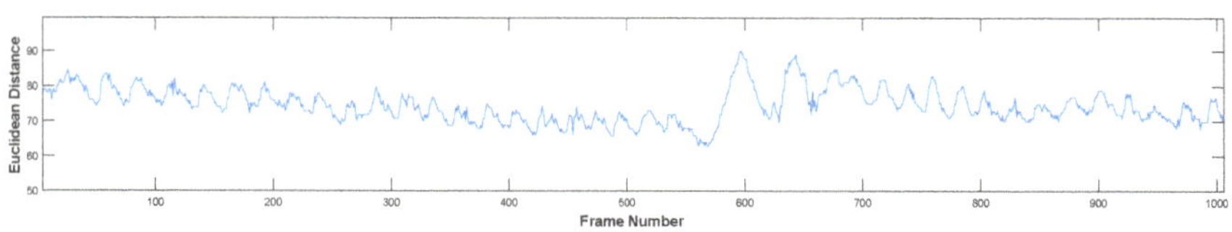

Figure 7. A chewing signal with many fake peaks caused by noise.

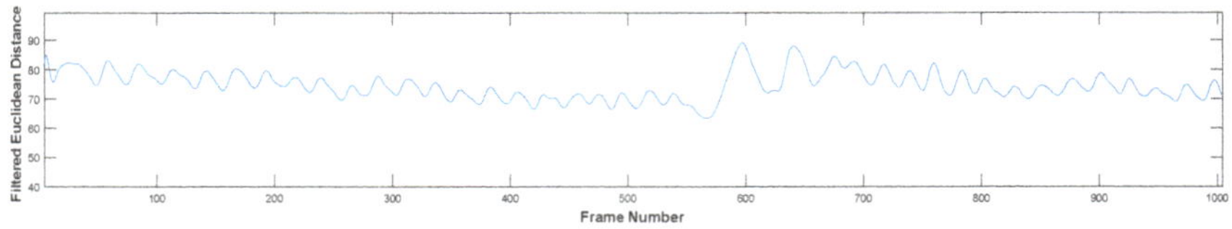

Figure 8. The same signal in Figure 7 after low pass filtration.

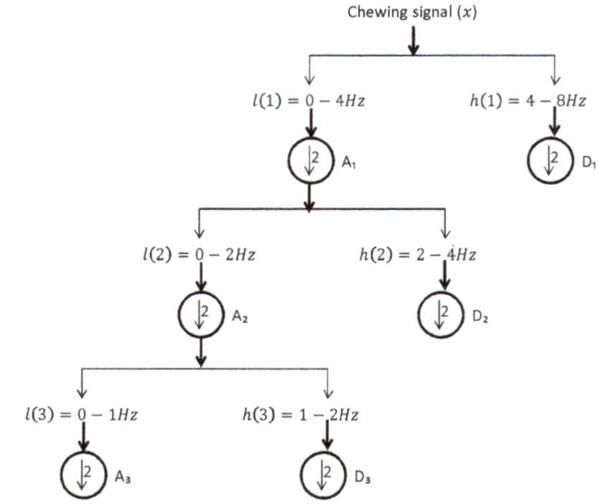

Figure 9. Three-level discrete wavelet decomposition.

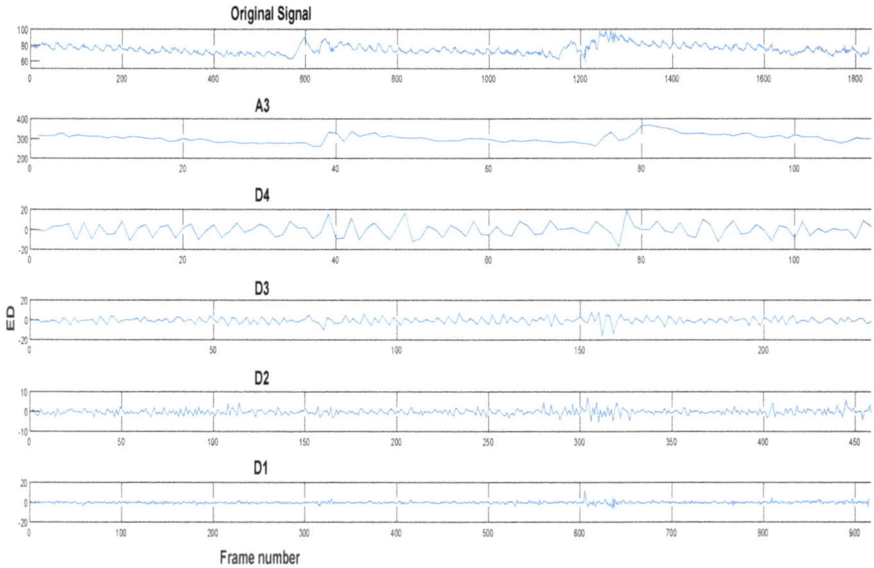

Figure 10. Four-level DWD of the signal in Figure 7.

3.5.5. Counting Chews

The output from either one of the two signal processing techniques (i.e., LPF and DWS) forms the basis for determining the number of chews. A peak detection algorithm was employed to detect the chewing markers. The algorithm works by finding every local maximum in the signal that is larger than the adjacent two neighboring points, where every peak represents one chew. The Minimum-Peak-Height (MPH) parameter for peak detection was set for LPF to half the average of all peak heights (PH), see Equation (3). For DWD and slow chewing videos, the MPH was set to half the average of PH see Equation (4). Equations (5) and (6) show the values of the MPH for the DWD processing of the normal and fast chewing speeds.

The MPH was set differently for the three chewing speed signals because it was observed that the mandible movement changes in response to different chewing speeds. The highest displacement occurred in the slow chewing speed signals. Thus, the chewing peaks were high in comparison to false peaks (i.e., noise). On the other hand, the mandible displacement was small in the fast chewing speed signals, so more of the peaks need to be counted. Figure 11 shows the application of the peak counting algorithm on the LPF-processed signal, and Figure 12 shows the results from the DWD output.

$$MPH_{LPF} = \frac{1}{2} \times \frac{1}{n} \sum_{i=0}^{n} P_H \tag{3}$$

$$MPH_{DWD\_slow} = \frac{1}{2} \times \frac{1}{n} \sum_{i=0}^{n} P_H \tag{4}$$

$$MPH_{DWD\_normal} = \frac{1}{3} \times \frac{1}{n} \sum_{i=0}^{n} P_H \tag{5}$$

$$MPH_{DWD\_fast} = \frac{1}{4} \times \frac{1}{n} \sum_{i=0}^{n} P_H \tag{6}$$

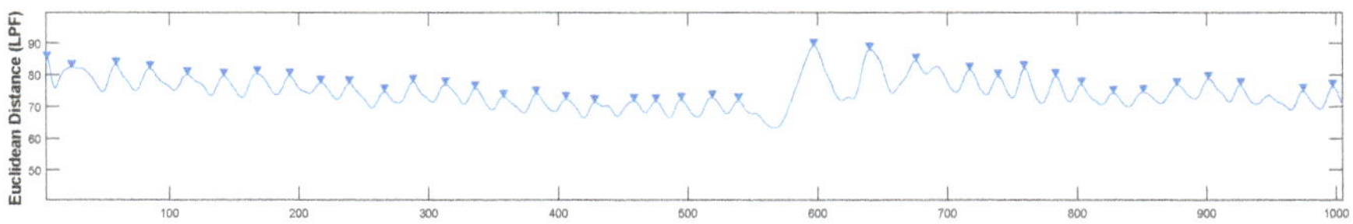

Figure 11. LPF output for counting chewing peaks in the processed signal.

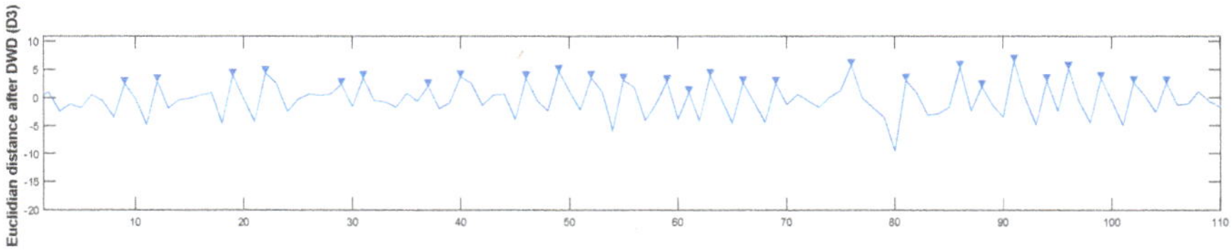

Figure 12. DWD output for counting chewing peaks in the processed signal.

4. Results and Evaluation

4.1. Complexity Analysis

As presented earlier, the proposed work relies on software-based methods as opposed to hardware solutions (i.e., dedicated sensors). Sensing and counting hardware maybe invasive but it provides less computationally intensive option. However, the approach used in this paper is based upon well-established practical methods with linear time complexity. The Viola-Jones face detector runs in linear time $O(N)$, where N is the number of pixels in the image. The calculations are done within a small region of interest in the integral image. Moreover, the Haar features are computed in constant time [38]. The next step is facial landmark detection, which uses the Kazemi and Sullivan [33]. Both this and the Viola-Jones algorithms are considered real-time algorithms with low complexity and high speed [39]. The third step computes the average Euclidean distance for 11 chin/jaw landmarks in each frame. At a frame rate of 30 fps, this computation is negligible. Next, the chewing signal is filtered using either LPF or DWD, with the later having linear time complexity [40]. The last step is counting peaks, which inspects the elements before and after each possible peak. Thus, it requires linear number of steps.

4.2. Performance Evaluation Metrics

The performance of the proposed methods was evaluated in terms of the absolute error (AE), mean absolute percentage error ($MAPE$), and root mean squared error ($RMSE$). Each one of these metrics provides a different insight into the accuracy of the counting algorithm. $RMSE$ tends to penalize large errors. On the other hand, AE and $MAPE$ are easier to interpret. In addition, $MAPE$ allows comparisons between varying chewing counts as the error is relative to the gold standard. Equations (7)–(9) to show the formulas for calculating these metrics.

$$AE = |Actual_{count} - Measured_{count}| \quad (7)$$

$$MAPE = \frac{1}{n}\sum_{1}^{n}\frac{|Actual_{count} - Measured_{count}|}{Actual_{count}} \times 100\% \quad (8)$$

$$RMSE = \sqrt{\frac{1}{n}\sum_{1}^{n}(Actual_{count} - Measured_{count})^2} \quad (9)$$

The Bland-Altman plot was used to measure the agreement between the proposed algorithms and the actual chew count as determine by each annotator. This is a graphical method that plots the difference between the calculated values and the gold standard values against the average of the two methods. Any two methods can be used interchangeably used if 95% of the data points are located within the limits of agreement, which are defined as the mean $\pm 1.96 \times SD$ [41].

4.3. Results

Table 2 shows the AE for the two signal processing methods. The average AE is lowest for the slow chewing speed for both LPF and DWD, although LP slightly outperforms DWD with an AE of 5.42 ± 4.61. Moreover, the error is higher for faster speeds. The same trend appears in Tables 3 and 4 for $MAPE$ and $RMSE$ respectively. Again, LPF achieved superior performance for normal chewing with 7.76% and 7.93 for $MAPE$ and $RMSE$, respectively.

Figure 13 show the Bland-Altman plot for the agreement between the proposed algorithm and the average of the three annotators (i.e., the gold standard) using LPF or DWD. The figures show that most of the points are within the lines of agreement. However, the algorithm needs improvement for faster chewing. Nonetheless, our method can be used interchangeably with the manual measuring techniques but provides the advantages of automated measurement and reliable results. This serves as an evidence of the accuracy and efficacy of the proposed approach.

Table 2. Performance comparison between LPF and DWD in terms of AE. SD stands for standard deviation.

Chewing Speed	**LPF**			**DWD**		
	AE_{avg}	AE_{avg}	$\pm SD$	AE_{avg}	AE_{avg}	$\pm SD$
Slow	5.42	0	4.61	5.72	0	4.8
Normal	7.47	0	6.85	7.45	0	6.85
Fast	9.84	0	9.55	10.32	0	10.42

Table 3. Performance comparison between LPF and DWD in terms of MAPE.

Chewing Speed	MAPE (LPF)	MAPE (DWD)
Slow	6.48%	9.09%
Normal	7.76%	7.03%
Fast	8.38%	8.31%

Table 4. Performance comparison between LPF and DWD in terms of RMSE.

Chewing Speed	RMSE (LPF)	RMSE (DWD)
Slow	5.56	7.64
Normal	7.93	7.09
Fast	13.03	13.43

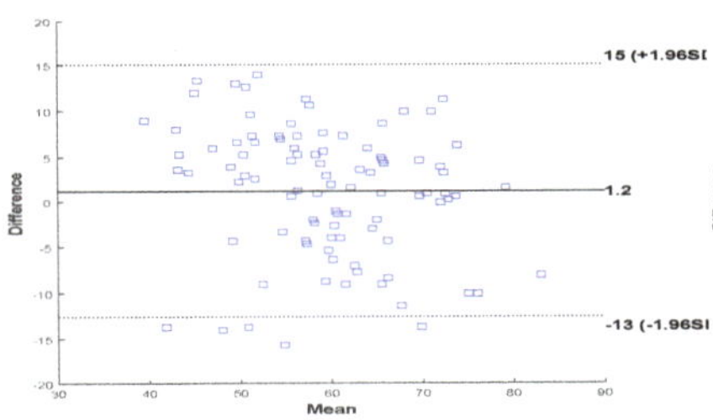

(**a**) Slow and LPF.

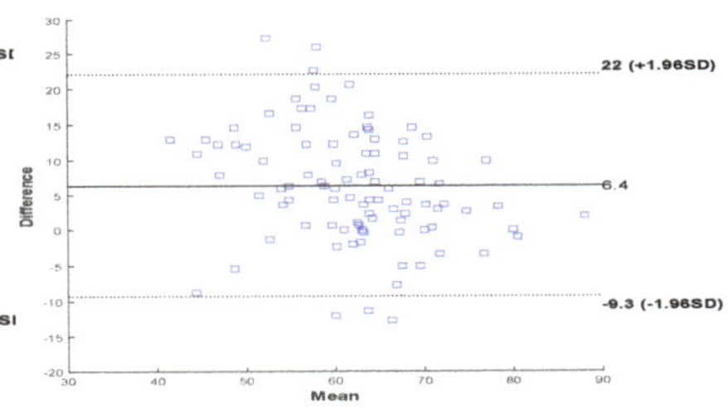

(**b**) Slow and DWD.

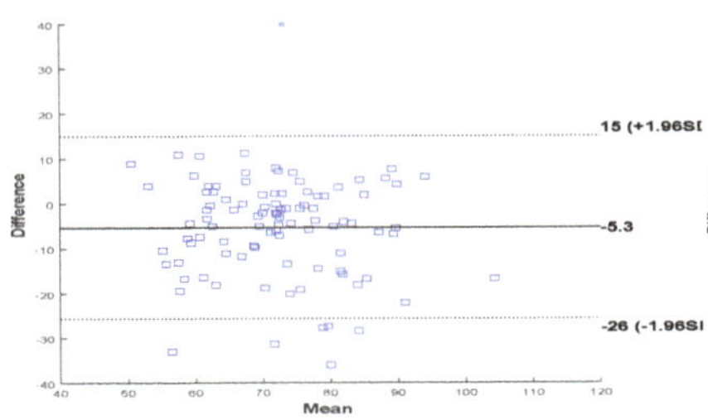

(**c**) Normal and LPF.

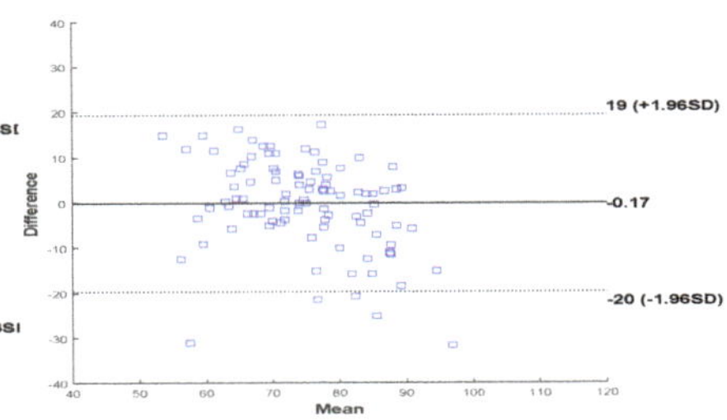

(**d**) Normal and DWD.

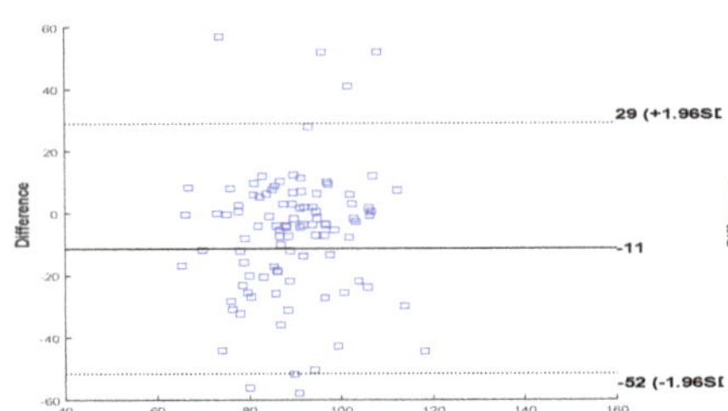

(**e**) Fast and LPF.

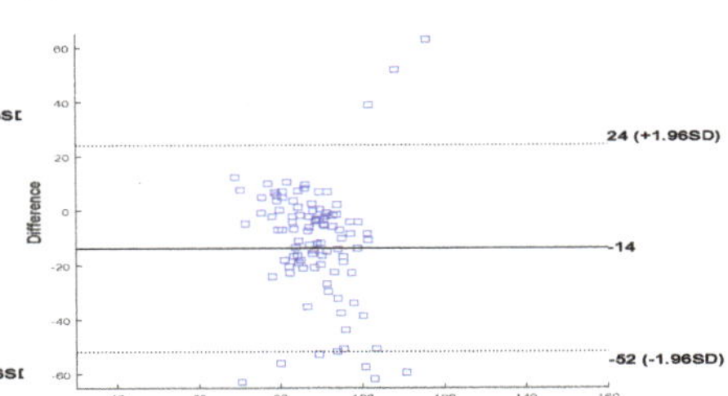

(**f**) Fast and DWD.

Figure 13. Bland-Altman plots for the chewing counts at the three speeds with LPF and DWD processing.

Table 5 shows a comparison to the related literature in terms of best average error, the counting method, and the number of subjects recruited by the researchers. The evaluation of the proposed approach in this paper is based on the largest number of subjects and achieved the least average error. Almost all of these approaches rely on dedicated hardware or signals extracted from this hardware. On the other hand, our work uses input from camera-equipped smart devices. Moreover, the number of subject recruited in most studies is small, which may result in overfitting of the proposed methods to the specific chewing pattern. Additionally, these studies did not test for different chewing speeds although multiple food types were used to record chewing cycles.

Table 5. Performance comparison to the related literature.

Study	Avg Error ± SD	Counting Method	No. of Subjects
Farooq and Sazonov [3]	10.40% ± 7.03%	Peak detection in manually annotated segments	30
	15.01%± 11.06%	Counting in ANN classified epochs	30
Farooq and Sazonov [22]	8.09% ± 7.16%	Piezoelectric strain sensor	5
	8.26% ± 7.51%	Piezoelectric strain sensor	5
Farooq and Sazonov [42]	9.66% ± 6.28%	Linear regression of piezoelectric sensor signal	10
Bedri et al. [24]	F1-score = 90.9%	Acoustic sensor	10
Cadavid et al. [27]	Avg agreement = 93%	SVM classification of AMM spectral features	37
Taniguchi et al. [43]	Precision = 0.958	Earphone sensor	6
Wang et al. [44]	12.2%	Triaxial accelerometer on the temporalis	4
Hossain et al. [26]	Mean accuracy 88.9% ±7.4%	Deep learning and affine optical flow	28
This paper	5.42% ± 4.61 (slow) 7.47% ± 6.85 (normal) 9.84% ± 9.55 (fast)	Image processing of chewing videos	100

5. Discussion

The work in this paper presents a method for the automatic counting of chewing from video recordings. The results from both the LPF and DWD approaches suggest that the proposed method can be used as an objective and accurate chewing counter. In comparison to the literature, the method was tested on a reasonably large number of subjects and chewing speeds.

In both signal processing techniques, the algorithm was used to estimate chew counts in manually annotated chewing clips and was able to achieve a best AE, MAPE, and RMS of 5.42 ± 4.61, 6.48%, and 5.56, respectively. However, this was achieved for slow chewing speeds. The same values for the normal chewing were 7.47 ± 6.85, 7.76%, and 7.93, respectively. Moreover, given that the human counting accuracy is typically 5.7% ± 11.2% [3], our results present an excellent objective and automated methodology for accurate chew counting. In addition, the results in Figure 11 show that the difference between the measured and annotated values to fall in the region over the mean, which may be explained by the tendency of the annotator to underestimate the chew count [3].

This study has several limitations. First, we did not experiment with different food types (e.g., hard, crunchy, crispy, tough, chewy, etc.). Second, the gold standard depends on the annotators, who-although trained- are subject to mistakes and underestimation [3]. It would have been more accurate to equip the participants with piezoelectric sensors, which could capture the chewing count more accurately. Third, the length of the videos clips was one minute, which was enough time to finish the piece of food provided to the subjects. Fourth, the collected data did not include videos with different out of plane rotation (i.e., pose) or in plane rotation (i.e., orientation) as a normal chewing posture was assumed. However, the Viola-Jones algorithm can detect faces that are tilted by ±15 degrees in plane and ±45 degrees out of plane [45]. Finally, we did not perform fine-grained annotation of the chewing clips, but this can be accomplished in future works. Annotating individual chews in the videos would allow elaborate technical analysis and the development of feature-based and artificial intelligence-based counting methods.

Nonetheless, the proposed approach has several merits. First, no extra hardware is required for the deployment and usability of the counting algorithm. Once the system is installed, researchers who are interested in studying the chewing behavior of subjects (e.g., children) can use it easily. It can be used in natural everyday settings (e.g., subjects are using their smartphone or any camera-equipped smart device). Second, the study used a reasonably large number of subjects and investigated a wide range of chewing speeds. In comparison, the number of subjects in the relevant literature was less than 50 [33,35]. Third, the accuracy of the model surpasses relevant literature without requiring extra hardware or intensive computation [3,19–21]. Finally, the algorithm displayed robustness against different subject ages, skin colors, facial hair, or gender.

6. Conclusions

Chewing is an important process in the digestive system with much research dedicated to studying the effects of chew speed, chewing rate, and bolus size on the human health (e.g., BMI). In addition, it has been found that chewing speed is associated with cognitive functions.

Recent proliferation of mobile smart devices, which are equipped with cameras and strong processing power, facilitated the development of many applications from a wide range of disciplines. Another aspect to consider is the health impacts of these devices, which are being used during everyday activities including eating. Thus, the work in this paper allows for the monitoring of the chewing behavior to enable researchers to further study human dietary habits while using smart devices.

In this research, an algorithm was developed to count the number of chews from eating video recordings. The input is processed using two well-known and established methods (i.e., LPF and DWD) followed by a peak counting algorithm. Performance evaluation results greatly improved on the existing literature. Moreover, the system allows for the natural measurement without the need for expensive or uncomfortable hardware. We expect this work to enable further studies into eating and weight disorders, especially those connected to smart devices.

Author Contributions: Conceptualization, S.A. and M.F.; methodology, S.A. and M.F.; software, S.A.; validation, M.F.; formal analysis, S.A. and M.F.; investigation, S.A. and M.F.; resources, S.A. and M.F.; data curation, S.A. and M.F.; writing—original draft preparation, M.F.; writing—review and editing, M.F.; visualization, S.A. and M.F.; supervision, M.F.; project administration, M.F. Both authors have read and agreed to the published version of the manuscript.

Funding: This research received no external funding.

Institutional Review Board Statement: The study was conducted according to the guidelines of the Declaration of Helsinki, and approved by the Institutional Review Board of Jordan University of Science and Technology (protocol code: 99/118/2018 and date of approval: 29 November 2018).

Informed Consent Statement: Informed consent was obtained from all subjects involved in the study. All study participants (or their parents in case of underage subjects) provided written informed consent to being included in the study and allowing their data to be shared. The data collection was carried out under the relevant guidelines and regulations. The authors have the right to share the data publicly and the data will be shared via a separate data article.

Data Availability Statement: The dataset generated during and/or analysed during the current study are available from the corresponding author on reasonable request. The dataset will be made public in a separate data article.

Acknowledgments: The authors would like to thank Taisir Eldos for his valuable comments.

Conflicts of Interest: The authors declare no conflict of interest.

Abbreviations

The following abbreviations are used in this manuscript:

BMI	Body Mass Index
EMG	Electromyography
ANN	Artificial neural networks
AMM	Active appearance model
IRB	Institutional review board
KAUH	King Abdullah University Hospital
ICC	Intra-class correlation coefficient
HF	Haar feature
ERT	ensemble of regression trees
ED	Euclidean distance
LPF	Low pass filter
DWD	Discrete wavelet decomposition
MPH	Minimum-Peak-Height
PH	Peak heights
AE	Absolute error
MAPE	Mean absolute percentage error
RMSE	Root mean squared error

References

1. Fairburn, C.G.; Harrison, P.J. Eating disorders. *Lancet* **2003**, *361*, 407–416. [CrossRef]
2. Fontana, J.M.; Higgins, J.A.; Schuckers, S.C.; Bellisle, F.; Pan, Z.; Melanson, E.L.; Neuman, M.R.; Sazonov, E. Energy intake estimation from counts of chews and swallows. *Appetite* **2015**, *85*, 14–21. [CrossRef]
3. Farooq, M.; Sazonov, E. Automatic Measurement of Chew Count and Chewing Rate during Food Intake. *Electronics* **2016**, *5*, 62. [CrossRef]
4. Fraiwan, M.; Almomani, F.; Hammouri, H. Body mass index and potential correlates among elementary school children in Jordan. *Eat. Weight.-Disord.-Stud. Anorexia Bulim. Obes.* **2021**, *26*, 629–638. [CrossRef] [PubMed]
5. Révérend, B.J.D.L.; Edelson, L.R.; Loret, C. Anatomical, functional, physiological and behavioural aspects of the development of mastication in early childhood. *Br. J. Nutr.* **2013**, *111*, 403–414. [CrossRef] [PubMed]
6. Grimm, E.R.; Steinle, N.I. Genetics of eating behavior: Established and emerging concepts. *Nutr. Rev.* **2011**, *69*, 52–60. [CrossRef] [PubMed]
7. Bellisle, F. Why should we study human food intake behaviour? *Nutr. Metab. Cardiovasc. Dis.* **2003**, *13*, 189–193. [CrossRef]
8. Okubo, H.; Murakami, K.; Masayasu, S.; Sasaki, S. The Relationship of Eating Rate and Degree of Chewing to Body Weight Status among Preschool Children in Japan: A Nationwide Cross-Sectional Study. *Nutrients* **2018**, *11*, 64. [CrossRef]
9. Li, J.; Zhang, N.; Hu, L.; Li, Z.; Li, R.; Li, C.; Wang, S. Improvement in chewing activity reduces energy intake in one meal and modulates plasma gut hormone concentrations in obese and lean young Chinese men. *Am. J. Clin. Nutr.* **2011**, *94*, 709–716. [CrossRef]
10. Zhu, Y.; Hollis, J.H. Increasing the Number of Chews before Swallowing Reduces Meal Size in Normal-Weight, Overweight, and Obese Adults. *J. Acad. Nutr. Diet.* **2014**, *114*, 926–931. [CrossRef]

11. Lepley, C.; Throckmorton, G.; Parker, S.; Buschang, P.H. Masticatory Performance and Chewing Cycle Kinematics—Are They Related? *Angle Orthod.* **2010**, *80*, 295–301. [CrossRef]
12. Spiegel, T. Rate of intake, bites, and chews—The interpretation of lean–obese differences. *Neurosci. Biobehav. Rev.* **2000**, *24*, 229–237. [CrossRef]
13. Chen, H.; Iinuma, M.; Onozuka, M.; Kubo, K.Y. Chewing Maintains Hippocampus-Dependent Cognitive Function. *Int. J. Med. Sci.* **2015**, *12*, 502–509. [CrossRef] [PubMed]
14. Chuhuaicura, P.; Dias, F.J.; Arias, A.; Lezcano, M.F.; Fuentes, R. Mastication as a protective factor of the cognitive decline in adults: A qualitative systematic review. *Int. Dent. J.* **2019**, *69*, 334–340. [CrossRef] [PubMed]
15. Lin, C. Revisiting the link between cognitive decline and masticatory dysfunction. *BMC Geriatr.* **2018**, *18*, 1–14. [CrossRef] [PubMed]
16. Hansson, P.; Sunnegårdh-Grönberg, K.; Bergdahl, J.; Bergdahl, M.; Nyberg, L.; Nilsson, L.G. Relationship between natural teeth and memory in a healthy elderly population. *Eur. J. Oral Sci.* **2013**, *121*, 333–340. [CrossRef]
17. Vu, T.; Lin, F.; Alshurafa, N.; Xu, W. Wearable Food Intake Monitoring Technologies: A Comprehensive Review. *Computers* **2017**, *6*, 4. [CrossRef]
18. Moraru, A.M.O.; Preoteasa, C.T.; Preoteasa, E. Masticatory function parameters in patients with removable dental prosthesis. *J. Med. Life* **2019**, *12*, 43–48. [CrossRef]
19. Rustagi, S.; Sodhi, N.S.; Dhillon, B. A study to investigate reproducibility of chewing behaviour of human subjects within session recordings for different textured Indian foods using electromyography. *Pharma Innov. J.* **2018**, *7*, 5–9.
20. Smit, H.J.; Kemsley, E.K.; Tapp, H.S.; Henry, C.J.K. Does prolonged chewing reduce food intake? Fletcherism revisited. *Appetite* **2011**, *57*, 295–298. [CrossRef]
21. Révérend, B.L.; Saucy, F.; Moser, M.; Loret, C. Adaptation of mastication mechanics and eating behaviour to small differences in food texture. *Physiol. Behav.* **2016**, *165*, 136–145. [CrossRef]
22. Farooq, M.; Sazonov, E. Comparative testing of piezoelectric and printed strain sensors in characterization of chewing. In Proceedings of the 2015 37th Annual International Conference of the IEEE Engineering in Medicine and Biology Society (EMBC), Milan, Italy, 25–29 August 2015.
23. Amft, O.; Kusserow, M.; Troster, G. Bite Weight Prediction From Acoustic Recognition of Chewing. *IEEE Trans. Biomed. Eng.* **2009**, *56*, 1663–1672. [CrossRef]
24. Bedri, A.; Li, R.; Haynes, M.; Kosaraju, R.P.; Grover, I.; Prioleau, T.; Beh, M.Y.; Goel, M.; Starner, T.; Abowd, G. EarBit. *Proc. ACM Interact. Mob. Wearable Ubiquitous Technol.* **2017**, *1*, 1–20. [CrossRef]
25. Papapanagiotou, V.; Diou, C.; Zhou, L.; van den Boer, J.; Mars, M.; Delopoulos, A. A novel approach for chewing detection based on a wearable PPG sensor. In Proceedings of the 2016 38th Annual International Conference of the IEEE Engineering in Medicine and Biology Society (EMBC), Orlando, FL, USA, 16–20 August 2016.
26. Hossain, D.; Ghosh, T.; Sazonov, E. Automatic Count of Bites and Chews From Videos of Eating Episodes. *IEEE Access* **2020**, *8*, 101934–101945. [CrossRef] [PubMed]
27. Cadavid, S.; Abdel-Mottaleb, M.; Helal, A. Exploiting visual quasi-periodicity for real-time chewing event detection using active appearance models and support vector machines. *Pers. Ubiquitous Comput.* **2011**, *16*, 729–739. [CrossRef]
28. Nyamukuru, M.T.; Odame, K.M. Tiny Eats: Eating Detection on a Microcontroller. In Proceedings of the 2020 IEEE Second Workshop on Machine Learning on Edge in Sensor Systems (SenSys-ML), Sydney, Australia, 21 April 2020.
29. Little, M.A.; Varoquaux, G.; Saeb, S.; Lonini, L.; Jayaraman, A.; Mohr, D.C.; Kording, K.P. Using and understanding cross-validation strategies. Perspectives on Saeb et al. *GigaScience* **2017**, *6*, gix020. [CrossRef] [PubMed]
30. Bartko, J.J. The Intraclass Correlation Coefficient as a Measure of Reliability. *Psychol. Rep.* **1966**, *19*, 3–11. [CrossRef]
31. Shrout, P.E.; Fleiss, J.L. Intraclass correlations: Uses in assessing rater reliability. *Psychol. Bull.* **1979**, *86*, 420–428. [CrossRef]
32. Viola, P.; Jones, M. Rapid object detection using a boosted cascade of simple features. In Proceedings of the 2001 IEEE Computer Society Conference on Computer Vision and Pattern Recognition (CVPR 2001), Kauai, HI, USA, 8–14 December 2001; pp. 511–518.
33. Kazemi, V.; Sullivan, J. One millisecond face alignment with an ensemble of regression trees. In Proceedings of the 2014 IEEE Conference on Computer Vision and Pattern Recognition 2014, Columbus, OH, USA, 23–28 June 2014; pp. 1867–1874.
34. Wilson, P.I.; Fernandez, J.D. Facial feature detection using Haar classifiers. *J. Comput. Sci. Coll.* **2006**, *21*, 127–133.
35. Rabiner, L. Approximate design relationships for low-pass FIR digital filters. *IEEE Trans. Audio Electroacoust.* **1973**, *21*, 456–460. [CrossRef]
36. Shensa, M. The discrete wavelet transform: Wedding the a trous and Mallat algorithms. *IEEE Trans. Signal Process.* **1992**, *40*, 2464–2482. [CrossRef]
37. Alafeef, M.; Fraiwan, M. Smartphone-based respiratory rate estimation using photoplethysmographic imaging and discrete wavelet transform. *J. Ambient Intell. Humaniz. Comput.* **2019**, *11*, 693–703. [CrossRef]
38. Ren, J.; Kehtarnavaz, N.; Estevez, L. Real-time optimization of Viola-Jones face detection for mobile platforms. In Proceedings of the 2008 IEEE Dallas Circuits and Systems Workshop: System-on-Chip- Design, Applications, Integration, and Software, Richardson, TX, USA, 19–20 October 2008; pp. 1–4. [CrossRef]
39. Bodini, M. A Review of Facial Landmark Extraction in 2D Images and Videos Using Deep Learning. *Big Data Cogn. Comput.* **2019**, *3*, 14. [CrossRef]
40. Barina, D. Real-time wavelet transform for infinite image strips. *J. Real-Time Image Process.* **2020**, *18*, 585–591. [CrossRef]

41. Bland, J.M.; Altman, D. Statistical methods for assessing agreement between two methods of clinical measurement. *Lancet* **1986**, *327*, 307–310. [CrossRef]
42. Farooq, M.; Sazonov, E. Linear regression models for chew count estimation from piezoelectric sensor signals. In Proceedings of the 2016 10th International Conference on Sensing Technology (ICST), Nanjing, China, 11–13 November 2016. [CrossRef]
43. Taniguchi, K.; Kondo, H.; Tanaka, T.; Nishikawa, A. Earable RCC: Development of an Earphone-Type Reliable Chewing-Count Measurement Device. *J. Healthc. Eng.* **2018**, *2018*, 1–8. [CrossRef] [PubMed]
44. Wang, S.; Zhou, G.; Ma, Y.; Hu, L.; Chen, Z.; Chen, Y.; Zhao, H.; Jung, W. Eating detection and chews counting through sensing mastication muscle contraction. *Smart Health* **2018**, *9*, 179–191. [CrossRef]
45. Viola, P.; Jones, M.J. Robust Real-Time Face Detection. *Int. J. Comput. Vis.* **2004**, *57*, 137–154.:visi.0000013087.49260.fb. [CrossRef]

sensors

MDPI

Article

Encoder-Decoder Architecture for Ultrasound IMC Segmentation and cIMT Measurement

Aisha Al-Mohannadi [1], Somaya Al-Maadeed [1,*], Omar Elharrouss [1] and Kishor Kumar Sadasivuni [2]

1 Department of Computer Science and Engineering, Qatar University, Doha P.O. Box 2713, Qatar; aishaalmohannadi@outlook.com (A.A.-M.); elharrouss.omar@gmail.com (O.E.)
2 Center for Advanced Materials, Qatar University, Doha P.O. Box 2713, Qatar; kishorkumars@qu.edu.qa
* Correspondence: s_alali@qu.edu.qa

Abstract: Cardiovascular diseases (CVDs) have shown a huge impact on the number of deaths in the world. Thus, common carotid artery (CCA) segmentation and intima-media thickness (IMT) measurements have been significantly implemented to perform early diagnosis of CVDs by analyzing IMT features. Using computer vision algorithms on CCA images is not widely used for this type of diagnosis, due to the complexity and the lack of dataset to do it. The advancement of deep learning techniques has made accurate early diagnosis from images possible. In this paper, a deep-learning-based approach is proposed to apply semantic segmentation for intima-media complex (IMC) and to calculate the cIMT measurement. In order to overcome the lack of large-scale datasets, an encoder-decoder-based model is proposed using multi-image inputs that can help achieve good learning for the model using different features. The obtained results were evaluated using different image segmentation metrics which demonstrate the effectiveness of the proposed architecture. In addition, IMT thickness is computed, and the experiment showed that the proposed model is robust and fully automated compared to the state-of-the-art work.

Keywords: carotid intima-media thickness; IMT; CCA; segmentation; deep learning; encoder-decoder model

Citation: Al-Mohannadi, A.; Al-Maadeed, S.; Elharrous, O.; Sadasivuni, K.K. Encoder-Decoder Architecture for Ultrasound IMC Segmentation and cIMT Measurement. *Sensors* **2021**, *21*, 6839. https://doi.org/10.3390/s21206839

Academic Editors: Ayman El-baz, Guruprasad A. Giridharan, Ahmed Shalaby, Ali H. Mahmoud and Mohammed Ghazal

Received: 31 August 2021
Accepted: 9 October 2021
Published: 14 October 2021

1. Introduction

The heart is an essential organ in the body, where its main job is to push the blood all around the human body. Furthermore, it is the main and central part of the cardiovascular system, which contains the blood vessels that form the blood circulation [1]. Moreover, cardiovascular diseases (CVDs) play a great role in the worldwide death toll, and this highlights the importance of early diagnosis of such disease. According to World Health Organization (WHO), CVD is the first cause of death in the world, taking 17.9 million lives each year [2].

According to the authors in [3], CVD is an abnormal illness that affects the heart and the blood vessels. With that being said, the authors in [4] highlighted that in their study of the worldwide deaths that were caused by CVDs, almost half of the deaths (48.5%) were associated with coronary heart disease, while strokes only took part in 20.8% of the population tested and the rest is for other diseases. Hence, it indicates the importance of preventing the progression of coronary heart disease.

In addition, some of the risk factors of CVDs could be due to high blood pressure or high cholesterol. As a result, a buildup of inflammatory cells known as plaques in the artery wall, resulting in blood limitation to the heart and lower oxygen intake, can be one of the main causes of such disease. This phenomenon is known as atherosclerosis. As a result, early detection of this condition could aid in reducing the advancement of atherosclerosis as well as heart failure. In Figure 1, the plaque buildup is usually seen in the common carotid artery (CCA) and the internal carotid artery (ICA).

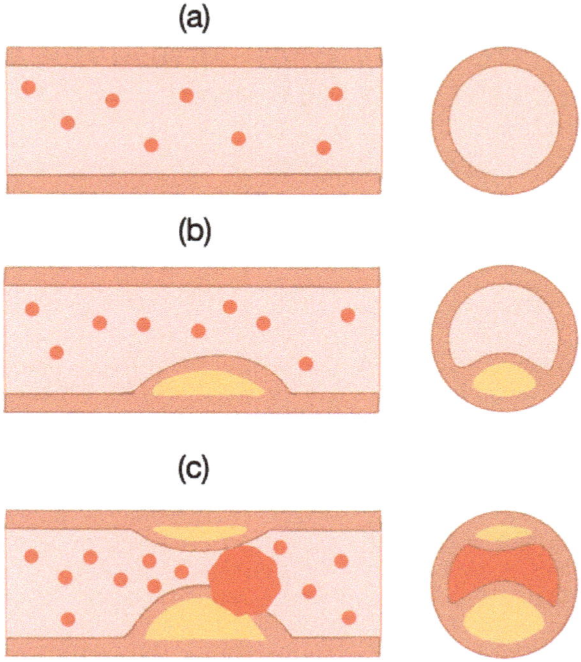

Figure 1. (**a**) Health artery, (**b**) formation of plaques in CCA, (**c**) atherosclerosis.

The carotid artery, which is made up of two blood vessels and has numerous components, including the internal, exterior, and common parts, is one approach to discover plaques in the arterial wall. Plaques can form in the interior segment of the carotid artery as well as the common blood vessels. Hence, plaques thicken the walls of these vessels, which is quantified as intima-media thickness (IMT). Thus, the difference between the lumen-initima (LI) and media adventitia (MA) walls can be measured to determine cIMT as a risk marker for early detection of heart disease [5]. Referring to a review done in [6], cIMT measures have shown to be able to predict CVD events independently of other risk variables; in fact, according to a study published in [7], it is a stronger predictor of strokes than other vascular disorders.

The carotid IMT test is a method of detecting IMT and diagnosing atherosclerosis that is carried out in clinics using an ultrasound instrument and is mostly performed by doctors. When the ultrasound image is obtained, the physician segments the IMT measurements manually. Another option is semi-automatic detection and segmentation, in which a physician locates the area of interest followed by automated segmentation of the artery walls. Furthermore, fully automated systems can detect and calculate cIMT without the need for a physician's intervention. This highlights one challenge: systems must be accurate in their calculations in order to provide a reasonable evaluation of the IMT measurement. When a fully automated model is implemented, it eliminates the need for physicians. Hence, it encourages the employment of portable devices.

Furthermore, detecting IMC and measuring it have proven difficult in some cases, where locating the artery walls and determining its boundaries can vary depending on the quality of the B-mode ultrasound images. Furthermore, ground truth points generated by physicians may contain some errors due to differences in inter and intra-observer readings.

Using deep learning techniques to diagnose such disease can be beneficial in many ways, namely, it can be deployed in portable devices, hence, help patients in self-diagnosing themselves. Additionally, it can reduce the load on doctors that might be examining and diagnosing each patient including the ones with no risks. Many applications have been conducted for cIMT segmentation and identification using deep learning and machine learning techniques, however, the accuracy of the cIMT estimation is arguable.

In this paper, we focus more on evaluating the encoder-decoder model on IMC segmentation along with finding the best hyper-parameters for the model. This is mainly done using encoder-decoder networks that aim to compress the data to a latent representation and decode it using another decoder network to decompress the image, where latent representation commonly contains the features of the image. Additionally, we train and test the model using the encoder-decoder architecture as well as a dataset from [8] with pre-processing and post-processing techniques. The main aim of this research is to perform segmentation of B-mode ultrasound images using deep learning encoder-decoder architecture.

In this work, the main purpose is to develop a system that is able to segment the IMT in the arterial walls using deep learning models. Thus, deep learning models, specifically encoder-decoder models are investigated. The main contributions of the research are summarized as the following,

- Provide a comprehensive review of convolutional autoencoder (CAE) applications as well as IMT segmentation applications.
- Develop a convolutional autoencoder model for carotid intima-media complex (IMC) segmentation and IMT measurement on B-mode ultrasound images.
- Evaluate the effectiveness of CAEs in variation with hyper-parameters.
- Find an optimal architecture for CAEs by comparing the effectiveness of models with state-of-the-art methods.

In addition, we focus on main research questions to be able to evaluate the outcome of our solution, such as, how does the encoder-decoder model improve carotid IMT segmentation as well as how is it unique from previous solutions. Finally, we examine if the encoder-decoder model is able to be effective with the data augmentation on the given dataset with a limited number of images.

The sections for the rest of the paper are divided as follows; in Section 2, we highlight the recent work applied for carotid IMT segmentation and classification, including the encoder-decoder applications as well. Then, in Section 3, we propose our solution and present the model architecture for the deep learning model along with the data preparation process. Whereas, in Section 4, we present the experimental setup along with the evaluation metrics and the results of the model. After that, in Section 5, the results are discussed and the main challenges are pointed out. Finally, we conclude and explain the future work in Section 6.

2. Related Work

This section introduces the previous methods done for carotid IMT segmentation, as well as medical applications using encoder-decoder models [9], where there is a considerable amount of literature on carotid artery IMT segmentation using deep learning, machine learning, and contour techniques. The sections are structured as follows; the encoder-decoder applications in the medical field are introduced briefly. Then, the segmentation techniques for cIMT are tackled, followed by identification of the shortcomings of the current literature that has been implemented regarding this work.

2.1. Medical Encoder-Decoder Applications

Currently, encoder-decoder models are growing in the medical imaging field, as they consist of many types including merged techniques such as stacked autoencoders (SAE), stacked denoising autoencoders (SDAE), stacked sparse autoencoders (SSAE), and convolutional variational autoencoders (CVAE). Many studies have been published on CVAE including medical applications to predict post-trauma health outcomes [10]. Another study was done by the authors of [11], which included using CVAE to automatically detect plant diseases, as well, the authors in [12] developed CVAE based system for electrocardiographic imaging (ECGI).

Several studies have been conducted for encoder-decoder models in medical applications namely, mortality risk prediction [13], as well as chest radiology improvement using denoising autoencoders [14]. Regarding image segmentation in the medical field, encoder-decoder models show a huge impact on the accuracy of applications comparing to other models. Thus, the authors of [15] claimed that their application for 3D image segmentation using CT scans shows improvement in results.

2.2. Carotid IMT Segmentation Applications

Many attempts have been made regarding carotid IMT segmentation and classification, however, only a few show competitive results given the fact that IMT segmentation is the most sensitive step as the thickness measurements depend on the accuracy of the IMT segmentation. The authors of [16] use support vector machines in order to train and segment the carotid IMT. In their method, they used 49 ultrasound images and divided them into two sets with 50% for training and the rest for testing. Their method provided 93% accuracy, and as for the IMT measurement, they found it to be 0.66 mm.

One of the first attempts for carotid segmentation was done by Loizou et al. (2013) [17], where they implemented a semi-automated snake-based segmentation system proper for complete CCA segmentation. Their method concentrated on estimating IMT measurements by manually defining the carotid plaque and diameter and then applying the snake algorithm to get the measurements. The dataset that was used for this algorithm was 300 2D ultrasound images. Their method did not result in a significant difference from the state-of-the-art, as it was limited to only manual readings.

Furthermore, the authors of [18] attempted to implement a fully automated segmentation system using adaptive snake's contour as well as level set segmentation. When comparing both techniques together the authors found out that the snake's contour method outperformed the level set segmentation. Another technique was developed by the authors of [19] that also does not depend on AI, their method included bulb edge detection and then segmental IMT measures are applied according to the detected edge. Their dataset consisted of 649 images that have between moderate and heavy lighting. They got a significantly low error in calculating the IMT measurement which is around 0.0106 mm and precision of merit that equals 98.23%.

Another technique was built by the authors of [20] that avoided the implementation of deep learning for IMT segmentation. The authors illustrated that they used wind-driven optimization technique for carotid IMT segmentation, as they focused on developing a fully automated region of interest (ROI) extraction as well as they used for intima-media complex a threshold-based method. Their results included an IMT measurement of 0.69 mm as they claimed that their method outperformed other work in the literature.

Experiments on IMT segmentation were not limited to non-AI only, where authors in [21] implemented a screening tool that integrates a two-stage artificial intelligence model for IMT and carotid plaque measurements, which consists of a CNN and fully convolutional network (FCN). The system goes through two deep learning models, as the first divides the CCA from the ultrasound images into two categories the rectangular wall and non-wall patches. Then, the region of interest is analyzed and fed to the second stage, where they identify some features to calculate the carotid IMT and the plaque total as well. Furthermore, their dataset consisted of 250 images, whereas their results while using the proposed AI model showed an error of IMT measurement that equals 0.0935 mm.

As investigations of IMT segmentation went on with deep learning and machine learning, the authors of [22] proposed a method for segmentation using CNN. Therefore, the researchers applied an algorithm that finds the ROI using the CNN architecture which includes eight layers. Moreover, they trained the network using 220 left and right CCA images for ROI localization. After that, the intima-media complex area is extracted in order to measure the IMT. The mean difference for IMT measurement is found to be 0.08 mm, where they had an accuracy of 89.99% for the CNN network.

Another research group [23] investigated IMT segmentation in video interpretation of IMT measurement using CNN. They performed CNN using six layers, and they claimed that they were able to achieve a low error rate in their measurements as they got a result of 2.1 mm error with only one failure for testing subjects. Furthermore, another technique was used by Joseph and Sivaprakasam (2020) [24], where they used double line echo patterns coming from the B-mode and A-mode ultrasound images to identify both arterial walls. Their method showed an error of IMT measurement that equals 0.18 mm.

Another combined method was implemented by researchers in [25], where they used deep learning for IMT measurement for patients with diabetes. Their method includes two stages, the first is the CNN network that is used for segmentation and the other is machine learning-based regression. Therefore, their output was the borders of the lumen intima and the media-adventitia which is used to calculate the carotid IMT. In their work, they used a dataset of 396 B-mode ultrasound images, as they got the result of the error for cIMT measurement to be around 0.126 mm. Researchers claimed that their method was 20% improved compared to other non-deep learning methods.

One more deep learning method was discussed by researchers in [26], where they used CNN with multiple hidden layers for image classification. They were able to test the network using 501 ultrasound images dataset and achieve an accuracy of 89.1% for IMT classification. The other method was developed by the authors of [27], where they used four classification algorithms for IMT measurement, the algorithms consisted of SVM with linear kernel, SVM with radial basis kernel, AdaBoost, and random forest. They evaluated their method using a dataset that consisted of 29 images, and they concluded that the best results were for the integrated random forest method which results in 80.4% sensitivity and 96.5% specificity.

One study has been made regarding IMT measurements using autoencoders and this was done by the authors of [28], their method included ROI prediction and then lumen-intima interface (LII) and media-adventitia interface (MAI) walls predictions in the predicted ROI, as their dataset consisted of 67 images. The authors claimed that they used extreme learning machines (ELM) along with autoencoders in order to distinguish which block is included in the ROI and which is not. Whereas the LII and MAI recognition was done using pixel classification. Moreover, they evaluated their IMC segmentation by using accuracy, specificity, sensitivity, and Matthews correlation coefficient (MCC). Their results used sensitivity and specificity for evaluating ROI prediction, on the other hand, accuracy and MCC were used LII and MAI. The final results were a mean IMT measurement of 0.625 ± 0.1673 mm, with an accuracy for LII of 99.30% and for MAI of 98.8%, and the MCC for LII and MAI was 98.03% and 97.05%, respectively.

Given the above methods, one research used autoencoders for IMT measurement which is the one done in [28]. Their findings were done using machine learning and autoencoders for ROI localization only, where they used another technique for IMT segmentation and recognition. Moreover, some limitations were identified, such as the fact that using semi-automated systems could lower the feature of having a portable system, also some methods used clinical instruments that are not portable. Furthermore, when compare to non-AI methods, we observe that errors found can be lower and accuracy can be enhanced further when using AI methods. To illustrate more, we conclude that work done in [25] has a lower error calculated in IMT measurement (0.126 mm) than the one in [24], which is 0.18 mm. Therefore, in our research, we focus on implementing a solution that is fully automated and supports portability along with taking into account segmentation metrics.

One more thing to point out is that Table 1 shows the different applications that have been done for IMT predictions including AI and non-AI techniques. However, comparing these applications together may not be fair since each application uses a different set of datasets, and the percentage of the dataset for training that was used is not the same. With that being said, we can make relative comparisons where we can point out the outcomes of each application given their architecture or method used. Thus, in this work, we did not compare our results quantitatively with the provided literature since different datasets are used. Instead, a comparison is only done with applications [8].

Table 1. Literature summary of cIMT segmentation applications.

Method	Dataset Size	Techniques	Metrics	Error in IMT (mm)
[16] (2018)	49	SVM	the correlation coefficient R, accuracy	0.01
[17] (2013)	300	snake's segmentation	Wilcoxon-sum test	0.01
[18] (2012)	100	snake's contour, level set segmentation	Wilcoxon-sum test	IMT SC: 0.12, LS: 0.09
[19] (2017)	D1: 172, D2: 649	bulb edge detection	precision accuracy, sensitivity, specificity	0.01603 ± 0.0031
[20] (2018)	D1: 100, D2: 25	wind driven optimization technique	The correlation coefficient R	-
[21] (2020)	250	CNN, FCN	correlation coefficient, Polyline distance metric (PDM),accuracy	0.0935 ± 0.0637
[22] (2018)	220	CNN	accuracy	0.08
[23] (2016)	92 videos	CNN	-	2.1
[24] (2020)	40	dignal processing	accuracy of RF frame sequqences with different SNR	0.18
[25] (2018)	396	FCN, CNN, regression	PDM, Precision of Merit (PoM)	0.126 ± 0.134
[26] (2019)	501	CNN	precision, recall, f1score, support	-
[27] (2017)	29	SVM	specificity, sensitivity, dice coefficient	-
[28] (2016)	67	ELM autoencoder	accuracy, specificity, sensitivity, Matthews correlation coefficient	0.1673

3. Proposed Method

Carotid artery detection and segmentation can be one of the important solutions for healthcare using medical imaging techniques. The lack of labeled large-scale datasets is one of the challenges that can be faced for this task. In the case of the carotid artery, one dataset was found with no labeling. Due to the fact that segmentation of regions of a medical image is very helpful for doctors to diagnose, a pre-processing technique on the original dataset is used to prepare this dataset for segmentation purposes. Then, using the proposed deep-learning-based model the carotid artery is segmented. To remove the false segmented pixels in the images a post-processing technique is applied using morphological operation. In this section, each step is described in detail.

3.1. Data Preparation

The dataset used for this paper is a dataset in [8]. It contains 100 carotid IMT B-Mode ultrasound images with their ground truth points determined by two clinical experts. In their work, Loizou et al. [8] highlighted that images were taken from 42 female and 58 male symptomatic patients aged between 26 and 95, where they produced longitudinal ultrasound images.

The images were obtained from the ATL HDI–3000 scanner (Advanced Technology Laboratories, Seattle, WA, USA), and were logarithmically compressed to produce images with 768 × 576 pixels resolution and 256 grey levels. The scanner has a multi-element ultrasound scan head with an operating frequency range of 4–7 MHz, an acoustic aperture of 10 × 8 mm, and a transmission focal range of 0.8–11 cm, with 64 elements fine pitch high-resolution, and 38 mm broadband array. Furthermore, the bicubic method was used to resize digital images to a standard pixel density of 16.66 pixels/mm.

Figure 2 illustrates three sample images from the dataset that we work within this paper. Given that the ultrasound image is all that is required, the frames in the samples that included patient information were removed as part of the pre-processing step.

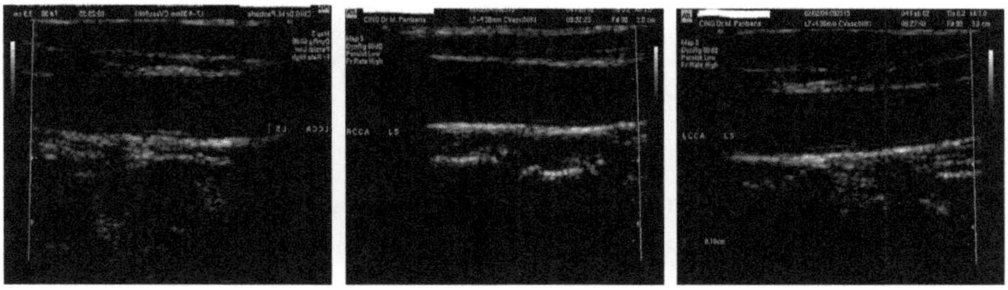

Figure 2. Three sample images from the dataset [8].

Similarly, the authors of [8] identified the IMT measurements from both experts with a number of techniques. They used speckle reduction, as well as normalization as pre-processing steps. In this research, we focus only on normalized images, hence, only IMT measurements for normalized images are used. Table 2 shows the expert's measurements for IMT in the case of normalized 100 images.

Table 2. Ground truth measurements for IMT in mm.

	Time 0	Time 12	Time 0	Time 12	Time 0	Time 12	Time 0	Time 12
Expert	Mean (Std)	Mean (Std)	Min (Std)	Min (Std)	Max (Std)	Max (Std)	Median (Std)	Median (Std)
1	0.68 (0.17)	0.68 (0.17)	0.52 (0.15)	0.52 (0.15)	0.85 (0.21)	0.85 (0.21)	0.66 (0.18)	0.66 (0.18)
2	0.61 (0.17)	0.57 (0.13)	0.54 (0.14)	0.47 (0.14)	0.7 (0.2)	0.66 (0.14)	0.61 (0.17)	0.61 (0.14)

The experts readings included two time periods one at time 0 months and the other at time 12 months. According to others in [8], this was done to test the intra-observer variability for the same expert. This means that the experts highlighted the carotid walls two times in different period of time for the same image in order to assess observer errors.

3.1.1. Pre-Processing

First of all, we took the raw images and removed the frames that were not of interest. After that, images were normalized and taken to be processed using Sobel and Prewitt gradient methods that are available built-in functions in MATLAB. We have examined them with other filters like the canny filter, however, given that it is an edge detector, the IMT region was identified as small, disconnected circles. Thus, it was not retrieving the features accurately. Then, we experimented with gradient images and found that they were able to distinguish the IMT region properly. Both methods produced gradient magnitude as well as gradient direction. For this implementation, we stored only the normalized gradient direction for both methods. After trying other filters, the gradient directional images were found to be the most accurate shows the cIMT more clearly than the rest of the images.

As for the ground truth points, we converted the points to binary images in order to input them as labels in the deep learning model, as well as to compare them with predicted images in the testing phase. In Figure 3, the original image along with the gradient images and the produced ground truth image are shown. Additionally, in order to train the model with data augmentation, the newly generated ground truth mask images were produced using lines that connects the ground truth manual points given in the dataset without using a threshold.

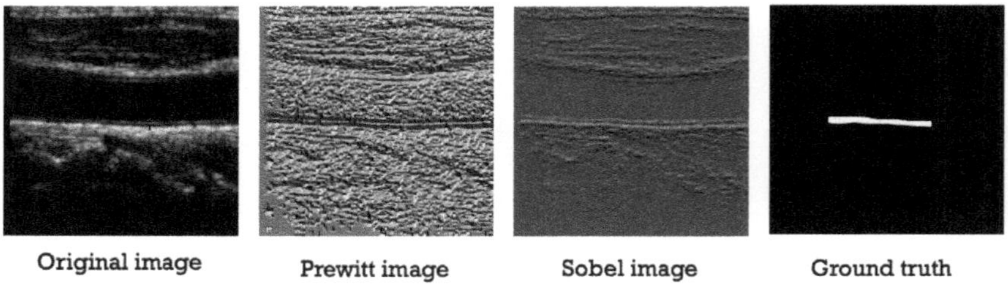

Figure 3. The pre-processing phase.

3.1.2. Data Augmentation

Data augmentation is mainly used when we have a small dataset and would like to increase the number of images in a given dataset [29]. Thus, it provides small operations that can give the ability to rotate, flip, shift, zoom, or translate a given image without changing its content. Hence, we keep the final image as the original image features. Moreover, in order to do data augmentation, we need to have binary mask images since we are changing the display of an image, then the given mask should go through the same process.

In this stage, we use special features to implement augmentation namely, rotation, width and height shift, and zoom. Table 3 shows the values used for the augmentation. The augmentation was done using ImageDataGenerator library in python, where it was used to augment both image and its binary mask.

Table 3. Data augmentation parameters.

Feature	Value
Rotation	10
Width shift	0.2
Height shift	0.2
Zoom	0.2

3.2. *Encoder-Decoder Architecture*

The introduction of deep learning techniques, such as convolutional neural networks, improved the image segmentation task in terms of the quality and quantity of segmented parts in an image. From the famous architecture that used CNNs layers for images segmentation, we can find SegNet [30] and U-Net [31] which are encoder-decoder-based models that achieved good results in semantic segmentation. Both architectures are capable of binary and multi-class segmentation, where binary image segmentation is much easier than colored image segmentation. Thus, we were inspired by the SegNet architecture to implement the proposed model for segmenting the carotid artery from ultrasound images. The proposed architecture used two inputs instead of the model's single input as used by U-Net and SegNet. A model's multiple input can assist in the extraction of useful information while allowing for multi-feature learning. The proposed model includes two encoders for feature extraction, a fusion layer, a decoder with upsampling, and convolutional layers to produce the final results.

Each encoder is implemented based on VGG-19 [32] backbone as SegNet, which is a series of (conv+BN+PReLU) layers with pooling layers and batch normalization (BN) [33]. The two encoders are merged by concatenating the feature maps of each encoder output. Like SegNet and U-Net, the proposed decoder employs blocks of upsampling (unpooling) and convolutional layers (upsampling+Conv+BN+PReLU). The encoder part's feature maps are converted into the final label by the decoder, which takes into account spatial restoration. The same structure used in the encoder is also used for the decoder by replacing the pooling layers with upsampling layers. Hence, the final architecture is shown in Figure 4. For the loss function, the SoftMax function is used to calculate the loss function:

$$loss = \frac{1}{N}\sum_{N=1}^{N}\sum_{i=1}^{k} y_j^i log(\frac{exp(p_j^i)}{\sum_{l=1}^{k} exp(p_j^l)}) \quad (1)$$

where N is the number of pixels in the input image, k is the number of classes and, for a specified pixel i; y_i denotes its label and the prediction vector.

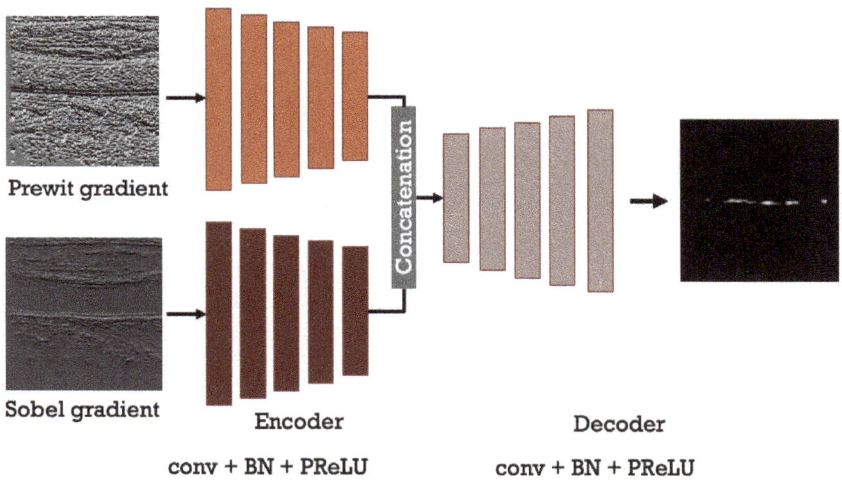

Figure 4. The model architecture used for the research solution.

For this paper, we use two components namely, the Sobel gradient direction image and Prewitt gradient direction image as inputs of the model. Additionally, these images went through pre-processing steps which are discussed in Section 3.1.1.

In the case of the segmentation process, it was mainly done by using 80% of the final dataset and converting it to both Sobel gradient and Prewitt gradient. These images were fed to the encoder-decoder architecture described in Figure 4. During the training phase, we trained the model multiple times in order to get the best performance and tune the hyper-parameters for better accuracy. Finally, the training was done using 50 epochs along with 10 steps per epoch, which means it increases the data augmentation for each epoch 10 times.

Furthermore, post-processing techniques were applied since the final segmented image had some noise that needed to be reduced and specific regions of interest (ROI) needed to be highlighted. For that, we used morphological opening, which removes any small noise in the image and can detect discontinued blobs. Additionally, we used morphological closing in order to avoid having a discontinued segmentation of the carotid artery IMT. The shape for the morphological operations was a rectangular shape with different sizes each time. Firstly, morphological close is applied with a size of [(2 ,30] in order to close the gaps between discontinued IMT. Then, morphological open with a size of [2 ,30] is applied to remove small noises from the image. Finally, morphological close is applied with a size of [3 ,30].

4. Experimental Results

This section tackles the setup and evaluation metrics that lead to the given results as well as an analysis of the produced results.

4.1. Experimental Setup

In order to implement the architecture and train it using the model described in Section 3.2, we use python programming language. We built and trained the model on NVIDIA GeForce GPU using Python. The implementation was done using Windows 10 operating system and the framework was done on Anaconda. Python version 2.7 was used for the training process. Keras and Tensorflow software packages were used to model and evaluate the results.

4.2. Evaluation Metrics

The evaluation of the deep learning model performance computed in the testing phase was based on the segmentation metrics [34,35]. These metrics are defined as follows:

- **Precision**: This calculates how close the values are to each other and how close they are to the true values.
- **Recall**: Also known as sensitivity. This is the ratio of the correct results by the overall correct data.
- **F1 Measure**: This is calculated using both precision and recall, where it gives an overall overview of the performance of the system.

$$F1\ Measure = \frac{2 * Precision * Recall}{Precision + Recall} \tag{2}$$

- **Sorensen Dice Coefficient**: This calculates the similarity of two samples and is mainly used to validate image segmentation algorithms. It is also more about the percentage of overlap between two images.

$$Dice = \frac{2 * TP}{2 * TP + FP + FN} \tag{3}$$

- **Jaccard Index**: This is the percentage of similarity for two images. It is similar to the Dice index, however, the Jaccard index takes into account true positive only once, while in the Dice Coefficient it does it twice.

$$Jaccard\ Index = \frac{TP}{TP + FP + FN} \tag{4}$$

We focus mainly about the F1 measure, Dice coefficient, and the Jaccard index in this work, as they mainly evaluate the similarity and the efficiency of the model and segmentation algorithm.

4.3. Evaluation

During the implementation of the deep learning model, we did extensive training as we ran the experiments various times with different numbers of epochs. This included changing the batch size as well as experimenting with the input images along with the pre-processing techniques.

Firstly, the training was done on the Prewitt and Sobel images as inputs with batch sizes equal to 32 and 8 as well as we included data augmentation in this phase. As a result, it was clear that the 32 batch size was not segmenting only the desired part and 8 batch size was more accurate. Thus, we trained the model using 8 batch size and augmentation in the second phase. Furthermore, we examined with changing input images as Prewitt and Sobel, and in the other experiment we made the inputs as the original image and Sobel image. However, the two gradient images were giving more accurate results. The first results were done using the architecture without batch normalization layers. We examined then the batch normalization layers on the final results and it gave preferable results than the outputs previously examined.

Similarly, Table 4 illustrates the trials that were done and how the parameters were changed. The last two trials included the batch normalization layer, which had the higher percentages in the final results explained in Table 5. In addition, in Table 6 the performance of each trial is provided.

Table 4. Experimental trials for hyper-parameter tuning.

Trial	Input 1	Input 2	Batch Size	Epochs	Steps/Epoch	Learning Rate	Augmentation
1	Prewitt	Sobel	32	50	-	0.0001	No
2	Prewitt	Sobel	8	50	-	0.0001	No
3	Prewitt	Sobel	8	15	5	0.0001	Yes
4	Original	Sobel	8	5	50	0.0001	Yes
5	Prewitt	Sobel	8	7	80	0.00001	Yes
6	**Prewitt**	**Sobel**	**8**	**50**	**10**	**0.00001**	**Yes**

Table 5. Evaluation of the experimental trials.

Trial	Input 1	Input 2	Batch Size	F1 Measure	Jaccard Index	Dice Coefficient
1	Prewitt	Sobel	32	-	50.77%	36.93%
2	Prewitt	Sobel	8	64.92%	45.65%	60.44%
3	Prewitt	Sobel	8	70.77%	45.43%	60.51%
4	Original	Sobel	8	67.63%	46.64%	61.31%
5	Prewitt	Sobel	8	73.63%	52.29%	66.07%
6	**Prewitt**	**Sobel**	**8**	**79.92%**	**60.24%**	**74.23%**

After tuning the hyper-parameters and decreasing the learning rate we were able to get the results shown in Figure 5.

In addition, the results show better similarity with the ground truth with little extension of the line. During the testing phase, we evaluate the model using three metrics discussed in Section 4.2. The results of the metrics are shown in Table 6.

According to the Jaccard index and the Dice coefficient, they show a similarity of the tested data with the binary masks. The highest percentage is the F1 measure, where it gives an overview of the performance of the system.

The results showed that the system has somewhat good performance, however, it can be further enhanced, where pre-processing or post-processing techniques need to be further enhanced. Results might not give the best accuracy due to the fact that the dataset is not very clean, as it was hard to work with.

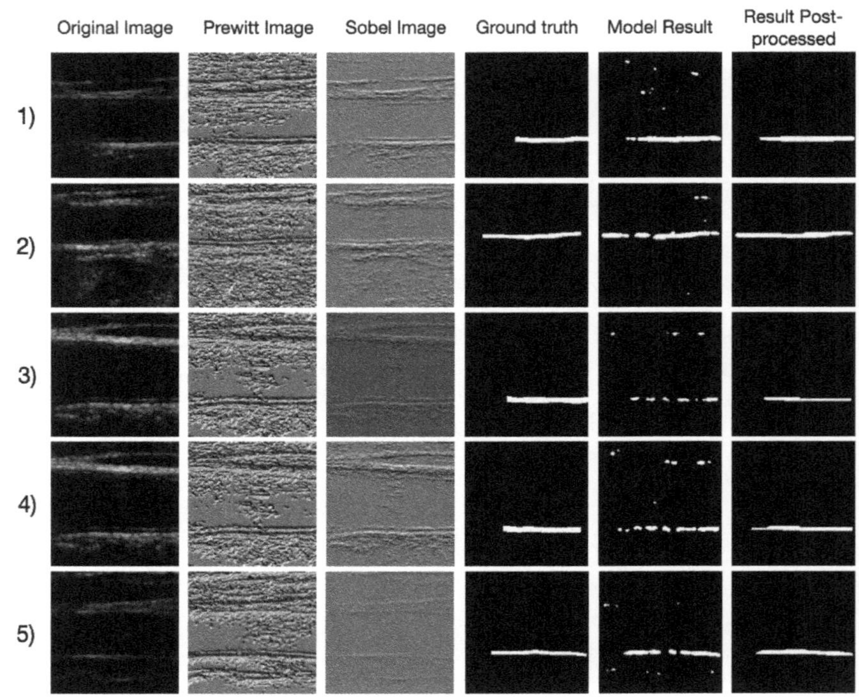

Figure 5. The results of five images for the final training.

Table 6. Improved model architecture results.

Metric	Proposed Model
F1 Measure	79.92%
Precision	81.18%
Recall	82.06%
Dice Coefficient	74.23%
Jaccard Index	60.24%

Moreover, we performed pixel calculations to get the thickness of the predicted IMT measurement. The calculations were made by calculating the distance from the upper boundary to the lower boundary. It was done using MATLAB functions bwdist(), as it calculates the vertical distance of a binary object. Additionally, the local max value was taken and then the mean value was calculated for all tested images to get the thickness as 2.989 pixels. Furthermore, converting pixels to mm we get 0.54 mm as the mean IMT measurement.

In comparison to the work done in [8], as well as the ground truth, Table 7 illustrates the error found in both the dataset and the proposed method compared to the ground truth. As explained before in Table 2, the ground truth IMT has been determined by two experts at a certain time. We observed from the table that the minimum IMT measurement in the proposed solution is smaller than the ground truth. This is due to some predictions where the IMT was not clear in the image, thus, the model was only able to distinguish a small part of the IMT. Furthermore, the median value of the proposed model is close to the reading for Expert 2 than the one in [8]. Regarding the max value, the proposed model was also able to achieve a similar thickness as Expert 2. With that being pointed out, the dataset was used in [8] had a semi-automated model, comparing our model to theirs, our results were better given the automation.

Table 7. Comparison of the results.

	Expert 1	Expert 2	Snake's Segmentation [8]	Proposed Solution
Normalized mean IMT measurement(mm) (std)	at time 0,12: 0.6 8 (0.17)	at time 0,12: 0.6 1 (0.17), 0.5 7 (0.13)	0.6 7 (0.13)	0.54
Error in mean IMT	-	-	Expert 1: at time 0,12: **0.01** , Expert 2: at time 0,12: **0.06,0.1**	Expert 1: at time 0,12: **0.14**, Expert 2: at time 0,12: **0.07,0.03**
Normalized IMT min(std)	at time 0,12: 0.5 2 (0.15)	at time 0,12: 0.54 (0.14), 0.47 (0.14)	0.51 (0.14)	0.18
Normalized IMT max(std)	at time 0,12: 0.8 5 (0.21)	at time 0,12: 0.7 (0.2), 0.66 (0.14)	0.86 (0.17)	0.71 (0.13)
Normalized IMT median(std)	at time 0,12: 0.6 6 (0.18)	at time 0,12: 0.61 (0.17), 0.61 (0.14)	0.66 (0.12)	0.60 (0.14)

5. Discussion and Challenges

Given the results discussed in Section 4, we were able to achieve a segmented region for the carotid IMT, which was then used to estimate the thickness. For this paper, we were able to train and test the images and compare them to the ground truth points.

During the implementation of this solution, many other architectures were investigated, including UNet segmentation using MATLAB. These models were trained using more than 50 epochs with no good results. Therefore, the encoder-decoder architecture was able to produce segmented output which achieved a good performance. The results of this model look promising and are good for future expansion.

One of the main challenges faced in this research is finding a good segmented and annotated dataset. We faced many issues to get a dataset and we were able to receive the dataset that we worked on. Moreover, the dataset was not clean enough to be processed, hence, it was time consuming to work on these images, where in some cases the IMT was not very clear. Thus, the output for these images from the model are discontinued parts of sections around the IMT. Additionally, the dataset has no recent studies, which makes it hard to compare between results.

According to the research questions described in Section 1, we can conclude now that the model was able to segment IMC fairly well. However, due to the lack of variety of images in the given dataset, it is not clear if the model can improve IMT segmentation. Thus, further research needs to be done regarding the dataset. Moving to the second question, the model chosen has not been used before for IMT segmentation and it has shown good results for this dataset and it is open for further improvements. We also observed from the trials and experimentation that 8 batch output with augmentation showed better segmentation than the one without augmentation. Hence, the data augmentation was effective on the dataset along with the encoder-decoder model.

In general, after comparing with the results found in [8], we identify that the proposed method is robust and fast and is fully automated compared to their semi-automated snake segmentation.

6. Conclusions and Future Direction

In conclusion, CVDs take millions of lives on a yearly basis, which means it is important to provide people with ways for early diagnosis of such a disease. Many implementations were done for such a problem using computer vision techniques for B-mode ultrasound images. In addition, we looked at recent work on carotid intima-media thickness segmentation and encoder-decoder applications. In this research, we investigated a deep learning model, specifically a convolutional autoencoder with two inputs for two encoders, and identified the optimum hyper-parameters and architecture that produced results that were similar to the dataset's provided ground truth. We trained the encoder-decoder architecture using 10 steps per epoch and 50 epochs and 80% of the dataset. We were able to obtain results of 79.92%, 74.23%, and 60.24% for the F1 Measure, Dice coefficient, and Jaccard index, respectively. We also calculated the IMT thickness, which was 0.54 mm. The model showed good performance with the lowest error of 0.03 mm, compared to the ground truth data.

Further enhancement could be done by experimenting with the optimized model along with other ultrasound B-mode carotid datasets, this would give an overview of the generality of such system and the performance given other images. Furthermore, we could experiment with different modern filters to input with the model and evaluate the performance. Our proposed system is highly recommended to be used along with a portable device that acquires ultrasound images and processes them in order to give patients the ability to early diagnose themselves.

Author Contributions: Conceptualization, A.A.-M., O.E., S.A.-M., and K.K.S.; data curation, A.A.-M.; formal analysis, A.A.-M.; investigation, A.A.-M., O.E., S.A.-M., and K.K.S.; methodology, A.A.-M., O.E., and S.A.-M.; project administration, S.A, and K.K.S.; software, A.A.-M.; supervision, S.A.-M.; validation, A.A.-M., O.E., S.A.-M., and K.K.S.; visualization, A.A.-M., and O.E.; writing—original draft, A.A.-M.; writing—review and editing, A.A.-M., O.E., S.A.-M., and K.K.S. All authors have read and agreed to the published version of the manuscript.

Funding: This publication was supported by Qatar University Internal Grant No. IRCC-2020-013 and Sultan Qaboos University through Grant # CL/SQU-QU/ENG/20/01, respectively. The findings achieved herein are solely the responsibility of the authors.

Institutional Review Board Statement: Not applicable.

Informed Consent Statement: Not applicable.

Data Availability Statement: Not applicable.

Conflicts of Interest: The authors declare no conflict of interest.

References

1. Yahaya, L.; David Oye, N.; Joshua Garba, E. A comprehensive review on heart disease prediction using data mining and machine learning techniques. *Am. J. Artif. Intell.* **2020**, *4*, 20. [CrossRef]
2. Cardiovascular Diseases. Available online: https://www.who.int/health-topics/cardiovascular-diseases (accessed on 20 February 2021).
3. Coronary Heart Disease. Available online: https://www.healthknowledge.org.uk/public-health-textbook/disease-causation-diagnostic/2b-epidemiology-diseases-phs/chronic-diseases/coronary-heart-disease (accessed on 20 February 2021).
4. Hamer, M.; O'Donovan, G.; Stamatakis, E. Association between physical activity and sub-types of cardiovascular disease death causes in a general population cohort. *Eur. J. Epidemiol.* **2018**, *34*, 483–487. [CrossRef]
5. Molinari, F.; Meiburger, K.M.; Saba, L.; Rajendra Acharya, U.; Ledda, M.; Nicolaides, A.; Suri, J.S. Constrained snake vs. conventional snake for carotid ultrasound automated IMT measurements on multi-center data sets. *Ultrasonics* **2012**, *52*, 949–961. [CrossRef] [PubMed]
6. Ravani, A.; Werba, J.; Frigerio, B.; Sansaro, D.; Amato, M.; Tremoli, E.; Baldassarre, D. Assessment and Relevance of Carotid Intima-Media Thickness (C-IMT) in Primary and Secondary Cardiovascular Prevention. *Curr. Pharm. Des.* **2015**, *21*, 1164–1171. [CrossRef]
7. Saxena, Y.; Saxena, V.; Mittal, M.; Srivastava, M.; Raghuvanshi, S. Age-Wise Association of Carotid Intima Media Thickness in Ischemic Stroke. *Ann. Neurosci.* **2017**, *24*, 5–11. [CrossRef] [PubMed]
8. Petroudi, S.; Loizou, C.; Pantziaris, M.; Pattichis, C. Segmentation of the Common Carotid Intima-Media Complex in Ultrasound Images Using Active Contours. *IEEE Trans. Biomed. Eng.* **2012**, *59*, 3060–3069. [CrossRef] [PubMed]
9. Elharrouss, O.; Subramanian, N.; Al-Maadeed, S. An encoder-decoder-based method for COVID-19 lung infection segmentation. *arXiv* **2020**, arXiv:2007.00861.
10. Cakmak, A.S.; Thigpen, N.; Honke, G.; Alday, E.P.; Rad, A.B.; Adaimi, R.; Chang, C.J.; Li, Q.; Gupta, P.; Neylan, T.; et al. Using Convolutional Variational Autoencoders to Predict Post-Trauma Health Outcomes from Actigraphy Data. *arXiv* **2020**, arXiv:cs.LG/2011.07406.
11. Zilvan, V.; Ramdan, A.; Suryawati, E.; Kusumo, R.; Krisnandi, D.; Pardede, H. Denoising Convolutional Variational Autoencoders-Based Feature Learning for Automatic Detection of Plant Diseases. In Proceedings of the 2019 3rd International Conference on Informatics and Computational Sciences (ICICoS), Semarang, Indonesia, 29–30 September 2019; pp. 1–6. [CrossRef]
12. Bacoyannis, T.; Krebs, J.; Cedilnik, N.; Cochet, H.; Sermesant, M. Deep Learning Formulation of ECGI for Data-Driven Integration of Spatiotemporal Correlations and Imaging Information. In *International Conference on Functional Imaging and Modeling of the Heart*; Springer: Cham, Switzerland, 2019; pp. 20–28. [CrossRef]

13. Alhassan, Z.; Budgen, D.; Alshammari, R.; Daghstani, T.; McGough, A.S.; Al Moubayed, N. Stacked Denoising Autoencoders for Mortality Risk Prediction Using Imbalanced Clinical Data. In Proceedings of the 2018 17th IEEE International Conference on Machine Learning and Applications (ICMLA), Orlando, FL, USA, 17–20 December 2018; pp. 541–546. [CrossRef]
14. Lee, D.; Choi, S.; Kim, H.J. Performance evaluation of image denoising developed using convolutional denoising autoencoders in chest radiography. *Nucl. Instrum. Methods Phys. Res. Sect. A* **2018**, *884*, 97–104. [CrossRef]
15. Sital, C.; Brosch, T.; Tio, D.; Raaijmakers, A.; Weese, J. 3D medical image segmentation with labeled and unlabeled data using autoencoders at the example of liver segmentation in CT images. *arXiv* **2020**, arXiv:eess.IV/2003.07923.
16. Nagaraj, Y.; Teja, A.; Narasimha, D. Automatic Segmentation of Intima Media Complex in Carotid Ultrasound Images Using Support Vector Machine. *Arab. J. Sci. Eng.* **2018**, *44*. [CrossRef]
17. Loizou, C.; Kasparis, T.; Spyrou, C.; Pantzaris, M. Integrated system for the complete segmentation of the common carotid artery bifurcation in ultrasound images. In *IFIP International Conference on Artificial Intelligence Applications and Innovations*; Springer: Berlin/Heidelberg, Germany, 2013; Volume 412, pp. 292–301. [CrossRef]
18. Christodoulou, L.; Loizou, C.P.; Spyrou, C.; Kasparis, T.; Pantziaris, M. Full-automated system for the segmentation of the common carotid artery in ultrasound images. In Proceedings of the 2012 5th International Symposium on Communications, Control and Signal Processing, Rome, Italy, 2–4 May 2012; pp. 1–6. [CrossRef]
19. Ikeda, N.; Dey, N.; Sharma, A.; Gupta, A.; Bose, S.; Acharjee, S.; Shafique, S.; Cuadrado-Godia, E.; Araki, T.; Saba, L.; et al. Automated Segmental-IMT Measurement in Thin/Thick Plaque with Bulb Presence in Carotid Ultrasound from Multiple Scanners: Stroke Risk Assessment. *Comput. Methods Programs Biomed.* **2017**, *141*. [CrossRef] [PubMed]
20. Madipalli, P.; Kotta, S.; Dadi, H.; Nagaraj, Y.; Asha, C.S.; Narasimhadhan, A.V. Automatic Segmentation of Intima Media Complex in Common Carotid Artery using Adaptive Wind Driven Optimization. In Proceedings of the 2018 Twenty Fourth National Conference on Communications (NCC), Hyderbad, India, 25–28 February 2018; pp. 1–6. [CrossRef]
21. Biswas, M.; Saba, L.; Chakrabartty, S.; Khanna, N.N.; Song, H.; Suri, H.S.; Sfikakis, P.P.; Mavrogeni, S.; Viskovic, K.; Laird, J.R.; et al. Two-stage artificial intelligence model for jointly measurement of atherosclerotic wall thickness and plaque burden in carotid ultrasound: A screening tool for cardiovascular/stroke risk assessment. *Comput. Biol. Med.* **2020**, *123*, 103847. [CrossRef] [PubMed]
22. Madian, N.; Sunder, T. Convolutional Neural Network for Segmentation and Measurement of Intima Media Thickness. *J. Med. Syst.* **2018**, *42*. [CrossRef]
23. Shin, J.Y.; Tajbakhsh, N.; Hurst, R.T.; Kendall, C.B.; Liang, J. Automating Carotid Intima-Media Thickness Video Interpretation with Convolutional Neural Networks. In Proceedings of the 2016 IEEE Conference on Computer Vision and Pattern Recognition (CVPR), Las Vegas, NV, USA, 27–30 June 2016; pp. 2526–2535. [CrossRef]
24. Raj, K.V.; Joseph, J.; Sivaprakasam, M. Automated Measurement of Compression-Decompression in Arterial Diameter and Wall Thickness by Image-Free Ultrasound. *Comput. Methods Programs Biomed.* **2020**, *194*, 105557. [CrossRef]
25. Biswas, M.; Kuppili, V.; Araki, T.; Edla, D.; Godia, E.; Saba, L.; Suri, H.; Omerzu, T.; Laird, J.; Khanna, N.; et al. Deep learning strategy for accurate carotid intima-media thickness measurement: An ultrasound study on Japanese diabetic cohort. *Comput. Biol. Med.* **2018**, *98*. [CrossRef]
26. Savaş, S.; Topaloglu, N.; Kazcı, Ö.; Koşar, P. Classification of Carotid Artery Intima Media Thickness Ultrasound Images with Deep Learning. *J. Med. Syst.* **2019**, *43*. [CrossRef]
27. Qian, C.; Yang, X. An Integrated Method For Atherosclerotic Carotid Plaque Segmentation In Ultrasound Image. *Comput. Methods Programs Biomed.* **2017**, *153*. [CrossRef]
28. Menchón-Lara, R.M.; Sancho-Gómez, J.L.; Bueno-Crespo, A. Early-stage atherosclerosis detection using deep learning over carotid ultrasound images. *Appl. Soft Comput.* **2016**, *49*, 616–628. [CrossRef]
29. Elharrouss, O.; Almaadeed, N.; Al-Maadeed, S.; Bouridane, A. Gait recognition for person re-identification. *J. Supercomput.* **2021**, *77*, 3653–3672. [CrossRef]
30. Khagi, B.; Kwon, G.R. Pixel-Label-Based segmentation of Cross-Sectional Brain MRI using Simplified SEGNET Architecture-Based CNN. *J. Healthc. Eng.* **2018**, *2018*, 1–8. [CrossRef] [PubMed]
31. Ronneberger, O.; Fischer, P.; Brox, T. U-net: Convolutional networks for biomedical image segmentation. In *International Conference on Medical Image Computing and Computer-Assisted Intervention*; Springer: Munich, Germany, 2015; pp. 234–241.
32. Simonyan, K.; Zisserman, A. Very deep convolutional networks for large-scale image recognition. *arXiv* **2014**, arXiv:1409.1556.
33. Ioffe, S.; Szegedy, C. Batch normalization: Accelerating deep network training by reducing internal covariate shift. In *International Conference on Machine Learning*; PMLR 37: Lille, France, 2015; pp. 448–456.
34. Elharrouss, O.; Abbad, A.; Moujahid, D.; Riffi, J.; Tairi, H. A block-based background model for moving object detection. *ELCVIA Electron. Lett. Comput. Vis. Image Anal.* **2016**, *15*, 17–31. [CrossRef]
35. Elharrouss, O.; Moujahid, D.; Elkah, S.; Tairi, H. Moving object detection using a background modeling based on entropy theory and quad-tree decomposition. *J. Electron. Imaging* **2016**, *25*, 061615. [CrossRef]

sensors

MDPI

Article

A Flow Sensor-Based Suction-Index Control Strategy for Rotary Left Ventricular Assist Devices

Lixue Liang [1], Kairong Qin [2], Ayman S. El-Baz [3], Thomas J. Roussel [3], Palaniappan Sethu [4], Guruprasad A. Giridharan [3,†] and Yu Wang [2,*,†]

1 School of Mechanical Engineering, Dalian University of Technology, No. 2 Linggong Road, Ganjingzi District, Dalian 116024, China; lixueliang@mail.dlut.edu.cn
2 School of Optoelectronic Engineering and Instrumentation Science, Dalian University of Technology, No. 2 Linggong Road, Ganjingzi District, Dalian 116024, China; krqin@dlut.edu.cn
3 Department of Bioengineering, University of Louisville, Louisville, KY 40292, USA; ayman.elbaz@louisville.edu (A.S.E.-B.); thomas.roussel@louisville.edu (T.J.R.); guruprasad.giridharan@louisville.edu (G.A.G.)
4 Department of Biomedical Engineering, School of Engineering, University of Alabama at Birmingham, 1075 13th St. S., Birmingham, AL 35294, USA; psethu@uabmc.edu
* Correspondence: yuwang0410@dlut.edu.cn
† These authors had equal credits.

Abstract: Rotary left ventricular assist devices (LVAD) have emerged as a long-term treatment option for patients with advanced heart failure. LVADs need to maintain sufficient physiological perfusion while avoiding left ventricular myocardial damage due to suction at the LVAD inlet. To achieve these objectives, a control algorithm that utilizes a calculated suction index from measured pump flow (SIMPF) is proposed. This algorithm maintained a reference, user-defined SIMPF value, and was evaluated using an in silico model of the human circulatory system coupled to an axial or mixed flow LVAD with 5–10% uniformly distributed measurement noise added to flow sensors. Efficacy of the SIMPF algorithm was compared to a constant pump speed control strategy currently used clinically, and control algorithms proposed in the literature including differential pump speed control, left ventricular end-diastolic pressure control, mean aortic pressure control, and differential pressure control during (1) rest and exercise states; (2) rapid, eight-fold augmentation of pulmonary vascular resistance for (1); and (3) rapid change in physiologic states between rest and exercise. Maintaining SIMPF simultaneously provided sufficient physiological perfusion and avoided ventricular suction. Performance of the SIMPF algorithm was superior to the compared control strategies for both types of LVAD, demonstrating pump independence of the SIMPF algorithm.

Keywords: left ventricular assist devices; sensor-based control; pump independent; suction index; physiological perfusion; suction prevention

Citation: Liang, L.; Qin, K.; El-Baz, A.S.; Roussel, T.J.; Sethu, P.; Giridharan, G.A.; Wang, Y. A Flow Sensor-Based Suction-Index Control Strategy for Rotary Left Ventricular Assist Devices. *Sensors* **2021**, *21*, 6890. https://doi.org/10.3390/s21206890

Academic Editor: James F. Rusling

Received: 2 September 2021
Accepted: 13 October 2021
Published: 18 October 2021

1. Introduction

Heart failure (HF) is a highly prevalent disease and a leading cause of mortality in the world, with approximately 2% of adults suffering from HF worldwide [1]. The most effective treatment for advanced HF is heart transplantation [2], but due to the limited number of available donor hearts, only a few thousand patients in the world receive heart transplantation every year, with more than 20% of waitlisted patients perishing before a donor heart becomes available [3]. Rotary left ventricular assist devices (LVAD), surgically implantable mechanical blood pumps, have been increasingly utilized as a long-term treatment for advanced HF patients. The pump inlet is attached to the apex of the left ventricle (LV) and the pump outlet is anastomosed to the aorta. The LVAD pumps blood from the LV to the aorta, alleviating the workload of the native heart, thereby serving as a bridge to transplantation or destination therapy [4,5]. Rotary LVADs have effectively replaced pulsatile LVADs since rotary LVADs are mechanically simpler, smaller, lighter weight, and have higher operating efficiencies. Additionally, rotary LVADs are more durable, showing improved survival rates compared to pulsatile LVADs [6,7].

LVADs must generate sufficient physiological perfusion as insufficient pump flow rates can lead to hypoperfusion, pulmonary edema, and volume overload of the native LV. Simultaneously, LVADs must also avoid suction due to over pumping, which can result in severe LV decompression and/or LVAD inflow obstruction. Suction events can trigger pump flow stoppage, LV collapse, myocardial damage, or induce myocardial arrhythmias, each of which may lead to potentially life-threatening events or death [8]. Pulsatile LVADs have low risk of LV suction due to phasic filling, which results in a higher preload sensitivity. In contrast, suction occurs commonly during the rotary LVAD support due to its lower preload sensitivity [9,10]. For example, 15 out of 19 patients with rotary LVAD support experienced suction events with 13 suction events per 1000 min of support [11]. Patients with rotary LVADs are also prone to suction during Valsalva maneuver, coughing, hypovolemia, and transient reduction in cardiac return [12]. Therefore, avoiding LV suction while providing adequate pump-augmented cardiac output (CO) during various levels of activity is critical for patients on LVAD support.

Suction detection algorithms based on a variety of pump signals for rotary LVADs have been proposed [13–16], however, these algorithms only detect suction events after they have occurred, which results in myocardial damage. Many physiological control strategies have also been developed that aim to reduce LV suction events [17–22], but some of these require the measurement of ventricular pressure and/or volume, which require sensors that are in contact with blood, and thus susceptible to thrombosis or failure, while others may not be able to generate sufficient perfusion during varying physiological conditions. Our group and others have developed sensorless algorithms [23–26] with model-based parameter estimation strategies. However, the performance of these algorithms may be adversely affected by changes in blood viscosity, friction forces, and device inertia [27]. Recently, non-model-based, sensorless control algorithms have been proposed [27,28], but the performance of the differential pump speed (ΔRPM) controller may be degraded by increased levels of measurement noise or with rapidly changing ventricular contractilities. Furthermore, obtaining the suction index (SI) from the pump speed (PS) cannot be pump-independent. Constant parameter-based control strategies by maintaining constant pump speed (CPS), LV end-diastolic pressure (LVEDP), mean aortic pressure (MAoP), and pressure head (ΔP) across the LVAD have also been proposed in the literature [29–31]. While these control algorithms can be effective in a limited set of conditions, they may not be adequate with changing physiologic demand conditions.

In this paper, a new pump-independent, flow sensor based control algorithm is proposed. In contrast to pressure and volume sensors, ultrasonic flow sensors are implanted outside the pump outflow graft and do not come in contact with blood. Flow sensors have been clinically implanted in patients with the HeartAssist 5 LVAD [32]. In this manuscript, we utilize the measured pump flow (PF) signal (e.g., SIMPF control) with 5% and 10% normally distributed noise added to the original signal. The feasibility of the control algorithm to sense the adequate level of perfusion and avoid suction was tested for two different types of rotary LVADs to test for pump independence. Performance of the proposed SIMPF control strategy was evaluated in silico under different simulated conditions and compared to other control algorithms that are clinically used or previously reported in the literature.

2. Methods

2.1. Modeling of the Biventricular Cardiovascular System

In this study, a validated and published model of a biventricular cardiovascular system was used to develop the SIMPF control algorithm. The lumped parameter model has previously been used for testing control algorithms, timing algorithms, and fault detection algorithms with different types of LVADs [27,33,34]. Four valves and twelve lumped parameter blocks constitute the model [28]. Amongst these blocks, nonlinear active elements include the left and right atrium and ventricles because their values of compliance were time-varying, and the other blocks had time-invariant compliance values. Each block was represented using the differential equation that described the rate of change of volume (V) as a function of resistance (R), and compliance (C), as follows:

$$\frac{dV_n}{dt} = F_n^{in} - F_n^{out} \tag{1}$$

$$\frac{dV_n}{dt} = \frac{V_{n-1}}{C_{n-1}R_{n-1}} - \frac{V_n}{C_n}\left(\frac{1}{R_{n-1}} + \frac{1}{R_n}\right) + \frac{V_{n+1}}{C_{n+1}R_n} \tag{2}$$

where in block n, dV_n/dt is the rate of volumetric change; F^{in} is blood flowing into the block n; and F^{out} is blood flowing out of the block n. A model of a rotary LVAD, which was an axial flow pump (AFP) or Deltastream mixed flow pump (DP2), was incorporated into this circulatory system model.

2.2. The Rotary LVAD Model

The model of the axial flow rotary LVAD is described by the following two ordinary differential equations:

$$J\frac{d\omega}{dt} = \frac{3}{2}K_B I - B\omega - a_0\omega^3 - a_1 F_p \omega^2 \tag{3}$$

$$\frac{dV_n}{dt} = \frac{V_{n-1}}{C_{n-1}R_{n-1}} - \frac{V_n}{C_n}\left(\frac{1}{R_{n-1}} + \frac{1}{R_n}\right) + \frac{V_{n+1}}{C_{n+1}R_n} \tag{4}$$

where the various model parameters (J, ω, K_B, I, B, a_0, a_1, F_p, b_0, b_1, and b_2) in Equations (3) and (4) and their associated values can be found in [35,36]. ω is the LVAD pump speed, the pump current (control variable) is represented by I, and F_p is the LVAD pump flow.

A mixed flow LVAD (DP2) model was also simulated in this study to demonstrate the pump independence of the SIMPF control algorithm. The model of DP2 was developed by Petrou et al. [37]:

$$\frac{d\omega}{dt} = \frac{1}{J(\omega)}\left(k_T I - g_1(\omega) + g_2\omega - g_3\omega^2 - g_4 F_p \omega\right) \tag{5}$$

$$\frac{dF_p}{dt} = -\frac{1}{F}\left(-\Delta P + f_1\omega^2 - f_2 F_P - f_3 F_p^2\right) \tag{6}$$

The various model parameters ($J(\omega)$, k_T, $g_1(\omega)$, g_2, g_3, g_4, f_1, f_2, f_3) in Equations (5) and (6) and their associated values can be found in [37]. Either AFP or DP2 was incorporated into the biventricular cardiovascular model to remove volume from the LV and to add volume to the aorta.

2.3. SIMPF Control Strategy

The SIMPF control strategy was developed to keep a single fixed setpoint and provide adequate COs for the circulatory system under varying physiological conditions, while preventing LV suction. In order to achieve this proposed control algorithm, the real-time SI was extracted with a sampling rate of 100 Hz and a moving window of 5 s [12,14]. The window was recalculated every 0.1 s:

$$SI = \frac{max\left[\frac{d(PF)}{dt}\right] - min\left[\frac{d(PF)}{dt}\right]}{max(PF)} \tag{7}$$

In this study, PF was measured using the flow sensor including 5% and 10% uniformly distributed measurement noise, and the implementation of the SIMPF control strategy depended on a gain scheduled PI controller. The following control law was used to update the pump current:

$$I = K_P(SI - SI_r) + K_I \int_0^t (SI - SI_r)dt \tag{8}$$

where the SI setpoint is represented by SI_r, and the proportional and integral coefficients are represented by K_P and K_I, respectively. These parameters can be determined *a priori* [38] and were unchanged during all test conditions in both pumps. In this study, the controller of AFP used 9, 0.07, and 0.014 for SI_r, K_P, and K_I, respectively, while the controller of DP2 set 5, 0.15, and 0.03 for SI_r, K_P, and K_I, respectively. Figure 1 shows the schematic of the proposed SIMPF control strategy and the related flowchart, respectively.

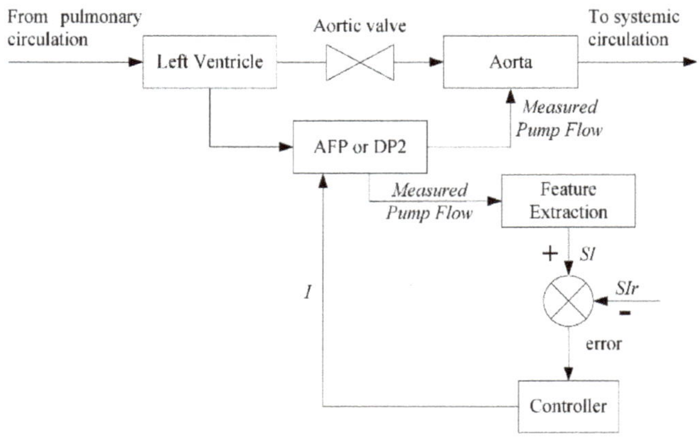

(**a**)

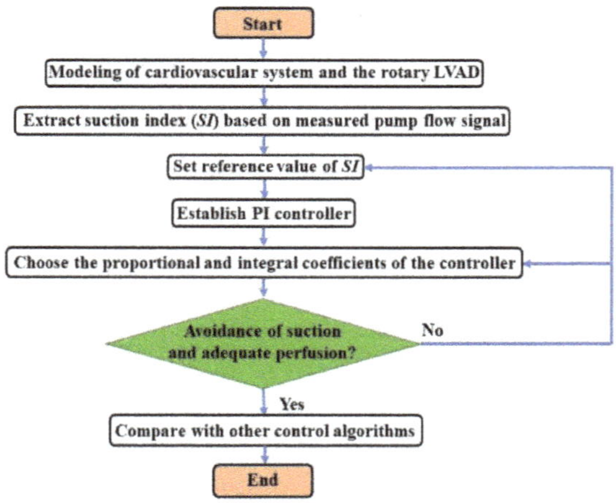

(**b**)

Figure 1. (**a**) Diagrammatic drawing of the proposed suction-index based measured pump flow (SIMPF) control algorithm. The measured pump flow (PF) signals were used to calculate suction index (*SI*) and fed to the PI controller with the reference *SI* (SI_r) for axial flow pump (AFP) and Deltastream mixed flow pump (DP2), respectively, which were surgically implanted from the left ventricular to the aorta. (**b**) Flowchart of the proposed *SI* control method.

2.4. Comparison with the Other Control Strategies

The SIMPF control strategy was compared to previously reported control strategies. (1) sensorless ΔRPM control that kept the actual ΔRPM above a fixed setpoint, $\Delta RPMr$. The actual ΔRPM was obtained using the difference between the maximum and minimum PS as described in [27]. The reference ΔRPM_r was set to 800 RPM for AFP to satisfy the physiological demands during rest (PF was 5 L/min), and K_P and K_I were 0.00025 and 0.00005, respectively. For DP2, ΔRPM_r was set to 150 RPM, K_P and K_I were 0.0004 and 0.00008, respectively. (2) Maintain a CPS [28]. The setpoint of PS was 10,452 RPM selected for AFP to provide sufficient physiological perfusion at rest, and K_P and K_I were 0.003 and 0.0006, respectively. In addition, the PS setpoint was 4338 RPM, and K_P and K_I were 0.006 and 0.0012 for DP2, respectively. This sensorless control method was regarded as CPS control, the current clinical standard. (3) Control the average ΔP from the LV to aorta across an LVAD, ΔP control. ΔP can be estimated using pump speed measurements with 2% noise, an extended Kalman filter (EKF) [39,40], and a second order polynomial Golay–Savitsky (GS) filter [41,42], which was established with a 17-point moving window. Low and high frequencies could be filtered with the GS filter by holding the maximum and minimum values [29]. The reference value of ΔP was set to 87 mmHg to meet the physiological perfusion of 5 L/min at rest, and K_P and K_I were 0.008 and 0.0016 for AFP and DP2, respectively. (4) Maintain a constant MAoP [30]. MAoP can be measured using a pressure sensor (sensor-based MAoP control). The reference MAoP was set as 100 mmHg to reach a total output of 5 L/min under rest condition. K_P and K_I were set to 0.007 and 0.0014, respectively, for both pumps. (5) Maintain an average LVEDP [31]. LVEDP can be measured using pressure sensors. The setpoint of LVEDP was 6.6 mmHg to match PF of 5 L/min under rest with K_P = 0.045 and K_I = 0.009 for both pumps. This sensor-based control method is referred to as the LVEDP control.

2.5. Simulation Description and Data Analysis

Several conditions were considered to quantify the overall performance of all the control algorithms: (1) rest and exercise; (2) rapid pulmonary vascular resistance (PVR) increase by eight-fold during rest and exercise; (3) rapid change in physiologic condition from rest to exercise and exercise to rest. Noise was included to simulate a uniformly distributed random variable up to ±5 to 10% of actual PF signals [27]. The simulated heart rates were 80 bpm during rest and 120 bpm during exercise. All the initial pump parameters were zero, approximating a realistic pump start condition.

MATLAB (MathWorks, Natick, MA, USA) was used for simulation, data reduction, and analysis including the calculation of PS, PF, CO, AoP, LVEDP, and left ventricular volume (LVV). The mean values in this simulation were calculated based on the final 20 cardiac cycles after the simulation reached a steady state. Instantaneous values of LV pressure less than 1 mmHg were considered to be a suction event [3,17,43].

3. Results

3.1. The Proposed SIMPF Control Algorithm

Figure 2 shows the extracted SI from the measured pump flow signals for both axial and mixed flow pumps, respectively. The extracted SI was initially high at low LVAD flow rates and reduced gradually to 9 ± 0.5 and 5 ± 0.3, which were close to the SIr setpoints for AFP and DP2, respectively, while PF, PS, and control variable increased. The proposed SIMPF control algorithm provided sufficient physiologic perfusion and avoided suction during various conditions (Tables 1 and 2). For AFP, the SIMPF control algorithm generated flow rates of 5 L/min and 8.2 L/min at rest and exercise (Table 1), respectively. Figures 3a–c and 4a–c demonstrate that the SIMPF control strategy successfully avoided LV suction under conditions when the PVR increased 8-fold and during step change from exercise to rest for AFP. The simulated results of DP2 were similar to AFP during almost all test conditions (Figures 5a–c and 6a–c). In addition, at rest, the root mean square errors (RMSE) of the measured values of pump flow rate were 2.4 mL/s (5% noise) and

4.8 mL/s (10% noise) for AFP, and 2.4 mL/s (5% noise) and 4.8 mL/s (10% noise) for DP2, respectively. At exercise, RMSE of the measured values of pump flow rate were 3.9 mL/s (5% noise) and 7.9 mL/s (10% noise) for AFP, and 3.8 mL/s (5% noise) and 7.9 mL/s (10% noise) for DP2, respectively.

Table 1. Performance comparison among the proposed SIMPF control strategy and other control algorithms during various test conditions with AFP.

	CO (L/min)	AoP (mmHg)	Min LVP (mmHg)	LVV (mL)	Mean PS (RPM)	Suction
		Healthy heart without LVAD support				
Rest	5.0	122/80	2.7	43/106	N/A	No
Exercise	8.6	121/74	2.8	42/114	N/A	No
		HF without LVAD support				
Rest	3.8	97/63	15.5	181/229	N/A	No
Exercise	6.8	95/58	15.4	178/234	N/A	No
		HF with AFP support at rest				
SIMPF control [1]	4.9	102/97	4.7	54/82	10,365	No
SIMPF control [2]	5.0	103/98	4.4	49/77	10,441	No
ΔRPM control	5.1	104/101	3.3	35/62	10,717	No
CPS control	5.0	103/97	4.4	49/78	10,448	No
ΔP control	5.0	103/97	4.4	50/78	10,447	No
MAoP control	5.0	103/99	4.1	46/74	10,506	No
LVEDP control	5.0	103/98	4.4	49/77	10,449	No
		HF with AFP support at exercise				
SIMPF control [1]	8.1	94/89	6.7	75/106	10,505	No
SIMPF control [2]	8.2	95/91	6.1	68/98	10,653	No
ΔRPM control	8.5	97/94	4.8	51/80	11,000	No
CPS control	8.1	94/88	7.0	79/109	10,450	No
ΔP control	8.7	99/96	3.5	36/64	11,276	No
MAoP control	9.0	101/99	2.2	20/47	11,590	No
LVEDP control	8.5	98/94	4.5	48/77	11,037	No
		HF with AFP support during 8-fold increase in PVR at rest				
SIMPF control [1]	4.3	90/85	1.2	46/68	9712	No
SIMPF control [2]	4.3	90/86	1.1	42/64	9800	No
ΔRPM control	4.4	90/87	0.8	37/58	9900	IS
CPS control	4.6	94/92	0.5	14/29	10,448	IS
ΔP control	4.6	93/91	0.6	17/34	10,355	IS
MAoP control	5.0	100/100	−1.8	−2/−1	11,065	CS
LVEDP control	4.2	89/84	2.3	54/77	9547	No
		HF with AFP support during 8-fold increase in PVR at exercise				
SIMPF control [1]	7.1	83/78	2.7	65/90	9867	No
SIMPF control [2]	7.2	84/79	2.3	58/83	10,013	No
ΔRPM control	7.3	85/81	1.4	51/75	10,176	No
CPS control	7.5	86/83	2.2	38/60	10,450	No
ΔP control	8.1	92/90	0.5	13/26	11,149	IS
MAoP control	8.9	100/100	−5.1	−13/−7	11,950	CS
LVEDP control	7.3	84/80	1.7	53/77	10,125	No

[1] With 5% noise. [2] With 10% noise.

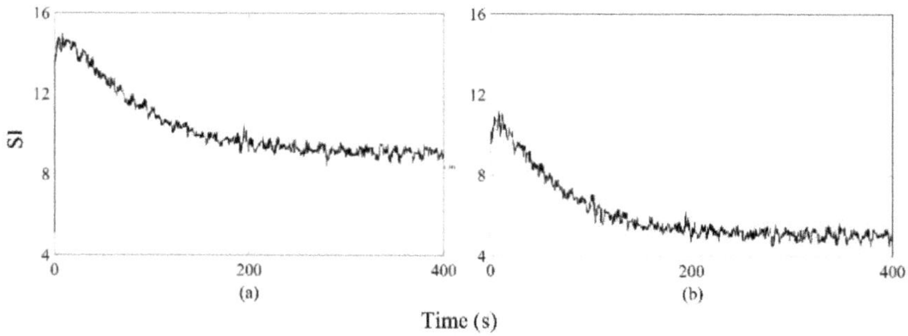

Figure 2. Measured pump flow signals were used to calculate *SI*, whose values gradually decreased and finally approached the setpoints of 9 for AFP (**a**) and 5 for DP2 (**b**), respectively.

Table 2. Performance comparison among the proposed SIMPF control strategy and other control algorithms during various test conditions with DP2.

	CO (L/min)	AoP (mmHg)	Min LVP (mmHg)	LVV (mL)	Mean PS (RPM)	Suction
			Healthy heart without LVAD support			
Rest	5.0	122/80	2.7	43/106	N/A	No
Exercise	8.6	121/74	2.8	42/114	N/A	No
			HF without LVAD support			
Rest	3.8	97/63	15.5	181/229	N/A	No
Exercise	6.8	95/58	15.4	178/234	N/A	No
			HF with DP2 support at rest			
SIMPF control [1]	5.0	102/98	4.2	50/76	4337	No
SIMPF control [2]	5.0	103/100	3.0	38/63	4419	No
Δ*RPM* control	5.1	104/101	3.2	35/60	4385	No
CPS control	5.0	102/98	4.5	51/77	4336	No
Δ*P* control	5.0	101/98	4.6	53/78	4326	No
MAoP control	5.0	102/99	4.2	47/74	4363	No
LVEDP control	5.0	102/98	4.5	51/77	4339	No
			HF with DP2 support at exercise			
SIMPF control [1]	8.0	92/89	7.4	85/112	4856	No
SIMPF control [2]	8.3	94/92	5.8	66/93	5023	No
Δ*RPM* control	8.1	92/90	6.9	78/105	4957	No
CPS control	7.3	84/80	12.0	142/169	4337	No
Δ*P* control	8.7	98/96	3.8	40/67	5268	No
MAoP control	9.0	101/100	2.3	21/47	5453	No
LVEDP control	8.5	96/94	4.6	50/77	5173	No
			HF with DP2 support during 8-fold increase in PVR at rest			
SIMPF control [1]	4.3	89/86	1.0	41/62	4048	No
SIMPF control [2]	4.4	91/88	0.5	32/51	4104	IS
Δ*RPM* control	4.4	90/87	−0.4	36/56	4067	IS
CPS control	4.7	95/93	0.3	11/24	4336	CS
Δ*P* control	4.6	93/91	0.6	18/34	4243	IS
MAoP control	5.0	100/100	−1.8	−3/−1	4566	CS
LVEDP control	4.2	88/84	2.4	56/77	3911	No
			HF with DP2 support during 8-fold increase in PVR at exercise			
SIMPF control [1]	7.1	81/78	3.0	70/92	4462	No
SIMPF control [2]	7.3	83/81	2.0	54/76	4616	No
Δ*RPM* control	6.9	79/76	1.5	82/105	4340	No
CPS control	6.9	79/76	5.9	83/106	4337	No
Δ*P* control	8.1	91/90	0.5	15/28	5101	IS
MAoP control	8.9	100/100	−5.1	−13/−8	5572	CS
LVEDP control	7.3	83/81	1.5	55/77	4604	No

[1] With 5% noise. [2] With 10% noise.

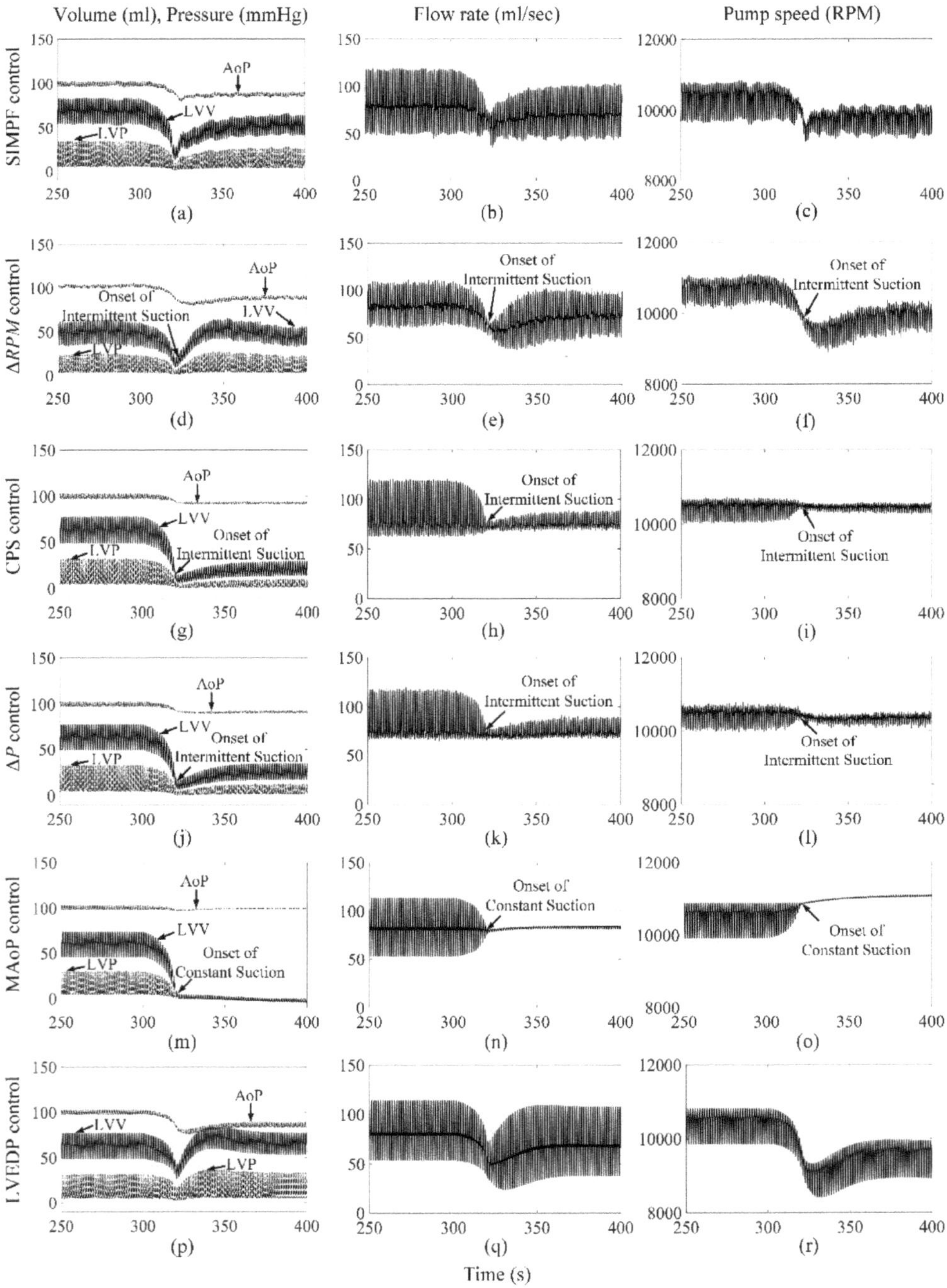

Figure 3. Comparison of performance among six control strategies at rest when the PVR increase eight times for AFP. The increase in PVR started when t = 300 s. (**a**–**c**) SIMPF control with 5% noise. (**d**–**f**) ΔRPM control. (**g**–**i**) CPS control. (**j**–**l**) ΔP control. (**m**–**o**) MAoP control. (**p**–**r**) LVEDP control. SIMPF and LVEDP control did not cause any LV suction. ΔRPM, CPS, and ΔP control induced intermittent suction. MAoP control induced constant suction.

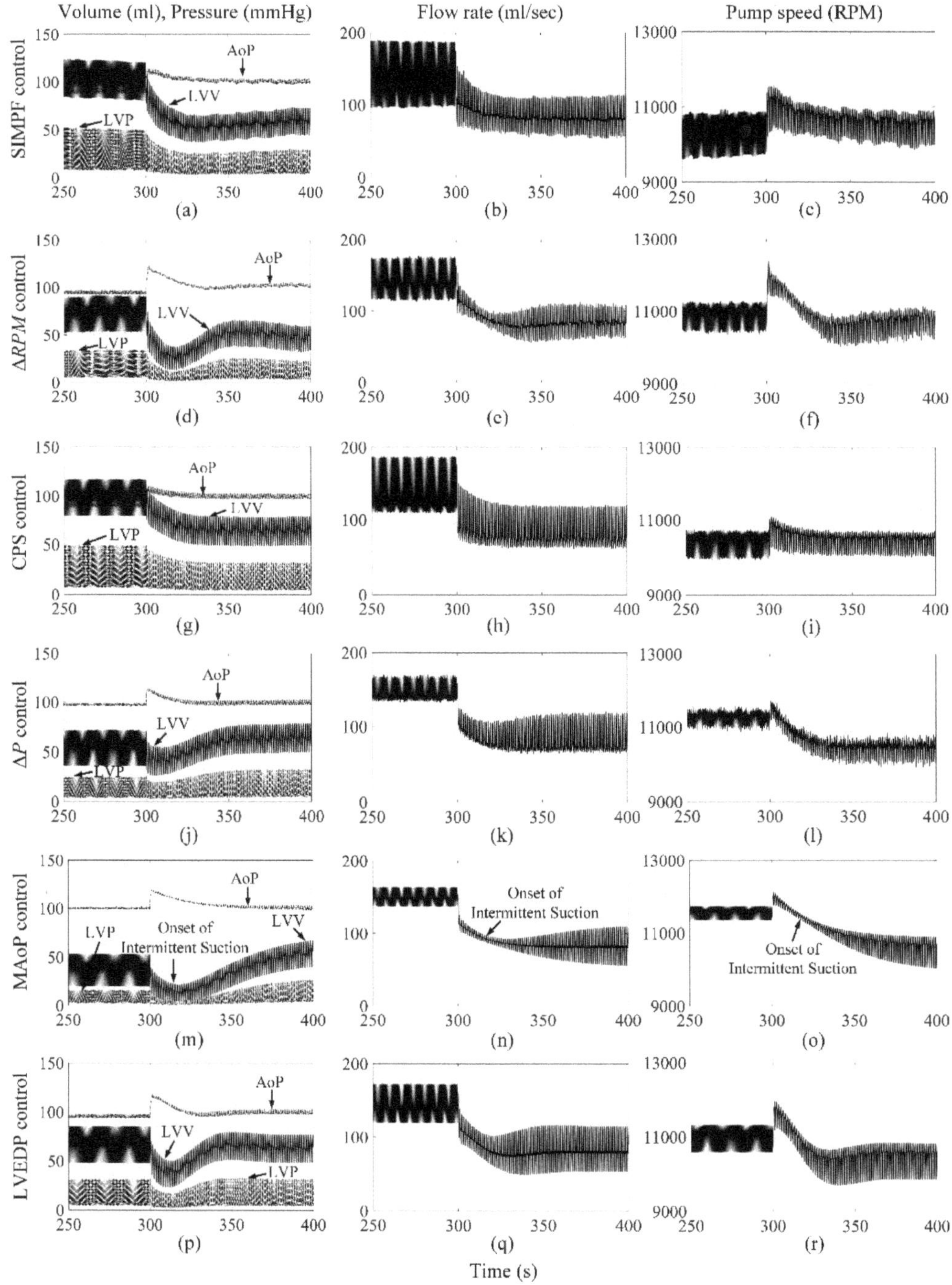

Figure 4. Comparison of performance among six control strategies under step change from exercise to rest for AFP. The transition started when t = 300 s. (**a**–**c**) SIMPF control with 5% noise. (**d**–**f**) ΔRPM control. (**g**–**i**) CPS control. (**j**–**l**) ΔP control. (**m**–**o**) MAoP control. (**p**–**r**) LVEDP control. Intermittent suction events were found for the MAoP control algorithm.

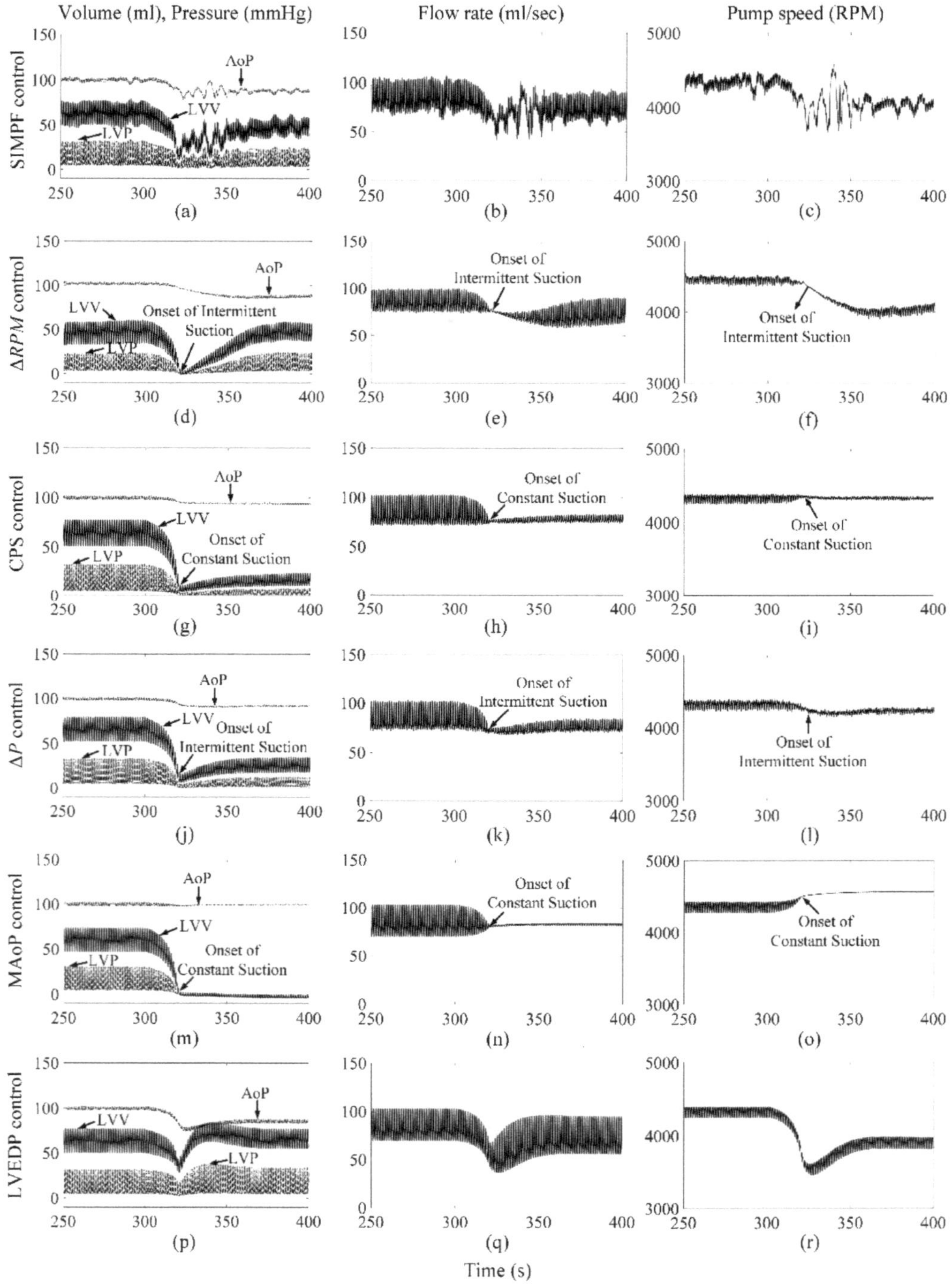

Figure 5. Comparison of performance among six control strategies at rest when the PVR increase eight times for DP2. The increase in PVR started when t = 300 s. (**a**–**c**) SIMPF control with 5% noise. (**d**–**f**) ΔRPM control. (**g**–**i**) CPS control. (**j**–**l**) ΔP control. (**m**–**o**) MAoP control. (**p**–**r**) LVEDP control. SIMPF and LVEDP control did not cause any LV suction. ΔRPM and ΔP control induced intermittent suction. CPS and MAoP control induced constant suction.

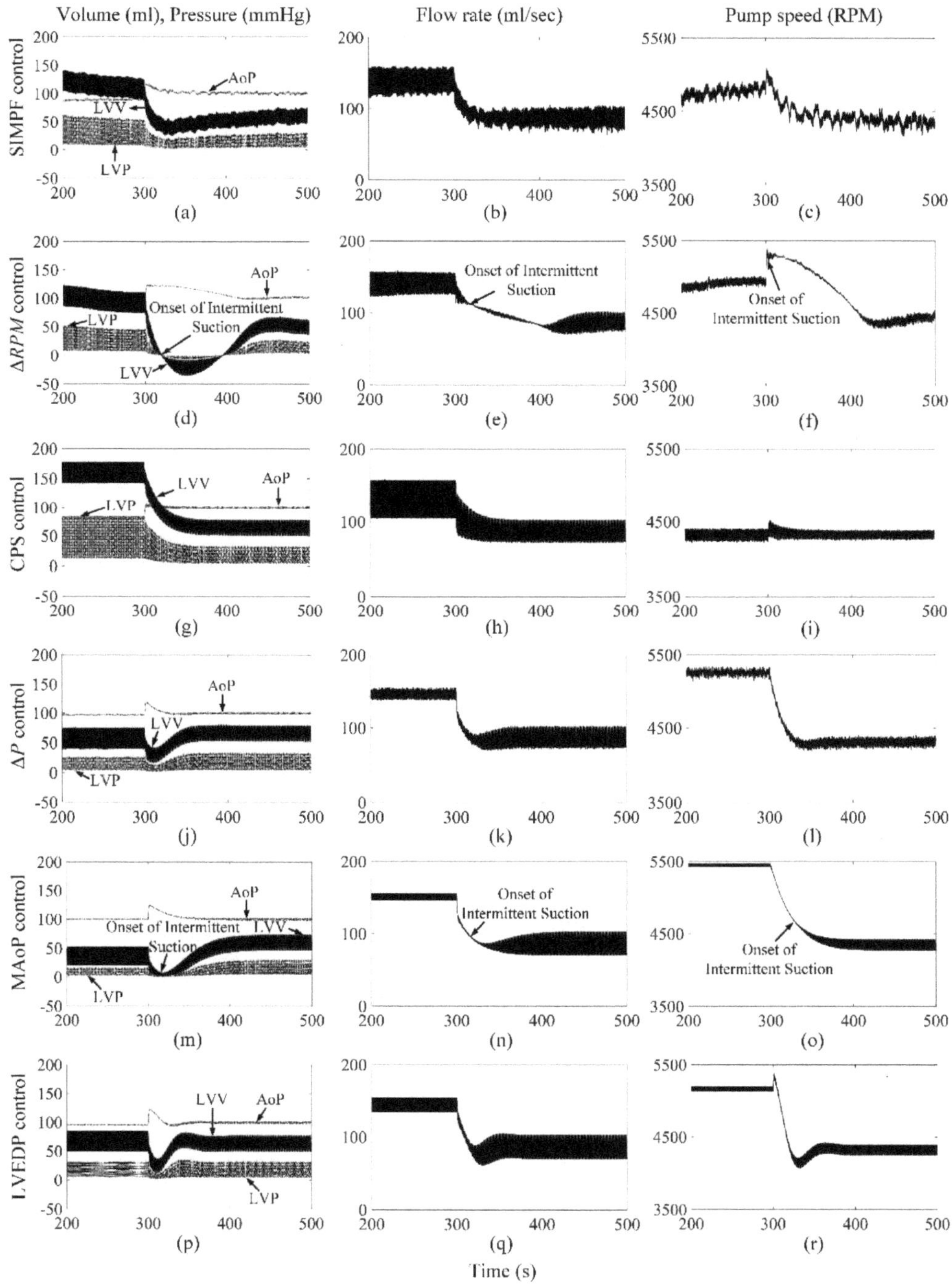

Figure 6. Comparison of performance among six control strategies under step change from exercise to rest for DP2. The transition started when t = 300 s. (**a**–**c**) SIMPF control with 5% noise. (**d**–**f**) ΔRPM control. (**g**–**i**) CPS control. (**j**–**l**) ΔP control. (**m**–**o**) MAoP control. (**p**–**r**) LVEDP control. Intermittent suction events were found for the ΔRPM and MAoP control algorithms.

3.2. ΔRPM Control Algorithm

The Δ*RPM* control algorithm successfully generated sufficient cardiac outputs and avoided LV suction events during rest and exercise conditions for both pumps (Tables 1 and 2). However, as shown in Figures 3d–f and 5d–f, an intermittent LV suction event occurred when the PVR was increased under rest, since the instantaneous LV pressure decreased to less than 1 mmHg. Meanwhile, no LV suction was found under exercise when the PVR was increased. The control algorithm could function effectively during the rapid step change from rest to exercise (no figures shown) and exercise to rest (Figure 4d–f) for AFP. However, for DP2, there was a serious intermittent LV suction event (~100 s), causing the minimum LVP to be −7.1 mmHg during the rapid transition from exercise to rest (Figure 6d–f).

3.3. CPS Control Algorithm

The CPS control strategy did not induce LV suction events without a change in PVR and provided adequate physiological perfusion during the rest condition (5.0 L/min) for both pumps. However, during exercise, the increase in pump flow was lower than that using any other control algorithm, especially for DP2 (Tables 1 and 2). Figure 3g–i also shows that this control algorithm caused intermittent LV suction at rest with AFP when the PVR was octupled compared to the normal activities of the patients. It caused constant suction with DP2, as shown in Figure 5g–i. Furthermore, the CPS control strategy did not trigger LV suction events during rapid condition change from rest to exercise (no figure shown) and exercise to rest (Figures 4g–i and 6g–i) and for both pumps.

3.4. ΔP Control Algorithm

Maintaining a fixed ΔP from LV to the aorta across AFP or DP2 provided physiological demands of 5.0 L/min and 8.7 L/min during rest and exercise conditions, respectively (Tables 1 and 2). However, intermittent suction events were observed at rest and during exercise with a rapid 8-fold increase in PVR (Figures 3j–l and 5j–i). No suction events were found during transitions between rest and exercise conditions.

3.5. MAoP Control Algorithm

For both pumps, the MAoP control algorithm guaranteed adequate end-organ perfusion at rest (5.0 L/min) and exercise (9.0 L/min) (Tables 1 and 2). However, MAoP control failed to adapt to sufficient end-organ perfusion under rest (Figures 3m–o and 5m–o) and exercise states when the PVR increased eight times, because the onset of constant suction was observed as the minimum value of LVP was negative. The controller also caused intermittent suction cases during the transition from exercise to rest (Figures 4m–o and 6m–o).

3.6. LVEDP Control Algorithm

The LVEDP control strategy increased the pump flow rate from 5.0 L/min to 8.5 L/min for both pumps when the physiologic condition changed from rest to exercise (Tables 1 and 2). No suction events were observed during all the tested conditions (Figure 3p–r, Figure 4p–r, Figures 5p–r and 6p–r).

In summary, based on all the simulation results, the proposed control algorithm is pump-independent and outperformed other control strategies for both axial and mixed flow pumps by avoiding suction and providing physiologic levels of perfusion.

4. Discussion

The computer simulation results demonstrated the feasibility and performance of the proposed SIMPF control strategy to autonomously regulate pump flow rates. The human circulatory system has highly non-linear dynamics including flow discontinuities due to the presence of valves, and highly variable physiological perfusion needs. Similarly, the LVAD pump dynamics are non-linear and depend on the design of the pump. LVAD support to the circulatory system has several requirements and constraints, which makes the design of a control algorithm highly challenging: (1) LVADs have low preload and afterload sensitivity; (2) appropriate amounts of flow to meet varying cardiac demand must be maintained for the functional capacity of patients; and (3) over-pumping and suction need to be avoided even during the rapid reduction in preload (e.g., Valsalva). The proposed SIMPF algorithm adequately met the conflicting demands of maintaining perfusion demand and avoided LV suction events under various simulated conditions. Notably, the SIMPF control algorithm was effective at avoiding suction even when PVR was increased resulting in a drastic reduction in preload. Similarly, quick step transitions between exercise and rest were also simulated to produce conditions that are conducive to causing suction events. The proposed SIMPF control algorithm measured pump flow with 5–10 percent uniformly distributed noise added to the PF signals, which were used to extract *SI*. Up to 10% noise was used as this is the maximum error for ultrasonic flow probes used clinically.

Axial flow and mixed flow pumps are two different types of pumps. Axial pumps are based on the Archimedes screw, where the flow of the liquid is along the axis of the impeller. Mixed flow is a centrifugal flow pump with a mixed flow impeller. In the DP2 pump, the fluid experiences both radial acceleration and lift, and exits the impeller nearly perpendicular to the axial direction. There are differences in pump dynamics between the axial flow pump and DP2 pump, and different sensitivities between the two devices to the pressure head (HQ curves). However, the proposed SIMPF algorithm was able to achieve similar results using both AFP and DP2, demonstrating the pump-independence of the proposed control method. The *SI* values between the two pumps were notably different, as expected due to their intrinsic differences causing differences in pump flow used to extract *SI*, and also because pump types are affected differently by the contractility of the native heart. The SIMPF algorithm requires the direct measurement of flow. Measuring LVEDP using pressure sensors can provide similar performance compared to the SIMPF control strategy. However, pressure measurements are prone to failure and long-term drift due to contact with blood. A sensor drift of even 2–3 mmHg can cause significant performance degradation and suction with the LVEDP control algorithm. Unlike pressure sensors, ultrasonic flow probes have been successfully used for long term LVAD flow measurements. When mounted on the outflow graft of an LVAD, the performance of ultrasonic flow probes is not significantly affected by tissue ingrowth. Unfortunately, flow probe measurement noise is unavoidable, and control algorithm performance degrades with increasing measurement noise. However, even with 10% noise, the algorithm prevented suction and provided physiologic perfusion. The chosen measurement noise levels (5–10%) were based on the levels reported for ultrasound flow probes. The performance of the control algorithm can be further improved by periodic calibration of the flow probe.

The SIMPF algorithm requires some level of native LV function to generate the variation in flow rate for *SI*. This native ventricular contractility is always present clinically. If ventricular asystole occurs, it would also result in the loss of right ventricular function and lead to mortality, even in the presence of adequate LVAD support. During exercise, an increase in preload due to venous return will increase native ventricular contractility due to the Frank–Starling mechanism. This increase in contractility will increase *SI*, which in turn will result in increased LVAD flow to meet the perfusion demand. Similarly, a reduction in LV contractility caused by reduced physiological demand would generate lower pump flow rates to prevent LV suction. A 5 s moving window was used in this study to minimize oscillations in *SI* values due to varying heart rates that are independent of physiological conditions. A shorter moving window will increase the speed of response, but may be more sensitive to noise and transient events.

The performance of the proposed SIMPF control strategy was superior compared to previously proposed control algorithms. It provided physiologically relevant cardiac outputs that were similar to other algorithms proposed in the literature, but was better at avoiding suction compared to the other sensor-based and sensorless control algorithms, especially when elevated PVR occurred briefly during the Valsalva maneuver or coughing.

Rapid and sustained PVR increase by eight-fold during rest and exercise does not occur in nature. This was done to demonstrate the robustness of the controller to avoid suction even under non-physiologic, extreme conditions. Furthermore, sensor based control algorithms are usually model-based and predict pressure heads and flows. They usually require *a priori* knowledge of the blood viscosity or can be erroneous in the case of inflow or outflow kinking or thrombus formation in the blood pump. While incorporating a flow sensor increases complexity, an actual measurement of flow obviates the need for estimation and improves the performance of the controller under inflow/outflow graft kinks or thrombus formation that occurs in patients implanted with LVAD. The flow probes that were previously implanted with DeBakey/Heart Assist 5 LVADs underwent rigorous durability testing prior to approval by the Food and Drug Administration and no flow probe failures have been reported during LVAD implants.

In this study, the in silico computer simulation model provided a meaningful initial step for early tested hypotheses, but it cannot replace mock flow loop studies, animal testing, and clinical trials. For instance, it cannot fully replicate the complex in vivo dynamics including tissue remodeling, autonomous regulation, and neurohumoral responses. The lumped parameter human circulatory system model has several inherent limitations due to assumptions of ideal heart valves, Newtonian blood, and ignores the effects of gravity and inertia. However, the in silico model demonstrated the feasibility control algorithms despite these limitations. Pre-clinical in vitro and in vivo experiments will be used to validate the SIMPF control algorithm.

5. Conclusions

A new flow sensor-based SIMPF control strategy was developed for rotary LVADs to provide adequate cardiac output and prevent LV suction. This proposed control strategy implemented the control objective using an effective *SI* extracted from the measured pump flow signal. Two different types of rotary LVADs were incorporated to quantify the performance of the SIMPF strategy, showing promising results. This algorithm is pump-independent and can be incorporated into existing LVAD control systems.

Author Contributions: Software, writing—original draft preparation, L.L.; Supervision, writing—review and editing, K.Q.; Formal analysis, validation, A.S.E.-B., T.J.R., and P.S.; Funding acquisition, writing—review and editing, G.A.G.; Conceptualization, funding acquisition, methodology, writing—review and editing, Y.W. All authors have read and agreed to the published version of the manuscript.

Funding: This research was funded by the LiaoNing Revitalization Talent Program of China (grant number XLYC1807016), the National Natural Science Foundation of China (grant number 32071314), and the National Institutes of Health R01 Grant (grant number R01HL151663).

Institutional Review Board Statement: Not applicable.

Informed Consent Statement: Not applicable.

Data Availability Statement: Data are made available through the corresponding author upon a reasonable request.

Conflicts of Interest: The authors declare no conflict of interest.

References

1. Metra, M.; Teerlink, J.R. Heart Failure. *Lancet* **2017**, *390*, 1981–1995. [CrossRef]
2. Mancini, D.; Lietz, K. Selection of cardiac transplantation candidates in 2010. *Circulation* **2010**, *122*, 173–183. [CrossRef]
3. Simaan, M.A.; Ferreira, A.; Chen, S.; Antaki, J.F.; Galati, D.G. A dynamical state space representation and performance analysis of a feedback-controlled rotary left ventricular assist device. *IEEE Trans. Control Syst. Technol.* **2009**, *17*, 15–28. [CrossRef]
4. Slaughter, M.S.; Rogers, J.G.; Milano, C.A.; Russell, S.D.; Conte, J.V.; Feldman, D.; Sun, B.; Tatooles, A.J.; Delgado, R.M., 3rd; Long, J.W. Advanced heart failure treated with continuous-flow left ventricular assist device. *N. Engl. J. Med.* **2009**, *361*, 2241–2251. [CrossRef]
5. Felix, S.E.A.; de Jonge, N.; Caliskan, K.; Birim, O.; Damman, K.; Kuijpers, M.; Tops, L.F.; Palmen, M.; Ramjankhan, F.Z. The role of long-term mechanical circulatory support in patients with advanced heart failure. *Neth. Heart J.* **2020**, *28*, 115–121. [CrossRef]

6. Carpenter, B.A.; Gonzalez, C.J.; Jessen, S.L.; Moore, E.J.; Thrapp, A.N.; Weeks, B.R.; Clubb, F.J., Jr. A brief review of ventricular assist devices and a recommended protocol for pathology evaluations. *Cardiovasc. Pathol.* **2013**, *22*, 408–415. [CrossRef]
7. Kirklin, J.K.; Pagani, F.D.; Kormos, R.L.; Stevenson, L.W.; Blume, E.D.; Myers, S.L.; Miller, M.A.; Baldwin, J.T.; Young, J.B.; Naftel, D.C. Eighth annual INTERMACS report: Special focus on framing the impact of adverse events. *J. Heart Lung Transplant.* **2017**, *36*, 1080–1086. [CrossRef]
8. Gross, C.; Shima, H.; Schlöglhofer, T.; Dimitrov, K.; Maw, M.; Riebandt, J.; Wiedemann, D.; Zimpfer, D.; Moscato, F. Continuous LVAD monitoring reveals high suction rates in clinically stable outpatients. *Artif. Organs* **2020**, *44*, E251–E262. [CrossRef] [PubMed]
9. Fukamachi, K.; Shiose, A.; Massiello, A.; Horvath, D.J.; Golding, L.A.R.; Lee, S.; Starling, R.C. Preload sensitivity in cardiac assist devices. *Ann. Thorac. Surg.* **2013**, *95*, 373–380. [CrossRef] [PubMed]
10. Giridharan, G.A.; Koenig, S.C.; Slaughter, M.S. Do axial-flow LVADs unload better than centrifugal-flow LVADs? *ASAIO J.* **2014**, *60*, 137–139. [CrossRef] [PubMed]
11. Vollkron, M.; Voitl, P.; Ta, J.; Wieselthaler, G.; Shima, H. Suction events during left ventricular support and ventricular arrhythmias. *J. Heart Lung Transplant.* **2007**, *26*, 819–825. [CrossRef] [PubMed]
12. Vollkron, M.; Schima, H.; Huber, L.; Benkowski, R.; Morello, G.; Wieselthaler, G. Development of a suction detection system for axial blood pumps. *Artif. Organs* **2004**, *28*, 709–716. [CrossRef]
13. Karantonis, D.M.; Lovell, N.H.; Ayre, P.J.; Mason, D.G.; Cloherty, S.L. Identification and classification of physiologically significant pumping states in an implantable rotary blood pump. *Artif. Organs* **2006**, *30*, 671–679. [CrossRef] [PubMed]
14. Karantonis, D.M.; Cloherty, S.L.; Lovell, N.; Mason, D.G.; Salamonsen, R.F.; Ayre, P. Noninvasive detection of suction in an implantable rotary blood pump using neural networks. *Int. J. Comput. Intell. Appl.* **2008**, *7*, 237–247. [CrossRef]
15. Wang, Y.; Simaan, M.A. A suction detection system for rotary blood pumps based on the Lagrangian support vector machine algorithm. *IEEE J. Biomed. Health Inform.* **2013**, *17*, 654–663. [CrossRef]
16. Tzallas, A.T.; Katertsidis, N.S.; Karvounis, E.C.; Tsipouras, M.G.; Rigas, G.; Goletsis, Y.; Zielinski, K.; Fresiello, L.; Di Molfetta, A.; Ferrari, G.; et al. Modeling and simulation of speed selection on left ventricular assist devices. *Comput. Biol. Med.* **2014**, *51*, 128–139. [CrossRef]
17. Gaddum, N.R.; Stevens, M.; Lim, E.; Fraser, J.; Lovell, N.; Mason, D.; Timms, D.; Salamonsen, R. Starling–Like Flow Control of a Left Ventricular Assist Device: In Vitro Validation. *Artif. Organs* **2014**, *38*, E46–E56. [CrossRef]
18. Rüschen, D.; Prochazka, F.; Amacher, R.; Bergmann, L.; Leonhardt, S.; Walter, M. Minimizing left ventricular stroke work with iterative learning flow profile control of rotary blood pumps. *Biomed. Signal Process. Control* **2017**, *31*, 444–451. [CrossRef]
19. Ochsner, G.; Wilhelm, M.J.; Amacher, R.; Petrou, A.; Cesarovic, N.; Staufert, S.; Röhrnbauer, B.; Maisano, F.; Hierold, C.; Meboldt, M.; et al. In vivo evaluation of physiologic control algorithms for left ventricular assist devices based on left ventricular volume or pressure. *ASAIO J.* **2017**, *63*, 568–577. [CrossRef]
20. Gregory, S.D.; Stevens, M.C.; Pauls, J.P.; Schummy, E.; Diab, S.; Thomson, B.; Anderson, B.; Tansley, G.; Salamonsen, R.; Fraser, J.F.; et al. In vivo evaluation of active and passive physiological control systems for rotary left and right ventricular assist devices. *Artif. Organs* **2016**, *40*, 894–903. [CrossRef]
21. Pauls, J.P.; Stevens, M.C.; Schummy, E.; Tansley, G.; Fraser, J.F.; Timms, D.; Gregory, S.D. In vitro comparison of active and passive physiological control systems for biventricular assist devices. *Ann. Biomed. Eng.* **2016**, *44*, 1370–1380. [CrossRef] [PubMed]
22. Bakouri, M. Physiological control law for rotary blood pumps with full-state feedback method. *Appl. Sci.* **2019**, *9*, 4593. [CrossRef]
23. Arndt, A.; Nüsser, P.; Graichen, K.; Müller, J.; Lampe, B. Physiological control of a rotary blood pump with selectable therapeutic options: Control of pulsatility gradient. *Artif. Organs* **2008**, *32*, 761–771. [CrossRef] [PubMed]
24. AlOmari, A.H.; Savkin, A.V.; Karantonis, D.M.; Lim, E.; Lovell, N.H. Non-invasive estimation of pulsatile flow and differential pressure in an implantable rotary blood pump for heart failure patients. *Physiol. Meas.* **2009**, *30*, 371–386. [CrossRef] [PubMed]
25. Ferreira, A.; Boston, J.R.; Antaki, J.F. A control system for rotary blood pumps based on suction detection. *IEEE Trans. Biomed. Eng.* **2009**, *56*, 656–665. [CrossRef]
26. Wang, Y.; Koenig, S.C.; Wu, Z.J.; Slaughter, M.S.; Giridharan, G.A. Sensorless Physiologic Control, Suction prevention, and Flow Balancing Algorithm for Rotary Biventricular Assist Devices. *IEEE Trans. Control Syst. Technol.* **2019**, *27*, 717–729. [CrossRef]
27. Meki, M.; Wang, Y.; Sethu, P.; Ghazal, M.; El-Baz, A.; Giridharan, G. A sensorless rotational speed-based control system for continuous flow left ventricular assist devices. *IEEE Trans. Biomed. Eng.* **2019**, *67*, 1050–1060. [CrossRef]
28. Liang, L.; Meki, M.; Wang, W.; Sethu, P.; El-Baz, A.; Giridharan, G.A.; Wang, Y. A suction index based control system for rotary blood pumps. *Biomed. Signal Process. Control* **2020**, *62*, 102057. [CrossRef]
29. Guruprasad, G.A.; Skliar, M. Physiological control of blood pumps using intrinsic pump parameters: A computer simulation study. *Artif. Organs* **2006**, *30*, 301–307.
30. Wu, Y.; Allaire, P.E.; Tao, G.; Olsen, D. Modeling, estimation, and control of human circulatory system with a left ventricular assist device. *IEEE Trans. Control Syst. Technol.* **2007**, *15*, 754–767. [CrossRef]
31. Bullister, E.; Reich, S.; Sluetz, J. Physiologic control algorithms for rotary blood pumps using pressure sensor input. *Artif. Organs* **2002**, *26*, 931–938. [CrossRef] [PubMed]
32. Demirozu, Z.T.; Arat, N.; Kucukaksu, D.S. Fine-tuning management of the Heart Assist 5 left ventricular assist device with two- and three-dimensional echocardiography. *Cardiovasc. J. Afr.* **2016**, *27*, 208–212. [CrossRef] [PubMed]

33. Ising, M.; Warren, S.; Sobieski, M.A.; Slaughter, M.S.; Koenig, S.C.; Giridharan, G.A. Flow modulation algorithms for continuous flow left ventricular assist devices to increase vascular pulsatility: A computer simulation study. *Cardiovasc. Eng. Technol.* **2011**, *2*, 90–100. [CrossRef]
34. Soucy, K.G.; Koenig, S.C.; Sobieski, M.A.; Slaughter, M.S.; Giridharan, G.A. Fault detection in rotary blood pumps using motor speed response. *ASAIO J.* **2013**, *59*, 410–419. [CrossRef]
35. Choi, S.; Boston, J.R.; Thomas, D.; Antaki, J.F. Modeling and identification of an axial flow blood pump. In Proceedings of the 1997 American Control Conference (ACC), Albuquerque, NM, USA, 6 June 1997; pp. 3714–3715.
36. Pillay, P.; Krishnan, R. Modeling, simulation and analysis of permanent-magnet motor drives, part II: The brushless DC motor drive. *IEEE Trans. Ind. Appl.* **1989**, *25*, 265–273. [CrossRef]
37. Petrou, A.; Kuster, D.; Lee, J.; Meboldt, M.; Daners, M.S. Comparison of flow estimators for rotary blood pumps: An in vitro and in vivo study. *Ann. Biomed. Eng.* **2018**, *46*, 2123–2134. [CrossRef]
38. Giridharan, G.A.; Skliar, M.; Olsen, D.B.; Pantalos, G.M. Modeling and control of a brushless DC axial flow ventricular assist device. *ASAIO J.* **2002**, *48*, 272–289. [CrossRef]
39. Jazwinski, A.H. *Stochastic Processes and Filtering Theory*; Academic Press: New York, NY, USA, 1970; pp. 277–281.
40. Picard, J. Efficiency of the extended Kalman filter for nonlinear systems with small noise. *SIAM J. Appl. Math.* **1991**, *51*, 843–885. [CrossRef]
41. Savitzky, A.; Golay, M.J.E. Smoothing and differentiation of data by simplified least squares procedures. *Anal. Chem.* **1964**, *36*, 1627–1639. [CrossRef]
42. Orfanidis, S.J. *Introduction to Signal Processing*; Prentice Hall: Upper Saddle River, NJ, USA, 1996; pp. 427–462.
43. Sen, A.; Larson, J.S.; Kashani, K.B.; Libricz, S.L.; Patel, B.M.; Guru, P.K.; Alwardt, C.M.; Pajaro, O.; Farmer, J.C. Mechanical circulatory assist devices: A primer for critical care and emergency physicians. *Crit. Care* **2016**, *20*, 1–20. [CrossRef]

sensors

MDPI

Article

Atrial Fibrillation Classification with Smart Wearables Using Short-Term Heart Rate Variability and Deep Convolutional Neural Networks

Jayroop Ramesh, Zahra Solatidehkordi, Raafat Aburukba * and Assim Sagahyroon

Department of Computer Science and Engineering, American University of Sharjah, Sharjah P.O. Box 26666, United Arab Emirates; jramesh@aus.edu (J.R.); g00059068@aus.edu (Z.S.); asagahyroon@aus.edu (A.S.)
* Correspondence: raburukba@aus.edu; Tel.: +971-6-5152956

Abstract: Atrial fibrillation (AF) is a type of cardiac arrhythmia affecting millions of people every year. This disease increases the likelihood of strokes, heart failure, and even death. While dedicated medical-grade electrocardiogram (ECG) devices can enable gold-standard analysis, these devices are expensive and require clinical settings. Recent advances in the capabilities of general-purpose smartphones and wearable technology equipped with photoplethysmography (PPG) sensors increase diagnostic accessibility for most populations. This work aims to develop a single model that can generalize AF classification across the modalities of ECG and PPG with a unified knowledge representation. This is enabled by approximating the transformation of signals obtained from low-cost wearable PPG sensors in terms of Pulse Rate Variability (PRV) to temporal Heart Rate Variability (HRV) features extracted from medical-grade ECG. This paper proposes a one-dimensional deep convolutional neural network that uses HRV-derived features for classifying 30-s heart rhythms as normal sinus rhythm or atrial fibrillation from both ECG and PPG-based sensors. The model is trained with three MIT-BIH ECG databases and is assessed on a dataset of unseen PPG signals acquired from wrist-worn wearable devices through transfer learning. The model achieved the aggregate binary classification performance measures of accuracy: 95.50%, sensitivity: 94.50%, and specificity: 96.00% across a five-fold cross-validation strategy on the ECG datasets. It also achieved 95.10% accuracy, 94.60% sensitivity, 95.20% specificity on an unseen PPG dataset. The results show considerable promise towards seamless adaptation of gold-standard ECG trained models for non-ambulatory AF detection with consumer wearable devices through HRV-based knowledge transfer.

Keywords: biomedical informatics; cardiovascular disease; deep learning; ECG; heart rate variability; machine learning; PPG; smartphones; smart wearables

Citation: Ramesh, J.; Solatidehkordi, Z.; Aburukba, R.; Sagahyroon, A. Atrial Fibrillation Classification with Smart Wearables Using Short-Term Heart Rate Variability and Deep Convolutional Neural Networks. *Sensors* **2021**, *21*, 7233. https://doi.org/10.3390/s21217233

Academic Editors: Ayman El-baz, Guruprasad A. Giridharan, Ahmed Shalaby, Ali H. Mahmoud and Mohammed Ghazal

Received: 3 September 2021
Accepted: 26 October 2021
Published: 30 October 2021

1. Introduction

Cardiovascular diseases (CVD) are the leading cause of death worldwide, with the World Health Organization (WHO) in 2016 estimated 17.9 million deaths annually [1]. CVD is a group of conditions that affect the heart's rhythm mechanical function, and electrical activity [2]. This is associated with an increased likelihood of strokes and heart failure. Timely detection through regular monitoring of CVD is necessary to improve the treatment process for heart conditions and lower the risk of mortality [3]. Cardiac arrhythmia is categorized under CVD and is characterized by the disordered electrical activity of the heart. An arrhythmia can manifest as irregularly rapid heart rhythms (tachycardia) or anomalous slow heart rhythms (bradycardia). AF is one of the most common types of cardiac arrhythmia. In this work, the focus is on the classification of (i) normal sinus rhythm (NSR), and (ii) atrial fibrillation (AF). Goldberger et al. [4] defines NSR as a rhythm with normal (1:1) atrioventricular conduction and a normal PR interval (the interval between atrial depolarization and ventricular depolarization) at a heart rate between 60 and 100 beats/min, although normal heart rates may vary between individuals. The work reported in [5] defines AF as an arrhythmia with uncoordinated atrial activation and characteristics of irregular beat-to-beat intervals, absence of repeating P waves (indicates atrial depolarization), and irregular atrial activity.

The common technique for the clinical diagnosis of cardiac arrhythmia is based on the electrocardiogram (ECG). The ECG is a test that uses skin level electrodes with built-in sensors to measure the heart's electrical activity and identify abnormal heart rhythms and additional pathological conditions [6]. However, despite the multi-faceted diagnostic nature of ECG, most dedicated ECG devices available currently are expensive and are typically used within clinical or limited ambulatory settings [7]. While wearable ECG devices are emerging commercially, individuals gravitate towards smart wearables that can serve general functions and are not only intended for health monitoring. Off-the-shelf smartphones and wearable devices that use photoplethysmography (PPG) sensors can serve as an affordable alternative to existing ECG devices, albeit as a supplementary approach for screening and not for conclusive diagnosis. PPG sensors are optical light sensors that record blood volume variations at sensitive peripheral sites of the human body, such as fingertips, wrist, and earlobes [8]. Moreover, PPG sensors are currently used extensively by fitness tracking applications to estimate the physiological events of heart rate and heart rate variability (HRV) [9]. PPG signals differ morphologically from ECG signals but exhibit similar characteristics as the HRV. This is termed as pulse rate variability (PRV). The advantages of PPG sensor-based consumer devices for cardiac arrhythmia monitoring are that they are relatively less obtrusive than their ECG counterparts. Their ubiquitous nature facilitates higher adoption by the general population. Despite these advantages, PPG recordings are more susceptible to noise saturation and variations in signal quality caused by user movement and skin tones [10].

The data features extracted from ECG and PPG heart signals to develop learning algorithms can be categorized as temporal or morphological [11]. Temporal features are the time-domain metrics such as the time between heartbeats. Many deep learning works in this area pursue the development of morphology-based models using the PPG segments or corresponding images to leverage the robustness and have generally superior performance in classification problems. However, there are significant challenges in developing PPG-based analytical models due to the limited public availability of universally reviewed benchmark databases, as opposed to the abundant ECG signals databases. Moreover, signal quality and noise saturation can corrupt the performance of the developed models. The manual annotation process for creating labeled datasets is complex and has the consistency issue of interrater variability [3]. Interrater variability arises when multiple expert annotators are involved in labeling heart rhythms manually. Different labels are assigned to the same data instance due to differences in their specific experiences. In practice, it is difficult to reach an agreement across multiple experts if the data are not ideally preprocessed and motion artifacts are not eliminated. This is the case with the PPG signal annotation efforts in most of the literature. Moreover, most developed algorithms in the literature are only applicable in controlled clinical settings, which hinders early prognosis accessibility to the general population.

Although there are inherent morphological differences between ECG and PPG-based signals, the studies reported in [12,13] have exhibited a high degree of correlation between the signals, especially their corresponding temporal HRV features. HRV measures the variation in terms of time between consecutive instantaneous heartbeats, measured through the ECG [9].

The PRV and HRV parameters, derived from ECG and PPG, respectively, exhibit similar properties under certain conditions. The properties have higher levels of agreement/equivalence when the PPG signals are not excessively situated with motion artifacts. Various predictive and detection models have been implemented using different HRV metrics with standard statistical and machine learning approaches [14–19]. However, there are considerably fewer deep learning-based models oriented towards usage in smartphones and wearable devices. Deep learning has recently emerged as an effective methodology for cardiac classification tasks [20]. The experiments reported in [21–24] have achieved successful ECG signal classification using ECG databases by implementing convolutional neural networks. However, the existing approaches are designed for use in controlled hospital settings.

This research addresses the scarcity of publicly available PPG datasets, limited reproducible approaches in the existing literature, and varying sensor specifications. This work proposes implementing a deep learning approach that utilizes the knowledge transfer paradigm for cross-domain generalizability by training a model on ECG databases and adapting the developed model for PPG signals-based AF classification. The commonality in the distribution of temporal features derived from HRV (ECG) and PRV (PPG) is leveraged as input features to implement a one-dimensional convolutional neural network for classifying NSR and AF rhythms. The motivation for this approach is to introduce generalizable deep learning models that can mitigate the challenges associated with purely PPG- based analytical models and facilitate close to real-time AF detection.

The contributions of this work are as follows:

- The incorporation of the state-of-the-art methods for ECG and PPG signal processing and HRV feature extraction from short length signals;
- The development of a deep learning model trained on HRV features derived from on gold standard ECG for classification of AF with PRV derived from PPG features through transfer learning;
- The evaluation of the developed model performance on three ECG datasets and a PPG dataset composed of wrist-worn wearable signals which achieved competitive results when compared to the recent literature;
- The implementation of a cloud-based platform and the evaluation of the developed model performance on PPG signals acquired from live subjects via smartphones.

This paper is organized as follows: Section 2 introduces the background of the concepts used in the analysis of this work, Section 3 details the proposed approach, Section 4 presents the obtained results of the model, Section 5 discusses the results, and is followed by the conclusion and future work in Section 6.

2. Background

2.1. Heart Activity Measures

The entire sequence of a single heartbeat, beginning with the initial atrial excitation and concluding with the exit from the ventricular chambers, is called PQRST and is shown in Figure 1. An electrical impulse travels through the heart during each heartbeat, causing the heart muscles to pump blood. After a flat line driven by the impulse traveling to the bottom heart chambers, the right and left atria (upper heart chambers) create the first wave, called P wave. The right and left ventricles (bottom chambers) make the next wave called the QRS complex, and the final T wave indicates the repolarization of the ventricles. The QRS complex is the peak shown in Figure 1. Variations in parameters obtained from ECG and PPG, such as the duration and rate of heartbeats, can help detect abnormal heart activity [6].

PPG is an optical light-based technique to measure the volumetric change of the heart. As the heart contracts, blood pressure in the left ventricle (bottom chambers) increases. This is reflected by an increased pressurized pulse of blood into the capillaries and arteries of the body, indicated by discoloration of the skin. An LED light measures the difference in the amount of light reflected from sensitive areas, where the arteries are close to the skin, such as fingertips or earlobes, which is then used to measure an individual's heart rate [25]. A typical waveform of the PPG signal and its characteristic parameters are shown in Figure 2, which are the systolic peak, pulse with and diastolic peak, and dicrotic notch. Smartphones and wearable devices are generally accurate in acquiring PPG signals when the user is at rest, but potential inaccuracies are introduced because of motion artifacts and diverse skin tones. Motion artifacts typically occur due to misplacement of sensors such that it does not make sufficient contact with the measurement site. Various skin tones affect the reflective properties of the optical light differently and therefore affect the accurate assessing of the changes in blood volume under the skin [26].

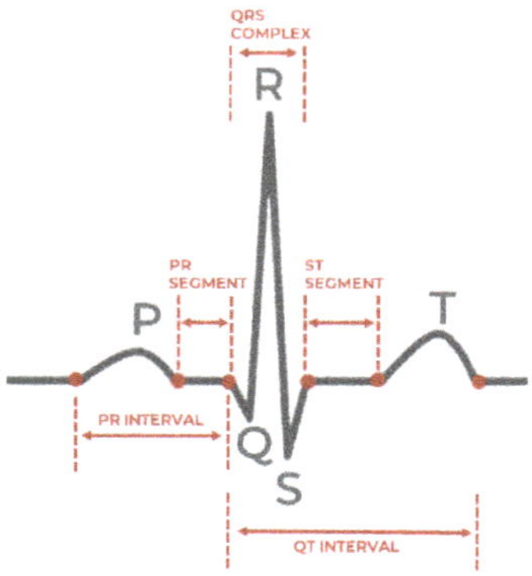

Figure 1. Single heartbeat sample with the QRS complex [4].

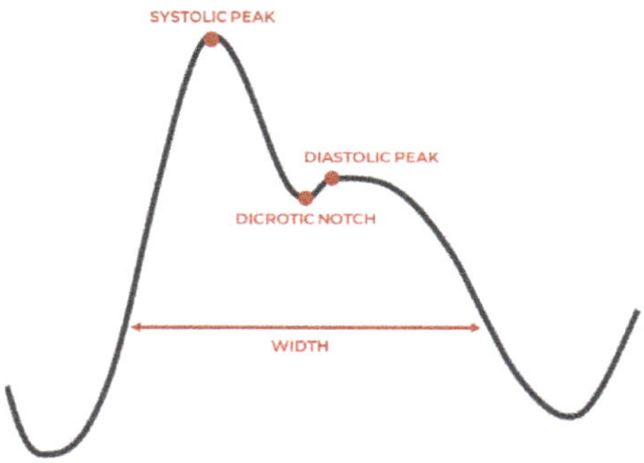

Figure 2. PPG waveform characteristics [3].

PPG has two peaks corresponding to the blood volume changes in the microvascular bed of tissue around the physical measurement site of the fingertips, earlobes, wrists, etc. Systolic peak is caused by the direct pressure wave traveling from the left ventricle to the body periphery (heart contraction). The diastolic peak reflects the pressure wave by arteries in the lower body (heart relaxation). The pulse width correlates with systemic vascular resistance, and the dicrotic notch reflects a transient increase in aortic pressure [27]. Although PPG is an indirect way to record the heart's activity, it has a high correlation with ECG signals. Its portability and relatively inexpensiveness make it a valuable alternative method to monitor cardiac activity [8].

2.2. Heartrate Variability

The HRV phenomenon is controlled by the Autonomous Nervous System (ANS) and is a direct result of the behavior of the primitive part: the parasympathetic nervous system. The brain processes information in the hypothalamus region, and the ANS sends signals to the rest of the body to either stimulate or relax different functions. Auto-responses from the ANS are elicited in the event of stress, fragmented sleep, unhealthy diets and other chemical or neural factors affecting a person's resting state. HRV is a non-invasive way to identify ANS imbalances, as when the nervous system is behaving unusually, the variation in the heartbeats is relatively more erratic. A higher HRV score generally indicates better cardiovascular fitness and resilience to stress. In comparison, a lower HRV score is associated with an increased risk of cardiovascular health and mental health concerns [9].

The primary feature used in HRV calculations is the time between each successive heartbeats, or the time between successive normal or abnormal QRS complexes/peaks in milliseconds, defined as the R-R peak interval. Estimation of the R-R interval involves first detecting the QRS complexes/peaks and subtracting the observed times of successive peaks. It should be noted that a distinction is made between R-R intervals, and the typically synonymous N-N interval, as the latter only accounts for normal-normal beats, while the former accounts for normal-normal, normal-abnormal, or abnormal-abnormal cases.

PRV is used to measure the similar inter-beat variation property with PPG signals, and this denotes the pulse-to-pulse variation in time. PRV quantifies approximately the same behavior as the intervals between successive R peaks or QRS complex observed in ECG with the systolic peak-to-systolic peak or diastolic peak-to-diastolic peak intervals.

Malik et al. [28] observed the potential of HRV in assessing the role of ANS fluctuations in normal healthy individuals and those with diseases. Relevant measures were selected from the previous research and used as HRV features for the scope of this work.

This work primarily uses the formulas shown by Equations (1) and (2) to calculate Root Mean Square of Successive Differences between the R-R intervals (rMSSD) [28] and Standard Deviation of RR intervals (SDRR) [28]:

$$rMSSD = \sqrt{\frac{\sum_{i=1}^{N-1} (RR_i - RR_{i+1})^2}{N-1}} \quad (1)$$

From Equation (1), N is the number of R-R intervals and RR_i is the location of the ith QRS complex/peak observed at a time in milliseconds.

$$SDRR = \sqrt{\frac{1}{N-1} * \sum_{j=1}^{N} (RR_j - \overline{RR})^2} \quad (2)$$

From Equation (2), N is the number of R-R intervals, RR_j is the location of the jth QRS complex/peak observed at a time in milliseconds.

The features of rMSSD and SDRR respectively reflect the number of fluctuations in heart rhythms and the degree of variation between heart beats. Hence, both are vital features to consider when aiming to predict the cardiovascular state. Various cardiac conditions were detected using short-term HRV features, with rMSSD, SDRR, and pRR50 being the most useful in predicting changes in parasympathetic activity and even being a possible indicator of cardiac mortality [29]. Additional HRV features are also included in Table 1 and used in this work. Those additional features include the coefficient of variation in R-R intervals (CVRR) and coefficient of variation in the differences of successive R-R intervals (CVSD), as they are features that improve the classification of CVD [30]. Researchers recorded PPG signals from the fingertips of subjects extracted PRV features, such as rMSSD, SDRR, and pRR50, compared them with the same features obtained from ECG to validate the accuracy, and found that the average error rate was less than 6% [30]. Another study used wearables to compare the time domain features (rMSSD, SDRR) of HRV extracted from ECG and PRV extracted from PPG signals and found that PPG signals can be used as an alternative source for HRV measurement [31]. The features used in this work are presented in Table 1.

Table 1. A summary of the HRV feature characteristics used in this work.

Feature	Domain	Description
R-R interval	Time	Times between each successive heartbeat, measured from one normal or abnormal R peak/QRS to the next in milliseconds.
rMSSD	Time	Square root of the mean of the sum of the squares between adjacent R-R intervals.
SDRR	Time	Standard deviation of R-R intervals in milliseconds.
meanRR	Time	Average value of the R-R interval in milliseconds.
CVRR	Time	Coefficient of variation in R-R intervals.
CVSD	Time	Coefficient of variation between successive R-R interval differences.
medianRR	Time	Median value in R-R intervals in milliseconds.
madRR	Time	Median value of R-R interval deviation in milliseconds.
mcvRR	Time	Median value of the coefficient of variation.
RR20	Time	Number of pairs of adjacent R-R intervals differing by more than 20 milliseconds.
pRR20	Time	Count of RR20 over a total number of R-R intervals.
RR50	Time	Number of pairs of adjacent R-R intervals differing by more than 50 milliseconds.
pRR50	Time	Count of RR50 over the total number of R-R intervals.

This relationship can be utilized to monitor individuals' cardiovascular health with off-the-shelf sensors for classifications and early detection of diseases. The commonality between the behavior of the HRV and PRV parameters can be utilized to enable generalized detection of AF across two different modalities: ECG and PPG. The model is trained on HRV features derived from ECG signals within the three ambulatory datasets. The model is tested and finetuned on PRV features derived from PPG signals within the wearable dataset.

For verification of the created dataset and its respective HRV values for different R-R interval measures, it was compared to the short-term normative values reported in [32], and the reference ranges for HRV from ECG recordings [33]. The HRV features of NN intervals, rMSSD, and SDRR were the most reported along with their normative ranges, and it is shown in Table 2. This comparison ensured that the extracted PRV features for real-time samples from the low-cost PPG sensors from wearables were within reasonable bounds of the ground truth cases and should remain valid for this experimentation.

Table 2. HRV Reference Ranges.

Feature	Range	Mean ± SD
RR interval (ms)	785–1160	926 ± 90
rMSSD (ms)	19–75	42 ± 15
SDRR (ms)	32–93	50 ± 16

3. Proposed Approach

The proposed approach has three main stages after the initial acquisition of datasets, as shown in Figure 3. The first stage involves preprocessing the signals in terms of filtering, peak detection, and feature extraction. The second involves the one-dimensional convolutional neural network (CNN) model development for binary classification between NSR and AF with temporal HRV features, and trained with the ECG datasets. The third stage involves model evaluation. The model evaluation is done on both the holdout testing on a subset from the ECG datasets and out-of-sample cross-domain testing instances from the PPG datasets. Each stage is detailed in the following subsections.

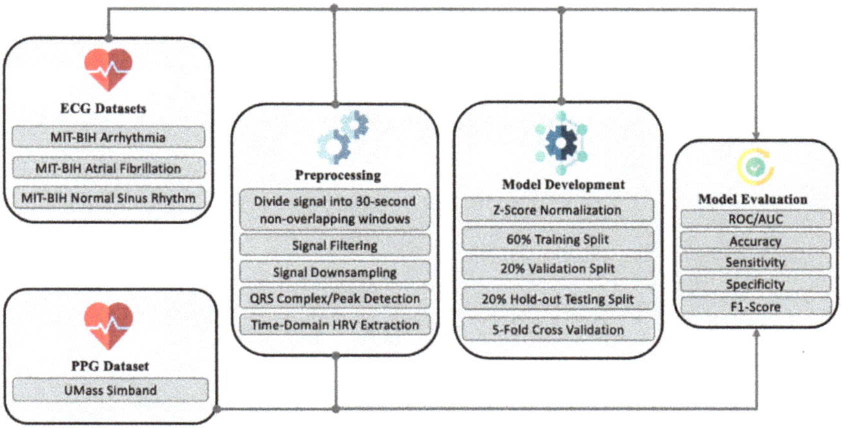

Figure 3. High-level view of the proposed approach.

3.1. ECG Datasets

NSR and AF rhythms are collected from three datasets [34]: MIT-BIH Normal Sinus Rhythm (NSR-DB), MIT-BIH Atrial Fibrillation (AF-DB), and MIT-BIH Arrhythmia (ARR-DB).

Using ambulatory ECG recorders, each record was acquired from patients referred to the Arrhythmia Laboratory at the Beth Israel Deaconess Medical Center, Massachusetts Institute of Technology. They are accessible via the Physiobank repository, a digital archive of well-characterized biomedical signals created by the United States National Institutes of Health for use by the research community [35].

AF-DB consists of 23 two-channel ECG recordings (sampled at 250 Hz), from subjects with paroxysmal atrial fibrillation, atrial flutter, AV junctional rhythm, and normal rhythms, with a typical recording bandwidth of approximately 0.1 to 40 Hz. NSR-DB consists of 18 two-channel ECG recordings (sampled at 128 Hz) from subjects with no significant arrhythmia or heart abnormalities. ARR-DB consists of 48 records, each containing two-channel ambulatory ECG signals of 30-min duration. Lead 1 channel ECG signals, which record the right ventricle and right atrium, are used in this work.

The signals in AF-DB have rhythm annotations indicating NSR and AF. Meanwhile, the signals in NSR-DB and ARR-DB have heartbeat annotations as well, in addition to rhythm annotations for AF and NSR. The annotations are provided in terms of a distinct beginning and end label pertaining to particular regions of the signals. The heartbeats in NSR-DB and ARR-DB follow the recommended standards of the Association for the Advancement of Medical Instrumentation [36]. Hence, the annotations/labels for each heartbeat in the NSR-DB and ARR-DB fall into multiple categories [37]. The beat superclasses and their corresponding beat annotations of interest in this work are N: (N, L, R, B) and S: A, a, J, S, j, e, n. While the primary focus is on heart rhythm classification, specific samples in the dataset are considered on a heartbeat segment basis for incorporating cases of atrial premature complexes (APC) [38]. The rationale for incorporating heart rhythms with high saturation levels of anomalous heartbeats is to contribute stochasticity (diversity) to the AF class. The expectation is that the dataset consisting of contiguous AF rhythms and AF rhythms interspersed with normal and other types of beats will allow for the eventual detection of varying anomalous rhythms that differ considerably from the purely NSR training samples [39,40].

3.2. PPG Dataset

The privately held UMass PPG database (UMass-DB) [41] collected by the University of Massachusetts Medical School was used for further testing to discover the strengths and weaknesses of the model. The authors of [42] granted access to this dataset and consists of

37 subjects, with 10 having AF. The PPG signals were recorded at a sampling frequency of 128 Hz from the Simband, smart wristwatch provided by Samsung, which has 8 PPG sensors, a triaxial accelerometer, an ECG lead, and a temperature sensor [42].

Figure 4 presents the typical characteristic heart rate rhythm samples from both datasets reflecting NSR and AF, respectively, across the ECG and PPG modalities. As observed from Figure 4a,c,e, NSR instance is a normal heart rhythm that maintains a steady rate with no irregularities. From Figure 4b,d,f, the AF instance is a sustained unsteady heart rhythm with rapid fluctuations.

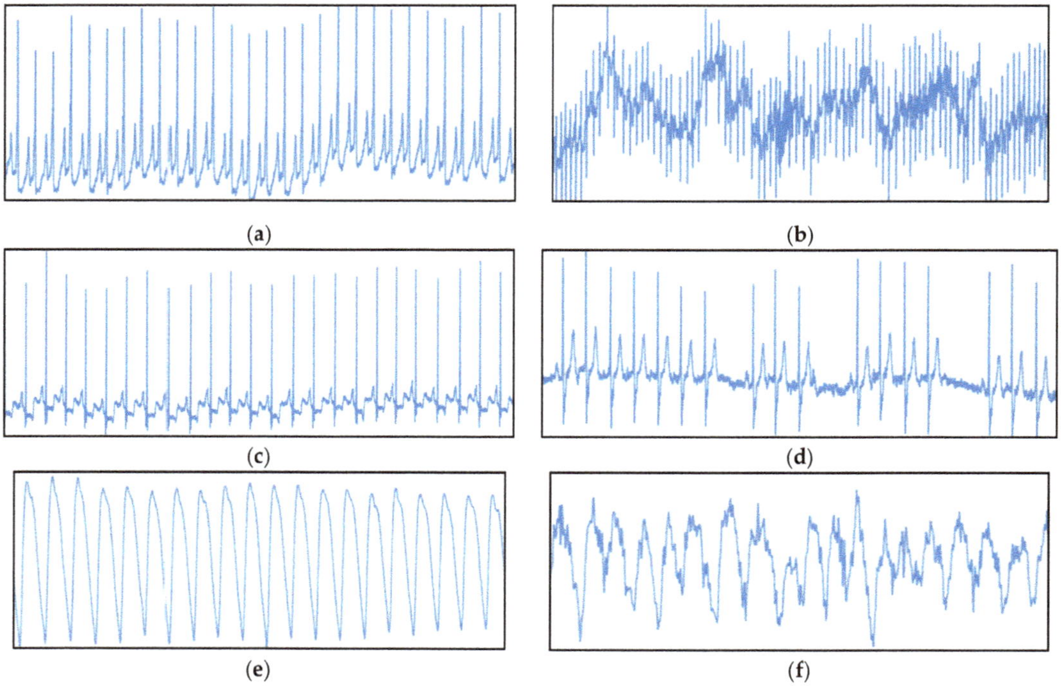

(a) (b) (c) (d) (e) (f)

Figure 4. Sample 30-s heart rhythm instances represented as raw amplitude (y-axis) against time (x-axis) from ECG datasets; (**a**) NSR ECG from AF-DB (Patient 4015); (**b**) AF ECG from AF-DB (Patient 4043); (**c**) NSR ECG from ARR-DB (Patient 100); (**d**) AF ECG from ARR-DB (Patient 222) and PPG dataset; (**e**) NSR PPG (Patient 4002); (**f**) AF PPG (Patient 4012).

3.3. Preprocessing

Initially, the signals with rhythm annotations of NSR and AF from AF-DB, ARR-DB, and NSR-DB were divided into 30-s samples with no-overlapping windows. The segmented 30-s signals retained the respective label of NSR or AF as multiple 30-s samples can be obtained from a single longer signal with the same annotation. In the case of ARR-DB, all signals with annotations corresponding to non-atrial complications, such as paced rhythms, ventricular bigeminy, trigeminy, tachycardia, were ignored.

Most AF contiguous data samples originated from the AF-DB, with approximately 3.6% being from the ARR-DB dataset. From the NSR database, 15% of the total NSR rhythm records were arbitrarily selected. Most NSR data originated from NSR-DB, followed by ARR-DB while AF-DB contributed only 5% of the total NSR samples. All the signals accounted for had the highest resolution in terms of QRS complex certainty.

In addition, signals with ARR-DB were examined further in terms of heartbeat saturation to determine the presence of excessive supraventricular activity, which is associated with an increased risk of developing atrial fibrillation [43]. The examined signals were annotated with APC, supraventricular tachyarrhythmia (SVTA), atrial couplets, or atrial flutter. As per AAMI standards, all considered heartbeats in the 30-s window derived from these signals belonged to the class N or S. The beats denoted by S can be referred to as supraventricular ectopic beats or premature beats. Although ectopic beats are mostly harmless, recent studies have shown that frequent repetitions of supraventricular ectopic behavior can indicate the presence of potential atrial abnormalities [44].

The criteria for judging the label of a 30-s rhythm are based on the saturation level of class S beats. If zero S beats are present, then it is ignored, and if over 50% of the beats are S with an annotation of a, *J*, *A*, *S*, *j*, *e*, or *n*, it is treated as an AF rhythm. The passage from heartbeat types to heart rhythms is not necessarily direct. Thus, this rule is to ensure that only segments consisting of non-isolated beats are treated as AF samples.

Individuals in real scenarios may not always exhibit signs of sustained arrhythmia. It is possible for a fluctuating pattern between normal rhythms, where relatively shorter (<30 s) intermittent periods of abnormal heart behavior associated with AF can be observed, and thereby contributing to AF risk stratification. Excessive ectopic activity can cause palpitations, light-headedness, and increased awareness of heartbeats [45]. For instance, patient 232 does not have any AF rhythm annotations, but has frequent ectopic runs. The cardiologists' notes associated with the annotated record of patient 232 report the presence of sick sinus syndrome, which is an abnormality in the right atrium of the heart. To address this case of potential variability in patients and boost the robustness in classification performance of the developed model, instances that are not solely NSR but anomalous to a considerable degree were treated as an AF class instance.

As per the findings of [27,46], a second-order Butterworth filter was applied with the bandpass frequencies of 8Hz–20Hz for removing baseline drift, motion artifacts and minimizing other ECG features such as the P and T waves. The signals of the MIT-BIH Arrhythmia, MIT-BIH NSR, and MIT-BIH AF databases have sampling rates of 360 Hz, 128 Hz, 250 Hz, respectively. Fast Fourier (FFT) resampling is applied to down-sample the signals to 50 Hz, as the signals from the three MIT-BIH databases have different original sampling rates. It, therefore, must have the same frequency before any further processing. The method reported in [46] achieves the highest signal-to-noise ratio and optimal QRS complex detection on the MIT-BIH databases instead of techniques such as the Pan Tompkins algorithm [47], and the former method is utilized to produce a list of the peaks necessary to derive the time-domain HRV features.

PPG signal filtering was conducted with a 3rd order Butterworth filter with 0.5 Hz and 8 Hz cutoffs to remove powerline interference, motion artifacts, and other saturated noise [48]. The UMass dataset signals were down-sampled from 128 Hz to 50 Hz using FFT resampling, similar to the approach executed in [42]. Systolic peak detection in the PPG signals utilized the algorithm outlined in [49], where two event-related moving averages with an offset threshold empirically yielded higher accuracy than the alternative techniques of Billauer [50], Li [48], and Zong [51].

The decision for down-sampling all signals to 50 Hz, instead of up-sampling any acquired signals to 128 Hz is based on two key factors. Firstly, most PPG based devices do not have a high sampling rate (~128 Hz), and vary from 60 Hz to 100 Hz based on the quality of the sensor and the battery levels of the device the sensor is embedded in. However, the minimum sampling frequency required is 50 Hz to derive reasonably accurate HRV and PRV parameters with a low margin of error from ECG and PPG signals, respectively [52,53]. Secondly, the computational overhead is reduced without a significant effect on the signal acquisition or processing aspects, which can extend the deployment of the proposed model in this work to resource-constrained wearable devices.

It is to be noted that the systolic peak detection algorithm for PPG signals proposed in [48] is a modified variant of the QRS peak detection algorithm for MIT-BIH database ECG signals proposed in [46]. This work performed filtering as per the recommended cutoff frequencies before applying the algorithm, as mentioned previously in this section. The general description of the algorithm reported in [46,48] is as follows:

(i) Consider a filtered signal $S[n]$, consisting of a sequence of n samples over a sampling period $T = 30$ s, as input to either the ECG variant of the algorithm or the PPG variant of the algorithm;
(ii) Detect R peaks in the ECG signals and systolic peaks in the PPG signals through a combination of potential block generation and thresholding;
(iii) Preprocess PPG systolic peak detection (step skipped for ECG R peak detection in the squaring phase), where large differences resulting from the systolic peak are emphasized, while the small differences caused by the diastolic peak, dicrotic notch, and saturated noise are suppressed;
(iv) In the potential block generation phase, regions of the signal $S[n]$ where peaks are likely to occur are demarcated in terms of the onset and offset points by two moving averages MA_{peak} and MA_{beat};
(v) MA_{peak} estimates the possible regions of R peak or systolic peak amplitude and MA_{beat} represents the amplitude in regions of a full heartbeat (RR peak, or systolic peak-to-systolic peak);
(vi) The window size W_1 of the MA_{peak} is selected based on a healthy adult's average duration of a QRS complex (100 milliseconds) or systolic peak (111 milliseconds) depending on the signal modality. The window size W_2 for the MA_{beat} is selected based on the average duration of one full heartbeat (525 ms) or systolic peak (667 ms) in a healthy adult [49]. The defined windows W_1 *and* W_2 bound the lower limit TH_1 and upper limits of the generated blocks, respectively;
(vii) The specific windowed regions where the amplitude values of MA_{peak} are greater than MA_{beat}, are selected as blocks of interest;
(viii) As a signal $S[n]$ can be saturated with noise and motion artifacts during acquisition, the thresholding phase eliminates blocks that are likely to hinder accurate peak detection. The threshold α specifies the anticipated width of a block, and any detected QRS complex or systolic peaks with width less than this threshold is rejected. An optional parameter β can be added to the threshold to consider minor deviations in peak width and either tighten or loosen the constraints on a rejected block;
(ix) The output of the algorithm is a list of peak locations and their corresponding times in milliseconds.

After performing the peak detection algorithm summarized in Algorithm 1, a list of peak locations and their occurrence times enables the estimation of RR intervals or systolic peak-to-systolic peak intervals. From the intervals, the time-domain HRV and PRV features are derived in terms of their statistical characteristics as described in Table 1.

Algorithm 1. Pseudocode of peak detection algorithm and feature detection for dataset ***D***.

FOR x_i in ***D*** (ECG or PPG data instance from dataset, where i = {0 . . . size(D))
Filtered signal $S[n]$ = BandpassFilter(x_i)
Let $peaklist = \{\}$ (Peak amplitudes)
Let $timelist = \{\}$ (Peak times)
Let $BlocksOfInterest = \{\}$
Let $y_i = \{\}$
Set W_1 = Average ECG or PPG peak duration
Set W_2 = Average ECG or PPG beat duration
Set MA_{peak} = MovingAverage($S[n]$, W_1)
Set MA_{beat} = MovingAverage($S[n]$, W_2)
Set threshold α = $W_1 + \beta$
FOR n = 1 to length(MA_{peak})
IF $MA_{peak}[n]$ > $MA_{beat}[n]$ **THEN**

$$BlocksOfInterest[n] = 1$$

ELSE

$$BlocksOfInterest[n] = 0$$

END IF
END FOR

FOR j = 0 to length(BlocksOfInterest)
IF $width(BlocksOfInterest[j]) \geq \alpha$ **THEN**
$peaklist[j]$ = max(BlockOfInterest[j])
$timelist[j]$ = time(BlockOfInterest[j])
ELSE;
reject block
END IF
END FOR
$\{rMSSD, \ldots, pRR50\}$ = Calculate HRV/PRV (peaklist, timelist)
Transformed data instance $y_i = \{rMSSD, \ldots, pRR50\}$
Save y_i to updated dataset $\overline{D}$
END FOR

Finally, Z-score normalization is performed on the derived features. All ECG and PPG datasets signal instances are fixed with zero mean (μ = 0), and unit standard deviation (σ = 1.) This step mitigates amplitude scaling issues, offset effects, and reduces drastic variability in the signal values. Table 3 presents total data samples of NSR and AF classes after pre-processing.

Table 3. Total data Samples of NSR and AF classes after preprocessing.

Dataset	NSR	AF
ARR-DB(ECG)	2365	190
NSR-DB (ECG)	7736	
AF-DB (ECG)	83	5060
Total (ECG)	10,184	5250
UMass-DB (PPG)	192	54

3.4. Model Development

The model developed in this work is a one-dimensional 12-layer CNN for the classification of NSR and AF. The proposed architecture for the CNN is depicted in Figure 5, outlining the input tier, model tier, and output tier. The model receives temporal HRV features extracted from ECG signals as input, propagates them through the neural network, and outputs a single output indicating whether the input instance belongs to NSR or AF class. A detailed summary of the CNN properties and parameters is listed in Table 4. The configuration of the layers and their respective parameters reported were attained after hyperparameter tuning through GridSearch.

A single model is selected after training and evaluation. It is trained and tested using the HRV features derived from ECG, and finetuned to classify AF with PRV features derived from PPG. Due to the inherent similarities between the statistical properties of HRV and PRV, this approximation makes it possible for a unified AF representation across two wearable modalities.

There are three types of layers within a CNN: convolutional, pooling, and fully connected layers. An instantiated convolutional layer detects local conjunctions of features from a preceding layer which can be either an input layer or another convolutional layer. The convolutional layer merges semantically similar input features into a single learned representation. It is to be noted that features in the context of the neural network imply semantic similarities or overarching patterns detected across the provided inputs (a unified vector of HRV features). Receptive fields in each convolutional layer focus on different aspects of the derived features to create their internal representation of the inputs. The property of shared weights ensures that general features common to all data samples are learned once and shared with the other convolutional layers in the network. Subsampling reduces the dimensionality of the data to identify the most significant features. This can be related to size (spatial) or time sequence (temporal). A set of weighted vectors known as a filter/kernel outputs feature maps based on local receptive fields at each layer. These feature maps usually hold general characteristic information inferred from input feature data samples at a particular layer by the neural network [54].

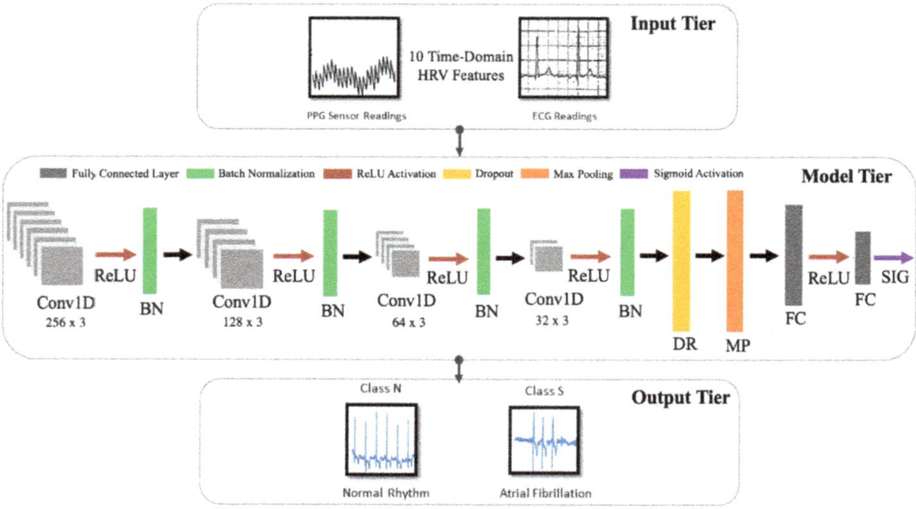

Figure 5. Architecture for the proposed CNN model.

Table 4. Summary of properties for the proposed CNN model.

Layers	Type	No. of Kernels	Kernel Size	Parameters
0—1	Conv1D	256	3	Activation = ReLU, Strides = 1
1–2	BatchNormalization	–	–	–
2–3	Conv1D	128	3	Activation = ReLU, Strides = 1
3–4	BatchNormalization	–	–	-
4–5	Conv1D	64	3	Activation = ReLU, Strides = 1
5–6	BatchNormalization	–	–	–
6–7	Conv1D	32	3	Activation = ReLU, Strides = 1
7–8	BatchNormalization	–	–	–
8–9	Dropout	–	–	Rate = 0.2
9–10	MaxPooling1D	–	–	Pooling Size = 2
–	Flatten	–	–	–
10–11	Dense	8	–	Activation = ReLU
11–12	Dense	1	–	Activation = Sigmoid

Each layer of the proposed CNN architecture and the components of activation and regularization presented in Figure 5 are described as follows:

1. Convolutional Layer (Conv1D): In this layer, a convolution operation using Equation (3) is performed by sliding the filter/kernel over the input features to obtain a feature map as the output.
$$c_m = \sum_{n=0}^{N-1} f_n k_{m-n} \tag{3}$$
From Equation (3), k, c, f, and N denote the inputs, filter/kernel, the output feature map, and the number of elements in input k, respectively. In the CNN model developed for this work, there are four convolutional layers with 256, 128, 64 and 32 filters, respectively. The filter dimensions used in this layer are 5 × 5, which yielded the best result.
2. Fully Connected Layer (FC): This layer compiles the results obtained from the preceding convolution and pooling layers to estimate an output classification label using Equation (4) [55]:
$$x_i = \sum_j w_{ji} y_j + b_i \tag{4}$$
From Equation (4), w and b denote weights and biases, respectively. Here, y is the output from a previous layer j and x is the output of the current layer i. In the CNN model developed in this work, there are two fully connected layers, with 8 and 1 neurons, respectively.
3. Pooling Layer (MaxPooling1D): In this layer, the maxpooling operation is a type of spatial sub-sampling method that decreases the size of the feature maps derived by the convolutional layers. This is performed to retain only the features contributing significantly to the internal knowledge representation of the CNN, which is learned through the training process. In the CNN model developed for this work, there is 1 pooling layer, with 32 filters after the final convolutional layer and the following dropout layer. The filter dimensions of the pooling size used in this layer are 2 × 2.
4. Activation Functions: This determines the firing threshold of neurons in the hidden layer based on the weighted sum of input and biases.
   - Rectified Linear Unit (ReLU) [56]: This is the activation function that is used in all three convolutional layers of the network. The Rectified Linear Unit produces 0, as an output $x < 0$, and then produces a linear output with slope 1, when $x > 0$. It introduces non-linearity and mitigates the vanishing gradient problem, which is where the lower layers of the network train slowly as the gradient of optimization decreases exponentially. This leads to sparse neuron activation, more straightforward output, and makes computations easier while preserving the significant receptive fields of the convolution layers.
   - Sigmoid [57]: An activation function used in the second fully connected layer, with 1 neuron. Sigmoid activation functions are monotonic and differentiable. Their mathematical property maps real number values to the [0, 1] range to render the output as a probability, given the particular set of transformed input HRV features. In this work, the binary classification output of 0 indicates that an instance belongs to the NSR class, and 1 means that it belongs to the AF class.
5. Regularization [58]: This is a technique to prevent overfitting. Overfitting limits the ability of the model to predict new data, which means the network has learned only the specific features of the training set, like memorization, and cannot perform generalization on similar data. To mitigate this, the following two methods were used after all four convolutional layers.
   - Batch Normalization (BN) [59]: This technique reduces the covariance shift, meaning that minor features differences that do not contribute heavily to the overall model performance will not be considered with high priority. Therefore, minor changes between the ranges of training data, validation data, or unseen data will not affect the classification performance and allow each layer to be more independent about certain input features.

- Dropout (DP) [60]: This technique randomly drops neurons and their connections to prevent neurons from co-adapting. This makes each neuron more responsible for capturing the overall data representation and contributing to the final output. The dropout rate, which reflects the percentage of random neurons to be dropped, was set to 0.2.

3.5. Training and Testing

The CNN model is trained with the back-propagation algorithm [54] with a mini-batch of 16. According to [61], taking a subset of the entire data for each epoch improved generalization performance and had a smaller memory footprint. An epoch is the number of times the training set passes through a neural network completing a feed-forward and back-propagation phase. In this work, the total number of epochs was 50. The Adaptive Moment Estimation (ADAM) [62] optimizer was used for effective training convergence.

From the dataset, 80% was randomly divided for training and validation, and 20% was used as the test set. The Stratified k-fold cross-validation strategy was implemented with k = 5 [63]. In each fold, the training and validation subset is randomly divided into 5 equal parts, where with cross-validation, each data instance is used for both training and validation. Stratified k-fold cross-validation ensures that the class distribution in each of the five equal parts remains consistent across iterations to address potential biases. This was conducted to observe the generalizability and variability of the developed model to reflect its performance with new data. The 20% testing subset serves as the holdout data that the model has not been trained/validated with.

4. Results

This section describes the environment setting, reports the achieved diagnostic performance measures of the proposed convolutional model neural network on the ECG training data and unseen PPG data. To assess the implementation feasibility of the developed model, it was interfaced with a smartphone application and integrated within a health monitoring context.

4.1. Implementation Environment

The proposed CNN algorithm was implemented on a workstation with Windows OS, an Intel Kabylake 2.80GHz processor (i7-7700HQ), and 16 GB of RAM. The time required for training and testing the CNN model with 50 epochs was approximately 4420.67 s. The deep learning platform employed in this work was Keras [64], a high-level neural networks framework with a Tensorflow backend [65]. The Waveform-Database Package (WFDB) published by Physionet was used to directly access the MIT-BIH Arrhythmia dataset [35], consisting of heart rhythm samples and their respective annotations. The Sklearn module was used for data preprocessing and normalization operations [66]. Neurokit (NK), a toolbox for statistics and neurophysiological signal processing, was used to extract the ECG and PPG time-series features [67].

4.2. Model Evaluation on ECG Datasets

The diagnostic performance measures of accuracy, sensitivity, specificity, F1-score, and AUC are evaluated on a holdout test set in each of the five folds. Accuracy is the proportion of true outputs with respect to all data instances. Sensitivity is the model's ability to classify data instances belonging to a certain class correctly. Specificity is the model's ability to correctly distinguish data instances that do not belong to specific classes. F1-score is the harmonic mean between precision (ratio of correctly distinguished positives over all predicted positive) and recall (sensitivity), and the area under the curve (AUC) measures the quality of binary classification outputs in terms of sensitivity against false positive rate. To develop high-fidelity biomedical models as the proposed approach, high sensitivity and specificity are vital. They gauge the model's ability to correctly detect patients with a certain cardiac arrhythmia and correctly detect patients without cardiac arrythmia [68].

To calculate the measures as in Equation (5), the model classification outputs must be quantified in terms of True Positives (TP), False Positives (FP), False Negatives (FN) and True Negatives (TN) [69].

$$\begin{aligned} Accuracy &= \frac{TP_{NSR}+TN_{NSR}}{TP_{NSR}+TN_{NSR}+FP_{NSR}+FN_{NSR}} \\ Sensitivity &= \frac{TP_{NSR}}{TP_{NSR}+FN_{NSR}} \\ Specificity &= \frac{TN_{NSR}}{TN_{NSR}+FP_{NSR}} \\ F1Score &= \frac{TP_{NSR}}{TP_{NSR}+(0.5*(FP_{NSR}+FN_{NSR}))} \end{aligned} \quad (5)$$

Let Y_j^i be the data instances where i is the true class, j is the predicted class, and $i,j \in \{NSR, AF\}$. Consider the class AF signifying atrial fibrillation rhythms, and then, its outputs are defined as follows:

- $TP_{AF} = Y_{AF}^{AF}$, denotes data instances correctly classified as AF;
- $FP_{AF} = Y_{AF}^{NSR}$, denotes data instances incorrectly classified as AF;
- $FN_{AF} = Y_{NSR}^{AF}$, denotes data instances incorrectly classified as non-AF classes;
- $TN_{AF} = Y_{ij}$, denotes $i,j \neq AF$, denotes data instances correctly classified as non-AF classes.

The aggregated scores across all 5 folds are summarized in Table 5, and exhibit a high AF classification performance. The true positive (TP_{AF}) rate is 96.90%, and the true negative TN_{AF} rate is 95.13%.

Table 5. Aggregated classification metrics across five-folds expressed as mean and standard deviation.

Accuracy (%)	Sensitivity (%)	Specificity (%)	F1-Score (%)	AUC (%)
95.50 ± 0.2	94.50 ± 1.8	96.00 ± 0.7	93.36 ± 0.4	95.3 ± 0.5

4.3. Model Evaluation on PPG Dataset

While evaluating the model on the PPG dataset, two scenarios are considered. In the first scenario, the weights of the pre-trained model were not updated through transfer learning. In the second scenario, the model was finetuned by retraining the PPG signals.

In the first scenario, the model correctly classified 170 out of 192 samples of NSR, and 42 out of 54 samples as AF. The true positive (TP_{AF}) rate is 77.80%, and the true negative (TN_{AF}) rate is 88.54%. The measures reported in Table 6 serves as an initial benchmark test to gauge the performance of the ECG HRV trained on PPG data that have not been encountered during training or validation by the CNN model.

Table 6. Performance measures of the ECG-trained model on the complete UMass-DB PPG signals before transfer learning.

Accuracy (%)	Sensitivity (%)	Specificity (%)	F1-Score (%)	AUC (%)
86.00	77.80	88.54	72.00	83.16

In the second scenario, the learned weights of the model are updated by using 75% of UMass-DB for (60%) training and (15%) validation, with 25% for holdout testing, following the Stratified k-fold cross-validation with k = 4. By employing this approach, the intention is to adapt the weights of the pre-trained CNN model with 75% of the PPG data instances, test its performance on the remaining 25% of the untrained PPG data instances. This was applied four separate times, such that every instance is used for training, validation, and testing independently without data leakage between the training/validation and the testing sets. The aggregated testing performance is reported in Table 7, where the model makes predictions on all instances fairly.

Table 7. Performance measures of the ECG-trained model on UMass-DB PPG signals after transfer learning folds expressed as mean and standard deviation.

Accuracy (%)	Sensitivity (%)	Specificity (%)	F1-Score (%)	AUC (%)
95.10 ± 2.9	94.6 ± 2.4	95.20 ± 6.5	89.34 ± 1.8	94.9 ± 4.10

After retraining, the average true positive (TP_{AF}) rate is 94.33% and the average true negative TN_{AF} rate is 95.20%.

This performance is considerably high as the model classifies instances from a different input modality (PPG), when it was trained using only ECG signals. A marginal increase in performance is observed when transfer learning is implemented. Type I and type II errors were also observed, at a lower degree, resulting in AF false positives and AF false negatives, as shown by the results in Tables 6 and 7. This indicates that the boundaries between the NSR and AF to a certain extent are not clearly distinct in both the ECG and PPG recordings. Factors, such as PPG sensor specifications, reliability, and quality, may contribute to the decreased classification measures compared to the training performance. It is to be noted that both the ECG training samples and the PPG samples were resampled using FFT at 50 Hz, 100 Hz, 128 Hz, 250 Hz and 360 Hz, corresponding to the different sampling rates of the original dataset recordings to see the differences in the achieved results. The conducted empirical experiments found that 50 Hz for all recordings yielded relatively similar performance when classifying PPG signals as ~128 Hz (the minimum sampling rate across all datasets).

4.4. Implementation and Testing

In addition to the validation conducted in Section 4.3, a prototype implementation was further developed and tested on live human subjects. The developed model was integrated within a health monitoring platform to test and ascertain its real-world performance. A smartphone application was designed to acquire PPG recordings, interface with the model, and retrieve predictions of AF from human subjects.

The system that implements the proposed CNN model presented in this work was realized by following the three-tier architecture for modularity, scalability, and testing. The model was deployed via a Python Flask [70] server with a Google Firestore [71] database on the same workstation. Figure 6 presents the smartphone application collecting the input from the sensor, i.e., raw PPG heart rhythm values and sending an HTTP POST request to the REST API server containing the recorded heart rhythm values. The smartphone application receives a response from the server (end-to-end response time ≈ 1.25 s) indicating whether the recording was NSR or AF.

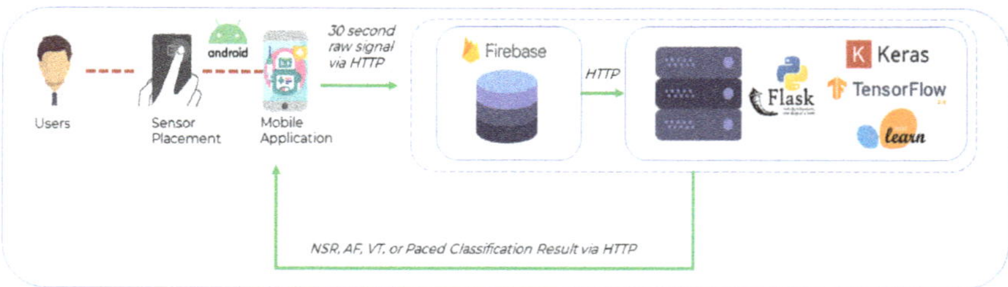

Figure 6. Implementation Architecture.

The PPG signals from most variations of optical sensors available in general-purpose smartphones and wearable devices can be used in the classification of AF after applying the techniques of filtering, down-sampling, peak detection, PRV extraction as outlined in Section 3.3. The specifications of the particular sensor used in this implementation are listed in Table 8 and have a maximum frequency of 100.0 Hz. The sensor type is 65,572 and is manufactured by MAXIM. The heart rate monitor LED measures the magnitude of the red light reflected from an individual's blood vessels at the measurement location, in the range of 0–350,000 (unitless). It operates on a 3.0 V to 5.5 V single supply voltage, with dimensions of 2.9 mm × 4.3 mm × 1.4 mm, and is integrated into portable or wearable devices. The devices used in the experiments were the Samsung S9, Samsung Note 8, and Samsung Note 9. M. Elgendi et al. [72] used Samsung 9th generation smartphones, the same ones used in this work.

Table 8. Sensor specifications for the smartphones used in this experiment.

Name	Vendor	Range	Voltage (V)	Type
HRMLED RED	MAXIM	0–350,000	3.0 V–5.5 V	65,572

The prototype implementation was successfully verified on the human subjects with the complete flow from signal acquisition to live AF classification following the same preprocessing techniques for filtering and resampling used for the UMass-DB PPG signals.

The human subjects were classified into healthy human subjects with no reported medical conditions, while the other was a heart patient from the Welcare Hospital Ernakulam, India. To record the heart rhythm, the subject is required to position their fingertip on the smartphone's heart rate sensor. Upon the detection of the PPG input signal, the smartphone application initiates the PPG value acquisition process. The healthy subject continues to hold their fingertip in place for 30 s, and then, the signal is transmitted to the server. The model classified one of the short length heart rhythms obtained at rest as NSR, as shown in Figure 7a. The heart patients' vitals are supervised through a bedside monitor by the doctor. Upon detecting an oncoming abnormality on the monitor, the patient is asked to place their finger on the smartphone and record a PPG signal. The result is shown in Figure 7b. The classification is saved in the cloud database under a specific entry for each subject, and the REST API server processes and responds to each acquired signal. This allows subjects and doctors to access historical records of the subject heart activity regularly.

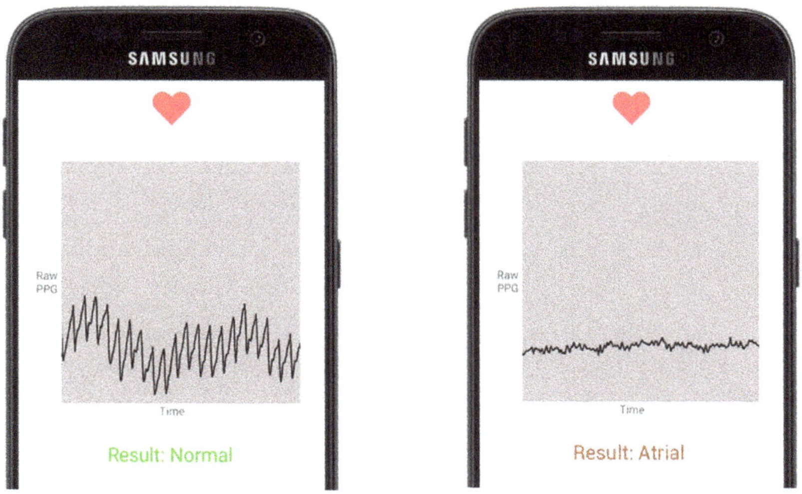

(**a**) (**b**)

Figure 7. Cardiac arrythmia classifications presented on a smartphone application by the model using live PPG readings from the fingertip smartphone sensor; (**a**) presents NSR Classification; (**b**) presents AF Classification.

The healthy subject underwent a Treadmill Stress Test in the clinical laboratory to observe the similarity in heartbeats and peak formations between an ECG and the PPG peak detection algorithm used in this work. The Treadmill Stress Test uses medical-grade multi-lead ECG to capture heart activity to measure cardiovascular health. A reference ECG signal was simultaneously collected to validate the PPG signal obtained from the smartphone sensors for the same 30 s. The resulting waveforms are shown in Figure 8a,b. Both Figure 8a,b estimate the same BPM, indicating potential consistency in the number of detected peaks.

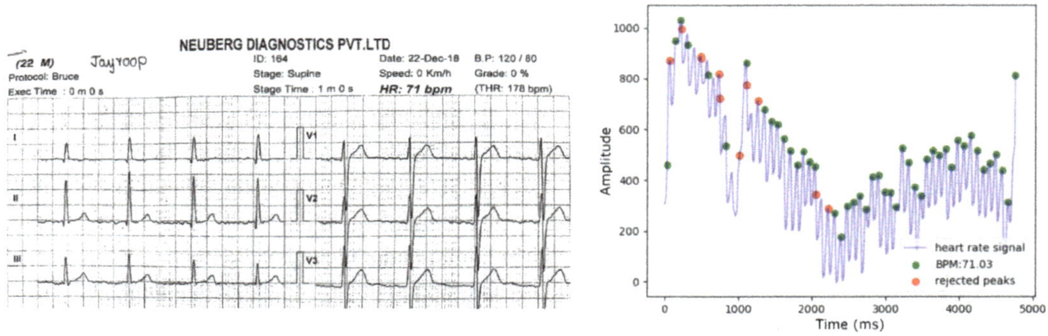

(a) (b)

Figure 8. Measured ECG vs. estimated PPG BPM comparison. (**a**) Reference ECG-measured BPM; (**b**) PPG-derived BPM by peak detection algorithm.

5. Discussion

This study explored the efficiency of using convolutional neural networks to classify short-length heart rhythms using the concept of HRV-derived features to generalize AF representation across both the ECG and PPG modality. In this paper, the proposed model is compared and contrasted with similar works in the literature. The primary contributions of this research are highlighted in the following subsections.

5.1. Comparison with Existing Works

Table 9 presents recent advances in the literature for short-length cardiac arrhythmia detection using one or more HRV features with applicability in portable devices.

Zhou et al. [17] employed a modified version of the Shannon entropy algorithm for AF detection by constructing symbolic sequences and probability distributions using ECG-based R-R intervals from the MIT AF database. This statistical approach was one of the first studies to discuss the possibility of deploying such approaches in portable devices. Islam et al. [73] presented a rhythm-based heartbeat normalization technique for improved ECG-based AF detection by measuring irregularities in a specified window of heartbeats. The datasets used for training and testing were the MIT-BIH AF database and MIT-BIH Arrhythmia, respectively. Cui et al. [18] proposed a similarity analysis and ensemble scheme that maps R-R intervals to binary symbolic sequences and compares the rank-frequencies to quantify the differences between AF and NSR using the ECG-based MIT-BIH AF database. Shashikumar et al. [74] presented one of the first and few works proposing cross-domain generalizability of cardiac arrhythmia models and used Bidirectional Recurrent Neural Network for AF detection from a single lead ECG. The researchers collected the ECG dataset from the University of Virginia Heart Station, United States, for training and collected the PPG dataset from the Emory Hospital and Grady Memorial Hospital, Atlanta, United States, for testing. They reported high classification performance for the cross-domain application using spectral features and R-R time series features with wavelet decomposition. Bashar et al. [75] utilized support vector machines on 30-s-long PPG signals for AF and NSR detection. They trained and tested on a custom-made PPG dataset and addressed noise saturation by using Butterworth filters. Tarniceriu et al. [76] implemented Markov models to detect AF and NSR by using R-R intervals as features and collected a dataset with a custom wearable prototype. Aliamiri et al. [77] employed an end-end deep learning PPG-based AF detection system that filters poor quality signals. They developed a convolution-recurrent hybrid model using waveform features on a custom-made PPG dataset that could effectively distinguish between AF and NSR. Tison et al. [78] conducted one of the first large-scale studies for passive AF detection using PPG-enabled smartwatches in collaboration with the University of California, San Francisco and Cardiogram. Cardiogram is an Apple watch application used to obtain heart rate data. The researchers used these collected data to implement a deep neural network with heuristic pretraining and R-R intervals as a feature set. Fallet et al. [79] utilized decision trees with waveform features and RR-intervals to classify AF and ventricular arrhythmia in 10-s-long PPG signals. The researchers created a PPG signal dataset from Lausanne University Hospital Switzerland and used a custom wearable prototype to test their results. Kwon et al. [80] employed a 1D CNN to process 30-s-long PPG signals to classify AF and NSR with a custom-made dataset.

Table 9. A comparison of recent works developed for CVD detection with machine learning and portable devices.

Author (Year)	Features	Approach	Modality	Accuracy (%)	Sensitivity (%)	Specificity (%)
This work	Temporal HRV	Convolutional Neural Networks	ECG; PPG	ECG = 95.50 PPG = 95.10	ECG = 94.50 PPG = 94.60	ECG = 96.00 PPG = 95.20
Zhou et al. [17] (2015)	R-R intervals	Shannon Entropy	ECG	97.89	97.37	98.44
Cui et al. [18] (2017)	R-R intervals	Ensemble Model	ECG	97.78	97.04	96.97
Shashikumar et al. [74] (2018)	R-R Intervals and waveform features	Bidirectional Recurrent Neural Networks	ECG; PPG	ECG = 94.00 PPG = 95.00	-	ECG = 95.00 PPG = 100.00
Bashar et al. [75] (2018)	R-R intervals and waveform features	Support Vector Machines	PPG	91.16	-	-
Tarniceriu et al. [76] (2018)	R-R Intervals	Markov Model	PPG	-	98.45	99.13
Aliamiri et al. [77] (2018)	Waveform features	Convolutional Recurrent Neural Networks	PPG	98.19	-	-
Tison et al. [78] (2018)	R-R Intervals	Neural Network	PPG	-	98.00	90.20
Fallet et al. [79] (2019)	R-R intervals and waveform features	Decision Trees	PPG	95.00	92.90	96.20
Kwon et al. [80] (2019)	R-R intervals	Convolutional Neural Network	PPG	97.58	99.32	95.85

The performance measures obtained in this work are competitive with the works reported previously. The existing research has achieved successful results in the domain, however, has a few limitations that the proposed approach in this paper addresses. Firstly, the PPG datasets are not gold-standard and are not publicly accessible to reproducible and further testing. In this work, the reputed MIT-BIH datasets are utilized for implementing a cross-domain generalizable model. The input features of HRV captures a holistic representation of cardiac activity, as they are the most consistent medium of commonality between ECG and the PRV aspect of PPG signals. Secondly, existing models trained on ECG signals cannot be applied to predict PPG directly due to the differences in their morphology. In most of the works, ECG-based models can only work with portable devices having ECG sensors, and the PPG based-models require custom wearable prototypes or hospital settings, except in [78]. Thirdly, the developed models are not trained with multiple datasets or assessed on unseen data, lowering the likelihood of being applicable in non-ambulatory settings. Lastly, this work provides a supplementary approach, wherein the time-domain HRV representations are extracted from larger public datasets instead of raw signals, which extends the applicability to both ECG and PPG derived from clinical devices or consumer wearables.

5.2. Research Impact

This work presents a generalizable approach that has the potential for sensor agnostic CVD classification. The model is trained on data acquired from the source ECG modality and finetuned by updating the learned parameters using data from the target PPG modality. There were 15,434 instances from the ECG datasets of both NSR and AF for training the model, while there were only 192 total instances from the PPG dataset. Through the development of models with large cohorts of data in the related domain of ECG and the use of transfer learning, the issue of limited, gold-standard data accessibility from consumer wearable devices can be resolved. This can enable healthcare providers to leverage such devices in conjunction with cardiac arrhythmia classification models for non-ambulatory cardiovascular prognosis in the general population.

Smart healthcare platforms are holistic systems that enable disease prevention, monitoring, diagnosis, and treatment and connect patients with medical professionals. These are significant risk factors for the progression of CVD in patients. Repeated detection of any cardiovascular impairments as indicated by the AF in this work can prompt a clinical checkup, thereby allowing for early treatment and outcome improvement. A systematic survey by Majumder et al. [81] of 11 smartphone cardiac monitoring applications showed that the majority of them used simple, static heart rate threshold-based risk stratification. Furthermore, the existing solutions were not designed to be part of a monitoring system that can interface with clinicians but rather limited to the device only within the scope of the testing setting. Kakria et al. [82] proposed a real-time cardiac health monitoring system with a patient and doctor portal for effective monitoring using a custom Bluetooth wearable device and smartphone. However, medical alerts sent to patients and users lacked specificity, as any heartbeat above or below a threshold is flagged as abnormal. Moreover, there were no considerations for noise saturation or adaptability to signals other than PPG. In resource-constrained settings such as inexpensive fitness bands, extracting only the features necessary instead of complete raw signal samples can prove to be more efficient, as demonstrated in this work.

A possible limitation stems from the fact that there appears to be an overlap between the samples of each class. This could be due to the differences in resting heart rates across individuals, general fitness levels, and the influence of underlying health conditions. A direct approach to boost the model's performance is to incorporate additional real ECG samples from more reputable datasets. Finally, spectral and non-linear HRV measures [83] can be added to the feature space to capture more robust representations of each class.

6. Conclusions

This work proposed a design and implementation of an explainable deep learning 1D-CNN model for use in smart healthcare systems with general-purpose devices such as smart wearables and smartphones. The 1D-CNN model classifies the NSR and AF from short length ECG or PPG signals using HRV features as inputs with the MIT-BIH ECG datasets.

The 1D-CNN model achieved overall classification performances with accuracy of 95.50%, sensitivity: 94.50%, specificity: 96.00%, F1-score: 93.40%, and AUC: 95.30% across a five-fold cross-validation approach. In comparison to other works in the literature, these performance measures are highly competitive and can be integrated into mobile health monitoring platforms with general-purpose devices. Thereby, the proposed approach is one of the first works to develop a cross-domain generalizable ECG-based model for deployment in smartphones and wearable devices.

Furthermore, the proposed methodology removes noise and motion artifacts from commercial PPG-sensors within a framework for health monitoring, thereby making early detection systems accessible for the general public. This approach brings to the forefront the applicability of ECG databases to enable machine learning to transform the PPG sensor readings from commercial devices. This can mitigate the issues of developing classification models that can only be used in controlled settings as well as increase the types of cardiac arrhythmia that can be observed from general-purpose devices and eliminate difficulties associated with creating custom PPG datasets for each study.

Subsequent research directions involve conducting a longitudinal study for exhaustive testing with users to attain additional empirical evidence supporting the real-world applicability of this approach, benchmarking the model against further gold-standard datasets, and extending the scope of the health monitoring framework.

Author Contributions: Conceptualization, J.R., R.A. and A.S.; data curation, J.R. and Z.S.; investigation, J.R. and Z.S.; methodology, J.R., R.A. and A.S.; software, J.R., Z.S. and R.A.; supervision, R.A. and A.S.; writing, J.R., Z.S., R.A. and A.S. All authors have read and agreed to the published version of the manuscript.

Funding: This research was partially funded by the American University of Sharjah faculty research grant FRG17-R-20. The work in this paper was supported, in part, by the Open Access Program from the American University of Sharjah. This paper represents the opinions of the author(s) and does not mean to represent the position or opinions of the American University of Sharjah.

Institutional Review Board Statement: No IRB required.

Informed Consent Statement: A consent has been obtained from the patient(s) to use this dataset for research purposes and publishing this paper.

Data Availability Statement: The ECG dataset adopted in this research is openly available in [Physionet] at https://doi.org/10.13026/C2F305, https://doi.org/10.13026/C2MW2D, and https://doi.org/10.13026/C2NK5R (accessed on 1 September 2021). The PPG dataset analyzed in this research is openly available in https://www.synapse.org/#!Synapse:syn23565056/wiki/608635 (accessed on 1 September 2021).

Conflicts of Interest: The authors declare no conflict of interest.

References

1. Cardiovascular Diseases. Available online: https://www.who.int/westernpacific/health-topics/cardiovascular-diseases (accessed on 16 December 2020).
2. Cardiovascular Disease. nhs.uk. 17 October 2017. Available online: https://www.nhs.uk/conditions/cardiovascular-disease/ (accessed on 16 December 2020).
3. Pereira, T.; Tran, N.; Gadhoumi, K.; Pelter, M.M.; Do, D.H.; Lee, R.J.; Colorado, R.; Meisel, K.; Hu, X. Photoplethysmography based atrial fibrillation detection: A review. *NPJ Digit. Med.* **2020**, 3, 3. [CrossRef]
4. Goldberger, A.L.; Goldberger, Z.D.; Shvilkin, A. Chapter 13-Sinus and Escape Rhythms. In *Goldberger's Clinical Electrocardiography (Ninth Edition)*; Goldberger, A.L., Goldberger, Z.D., Shvilkin, A., Eds.; Elsevier: Amsterdam, The Netherlands, 2018; pp. 122–129.
5. Field, M.E. Chapter 35—Atrial Fibrillation. In *Cardiology Secrets*, 5th ed.; Levine, G.N., Ed.; Elsevier: Amsterdam, The Netherlands, 2018; pp. 323–329.
6. Electrocardiogram (ECG or EKG). www.heart.org. Available online: https://www.heart.org/en/health-topics/heart-attack/diagnosing-a-heart-attack/electrocardiogram-ecg-or-ekg (accessed on 9 October 2021).
7. Sagahyroon, A. Remote patients monitoring: Challenges. In Proceedings of the 2017 IEEE 7th Annual Computing and Communication Workshop, Las Vegas, NV, USA, 9–11 January 2017.
8. Measuring the Heart—How Does ECG and PPG Work? iMotions, 21 March 2017. Available online: https://imotions.com/blog/measuring-the-heart-how-does-ecg-and-ppg-work/ (accessed on 28 July 2021).
9. MD, M.C. Heart Rate Variability: A New Way to Track Well-Being. Harvard Health Blog. 22 November 2017. Available online: https://www.health.harvard.edu/blog/heart-rate-variability-new-way-track-well-2017112212789 (accessed on 4 June 2020).
10. Neurosky.com. 2019. Available online: http://neurosky.com/wp-content/uploads/2016/06/TOF-side-by-side-competitor-comparison.pdf (accessed on 17 June 2020).
11. Paradkar, N.; Chowdhury, S.R. Cardiac arrhythmia detection using photoplethysmography. In Proceedings of the 2017 39th Annual International Conference of the IEEE Engineering in Medicine and Biology Society (EMBC), Jeju, Korea, 11–15 July 2017; pp. 113–116. [CrossRef]

12. Koshy, A.N.; Sajeev, J.K.; Nerlekar, N.; Brown, A.J.; Rajakariar, K.; Zureik, M.; Wong, M.C.; Roberts, L.; Street, M.; Cooke, J.; et al. Utility of photoplethysmography for heart rate estimation among inpatients. *Intern. Med. J.* **2018**, *48*, 587–591. [CrossRef] [PubMed]
13. Millán, C.A.; Girón, N.A.; Lopez, D.M. Analysis of Relevant Features from Photoplethysmographic Signals for Atrial Fibrillation Classification. *Int. J. Environ. Res. Public Health* **2020**, *17*, 498. [CrossRef]
14. Aschbacher, K.; Yilmaz, D.; Kerem, Y.; Crawford, S.; Benaron, D.; Liu, J.; Eaton, M.; Tison, G.H.; Olgin, J.E.; Li, Y.; et al. Atrial fibrillation detection from raw photoplethysmography waveforms: A deep learning application. *Hear. Rhythm O2* **2020**, *1*, 3–9. [CrossRef]
15. Alian, A.A.; Shelley, K.H. Photoplethysmography. *Best Pract. Res. Clin. Anaesthesiol.* **2014**, *28*, 395–406. [CrossRef]
16. Charlton, P.; Bonnici, T.; Tarassenko, L.; Alastruey, J.; Clifton, D.A.; Beale, R.; Watkinson, P. Extraction of respiratory signals from the electrocardiogram and photoplethysmogram: Technical and physiological determinants. *Physiol. Meas.* **2017**, *38*, 669–690. [CrossRef] [PubMed]
17. Zhou, X.; Ding, H.; Wu, W.; Zhang, Y. A Real-Time Atrial Fibrillation Detection Algorithm Based on the Instantaneous State of Heart Rate. *PLoS ONE* **2015**, *10*, e0136544. [CrossRef] [PubMed]
18. Cui, X.; Chang, E.; Yang, W.-H.; Jiang, B.C.; Yang, A.C.; Peng, C.-K. Automated Detection of Paroxysmal Atrial Fibrillation Using an Information-Based Similarity Approach. *Entropy* **2017**, *19*, 677. [CrossRef]
19. Dash, S.; Chon, K.H.; Lu, S.; Raeder, E.A. Automatic real time detection of atrial fibrillation. *Ann. Biomed. Eng.* **2009**, *37*, 1701–1709. [CrossRef]
20. Tateno, K.; Glass, L. Automatic detection of atrial fibrillation using the coefficient of variation and density histogram of NN and NN intervals. *Med. Biol. Eng. Comput.* **2001**, *39*, 664–671. [CrossRef]
21. Hagiwara, Y.; Fujita, H.; Oh, S.L.; Tan, J.H.; Tan, R.S.; Ciaccio, E.J.; Acharya, U.R. Computer-aided diagnosis of atrial fibrillation based on ECG Signals: A review. *Inf. Sci.* **2018**, *467*, 99–114. [CrossRef]
22. Yıldırım, Ö.; Pławiak, P.; Tan, R.S.; Acharya, U.R. Arrhythmia detection using deep convolutional neural network with long duration ECG signals. *Comput. Biol. Med.* **2018**, *102*, 411–420. [CrossRef]
23. Acharya, U.R.; Oh, S.L.; Hagiwara, Y.; Tan, J.H.; Adam, M.; Gertych, A.; Tan, R.S. A deep convolutional neural network model to classify heartbeats. *Comput. Biol. Med.* **2017**, *89*, 389–396. [CrossRef]
24. Kiranyaz, S.; Ince, T.; Gabbouj, M. Personalized Monitoring and Advance Warning System for Cardiac Arrhythmias. *Sci. Rep.* **2017**, *7*, 9270. [CrossRef] [PubMed]
25. Ramos, G.; Alfaras, M.; Gamboa, H. Real-Time Approach to HRV Analysis. In Proceedings of the 11th International Joint Conference on Biomedical Engineering Systems and Technologies, Funchal, Madeira, Portugal, 19–21 January 2018; pp. 208–215.
26. Bent, B.; Goldstein, B.A.; Kibbe, W.A.; Dunn, J.P. Investigating sources of inaccuracy in wearable optical heart rate sensors. *NPJ Digit. Med.* **2020**, *3*, 18. [CrossRef] [PubMed]
27. Elgendi, M. On the Analysis of Fingertip Photoplethysmogram Signals. *Curr. Cardiol. Rev.* **2012**, *8*, 14–25. [CrossRef] [PubMed]
28. Malik, M.; Camm, A.J.; Bigger, J.T.; Breithardt, G.; Cerutti, S.; Cohen, R.J.; Coumel, P.; Fallen, E.L.; Kennedy, H.L.; Kleiger, R.E.; et al. Heart rate varia-bility. Standards of measurement, physiological interpretation, clinical use. *Eur. Heart J.* **1996**, *17*, 354–381. [CrossRef]
29. Smith, A.-L.; Owen, H.; Reynolds, K. Heart rate variability indices for very short-term (30 beat) analysis. Part 1: Survey and toolbox. *J. Clin. Monit.* **2013**, *27*, 569–576. [CrossRef]
30. Lu, S.; Zhao, H.; Ju, K.; Shin, K.; Lee, M.; Shelley, K.; Chon, K.H. Can Photoplethysmography Variability Serve as an Alternative Approach to Obtain Heart Rate Variability Information? *J. Clin. Monit.* **2007**, *22*, 23–29. [CrossRef] [PubMed]
31. Jeyhani, V.; Mahdiani, S.; Peltokangas, M.; Vehkaoja, A. Comparison of HRV parameters derived from photoplethys-mography and electrocar-diography signals. In Proceedings of the 2015 37th annual international conference of the IEEE engineering in medicine and biology society (EMBC), Milan, Italy, 25–29 August 2015; pp. 5952–5955.
32. Shaffer, F.; Ginsberg, J.P. An Overview of Heart Rate Variability Metrics and Norms. *Front. Public Health* **2017**, *5*, 258. [CrossRef] [PubMed]
33. O'Neal, W.T.; Chen, L.; Nazarian, S.; Soliman, E.Z. Reference ranges for short-term heart rate variability measures in individuals free of cardiovascular disease: The Multi-Ethnic Study of Atherosclerosis (MESA). *J. Electrocardiol.* **2016**, *49*, 686–690. [CrossRef] [PubMed]
34. Moody, G.B.; Mark, R.G. The impact of the MIT-BIH Arrhythmia Database. *IEEE Eng. Med. Biol. Mag.* **2001**, *20*, 45–50. [CrossRef]
35. Goldberger, A.L.; Amaral, L.A.N.; Glass, L.; Hausdorff, J.M.; Ivanov, P.C.; Mark, R.G.; Mietus, J.E.; Moody, G.B.; Peng, C.-K.; Stanley, H.E. PhysioBank, PhysioToolkit, PhysioNet. *Circulation* **2000**, *101*, e215–e220. [CrossRef]
36. American Association of Medical Instrumentation. ANSI/AAMI EC57: 2012—Testing and Reporting Performance Results of Cardiac Rhythm and ST Segment Measurement Algorithms. In *American National Standard*; Association for the Advancement of Medical Instrumentation (AAMI): Washington, DC, USA, 2013.
37. Teijeiro, T.; Felix, P.; Presedo, J.M.R.; Castro, D. Heartbeat classification using abstract features from the abductive interpretation of the ECG. *IEEE J. Biomed. Health Inform.* **2016**, *22*, 409–420. [CrossRef]
38. Proenca, T.; Carvalho, M.M.; Pinto, R.A.; Resende, C.; Grilo, P.; Torres, S.; Paiva, M.; Lebreiro, A.; Campelo, M.; Rema, J.; et al. Supraventricular ectopic activity as a predictor of atrial fibrillation—what we didn't see 10 years ago. *Eur. Heart J.* **2020**, *41*, ehaa946-2422. [CrossRef]

39. Sörnmo, L.; Laguna, P. *Bioelectrical Signal Processing in Cardiac and Neurological Applications*; Academic Press: Cambridge, MA, USA, 2005; pp. 411–452. [CrossRef]
40. Rajoub, B. *Biomedical Signal Processing and Artificial Intelligence in Healthcare*; Academic Press: Cambridge, MA, USA, 2020; pp. 91–112. [CrossRef]
41. Han, D.; Bashar, S.K.; Mohagheghian, F.; Ding, E.; Whitcomb, C.; McManus, D.D.; Chon, K.H. Premature Atrial and Ventricular Contraction Detection using Photoplethysmographic Data from a Smartwatch. *Sensors* **2020**, *20*, 5683. [CrossRef] [PubMed]
42. Bashar, S.K.; Han, D.; Hajeb-Mohammadalipour, S.; Ding, E.; Whitcomb, C.; McManus, D.D.; Chon, K.H. Atrial Fibrillation Detection from Wrist Photoplethysmography Signals Using Smartwatches. *Sci. Rep.* **2019**, *9*, 11452. [CrossRef]
43. Binici, Z.; Intzilakis, T.; Nielsen, O.W.; Køber, L.; Sajadieh, A. Excessive Supraventricular Ectopic Activity and Increased Risk of Atrial Fibrillation and Stroke. *Circulation* **2010**, *121*, 1904–1911. [CrossRef] [PubMed]
44. Ding, E.Y.; Han, D.; Whitcomb, C.; Bashar, S.K.; Adaramola, O.; Soni, A.; Saczynski, J.; Fitzgibbons, T.P.; Moonis, M.; Lubitz, S.A.; et al. Accuracy and Usability of a Novel Algorithm for Detection of Irregular Pulse Using a Smartwatch Among Older Adults: Observational Study. *JMIR Cardio* **2019**, *3*, e13850. [CrossRef] [PubMed]
45. Ebrahimi, Z.; Loni, M.; Daneshtalab, M.; Gharehbaghi, A. A review on deep learning methods for ECG arrhythmia classification. *Expert Syst. Appl. X* **2020**, *7*, 100033. [CrossRef]
46. Elgendi, M.; Jonkman, M.; Boer, F.D. Frequency bands effects on QRS detection. In Proceedings of the BIOSIGNALS 2010—Proceedings of the 3rd International Conference on Bioinpsired Systems and Signal Processing, Valencia, Spain, 20–23 January 2010; pp. 428–431.
47. Pan, J.; Tompkins, W.J. A Real-Time QRS Detection Algorithm. *IEEE Trans. Biomed. Eng.* **1985**, *BME-32*, 230–236. [CrossRef]
48. Li, B.N.; Dong, M.C.; Vai, M.I. On an automatic delineator for arterial blood pressure waveforms. *Biomed. Signal Process. Control* **2010**, *5*, 76–81. [CrossRef]
49. Elgendi, M.; Norton, I.; Brearley, M.; Abbott, D.; Schuurmans, D. Systolic Peak Detection in Acceleration Photoplethysmograms Measured from Emergency Responders in Tropical Conditions. *PLoS ONE* **2013**, *8*, e76585. [CrossRef]
50. Billauer, E. Peakdet: Peak Detection Using MATLAB. Available online: http://billauer.co.il/peakdet.html (accessed on 7 July 2021).
51. Zong, W.; Heldt, T.; Moody, G.; Mark, R. An open-source algorithm to detect onset of arterial blood pressure pulses. In Proceedings of the Computers in Cardiology, Thessaloniki, Greece, 21–24 September 2003; pp. 259–262. [CrossRef]
52. Mahdiani, S.; Jeyhani, V.; Peltokangas, M.; Vehkaoja, A. Is 50 Hz High Enough ECG Sampling Frequency for Accurate HRV Analysis? The work was partially funded by the Finnish Funding Agency for Technology and Innovation (TEKES) as a part of project VitalSens (decision ID 40103/14). In Proceedings of the 2015 37th Annual International Conference of the IEEE Engineering in Medicine and Biology Society (EMBC), Milan, Italy, 25–29 August 2015; pp. 5948–5951. [CrossRef]
53. Béres, S.; Hejjel, L. The minimal sampling frequency of the photoplethysmogram for accurate pulse rate variability parameters in healthy volunteers. *Biomed. Signal Process. Control* **2021**, *68*, 102589. [CrossRef]
54. LeCun, Y.; Bengio, Y. Convolutional networks for images, speech, time series. In *The handbook of Brain Theory and Neural Networks*; MIT Press: Cambridge, MA, USA, 1998; pp. 255–258.
55. Goodfellow, Y.; Bengio, A. *Courville, Deep Learning*; MIT Press: Cambridge, MA, USA, 2016.
56. Agarap, A.F. Deep Learning using Rectified Linear Units (ReLU). *arXiv* **2019**, arXiv:1803.08375.
57. Han, J.; Moraga, C. The influence of the sigmoid function parameters on the speed of back-propagation learning. In *From Natural to Artificial Neural Computation*; Springer: Berlin/Heidelberg, Germany, 1995; pp. 195–201. [CrossRef]
58. Nielsen, M.A. *Neural Networks and Deep Learning*; Determination Press: San Francisco, CA, USA, 2015.
59. Ioffe, S.; Szegedy, C. Batch Normalization: Accelerating Deep Network Training by Reducing Internal Covariate Shift. *arXiv* **2015**, arXiv:2.03167.
60. Srivastava, N.; Hinton, G.; Krizhevsky, A.; Sutskever, I.; Salakhutdinov, R. Dropout: A Simple Way to Prevent Neural Networks from Over-fitting. *J. Mach. Learn. Res.* **2014**, *15*, 1929–1958.
61. Masters, D.; Luschi, C. Revisiting Small Batch Training for Deep Neural Networks. *arXiv* **2018**, arXiv:1804.07612.
62. Kingma, D.P.; Ba, J. Adam: A Method for Stochastic Optimization. *arXiv* **2017**, arXiv:1412.6980 [cs].
63. Kohavi, R. A study of cross-validation and bootstrap for accuracy estimation and model selection. In Proceedings of the 14th International Joint Conference on Artificial Intelligence—Volume 2, Montreal, QC, Canada, 20–25 August 1995; pp. 1137–1143.
64. Chollet, F. Keras. 2015. Available online: https://github.com/fchollet/keras (accessed on 24 April 2021).
65. Abadi, M.; Barham, P.; Chen, J.; Chen, Z.; Davis, A.; Dean, J.; Devin, M.; Ghemawat, S.; Irving, G.; Isard, M.; et al. TensorFlow: A System for Large-Scale Machine Learning. In Proceedings of the Proceedings of the 12th USENIX Conference on Operating Systems Design and Implementation, Savannah, GA, USA, 2–4 November 2016; pp. 265–283.
66. Virtanen, P.; Gommers, R.; Oliphant, T.E.; Haberland, M.; Reddy, T.; Cournapeau, D.; Burovski, E.; Peterson, P.; Weckesser, W.; Bright, J.; et al. SciPy 1.0: Fundamental Algorithms for Scientific Computing in Python. *Nat Methods* **2020**, *17*, 261–272. [CrossRef]
67. Makowski, D. *NeuroKit: A Python Toolbox for Statistics and Neurophysiological Signal Processing (EEG, EDA, ECG, EMG...)*; Memory and Cognition Lab' Day: Paris, France, 2016.
68. Wong, H.B.; Lim, G.H. Measures of Diagnostic Accuracy: Sensitivity, Specificity, PPV and NPV. *Proc. Singap. Health* **2011**, *20*, 316–318. [CrossRef]
69. Tharwat, A. Classification assessment methods. *Appl. Comput. Inform.* **2018**, *17*, 168–192. [CrossRef]

70. Welcome to Flask—Flask Documentation (1.1.x). Available online: https://flask.palletsprojects.com/en/1.1.x/ (accessed on 12 March 2021).
71. Cloud Firestore | Firebase. Available online: https://firebase.google.com/docs/firestore (accessed on 16 March 2021).
72. Elgendi, M.; Fletcher, R.; Liang, Y.; Howard, N.; Lovell, N.H.; Abbott, D.; Lim, K.; Ward, R. The use of photoplethysmography for assessing hypertension. *NPJ Digit. Med.* **2019**, *2*, 60. [CrossRef] [PubMed]
73. Islam, S.; Ammour, N.; Alajlan, N.; Aboalsamh, H. Rhythm-based heartbeat duration normalization for atrial fibrillation detection. *Comput. Biol. Med.* **2016**, *72*, 160–169. [CrossRef]
74. Shashikumar, S.P.; Shah, A.J.; Clifford, G.D.; Nemati, S. Detection of Paroxysmal Atrial Fibrillation using Attention-based Bidirectional Recurrent Neural Networks. *arXiv* **2018**, arXiv:1805.09133. Available online: http://arxiv.org/abs/1805.09133 (accessed on 10 October 2021).
75. Bashar, S.K.; Han, D.; Soni, A.; McManus, D.D.; Chon, K.H. Developing a novel noise artifact detection algorithm for smartphone PPG signals: Preliminary results. In Proceedings of the 2018 IEEE EMBS International Conference on Biomedical Health Informatics (BHI), Las Vegas, NV, USA, 4–7 March 2018; pp. 79–82. [CrossRef]
76. Tarniceriu, A.; Harju, J.; Yousefi, Z.R.; Vehkaoja, A.; Parak, J.; Yli-Hankala, A.; Korhonen, I. The Accuracy of Atrial Fibrillation Detection from Wrist Photoplethysmography. A Study on Post-Operative Patients. In Proceedings of the 2018 40th Annual International Conference of the IEEE Engineering in Medicine and Biology Society (EMBC), Honolulu, HI, USA, 18–21 July 2018; pp. 1–4. [CrossRef]
77. Aliamiri, A.; Shen, Y. Deep learning based atrial fibrillation detection using wearable photoplethysmography sensor. In Proceedings of the 2018 IEEE EMBS International Conference on Biomedical Health Informatics (BHI), Las Vegas, NV, USA, 4–7 March 2018; pp. 442–445. [CrossRef]
78. Tison, G.; Sanchez, J.M.; Ballinger, B.; Singh, A.; Olgin, J.E.; Pletcher, M.J.; Vittinghoff, E.; Lee, E.S.; Fan, S.M.; Gladstone, R.A.; et al. Passive Detection of Atrial Fibrillation Using a Commercially Available Smartwatch. *JAMA Cardiol.* **2018**, *3*, 409–416. [CrossRef]
79. Fallet, S.; Lemay, M.; Renevey, P.; Leupi, C.; Pruvot, E.; Vesin, J.-M. Can one detect atrial fibrillation using a wrist-type photoplethysmographic device? *Med Biol. Eng. Comput.* **2018**, *57*, 477–487. [CrossRef]
80. Kwon, S.; Hong, J.; Choi, E.-K.; Lee, E.; Hostallero, D.E.; Kang, W.J.; Lee, B.; Jeong, E.-R.; Koo, B.-K.; Oh, S.; et al. Deep Learning Approaches to Detect Atrial Fibrillation Using Photoplethysmographic Signals: Algorithms Development Study. *JMIR mHealth uHealth* **2019**, *7*, e12770. [CrossRef]
81. Majumder, S.; Deen, M.J. Smartphone Sensors for Health Monitoring and Diagnosis. *Sensors* **2019**, *19*, 2164. [CrossRef]
82. Kakria, P.; Tripathi, N.K.; Kitipawang, P. A Real-Time Health Monitoring System for Remote Cardiac Patients Using Smartphone and Wearable Sensors. *Int. J. Telemed. Appl.* **2015**, *2015*, 373474. [CrossRef] [PubMed]
83. Huikuri, H.V.; Perkiömäki, J.S.; Maestri, R.; Pinna, G.D. Clinical impact of evaluation of cardiovascular control by novel methods of heart rate dynamics. *Philos. Trans. R. Soc. A Math. Phys. Eng. Sci.* **2009**, *367*, 1223–1238. [CrossRef] [PubMed]

sensors

MDPI

Article

Non-Contact Spirometry Using a Mobile Thermal Camera and AI Regression

Luay Fraiwan [1,2,*], Natheer Khasawneh [3], Khaldon Lweesy [2], Mennatalla Elbalki [1], Amna Almarzooqi [1] and Nada Abu Hamra [1]

1 Department of Electrical, Computer and Biomedical Engineering, Abu Dhabi University, Abu Dhabi 55991, United Arab Emirates; 1065023@students.adu.ac.ae (M.E.); 1065804@students.adu.ac.ae (A.A.); 1064647@students.adu.ac.ae (N.A.H.)
2 Department of Biomedical Engineering, Jordan University of Science and Technology, Irbid 2210, Jordan; klweesy@just.edu.jo
3 Department of Software Engineering, Jordan University of Science and Technology, Irbid 2210, Jordan; knatheer@just.edu.jo
* Correspondence: fraiwan@just.edu.jo

Abstract: Non-contact physiological measurements have been under investigation for many years, and among these measurements is non-contact spirometry, which could provide acute and chronic pulmonary disease monitoring and diagnosis. This work presents a feasibility study for non-contact spirometry measurements using a mobile thermal imaging system. Thermal images were acquired from 19 subjects for measuring the respiration rate and the volume of inhaled and exhaled air. A mobile application was built to measure the respiration rate and export the respiration signal to a personal computer. The mobile application acquired thermal video images at a rate of nine frames/second and the OpenCV library was used for localization of the area of interest (nose and mouth). Artificial intelligence regressors were used to predict the inhalation and exhalation air volume. Several regressors were tested and four of them showed excellent performance: random forest, adaptive boosting, gradient boosting, and decision trees. The latter showed the best regression results, with an R-square value of 0.9998 and a mean square error of 0.0023. The results of this study showed that non-contact spirometry based on a thermal imaging system is feasible and provides all the basic measurements that the conventional spirometers support.

Keywords: thermal camera; non-contact spirometry; artificial intelligence regression; respiration signal; respiration rate mobile application

Citation: Fraiwan, L.; Khasawneh, N.; Lweesy, K.; Elbalki, M.; Almarzooqi, A.; Abu Hamra, N. Non-Contact Spirometry Using a Mobile Thermal Camera and AI Regression. *Sensors* **2021**, *21*, 7574. https://doi.org/10.3390/s21227574

Academic Editor: Giacomo Oliveri

Received: 30 September 2021
Accepted: 6 November 2021
Published: 15 November 2021

1. Introduction

Pulmonary diseases such as asthma, chronic obstructive pulmonary disease (COPD), pneumonia, bronchitis, pleural effusion, and lung fibrosis affect tens of millions of people all over the world [1]. The monitoring of respiratory function is of great importance in diagnosing these diseases. One of the most widely used methods of diagnosing and assessing the progression of respiratory diseases is spirometry. In conventional spirometry, the patient wears a mouthpiece for breathing and puts on a nose clip. The patient is instructed to breathe in a certain procedure so that several parameters can be measured during the breathing protocol. The patient is instructed to inhale and exhale into the spirometer mouthpiece at a certain breathing rate and force, then the spirometer calculates the breathing rate and the volumes of inhaled and exhaled air during the measurement procedure. As an example of using the spirometer in clinical procedures to diagnose obstructed airways, the ratio of the forced expiratory volume in one second (FEV1) to the forced vital capacity (FVC) (i.e., FEV1/FVC) is measured, where FEV1 represents the maximum amount of air the subject can exhale in 1 s and FVC represents the greatest volume of air the subject can exhale after a deep inhale [2]. A low FEV1/FVC value means that the amount of air that the airways can quickly exhale out of the lungs is reduced, which indicates that the airways are obstructed [3,4], while an increase in the FEV1/FVC value results in a restrictive condition that affects the ability to inhale. According to the American thoracic society, an FEV1/FVC value of 0.7 or above is considered normal for adults, while a value of 0.85 or above is considered normal for children aged 5 to 18 years [5].

The current techniques that are used for spirometry can be classified into two categories: contact spirometry and non-contact spirometry. Contact spirometry is the traditional and the most common method in clinical practice. This conventional way of performing spirometry can be uncomfortable for patients, since it requires them to keep the spirometer in their mouth for up to 30 min. Moreover, after each patient use, the spirometry mouthpiece is subjected to a sterilization procedure to prevent any cross-infection among the patients. There have been several techniques developed for non-contact spirometry. Most of these techniques depend on body movement detection [6,7], photoplethysmography (PPG) [8], and imaging techniques. Droitcour et al. [6] and Mostov et al. [9] used Doppler radar to measure the movement of the body due to heart and respiration signals. For this, they used a high-quality CMOS Doppler radar sensor and verified their results against standard heart and respiration devices. An image-based system was used by Lin et al. [10], where they developed a method based on harmonic analysis of body motion to detect changes in the respiration rate pattern. The second category of non-contact spirometry techniques is based on signal analysis of the PPG signals. In this category, the change in blood volume in the blood vessels is measured by observing changes in light absorption. The measured PPG signal is normally modulated by the respiratory signal (activity) due to movement of the chest cavity during blood flow. These techniques that are based on the analysis of PPG signals are normally based on signal processing techniques and can provide only frequency information about respiration without any information about the changes in the lung volume. Madhav et al. [8] used a modified method of principal component analysis (PCA) to separate the heart activity from the respiration activity. The recorded PPG signal was acquired by a pulse oximeter. Another study depending on ambient light for the recording of the PPG signal was performed by Verkruysse et al. [11]. They used harmonic analysis for extraction of the different components of the PPG signal including the respiration activity. Al-Naji et al. [12] used an ultrasonic PING sensor and PIC18F45 microcontroller to monitor the normal and abnormal breathing activity of the subjects continuously and instantaneously at different distances. The third category of non-contact spirometry techniques is based on thermal imaging, where measurement of the respiration activity is performed through monitoring the changes in the air temperature during inhalation and exhalation [13,14]. Murthy and Pavlidias used a highly sensitive imaging system in their measurements [14]. They used a statistical model of the recorded image to extract respiratory breathing information. Another study by Murphy et al. [15] evaluated the airflow rate using a thermal imaging system.

Most of the non-contact techniques mentioned in the literature do not provide complete respiratory values as the conventional method does, such as the volume of air inhaled and exhaled during the measurement protocols [6,8–10,14,16,17]. Moreover, most times, they require sophisticated techniques, a special setup, and special hardware, while conventional spirometry is considered simple and cheap, with the only disadvantage of requiring direct contact with the patient, which could produce cross-infection and discomfort. Therefore, any non-contact spirometry system should address these issues. This present work provides a feasibility study of using a mobile thermal camera to replace the conventional spirometer for measurements of the respiration rate and the volume of inhaled and exhaled air in and out of the lungs. The purpose of this study was to build a simple non-contact respiratory measurement system using a mobile thermal camera. The targeted measurements included the respiration rate and the volume of inhaled and exhaled air based on artificial intelligence (AI) regressors.

2. Materials and Methods

The complete structure of the proposed study is shown in Figure 1. A mobile phone, with a thermal camera connected to it, was used to acquire thermal images from the face of the subject using a mobile application that was built specifically for this purpose. The mobile application extracts the respiration signal and exports it to a back-end server for further spirometry analysis of the inhaled and exhaled air volumes, which was performed based on the AI regression approach. The spirometry measurements were carried out using a conventional spirometer.

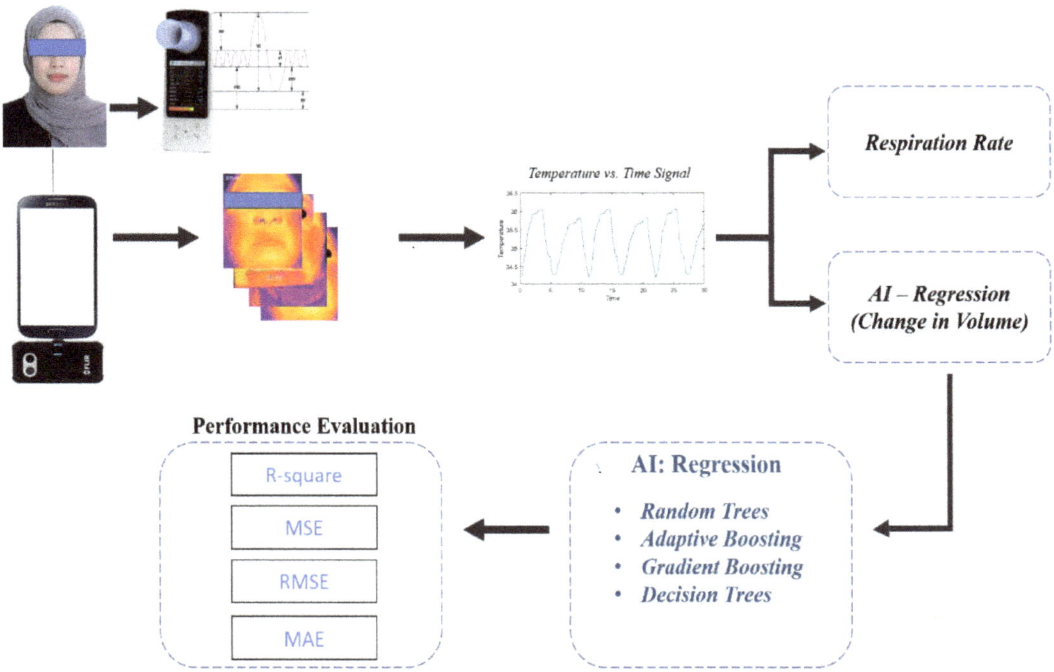

Figure 1. Graphical abstract of the proposed work.

2.1. Thermal Image Acquisition System

The thermal image acquisition system consisted of a mobile phone (Samsung S6) with an Android platform and a FLIR I thermal camera [18]. The camera produced images with thermal resolution of 160 × 120 pixels with a pixel size of 12 microns. Its accuracy was around 3 °C or ±5% of difference between the ambient and the scene temperature. Both still and video thermal images could be recorded, with video images recorded at a rate of 9 frames per second. A special application that used the FLIR I software development kit (SDK) (available at https://developer.ir.com/mobile/ironesdk/, accessed on 10 October 2021) was built for image acquisition. Moreover, the application used the OpenCV android SDK library for image processing. The image acquisition rate was fully controlled by the FLIR I SDK, with a static value of 9 frames per second. The application detected the region of interest (the area under the nose or the mouth) initially using a regular camera image and calculated the average temperature in that region. The application also specified the duration of the recording; a default duration of 20 s was used initially. The recorded signal of temperature versus time was displayed by the application and transmitted to a PC for further spirometry measurements.

2.2. Respiration Rate Measurement

The mobile application that was built for this study was used for two purposes: the first one was to record and transmit the respiration signal vs. time to a PC for further measurements, and the second one is was calculate the respiration rate from the recorded signal by finding the number of peaks (local maxima) in that signal divided by the duration of the recording. The mobile application indicated whether the respiration rate was normal (15–24 breaths/min) or abnormal. The flow chart of the mobile application is shown in Figure 2.

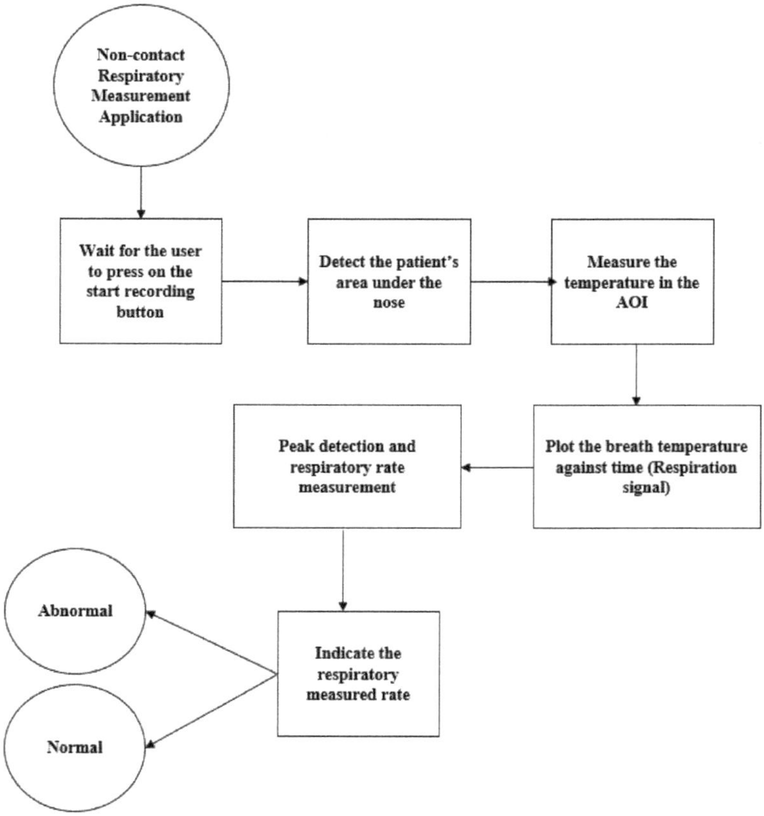

Figure 2. Mobile application workflow diagram.

2.3. Spirometry Measurements

The spirometry measurement approach adopted in this work was an artificial intelligence system based on regression trees. The system's plan of operation is shown in Figure 3. To be able to build such a system, a conventional spirometer was used to provide data about the change in lung volume during measurements. These measurements provided the ground truth for the training and testing of the AI system. The spirometer used in this study was a Contec SP80 healthcare portable medical patient spirometer (shown in Figure 4) [19]. Data were acquired from different subjects, where each time, the change in lung volume during the respiration protocol was recorded.

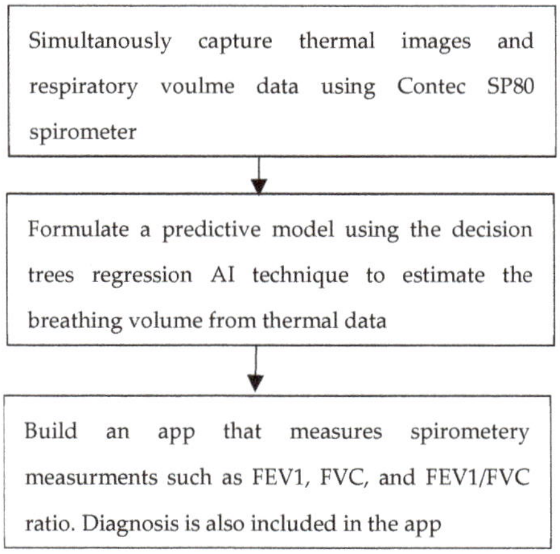

Figure 3. Plan of the spirometry measurement system.

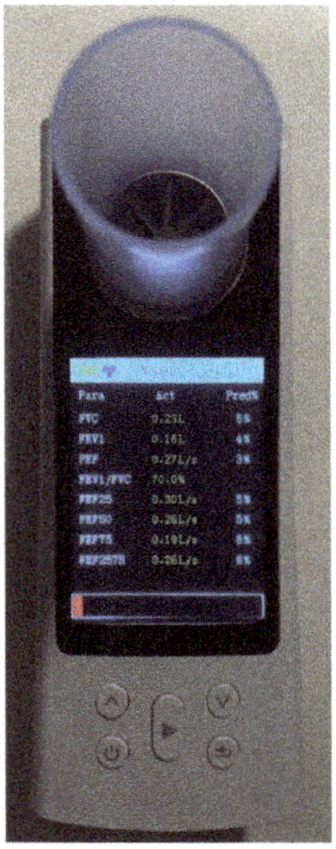

Figure 4. SP80B spirometer, Contec Medical Systems.

2.3.1. Subject

The measurements used in this study were taken from 18 subjects. The age of the subjects ranged from 16 to 28 years, with an average age of 22.5. The subjects' mass was in the range of 54 to 90 kg, with an average value of 67.5 kg, while their height was in the range of 159 to 188 cm, with an average value of 167 cm.

2.3.2. Regression Models

The recorded signals of temperature versus time were used to build a regression model to predict the value of the change in volume during the respiration protocol. Several regression tree models were tested for this work. The workflow of the proposed model is shown in Figure 5.

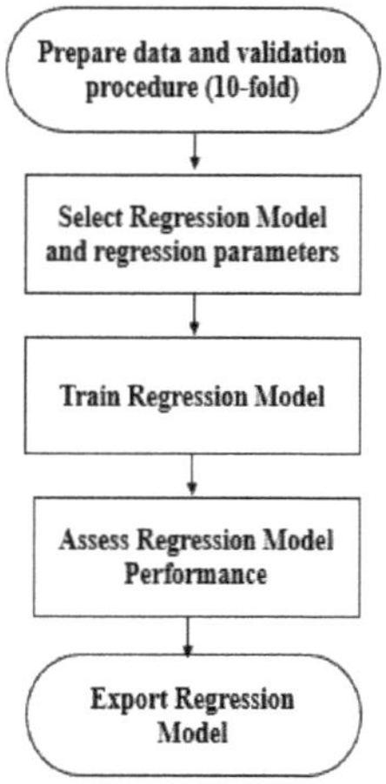

Figure 5. General workflow for the regression procedure.

– Decision Trees Regressor

Decision trees (DT) were first introduced by Breiman et al. in 1984 [20]. This method is widely used due to its simplicity and efficiency. The learner uses a decision tree as a predictive model for the output. The decision tree is constructed based on the recorded signal, which is considered as a feature vector (observation) for training and testing the trees. It basically splits the training dataset into smaller and smaller subsets, while simultaneously developing the corresponding decision tree in an incremental manner. The DT normally works as a top-down scheme, where each observation is used to measure the output based on a certain measure such as Gini impurity, information gain, and variance reduction. To predict a particular data point, the algorithm runs through the complete decision tree by answering "true/false" questions at every node, until arriving at the leaf node which represents the outcome. Most importantly, the same procedure is iterated multiple times to increase the accuracy of prediction. The major advantage of DT is the simplicity and the ability to handle numeric variables (regression), while the major disadvantage is the sensitivity to noise in the observations, which may cause a large variation in the decision trees and hence increase the error in the predictions [21].

– Random Forest Regressor

The random forest classifier and regressor was first introduced by Breiman in 2001 and has been subjected to several improvements since then [20,22]. The random forest is a supervised machine learning technique that deploys multiple trees running in parallel during the training stage with no interaction among the trees. The outputs of all trees are aggregated to calculate the final output of the random forest regressor. If the vector x contains N features such that $x = [x_1, x_2, \ldots, x_N]$, these features are used to predict the output for a given input feature. The vector X in this study represents the thermal respiration signal recorded during the measurement protocol. The signal is used to build a predictive model to predict the value of the respiration volume. If the true measured volume is V, then the predicted volume is $\widetilde{V}$.

This algorithm works in the following steps: firstly, it selects uncorrelated and random sub-samples from the training dataset and builds up a separate decision tree for each sub-sample. Next, to predict a particular data point, it extracts a prediction result from every decision tree. Lastly, it applies a vote procedure to all available prediction results and declares the prediction result with the greatest number of votes as the final predication. In random forests regression, the voting is the average prediction of each tree; $\widetilde{V}_i$ is the output for of an individual tree i. If there are M trees in the random forests regressor, then the final output of the is calculated as:

$$\widetilde{V} = \frac{1}{M}\sum_{i=1}^{M}\widetilde{V}_i$$

Some of the advantages of the random forest regressor include its efficiency in handling large databases, its accuracy in performing classification and regression, and its accuracy in the case of missing data points. The main weakness of the random forest regressor is overfitting in the presence of noisy training data.

– Gradient and Adaptive Boosting Regressors

Boosting classifiers and regressors start the learning process using weak classifiers and regressors such as decision trees. They modify these weak learners to make them strong learners by trying to improve the initial model. In boosting techniques, multiple individual models are trained in a sequential way, while every successive model keeps on learning from mistakes of its predecessor model. There are several techniques for this procedure, with the most common ones being gradient boosting (GB) and adaptive boosting (AdaBoost) [21,23]. In the gradient boosting technique, several models (decision trees) are trained either in an additive or sequential manner. The learner tries to identify the weaknesses of the weak model using the gradients of the loss functions; the performance measure of the regressor used in this work was the mean square error. The different models are updated on the basis of the gradient of the loss function, and weak learners are improved. The gradient boosting regressor works as follows: firstly, it trains a decision tree with an original training dataset and extracts predictions from the trained decision tree. It then computes the residual error of the trained decision tree and stores its value as a variable Y. To keep on learning from previous mistakes, the next stage will utilize the calculated residual error of each stage. It repeats the same procedure for a prespecified number of trees to train the model. To predict a particular data point, it simply adds up the prediction results of all trees. In the adaptive boosting technique, the learner identifies the weak classifier (trees) using the cost function, modifies them to enhance their performance, and builds a second regression model based on these analyses. The process continues until an accurate model is completed or a certain number of models has been reached. Similar to the gradient boosting technique, firstly, it trains a simple decision tree with the original training dataset. It computes the weighted error rate (number of false predictions out of total predictions) for the decision tree. It then calculates the weight of the decision tree in the ensemble and updates the weights of all misclassified data points (wrong predictions). Lastly, it repeats the same procedure for a prespecified number of trees to train the model. To predict a particular data point, the adaptive boosting algorithm multiplies the tree's weight by the tree's prediction and adds up all the trees. Consequently, the tree with the highest weighting will be the most significant influencer of the final prediction.

2.3.3. Performance Measures

The performance of the different regressors was evaluated based on four different measures: the coefficient of determination or R-squared (R^2), the mean square error (MSE), the root means square error (RMSE), and the mean absolute error (MAE). These performance measures were calculated during the regression procedure based on 10-fold cross-validation.

The R-squared value is a statistical measure of how close the predicted data using the regression model are to the true measured value of the spirometer, based on the sum of squared errors [24,25]. It is given by:

$$R^2 = 1 - \frac{SS_{res}}{SS_{total}} \quad (1)$$

where SS_{total} and SS_{res} are given by:

$$SS_{total} = \sum_{i=1}^{n}(y_i - \overline{y}) \tag{2}$$

$$SS_{res} = \sum_{i=1}^{n}(y_i - \hat{y}_i) \tag{3}$$

where y_i is the volume measured using the spirometer (the ground truth), $\overline{y}$ is the average value of the measured values, $\hat{y}_i$ is the predicted regression model volume, and n is the number of signals tested (sample size).

The *MSE* is a measure of the average error between the measured and the predicted values and is given by:

$$MSE = \frac{1}{n}\sum_{i=1}^{n}(y_i - \hat{y}_i) \tag{4}$$

The *RMSE* is the square root of mean square error and is given by:

$$RMSE = \sqrt{\frac{1}{n}\sum_{i=1}^{n}(y_i - \hat{y}_i)} \tag{5}$$

The *MAE* is a measure of the absolute error between the measured and the predicted volumes. It is given by:

$$MAE = \frac{1}{n}\sum_{i=1}^{n}|y_i - \hat{y}_i| \tag{6}$$

3. Results

The complete proposed system was implemented using a mobile application with the functionality illustrated in Figure 6. The system can provide two types of measurements: the first one is the respiration rate and the second one is the respiration volume measurement, which depends on the measurement protocol. Three volume measurements were programmed in the app: the normal respiration volume (tidal volume), the functional reserve capacity (FVC) or deep breathing, and the FEV1/FVC ratio.

3.1. Respiration Signal and Respiration Rate Measurements

This module was implemented as a mobile app with a workflow described in Figure 2. The application was programmed using Java programming language in the environment of the Android studio. Thermal image acquisition was performed using the mobile thermal camera software development kit, and facial recognition and the area of interest were implemented using the OpenCV image processing library. Figure 7 shows the interface of the mobile application with the respiration rate measurement and the respiration signal. The two measurements were recorded at a distance of around 20 cm from the subject's face with a duration of 20 s as a default value. The recording was carried out at room temperature (23 °C).

The recorded respiration signal was exported to a back-end server for further measurements. Figure 8 shows an example of these recordings at three different respiration rates.

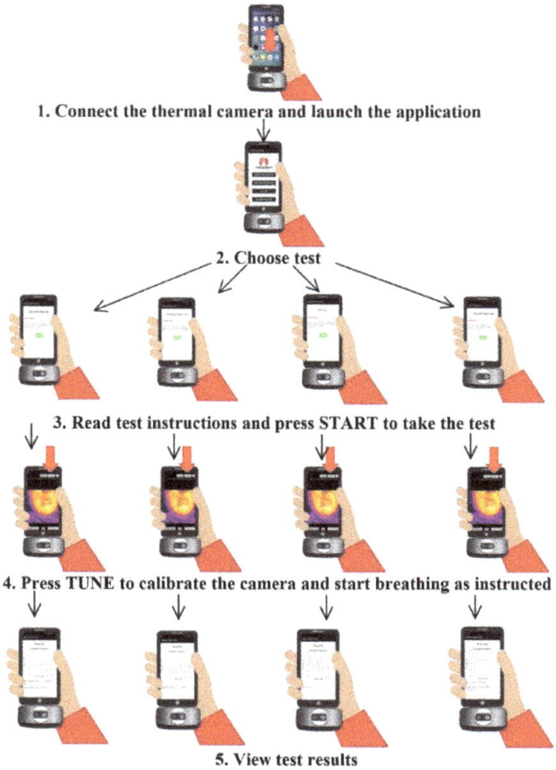

Figure 6. Mobile application functionality of the proposed system.

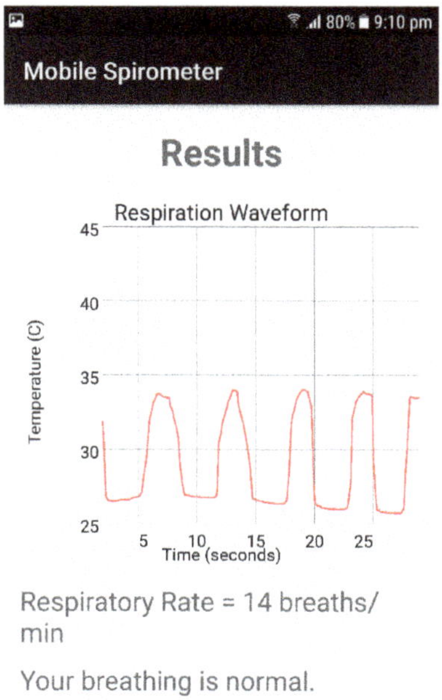

Figure 7. The interface of the mobile application for respiration rate measurements.

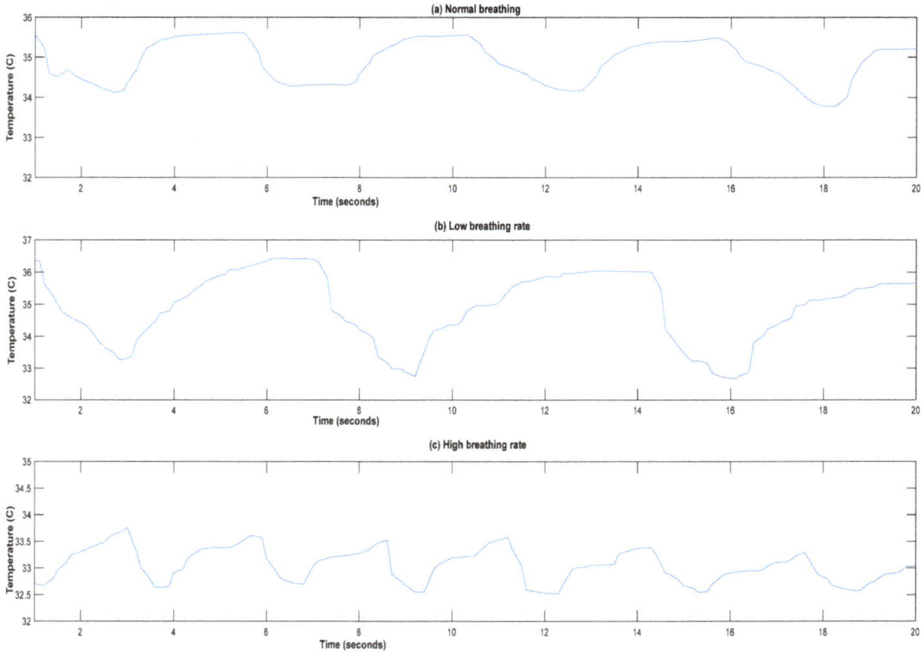

Figure 8. Respiration signal recorded at different rates: (**a**) normal breathing rate, (**b**) low breathing rate, and (**c**) high breathing rate.

To explore the effect of the camera distance from the subject's head, four respiration signals were recorded at 10 cm, 30 cm, 60 cm, and 100 cm, as shown in Figure 9.

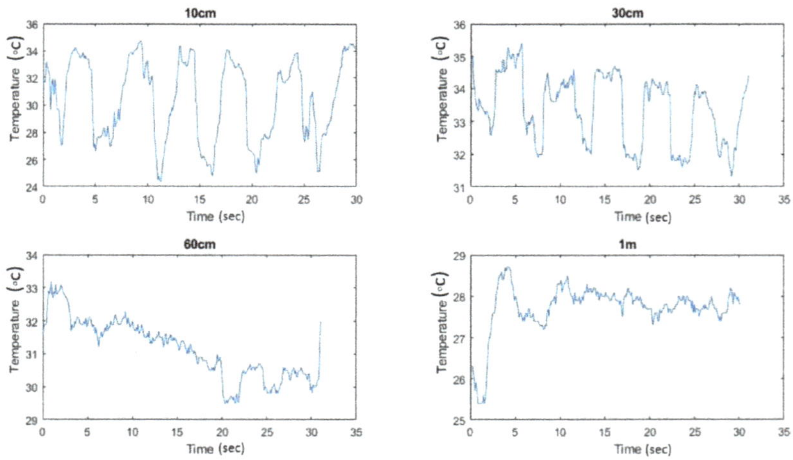

Figure 9. Respiration signals recorded at 10 cm, 30 cm, 60 cm, and 100 cm.

3.2. Spirometry Measurement System

The spirometry measurement system was completely performed in the Python 3.7 programming environment. The package Scikit-learn 0.24.1 was used for this purpose [25]. The four regression models mentioned earlier were considered. The regression testing and training were carried out using a 10-fold cross-validation technique. The performance of the regression of four techniques is listed in Table 1. The performance measures indicated that the decision trees, along with the gradient boosting regression methods, had better performance in comparison with the other two methods, with slightly superior performance for the decision trees.

Table 1. Summary of the regression methods used.

Performance Measure/ Regression Method	Random Forest	Gradient Boosting	Adaptive Boosting	Decision Trees
R-square	0.9409	0.9948	0.9558	0.9998
Mean absolute error	0.1886	0.0532	0.1724	0.0023
Mean squared error	0.0670	0.0049	0.0423	0.0002
Root mean squared error	0.2484	0.0687	0.2054	0.0088

Testing of the proposed methods was carried out using a 10-fold cross-validation procedure. Figure 10 shows the agreement between the predicted change in volume of the method in comparison with the measured spirometer value. A perfect agreement is indicated by a line of a slope of 1. The performance of the decision trees method is evident in Figure 8c and the performance measures in Table 1.

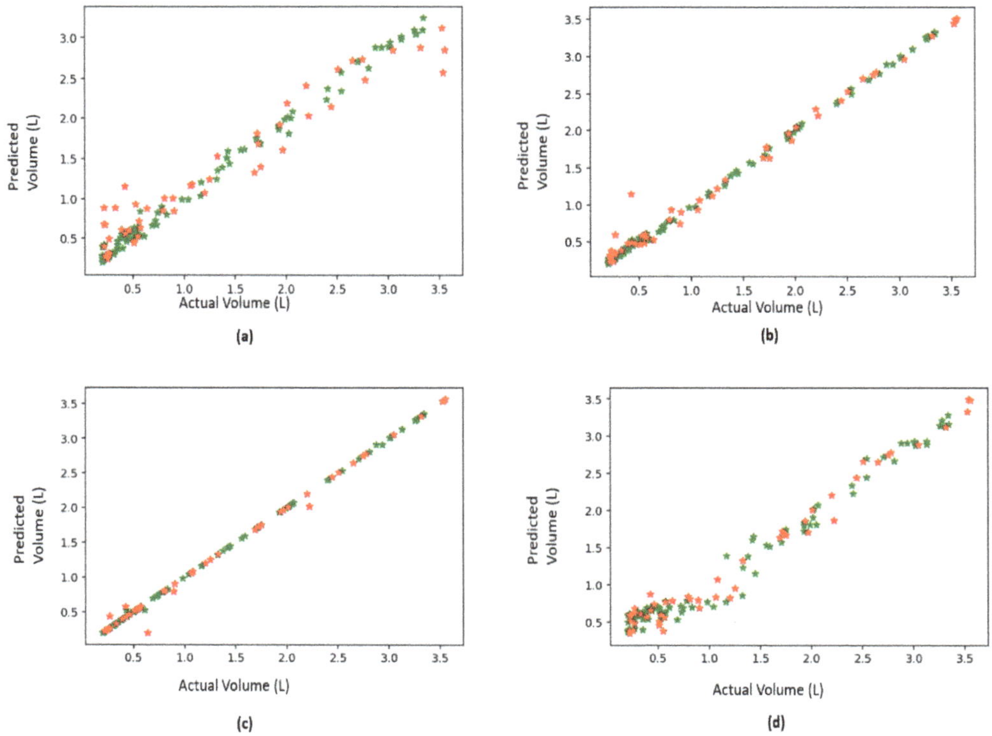

Figure 10. Results of the 10-fold cross-validation testing procedure: (**a**) random forests regressor, (**b**) gradient boost regressor, (**c**) decision trees regressor, and (**d**) adaptive boosting regressor.

3.3. Spirometry System Testing

The complete proposed system was tested for volume measurements with several breathing volumes and compared with the reading provided by the conventional spirometer. The first test was performed on a normal subject with a normal breathing rhythm. As shown in Figure 11, a breathing volume of 0.55 L was recorded using the mobile spirometer application, while the conventional spirometer recorded a breathing volume of 0.59 L. Another breathing test was performed to measure the FVC of a normal subject. The proposed system showed a measured volume of 3.01 L, which was exactly the same volume measured by the conventional spirometer. The measurements are shown in Figure 12.

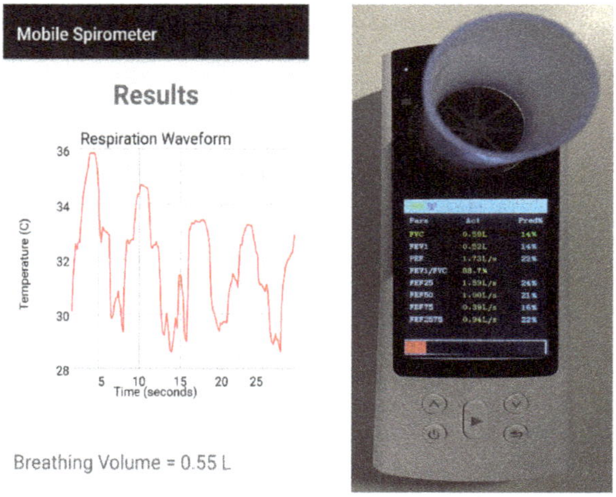

(**a**) (**b**)

Figure 11. Measured normal breathing volume (tidal volume) (**a**) using the mobile application with a thermal camera and (**b**) using the conventional spirometer.

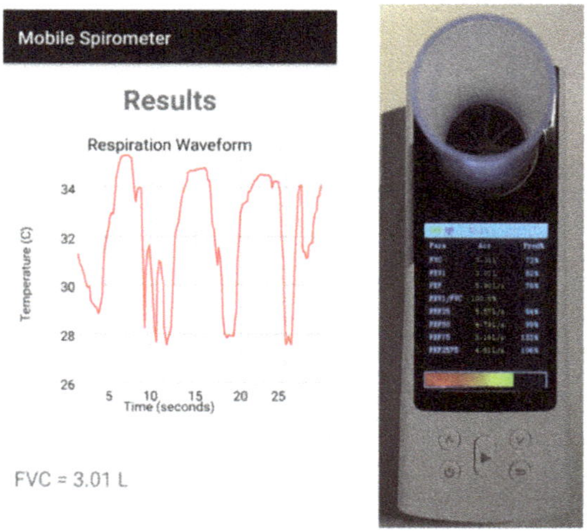

(a) (b)

Figure 12. FVC test measurement: (**a**) mobile app reading; (**b**) conventional spirometer reading.

The last measurement test was the FEV1/FVC ratio. The FVC was measured as mentioned previously, while the FEV1 was measured based on the change in respiration volume with time (1 s). Figure 13 shows the FEV1/FVC measurement using both the mobile app and the Contec spirometer.

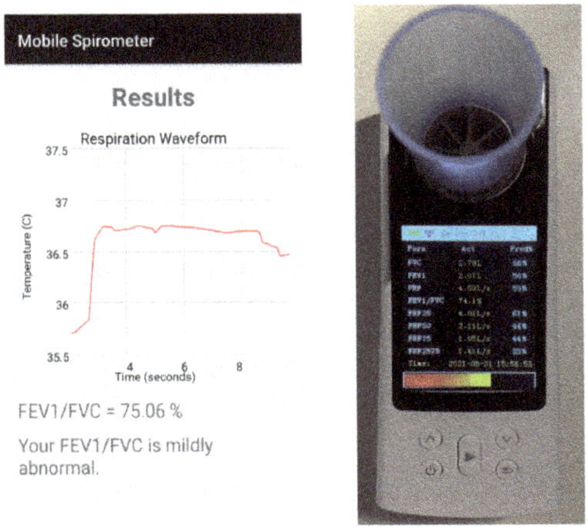

(a) (b)

Figure 13. FEV1/FVC measurement (**a**) using the mobile app and (**b**) using the Contec spirometer.

4. Discussion

This work presents a feasibility study for respiratory measurements using a mobile thermal camera. The measurements were made by a first-generation FLIR I mobile thermal camera. Although there are more advanced thermal cameras now, due to the need for temperature monitoring because of the COVID-19 pandemic, the camera provided good results for respiration rate measurements at a close distance. The FLIR I is a very basic first-generation mobile thermal camera with low resolution compared with other advanced cameras. The camera provides the highest possible accuracy by automatically calibrating itself according to the scene temperature by calculating the emissivity of the objects, the reflected temperature, and the distance; it then returns the actual temperature of the object. The accuracy of the recorded temperature was reported in the literature to be around 3 °C [26]. The effect of the measurement accuracy was minimized in this study for two reasons: first, we measured the average temperature of the area of interest and not pixel by pixel temperature, which resulted in reducing errors in the measured temperature. The second reason is that the measured signal represents the change in temperature and not the actual temperature, which cancels the effect of errors that may appear during the calibration of the camera.

In the current study, the distance was around 20 cm; greater distances resulted in degradation of the signal quality, as shown in Figure 6. Therefore, higher-quality cameras may result in a better respiration signal and thus better measurements at higher distances. One of the most promising applications of respiratory rate measurements is sleep apnea (cessation of breathing). The mobile thermal camera, along with the mobile application, could provide a non-contact and hassle-free system to detect apnea during sleep, as the current clinical apnea monitoring system requires wiring to the patient's body.

The FLIR I thermal camera has an image acquisition rate of nine frames per second; therefore, the average temperature has a sampling rate of 9 Hz. The respiration rate varies with age and the maximum breathing rate can reach up to 55 breaths per minutes in neonates [27]. This means that the maximum breathing frequency is 1.1 Hz and therefore, the current image acquisition rate of the FLIR I is enough to provide a faithful representation of the respiration waveform. At the same time, higher imaging rates would provide a better representation of the respiration signal and hence better performance.

The change in the lung volume (spirometry) measurement was performed using an AI approach based on different regression models. The decision trees regressor showed excellent performance in predicting the change in volume due to respiration, with a mean R-square value of 0.9998 and a mean square error of 0.0023, as listed in Table 1. Moreover, the AI system was built (training and testing) using a range of volumes (0.2 L to 3.5 L), which makes it appropriate for a wide range of subjects and ages. Several studies have adopted a non-contact approach for respiration measurements [8,28,29]. Brieva et al. [30] estimated the respiratory rate using a Hermite magnification technique and a convolutional neural network (CNN). Their contactless system monitored the subjects' chest movements with and without an ROI (region of interest), and they evaluated the performance of their methods using the mean average error. With and without an ROI, the respiratory rate was estimated with a mean average error of 1.83 ± 1.61% and 3.28 ± 3.33%, respectively. Liu et al. [31] proposed an imaging-based approach to determine spirometry parameters such as FEV1, FVC, and PEF. They captured images of the subjects' faces and shoulders during inspiration and expiration using a webcam. Their method showed fair performance, with a root mean square error of 0.27, 0.18, and 0.56 and an average error of 8.5%, 6.9%, and 7.7% for FEV1, FVC, and PEF, respectively. However, using infrared thermography, Pereira et al. [32] estimated the breathing rate with a mean absolute error of 0.33, 0.55, and 0.96 bpm (breaths per minute). One of the most recent studies is the study by Schoun et al. [28]. They used an in-vitro benchtop thermal imaging setup to acquire simulated measurements. They used a recurrent network model (AI) to predict the respiration signal, and from the predicted signal, they made respiration measurements. Using RMSE, their LSTM neural network predicted the expiratory volume from human tests with an average error of 10.61%. However, in this study, the change in volume due to respiration was predicted directly using AI regression models.

5. Conclusions and Future Work

The current study presents a successful approach for respiratory measurements of the respiration rate and volume change. It could provide a means for a non-contact, continuous, and accurate method for the monitoring of chronic and acute pulmonary diseases. However, more steps forward are still needed to improve the quality of the thermal signal measurements by using a more advanced thermal camera and probably more advanced image processing techniques for detection of the area of interest in the face. Advanced thermal cameras can provide better signal quality at longer distances and, at the same time, better image quality. Moreover, an increase in the image acquisition rate should significantly improve the proposed system. This study could also be further developed to be used for simultaneous multiple subject monitoring and measurements, especially with the current COVID-19 pandemic. This study could also be tested in a clinical setup with diseases such as asthma, chronic obstructive pulmonary disease (COPD), and pneumonia. Moreover, this study could be performed against different temperature background temperatures to check the reliability of the measurements in a neutral thermal zone. This will require a special setup that can produce different thermal background temperatures.

Author Contributions: Conceptualization, L.F.; methodology, L.F., K.L. and N.K.; software, N.K., M.E., A.A. and N.A.H.; validation, L.F.; formal analysis, L.F. and N.K.; investigation, L.F., M.E., A.A. and N.A.H.; resources, L.F. and N.K.; writing—original draft preparation, L.F.; writing—review and editing, M.E. and K.L.; visualization, L.F. and N.K.; supervision, L.F.; project administration, L.F.; funding acquisition, L.F. All authors have read and agreed to the published version of the manuscript.

Funding: This research was funded by Abu Dhabi University research office.

Institutional Review Board Statement: The study was conducted according to the guidelines of the Declaration of Helsinki and approved by the Institutional Review Board of Abu Dhabi University (File Number: CoE-21-06-019, 27 June 2021).

Informed Consent Statement: Informed consent was obtained from all subjects involved in the study.

Acknowledgments: The authors would like to thank Eng. Tasnim Basmaji for her help and support during the entire period of the project.

Conflicts of Interest: The authors declare no conflict of interest.

References

1. Athanazio, R. Airway disease: Similarities and differences between asthma, COPD and bronchiectasis. *Clinics* **2012**, *67*, 1335–1343. [CrossRef]
2. Ponce, M.C.; Sharma, S. *Pulmonary Function Tests*; Springer: Berlin/Heidelberg, Germany, 2021; pp. 11–20.
3. Mannino, D.M.; Buist, A.S.; Vollmer, W.M. Chronic obstructive pulmonary disease in the older adult: What defines abnormal lung function? *Thorax* **2007**, *62*, 237–241. [CrossRef] [PubMed]
4. Güder, G.; Brenner, S.; Angermann, C.E.; Ertl, G.; Held, M.; Sachs, A.P.; Lammers, J.W.; Zanen, P.; Hoes, A.W.; Störk, S.; et al. GOLD or lower limit of normal definition? A comparison with expert-based diagnosis of chronic obstructive pulmonary disease in a prospective cohort-study. *Respir. Res.* **2012**, *13*, 13. [CrossRef] [PubMed]
5. Thomas, E.T.; Guppy, M.; Straus, S.E.; Bell, K.J.L.; Glasziou, P. Rate of normal lung function decline in ageing adults: A systematic review of prospective cohort studies. *BMJ Open* **2019**, *9*, e028150. [CrossRef]
6. Droitcour, A.D.; Boric-Lubecke, O.; Kovacs, G.T.A. Signal-to-Noise Ratio in Doppler Radar System for Heart and Respiratory Rate Measurements. *IEEE Trans. Microw. Theory Tech.* **2009**, *57*, 2498–2507. [CrossRef]
7. Shao, D.; Yang, Y.; Liu, C.; Tsow, F.; Yu, H.; Tao, N. Noncontact Monitoring Breathing Pattern, Exhalation Flow Rate and Pulse Transit Time. *IEEE Trans. Biomed. Eng.* **2014**, *61*, 2760–2767. [CrossRef]
8. Madhav, K.V.; Ram, M.R.; Krishna, E.H.; Komalla, N.R.; Reddy, K.A. Robust Extraction of Respiratory Activity from PPG Signals Using Modified MSPCA. *IEEE Trans. Instrum. Meas.* **2013**, *62*, 1094–1106. [CrossRef]
9. Mostov, K.; Liptsen, E.; Boutchko, R. Medical applications of shortwave FM radar: Remote monitoring of cardiac and respiratory motion. *Med. Phys.* **2010**, *37*, 1332–1338. [CrossRef] [PubMed]
10. Lin, K.; Chen, D.; Tsai, W. Image-Based Motion-Tolerant Remote Respiratory Rate Evaluation. *IEEE Sens. J.* **2016**, *16*, 3263–3271. [CrossRef]
11. Verkruysse, W.; Svaasand, L.O.; Nelson, J.S. Remote plethysmographic imaging using ambient light. *Opt. Express* **2008**, *16*, 21434–21445. [CrossRef]
12. Al-Naji, A.; Al-Askery, A.J.; Gharghan, S.K.; Chahl, J. A system for monitoring breathing activity using an ultrasonic radar detection with low power consumption. *J. Sens. Actuator Netw.* **2019**, *8*, 32. [CrossRef]
13. Huang, Y.P.; Young, M.S.; Tai, C.C. Noninvasive respiratory monitoring system based on the piezoceramic transducer's pyroelectric effect. *Rev. Sci. Instrum.* **2008**, *79*, 35103. [CrossRef]
14. Murthy, R.; Pavlidis, I. Noncontact measurement of breathing function. *IEEE Eng. Med. Biol. Mag.* **2006**, *25*, 57–67. [CrossRef] [PubMed]
15. Murthy, J.N.; Van Jaarsveld, J.; Fei, J.; Pavlidis, I.; Harrykissoon, R.I.; Lucke, J.F.; Faiz, S.; Castriotta, R.J. Thermal Infrared Imaging: A Novel Method to Monitor Airflow During Polysomnography. *Sleep* **2009**, *32*, 1521–1527. [CrossRef] [PubMed]
16. Drummond, G.B.; Duffy, N.D. A video-based optical system for rapid measurements of chest wall movement. *Physiol. Meas.* **2001**, *22*, 489–503. [CrossRef]
17. Chon, K.H.; Dash, S.; Ju, K. Estimation of Respiratory Rate From Photoplethysmogram Data Using Time–Frequency Spectral Estimation. *IEEE Trans. Biomed. Eng.* **2009**, *56*, 2054–2063. [CrossRef]
18. Teledyne FLIR. Available online: https://www.flir.com/products/flir-one-pro/ (accessed on 25 October 2021).
19. Contec Medical. Available online: https://contecmed.eu/products/sp80b-bluetooth-digital-spirometer-lung-function-breathing-pulmonary-diagnostic?_pos=1&_sid=28dfd9d6c&_ss=r (accessed on 24 October 2021).
20. Breiman, L.; Friedman, J.; Stone, C.J.; Olshen, R.A. *Classification and Regression Trees*; CRC Press: Boca Raton, FL, USA, 1984.
21. Hastie, J.F.T. Robert Tibshirani. In *The Elements of Statistical Learning*; CRC Press: Boca Raton, FL, USA, 2009.
22. Geurts, P.; Ernst, D.; Wehenkel, L. Extremely randomized trees. *Mach. Learn.* **2006**, *63*, 3–42. [CrossRef]
23. Friedman, J.H. Greedy Function Approximation: A Gradient Boosting Machine. *Ann. Stat.* **2001**, *29*, 1189–1232. [CrossRef]
24. Devore, J.L. *Probability and Statistics for Engineering and the Sciences*, 8th ed.; Cengage Learning: Boston, MA, USA, 2011.
25. Scikit-Learn, Machine learning in Python. Available online: https://scikit-learn.org/stable/ (accessed on 25 October 2021).
26. Fraiwan, L.; AlKhodari, M.; Ninan, J.; Mustafa, B.; Saleh, A.; Ghazal, M. Diabetic foot ulcer mobile detection system using smart phone thermal camera: A feasibility study. *Biomed. Eng. Online* **2017**, *16*, 117. [CrossRef] [PubMed]
27. Al-Naji, A.A.; Chahl, J. Detection of Cardiopulmonary Activity and Related Abnormal Events Using Microsoft Kinect Sensor. *Sensors* **2018**, *18*, 920. [CrossRef]
28. Schoun, B.; Transue, S.; Halbower, A.C.; Choi, M.-H. Non-contact tidal volume measurement through thin medium thermal imaging. *Smart Health* **2018**, *9–10*, 37–49. [CrossRef]
29. L-Khalidi, F.Q.A.; Saatchi, R.; Burke, D.; Elphick, H. Facial tracking method for noncontact respiration rate monitoring. In Proceedings of the 2010 7th International Symposium on Communication Systems, Networks Digital Signal Processing (CSNDSP 2010), Newcastle Upon Tyne, UK, 21–23 July 2010; pp. 751–754. [CrossRef]
30. Brieva, J.; Ponce, H. A Contactless Respiratory Rate Estimation Method Using a Hermite Magnification Technique and Convolutional Neural Networks. *Appl. Sci.* **2020**, *10*, 607. [CrossRef]
31. Liu, C.; Liu, C.; Yang, Y.; Tsow, F.; Shao, D.; Tao, N. Noncontact spirometry with a webcam. *J. Biomed. Opt.* **2021**, *22*, 57002. [CrossRef] [PubMed]
32. Pereira, C.B.; Yu, X.; Czaplik, M.; Blazek, V.; Leonhardt, S. Remote monitoring of breathing dynamics using infrared thermography. *Biomed. Opt. Express* **2015**, *6*, 1373–1384. [CrossRef] [PubMed]

sensors

Article

Brain Strategy Algorithm for Multiple Object Tracking Based on Merging Semantic Attributes and Appearance Features

Mai S. Diab [1,2,*], Mostafa A. Elhosseini [3,4], Mohamed S. El-Sayed [1] and Hesham A. Ali [3,5]

1 Faculty of Computer & Artificial Intelligence, Benha University, Benha 13511, Egypt; ms4elsayed@fci.bu.edu.eg
2 Intoolab Ltd., London WC2H 9JQ, UK
3 Computers Engineering and Control System, Faculty of Engineering, Mansoura University, Mansoura 35516, Egypt; melhosseini@mans.edu.eg (M.A.E.); h_arafat_ali@mans.edu.eg (H.A.A.)
4 College of Computer Science and Engineering in Yanbu, Taibah University, Madinah 46421, Saudi Arabia
5 Faculty of Artificial Intelligence, Delta University for Science and Technology, Mansoura 35511, Egypt
* Correspondence: may.mossoua@fci.bu.edu.eg

Abstract: The human brain can effortlessly perform vision processes using the visual system, which helps solve multi-object tracking (MOT) problems. However, few algorithms simulate human strategies for solving MOT. Therefore, devising a method that simulates human activity in vision has become a good choice for improving MOT results, especially occlusion. Eight brain strategies have been studied from a cognitive perspective and imitated to build a novel algorithm. Two of these strategies gave our algorithm novel and outstanding results, rescuing saccades and stimulus attributes. First, rescue saccades were imitated by detecting the occlusion state in each frame, representing the critical situation that the human brain saccades toward. Then, stimulus attributes were mimicked by using semantic attributes to reidentify the person in these occlusion states. Our algorithm favourably performs on the MOT17 dataset compared to state-of-the-art trackers. In addition, we created a new dataset of 40,000 images, 190,000 annotations and 4 classes to train the detection model to detect occlusion and semantic attributes. The experimental results demonstrate that our new dataset achieves an outstanding performance on the scaled YOLOv4 detection model by achieving a 0.89 mAP 0.5.

Keywords: multiple object tracking; data association; dataset; deep learning; semantic attribute

Citation: Diab, M.S.; Elhosseini, M.A.; El-Sayed, M.S.; Ali, H.A. Brain Strategy Algorithm for Multiple Object Tracking Based on Merging Semantic Attributes and Appearance Features. *Sensors* **2021**, *21*, 7604. https://doi.org/10.3390/s21227604

Academic Editors: Ayman El-baz, Guruprasad A. Giridharan, Ahmed Shalaby, Ali H. Mahmoud and Mohammed Ghazal

Received: 8 October 2021
Accepted: 11 November 2021
Published: 16 November 2021

1. Introduction

Object tracking is of great interest to researchers because of its numerous computer vision applications such as robot navigation, self-driving, and smart surveillance. It attempts to give a unique ID for every object throughout all frames. However, many fundamental challenges abound regarding the development of a robust object tracking model. These include unpredictable changes in the background and the appearance of objects, full or partial occlusion, and data association. Over the years, researchers have developed robust algorithms to address these challenges. Their methods, however, have not solved one of the main problems in MOT, which is occlusion. Moreover, their algorithms have not reached human brain performance because not many have studied how the human brain deals with such challenges.

The human brain can identify both stationary and dynamic objects. Moreover, it can effortlessly perform vision processes, including activity recognition, image compression, and motion analysis. Therefore, we believe that the uncertainty in the tracking problem could be solved by developing an object tracking algorithm that can mimic the human brain. Merging researchers' efforts in the neuroscientific community who have studied the approaches used by the human brain to track objects in real-time and researchers' attempts in the computer vision community are needed to improve MOT models. This is what we have achieved in this paper.

In neuropsychology, the cognitive function of recognising people includes simultaneous routes of information and multiple processing stages. Models of these multiple processing stages have been provided from neuropsychological data obtained from case reports. According to research on young adults [1], humans can simultaneously recognise objects and extract meaning from what they see in the first half-second—but what part of the brain is responsible for this? Researchers in neuroscience have used advanced techniques to identify the brain areas that are involved in object tracking, for instance, magnetoencephalography (MEG), whole-brain functional magnetic resonance imaging (fMRI), and electrocorticography (ECoG) [2,3]. It has been found that this ability involves continuous activity within the anteromedial temporal cortex through the ventral temporal cortex [3]. While visual input is processed through this pathway, it has been found that it is transformed into an initial semantic representation (plants, animals) [4]. This happens in the inferior temporal cortex, before specific semantic representation emerges (rose, cat) in the anteromedial temporal cortex. Another conclusion drawn by [4] is that people recognition includes many attributes, such as the perception of faces, whole bodies, emotional expressions, clothes, gait, and individual marks. In other words, with these biological processors, humans can transform object representations or visual inputs into a format that is easily understood and extractable, regardless of the viewing conditions; this is the semantic attribute. In our algorithm, we aimed to design a tracker that mimics the working principle of the brain to enhance the performance of computer vision state-of-the-art algorithms. Our tracker is motivated by contemporary cognitive psychology. It combines an appearance feature vector (inspired from computer vision algorithms) and a semantic attribute (inspired by cognitive psychology) to represent the object. The appearance feature vector is used to track targets with no occlusion, while the semantic attributes are used to prevent incorrect tracking of an occluded object.

This research proposes novel brain-based MOT algorithms based on eight human brain concepts. Our approach, which resolves the frame-by-frame association problem, is novel; it combines appearance feature vectors and several semantic attributes (trousers, shirts, men, and women) to recognise objects. The main contributions are three-fold:

- We introduced a new dataset, PGC (Pedestrians' Gender and Clothes Attributes), including a total of 40,000 images with more than 190,000 annotations for four classes (trousers, shirts, men, and women). We intend to ensure that the datasets are available and accessible to the public so that other researchers can benefit from our dataset and continue from where we ended. The reasons behind introducing our dataset as a main contribution are explained in Section 3.
- After evaluating our dataset by comparing it with an open dataset with the same classes using the same detection model, the results show that our PGC dataset facilitates the learning of robust class detectors with much a better generalisation performance.
- We introduced and evaluated a novel MOT algorithm that mimics the human brain, addresses occlusion problems, and improves the state-of-the-art performance on standard benchmark datasets.

The remainder of this paper is organised as follows: the next section explores various previous brain-inspired MOT algorithms. Section 3 presents the proposed method in detail. A quantitative evaluation for our algorithm (Merging Semantic Attributes and Appearance Feature MSA-AF), compared to five state-of-the-art algorithms, has been introduced in Section 4. Section 5 shows our algorithm's limitations, while Section 6 presents what went wrong in our dataset. Section 7 concludes.

2. Related Work

Multiple object tracking has long been a widespread topic in computer vision, with a large number of publications. Over the last few years, researchers have put forward several brain-inspired tracking algorithms. However, these algorithms can only adopt one of the key cognitive effects used by the human brain, such as memory and attention, instead of imitating the entire process [5,6]. Other algorithms have integrated powerful tools that mimic the human nervous system to tackle the occlusion problem, such as deep neural networks (DNNs) [7], artificial neural networks (ANNs) [8], recurrent neural networks (RNNs) [9], and convolutional neural networks (CNNs) [10]. These networks can simulate the processes used by the human brain to identify, store, or process information. However, according to the research findings of [11], ANNs are fundamentally different from biological neural networks (BNNs) in many ways. For instance, cortical neurons in BNN and artificial neurons in ANN communicate to each other differently. BNN's neurons are organised in a goal-driven manner, unlike ANN's neurons. Additionally, training is not needed in BNNs, unlike ANNs, in which the weight of the neural connections needs to be trained to obtain better results.

The question that emerges here is how can we judge the degree to which a model agrees with biological outcomes? Despite no definite answer to this question in the literature, we will try to find answers using findings from the cognitive neuroscience of MOT and what these computer vision trackers have introduced in their models.

Researchers in cognitive science and neuroscience have executed many studies to examine the cognitive mechanism behind MOT. According to their outcomes, MOT tasks focus on visual attention in early cognitive processing, while in later cognitive processing, visual short-term and working memory have been used [12]. Thus, we categorised the computer vision algorithms that imitate brain functions in their designs into two categories: memory-based algorithms and attention-based algorithms. We will cite a few MOT algorithms based on visual attention and short and long memory without being exhaustive.

Visual attention helps humans analyse complex scenes promptly and dedicate their limited cognitive and perceptual resources to the most relevant subsets of sensory data. Some human brain-inspired algorithms that achieved high accuracy predicted what part humans will attend to in an unobserved image. One of the best models for predicting fixation over images and videos is the decision theoretical model [13], which has shown promising results on the PASCAL 2006 dataset using the discriminant saliency model for visual recognition. This model has explained basic behavioural data that other models have explored less. In computer vision, attention is a convenient method for recognising targets by discriminating them from each other and the background. In [14], dual matching attention networks (DMAN) with a temporal and spatial attention mechanism strategy is proposed to allow the model to focus on matching similarity between each part of a pair of images.

The temporal attention network aims to investigate different observations in the trajectory by allocating different degrees of attention to them. The spatial attention module allows the network to focus on the matching patterns. Unlike [14], in which their attention model relies on only two aspects, [15] the temporal attention network focuses on four attention aspects to track the target. Two of these attention aspects are common with [14], which are temporal and spatial attention. The other two are layer-wise and channel-wise attention. However, the limitation of [15] is that their algorithm needs offline training to support feature selection in online tracking. Even though attention helps to tackle challenges such as background variability and variable target appearance, it suffers from occlusion due to its adaptability to variation. When a target is gradually occluded by an occluder, the algorithm misses the target because it tends to acknowledge it as a change in target appearance. Memory could be used to handle the occlusion by retaining the appearance information from the targets. [16] implement their network with long short-term memory (LSTM) units that improve their algorithm's performance.

Visual memory is an essential cognitive mechanism that the human brain uses to deal with partial and full occlusion and to overcome variable target appearances. Makovski and Jiang [17] proved in their studies that the reason behind the observer's recovery from any errors during tracking was the storing of surface properties inside the visual working memory. In [12], they propose a general theoretical framework for viewing human memory. They divide the memory model into three stages: the sensory register, the short-term store, and the long-term store. Many researchers in computer vision have used this theory to introduce brain-memory-inspired MOT [18,19]. In [18], they established a memory model to handle the main challenges in MOT by using the human brain three-stage memory theory [12]. Using this model, they proposed a template updating modelling algorithm that can remember and forget the target's appearance. Their experimental results are promising for tackling sudden changes in appearance and occlusion. In [19], they are inspired by the same three-stage memory model. However, the three-stage memory model in this work aimed to find the right match between the appearance and the object by integrating the model into a multiagent coevolutionary process. Each agent can forget and remember the object's appearance via its own experience through its memory system. Other researchers have used different strategies employing long short-term memory (LSTM) instead, such as [20–22]. Ref [20], introduced an algorithm based on deep reinforcement learning followed by the LSTM unit. Their track-by-detection algorithm detects the object and then applies an association model to solve the tracking problem. LSTM is used in the data association stage to address changes in appearance and occlusion. The experimental results of [20] show that their tracker is successful in handling scale changes, occlusion, and appearance similarity most of the time. However, their tracker faced some failures in some cases. For example, when the brightness of the environment changes, the detector fails to detect the object, leading to the tracker's failure.

All algorithms introduced in this section are based only on attention or memory modules, added to their algorithm to imitate the human visual role. Although attention is undoubtedly involved in feature extraction and memory is involved in retaining extracted information, they are rarely used together in the same algorithm. In MSA-AF, we used not only both modules, but also six other strategies inspired by the human brain. We introduced the advantages and limitations of both models, memory and attention, in Table 1.

Table 1. Human brain-inspired algorithms.

Type of Brain Inspiration	Contributions	Advantages and Limitations
Visual attention	Gao et al. [13] Zhu et al. [14] Chen et al. [15]	Most attention-based algorithms can handle variability in background and object appearance. However, this adaptation makes these algorithms suffer from occlusion.
Visual memory	Qi et al. [18] Wang et al. [19] Jiang et al. [20] Kim et al. [21] Wang et al. [22]	Memory-based algorithms can successfully handle occlusion and data association, but they need to formulate vital parameters to decide what to remember and what to forget.

3. Proposed Algorithm

In this section, our tracking algorithm has been presented, which uses the outcomes from the neuroscience researchers' community to imitate the human brain. What is critical in our work is to translate these biological findings into a computer vision algorithm. Both the neuroscience and computer vision communities share a general framework that focuses on the importance of memory, attention, and motion prediction to handle the MOT problem. To the best of our knowledge, no algorithms use all eight of the human brain strategies introduced in Table 2 as their building blocks. In contrast, our work was inspired by eight main findings from neuroscience research as building blocks to build MSA-AF. Table 2 shows these modules and how they inspired our algorithm. Integrating the eight modules together is undoubtedly ambitious, leading to improvements in the state-of-the-art MOT algorithms. However, strategies 4 and 8 from Table 2 played the most critical role in the final association stage, as discussed in more detail later on in this section.

Table 2. Eight human brain strategies behind our algorithm.

	Eight Human Brain Strategies to Handle Object Tracking	How MSA-AF Simulated These Strategies
1	Tracking in the human brain is a two-stage process; the first stage is for location processing, while the second stage is for identity processing [2].	MSA-AF is a tracking-by-detection algorithm. The first stage is detection (location process), then association (identifying process).
2	Experimental results by [23] suggest that the human brain uses motion prediction to handle the tracking problem.	MSA-AF used Kalman to predict the next position of the object.
3	Neural representation is needed to achieve particular goals in scenes, e.g., recognition [1].	MSA-AF used pre-trained CNN to compute the Bbox appearance descriptor in [24].
4	Neural representations reflect stimulus attributes in low-level visual areas and perceptual outcomes in high-level visual areas [4].	MSA-AF used semantic attributes (man, woman, shirt, trouser).
5	Experimental results by [17] conclude that the observer's recovery from any errors during tracking was by storing surface properties in the visual working memory.	MSA-AF used the long-memory theory to save all information about each target and retrieve it when it is more needed, usually when the object is in an occlusion state.
6	The brain provides more attentional resources when objects are in a crowded scene, with a higher chance of being lost when target switching conditions happen [25].	Using (4), MSA-AF can decide if any object is in an occlusion situation or not. If yes, MSA-AF gives more attention to this object by using semantic information.
7	The human brain uses optimised features to discriminate targets better and retrieve them faster and more efficiently [2].	MSA-AF uses appearance information to discriminate the object.
8	When the possibility of confusing targets increases, it is suggested that human subjects benefit from rescue saccades (saccades toward targets that are in a critical situation) to avoid incorrect associations [26,27].	Final association decision at MSA-AF, Section 3 imitates this concept.

The basic flow chart of the tracking algorithm we implemented in this work is illustrated in Figure 1. Our focus was on handling the existing challenges facing state-of-the-art algorithms, the most important of which was occlusion. The first building block in our algorithm is detection, which takes a frame and gives us the bounding boxes (Bbox) of the four classes (man, woman, shirt, trouser) inside the image. Then, the second block will take the Bbox from the previous frame, apply the Kalman filter [26] to predict their new position in the current frame, and then apply the cosine metric learning method for learning a feature space to associate the detection with the objects. The last three building blocks distinguish MSA-AF from any other MOT in the field of computer vision, which is similar to how human logic works to solve a tracking problem. This occurred by transferring the information in the image into semantic information that is saved in the memory for retrieval when it is needed. This brings us to the last building block, which uses the saved semantic information to decide whether occlusion is happening or not and how to deal with it. The rest of this section will introduce the logic behind each building block and how all are connected to imitate the human brain and improve the performance of recent MOT algorithms.

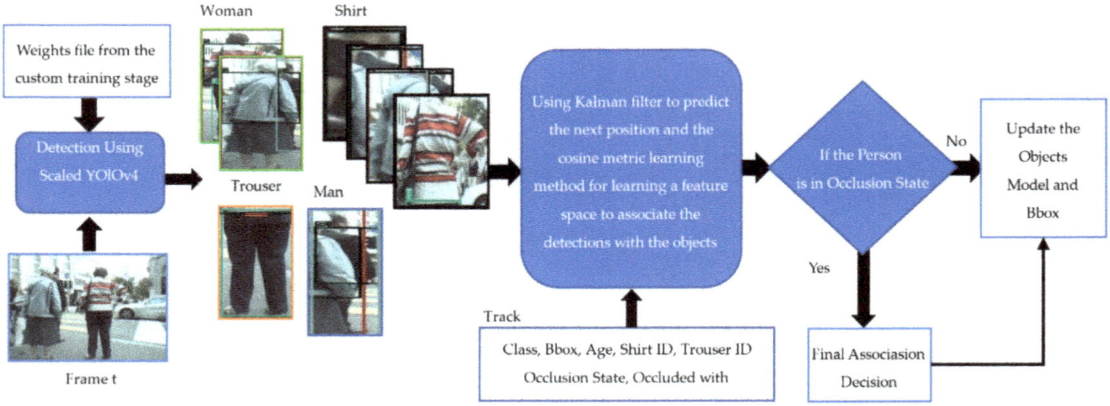

Figure 1. Overview of MSA-AF starting from the detection step, which feeds into the first association step. The final association step will be used in cases of occlusion. Track 1 to Track n represents the model of the object that has been tracked in the previous frames. A class could be 0, 1, 2, or 3, representing man, woman, shirt, and trousers. Bbox has x,y,h,w of the object's bounding box, in which (x,y) represents the centre point, h is the height, and w is the width. The occlusion state is a binary number: '1' if the object is in an occlusion state and '0' if not. Occluded with has the ID of the object that was occluded. Age is the number of frames in which the object is successfully tracked. Finally, Semantic information includes much information that will be described in detail in Section 3. The original image is taken from the MOTChalleng dataset [28].

3.1. Detection

Without exaggerating, we can say that the detection step is essential for any tracking-by-detection algorithm such as ours. Missing, false, or non-accurate detection will lead to poor MOT performance; consequently, more time is spent on this stage to secure a good foundation for our algorithm. Some algorithms assume that they have the detections needed to focus on the tracking step, such as in [24]. Three crucial questions need to be answered to deal with the detection step successfully: What classes do we need to detect? What is the detection model that will be used? Do we have a good dataset for the training? All these questions will be answered in this section. Figure 2 depicts the different phases used to ensure a reliable output from the detection stage.

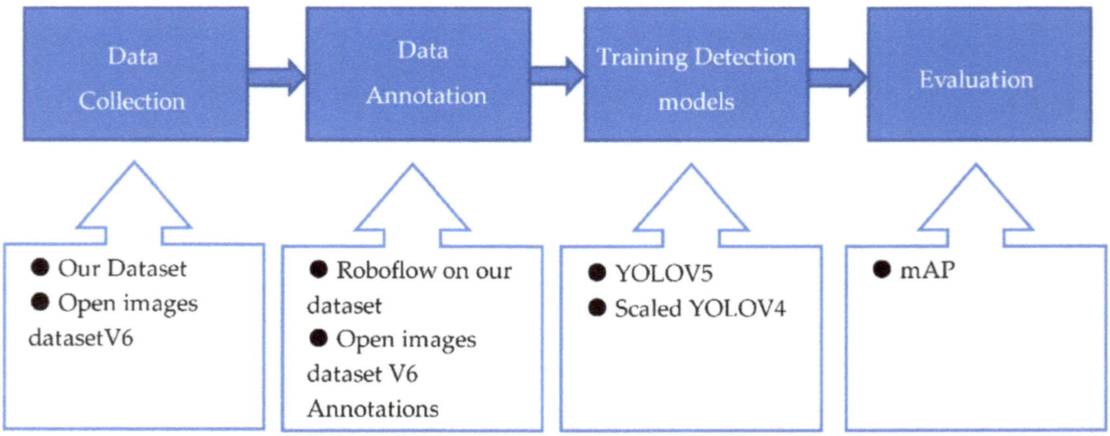

Figure 2. Steps that have been used to assert a high-performance detection model. Each phase included all options that we used for the comparison in order to get the best detection results.

3.1.1. Classes

In any MOT algorithm that deals with people, the person is the class that needs to be detected. In MSA-AF, as we imitate the human brain, we use a different approach. Biological evidence shows that the human brain transforms the visual input into an initial and then a specific semantic attribute [4]. We employ the person reidentification approach used in multi-camera networks to find a semantic attribute representing a person. This approach identifies the best attributes for recognising a person and helps an operator to track, search, and locate the target object. For example, in the Van Koppen and Lochun [29] survey, over 1313 human descriptions were collected from individuals who witnessed a robbery incident. They found that of the 43 categories identified, only 30% of the eyewitnesses accurately described all nine categories. The categories included skin colour, hair type, height, gender, appearance (which includes race), accent, hair colour, build, and age.

Similarly, Sporer [30] examined 139 descriptions provided by 100 witnesses. He discovered that of all the descriptions, 31% mentioned clothing information, 29.6% detailed facial features, 22% contained information on movement features and physical attributes (height, race, and age), and 5% included personality information. After considering the findings of these two studies, we selected clothes (trousers and shirt) and gender (man and women) as our semantic attributes. We will reserve the term semantic information units to refer to the trouser, shirt, man, woman semantic attributes.

3.1.2. Dataset

The training dataset can be defined as the initial data used to develop the machine learning model. A high-quality training dataset, without a doubt, is the critical item for any machine learning system. Most performance detection models can be rendered useless without high-quality and quantity training datasets.

After deciding what classes we needed to detect, we searched for a dataset to train the detection model with the same classes. However, we could not find any dataset with shirt, trouser, man, and woman classes that could benefit our algorithm. Thus, we built the PGC dataset not only to serve our algorithm, but also to benefit other researchers.

Uniqueness: We argue that there is no existing state of the art dataset like the PGC dataset. Existing datasets either have the person as a single class, such as MSCOCO [31], or recognise pedestrian attributes, such as PETA [32]. MSCOCO, like most detection datasets, has many different classes (81)—one of them representing a person, without any classes representing any details about the person. In contrast, like all pedestrian attribute datasets, the PETA dataset works on a set of images that show only one person and annotate a set of binary attributes to this person. Lable (upperBodyBlack, lowerBodyGrey, hairBlack, footwearWhite, lowerBodyCasual, lowerBodyJeans, personalLess30, personalMale) is one example of annotation in the PETA dataset. As we can see, this gives information about the person rather than where these attributes are in the image. On the other hand, PGC has four classes that represent attributes used by the human brain to identify a person, with the location of each attribute inside the image. Add to that the uniqueness of the PGC in the process of acquiring, annotating, and testing that will be discussed later in this section.

Usage: The PGC dataset can serve many fields in computer vision. For instance, pedestrian reidentification, detection and tracking research. Moreover, PGC can be integrated with different types of clothes instead of only shirts and trousers to serve fashion research. High-quality training data is a daunting task, so the quality and quantity could be compromised to speed up the procedure. In contrast, we prioritise quality over speed throughout the collection the annotation stages of this study.

At the data collection level, diversity is the main factor that leads to high-quality data. Representation bias is one of 23 types of bias introduced by [33] that could lead to unfairness in machine learning. For instance, [34] remark that some datasets such as IJB-A [35], which compiled 79.6% lighter-skinned faces with just 4.4% of images from dark-skinned female faces, show bias. Algorithms that rely on these datasets suffer from bad performance, due to the representation bias in the training data. Therefore, we considered diversity and quantity when collecting 30,000 images from the web and 10,000 from the PETA [32] dataset. To ensure that the PGC dataset includes all scenarios in the real world, we searched for specific events and a specific group of people; dark-skinned, light-skinned, man, woman, Asian, man or woman with headcover, Arab, old, and young people are examples of a diverse group of people we searched to include in our dataset. Another critical factor in our search is the scene's background, such as indoor, outdoor, night, or morning. The position of the person is a consistently underestimated factor in any pedestrian dataset. Therefore, it is essential for the training dataset to have all possible body positions such as standing, sitting, walking, running, side-view, back-view, front-view, high camera angle, entire body, and upper body part. Additionally, a wide range of image resolutions in any dataset makes the model robust to any movement in the camera or even to poor resolution images. Finally, we were eager to include images with occlusion as much as possible, which helped us handle the occlusion in the tracking step. Although applying a diversity search in the PGC dataset did slow the collection process, its outcome is outstanding, as shown in Section 4. The image collection in Figure 3 has been taken from the output of the scaled YOLOv4 detection model on our dataset. It is a random selection taken by the detection model for testing. As we can see, it shows the diversity of our dataset.

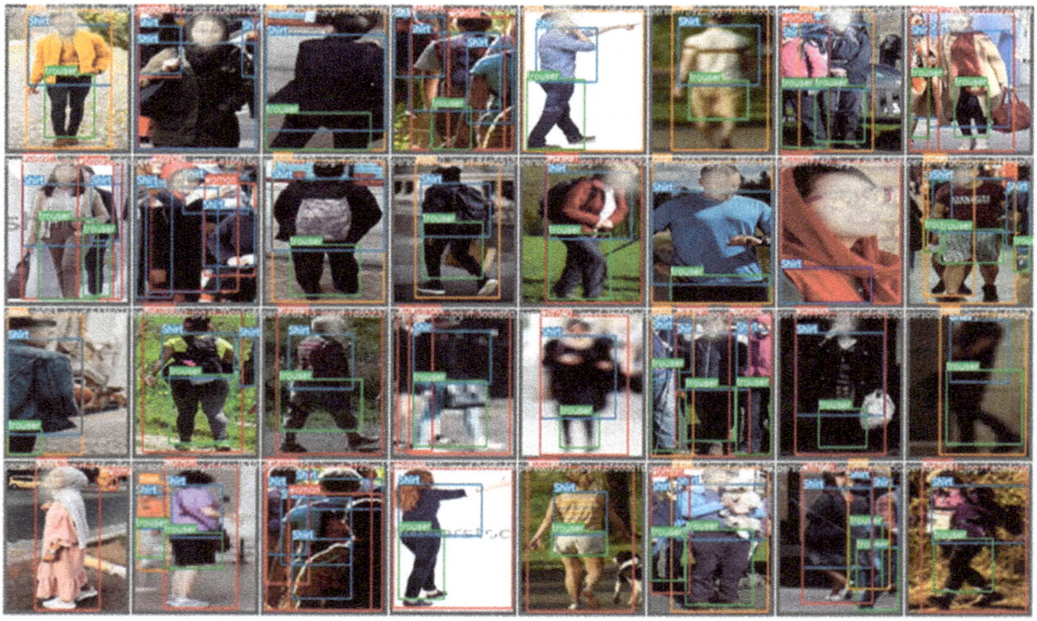

Figure 3. Images sample taken randomly from our dataset by Scaled Yolov4 to use in the training step; we did not choose any of them. These images prove the diversity of the PGC dataset, and it contains women, men, Arab women, Asian women, Black men, crowded scene, a single person scene, bluer scene, indoor scene, outdoor scene, back view, and front view.

Data annotation is the most critical and time-consuming step in the detection process. Two main factors are needed to achieve high-quality annotations: annotation tools and rules to guide the annotation procedure. We have used the Roboflow [16] tool to annotate our dataset. Using Roboflow made the process of annotation easier and faster. While the annotation tools speed up the process, the annotation rules increases its quality. Appendix A shows the annotation process and regulations that have been applied to our dataset. The main rule that needs to be known is that shirt class does not mean only shirts, but any clothes on the upper body such as a coat, jacket, sweater, or T-shirt. Same with the trousers, which could be shorts, leggings, jeans. Although this could be a limitation to our dataset, it would be possible for any researcher to change the labels on the shirts annotation to any other clothes they aim to investigate in their work. Including a wide range of clothes in one class has benefited our tracking algorithm.

Regarding dataset size, the most common question for researchers is how many images are needed to train the model? There is no magical equation regarding the dataset size that could tell us how many images are needed to train a detection model. However, it is a common understanding that having more training data leads to better performance. We discovered how much training data we needed by building the detection model at first with 10,000 images and checked how it performed. Then we increased it by another 10,000 until we reached our target performance. We stopped collecting data after 40,000 images, as that is when the model performance reached our desired performance.

To sum up, in the field of computer vision, and especially object detection, a good quality dataset is the core of any successful model, which make a good quality dataset a contribution that aims to improve the model performance. However, the scope of the time needed to organize, annotate, and clean the dataset still tends to be underestimated. Five remarkable criteria that show how PGC dataset contributes to the state of the art are introduced next: (1) the PGC dataset is unique—no other dataset in object detection or object tracking works using pedestrian attributes such as man, woman (using all of the body, not only faces), shirt and trouser. All known datasets, such as MSCOCO and PASCAL, works on the whole person as a single entity. (2) Rich annotation: almost all images have at least three classes out of four. (3) Large size: not only the number of images matters but also the number of annotations per class; our dataset has 190,000 annotations in 40,000 images for only four classes. Figure 4 shows the number of annotations for each class. (4) High diversity: we spent a lot of time introducing deliberately selected images; Figure 3 is proof of our dataset diversity. (5) Balance between classes: Figure 4 shows how PGC dataset classes were balanced, in which men and women were represented equally, with 34,163 women and 35,252 men.

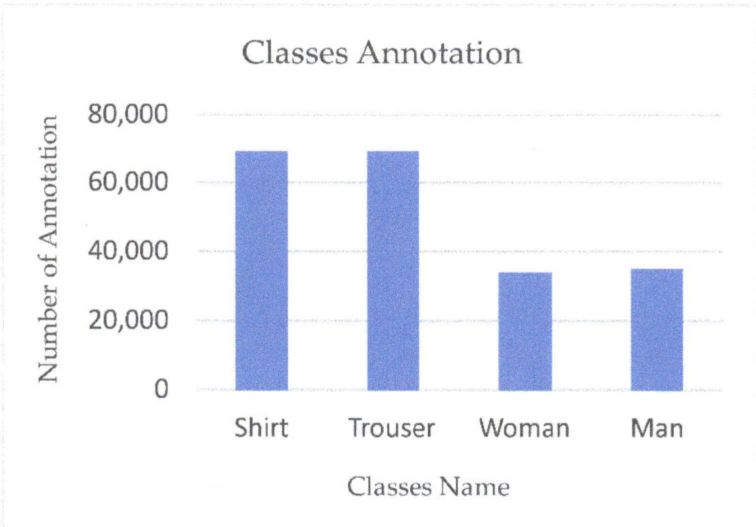

Figure 4. PGC class annotation balance.

3.1.3. Detection Model

Recent advances in methods for object detection are one of the main factors responsible for the success of MSA-AF. Tracking-by-detection algorithms such as ours rely on the quality of the detection model. Therefore, we searched for a detection model that achieves high performance at a reasonable speed. Deep neural network-based detection [36–39] showed a high performance compared to state-of-the-art detection algorithms. Region-based convolutional neural network (R-CNN)-based detection algorithms use the region to recognise the object inside the image. These algorithms do not look at all images, but only at the parts with a higher chance of containing the object. Unlike R-CNN-based detection algorithms, the YOLO family take the entire image in one run and predict the bounding boxes, as well as the class probability for these boxes. The YOLO family is commonly used for real-time detection, as it can process 45 frames per second.

This method was first described in 2015 [38], and many versions have been released since then, up until the latest version, published in November 2020 [40]. Not all versions of YOLO are published in a paper, such as YOLOv5; neither do they all have the same authors. Figure 5 summarises the performance and the timeline of all these versions; to conclude, we choose two of these versions for comparison, and finally choose just one of them. The results of our experiment in Section 4 between YOLOv5 and scaled YOLOv4 [41] shows that scaled YOLOv4 showed promising results for our dataset. Thus, scaled YOLOv4 was used as the detection model in MSA-AF.

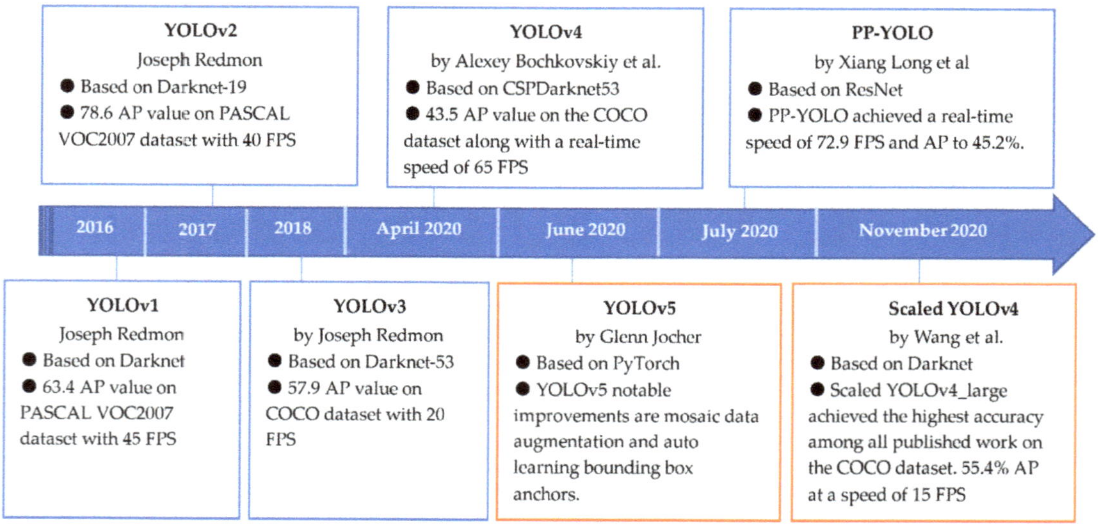

Figure 5. Timeline and performance comparison between members of the YOLO family.

3.2. First Association Stage

The main target of this stage is to decide whether the detection, which is the output from the scaled Yolov4, is associated with an existing track from previous frames or not. If the tracks did not associate with any detections, they would be added to the unassociated tracks list—the same with detections that did not associate with any existing tracks, which would be added to the unassociated detections list. While the first association stage deals with associated tracks and detection, both unassociated tracks and detections will be solved during the next stage—the final association stage.

Firstly, we need to predict the new position of the tracks in the current frame using the Kalman filter, and then build association cost metrics that will be used to solve the first stage of association between the detections and the predicted tracks. The output of this stage will guide the next step, where the final association decision will be made.

Prediction is an essential step that the human brain uses to track an object [25]. The Kalman filter has been used to predict the new position in many MOT algorithms due to its simplicity, versatility, and effectiveness. The complete mathematical derivations and formulation of the Kalman filter are beyond the scope of our paper. What we need to acknowledge is the dynamic model of target motion that the Kalman filter will use. The constant velocity model is suited for use in our framework as people hardly ever leave a constant velocity. In this model, we assume that the velocity is constant during the tracking so that we can predict the new position of the target easily using the Bbox location and the velocity information.

In the first association stage, the association cost metric has been used to decide which list from the three lists mentioned earlier the tracks and detections belong to. We know from cognitive study findings that the human brain uses all available information, such as appearance information, to discriminate an object [2]. Consequently, we decided to use appearance information to discriminate targets from each other rather than to discriminate them from backgrounds. CDA-DDAL [42] and DeepSort [24] learned the appearance features from the PETA reidentification task; we used the association metric from Deep sort [24]. Wojke et al. [24] used the person reidentification task to increase discrimination by applying the deep feature extractor from a wide residual network (WRN). The primary motive behind using the deep appearance description from Wojk et al. is that their network obtained a competitive performance for online tracks in real-time speed. Although appearance information can represent and discriminate the objects effectively, alone it is not enough. Adding spatial information is essential for forming a robust association cost metric. The Mahalanobis distance (1) between the predicted Kalman state of the tracks and the detection measure *KD(i,j)* will represent the spatial information, while the cosine distance (2) between the appearance information of the tracks and the detections *AD(i,j)* will represent the appearance information. Equation (3) shows this combination, which we believe would be representative enough at this stage.

$$KD(i,j) = \frac{(d_j - \mu_i)^T}{S_i(d_j - \mu_i)} \tag{1}$$

where $KD(i,j)$ represent the Mahalanobis distance of detections Bbox d_j from ith tracks with mean μ_i. The covariance matrix is S.

$$AD(i,j) = \min\left\{1 - r_j^T r_k^{(i)} \middle| r_k^{(i)} \in R_i\right\} \tag{2}$$

where $AD(i,j)$ is the smallest cosine distance between the jth detections and ith tracks, and r_j^T represents the appearance distributor of detections d_j, while $r_k^{(i)}$ is the appearance descriptor of the last k associations, which is sets at 100 [24].

$$A_{i,j} = \lambda KD(i,j) + (1 - \lambda)AD(i,j) \tag{3}$$

$A_{i,j}$ represents the association cost metric which combines the appearance and spatial representation of the object, while λ allows us to control the impact of each metric on the overall cost metrics.

Solving the association problem by using the Hungarian algorithm on the association cost metrics is the last step in this stage, generating three lists—the first list includes all detections and tracks associated with each other. The second list will consist of the tracks that did not associate with any detections in the current frame. The third list includes the detections that did not match with any tracks. In [24], they deleted the tracks in the second list if they exceeded a certain age and created a new track for all detections in the third list. However, not all unassociated tracks exiting from the scene are deleted; they could be in a long-occlusion. Moreover, not all unassociated detections are new tracks; they could be long-term occluded tracks reappearing in the scene. This was the reason for introducing the last decision stage, which solved all these questions using the attributes.

3.3. Final Association Stage

Semantic attributes have been used in many detection algorithms [43]. However, they have never been used to solve occlusion in MOT algorithms, to the best of our knowledge. Additionally, semantic attributes play a significant role in the human brain by discriminating targets during tracking [3]. We used these semantic attributes in MSA-AF during the final association decision for those two reasons: not only to detect the presence of occlusion but also to solve the occlusion problem. E. Jefferies [44] raised an essential question regarding the organisation of semantic attributes: how is semantic information linked together in our brain to generate a unitary experience of a person? In neuropsychology, there are two principles regarding the organisation of semantic information: semantic hub and distributed only. In the semantic hub model, the access to knowledge occurs through a semantic hub, which causes an inability to link any semantic information if damage occurs to the central hub [45]. On the other hand, the distributed-only model suggests that different types of semantic information interact directly without central hub [46]. We combined both models to benefit our algorithm as follows: The central hub will be the person track, which will contain all semantic, appearance, and spatial information, with direct access to all other semantic attributes (man, woman, shirt, trouser). At the same time, direct interactions between semantic attributes are necessary in case of any disappearance of these attributes. Figure 6 shows the relationship between these attributes and the central hub. The direct interactions between the four semantic attributes are the key step in this stage. In other words, how can we decide which shirt belongs to which person? In a normal situation where no occlusion occurs, bounding box overlap could be enough to make that decision. However, in the occlusion situation, more than one shirt could overlap with the same person. For this reason, we introduced a metric called intersection over attribute (IOA); this attribute here could be a shirt or trouser. Most MOT algorithm use intersection over union (IOU), which only indicates the overlap between Bboxes but does not give any information about occlusion.

$$\text{IOA} = \frac{\text{Area of Overlap}}{\text{Area of Attribute}} \tag{4}$$

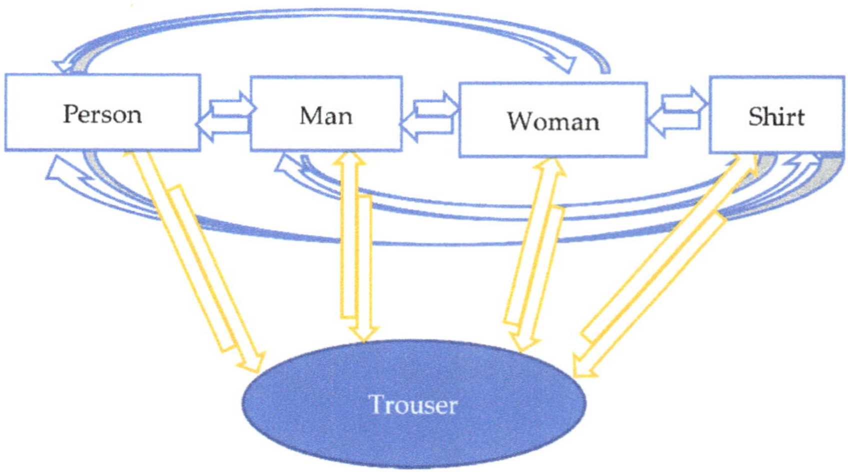

Figure 6. A combination of distributed-only and semantic hub for controlling the relationship between attributes.

IOA not only tells us which attributes belong to which person but can also be used to identify if the person is in an occlusion state or not. The ratio of the overlap between a person and an attribute (shirt or trouser), and the attribute area IOA, would be close to one if all of the attribute's bounding box is inside the person's bounding box. In this case, the shirt will be linked to that person as their shirt (see Figure 7a). In the occlusion state, the IOA will be less than 0.9 and more than 0.4, meaning that the person overlapped with parts of these attributes. An example of the three stages of occlusion that define the final decision is shown in Figure 7.

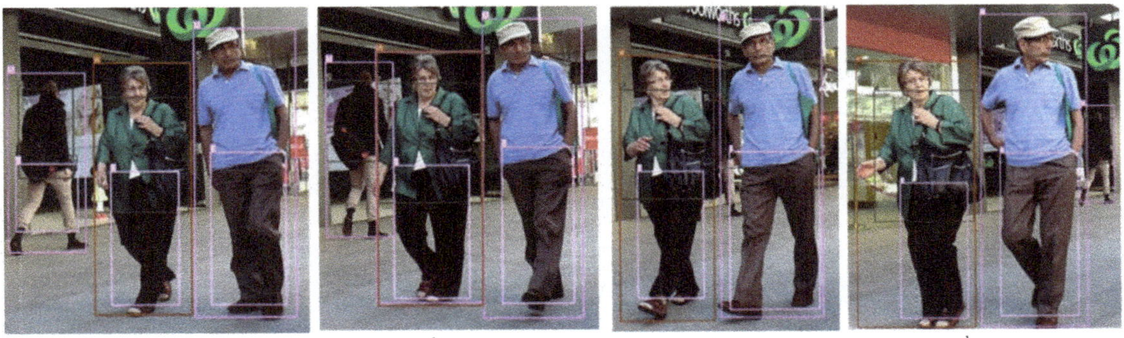

a b c d

Figure 7. Four images taken from our detection outputs to demonstrate the occlusion phases. The original image is taken from the MOTChalleng dataset [28]. Before occlusion state (**a**), in occlusion state (**b**,**c**), and after occlusion state (**d**).

The skeleton outline for using IOA in the final association decision is detailed in Algorithms 1–3. In the three algorithms, Tr refers to track IDs from the Associated_Man_list and the Associated_Woman_list, and Sh refers to the shirt IDs from the associated_shirt_list. At the same time, Sh.Track_bbox refers to the Bbox of the person that a shirt belongs to and the Tr.Shirt_bbox refers to the Bbox of the shirt belong to the person. Tr.Shirt_age counts how many frames the shirt of this person has been tracked in, Sh.Tracks_age counts how many frames the person linked to this shirt has been tracked in, and Sh.Occlusion_age counts how many frames the shirt was occluded in. Tr.Occlusion_status indicates if the person is in an occlusion situation or not, while Sh.Occlusion_status shows if the shirt is in an occlusion situation or not, and Sh.Occluded_with gives the ID of the person that occluded with that shirt. Finally, time_since_update gives the number of frames in which the person did not update.

Algorithm 1 Associated tracks and detection list

Input: List of associated tracks and detections
Output: Detecting occlusion state and save semantic attribute

```
For Tr in Associated_Man _Woman_list
    For Sh in Associated_Shirt_list
        IOA = Intersection_over_ShirtArea(Tr,Sh)
            If  IOA > 0.9
                If Tr.Shirt_id = Shirt_id and Sh.Track_id = Track_id
                    update Sh.Track_bbox & Tr.Shirt_bbox
                    Tr.Shirt_age = + 1
                    Sh.Track_age = + 1
                Else
                    Tr.Occlusion_status = true
                    Sh.Occlusion_status = true
                    Sh.Occluded_with = Tr.id
            else
                If IOA > 0.4
                    Tr.Occlusion_status = true
                    Sh.Occlusion_status = true
                    Sh.Occluded_with = Tr.id
```

Algorithm 2 Unassociated tracks list

Input: List of unassociated tracks
Output: Updated model

```
For Tr in unmatched_Person
        If Tr.Occlusion_status == true
                Tr.Occlusion_age = + 1
                time_since_update = + 1
                If Tr.Shirt_id in matches_Shirt
                        update   Tr.Shirt_bbox
                        Sh.Track_age = 0
                        Sh.Track_Occlusion_age = + 1
                        Shirt_age = + 1
                Else
                        Tr.Occlusion_age = + 1
                        time_since_update = + 1
        Else
          time_since_update = + 1
```

Algorithm 3 Unassociated detections list

Input: List of unassociated detections
Output: Retrieve the obj ID after appearing from occlusion

```
For Det in unmatched_detection_person
For Sh in matches_Shirt
        IOS = Intersection_over_ShirtArea (Det,Sh)
        If IOS > 0.9
                If Tr.Occlusion_age (Sh.Track_id) > 1
                        Tr.Occlusion_age (Sh.Track_id) = 0
                        Tr.age = 1
                        Track.update (Sh.Track_id.kf, Det)
                        Sh.Track.bbox = Det.bbox
                        Assosiated = True
                If Tr.time_since_updated > 0
                        Tr.time_since_updated = 0
                        Tr.age = 1
                        Track.update (Sh.Track_id.kf, Det)
                        Sh.Track.bbox = Det.bbox
                        Assosiated = True
If Assosiated = False
      initiate_track (Det (Det_idx],classes (Det_idx].item())
```

Each algorithm from the three has a different input list: associated tracks and detections list, unassociated tracks list, and unassociated detections list. We will work on each list separately to collect as much information as possible to feed to the main hub, which is the person, then take a suitable final decision depending on this information. The algorithm for each list will be repeated for the trousers too. As we can see from Algorithm 1, IOA has been calculated in line 3 to define whether a shirt belongs to that track or not, then this information was added to the person track. Moreover, the occlusion state will also be detected in line 9.

Algorithm 2 deals with tracks that disappeared in the current frame; this could be occlusion or a detection step problem. In Section 3, we introduced our scheme to ensure a high-quality output from the detection stage. However, what if the detection model fails to detect an object for a few frames or detects the object inaccurately? How will our algorithm solve such a problem? In this case, we need to know the reason for the disappearance to make the right decision. To that end, the information that we collected in Algorithm 1 was used, plus the age of the track, to decide whether we needed to forget this track, delete it, or keep it until it appears again. This step is what distinguishes MSA-AF. The knowledge of the occlusion state of the track will make us not rush to delete these tracks, even if the age exceeds the threshold age, as in line 3.

Even if the tracks are not in an occlusion state, they could disappear because of the detection problem. Therefore, we keep updating the tracks state for several frames to keep identifying the tracks when the detector model detects them again. We will keep track of the shirt and the trousers that belong to this person (line 6) if they are still detected, which is the case in Figure 7c.

Algorithm 3 includes the final decision concerning whether any unassociated detection is a new person, to create a new track; a person coming out of full or partial occlusion; or if that detection was a track missed due to a detection problem. Line 4 in Algorithm 3 finds the IOA between the unassociated person and the shirts in the associated detection, to see if they belong to that person or not.

4. Experiment Results

In this section, the results of our tracking algorithm and dataset will be introduced. Moreover, the comparison between the detection model we used and the nearest competitive model was presented, to prove that the model we used gives the best MT (mostly tracker metric).

4.1. Performance Metrics

Detection models are usually tested using precision, recall, and mAP at 0.5 or 0.5–0.95. Precision is the positive prediction value (of all the positive predictions, how many are true positive predictions). The recall metric is the true positive rate (of all the actual positives, how many are true positive predictions). These are then plotted to get a PR (precision-recall) curve; the area under the PR curve is called average precision (AP). Now we have AP per class; mAP is the averaged AP over all the object categories. Therefore, all detection models seek a high mAP value.

Regarding tracking performance metrics, defining the metrics that can say if MSA-AF solved the tracking problem in videos better than state-of-the-art algorithms is a challenge by itself. MOTChallenege [28] uses many metrics to evaluate the benchmark performance of MOT algorithms. We have used eight of these metrics to evaluate our algorithm. Multiple objects tracking accuracies (MOTA) [47] measure three errors: identity switches, missed targets, and false positives. In contrast, multiple objects tracking precision (MOTP) [47] measures the misalignment between the predicted Bbox and the annotated Bboxes. ID F1 [48] combines ID precision and ID recall by measuring the correctly identified and computed detection ratio and the ground truth average number. Ground truth trajectories covered by track trajectory for more than 80% of their life span were measured as the most tracked target (MT). In contrast, mostly lost (ML) measures the ground truth trajectory, covered for less than 20% of its life span by the track trajectory. Rcll is the ratio of correctly identified detections to the total number of ground truth boxes, and Prcn is the ratio of true positive TPs to the addition of true positives and false negatives. Finally, the FAF is the average number of false alarms per frame.

4.2. Detection Performance

Any detection algorithm's output depends on two main factors: the dataset and the detection model. Here, we will take each factor and show how it affected the overall performance of our MOT algorithm.

4.2.1. Dataset

The PGC dataset can be used in visual surveillance research on pedestrian detection, tracking, fashion projects, and reidentification. The key challenge of evaluating our dataset on the detection model is that we cannot know how it will perform until we test the model on new data that the model was not trained on. Therefore, we divided our dataset into a training set and a validation set. Then, the loss function for the two sets was evaluated, as shown in Figure 8; the smaller the loss, the better the classification performance.

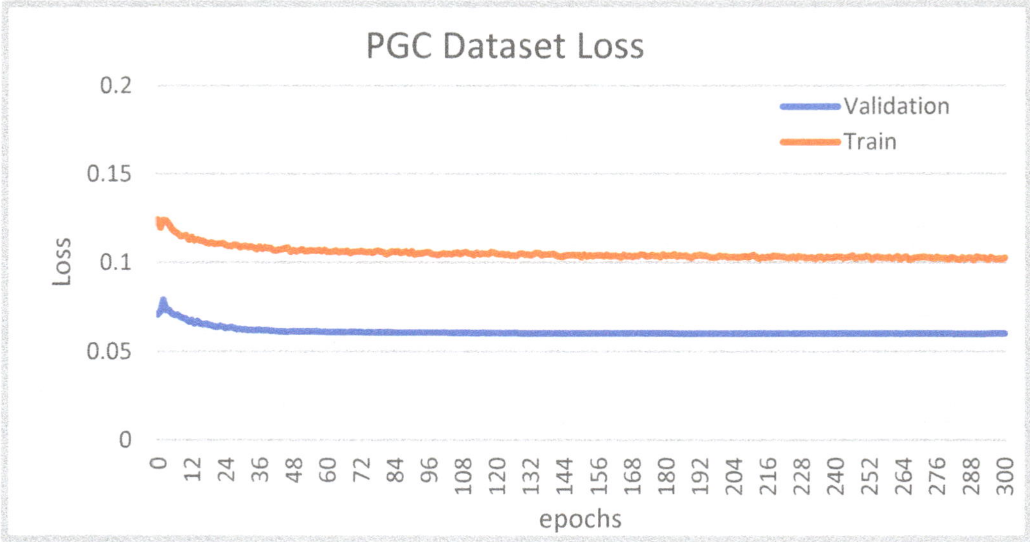

Figure 8. Our dataset loss plots for the training and validation sets.

Based on this diagram, it is clear that our model does not show any signs of overfitting. First, as the validation loss plot decreases, so does the training loss plot, while there is a small gap between the two. Second, there is no infliction point on the validation loss plot, which indicates that the training process did not receive sufficient experience with the data. Thus, the model still fits well.

In order to avoid overfitting, which resulted from the search for the perfect fit, the training ended at 300 epochs, based on early stopping.

Compared with the training set, the validation set had a smaller loss. Along with the early stopping criteria, YOLO uses a regularization approach to help regularize the model.

It could be a surprise that the loss of the validation set is less than that of the training set. The reason behind this is that the regularization loss did not add to the validation loss, but only to the training loss. YOLO uses a regularization method—batch normalization—after its convolutional layers to help regularize the model, which improves the mAP by 2%.

After proving that our dataset was not biased and did not overfit the model, we started to search how can we compare the PGC dataset to another dataset. Looking for how the most famous dataset in the field of object detection compared their datasets with others and imitating that was the best fit for our work. The extensive dataset, MSCOCO [31], has played an essential role in boosting object detection and tracking research—especially in person detection—by including more than 700,000 instances of the person category. Another dataset widely used in detection models is the Pascal VOC 2012 dataset, which has 17,118 images across 20 object classes with 13,168 person annotations [49]. Although MSCOCO has way more person instances in their dataset than PASCAL, PASCAL outperforms MSCOCO in 6 categories out of 20, including the person category. MSCOCO's results confirm that the annotation number could not be the main or the only factor differentiating the dataset. MSCOCO compared their dataset performance to the PASCAL VOC 12 dataset performance by using both datasets to train the same detection model; then, they used the performance differences of the model across the two datasets for comparison. The way MSCOCO compares their dataset has been used to examine our dataset and demonstrate its high quality. We have used scaled YOLOv4 as the detection model for measuring PGC dataset performance, for reasons given in Section 3.

The challenge in this evaluation was finding a dataset with the same classes we used (man, woman, shirt, trouser). As we mentioned previously, all known datasets have worked on persons as single entities, without any semantic attributes. The only option we had for evaluating our dataset was to collect the same amount of images, 40,000, with the same classes from the Open Images DatasetV6 [50]. Then, we trained scaled YOLOv4 using both datasets and compared their performance. However, Images DatasetV6 had only 23,000 images with our four classes. Therefore, we compared 23,000 images from our dataset with 23,000 from Image DatasetV6 to have a fair comparison. Figure 9 shows how PGC dataset classes are more balanced than Open Images Dataset V6 classes. Figure 10 shows the success of our dataset in outperforming every single metric—even the training time, as discussed next. Using the clarification at the performance metrics subsection, the higher the precision, recall, and mAP, the higher the model's performance. Our dataset gains higher precision, recall, and mAP. The mAP value of our dataset at 0.5 and 0.5–0.95 proves how rich, reliable, and robust our dataset is. The PGC dataset performs equally well in the four classes, unlike most big datasets that outperform in one class more than others; this is due to the balance. Figure 11 demonstrates the performance of the four classes in the YOLOv5 model.

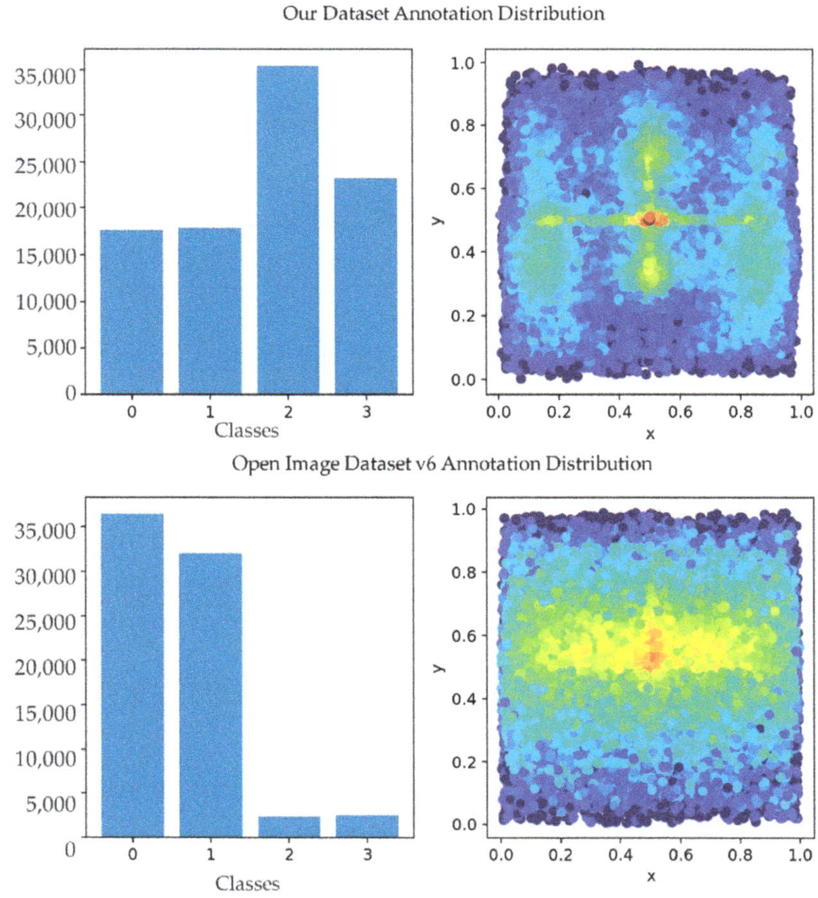

Figure 9. Comparison of class representation between the PGC dataset and open v6.

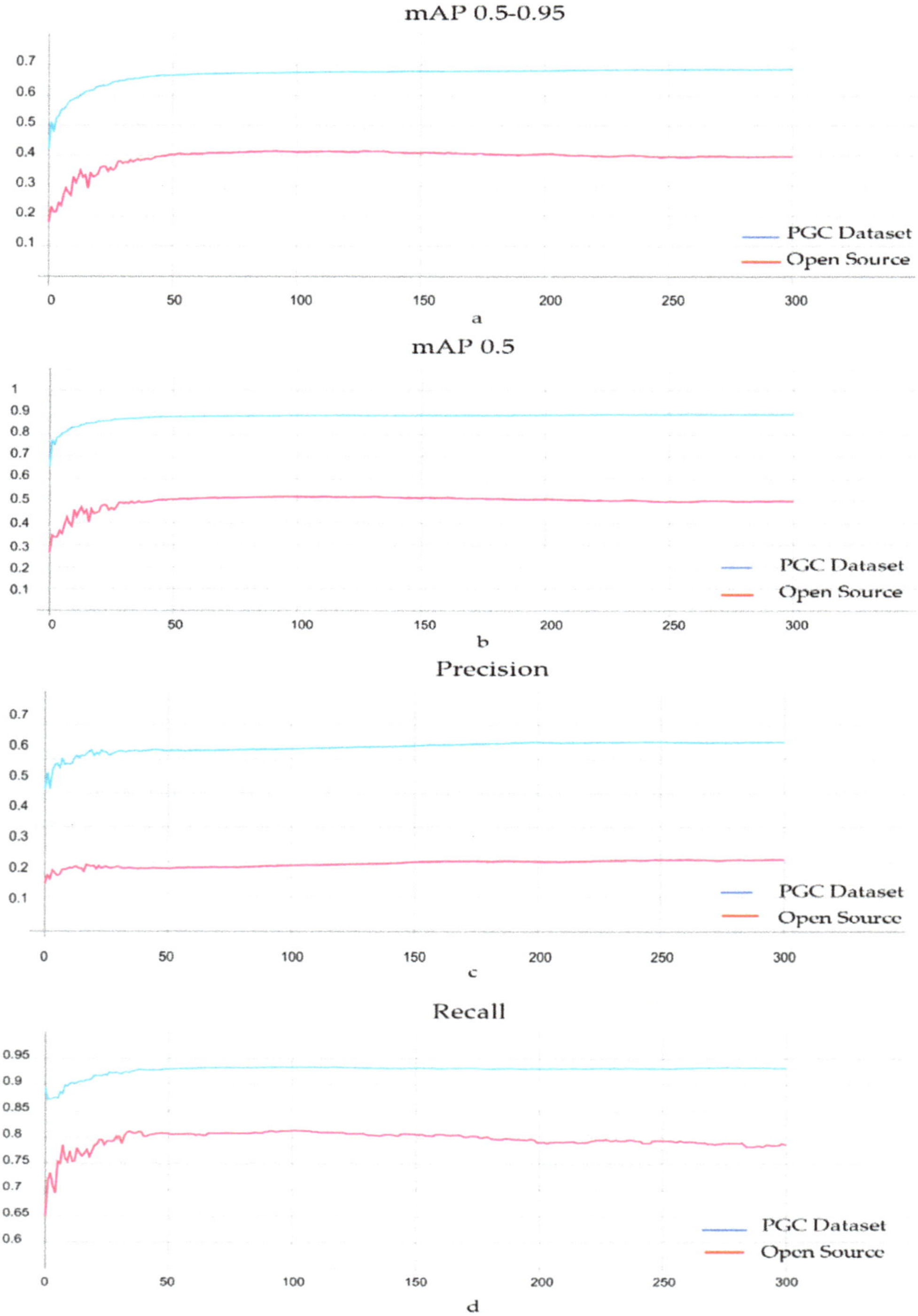

Figure 10. Four evaluation metrics, mAP 0.5–0.95 (**a**), mAP 0.5 (**b**), Recall (**c**), and Precision (**d**), that have been used to measure the performance of the PGC dataset and open dataset v6, after being used to train scaled YOLOv4. TensorBoard was used to create these graphics.

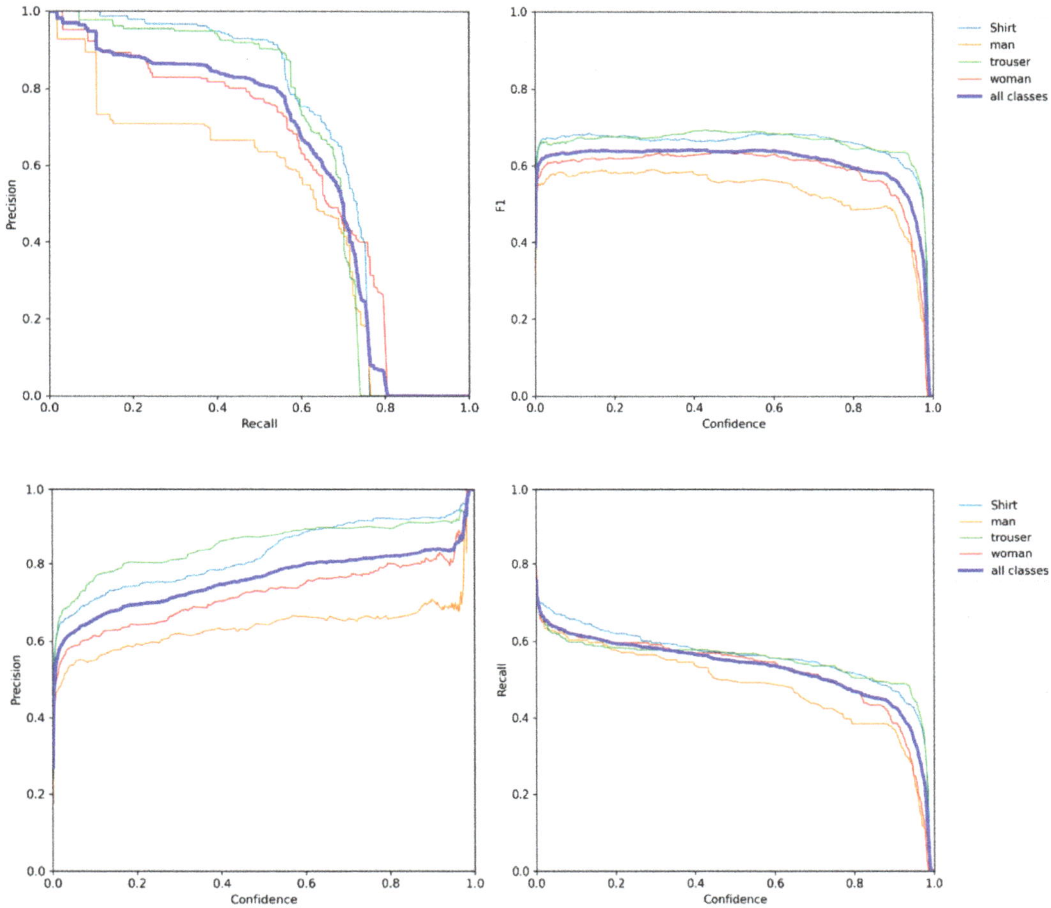

Figure 11. The performance metrics Precision, Recall, f1, and Precision-Recall of the four classes when the PGC dataset had been used to train YOLOv5. The YOLOv5 model was used to create these graphics.

Table 3 shows a comparison between the PGC dataset and the Open Images Dataset V6 across performance metrics, plus the training time. We used an intel core i7 computer with 64GB Ram and NIVIDA GeForce RTX2070 to train the detection models.

Table 3. Dataset Performance comparison with open image datasetv6 on scaled yolov4.

	Training Time	mAP 0.5	mAP 0.5–0.95	Precision	Recall
Open Images Dataset V6	3 d 5 h 11 min	0.4999	0.3983	0.2079	0.7867
PGC Dataset (ours)	**3 d 1 h 27 min**	**0.8924**	**0.6862**	**0.5487**	**0.9321**

4.2.2. Detection Model

Scaled YOLOv4, YOLOv5l, YOLOv5m, and YOLOv5s have been tested using the PGC dataset, in order to choose one of them for use in our MOT Algorithm. The reason behind using these four models is introduced in detail in Section 3. Although the training time of scaled YOLOv4 is much longer than the training time of the YOLOv5 family, the outstanding performance of scaled YOLOv4 on the PGC dataset is worth the long training time. While scaled YOLOv4 took 3 d 1 h 27 min 6 s to train 300 epochs, YLOLv5l took 1 h 23 min 12 s, YOLOv5m took 55 min 24 s, and YOLOv5s took 34 min 19 s. Figure 12 shows the performance of the four models using two metrics: mAP 0.5 and mAP 0.5–0.95. As a result of this comparison, scaled YOLOv4 with 0.8924 mAP was chosen as the detection model for MSA-AF.

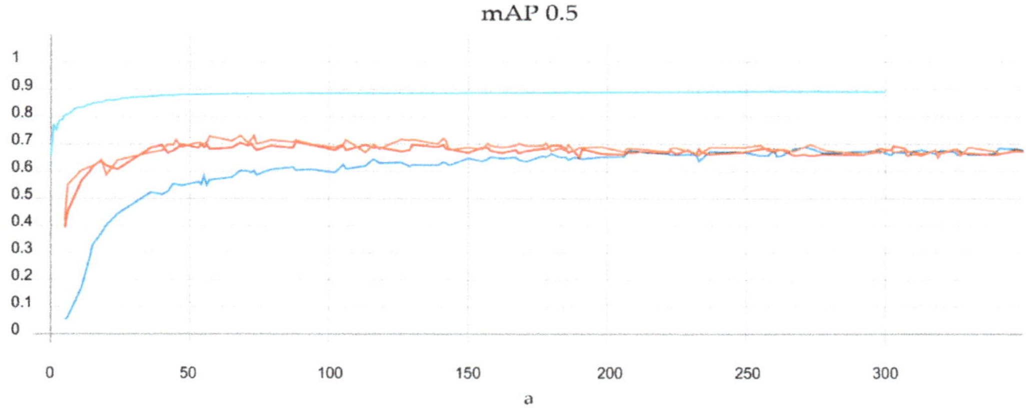

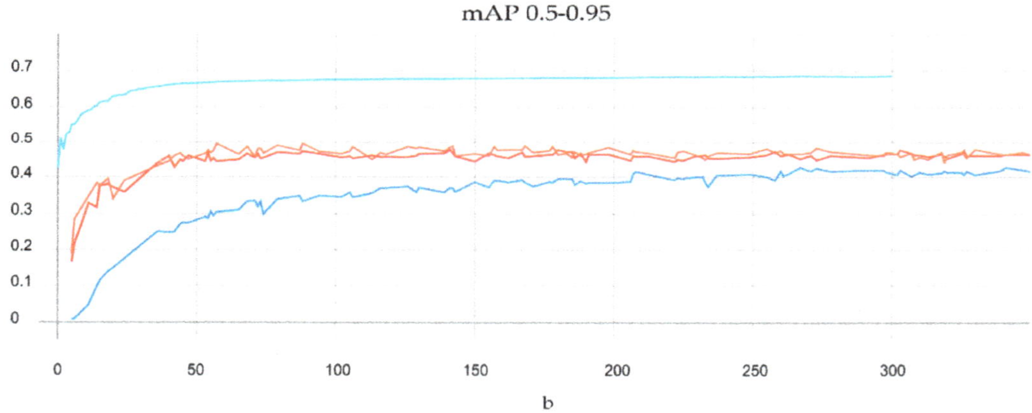

Figure 12. Performance of the four models, Scaled YOLOv4, YOLOv5l, YOLOv5s, and YOLOv5m using two metrics, mAP 0.5 (**a**) and mAP 0.5–0.95 (**b**). TensorBoard was used to create these graphics.

4.3. Tracking Performance

We tested MSA-AF on MOT17 and MOT20 challenges. Each challenge had several videos with zoomed-in and zoomed-out scenes. However, all videos in the MOT20 dataset had a crowded scene, unlike MOT17.

To evaluate the performance of our algorithm, we compared our results with five other MOT algorithms. LPC_MOT [51] introduced a proposal-based MOT learnable framework, while MPNTrack [52] used deep learning for feature extraction and association. GNN-Match [53] used graph convolutional neural networks (GCNN) on top of convolutional-based features for object association. At the same time, Tracktor++v2 [54] takes advantage of a detector's regression head to perform temporal realignment of the object's Bbox. The concepts of SORT17 [55] have been used in MSA-AF, which use Kalman filtering in the image space and the Hungarian method on the association metric to solve the association problem. Table 4 illustrates the comparison between the performance of these five algorithms and ours on the MOT17 dataset. As shown in Table 4, our algorithm achieved state-of-the-art results, especially in MOTP, ML, and FAF. We attribute this performance to our dataset, which provides high-quality detections to the first and final association decision. Moreover, our final association decision model decreased the number of lost tracks, leading our algorithm to have the lowest ML.

Table 4. Performance comparison with five state-of-the-art algorithms on MOT17.

MOT17	↑MOTA	↑IDF1	↑MOTP	↑MT	↓ML	↑Rcll	↑Prcn	↓FAF
LPC_MOT [51]	**59**	**66.8**	78	**29.9**	33.9	63.3	93.9	1.3
MPNTrack [52]	58.8	61.7	78.6	28.8	33.5	62.1	95.3	1
GNNMatch [53]	57.3	56.3	78.6	24.4	33.4	60.1	96	0.8
Tracktor++v2 [54]	53.5	52.3	78	19.5	36.6	56	**96.3**	**0.7**
SORT17 [55]	43.1	39.8	77.8	12.5	42.3	49.0	90.7	1.6
MSA-AF (Ours)	44.4	37.1	**80.1**	13	**30.25**	50.6	89.55	**0.7**

On the other hand, Table 5 compares the same algorithms, using the same evaluation metrics but on a more challenging dataset, to MOT20. All MOT20 videos have a crowded scene, and the pedestrians are too far from the camera, as shown in Figure 13. Using the MOT20 dataset makes the job of our algorithm much harder, because it relies on detecting semantic attributes, which could be a challenge in most MOT20 videos. However, MSA-AF did surprisingly well in the MOT20 dataset. Although the performance of MSA-AF on the MOT20 dataset is not as good as on MOT17, it still has the best MT and ML. These results prove that the robustness of our final association stage is high.

Table 5. Performance comparison with five state-of-the-art algorithms on MOT20.

MOT20	↑MOTA	↑IDF1	↑MOTP	↑MT	↓ML	↑Rcll	↑Prcn	↓FAF
LPC_MOT [51]	56.3	**62.5**	79.7	34.1	25.2	**58.8**	96.3	2.6
MPNTrack [52]	**57.6**	59.1	79	38.2	22.5	61.1	94.9	3.8
GNNMatch [53]	54.5	49	79.4	32.8	25.5	56.8	96.9	2.1
Tracktor++v2 [54]	52.6	52.7	**79.9**	29.4	26.7	54.3	**97.6**	**1.5**
SORT17 [55]	42.7	45.1	78.5	16.7	26.2	48.8	90.2	6.1
MSA-AF (Ours)	45.3	36.4	77.6	**40**	**19**	54.8	86.8	4.36

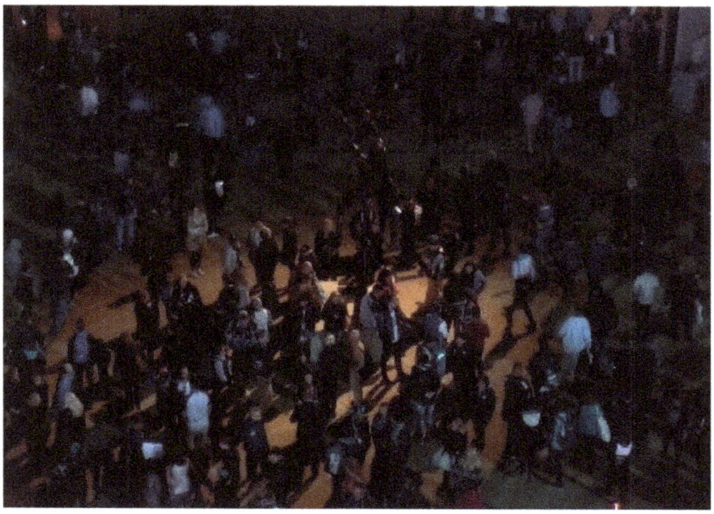

Figure 13. A sample from the MOT20-04 video [28].

It is worth mentioning here why we believe that MSA-AF is competitive with the results of the other algorithm. First, as shown in Table 4, MSA-AF dominated at MOTP, ML, and FAF metrics. Second, although the other five algorithms that we compared MSA-AF with from MOTChallenge use given detection as an input instead of detecting the object, it exceeds SORT17 [55] MOTA result. Furthermore, the proposed algorithm is capable of yielding solutions, which could be the start to a new pathway in the field of object tracking.

5. Limitations of the Study

This paper addressed only four semantic attributes, which could increase in future work by relabeling the shirts and trousers to include more clothes types. For instance, trousers can be relabelled to 'jeans, shorts, leggings, or sweatpants', and shirts can be relabelled to 'blouse, T-shirt, crop top, blazer, jacket, or hoodie'. Thus, pedestrian attribute detection algorithms would benefit from our dataset as much as object detection algorithms. Moreover, it could be a start to fashion-based detection. Additionally, MSA-AF did not give the same performance in videos with zoomed-out scenes, where people's appearance is rarely informative. This could be handled by adding more images to our dataset with a zoomed-out scene. Finally, as our algorithm is a tracking-by-detection algorithm, tracking performance relies on the detector's output. Although our dataset increased the overall detector performance, failing to detect an object is still an issue. When the detector fails to detect an object, the tracker fails to track it, which increases false negatives. On the other hand, the five algorithms we compared our results with use a publicly provided detection set from MotChallenge as their input. This caused low MOTA and IDF1 in our algorithm compared to their algorithms.

6. What Went Wrong

After training scaled YOLOv4 on our dataset, we found some confusion between the shirts and the man and woman class. In other words, many man-classed objects were detected as man and shirt simultaneously, which confused our algorithm. When we looked back to the PGC dataset annotation, in some cases such as occlusion or a person raising their hand, the shirt Bbox included faces, confusing the detection model and making it think that any person could be shirt too (see Appendix A). We went back to the 40,000 images in our dataset to handle this problem and resized the shirt Bbox, so that no faces were included inside it. After that, we retrained scaled YOLOv4, which solved the problem.

7. Conclusions

This paper has presented a novel MOT algorithm that imitates the human brain in eight different areas, and a new dataset of 40,000 images and more than 190,000 annotations to serve the computer vision community. Opening the doors to more human brain-inspired algorithms that would change the way in which the tracking problem has previously been solved is one of the goals of this paper. In addition, there are encouraging directions for future annotations on the PGC dataset that would benefit a wide range of researchers. Finally, we presented our results on challenging videos from the MOTChallenge benchmark, where we measured the quantitative performance of MSA-AF compared to five of the most recent state-of-the-art trackers. These results show our algorithm's impact on creating a stable tracker by decreasing the ML metric and increasing the MOTP at the same time. Moreover, our dataset gained 0.89 mAP compared to the 0.49 mAP from open image dataset v6.

Author Contributions: Methodology, M.S.D.; Software, M.S.D.; Supervision, M.A.E., M.S.E.-S. and H.A.A.; Validation, M.A.E., M.S.E.-S. and H.A.A.; Writing—original draft, M.S.D.; Writing—review & editing, M.A.E. and H.A.A. All authors have read and agreed to the published version of the manuscript.

Funding: This research received no external funding.

Institutional Review Board Statement: Not applicable.

Informed Consent Statement: Not applicable.

Data Availability Statement: Not applicable.

Conflicts of Interest: The authors declare no conflict of interest.

Appendix A

Using the Roboflow annotation tool, we have drawn a rectangle (Bbox) around all shirts, trousers, men and women at each image in our dataset and labelled them (shirt, trouser, man, woman). While annotating our dataset, we needed to implement some rules onto all the images. These rules helped us to recognise a problem with our MOT algorithm, when we found that the detection model detects some man and woman-classed objects as shirts. We added rule 6 to solve this problem.

1. Creating tight bounding boxes without taking any parts from the object.

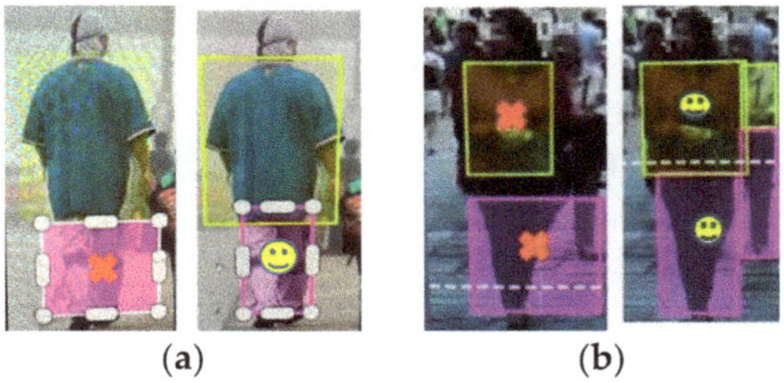

Figure A1. (**a**) how to annotate a trouser without including part of the background, (**b**) the all shirt should be included inside the Bbox.

2. Labelling all objects we could see in the image unless the appeared part was too small.

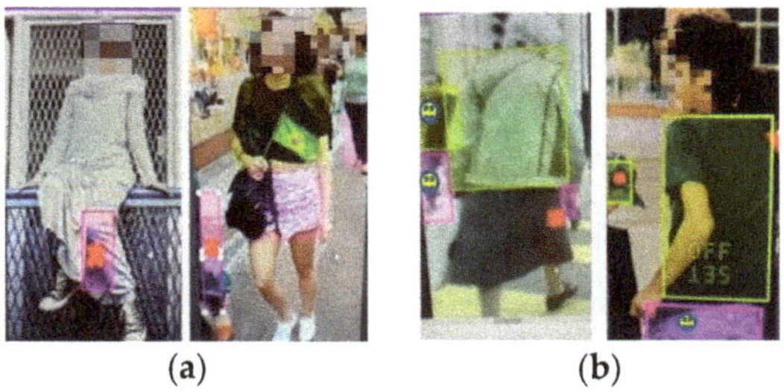

Figure A2. (**a**) don't annotate the trouser if only a small part is shown, (**b**) Annotate the shirt and trouser, even if they appeared in the background.

3. Label occluded (hidden partially behind another object), annotating the visible part only.

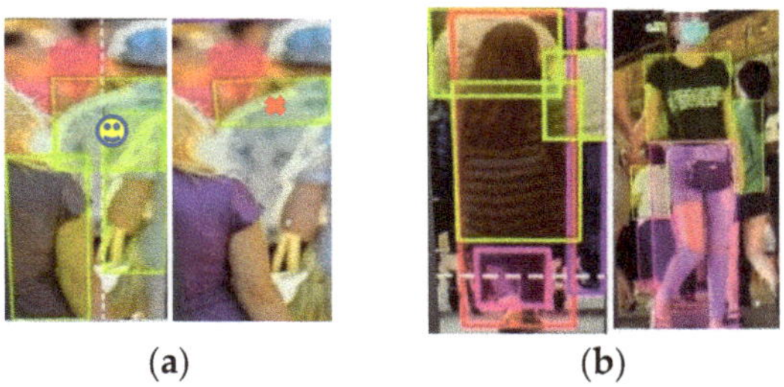

Figure A3. (**a**) shows how to annotate a shirt if part of it was occluded behind another person, (**b**) shows more crowded scene and how to annotate occluded objects.

4. Be careful with the empty Bounding boxes that you may draw by mistake. Always count the annotated bounding boxes and make sure that there are no extra free boxes.

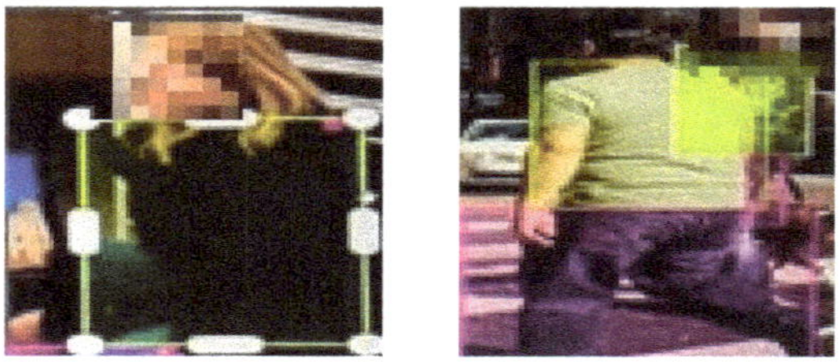

(a) (b)

Figure A4. In (**a**) and (**b**), there is a false positive Bbox in the right corner of the shirt.

5. Shirt class includes any clothes on the upper body (blazer, short dress, T-shirt, blouse); trouser includes shorts too.

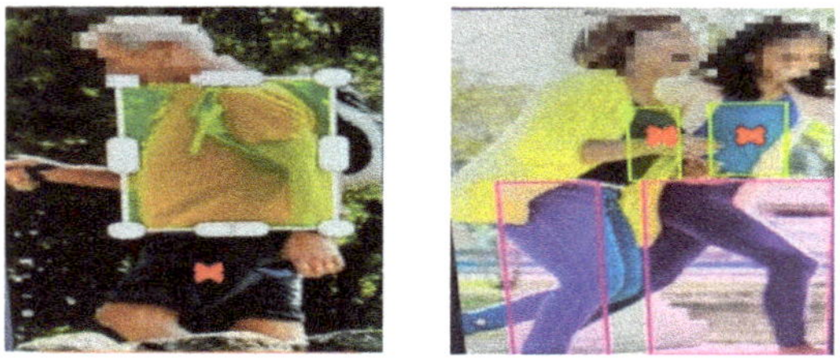

(a) (b)

Figure A5. (**a**) shorts should be annotated as trouser, (**b**) class shirt means any clothes in the upper body part.

6. We added this rule later in the work: Make sure that no shirt or trouser includes any part from the person's face as this will cause confusion to the model, and it will label any Bbox with a face as a shirt.

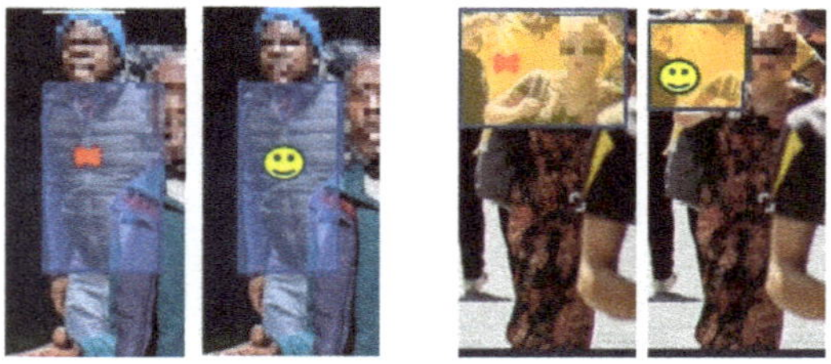

(a) (b)

Figure A6. In (**a**) and (**b**), You can cut part of the shirt if it includes another person's face.

References

1. Leonardelli, E.; Fait, E.; Fairhall, S.L. Temporal dynamics of access to amodal representations of category-level conceptual information. *Sci. Rep.* **2019**, *9*, 239. [CrossRef]
2. Lyu, C.; Hu, S.; Wei, L.; Zhang, X.; Talhelm, T. Brain Activation of Identity Switching in Multiple Identity Tracking Task. *PLoS ONE* **2015**, *10*, e0145489. [CrossRef] [PubMed]
3. Rupp, K.; Roos, M.; Milsap, G.; Caceres, C.; Ratto, C.; Chevillet, M.; Crone, N.E.; Wolmetz, M. Semantic attributes are encoded in human electrocorticographic signals during visual object recognition. *NeuroImage* **2017**, *148*, 318–329. [CrossRef]
4. Ardila, A. People recognition: A historical/anthropological perspective. *Behav. Neurol.* **1993**, *6*, 99–105. [CrossRef]

5. Hong, Z.; Chen, Z.; Wang, C.; Mei, X.; Prokhorov, D.; Tao, D. MUlti-Store Tracker (MUSTer): A cognitive psychology inspired approach to object tracking. In Proceedings of the IEEE Computer Society Conference on Computer Vision and Pattern Recognition, Boston, MA, USA, 7–12 June 2015; pp. 749–758. [CrossRef]
6. Song, Y.; Zhao, Y.; Yang, X.; Zhou, Y.; Wang, F.N.; Zhang, Z.S.; Guo, Z.K. Object detection and tracking algorithms using brain-inspired model and deep neural networks. *J. Phys. Conf. Ser.* **2020**, *1507*, 092066. [CrossRef]
7. Zhang, S.; Lan, X.; Yao, H.; Zhou, H.; Tao, D.; Li, X. A Biologically Inspired Appearance Model for Robust Visual Tracking. *IEEE Trans. Neural Netw. Learn. Syst.* **2016**, *28*, 2357–2370. [CrossRef]
8. Yoon, K.; Kim, D.Y.; Yoon, Y.-C.; Jeon, M. Data Association for Multi-Object Tracking via Deep Neural Networks. *Sensors* **2019**, *19*, 559. [CrossRef]
9. Zhang, K.; Liu, Q.; Wu, Y.; Yang, M.-H. Robust Visual Tracking via Convolutional Networks without Training. *IEEE Trans. Image Process.* **2016**, *25*, 1779–1792. [CrossRef] [PubMed]
10. Dequaire, J.; Ondrúška, P.; Rao, D.; Wang, D.; Posner, I. Deep tracking in the wild: End-to-end tracking using recurrent neural networks. *Int. J. Robot. Res.* **2017**, *37*, 492–512. [CrossRef]
11. Kamkar, S.; Ghezloo, F.; Moghaddam, H.A.; Borji, A.; Lashgari, R. Multiple-target tracking in human and machine vision. *PLoS Comput. Biol.* **2020**, *16*, e1007698. [CrossRef]
12. Atkinson, R.; Shiffrin, R. Human Memory: A Proposed System and its Control Processes. In *Psychology of Learning and Motivation—Advances in Research and Theory 2*; Academic Press: Cambridge, UK, 1968; Volume 2, pp. 89–195. [CrossRef]
13. Gao, D.; Han, S.; Vasconcelos, N. Discriminant Saliency, the Detection of Suspicious Coincidences, and Applications to Visual Recognition. *IEEE Trans. Pattern Anal. Mach. Intell.* **2009**, *31*, 989–1005. [CrossRef]
14. Zhu, J.; Yang, H.; Liu, N.; Kim, M.; Zhang, W.; Yang, M.-H. Online Multi-Object Tracking with Dual Matching Attention Networks. In Proceedings of the European Conference on Computer Vision (ECCV), Munich, Germany, 8–14 September 2018; pp. 379–396. [CrossRef]
15. Chen, B.; Li, P.; Sun, C.; Wang, D.; Yang, G.; Lu, H. Multi attention module for visual tracking. *Pattern Recognit.* **2018**, *87*, 80–93. [CrossRef]
16. Dwyer, B.; Nelson, J. Roboflow (Version 1.0). 2021. Available online: https://roboflow.com (accessed on 11 November 2021).
17. Makovski, T.; Jiang, Y.V. The role of visual working memory in attentive tracking of unique objects. *J. Exp. Psychol. Hum. Percept. Perform.* **2009**, *35*, 1687–1697. [CrossRef]
18. Qi, Y.; Wang, Y.; Xue, T. Brain Memory Inspired Template Updating Modeling for Robust Moving Object Tracking Using Particle Filter. In Proceedings of the International Conference on Brain Inspired Cognitive Systems, Shenyang, China, 11–14 July 2012; pp. 112–119. [CrossRef]
19. Wang, Y.; Qi, Y.; Li, Y. Memory-Based Multiagent Coevolution Modeling for Robust Moving Object Tracking. *Sci. World J.* **2013**, *2013*, 793013. [CrossRef]
20. Jiang, M.-X.; Deng, C.; Pan, Z.-G.; Wang, L.-F.; Sun, X. Multiobject Tracking in Videos Based on LSTM and Deep Reinforcement Learning. *Complexity* **2018**, *2018*, 4695890. [CrossRef]
21. Kim, C.; Li, F.; Rehg, J.M. Multi-object Tracking with Neural Gating Using Bilinear LSTM. In Proceedings of the European Conference on Computer Vision (ECCV), Munich, Germany, 8–14 September 2018; pp. 200–215. [CrossRef]
22. Wang, D.; Fang, H.; Liu, Y.; Wu, S.; Xie, Y.; Song, H. Improved RT-MDNet for panoramic video target tracking. *Harbin Gongye Daxue Xuebao J. Harbin Inst. Technol.* **2020**, *52*, 152–160. [CrossRef]
23. Grill-Spector, K.; Malach, R. The Human Visual Cortex. *Annu. Rev. Neurosci.* **2004**, *27*, 649–677. [CrossRef]
24. Wojke, N.; Bewley, A.; Paulus, D. Simple online and realtime tracking with a deep association metric. In Proceedings of the 2017 IEEE International Conference on Image Processing (ICIP), Beijing, China, 17–20 September 2017; pp. 3645–3649.
25. Iordanescu, L.; Grabowecky, M.; Suzuki, S. Demand-based dynamic distribution of attention and monitoring of velocities during multiple-object tracking. *J. Vis.* **2009**, *9*, 1. [CrossRef] [PubMed]
26. Welch, G.; Bishop, G. An Introduction to the Kalman Filter. *Practice* **2006**, *7*, 1–16.
27. Haller, S.; Bao, J.; Chen, N.; He, J.C.; Lu, F. The effect of blur adaptation on accommodative response and pupil size during reading. *J. Vis.* **2010**, *10*, 1. [CrossRef]
28. MOT Challenge. Available online: https://motchallenge.net/ (accessed on 16 May 2021).
29. Van Koppen, P.J.; Lochun, S.K. Portraying perpetrators: The validity of offender descriptions by witnesses. *Law Hum. Behav.* **1997**, *21*, 661–685. [CrossRef]
30. Sporer, S.L. An archival analysis of person descriptions. In *Biennial Meeting of the American Psychology-Law Society*; American Psychology-Law Society: San Diego, CA, USA, 1992.
31. Lin, T.-Y.; Maire, M.; Belongie, S.; Hays, J.; Perona, P.; Ramanan, D.; Dollár, P.; Zitnick, C.L. Microsoft COCO: Common Objects in Context. In *Lecture Notes in Computer Science (Including Subseries Lecture Notes in Artificial Intelligence and Lecture Notes in Bioinformatics)*; Springer: Berlin/Heidelberg, Germany, 2014. [CrossRef]
32. Deng, Y.; Luo, P.; Loy, C.C.; Tang, X. Pedestrian Attribute Recognition At Far Distance. In Proceedings of the 2014 ACM Conference on Multimedia. Association for Computing Machinery, Orlando, FL, USA, 3–7 November 2014; pp. 789–792. [CrossRef]
33. Mehrabi, N.; Morstatter, F.; Saxena, N.; Lerman, K.; Galstyan, A. A Survey on Bias and Fairness in Machine Learning. *ACM Comput. Surv.* **2021**, *54*, 1–35. [CrossRef]

34. Buolamwini, J. Gender Shades: Intersectional Accuracy Disparities in Commercial Gender Classification. In Proceedings of the the 1st Conference on Fairness, Accountability and Transparency, New York, NY, USA, 23–24 February 2018.
35. Klare, B.F.; Klein, B.; Taborsky, E.; Blanton, A.; Cheney, J.; Allen, K.; Grother, P.; Mah, A.; Burge, M.; Jain, A.K. Pushing the frontiers of unconstrained face detection and recognition: IARPA Janus Benchmark A. In Proceedings of the IEEE Conference on Computer Vision and Pattern Recognition, Boston, MA, USA, 7–12 June 2015; pp. 1931–1939. [CrossRef]
36. Forsyth, D. Object Detection with Discriminatively Trained Part-Based Models. *Computer* **2014**, *47*, 6–7. [CrossRef]
37. Hosang, J.; Benenson, R.; Schiele, B. Learning Non-maximum Suppression. In Proceedings of the 2017 IEEE Conference on Computer Vision and Pattern Recognition (CVPR), Honolulu, HI, USA, 21–26 July 2017; pp. 6469–6477. [CrossRef]
38. Redmon, J.; Divvala, S.; Girshick, R.; Farhadi, A. You Only Look Once: Unified, Real-Time Object Detection. In Proceedings of the IEEE Computer Society Conference on Computer Vision and Pattern Recognition, Las Vegas, NV, USA, 27–30 June 2016; pp. 779–788.
39. Viola, P.; Jones, M. Rapid object detection using a boosted cascade of simple features. In Proceedings of the 2001 IEEE Computer Society Conference on Computer Vision and Pattern Recognition, Kauai, HI, USA, 8–14 December 2001. [CrossRef]
40. Bochkovskiy, A.; Wang, C.-Y.; Liao, H.-Y.M. YOLOv4: Optimal Speed and Accuracy of Object Detection. *arXiv* **2020**, arXiv:2004.10934.
41. Wang, C.-Y.; Bochkovskiy, A.; Liao, H.-Y.M. Scaled-YOLOv4: Scaling Cross Stage Partial Network. In Proceedings of the IEEE/CVF Conference on Computer Vision and Pattern Recognition, Nashville, TN, USA, 19–25 June 2021; pp. 13024–13033. [CrossRef]
42. Bae, S.-H.; Yoon, K.-J. Confidence-Based Data Association and Discriminative Deep Appearance Learning for Robust Online Multi-Object Tracking. *IEEE Trans. Pattern Anal. Mach. Intell.* **2017**, *40*, 595–610. [CrossRef]
43. Mottaghi, R.; Chen, X.; Liu, X.; Cho, N.-G.; Lee, S.-W.; Fidler, S.; Urtasun, R.; Yuille, A. The Role of Context for Object Detection and Semantic Segmentation in the Wild. In Proceedings of the 2014 IEEE Conference on Computer Vision and Pattern Recognition, Columbus, OH, USA, 23–28 June 2014; Institute of Electrical and Electronics Engineers (IEEE): Piscatway, NY, USA, 2014; pp. 891–898.
44. Jefferies, E. The neural basis of semantic cognition: Converging evidence from neuropsychology, neuroimaging and TMS. *Cortex* **2013**, *49*, 611–625. [CrossRef]
45. Gainotti, G. The organization and dissolution of semantic-conceptual knowledge: Is the 'amodal hub' the only plausible model? *Brain Cogn.* **2011**, *75*, 299–309. [CrossRef]
46. Franconeri, S.; Jonathan, S.; Scimeca, J. Tracking Multiple Objects Is Limited Only by Object Spacing, Not by Speed, Time, or Capacity. *Psychol. Sci.* **2010**, *21*, 920–925. [CrossRef]
47. Bernardin, K.; Stiefelhagen, R. Evaluating Multiple Object Tracking Performance: The CLEAR MOT Metrics. *EURASIP J. Image Video Process.* **2008**, *2008*, 246309. [CrossRef]
48. Ristani, E.; Solera, F.; Zou, R.; Cucchiara, R.; Tomasi, C. Performance Measures and a Data Set for Multi-target, Multi-camera Tracking. In Proceedings of the European Conference on Computer Vision, Amsterdam, The Netherlands, 11–14 October 2016; pp. 17–35. [CrossRef]
49. Benchmarking the Major Cloud Vision AutoML Tools. Available online: https://blog.roboflow.com/automl-vs-rekognition-vs-custom-vision/ (accessed on 3 April 2021).
50. Open Images V6—Description. Available online: https://storage.googleapis.com/openimages/web/factsfigures.html (accessed on 14 May 2021).
51. Dai, P.; Weng, R.; Choi, W.; Zhang, C.; He, Z.; Ding, W. Learning a Proposal Classifier for Multiple Object Tracking. In Proceedings of the IEEE/CVF Conference on Computer Vision and Pattern Recognition, Nashville, TN, USA, 19–25 June 2021; pp. 2443–2452. [CrossRef]
52. Braso, G.; Leal-Taixe, L. Learning a Neural Solver for Multiple Object Tracking. In Proceedings of the IEEE Computer Society Conference on Computer Vision and Pattern Recognition, Seattle, WA, USA, 16–18 June 2020; pp. 6246–6256. [CrossRef]
53. Papakis, I.; Sarkar, A.; Karpatne, A. GCNNMatch: Graph Convolutional Neural Networks for Multi-Object Tracking via Sinkhorn Normalization. *arXiv* **2020**, arXiv:2010.00067.
54. Bergmann, P.; Meinhardt, T.; Leal-Taixe, L. Tracking Without Bells and Whistles. In Proceedings of the IEEE International Conference on Computer Vision, Seoul, Korea, 27 October–2 November 2019. [CrossRef]
55. Bewley, A.; Ge, Z.; Ott, L.; Ramos, F.; Upcroft, B. Simple online and realtime tracking. In Proceedings of the 2016 IEEE International Conference on Image Processing (ICIP), Phoenix, AZ, USA, 25–28 September 2016; pp. 3464–3468. [CrossRef]

sensors

MDPI

Article

The Role of Diffusion Tensor MR Imaging (DTI) of the Brain in Diagnosing Autism Spectrum Disorder: Promising Results

Yaser ElNakieb [1,†], Mohamed T. Ali [1,†], Ahmed Elnakib [1], Ahmed Shalaby [1], Ahmed Soliman [1], Ali Mahmoud [1], Mohammed Ghazal [2], Gregory Neal Barnes [3], and Ayman El-Baz [1,*]

1 Bioengineering Department, University of Louisville, Louisville, KY 40292, USA; y.elnakieb@louisville.edu (Y.E.); mtali003@louisville.edu (M.T.A.); aaelna02@louisville.edu (A.E.); ahmed.shalaby@louisville.edu (A.S.); ahmed.soliman@louisville.edu (A.S.); ahmahm01@louisville.edu (A.M.)
2 Department of Electrical and Computer Engineering, Abu Dhabi University, Abu Dhabi 59911, United Arab Emirates; mohammed.ghazal@adu.ac.ae
3 Department of Neurology Pediatric Research Institute, University of Louisville, Louisville, KY 40202, USA; gregory.barnes@louisville.edu
* Correspondence: aselba01@louisville.edu
† These authors contributed equally to this work.

Abstract: Autism spectrum disorder (ASD) is a combination of developmental anomalies that causes social and behavioral impairments, affecting around 2% of US children. Common symptoms include difficulties in communications, interactions, and behavioral disabilities. The onset of symptoms can start in early childhood, yet repeated visits to a pediatric specialist are needed before reaching a diagnosis. Still, this diagnosis is usually subjective, and scores can vary from one specialist to another. Previous literature suggests differences in brain development, environmental, and/or genetic factors play a role in developing autism, yet scientists still do not know exactly the pathology of this disorder. Currently, the gold standard diagnosis of ASD is a set of diagnostic evaluations, such as the Autism Diagnostic Observation Schedule (ADOS) or Autism Diagnostic Interview–Revised (ADI-R) report. These gold standard diagnostic instruments are an intensive, lengthy, and subjective process that involves a set of behavioral and communications tests and clinical history information conducted by a team of qualified clinicians. Emerging advancements in neuroimaging and machine learning techniques can provide a fast and objective alternative to conventional repetitive observational assessments. This paper provides a thorough study of implementing feature engineering tools to find discriminant insights from brain imaging of white matter connectivity and using a machine learning framework for an accurate classification of autistic individuals. This work highlights important findings of impacted brain areas that contribute to an autism diagnosis and presents promising accuracy results. We verified our proposed framework on a large publicly available DTI dataset of 225 subjects from the Autism Brain Imaging Data Exchange-II (ABIDE-II) initiative, achieving a high global balanced accuracy over the 5 sites of up to 99% with 5-fold cross validation. The data used was slightly unbalanced, including 125 autistic subjects and 100 typically developed (TD) ones. The achieved balanced accuracy of the proposed technique is the highest in the literature, which elucidates the importance of feature engineering steps involved in extracting useful knowledge and the promising potentials of adopting neuroimaging for the diagnosis of autism.

Keywords: autism spectrum disorder (ASD); DTI; neuroimaging; ABIDE-II; diagnosis

Citation: ElNakieb, Y.; Ali, M.; Elnakib, A.; Shalaby, A.; Soliman, A.; Mahmoud, A.; Barnes, G.; El-Baz, A. The Role of Diffusion Tensor MR Imaging (DTI) of the Brain in Diagnosing Autism Spectrum Disorder: Promising Results. *Sensors* **2021**, *21*, 8171. https://doi.org/10.3390/s21248171

Academic Editor: Loris Nanni

Received: 10 November 2021
Accepted: 4 December 2021
Published: 7 December 2021

1. Introduction

Autism spectrum disorder (ASD), famously known as just autism, is a pervasive developmental disorder manifested as problems in social interactions and communications, both verbal and non-verbal [1–3]. While there are no fully known causes of autism etiology, many hypotheses and theories exist. Regardless of the minutiae, it is believed that autism is a complex interaction between different genetic and environmental factors [4]. Current approved diagnosis techniques require significant clinical experience, assessing different aspects via a standard testing/scoring system, such as the ADOS [5] or ADI-R [6]. Those tests are subjective and can be time consuming and challenging, with limited accuracy of around 80–85% [7]. Furthermore, clinicians may not always agree with the results of those tests [8]. This is our main motivation for developing a neuroimaging-based alternative that can provide a non-subjective evaluation that may help clinicians reach a faster, more reliable diagnosis. Previous neurobiological studies investigated connections between ASD and underlying structure, trying to describe brain abnormalities associated with autism traits. Since the emergence of MRI, plenty of studies appeared to investigate connections between ASD and underlying brain features, either shape and volume features using structural MRI [9], or white matter (WM) diffusivity [10] anomalies using DTI, while others performed correlations of ASD with either task-based or resting-state functionality [11] using functional MRI (fMRI). In this paper, we will introduce our DTI-based algorithm for assessing ASD with the help of the ABIDE-II dataset.

DTI has been gaining rising popularity through the past couple of decades, especially for brain related disorders, as it provides a non-invasive way of characterizing the connective tracts inside the brain between different areas. It quantifies the diffusion patterns inside the white matter (WM). White matter mainly consists of axons of neurons (nerve fibers), and with the human brain containing hundreds of billions of neurons, the structure of WM is truly complex. The WM represents the axonal fibers carrying neural signals between various brain regions and between the brain and spinal cord through the brainstem. The organization of such a complex network contains a wealth of information; still, the current resolution for conventional MRI technologies cannot capture such small details, which are typically less than a micrometer to only few micrometers. Nevertheless, DTI provides diffusion measures that gives information about the tractography of the brain.

DTI's most used parameters [12] include fractional anisotropy (FA), mean diffusivity (MD), and sometimes also "radial" and "axial" diffusivities. These parameters actually describe the diffusion of water inside the brain, and since water diffusion is restricted outside of fiber tracts, this translates into indirect information regarding the micro-structure and connectivity of WM [13]. Additionally, some derived features are also used to characterize other diffusion measures in WM tracts, such as tensor trace, skewness, rotational invariance, and many others [14]. Abounding previous literature has noted WM abnormalities associated with autism, often as differences in WM micro-architecture across some local brain areas. For instance, differences in FA values were reported by Wolff et al. [15] between ASD and typically developed (TD) infants. Using DTI, Barnea et al. [11] compared WM structure of ASD to normal TD, accounting for IQ, age and gender. They reported reduced FA in areas affiliated with social cognition in ASD, but found no difference for MD values. The role of MD values was identified by Alexander et al. [10], as they reported reduced FA values backed by an overall increase in MD across the corpus callosum for ASD vs. non-ASD individuals. Lee et al. [16] also reported higher MD values accompanied with reduced FA in autistic subjects, as well as higher radial diffusivity. In [17], a sample of 38 infants from the Infant Brain Imaging Study (IBIS) were used for the diagnosis of autism using spherical harmonics. Another study of ASD children [18] found, again, significantly lower FA in ASD subjects and correspondingly greater MD in frontal lobe WM. A separate study of 45 autistic subjects and 30 TDs manifested diagnostic potential when the authors split ASD to language impaired and non-language impaired groups based on FA and MD, achieving an accuracy of up to 80% [19].

Aside from classical analysis studies, plenty of studies have employed ML techniques for ASD classification. The whole ABIDE-I f-MRI dataset was tested with a refined deep learning model that was introduced by Heinsfeld et al. [20] that exceeded the previous state-of-the-art performance, achieving 70% accuracy. Khosla [21] presented another deep learning algorithm using a volumetric convolutional neural network that fits non-linear predictive models on 3D resting state fMRI (rs-fMRI) input and recorded a classification accuracy of up to 73% on ABIDE-I rs-fMRI data. In [22], the authors proposed framework exploiting features from both structural MRI (sMRI) and fMRI applied on 185 subjects from the National Database for Autism Research (NDAR), achieving 81% accuracy fusing both modalities. While most of those works relied on sMRI and/or fMRI, the focus of our paper is using DTI. DTI micro-architectural features were incorporated in another large recent study on 263 NDAR subjects for the diagnosis of autism, achieving accuracy of up to 73% [23]. Up to now, most of the published work regarding autism classification used ABIDE-I, and very few studies used newer ABIDE-II data [21,24–26]. One study used one site of ABIDE-II only (San Diego State University cohort), and employed both fMRI and DTI imaging modalities using connectome features, accomplishing an accuracy of 72% [27]. We emphasize that the need to use more than one modality implicates added cost and scanning time. Another key contribution of this work is finding a best-fit dimensionality reduction technique. Having a very large feature space (p) with limited sample space, or subjects, in our case (n), is commonly known as the curse of dimensionality [28], which causes increased complexity of the models that easily results in overfitting, with less learning captured by the model. This phenomenon is very common with MRI imaging and medical data, where we have piles of data fields for a few number of patients, and sometimes is not handled correctly. The standard way to handle those data is by exploiting some sort of feature reduction algorithms such as linear discriminant analysis (LDA) [29], principal component analysis (PCA) [30], or auto-encoders [20]. The common shortcoming is that they usually do not keep the interpretation of the original feature in the new feature space, making it hard to explain clinical connections for any classification decision, and thus, making it less attractive for a practical medical use. The feature reduction method needs to help clinicians make an informative decision and aid in understanding the pathological abnormalities of the brain of autistic subjects. Our work investigates the recursive feature elimination (RFE) technique, which recursively eliminates the least contributing features for classification, ending with a best subset. We extensively carried out plethora of experiments to reach a near-optimal configuration that led to the best classification, as validated on our dataset.

Despite the numerous studies of autism-related changes in white matter integrity, the objective of this work is to implement a comprehensive ML-CAD system that, besides its ability to classify ASD vs. TD subjects, identifies brain areas correlated with autism, and was validated on a big, publicly available dataset using DTI data. The proposed algorithm employed a thorough feature selection using recursive feature elimination with cross-validation (RFE-CV) using four different kernels (SVM with linear kernel (LSVM), random forest (RF), and logistic regression (LR), either with a l_1-norm (LR1), or LR with l_2-norm (LR2)), and performed hyper-parameter optimization on eight different classification techniques. The best candidate configurations were validated using random splits of different k-folds' cross-validation to identify the global ML model alongside the global imaging bio-markers associated with ASD. Our main motivation behind this work is to present a reliable system that can help physicians better understand individuals with autism, allowing earlier and more personalized treatment plans. The rest of this paper is organized as follows: Section 2 presents the details of the pipeline of the proposed algorithm, while the experimental results are introduced in Section 3 for the ABIDE-II diffusion MRI data. Finally, Section 4 provides a discussion and the conclusions of the paper.

2. Methodology

A visualization of the pipeline of the whole framework is presented in Figure 1. It starts with pre-processing of each subject's input volumes, and is then followed by DTI parameter calculations, feature extraction and mapping to a WM atlas to get local features. This is followed by using two different feature representations, to be used in feature selection and classification steps. The following subsections provide details of these multi-stage processes until reaching a final diagnosis.

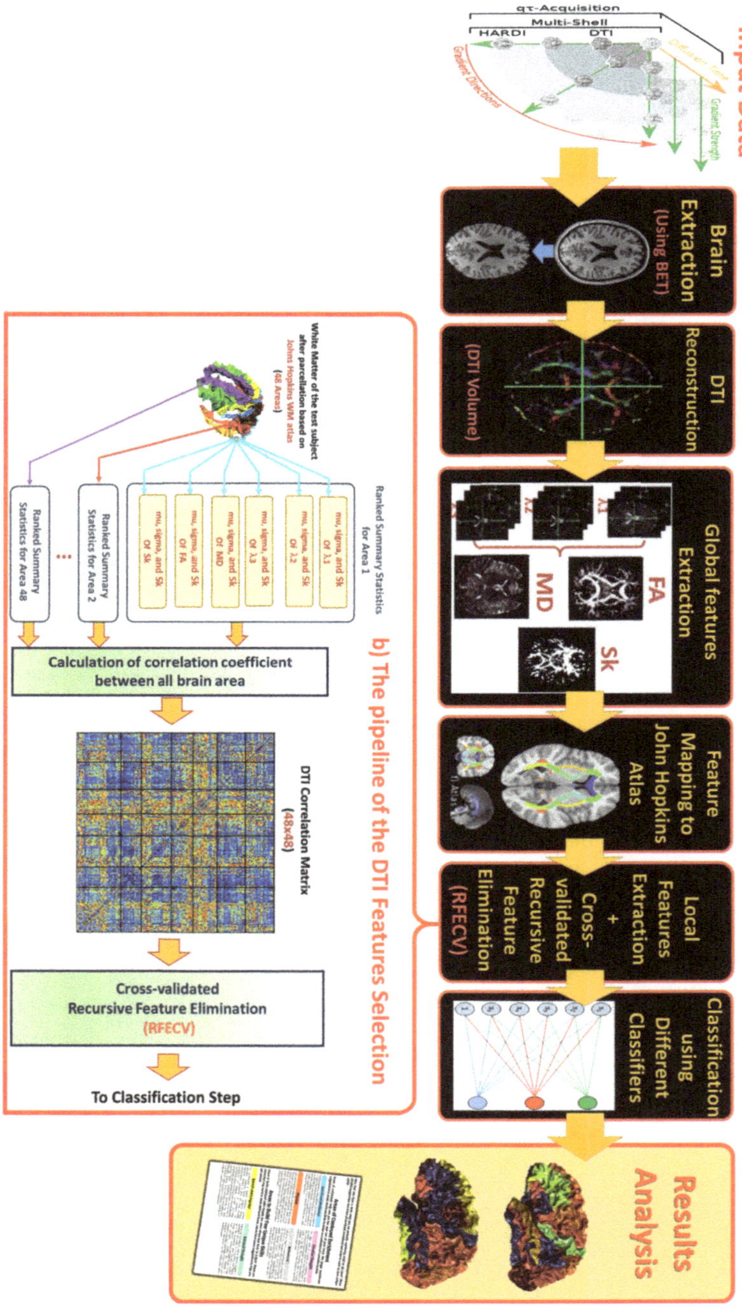

Figure 1. (**a**) Pipeline of the DTI-diagnosis algorithm. (**b**) Usage of the new derived feature representation $\hat{F}$ and feature selection before classification.

2.1. Data Used

This work utilized DTI data from the Autism Brain Imaging Data Exchange (ABIDE)-II dataset. ABIDE-II is a recent publicly available dataset that aggregates MRI data (sMRI, fMRI, and DTI) for autism studies across different multiple sites. ABIDE-II contains data from around 19 sites for more than 1000 subjects; half of them are autistic individuals. Working on a publicly available dataset facilitates replicating results and increases the reliability of our findings. ABIDE-II is considered a large dataset, which increases the power of our study. We selected datasets that involved DTI data, which included 6 datasets, namely: Barrow Neurological Institute (BNI), NYU Langone Medical Center 1 (NYU1), NYU Langone Medical Center sample 2 (NYU2), San Diego State University (SDSU), Institut Pasteur and Robert Debré Hospital (IP), and Trinity Centre for Health Sciences (TCD). IP DTI data bvals (diffusion gradient strength per volume values) and bvecs (diffusion gradient directions per volume values) were missing a value, so we excluded it, and used the remaining five sites. Those 5 sites originally had 284 subjects with DTI imaging data, and ended with 225 subjects of them after cleaning the data, on which we applied the steps of our pipeline, as we will elaborate on in the next subsections.

2.2. *Pre-Processing*

2.2.1. Input Image Preparation

After deciding which sites to work on, we downloaded their available data, which came organized as folders labeled by subject ID containing imaging data. We located subjects that had DTI data, copying the relevant image nii files along with bvals and bvecs to the working directory to be pre-processed.

2.2.2. Skull Stripping

The goal of the skull stripping step is to remove non-brain tissues (e.g., skull, scalp, dura, ...) from the image volumes, extracting only the brain. This automated process was implemented using the brain extraction tool (BET) algorithm [31] from FSL tools, generating the binary masks and using default parameters with a fractional intensity threshold of 0.25.

2.2.3. Eddy Current Correction

Eddy currents are induced currents due to gradient fields in the x, y, z directions that result in visible image artifacts that usually blur the boundaries between gray and white matter. Diffusion-weighted imaging is usually affected by this phenomenon, and an eddy current correction step is commonly implemented. For this purpose, we used the eddy current correction tool 'eddy' available through FSL [32] to correct for both common artifacts, including adjusting for induced currents and also for subject movement during the scan, across sections.

2.3. *Feature Calculation*

After having the diffusion-weighted volumes cleaned of non-brain tissues and common artifacts, we run DTI calculations to get the DTI diffusion tensor, its eigenvalues, and other metrics. For each voxel, diffusion can be represented by a 3 by 3 tensor, which describes the diffusion pattern at each point in 3D space. From this tensor, a more common metric, namely eigenvalues, is used to represent the magnitude of diffusion along 3 major perpendicular directions of its eigenvectors. The largest eigenvalue, λ_1, along with its eigenvector, v_1, represent the magnitude and direction of the primary direction of diffusion (along the fiber tract), while the other two represent radial diffusion perpendicular to the main one [33]. Other derived metrics, such as fractional anisotropy, mean diffusivity, skewness, and many others are commonly used to represent other characteristics of the diffusion. In our work, we included the following 6 metrics to describe our white matter micro-architecture:

1. Fractional anisotropy (FA): Measures the degree of anisotropy of the diffusion, with zero representing completely isotropic diffusion, and one representing a directional diffusion [33];
2. Mean diffusivity (MD): Average magnitude of diffusion at each point, independent of the direction. $MD = \frac{1}{3}\sum_{i=1}^{3}\lambda_i$;

3. Axial diffusivity (AD): Magnitude of diffusion along the major axis; AD $= \lambda_1$;
4. & 5. Radial diffusivities: Magnitude of diffusion along the two perpendicular axes to AD: RDs = $[\lambda_2, \lambda_3]$;
6. Tensor skewness: A higher order moment of diffusion, revealing more information not captured by lower order ones. [14];
TSkew $= \frac{1}{3}\sum_{i=1}^{3}(\lambda_i - MD)^3$.

For the first five features, the dtifit tool, part of the FSL package, was used to calculate the diffusion tensors along with eigenvalues, eigenvectors, FA, and MD. Tensor skewness (Tskew) was calculated using Matlab 2021a, as it was not provided through the previous tool. At this point, each subject is represented by six volumes, each comprising hundreds of thousands of raw voxel values.

Data Cleaning

In the previous parts of the pipeline, some subjects failed during volume size validation, BET and DTI calculations, or regional feature extraction, either with an error in the prepossessing or yielding a non-complete brain, identified by having more zero values, or "blanks", than it should. Excluding those subject from further processing, we ended up with 225 subjects that will be used for the rest of this work. Subject IDs along with age, label, IQ, and gender for all subjects used in this study are provided as a Supplemental Material, Table S3.

2.4. Atlas-Based Segmentation

Having each subject represented by its six volumes per voxel feature, now we need to assign those features to local brain areas. For this purpose, the white matter atlas ICBM-DTI-81, defined by Johns Hopkins University [34], is used. The JHU ICBM-DTI-81 WM atlas uses ICBM coordinates and defines 48 white matter areas. Those areas were originally hand-segmented from the average of diffusion MRI tensors of different 81 subjects. To locate local anatomical regions in each subject space, we implemented an atlas-based segmentation approach, where we preformed atlas registration for area localization. Registration from the atlas space to subject's space was performed in two iterations: a rigid transformation then an affine transformation. The objective of the rigid registration in the first iteration is just to find an initial alignment, not changing the size or shape, that will be used for next step. Then, an affine transformation is found to improve upon the initial estimation by providing a higher degree of freedom for a more generic linear transformation that enables the object's size and shape to be adjusted. This two-step registration task was implemented using DTI-TK software [35] using normalized mutual information measures with a 4 mm $\times$ 4 mm $\times$ 4 mm sampling distance and 1% tolerance. DTI-TK also enables interoperability with FSL software used in preprocessing. The found transformation was then applied to atlas labels, hence providing WM areas mask at each subject space. Those masks were used to define local features for those 48 areas. This segmentation technique provides a fast automated solution, enabling easy application to new subjects or datasets, with less error.

2.5. Feature Representation

At this point, each subject is represented by six features per 48 areas. Each of those features are per-voxel raw features, and their length, in tens of thousands, varies between areas. The first step is to convert those raw features into a better representation with the goal of reducing the number while keeping the most important aspects capturing underlying information. For this purpose, we replaced per-voxel features of each area with three summary statistics of underlying distribution, namely, the mean (μ), standard deviation (σ), and skewness (sk), where μ aims to the capture central tendency, σ captures the dispersion of values around this mean, and sk aims to measure the asymmetry of the data around this mean. At the end of this step, our feature matrix F, for each subject i, can be represented as a 48 by 18 matrix, as follows:

$$F_i = \begin{bmatrix} \mu_{FA_1} & \sigma_{FA_1} & sk_{FA_1} & \cdots & sk_{Tskew_1} \\ \mu_{FA_2} & \sigma_{FA_2} & sk_{FA_2} & \cdots & sk_{Tskew_2} \\ \vdots & \vdots & \vdots & \ddots & \vdots \\ \mu_{FA_{48}} & \sigma_{FA_{48}} & sk_{FA_{48}} & \cdots & sk_{Tskew_{48}} \end{bmatrix}$$

where F_i is the feature matrix for subject i using the first feature representation described above. Each element in this matrix is a summary statistic (baseline: $\mu/\sigma/sk$) for one of the six features (subscript: FA/MD/Tskew) for an area from 1 to 48 (sub-subscript index).

2.5.1. Feature Engineering

Instead of directly using per-area summary statistics features, we developed an enhanced representation that captures latent relative relationships between brain areas. We calculated Pearson correlation coefficient between each pair of brain areas l, m, and use this correlation matrix as our feature matrix. Therefore, for each subject i, $\rho_{l,m} = corr(F_i(l,:), F_i(m,:))$. Although this step increased the number of features per subject slightly [from 48 × 18 = 864 to (48 × 47/2) = 1128], it helped in boosting the performance of the classification, as we will see in the results. This novel representation, using interactions, is considered a key contribution that helped in improving the performance. The new second feature matrix F_{2_i} for subject i is now represented by:

$$F_{2\_i} = \begin{bmatrix} \rho_{1,1} & \rho_{1,2} & \cdots & \rho_{1,48} \\ \rho_{2,1} & \rho_{2,2} & \cdots & \rho_{2,48} \\ \vdots & \vdots & \ddots & \vdots \\ \rho_{48,1} & \rho_{48,2} & \cdots & \rho_{48,48} \end{bmatrix}$$

where each element in this matrix $\rho_{i,j}$ is a correlation between the summary statistics vectors of the two areas i, j. We highlight that only the upper triangle (U) of this new feature matrix (or lower L, because of symmetry) is used in subsequent steps, as the rest is redundant because of symmetry. Serializing those 1128 features, we can represent the final feature matrix for all 225 subjects as $\hat{F}$ with size 225 × 1128, where each row is the concatenated calculated correlations for one subject. Figure 1b illustrates those steps. In addition to the data matrix, we have another column vector y denoting the labels of each subject, whether ASD (y_i = 1) or TD (y_i = 0).

$$y = \begin{bmatrix} y_1, & y_2, & y_3, & \cdots, & y_{225} \end{bmatrix}$$

2.5.2. Feature Reduction: RFE-CV

The feature space (1128 correlations) is quite large relative to our sample size (225 subjects). As we discussed earlier, the number of features relative to the number of subjects needs to be reduced, keeping the most informative features. While many feature reduction techniques, such as linear discriminant analysis, principal component analysis, or autoencoders, can perform this task, they transform the feature space into a new one that does not preserve the meanings of the original features. Building classification systems based on those new ambiguous features would sophisticate the ability to understand any clinical reasoning of classification results, hence making it less beneficial and reasonable to physicians in generating an informative decision or understanding the underlying pathological abnormalities of an autistic brain. We employed the recursive feature elimination (RFE) technique, where only a subset of features is selected. RFE is a feature selection algorithm based on feature ranking with recursive feature elimination. The principle behind RFE is fitting a classification model, ranking the features by the model's scoring, then eliminating the weakest features recursively to find the optimal number of features to be selected. Cross validation is used with RFE (RFE-CV), where data is split into k-folds, features are scored based on different data subsets, and then the best scoring across the k-folds is selected. The target optimization scoring metric (whether accuracy, balanced accuracy, $f1$, weighted

$f1$, precision, recall, ...) can be specified, and here, we used balanced accuracy with $k = 10$ folds for optimization. The algorithm then finds the optimal n significant features to be selected that maximizes the average classification performance according to the target metric [36,37]. To find the best architecture of RFE-CV that best fits our problem, we tested four types of RFE-CV classifiers as kernels, namely linear SVM (LSVM), random forest (RF), logistic regression (LR) with l_1-norm (LR1), and LR with l_2-norm (LR2), on the two feature representations we have (original summary statistics F_i of 225×864 and correlations F_{2_i} of 225×1128). Thus, we obtained estimates using four different models, each selecting features according to its classifier independently, and providing average cross-validated scores for 10-folds; then we evaluated the performance of eight models to select which model to use for further processing.

2.6. Classification

After having n selected features for each of 8 models representing the top prominent features for distinguishing autistic brains, we set up a system of machine learning classifiers. We tested eight different classifier types, and performed hyper-parameter optimization for each one to end up with best parameter classifier model in terms of accuracy. We included both linear and non-linear classifiers to test both types of relationships between the two classes. The set of used classifiers are: (1) linear SVM (LSVM), (2) logistic regression (LR), (3) passive aggressive classifier (PAGG), (4) SVM with radial-basis kernel (RBF-SVM), (5) Gaussian naive Bayes (GNB), (6) random forest (RF), (7) XGboost (XGB), and (8) neural networks (NN). Classifiers 1–3 are linear classifiers, while the rest are non-linear. Classifiers 6 and 7 are ensemble-based classifiers, and for NN we included both shallow and deep configurations in our hyper-parameter search. For hyper-parameter optimization, after we selected only n features according to the previous RFE-CV step, we tested a set of different parameters with different ranges for each classifier. For this purpose, the input data is split into five folds to determine the best performance according to the average across those five folds. Therefore, for each classifier, using the selected features only, the following steps were performed: (i) split data into five folds, use four for training and one for testing each time, and for each parameters configuration, store the performance of the classifier for each fold; (ii) The balanced accuracy scoring is used to decide the best configuration; (iii) The best performing classifier is selected, and the hyper parameters along with its maximum average cross-validated score, and also standard deviation over folds, are highlighted. Table 1 shows the set of used hyper-parameters in the search associated with each classifier and their ranges. Algorithm 1 illustrates a step-by-step guide of the full implemented algorithm, and Figure 1 summarizes a graphical illustration of the pipeline of the entire system.

Table 1. Used hyper-parameter values in a cross-validated grid search. Names between parentheses are parameter names in the ML package.

Classifier	Hyper-Parameter	Range/ Values
(1) LSVM	Regularization (C)	0.1, 1, 5, 10
	Loss function (loss)	L1, L2
	Penalization strategy (penalty)	squared_hinge, hinge
(2) LR	Penalization strategy (penalty)	L1, L2 elastic
	Regularization (C)	0.1, 1, 5, 10
	Solver algorithm (solver)	newton-cg, lbfgs, liblinear, sag, saga
(3) PassiveAgressive	Regularization (C)	0.1, 1, 5, 10
	N idle iteration before stop (n_iter_no_change)	1, 5, 10
(4) Nonlinear-SVM	Regularization (C)	0.1, 1, 5, 10
	Kernel used (kernel)	rbf, poly, sigmoid
	Polynomial kernel degree (degree)	2–6
	Kernel coefficient (gamma)	scale, auto
	Independent term in kernel function (coef0)	0.0, 0.01, 0.1, 1, 5, 10, 50, 100

Table 1. *Cont.*

Classifier	Hyper-Parameter	Range/ Values
(5) GNB	Default parameters	priors = None, var_smoothing = 1×10^{-9}
(6) RF	Number of features to consider when looking for the best split (max_features)	auto, sqrt, log2
	Number of trees in the forest (n_estimators)	50, 100, 200, 500, 1000
	Function to measure the quality of a split (criterion)	gini, entropy
	Bootstrap samples when building trees (bootstrap)	True, False
	Min # of samples required to split an internal node (min_samples)	1, 2, 5, 10
(7) XGB	Which booster to use (booster)	gbtree, gblinear, dart
	Learning rate (learning_rate)	0.001, 0.01, 0.1, 0.3, 0.5, 1
	Min loss reduction required to make a further partition on a leaf node (gamma)	0, 0.1, 0.5, 1, 1.5, 2, 5, 20, 50, 100
	Min sum of instance weight needed in a child (min_child_weight)	0.1,0.5, 1, 5, 10
	Subsample ratio of columns when constructing each tree (colsample_bytree)	0.6, 0.8, 1.0
	L2 regularization term on weights (lambda)	0, 0.001, 0.5, 1, 10
	L1 regularization term on weights (alpha)	0, 0.001, 0.5, 1, 10
(8) NN	Hidden layer sizes (hidden_layer_sizes)	(150,100,50,), (100,50,25,), (100,)
	Activation function (activation)	tanh, relu, logistic
	Solver used for weight optimization (solver)	lbfgs, sgd, adam
	L2 regularization penalty (alpha)	0.0001,0.001,0.01, 0.05, 0.1, 0.5
	Initial learning rate (learning_rate)	constant, adaptive
	Exponential decay rate for estimates of first moment vector in adam (beta_1)	0, 0.001, 0.01, 0.1, 0.3, 0.5, 0.9
	Exponential decay rate for estimates of second moment vector in adam (beta_2)	0, 0.001, 0.01, 0.1, 0.3, 0.5, 0.9

Algorithm 1 Diffusion tensor autism diagnosis algorithm.

$\forall$ **subject's data files: (NII+bval+bvec)** :
1. Check for errors, check bval and bvec files.
2. run pre-processing modules:
(i) Run skull stripping using brain extraction tool (BET).
(ii) Run FSL's eddy current correction tool.
(iii) Register the DTI IIT Human Brain Atlas to each subject space using DTI-TK tool, save transformations.
(iv) Recheck for any generated errors or deformations.
3. Feature Calculations:
(i) Use FSL to calculate DTI tensor, scale units, calculate RDs, AD, FA, MD, Tskew volumes.
(ii) Apply resulted transformation on the JHU atlas labels to generate masks.
(iv) Use registered masks to extract each feature for each WM region.
(v) Calculate summary statistics (μ, σ, Sk) for each area for each feature (λ_1,λ_2,λ_3,FA,MD, Tskew), rank feature values across the different 48 brain areas, get a concatenated feature vector (3*6). Create feature matrix F to be used as a first variant of the input data matrix X.
(vi) Calculate correlations between feature vectors of each two areas to create feature matrix F_2.
(vii) From F_2: remove redundant correlations (L and diagonal) and concatenate U to create $\hat{F}$ to be used as a second variant of the input data matrix X.
4. RFECV feature selection: for each feature representation, and for each RFE-CV kernel:
(i) Split input data X, labels y into k folds. Each time use one fold as X_{test}, y_{test}, rest as X_{train}, y_{train}.
(ii) Train the classifier using each X_{train}, y_{train}.
(iii) Get the balanced accuracy score of the trained classifier using X_{test}, y_{test}.
(iv) Calculate the cross-validated score and sort features based on importance.
(v) Remove the least important features from X matrices, and repeat the steps from (i) to (v) until only one feature exists.
(vi) Determine the n features that provided the best cross-validated score along with its hyper-parameters to be used for each of the kernels.
5. Classification:
$\forall$ classifier, for each configuration of hyper-parameters:
(i) Split reduced X_{select}, with n selected features, into k folds, along with y.
(ii) Calculate the cross-validated score for each hyper-parameter's configuration.
(iii) Determine best hyper-parameter configuration in terms of score for each classifier.
(iii) Find the best classifier/parameters, along with its used n features.

3. Results

As discussed in the data subsection, the ABIDE-II dataset [38] was used for the testing and validation of the above-mentioned methodology. ABIDE-II [38] provides hundreds of subjects' brain imaging data (structural MRI, functional MRI, and DTI) to enhance research in autism spectrum disorder (ASD). DTI data used are only from the following five sites: IP, NYU1, NYU2, TCD, and SDSU. Diffusion-weighted MRI (dwMRI) scans for a total of 225 subjects were used: 125 ASDs and 100 TDs, with age ranges between 5.128 years and 46.6 years.

The four types of RFE-CV kernels (LSVM, LR1, LR2, and RF) were used to select features from the two different representations (summary statistics F, and correlations $\hat{F}$), and those features were used to train and test eight types of classifiers (LSVM, LR, PAGG, RBFSVM, GNB, RF, XGB, and NN). The hyper-parameter optimization step was carried out for each combination of [feature-RFECV kernel-classifier], using a grid search over the list of hyper-parameters on Table 1 with five-fold cross validation with the help of the GridSearchCV scikit learn toolkit. The aim of this search was to identify the best RFE-CV kernel in terms of accuracy, to be used for the final classification/validation stage. Based on the results of those 64 sets of combinations, we identified which setting best suits our data, then we investigated it with more validations, changing the splits and varying the number of folds.

Tables S1 and S2 in the Supplementary Materials show the full details of this round of experiments for both feature representations: summary statistics F and correlations $\hat{F}$, respectively. We notice that both LR1 and LR2 kernels almost failed to provide representative features in terms of accuracy results (accuracy ~60%). While the RF kernel provided us with moderate results (mostly above 70%), LSVM was the one we were searching for, achieving accuracies of up to 99% with $\hat{F}$ features. More importantly, we highlight that using our novel feature representation $\hat{F}$, we were able to achieve this high boost in classification results. To show which types of features were more representative, we show the histogram of the occurrence of each type of summary statistics appearing in selected features from F with LSVM RFE-CV used in Figure 2. The figure illustrates the efficacy of adding SK feature which appeared as important as the common FA metric, and points out coice of skewness as a relevant summary statistic.

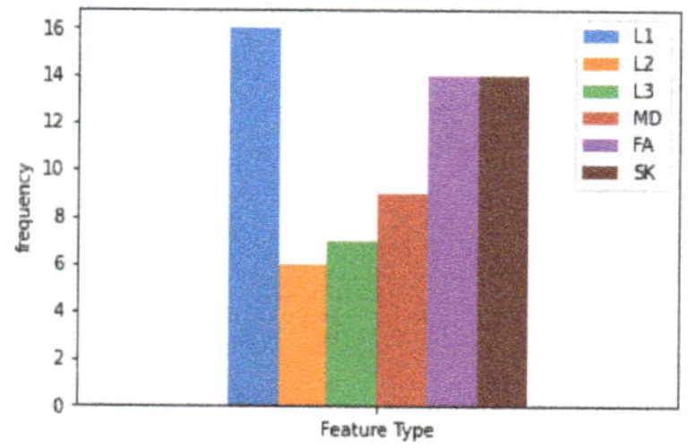

(a)

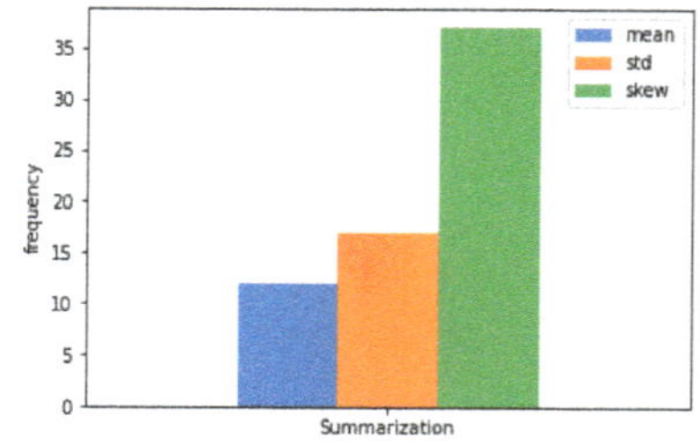

(b)

Figure 2. Histogram of types of selected summary statistic features. (**a**) for the occurances of each feature type, (**b**) for summary statistics occurrences.

Following these results, we will only use the LSVM RFE-CV kernel with $\hat{F}$ representation (correlations) for further investigations, as it shows better performance. We will fix the hyper-parameters of the eight classifiers to the ones we previously found on the first set of experiments (Table 2), and randomly re-split different settings of k-fold cross validation, with k = [2, 4, 5, 10], to test whether the achieved performance is highly dependent on the split and/or the subjects of previous experiment and see the effect of changing the proportion of train/test on the results.

Table 2. The fixed hyper-parameters found to optimize performance on the set of tested classifiers.

lSVM	{'penalty': 'l2', 'loss': 'hinge', 'C': 1}
pagg	{'n_iter_no_change': 5, 'C': 0.1}
LR	{'solver': 'newton-cg', 'penalty': 'none', 'C': 0.1}
XGB	{'reg_lambda': 0.001, 'reg_alpha': 0, 'min_child_weight': 10, 'learning_rate': 1, 'gamma': 0.1, 'colsample_bytree': 0.6, 'booster': 'gblinear'}
GNB	defaults
SVC	{'kernel': 'poly', 'gamma': 'scale', 'degree': 3, 'coef0': 5, 'C': 0.1}
Rf	{n_estimators': 50, 'min_samples_split': 2, 'min_samples_leaf': 0.1, 'max_features': 'sqrt', 'criterion': 'entropy', 'bootstrap': False}
nn	{'solver': 'adam', 'learning_rate': 'adaptive', 'hidden_layer_sizes': (100,), 'beta_2': 0.5, 'beta_1': 0.5, 'alpha': 0.0001, 'activation': 'logistic'}

Table 3 shows the final diagnostic accuracies of our proposed framework using our novel feature representation with the help of RFE-CV with the LSVM kernel, and Table 4 shows the area under the curve for each of the classifiers across different k-folds. Without a new optimization, using the same settings, and on new sets of random splits, our innovative algorithm was still able to provide up to 99% accuracy, which clearly manifested the strength of the presented algorithm.

Table 3. Mean accuracy ± standard deviation across the k-folds, with $k = 2, 4, 5, 10$.

	$k = 2$	$k = 4$	$k = 5$	$k = 10$
LSVM	0.92 ± 0.018	0.991 ± 0.015	0.999 ± 0.002	0.999 ± 0.002
pagg	0.893 ± 0.018	0.951 ± 0.037	0.96 ± 0.026	0.982 ± 0.03
LR	0.902 ± 0.0	0.964 ± 0.018	0.978 ± 0.02	0.991 ± 0.018
XGB	0.556 ± 0.011	0.604 ± 0.021	0.591 ± 0.041	0.609 ± 0.119
GNB	0.644 ± 0.025	0.618 ± 0.079	0.613 ± 0.08	0.684 ± 0.133
RBF-SVM	0.511 ± 0.038	0.529 ± 0.021	0.573 ± 0.022	0.582 ± 0.076
RF	0.609 ± 0.02	0.591 ± 0.04	0.591 ± 0.05	0.596 ± 0.054
NN	0.871 ± 0.004	0.969 ± 0.019	0.973 ± 0.026	0.964 ± 0.034

Table 4. Calculated area under the curve for each classifier across the k-folds, with $k = 2, 4, 5, 10$.

	$k = 2$	$k = 4$	$k = 5$	$k = 10$
LSVM	0.919	0.991	0.999	0.999
pagg	0.891	0.948	0.959	0.982
LR	0.9	0.962	0.977	0.991
XGB	0.543	0.593	0.583	0.606
GNB	0.644	0.618	0.608	0.683
RBF-SVM	0.509	0.529	0.565	0.575
RF	0.571	0.549	0.548	0.552
NN	0.873	0.969	0.975	0.963

Figure3 illustrates the importance of the top selected features by our RFE-CV LSVM kernel. The bars in blue on the left indicate high negative correlation importance with our positive class (autism), while the ones in dark orange on the right indicates a positive importance coefficient. The longer the bars, the higher the coefficient, indicating more importance for features of this brain-area pair. Table 5 lists the name of the top twelve feature-pairs as ranked by our selection algorithm for easier identification. We can see that most of those brain areas already appear in the literature as correlating with the ASD phenotype.

We already see some areas appear more than once in the top 12 pairs; we will discuss the importance of the highlighted brain areas more in the following section, Discussion.

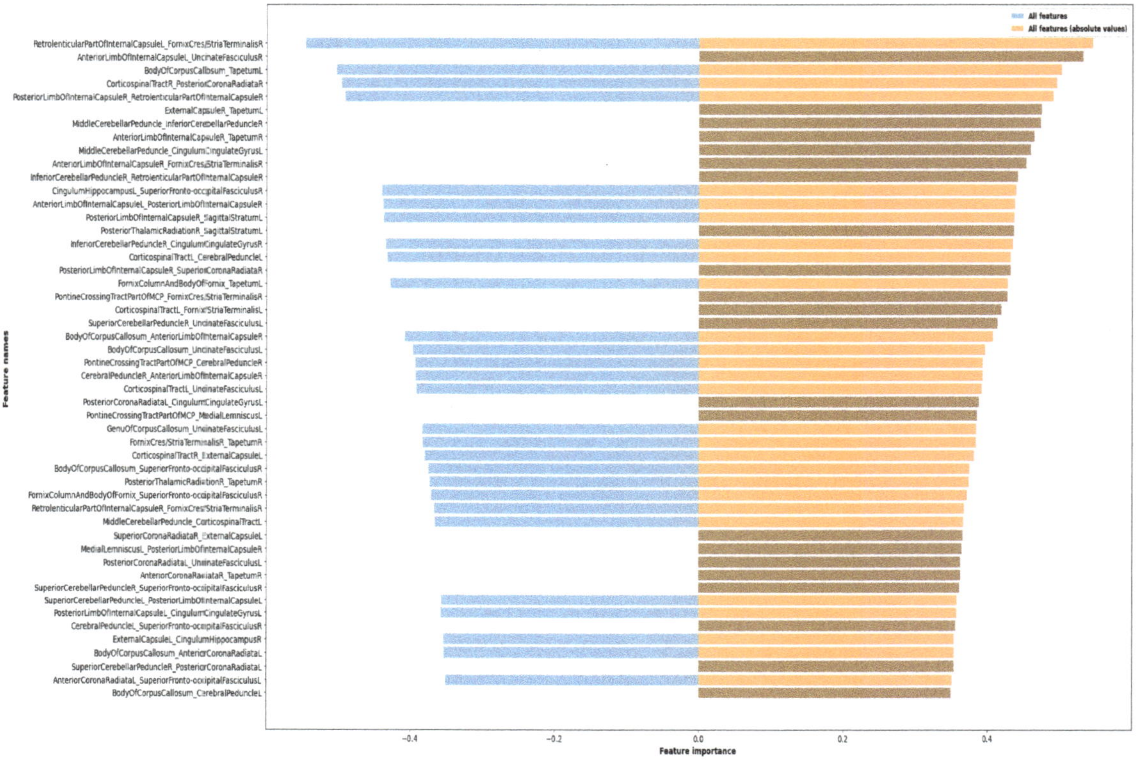

Figure 3. Sorted coefficient of importance for the top 50 selected features of the area pairs correlations.

Table 5. Top 12 WM brain area pairs which feature correlations were highly ranked through RFE-CV selection. L or R at the end stands for the left or right hemispheres, respectively.

Retrolenticular Part of Internal Capsule L	&	Fornix Cres/ Stria Terminalis
Anterior Limb of Internal Capsule L	&	Uncinate Fasciculus R
Body of Corpus Callosum	&	Tapetum L
Corticospinal Tract R	&	Posterior Corona Radiata R
Posterior Limb of Internal Capsule R	&	Retrolenticular Part Of Internal Capsule R
External Capsule R	&	Tapetum L
Middle Cerebellar Peduncle	&	Inferior Cerebellar Peduncle R
Anterior Limb of Internal Capsule R	&	Tapetum R
Middle Cerebellar Peduncle	&	Cingulum Cingulate Gyrus L
Anterior Limb of Internal Capsule R	&	Fornix Cres /StriaTerminalis R
Inferior Cerebellar Peduncle R	&	Retrolenticular Part Of Internal Capsule R
Cingulum Hippocampus L	&	Superior Fronto-occipital Fasciculus R

4. Discussion and Conclusions

The proposed technique adopted in this study introduced a novel feature representation applied to a large number of subjects obtained from a publicly available dataset. We performed extensive experimentation to validate the results introduced through this paper, as well as paved the path for developing new frameworks that may benefit from our novel algorithm. In addition to the achieved promising results, in terms of high cross-validated balanced accuracy, we introduced the notion of interaction between brain areas' micro-connectivity and its viability of reaching a better classification of autism. More importantly, we identified the brain-area pairs that mostly contributed to reaching the final decision. We highlight that those identified brain areas in Table 5 align with the corpus of findings from previous literature studying autism impairments. The uncinate fasciculus (uc) is a fiber pathway through the external capsule (ec) which links the ventral frontal cortex, in particular Brodmann areas 11 and 47, with the temporal pole, and differences in it were revealed in [39,40]. On the other hand, the middle cerebellar peduncle (mcp) carries signals from the cerebral cortex and subcortical regions, via the pontine nuclei, into the cerebellar cortex. The internal capsule (ic) microstructure was found to undergo an atypical developmental trajectory in autistic patients, manifested as increased connectivity from childhood to adulthood [41]. All parts cited in this study of the ic are involved in autism [41–45], and DTI changes have been correlated with autistic behaviors, including inattention, self injury, repetitive behaviors, and social deficits. In general, all white matter tracts identified here (Table 5, Figure 3) connect cortical (sensory motor cortex, frontal/occipital lobes, cingulate) and subcortical regions (thalamus, hippocampus, cerebellum), thereby contributing to deficits (inattention, self injury, repetitive behaviors, motor, social, memory, emotional regulation, and sensory impairments) found in autistic individuals [41–43]. Shukla et al. [45] identified reduced FA and increased RD in the ic and corpus callosum (cc) in children with autism. They also spotted increased MD in anterior and posterior limbs of ic. Significant differences in the AD of the stria terminalis (st) was reported by Yamagata et al. [46] between ASD and TD individuals. Reduced FA and increased RD of st was also reported in [40], and higher AD of st in TD children was noted in [43]. Differences in middle, inferior, and superior cerebellar peduncles [45,47–49] and the corpus callosum [43,45,47,50] were also reported in those previous studies.

The tapetum WM is part of the splenium fibers around the cc, providing connectivity between the temporal lobe, and was found to play a role in different mental disorders [51]. Reduced FA, increased RD, and decreased AD of the tapetum has been reported in ASD. Abnormalities in the corticospinal tract, corona radiata, external capsule, cingulum cingulate cyrus, cingulum hippocampus, and superior fronto-occipital fasciculus were noted in previous studies [13,23,40,42,44,49,52–56]. We stress that our findings are for brain regions' interactions with others, following the idea of disrupted connectivity introduced by Vasa et al., and work normally when done in functional MRI experiments. In [57], Vasa et al. reviewed some of the current structural and functional connectivity ASD data to examine the "disrupted connectivity" theory. They identified and highlighted many confounding factors in the literature that could have affected this conclusion.

In conclusion, the classification framework presented accomplishes many objectives. It provides a high state of the art balanced accuracy on a public dataset, and interpretability, not only in providing a ASD/TD diagnosis, but also in identifying what areas contributes to such a classification. Those spotted brain areas can be reported early with the framework's diagnosis to the physician, who can now make better informed decisions. We believe that this is an important aspect that would lead to a better understanding of the brain abnormalities associated with autism. The system we present is also scalable: adding more subjects that can be preprocessed and feature calculated independently, and fusion of an extra modality, such as structural MRI features or resting state functional MRI for the same subject, can be easily integrated. On the other hand, we stress that the robust results were obtained and validated using only five ABIDE-II sites, and adding more datasets should guarantee generalizability of our proposed framework, which can be a good direction for future work. Moreover, more sophisticated medical interpretation is needed not only to map those affected brain areas to TD vs. ASD, but also to correlate them with ADOS or similar scores, allowing more distinction per scored module. This may need integration with other imaging modalities such as sMRI or fMRI to incorporate different aspects (shape and functionality) to our classification framework, progressing towards an integrated system for autism assessment and providing better interpretation and understanding of underlying personalized diagnosis.

Supplementary Materials: The following are available at https://www.mdpi.com/article/10.3390/s21248171/s1, Table S1: contains accuracy results for F representation, for different RFE-CV kernels. Table S2: contains accuracy results for $\hat{F}$ representation, for different RFE-CV kernels. Table S3: subjects' demographics: subject IDs, along with age, label, IQ, and gender, and also the summary of those demographics for each group.

Author Contributions: Conceptualization, Y.E., M.T.A., A.E., A.S. (Ahmed Shalaby), A.S. (Ahmed Soliman), A.M., M.G., G.N.B. and A.E.-B.; methodology, Y.E., M.T.A., A.E., A.S. (Ahmed Shalaby), A.S. (Ahmed Soliman), A.M., M.G., G.N.B. and A.E.-B.; project administration, A.E.-B.; software, Y.E. and M.T.A.; supervision, G.N.B. and A.E.-B.; validation, G.N.B.; visualization, Y.E. and A.S. (Ahmed Shalaby); writing—original draft, Y.E.; writing—review & editing, Y.E., M.T.A., A.E., A.S. (Ahmed Shalaby), A.S. (Ahmed Soliman), A.M., M.G., G.N.B. and A.E.-B. All authors have read and agreed to the published version of the manuscript.

Funding: This research received no external funding.

Institutional Review Board Statement: Ethical review and approval were waived for this study due to being previously approved by local IRBs for each site.

Informed Consent Statement: Not applicable.

Data Availability Statement: This work uses DTI data from the ABIDE-II dataset, publicly available at http://fcon_1000.projects.nitrc.org/indi/abide/abide_II.html (accessed on 10 November 2021). DTI data were used from the downloaded sites of BNI, NYU1, NYU2, SDSU, and TCD. The website also contains phenotypic files for each site, as well as the DTI scanning parameters.

Conflicts of Interest: The authors declare no conflict of interest.

Abbreviations

The following abbreviations are used in this manuscript:

DTI	Diffusion tensor imaging
MRI	Magnetic resonance imaging
ASD	Autism spectrum disorder
ADOS	Autism Diagnostic Observation Schedule
ADI-R	Autism Diagnostic Interview-Revised
ABIDE	Autism Brain Imaging Data Exchange

References

1. American Psychiatric Association. *Diagnostic and Statistical Manual of Mental Disorders*, 5th ed.; (DSM-5); American Psychiatric Association: Arlington, TX, USA, 2013.
2. Casanova, M.F.; El-Baz, A.; Suri, J.S. *Autism Imaging and Devices*; CRC Press: Boca Raton, FL, USA, 2017.
3. Ismail, M.M.; Keynton, R.S.; Mostapha, M.M.; ElTanboly, A.H.; Casanova, M.F.; Gimel'farb, G.L.; El-Baz, A. Studying autism spectrum disorder with structural and diffusion magnetic resonance imaging: A survey. *Front. Hum. Neurosci.* **2016**, *10*, 211. [CrossRef]
4. Muhle, R.; Trentacoste, S.V.; Rapin, I. The genetics of autism. *Pediatrics* **2004**, *113*, e472–e486. [CrossRef] [PubMed]
5. Lord, C.; Risi, S.; Lambrecht, L.; Cook, E.H.; Leventhal, B.L.; DiLavore, P.C.; Pickles, A.; Rutter, M. The Autism Diagnostic Observation Schedule—Generic: A standard measure of social and communication deficits associated with the spectrum of autism. *J. Autism Dev. Disord.* **2000**, *30*, 205–223. [CrossRef]
6. Lord, C.; Rutter, M.; Le Couteur, A. Autism Diagnostic Interview-Revised: A revised version of a diagnostic interview for caregivers of individuals with possible pervasive developmental disorders. *J. Autism Dev. Disord.* **1994**, *24*, 659–685. [CrossRef] [PubMed]
7. Falkmer, T.; Anderson, K.; Falkmer, M.; Horlin, C. Diagnostic procedures in autism spectrum disorders: A systematic literature review. *Eur. Child Adolesc. Psychiatry* **2013**, *22*, 329–340. [CrossRef] [PubMed]
8. Hayes, J.; Ford, T.; McCabe, R.; Russell, G. Autism diagnosis as a social process. *Autism* **2021**.
9. Brieber, S.; Neufang, S.; Bruning, N.; Kamp-Becker, I.; Remschmidt, H.; Herpertz-Dahlmann, B.; Fink, G.R.; Konrad, K. Structural brain abnormalities in adolescents with autism spectrum disorder and patients with attention deficit/hyperactivity disorder. *J. Child Psychol. Psychiatry* **2007**, *48*, 1251–1258. [CrossRef] [PubMed]
10. Alexander, A.L.; Lee, J.E.; Lazar, M.; Boudos, R.; DuBray, M.B.; Oakes, T.R.; Miller, J.N.; Lu, J.; Jeong, E.K.; McMahon, W.M.; et al. Diffusion tensor imaging of the corpus callosum in Autism. *Neuroimage* **2007**, *34*, 61–73. [CrossRef] [PubMed]

11. Barnea-Goraly, N.; Kwon, H.; Menon, V.; Eliez, S.; Lotspeich, L.; Reiss, A.L. White matter structure in autism: Preliminary evidence from diffusion tensor imaging. *Biol. Psychiatry* **2004**, *55*, 323–326. [CrossRef]
12. O'Donnell, L.J.; Westin, C.F. An introduction to diffusion tensor image analysis. *Neurosurg. Clin.* **2011**, *22*, 185–196. [CrossRef]
13. Shukla, D.K.; Keehn, B.; Müller, R.A. Tract-specific analyses of diffusion tensor imaging show widespread white matter compromise in autism spectrum disorder. *J. Child Psychol. Psychiatry* **2011**, *52*, 286–295. [CrossRef] [PubMed]
14. Basser, P.J. New histological and physiological stains derived from diffusion-tensor MR images. *Ann. N. Y. Acad. Sci.* **1997**, *820*, 123–138. [CrossRef] [PubMed]
15. Wolff, J.J.; Gu, H.; Gerig, G.; Elison, J.T.; Styner, M.; Gouttard, S.; Botteron, K.N.; Dager, S.R.; Dawson, G.; Estes, A.M.; et al. Differences in white matter fiber tract development present from 6 to 24 months in infants with autism. *Am. J. Psychiatry* **2012**, *169*, 589–600. [CrossRef] [PubMed]
16. Lee, J.E.; Bigler, E.D.; Alexander, A.L.; Lazar, M.; DuBray, M.B.; Chung, M.K.; Johnson, M.; Morgan, J.; Miller, J.N.; McMahon, W.M.; et al. Diffusion tensor imaging of white matter in the superior temporal gyrus and temporal stem in autism. *Neurosci. Lett.* **2007**, *424*, 127–132. [CrossRef]
17. Mostapha, M.; Casanova, M.F.; Gimel'farb, G.; El-Baz, A. Towards non-invasive image-based early diagnosis of autism. In *Proceedings of the International Conference on Medical Image Computing and Computer-Assisted Intervention*; Springer: Berlin/Heidelberg, Germany, 2015; pp. 160–168.
18. Sundaram, S.K.; Kumar, A.; Makki, M.I.; Behen, M.E.; Chugani, H.T.; Chugani, D.C. Diffusion tensor imaging of frontal lobe in autism spectrum disorder. *Cereb. Cortex* **2008**, *18*, 2659–2665. [CrossRef]
19. Ingalhalikar, M.; Parker, D.; Bloy, L.; Roberts, T.P.; Verma, R. Diffusion based abnormality markers of pathology: Toward learned diagnostic prediction of ASD. *Neuroimage* **2011**, *57*, 918–927. [CrossRef]
20. Heinsfeld, A.S.; Franco, A.R.; Craddock, R.C.; Buchweitz, A.; Meneguzzi, F. Identification of autism spectrum disorder using deep learning and the ABIDE dataset. *NeuroImage Clin.* **2018**, *17*, 16–23. [CrossRef]
21. Khosla, M.; Jamison, K.; Kuceyeski, A.; Sabuncu, M.R. 3D convolutional neural networks for classification of functional connectomes. In *Deep Learning in Medical Image Analysis and Multimodal Learning for Clinical Decision Support*; Springer: Berlin/Heidelberg, Germany, 2018; pp. 137–145.
22. Dekhil, O.; Ali, M.; El-Nakieb, Y.; Shalaby, A.; Soliman, A.; Switala, A.; Mahmoud, A.; Ghazal, M.; Hajjdiab, H.; Casanova, M.F.; et al. A personalized autism diagnosis cad system using a fusion of structural mri and resting-state functional mri data. *Front. Psychiatry* **2019**, *10*, 392. [CrossRef] [PubMed]
23. Elnakieb, Y.A.; Ali, M.T.; Soliman, A.; Mahmoud, A.H.; Shalaby, A.M.; Alghamdi, N.S.; Ghazal, M.; Khalil, A.; Switala, A.; Keynton, R.S.; et al. Computer Aided Autism Diagnosis Using Diffusion Tensor Imaging. *IEEE Access* **2020**, *8*, 191298–191308. [CrossRef]
24. Lu, L.; Chen, T.; Chen, Y.; Yuan, M.; Gerstein, M.; Li, T.; Liang, H.; Froehlich, T. Towards developing a practical artificial intelligence tool for diagnosing and evaluating autism spectrum disorder: A study using multicenter ABIDE II datasets. *JMIR Med. Inform.* **2020**, *8*, e15767. [CrossRef]
25. Farooq, H.; Chen, Y.; Georgiou, T.T.; Tannenbaum, A.; Lenglet, C. Network curvature as a hallmark of brain structural connectivity. *Nat. Commun.* **2019**, *10*, 4937. [CrossRef] [PubMed]
26. Fredo, A.J.; Jahedi, A.; Reiter, M.; Müller, R.A. Diagnostic classification of autism using resting-state fMRI data and conditional random forest. *Age* **2018**, *12*, 6–41.
27. Crimi, A.; Dodero, L.; Murino, V.; Sona, D. Case-control discrimination through effective brain connectivity. In Proceedings of the 2017 IEEE 14th International Symposium on Biomedical Imaging (ISBI 2017), Melbourne, Australia, 18–21 April 2017; pp. 970–973.
28. Bellman, R. Dynamic programming. *Science* **1966**, *153*, 34–37. [CrossRef]
29. Haar, S.; Berman, S.; Behrmann, M.; Dinstein, I. Anatomical abnormalities in autism? *Cereb. Cortex* **2016**, *26*, 1440–1452. [CrossRef] [PubMed]
30. Sen, B.; Borle, N.C.; Greiner, R.; Brown, M.R. A general prediction model for the detection of ADHD and Autism using structural and functional MRI. *PLoS ONE* **2018**, *13*, e0194856. [CrossRef] [PubMed]
31. Smith, S.M. Fast robust automated brain extraction. *Hum. Brain Mapp.* **2002**, *17*, 143–155. [CrossRef]
32. Bodammer, N.; Kaufmann, J.; Kanowski, M.; Tempelmann, C. Eddy current correction in diffusion-weighted imaging using pairs of images acquired with opposite diffusion gradient polarity. *Magn. Reson. Med.* **2004**, *51*, 188–193. [CrossRef]
33. Alexander, A.L.; Lee, J.E.; Lazar, M.; Field, A.S. Diffusion tensor imaging of the brain. *Neurotherapeutics* **2007**, *4*, 316–329. [CrossRef]
34. Mori, S.; Wakana, S.; Van Zijl, P.C.; Nagae-Poetscher, L.M. *MRI Atlas of Human White Matter*; Elsevier: Amsterdam, The Netherlands, 2005.
35. Wang, Y.; Gupta, A.; Liu, Z.; Zhang, H.; Escolar, M.L.; Gilmore, J.H.; Gouttard, S.; Fillard, P.; Maltbie, E.; Gerig, G.; et al. DTI registration in atlas based fiber analysis of infantile Krabbe disease. *Neuroimage* **2011**, *55*, 1577–1586. [CrossRef] [PubMed]
36. Guyon, I.; Weston, J.; Barnhill, S.; Vapnik, V. Gene selection for cancer classification using support vector machines. *Mach. Learn.* **2002**, *46*, 389–422. [CrossRef]
37. Pedregosa, F.; Varoquaux, G.; Gramfort, A.; Michel, V.; Thirion, B.; Grisel, O.; Blondel, M.; Prettenhofer, P.; Weiss, R.; Dubourg, V.; et al. Scikit-learn: Machine Learning in Python. *Mach. Learn.* **2011**, *12*, 2825–2830.

38. Di Martino, A.; O'connor, D.; Chen, B.; Alaerts, K.; Anderson, J.S.; Assaf, M.; Balsters, J.H.; Baxter, L.; Beggiato, A.; Bernaerts, S.; et al. Enhancing studies of the connectome in autism using the autism brain imaging data exchange II. *Sci. Data* **2017**, *4*, 1–15. [CrossRef]
39. Panesar, S.S.; Yeh, F.C.; Deibert, C.P.; Fernandes-Cabral, D.; Rowthu, V.; Celtikci, P.; Celtikci, E.; Hula, W.D.; Pathak, S.; Fernández-Miranda, J.C. A diffusion spectrum imaging-based tractographic study into the anatomical subdivision and cortical connectivity of the ventral external capsule: Uncinate and inferior fronto-occipital fascicles. *Neuroradiology* **2017**, *59*, 971–987. [CrossRef]
40. Kleinhans, N.M.; Pauley, G.; Richards, T.; Neuhaus, E.; Martin, N.; Corrigan, N.M.; Shaw, D.W.; Estes, A.; Dager, S.R. Age-related abnormalities in white matter microstructure in autism spectrum disorders. *Brain Res.* **2012**, *1479*, 1–16. [CrossRef]
41. McLaughlin, K.; Travers, B.G.; Dadalko, O.I.; Dean III, D.C.; Tromp, D.; Adluru, N.; Destiche, D.; Freeman, A.; Prigge, M.D.; Froehlich, A.; et al. Longitudinal development of thalamic and internal capsule microstructure in autism spectrum disorder. *Autism Res.* **2018**, *11*, 450–462. [CrossRef]
42. Saaybi, S.; AlArab, N.; Hannoun, S.; Saade, M.; Tutunji, R.; Zeeni, C.; Shbarou, R.; Hourani, R.; Boustany, R.M. Pre-and post-therapy assessment of clinical outcomes and white matter integrity in autism Spectrum disorder: Pilot study. *Front. Neurol.* **2019**, *10*, 877. [CrossRef]
43. Vogan, V.; Morgan, B.; Leung, R.; Anagnostou, E.; Doyle-Thomas, K.; Taylor, M. Widespread white matter differences in children and adolescents with autism spectrum disorder. *J. Autism Dev. Disord.* **2016**, *46*, 2138–2147. [CrossRef]
44. Bashat, D.B.; Kronfeld-Duenias, V.; Zachor, D.A.; Ekstein, P.M.; Hendler, T.; Tarrasch, R.; Even, A.; Levy, Y.; Sira, L.B. Accelerated maturation of white matter in young children with autism: A high b value DWI study. *Neuroimage* **2007**, *37*, 40–47. [CrossRef]
45. Shukla, D.K.; Keehn, B.; Lincoln, A.J.; Müller, R.A. White matter compromise of callosal and subcortical fiber tracts in children with autism spectrum disorder: A diffusion tensor imaging study. *J. Am. Acad. Child Adolesc. Psychiatry* **2010**, *49*, 1269–1278.
46. Yamagata, B.; Itahashi, T.; Nakamura, M.; Mimura, M.; Hashimoto, R.I.; Kato, N.; Aoki, Y. White matter endophenotypes and correlates for the clinical diagnosis of autism spectrum disorder. *Soc. Cogn. Affect. Neurosci.* **2018**, *13*, 765–773. [CrossRef]
47. Brito, A.R.; Vasconcelos, M.M.; Domingues, R.C.; Hygino da Cruz Jr, L.C.; Rodrigues, L.d.S.; Gasparetto, E.L.; Calçada, C.A.B.P. Diffusion tensor imaging findings in school-aged autistic children. *J. Neuroimaging* **2009**, *19*, 337–343. [CrossRef]
48. Sivaswamy, L.; Kumar, A.; Rajan, D.; Behen, M.; Muzik, O.; Chugani, D.; Chugani, H. A diffusion tensor imaging study of the cerebellar pathways in children with autism spectrum disorder. *J. Child Neurol.* **2010**, *25*, 1223–1231. [CrossRef]
49. Cheng, Y.; Chou, K.H.; Chen, I.Y.; Fan, Y.T.; Decety, J.; Lin, C.P. Atypical development of white matter microstructure in adolescents with autism spectrum disorders. *Neuroimage* **2010**, *50*, 873–882. [CrossRef]
50. Barnea-Goraly, N.; Lotspeich, L.J.; Reiss, A.L. Similar white matter aberrations in children with autism and their unaffected siblings: A diffusion tensor imaging study using tract-based spatial statistics. *Arch. Gen. Psychiatry* **2010**, *67*, 1052–1060. [CrossRef]
51. Lee, S.W.; Lee, A.; Choi, T.K.; Kim, B.; Lee, K.S.; Bang, M.; Lee, S.H. White matter abnormalities of the tapetum and their associations with duration of untreated psychosis and symptom severity in first-episode psychosis. *Schizophr. Res.* **2018**, *201*, 437–438. [CrossRef]
52. Payabvash, S.; Palacios, E.M.; Owen, J.P.; Wang, M.B.; Tavassoli, T.; Gerdes, M.; Brandes-Aitken, A.; Cuneo, D.; Marco, E.J.; Mukherjee, P. White matter connectome edge density in children with autism spectrum disorders: Potential imaging biomarkers using machine-learning models. *Brain Connect.* **2019**, *9*, 209–220. [CrossRef]
53. Groen, W.B.; Buitelaar, J.K.; Van Der Gaag, R.J.; Zwiers, M.P. Pervasive microstructural abnormalities in autism: A DTI study. *J. Psychiatry Neurosci. JPN* **2011**, *36*, 32. [CrossRef]
54. Karahanoğlu, F.I.; Baran, B.; Nguyen, Q.T.H.; Meskaldji, D.E.; Yendiki, A.; Vangel, M.; Santangelo, S.L.; Manoach, D.S. Diffusion-weighted imaging evidence of altered white matter development from late childhood to early adulthood in autism spectrum disorder. *Neuroimage Clin.* **2018**, *19*, 840–847. [CrossRef]
55. Itahashi, T.; Yamada, T.; Nakamura, M.; Watanabe, H.; Yamagata, B.; Jimbo, D.; Shioda, S.; Kuroda, M.; Toriizuka, K.; Kato, N.; et al. Linked alterations in gray and white matter morphology in adults with high-functioning autism spectrum disorder: A multimodal brain imaging study. *NeuroImage Clin.* **2015**, *7*, 155–169. [CrossRef] [PubMed]
56. Rane, P.; Cochran, D.; Hodge, S.M.; Haselgrove, C.; Kennedy, D.; Frazier, J.A. Connectivity in autism: A review of MRI connectivity studies. *Harv. Rev. Psychiatry* **2015**, *23*, 223. [CrossRef]
57. Vasa, R.A.; Mostofsky, S.H.; Ewen, J.B. The disrupted connectivity hypothesis of autism spectrum disorders: Time for the next phase in research. *Biol. Psychiatry Cogn. Neurosci. Neuroimaging* **2016**, *1*, 245–252. [CrossRef] [PubMed]

sensors

Article

Feature-Based Fusion Using CNN for Lung and Heart Sound Classification †

Zeenat Tariq *,‡, Sayed Khushal Shah ‡ and Yugyung Lee

Department of Computer Science and Electrical Engineering, University of Missouri-Kansas City, Kansas City, MO 64110, USA; sayed.shah@unt.edu (S.K.S.); leeyu@umkc.edu (Y.L.)
* Correspondence: zeenat.tariq@unt.edu
† This paper is an extended version of "Automatic Multimodal Heart Disease Classification using Phonocardiogram Signal" by Tariq, Z.; Shah, S.K.; Lee, Y., published in the Proceedings of 2020 IEEE International Conference on Big Data (Big Data) and "Multimodal Lung Disease Classification using Deep Convolutional Neural Network" by Tariq, Z.; Shah, S.K.; Lee, Y., published in the Proceedings of 2020 IEEE International Conference on Bioinformatics and Biomedicine (BIBM).
‡ These authors contributed equally to this work.

Abstract: Lung or heart sound classification is challenging due to the complex nature of audio data, its dynamic properties of time, and frequency domains. It is also very difficult to detect lung or heart conditions with small amounts of data or unbalanced and high noise in data. Furthermore, the quality of data is a considerable pitfall for improving the performance of deep learning. In this paper, we propose a novel feature-based fusion network called FDC-FS for classifying heart and lung sounds. The FDC-FS framework aims to effectively transfer learning from three different deep neural network models built from audio datasets. The innovation of the proposed transfer learning relies on the transformation from audio data to image vectors and from three specific models to one fused model that would be more suitable for deep learning. We used two publicly available datasets for this study, i.e., lung sound data from ICHBI 2017 challenge and heart challenge data. We applied data augmentation techniques, such as noise distortion, pitch shift, and time stretching, dealing with some data issues in these datasets. Importantly, we extracted three unique features from the audio samples, i.e., Spectrogram, MFCC, and Chromagram. Finally, we built a fusion of three optimal convolutional neural network models by feeding the image feature vectors transformed from audio features. We confirmed the superiority of the proposed fusion model compared to the state-of-the-art works. The highest accuracy we achieved with FDC-FS is 99.1% with Spectrogram-based lung sound classification while 97% for Spectrogram and Chromagram based heart sound classification.

Keywords: lung sound detection; heart sound detection; convolutional neural network; model fusion; multi-features

Citation: Tariq, Z.; Shah, S.K.; Lee, Y. Feature-Based Fusion Using CNN for Lung and Heart Sound Classification. *Sensors* **2022**, 22, 1521. https://doi.org/10.3390/s22041521

Academic Editors: Ayman El-Baz, Guruprasad A. Giridharan, Ahmed Shalaby, Ali H. Mahmoud and Mohammed Ghazal

Received: 29 December 2021
Accepted: 14 February 2022
Published: 16 February 2022

1. Introduction

Cardiovascular and respiratory disease are the top two global causes of death according to World Health Organization [1]. Furthermore, the Centers for Disease Control and Prevention reported heart disease is the leading cause of death (one in every four deaths) for adults in the United States. In particular, there is an increased risk of severe COVID-19 infection of that individual with certain medical conditions, such as heart diseases or chronic obstructive pulmonary disease (COPD) [2].

The expenses of health care have been rapidly increased in the United States [3]. Due to the rapid surge of medical care costs, many people cannot afford health care and may have proper medical treatment. A physician can diagnose using a standard clinical stethoscope by hearing sounds from the human body. An auscultatory method has been applied widely by physicians to examine lung sounds associated with different respiratory symptoms. The auscultatory process has been the easiest way to diagnose patients with respiratory diseases, such as pneumonia, asthma, and bronchiectasis [4]. However, the sound quality is quite a noise or too weak to hear, sometimes due to the complexity of the sound patterns and characteristics. Thus, the manual process takes much time and effort for a physician to detect the condition using a stethoscope accurately [5]. For example, wheezing sounds could not accurately be identified in a series of the pulmonary disease sounds [6].

Similarly, the physicians use cardiac auscultation to evaluate cardiac functions and detect diseases [7]. However, it is a difficult task to manage this method manually at present. A signal produced by these heart sounds is recorded and is known as Phonocardiography (PCG). These signals are highly potent for detecting various heart diseases and are not costly, unlike the electrocardiogram (ECG) signals identified through machines. However, it takes much time to analyze the signals. Hence, deep learning analytic may play an essential role in interpreting the sound signals where corrective measures can be made for physicians' diseases.

There have been significant recent advances in deep learning and the potential of the deep learning model for various medical applications. Recently, there has been increasing attention for the classification of human body sounds for clinical conditions in the medical domain [8–10]. Advanced technologies are essential to achieving the improvement of lifestyle and health care. Some of these applications are ambient assisted living systems [11,12], fall detection [13], voice disorders [14], and heart condition detection [15]. These systems are useful in the early detection of different types of disease through human body sounds, which ultimately improves healthcare. More specifically, an extensive investigation in a partnership among researchers, health care providers, and patients is integral to bringing precise and customized treatment strategies in taking care of various diseases.

Recently, an electronic stethoscope, similar to the design of standard clinical stethoscopes, was designed to enhance the quality of body sounds through filtering or amplification and then extract features from the sounds for the automatic diagnosis of heart or lung conditions using deep learning algorithms. If a deep learning-based diagnosis of heart or lung disease can increase precision and productivity, we can reduce healthcare costs and improve healthcare quality. Moreover, deep learning is a branch derived from machine learning. It allows the computational models, which consist of several layers of processing used to learn the data representations over multiple levels of abstractions. It has attracted a lot of attention due to its high performance in classification. These learning techniques are among the fastest-growing fields at present in the area of audio classification [16]. Some studies reported that the deep learning models outperform humans due to the ability to filter the noise and intensive learning ability [17,18].

The human body sounds for classification are too complicated to understand the hidden patterns of data. The image-based sound classification was introduced to effectively captures the diverse patterns in the dataset [19–21]. As image-based sound classification was introduced, more diverse fusion approaches were also introduced to improve the performance of classification. These methods include the modality-based fusion [22], feature level fusion [23], network-level fusion [24,25] and methodology-based fusion [26]. Among various fusion techniques for sound classification, the most popular are those based on features and multi-modality. However, not much work has been conducted on the general fusion approach, such as network-level fusion using multi-features, which can apply to more diverse datasets or applications.

This paper proposes a novel convolutional neural network model-based fusion called "Fusion-based Disease Classification (FDC)". The model architecture is shown in Figure 1. Our contribution to this paper can be summarized as follows:

- We designed a feature-based fusion model (FDC-FS) transferred from the three feature-based convolutional neural network models to classify lung and heart disease.
- We found that it is more effective to classify heart or lung diseases with images transformed from three different sound features, i.e., Spectrogram, MFCC, and Chromagram (shown in Figures 2 and 3).

- The three types of data augmentation, such as Noise, Pitch-Shift, and Time-Stretch, have been effectively applied to the audio dataset for optimal deep learning training and testing performance.
- A comprehensive experimental results with the lung and heart sound datasets confirmed the superiority of the proposed FDC model over the state-of-the-art methods.

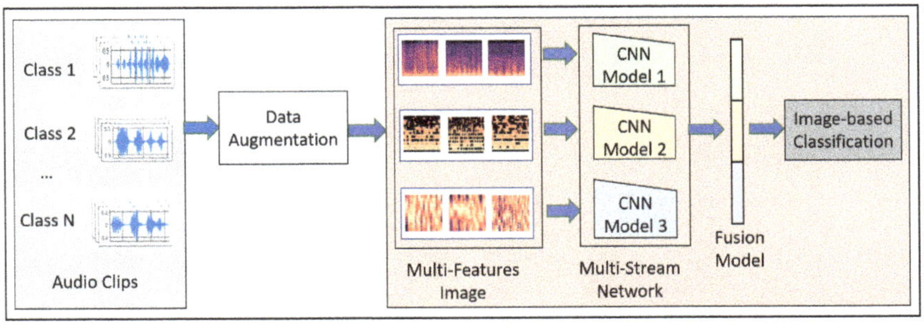

Figure 1. Fusion-Based Disease Classification Architecture.

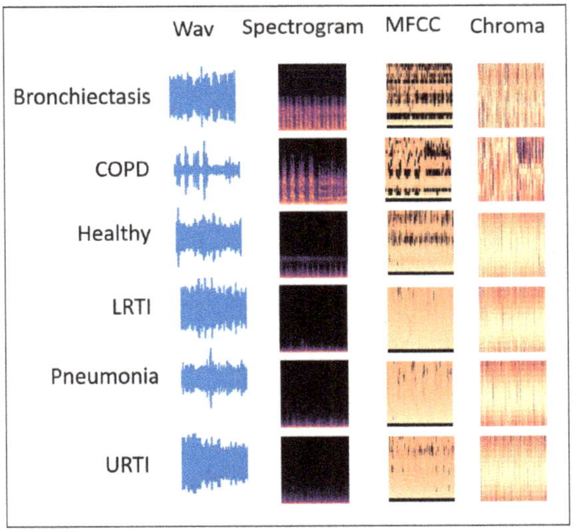

Figure 2. Lung Sound Features: (1) Wav (2) Spectrogram (3) MFCC (4) Chromagram.

The remainder of the paper is organized as follows: Section 2 describes the related work on different deep learning models and lung and heart disease classification techniques. Section 4 discusses the methodology of the proposed model, FDC-FS. Section 4 describes the results and evaluation of the classification model. Section 5 discusses the state-of-the-art comparison for both lung and heart datasets. Finally, Section 6 presents the conclusion and future work.

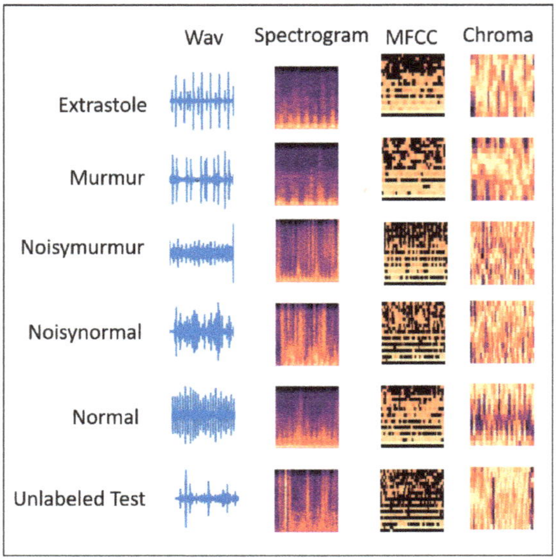

Figure 3. Heart Sound Features: (1) Wav (2) Spectrogram (3) MFCC (4) Chromagram.

2. Related Work

2.1. Lung Disease Classification

Rocha et al. [27] developed classification models for the diagnosis of chest conditions using a stethoscope for the environmental sounds. First, they created a database of lung sounds, which consisted of 920 samples for different categories (i.e., COPD, Healthy, etc.). The second task of the challenge was to extract the features and classify the sounds according to the nature of sound (Wheezes, Crackles, or both). Finally, they conducted feasibility studies on machine learning algorithms, such as support vector machine (SVM) and artificial neural networks (ANN) using features, such as MFCC, spectral features, energy, entropy, and wavelet coefficients. However, they have not overcome the data issues. Unlike this study, we extracted multiple image features from the same datasets, improved the data issues using data augmentation techniques, and obtained better results.

Several data augmentation techniques were applied to classify lung diseases using sounds [28–31]. Dalal et al. [32] explored four machine learning approaches for lung sound classification using lung dataset [33]. This study used data augmentation and extracted Spectrogram, MFCC, and LBP features using multiple machine learning algorithms, such as Support Vector Machine (SVM), K-Nearest Neighbor (KNN), Gaussian Mixture Model (GMM), and Convolutional Neural Network (CNN). Among these models, CNN outperformed all other classifiers with an accuracy of approximately 97%. However, their machine use was very high, applying almost 1 million or more epochs. On the contrary, we achieved higher accuracy than the study, with very low machine use and only 100 epochs with low parameter consumption.

The review in [34] mentioned several feature extraction and classification techniques for obstructive pulmonary diseases such as COPD and asthma. The process involves several traditional and deep learning classification techniques, such as K-Nearest Neighbor (KNN), Artificial Neural Network (ANN), Deep Neural Network (DNN), and Convolutional Neural Network (CNN) and feature extraction through signals such as Fast Fourier Transform (FFT), Short Time Fourier Transform (STFT), Spectrogram, and wavelet transform. For example, the best accuracy for CNN was approximately 95%.

Hai et al. [35] proposed a novel solution for lung sound classification using a publicly available dataset. The dataset was divided into three categories such as wheezes, crackles, and normal sounds. They proposed a detection method using optimized S-transformed (OST) and deep residual networks (ResNets). They performed preprocessing on the audio samples using OST for rescaling the features for ResNets and used a visual-based approach. Their experimental results showed the best multi-classification model with accuracy (98.7%).

Fateh et al. [36] proposed a pre-trained CNN model to extract deep features using the ICBHI challenge dataset. The dataset consists of crackles, wheezes, normal, and wheezes plus crackles categories. First, they used the visual approach with spectrogram images generated from lung sounds by extracting the features. Then, they used the deep features as the input of the Linear Discriminant Analysis (LDA) classifier using the Random Subspace Ensembles (RSE) method. As a result, their model improved the classification accuracy from 5% compared to the existing methods.

Demir et al. [37] proposed two approaches using CNN for the classification of lung diseases using the ICBHI lung sound dataset. The dataset consists of 4 classes with 6898 recordings. First, they converted the lung sounds to spectrogram images using the Short Time Fourier transform (STFT) method. Their first approach is classifying with the SVM based on the features extracted from a pre-trained CNN model. Then, the pre-trained CNN model was fined tuned using the transfer learning method for spectrogram images. The best accuracy for the proposed first and second methods are 65.5% and 63.09%, respectively.

Samiul et al. [38] proposed a lightweight CNN model for detecting respiratory diseases through lung sounds. They designed a hybrid scalogram-based approach using the ICBHI 2017 lung sound dataset by using the empirical mode decomposition (EMD) and the continuous wavelet transform (CWT). As a result, the three-class chronic and the six-class pathological classification accuracy were 98.2% and 98.72%, respectively, with 3M trainable parameters. However, we achieved a better accuracy with lower trainable parameters.

Elmar et al. [39] presented an approach for multi-channel lung sound classification using spectral, temporal, and spatial information. They proposed a convolutional recurrent neural network (CRNN) using spectrogram features to classify lung sounds collected from 16 channel recording devices. Their CRNN model obtained an F1-score of 92% for the binary classification.

Luay et al. [40] proposed homogeneous ensemble learning methods to perform multi-class classification of respiratory diseases. They also used the ICBHI challenge dataset, including 1176 recordings and 308 clinically obtained lung sounds. They used entropy features for machine learning models such as SVM, KNN, and Decision Tree. Among these three models, SVM received the best average accuracy of 98.20%.

2.2. Heart Disease Classification

Potes et al. [41] proposed a feature-based ensemble technique for the classification of normal vs. abnormal heart sounds. First, they extracted 124 time-frequency features such as MFCC from the phonocardiogram (PCG) signals. Then, they used the combination of AdaBoost classifier and CNN classifier to classify the heart sounds. The overall accuracy achieved was 86%. Zhang et al. [42] proposed a method for heart sound classification using a convolutional neural network (CNN). The spectrogram features were extracted from the cycles of sound signals for different positions of pre-trained CNN, and the classification model was based on a support vector machine (SVM). They reported the precision of 77% and 71% for the two datasets with 4 and 3 classes, respectively.

Bozkurt et al. [43] focused on segmentation and time-frequency components for the CNN-based designs. The Mel-spectrogram and MFCC features were extracted from heart sound data using the PhysioNet dataset [44]. They also performed the data augmentation by changing the sampling rate with a random value in range. The overall accuracy achieved was 81.50%. Shu et al. [45] proposed a novel deep WaveNet model for the classification of heart sounds. They used the dataset, composed of five categories with the 1000 PCG recordings, and obtained the overall highest training accuracy of 97%. Muqing et al. [46] proposed a combined model with a convolutional neural network (CNN) and recurrent neural network (RNN) based on the MFCC features for heart sound classification. Their results for the heart sound classification with pathological or non-pathological categories showed the accuracy of 98% with the PhysioNet database.

The authors [47] evaluated the challenges and future directions in the application of supervised learning to cardiovascular beats analysis in order to provide a critical guidance for future research. Despite substantial advancements in this domain, there are still constraints due to a lack of available datasets, inadequate learning, and a paucity of effective algorithms. Our study's major objective is to increase the validity of heart sound recognition. The present investigation included an in-depth analysis and evaluation of recent deep learning methods, with a concentration on the convolutional neural network (CNN) and recurrent neural network (RNN) techniques that have evolved progressively over the last several years.

Acharya et al. [48] proposed Convolutional Neural Network having nine layers for the classification of heart heartbeat signals, such as non-ectopic, supraventricular ectopic, ventricular ectopic, fusion, and unknown beats. Oh et al. [49] developed hybrid models, i.e., multiple layers of CNN and max-pooling and LSTM as the end layer, to extract the temporal information from the features from the ECG dataset and classify arrhythmia from ECG segments. Rajpurkar et al. [50] developed a 34-layer CNN model for the diagnosis of heart diseases such as arrhythmia with the ECG data, recorded with a single lead heart monitor. However, some issues arise in deep learning modeling with the data, including the limited amount of data for heart conditions, low quality with noise, and significant data variations. We also faced similar problems and addressed them in our work.

3. Methodology

We discuss the overall design goals for the FDC network (shown in Figure 1). The modeling process of FDC includes five stages. First, we apply data augmentation techniques onto the audio data to handle the data issues and improve heart and lung condition detection accuracy. Second, we extract the three types of unique and dominant features inherent from the audio data, i.e., Spectrogram, Mel-frequency cepstral coefficient (MFCC), and Chromagram. Third, we convert the extracted features in the form of the images and generate the feature vectors of the audio images in a color format. Fourth, we feed the image feature vector into the especially designed three convolutional neural network models (FDA-1, FDA-2, FDA-3). Finally, The fusion network model (FDA-FS) fuses these three models to optimize the learning performance for the heart and lung sound datasets.

3.1. Rationale of Design

The rationales of the FDC framework design are as follows: First, it is to enable the effective selection of features from the heart and lung sound data, which are highly noise and unbalanced. Several discrepancies existed in the datasets' sources. We did not, however, cut or change the audio input; rather, we extracted the most salient qualities or patterns from the complete dataset. Second, it can transform the audio features into consistent and reliable forms, i.e., audio images. FDC supports a multi-modality capability of audio and image in feature extraction, modeling, and inferencing. Third, it is to design the three different network models to effectively learn unique and dominant features. Finally, it is to transfer learning by fusing the three network models into one model to improve the learning performance in lung and heart condition detection.

The differences between the samples of the signals (audio) and images of the same signals are significant, although they are from the same sources. Thus, different modeling techniques are needed to support the multi-modality. For example, if one is talking in a visual context, it means that sound is transparent while the image is considered as non-transparent (opaque) [51]. The pixel formation shows that whatever is the position of an object belongs to the same category. However, audio cannot quickly identify where it belongs due to its observed frequency in spectrogram features. The audio spectrogram depends on the magnitude of the frequency. Therefore, it is not easy to process the object or its combination in a sequence manner, and it is challenging to identify the simultaneous sounds represented in the spectrogram features.

When a neural network uses images for classification, it considers the sharing weights available from the images in two dimensions, i.e., the X and Y-axis. Thus, the image will carry the same information if it is stretched or repositioned regardless of the position and presence. However, in audio, the two-dimensional data represents the frequency and time. Therefore, if the audio is moved horizontally or vertically, the meaning of the audio can changes. Furthermore, even the spatial features of the sound can change if we increase or decrease the pitch. Therefore, the intentionally introduced invariance can change the meaning, and the neural network will not perform well as it should perform on the trained and augmented data.

In the image format, the extracted pixels can assume that the image belongs to the same class, while in audio, this is not true. Audio is composed of periodic sounds that are composed of frequency and harmonics. The harmonics are spaced apart from each other according to their nature. The combination of these harmonics usually determines the sound's timbre. Suppose we assume from the physical point of view. In that case, the audio played to the audience will examine the type of sound only, while images typically contain a lot of parallel static information. The image classification depends on image features, such as brightness and resolution, among other features.

The design of the fusion-based FDC framework can be justified in terms of the classification effectiveness in terms of three perspectives: (1) Extracting features from the complex audio data of the time and frequent by transformation from audio to images. (2) Designing three specific deep neural networks to optimize their learning performance depending on their unique and dominant features. (3) Optimizing the learning performance through a fusion model by combining the three different models.

3.2. Data Augmentation

Deep learning relies on a large amount of data for more accurate classification. Therefore, we used several augmentation techniques for better classification, out of which we selected the best three methods, including background noise, time stretching, and pitch shifting. We designed these techniques to address the problems in the lung and heart audio classification.

We examined a range of alternative data augmentation techniques. Using a heuristic approach to produce the ideal output, we investigated and validated the augmentation. The experiments attempted to multiply the original file's size tenfold and determined the highest degree of performance. We required a consistent level of research across all models and data, which is why the initial data set was tenfold augmented.

3.2.1. Noise Distortion

We considered adding random noise to the audio samples to avoid overfitting during training. In this type, noise clips were randomly sampled [52] to be linearly mixed with the input signal represented as y'. α is used to describe random weights along with specific factors that are denoted by U as shown in Equation (1).

$$\begin{aligned} &Random-Weights : \alpha \sim_U [0.001, 0.005] \\ &Input-Signal : y' \leftarrow (1-\alpha)\cdot y + \alpha \cdot y_{\text{noise}} \end{aligned} \tag{1}$$

3.2.2. Time Stretching

Scaling the audio data horizontally by some stretching factor such as $a\_st > 0$ helps in increasing the size of the data for efficient classification. We applied time stretch (st) on the audio samples, which were later converted to images. It is to check if the meaning of the data remains the same as image data does not lose the information but changing the position of audio or slowing down the position as we generate the Spectrograms. We considered four different types of time stretch factor $n \in \{0.5, 0.7, 1.2, 1.5\}$.

3.2.3. Pitch Shifting

In this data augmentation technique, the audio samples' pitch is either decreased or increased by four values (semitones) [53]. We assume that with the pitch shifting factor a_s, the artificial training data generated is $Naug$ times larger than the original lung or heart sound data. The duration of audio samples is kept constant, like the actual audio samples, i.e., 10–90 s. For our experimentation, the value changed in semitones were in the interval $[-a_s, a_s]$ for each signal. Factors of pitch shift are $n \in \{-3.5, -2.5, 2.5, 3.5\}$ semitones.

3.3. *Feature Extraction*

We used the two datasets, i.e., lung and heart sound (for six categories for each in the lung dataset and the heart dataset). These datasets consist of sound clips that vary from 10 s to 90 s. However, to incorporate the consistent data in making a more accurate prediction model, we used the sliding window technique to make each clip of 3 s. The window size (i.e., 3 s) for optimal learning was chosen using a heuristic based on the distribution of signals from a small subset of the PCG input. Utilizing the spectrogram, MFCC, and chromagram approaches, we retrieved audio characteristics from the given input. Metadata describing the location of heart sounds or signal synchronization, as well as other insights, enabled the effective extraction of the different properties gained by these extraction strategies on the three-second PCG segments. The feature vectors of the extracted features for these three types are converted as JPG images in the dimension of [128 × 128] using the CV2 image and NumPy libraries.

3.3.1. Spectrogram Generation

We used the spectrogram to generate a visual representation of a signal in the time-frequency domain. These are generated by the application of the short-time Fourier transform (STFT) [54]. According to the theorem, a single Fourier analysis may not see a nonstationary signal's spectrum variation. The Fourier transform can be used to determine the frequency and sequence of signals and their changes over time. Hence, the spectrogram considers the stationary signal by computing the Fourier transform of the segmented signal into slices. The spectrogram can be calculated as:

$$\mathrm{STFT}_x^f(t,f) = \int_{\infty}^{\infty} [x(t)w(t-\tau)e^{-j2\pi ft}dt \tag{2}$$

where $x(t)$ is the time-domain signal, τ is the time localization of STFT, and $w(t-\tau)$ is a window function to cut and filter the signal. The length of the window function must be selected and adjusted according to the signal's length because it affects the time and frequency resolution [55]. The window size was determined using a heuristic based on the distribution of signals from a small subset of the input. To do this, we considered all possible window sizes and other criteria for selecting audio features in STFT. It should be noted, however, that the input data included just three seconds of each PCG signal. As a result, the maximum permissible window size was 3. The spectrogram was converted into a grayscale image, and the image will be used to generate a feature vector that will be feed for deep learning.

The scaling process is applied to the spectrogram to expand the values range between 0 and 255 because the range of the spectrogram is usually comprehensive. The method of scaling is done in a linear manner, which can be expressed as follows:

$$S(m,n) = \frac{|Spec(m,n)|}{max|Spec|} \times 255 \tag{3}$$

where $Spec(m, n)$ is the value of the spectrogram and $S(m, n)$ is the expanded value from a spectrogram.

3.3.2. Mel-Frequency Cepstral Coefficient

The Mel-frequency Cepstral Coefficient (MFCC) coefficients are a set of discrete cosine transform (DCT) derived from a type of cepstral representation of the audio clip. The frequency warping allows a better representation of sound by containing the difference between the cepstrum and the Mel-frequency cepstrum. It computed through logarithmic spectrum scale after it was transformed to the Mel scale [56] calculated as:

$$\mathrm{mel}(f) = 2595 \log_{10}\left(1 + \frac{f}{700}\right) \tag{4}$$

For the input signal $y(n)$, an N-point discrete Fourier transformation (DFT) is given as:

$$Y(k) = \sum_{n=1}^{M} y(n) \cdot e^{\left(\frac{-j2\pi nk}{M}\right)} \tag{5}$$

MFCCs are commonly derived as follows: first, we obtain the spectrum by taking the Fourier to transform to a signal. Second, we map the spectrum onto the Mel scale and then take a log-based transform of the Mel-frequency scaled spectrums. Finally, we take the discrete cosine transform of the Mel-log-frequency scaled spectrums and amplitude the spectrum.

3.3.3. Chromagram

Chromagram features or Chromagram are Pitch Class Profile whose pitches can be meaningfully categorized. The Chromagram technology was applied to generate a robust set of acoustic features by capturing harmonic and melodic characteristics of music in a signal whose pitches can be classified in the categories of lung or heart sounds. Since the heart and lung sounds have subtle differences in pitch, Chromagram has features that make it a good source of lung and heart sound classification.

3.4. Classification Model

3.4.1. Overview of the FDC Model

Convolutional neural network (CNN) has been recognized as a popular and powerful deep neural network model in audio and image classification applications. We developed a fusion model based on CNN-based architecture for heart and lung disease classification. Our model is a 2D CNN model composed of the input layer, convolutional 2D layer, max-pooling layer, and fully connected layers. The invention is a fusion model, FDC-FS, by combining multi-featured models, including FDC-1, FDC-2, and FDC-3. The fusion was conducted on their final layer to append all model parameters. The three models FDC-1, FDC-2, FDC-3, were trained concurrently and independently. After completing the single model development process, we combined the models to generate the FDC-FS fusion model. The general hyper-parameters are shown in Table 1. The detailed description of each model in given in Sections 3.4.2–3.4.5. These four models' (FDC-1, FDC-2, FDC-3, FDC-FS) accuracy was summarized in Section 4.

There are two essential components in the design of multi-feature models with CNNs. (1) the feature extractor collected features (Spectrogram, MFCC, and Chromagram) from the audio signals and transformed the features into images to generate visual feature vectors. (2) Each model (FDC-1, FDC-2, FDC-3) was uniquely designed to optimize learning for the specific features (Spectrogram, MFCC, and Chromagram), respectively, which is composed of multiple convolutional and pooling layers, activation, and fully connected layers with several hidden units. Finally, the fusion model was built by composing the features from these three models. After the models were trained, the visual feature vectors of the input signals were classified by the models into their appropriate categories.

Table 1. FDC Model Hyper-parameters.

Model.	Batch Size	# of Layers	# of Hidden Layers	# of Epochs	Dropout
Original Data					
FDC-1	64	3	2	50	0.5
FDC-2	64	2	2	50	0.5
FDC-3	64	8	1	50	0.5
FDC-FS	64	13	3	50	0.5
Augmented Data					
FDC-1	128	3	2	30	0.5
FDC-2	128	2	2	30	0.5
FDC-3	128	8	1	30	0.5
FDC-FS	128	13	3	30	0.5

The mathematical form of the convolutional layers is given in Equations (6) and (7)

$$[x^{l}_{i,j,k} = \sum_{a}\sum_{b}\sum_{c} w^{(l-1,f)}_{i,j,k} y^{(l-1)}_{i+a,j+b,k+c} + bias^{f}] \tag{6}$$

$$[y^{l}_{i,j,k} = \sigma(x^{(l)}_{i,j,k})] \tag{7}$$

The output layer is represented by $y^{l}_{i,j,k}$ where as the 3-dimensional input tensor is denoted by i, j, k. The weights for the filters are denoted by $w^{(l)}_{i,j,k}$ and $\sigma(x^{(l)}_{i,j,k})$ describes the sigmoid function for linear activation. The fully connected is the final layer represented by Equations (8) and (9).

$$[x^{(l)}_{i} \sum_{j} w^{l-1}_{i,j} y^{l-1}_{j} + bias^{l-1}_{j}] \tag{8}$$

$$[y^{l}_{i,j,k} = \sigma(x^{l}_{i,j,k})] \tag{9}$$

Our fusion model FDC-FS is composed of three different models, such as FDC-1, FDC-2, and FDC-3. They consist of the convolutional layers enclosed by the max pool layer, followed by fully connected layers, including dropout, batch Normalization, rectified linear units (ReLU), and LeakyReLU. During the extraction of features, we used the window size and hop size of 23 ms. As the sound clips vary between 3 and 5 s, that is why we kept the extraction to 3 s to make every bit of the sound clip usable. In addition, we reshaped the input taken from the sound clips to $X \in R^{128\times128}$ shape. Further, we sent these reshaped features to the classifier to predict heart or lung diseases.

3.4.2. FDC-1 Model

The FDC-1 model is designed for the classification based on the image feature vector of the three audio features (Spectrogram, MFCC, and Chromagram) for the given datasets, using convolutional neural network architecture with a total of five layers. Among the five layers, 3 are convolutional layers, and 2 are dense layers. We considered rectified linear units (ReLU) as the activation function between layers, a max-pooling is also applied, and we also used dropout in different layers to avoid overfitting. The total number of trainable parameters based on the five layers of architecture is 241,174 (0.24 M). The hyper-parameters are shown in Table 2.

The first layers of the FDC-1 model consist of 24 filters with a 5×5 receptive field. The layer is also followed by a (4×2) strided max-pooling function. The activation function used in this layer is rectified linear units (ReLU). The second layer of FDC-1 is composed of 48 filters with 5×5 receptive files. It is followed by 4×2 strided Max Pooling and ReLU activation. The padding for these layers is kept as "valid". The third layer of FDC-1 consists of 48 filters with 5×5 receptive fields. The layers have "valid" padding, which is followed by the ReLU activation function. After the activation, the output is flattened, and the dropout of factor "0.5" is applied to avoid overfitting the output from layer to layer. The fourth layer is the first dense layer which is also called the hidden layer. It consists of 64 hidden units followed by ReLU activation and dropout rate of 0.5 to avoid overfitting the output result to the next layer. The fifth layer is a final dense layer that consists of output units. The output units are always equal to the number of classes used in the dataset. The last layer is followed by the "Softmax" activation function.

Table 2. FDC-1 Model Hyper-parameters.

Layer (Type)	Output Shape	Param #
Conv2D	(None, 124, 124, 24)	624
MaxPooling2D	(None, 31, 62, 24)	0
Activation	(None, 31, 62, 24)	0
Conv2D	(None, 27, 58, 48)	28,848
MaxPooling2D	(None, 6, 29, 48)	0
Activation	(None, 6, 29, 48)	0
Conv2D	(None, 2, 25, 48)	57,648
Activation	(None, 2, 25, 48)	0
Flatten	(None, 2400)	0
DropOut	(None, 2400)	0
Dense	(None, 64)	153,664
Activation	(None, 64)	0
DropOut	(None, 64)	0
Dense	(None, 6)	650
Activation	(None, 6)	0
Total Parameters: 241,174		
Trainable Parameters: 241,174		
Non-Trainable Parameters: 0		

3.4.3. FDC-2 Model

The FDC-2 model is designed for classification based on the image feature vector of the three audio features (Spectrogram, MFCC, and Chromagram) for the given datasets. It is based on a convolutional neural network architecture consisting of 4 layers, including two convolutional layers, two hidden layers, and an L2 regularizer on the first layers to reduce likelihood and bias among the inputs. In addition, this model consists of Max Pooling to reduce unwanted features for training, dropout to avoid overfitting, ReLU, and Softmax activation. Feature vector flattening is also considered to convert 2-dimensional features to 1-dimensional features. The total number of trainable parameters based on the four layers of architecture is 879,430 (0.87 M). The overall hyper-parameters are shown in Table 3.

In the first layers of FDC-2, the layers take 32 filters with 3×3 receptive files. The first layers also consist of the L2 regularizer norm with the value of "0.0005". Then, Strided Max Pooling of 4×2 follows it. Finally, ReLU is used as an activation function. FDC-2 takes 48 filters with 3×3 receptive filed and "valid" padding in the second layer. It is pursued by the ReLU activation function and Max Pooling of 4×2. After all the operations above, the 2-Dimensional input is flattened to 1-Dimensional and passed on to the hidden layers, i.e., dense layers. A dropout follows the flatten with a rate of 0.5 to avoid overfitting the input. The third layer is the first hidden (dense) layer of FDC-2 with hidden units of 64, followed by ReLU activation and dropout with a rate of 0.5. The fourth layer is a dense layer consisting of the output units, which is equal to the number of classes available in the dataset. The final activation function is Softmax.

Table 3. FDC-2 Model Hyper parameters.

Layer (Type)	Output Shape	Param #
Conv2D	(None, 126, 126, 32)	320
Activation	(None, 126, 126, 32)	0
MaxPooling2D	(None, 31, 63, 32)	0
Conv2D	(None, 29, 61, 64)	18,496
Activation	(None, 29, 61, 64)	0
MaxPooling2D	(None, 7, 30, 64)	0
Flatten	(None, 13,440)	0
Dropout	(None, 13,440)	0
Dense	(None, 64)	860,224
Activation	(None, 64)	0
Dropout	(None, 64)	0
Dense	(None, 6)	650
Activation	(None, 6)	0
Total Parameters: 879,430		
Trainable Parameters: 879,430		
Non-Trainable Parameters: 0		

3.4.4. FDC-3 Model

The FDC-3 model is designed for the classification based on the image feature vector of the three audio features (Spectrogram, MFCC, and Chromagram) for the given datasets,

focused more on in-depth training and eventually reducing the number of trainable parameters. This model is composed of 8 convolutional layers and one dense layer. The layers consist of padding, ReLU, softmax activation, Max Pooling, Global Average Pooling, Batch Normalization, and dropout. The Batch Normalization is used to train the model intensely, and in return, it standardizes the input in a layer for each mini-batch. Hence, it has a perfect effect on the learning process, reducing the number of trainable parameters. The total number of trainable parameters based on the nine-layer architecture given below is 362,214 (0.36 M). FDC-3 hyper-parameters are shown in Table 4 in details.

The first and second layers of FDC-3 have 32 filters with 3 × 3 receptive fields and some padding and ReLU as activation function. Both layers also consist of 2 × 2 strided Max Pooling. Batch Normalization follows both layers to perform deep training and reduce the trainable parameters. However, the second layer is following by a dropout of 0.25 to overfitting the input to the next layer. The third-to-sixth layers of FDC-3 are the same as the first and second layers, but the third-to-sixth layers take 64 filters with 3 × 3 receptive fields. They use the same strided max-pooling, padding, activation, dropout, and Batch Normalization for deep training. The seventh and eighth layers of FDC-3 take 128 filters with 3 × 3 receptive files, followed by the same padding and ReLU activation function. Batch Normalization follows the activation function in both layers. However, the eighth layer is followed by the dropout of rate 0.25. Finally, the last convolutional layer is also followed by Global Average Pooling before the input is ready for output classification. The ninth layer is the final and only the dense layer in this architecture, consisting of output units equal to the number of classes in the dataset.

Table 4. FDC-3 Model Hyper-Parameters.

Layer (Type)	Output Shape	Param #
Conv2D	(None, 128, 128, 32)	320
BatchNormalization	(None, 128, 128, 32)	128
Conv2D	(None, 126, 126, 32)	9248
BatchNormalization	(None, 126, 126, 32)	128
MaxPooling2D	(None, 63, 63, 32)	0
Dropout	(None, 63, 63, 32)	0
Conv2D	(None, 63, 63, 32)	18,496
BatchNormalization	(None, 63, 63, 32)	256
Conv2D	(None, 61, 61, 64)	36,928
BatchNormalization	(None, 61, 61, 64)	256
MaxPooling2D	(None, 31, 31, 64)	0
Dropout	(None, 31, 31, 64)	0
Conv2D	(None, 31, 31, 64)	36,928
BatchNormalization	(None, 31, 31, 64)	256
Conv2D	(None, 29, 29, 64)	36,928
BatchNormalization	(None, 29, 29, 64)	256
MaxPooling2D	(None, 15, 15, 64)	0
Dropout	(None, 15, 15, 64)	0
Conv2D	(None, 15, 15, 64)	73,856
BatchNormalization	(None, 15, 15, 64)	512
Conv2D	(None, 13, 13, 128)	147,584
BatchNormalization	(None, 13, 13, 128)	512
MaxPooling2D	(None, 7, 7, 128)	0
Dropout	(None, 7, 7, 128)	0
GlobalAveragePooling	(None, 128)	0
Dense	(None, 6)	1290
Activation	(None, 6)	0
Total Parameters: 363,366		
Trainable Parameters: 362,214		
Non-Trainable Parameters: 1152		

3.4.5. FDC-FS Model

The FDC-FS model is a fusion model resulting from transfer learning from all three models (FDC-1, FDC-2, FDC-3). Its architecture is composed of the softmax activation and dense layers consisting of the output units equal to the number of classes in the dataset at the last layer. Therefore, FDC-FS is composed of 13 convolutional layers and 3 dense layers model, more specifically three convolutional layers from FDC-1, two convolutional layers from FDC-2, eight convolutional layers from FDC-3, one dense layer from FDC-1, and one dense layer from FDC-2, and a final dense layer of an output unit. The FDC-FS's total trainable parameters for six classes are 1,482,806 (1.4 M). Table 5 shows the hyper-parameters of the final convolutional architecture, which is a fusion of our novel three architectures shown in Figure 4.

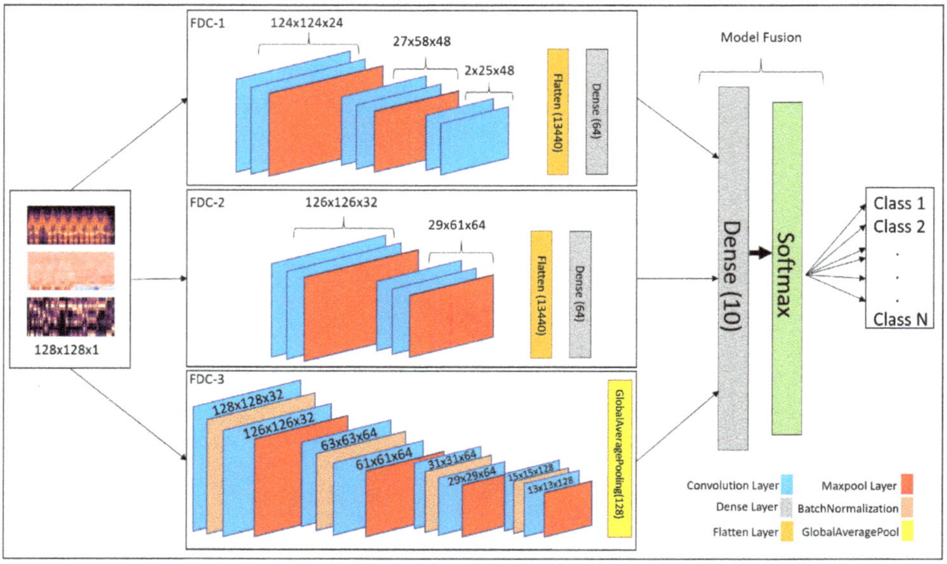

Figure 4. Overall FDC-FS Architecture Composed of FDC-1, FDC-2, and FDC-3.

Table 5. FDC-FS Model Hyper-Parameters.

Layer (Type)	Output Shape	Param #
Input	(None, 128, 128, 1)	0
Conv2D	(None, 128, 128, 32)	320
BatchNormalization	(None, 128, 128, 32)	128
Conv2D	(None, 126, 126, 32)	9248
BatchNormalization	(None, 126, 126, 32)	128
MaxPooling2D	(None, 63, 63, 32)	0
DropOut	(None, 63, 63, 32)	0
Conv2D	(None, 63, 63, 64)	18,496
BatchNormalization	(None, 63, 63, 64)	256
Conv2D	(None, 61, 61, 64)	36,928
BatchNormalization	(None, 61, 61, 64)	256
MaxPooling2D	(None, 31, 31, 64)	0
DropOut	(None, 31, 31, 64)	0
Conv2D	(None, 124, 124, 24)	624
Conv2D	(None, 31, 31, 64)	36,928
MaxPooling2D	(None, 31, 62, 24)	0
BatchNormalization	(None, 31, 31, 64)	256
Activation	(None, 31, 62, 24)	0
Conv2D	(None, 126, 126, 32)	320
Conv2D	(None, 29, 29, 64)	36,928
Conv2D	(None, 27, 58, 48)	28,848
Activation	(None, 126, 126, 32)	0

Table 5. *Cont.*

Layer (Type)	Output Shape	Param #
BatchNormalization	(None, 29, 29, 64)	256
MaxPooling2D	(None, 6, 29, 48)	0
MaxPooling2D	(None, 31, 63, 32)	0
MaxPooling2D	(None, 15, 15, 64)	0
Activation	(None, 6, 29, 48)	0
Conv2D	(None, 29, 61, 64)	18,496
DropOut	(None, 15, 15, 64)	0
Conv2D	(None, 2, 25, 48)	57,648
Activation	(None, 29, 61, 64)	0
Conv2D	(None, 15, 15, 128)	73,856
Activation	(None, 2, 25, 48)	0
MaxPooling2D	(None, 7, 30, 64)	0
BatchNormalization	(None, 15, 15, 128)	512
Flatten	(None, 2400)	0
Flatten	(None, 13,440)	0
Conv2D	(None, 13, 13, 128)	147,584
DropOut	(None, 2400)	0
DropOut	(None, 13,440)	0
BatchNormalization	(None, 13, 13, 128)	512
Dense	(None, 64)	153,664
Dense	None, 64)	860,224
MaxPooling2D	(None, 7,7, 128)	0
Activation	(None, 64)	0
Activation	(None, 64)	0
DropOut	(None, 7, 7, 128)	0
DropOut	None, 64)	0
DropOut	None, 64)	0
GlobalAveragePoolinh2D	(None, 128)	0
Concatenate	(None, 256)	0
Dense	(None, 6)	1542
Total Parameters: 1,483,958		
Trainable Parameters: 1,482,806		
Non-Trainable Parameters: 1152		

4. Result and Evaluation

We conducted comprehensive experiments for the FDC models using the lung and heart sound datasets [27,57]. We now present the results obtained from the experiments with the three FDC models and the fusion model (FDC-FS) using the original and augmented datasets of the lung and heart datasets. The results includes the accuracy, loss, and class-wise accuracy for original and augmented datasets. The experimental results have been obtained as compared to the state-of-the-art methods.

4.1. Experimental Setup

We conducted most of the experimentations using Google research collaboratory with 12 GB NVIDIA Tesla K80. For the data augmentation and feature extraction, we used the NVIDIA GeForce ® GTX 1080 Ti, packed with 11 Gbps GDDR5X memory and an 11 GB frame buffer. The number of epochs was set at 50 while avoiding overfitting, and a batch size of 64 was considered. However, for the training for the augmented datasets, the epochs were set at 30 with a 128 batch.

The model training was set to 80% training and 20% testing. From the 80% training data, we further split it into 80% training and 20% validation (64% training, 16% validation, 20% testing). This is to note here that testing data are not a subset of training data. After the data were split, the testing data was never seen by the previous model. We reported classification accuracies for training and testing. The class-wise accuracy was also reported for four different models (FDA-1, 2, 3 & FS), two types of data (original and augmented), and for two different datasets (lung and heart sound). We observed that FDC-FS performed the best compared to others.

4.2. Dataset

Heart Sound Dataset: The heart dataset consists of 656 audio recordings for different heart classes such as *Extrastole, Murmur, Noisy Murmur, Noisy Normal, Normal, Unlabeled test*. The author of the dataset [57] made this dataset public for two challenges, using an iPhone app and a digital stethoscope. The initial dataset has both clean and noisy data without any data synthesis. To increase the accuracy of the data, data augmentation techniques were added to the initial heard sound samples. After applying the data augmentation to the initial data, the total number of files increased to 7216 as shown in Table 6.

Lung Sound Dataset: The research team from Greece and Portugal created the lung dataset [27]. There are 920 annotated recordings, ranging from 10 s to 90 s (the total of 5.5 h), obtained from 126 patients using a digital stethoscope. Unfortunately, the complete dataset was not released. Therefore, the publicly available dataset used for lung sound classification modeling is mainly limited in data amount and sound quality. To overcome the data issues, we applied two approaches to balance the dataset: (1) The "Synthetic Minority Oversampling Technique (SMOTE)" replicates the same sample several times to balance the dataset with other classes. Most of the state-of-the-art research use SMOTE in their works. The second approach is to consider weighted average as our testing accuracy for the models. We further applied data augmentation techniques to generate synthesized data. Table 7 shows the amount of the original and augmented data. We removed the *Asthma* category having only a single recording from the dataset. The number of the original recordings was 919 for six categories (*Bronchiectasis, COPD, Health, LRTI, Pneumonia, URTI*) while the number of augmented recordings are 10,109.

Figure 5 shows the t-Distributed Stochastic Neighbor Embedding (t-SNE) visualization for heart and lung sound dataset. It can be seen that the Lung dataset is very dispersed, and classes are mixed up with each other.

Table 6. Heart Sound Dataset: Original and Augmented Data.

ID	Category	Ori. Data	Aug. Data
1	Extra Systole	46	506
2	Normal	200	2200
3	Noisy Normal	120	1320
4	Murmur	66	726
5	Noisy Murmur	29	319
6	Unlabelled Test	195	2145
	Total	**656**	**7216**

Table 7. Lung Sound Dataset: Original and Augmented Data.

ID	Category	Ori. Data	Aug. Data
1	Bronchiectasis	29	319
2	COPD	785	8635
3	Health	35	385
4	LRTI	2	22
5	Pneumonia	37	407
6	URTI	31	341
	Total	**919**	**10,109**

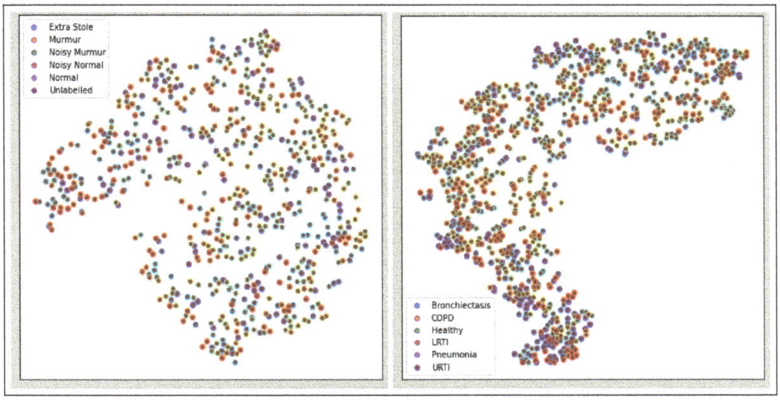

Figure 5. t-SNE Visualization: Heart Sound Dataset and Lung Sound Dataset.

4.3. Classification Results and Evaluations

Results on Original Lung Dataset: Based on the setup explained above, we obtained the accuracy performance for the four models (FDC-1, FDC-2, FDC-3, and FDC-FS). FDC-FS model obtains the highest accuracy model in all three feature cases. Specifically, the highest accuracy is achieved by Spectrogram 97%, while MFCC reported accuracy of 91% and Chromagram reported accuracy of 95%. Table 8 offers the accuracy of the lung original dataset. The classification results for the original lung dataset are shown in Figure 6. Class-wise accuracy for all models based on the original lung dataset is shown further on in this paper.

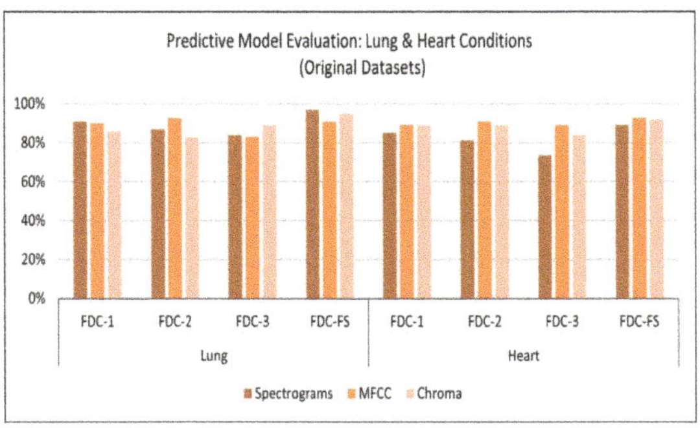

Figure 6. Accuracy for Lung/Heart Condition Detection (Original Dataset).

Results on Original Heart Dataset: Our experimental results are based on 50 epochs and 64 batch sizes and the categorical cross-entropy for the data validation. The average times taken for training the model were from 7 s to 1 min for the FDC models. Table 8 offers the accuracy of the heart original dataset. The classification results for the original heart dataset are shown in Figure 6. During the training and testing, we observed that FDC-FS performed the best compared to all others; specifically, we obtained the highest accuracy of 93% for MFCC. For the individual feature-model evaluation, the highest accuracy of Spectrogram was 85% with FDC-1; for MFCC, it was 91% with FDC-2. Chromagram was the accuracy of 89% with FDC-1 and FDC-2.

Table 8. Lung & Heart Condition Detection with Original Data (Testing Average Accuracy).

	Lung Sound Classification				Heart Sound Classification			
Features	**FDC-1**	**FDC-2**	**FDC-3**	**FDC-FS**	**FDC-1**	**FDC-2**	**FDC-3**	**FDC-FS**
Spectrogram	91%	87%	84%	97%	85%	81%	73.5%	89%
MFCC	90%	93%	83%	91%	89%	91%	89%	93%
Chromagram	86%	83%	89%	95%	89%	89%	84%	92%

Results on Augmented Lung Dataset: We achieved very impressive accuracy from the experiments with the augmented lung dataset that outperformed all state-of-the-art research. The highest accuracy was conducted by the FDC-FS model, which is the fusion of FDC-1, FDC-2, and FDC-FS. The weighted accuracy for the FDC-FS model for Spectrogram is 99.1%, the accuracy of 99% for MFCC, and 98.4% for Chromagram. Notably, it has been improved approximately 2%, 8%, 3% in Spectrogram, MFCC, and Chromagram, compared to the accuracy performance with the original data. The results for the augmented lung dataset are shown in Table 9 and Figure 7. The learning and validation graphs for learning and loss are shown in Figure 8.

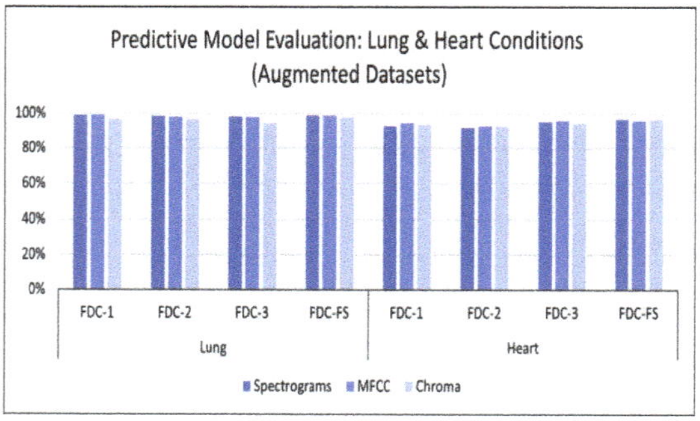

Figure 7. Accuracy for Lung/Heart Condition Detection (Augmented Dataset).

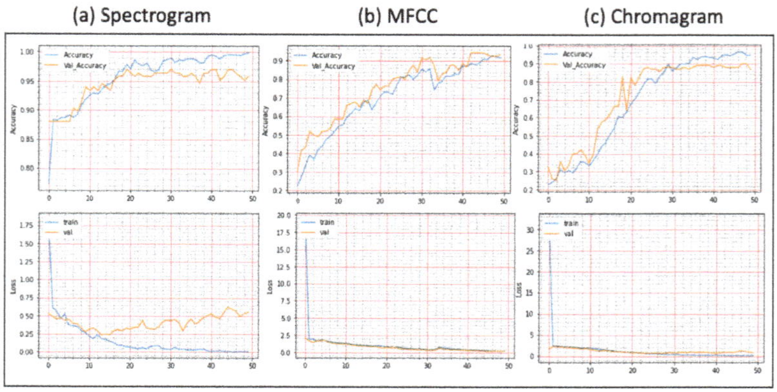

Figure 8. Lung Condition Classification (Accuracy vs. Loss): The Fusion Network Model (FDC-FS) was Evaluated with Three Features: (**a**) Spectrogram, (**b**) MFCC, (**c**) Chromagram.

Table 9. Lung & Heart Condition Detection with Original Data (Testing Average Accuracy).

	Lung Sound Classification				Heart Sound Classification			
Features	FDC-1	FDC-2	FDC-3	FDC-FS	FDC-1	FDC-2	FDC-3	FDC-FS
Spectrogram	99%	98.6%	98.3%	99.1%	93%	92%	95.5%	97%
MFCC	99.3%	98%	98.2%	99%	95%	93%	96%	96%
Chromagram	97%	97%	95%	98.4%	94%	93%	95%	97%

Results on the Augmented Heart Dataset: For the augmented heart data experiments, we observed that FDC-2 obtained the shortest training time of 42 s for MFCC, and FDC-FS took the longest time of 4 min and 11 s for Chromagram. The FDC-FS model obtained the highest accuracy of 97% with Spectrogram and Chromagram and 96% with MFCC. From the individual model evaluation, FDC-3 obtained the highest accuracy of 96% with MFCC. It is because the FDC-3 model is bigger/deeper compared to the other two models. The learning graphs of the heart dataset for the FDC-FS model are shown in Figure 9. The overall performance of the models is given in Table 9.

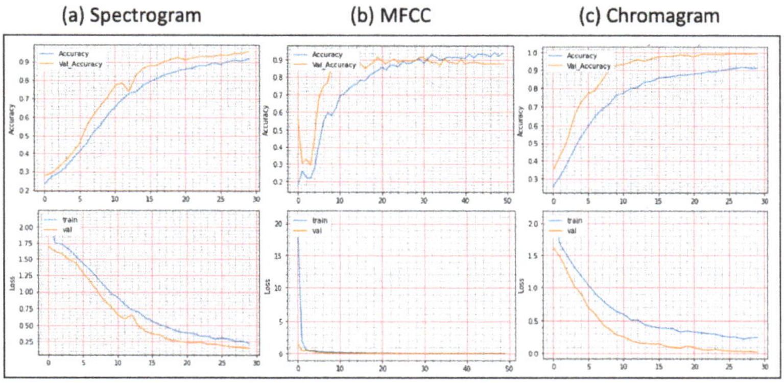

Figure 9. Heart Condition Classification (Accuracy vs. Loss): The Fusion Network Model (FDC-FS) was Evaluated with Three Features: (**a**) Spectrogram, (**b**) MFCC, (**c**) Chromagram.

Results on Class-wise Accuracy for Lung and Heart Datasets: Class-wise accuracy for all models based on the augmented lung dataset is also shown in Figure 10 and Table 10. We obtained the highest class-wise accuracy for the COPD category based on the Spectrogram and MFCC features. For the class-wise accuracy, the highest accuracy is reported by the FDC-FS model as shown in Figure 11 and Table 11. The heart data were unbalanced but showed consistent data patterns and characteristics among categories. Thus, as the average accuracy and weighted average accuracy were similar, we constantly reported the weighted accuracy strategy. As the heart data are similar to the musical dataset, MFCC and Chromagram performed better than Spectrogram. On the other hand, Spectrogram performed very well in FDC-FS for both the heart and lung datasets. Our results are very competitive even with the state-of-the-art approaches, even with a small and reduced number of measurements.

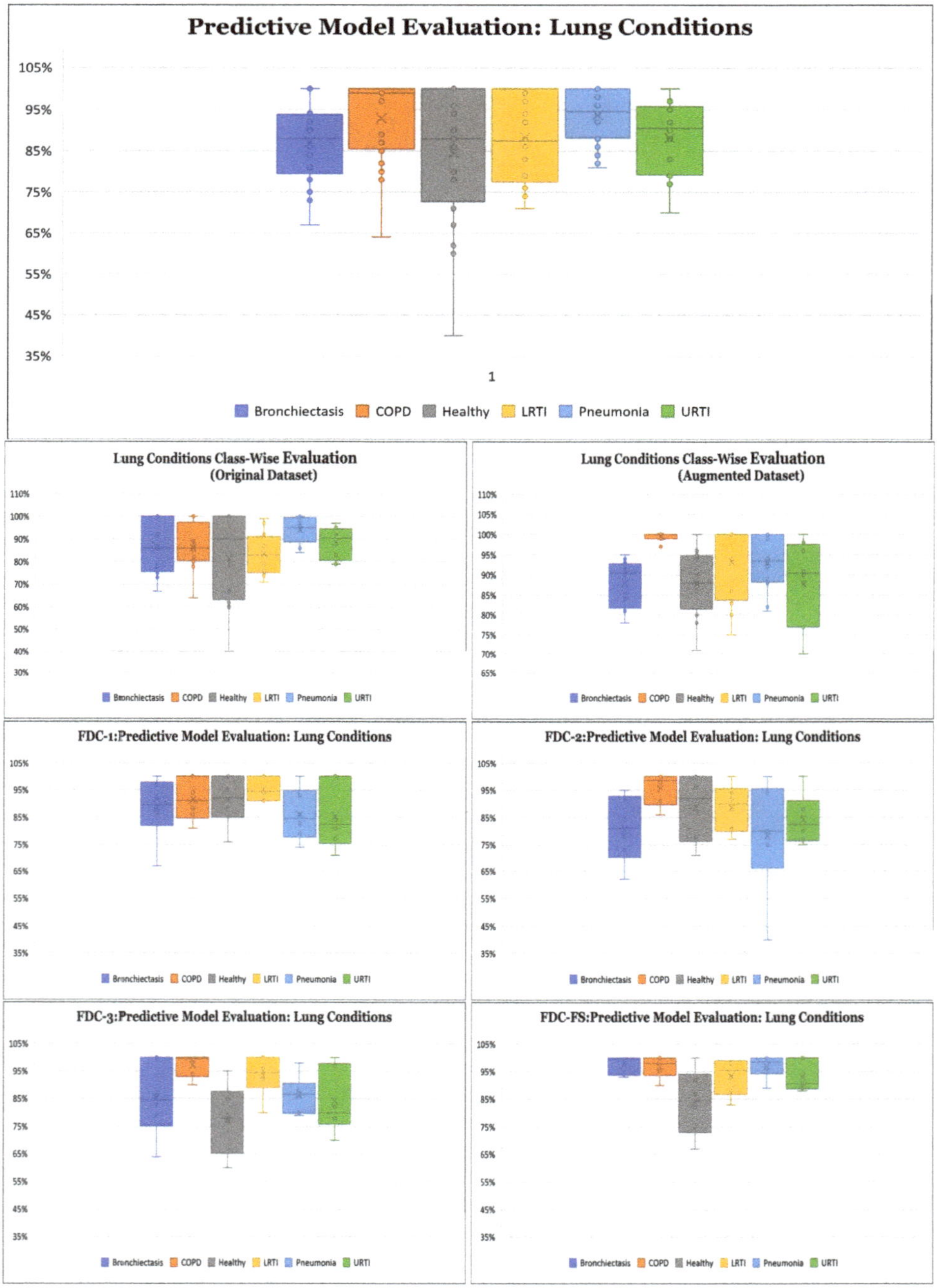

Figure 10. Class Wise Accuracy for Lung Condition Detection.

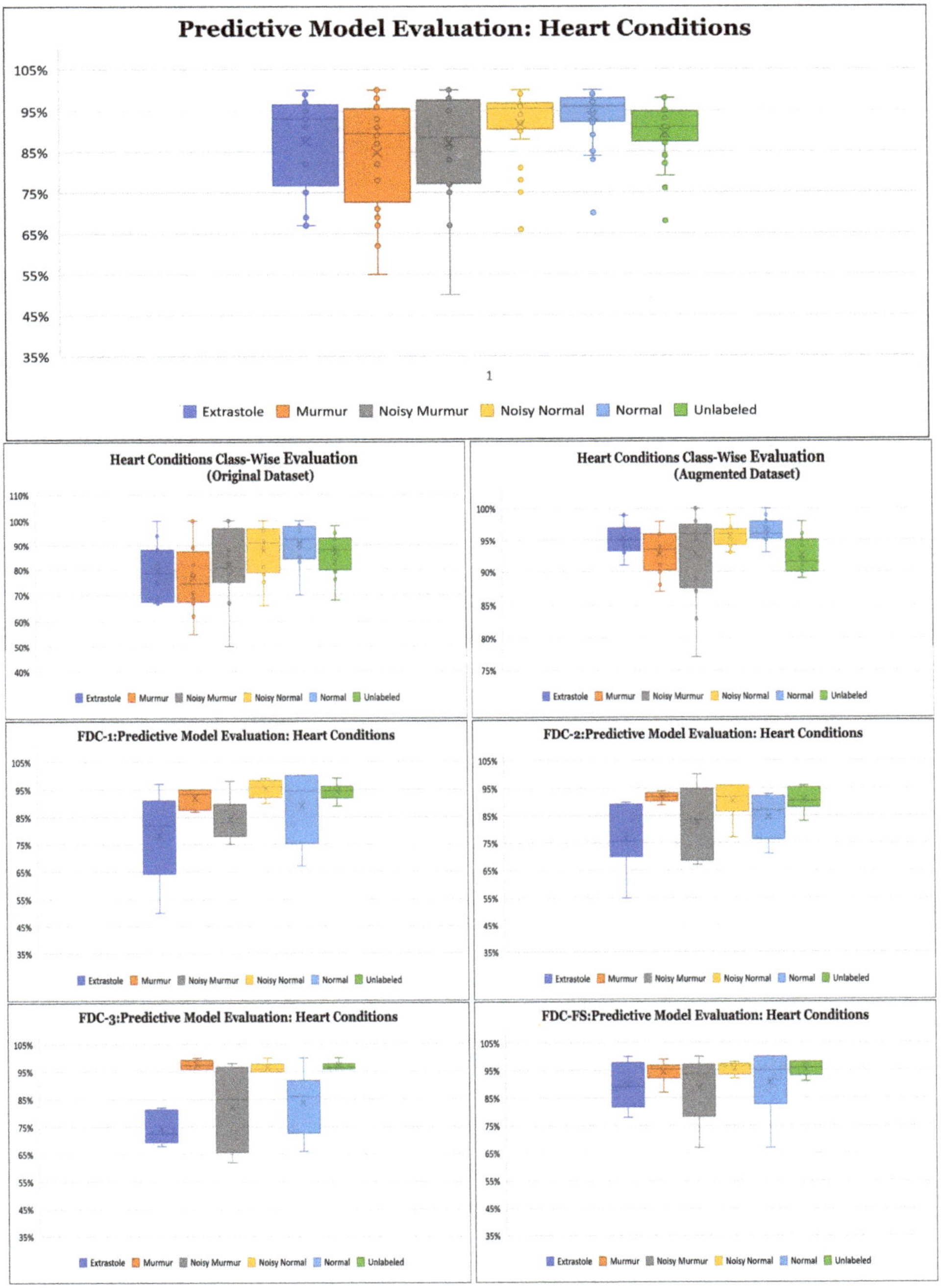

Figure 11. Class Wise Accuracy for Heart Condition Detection.

Table 10. Class Wise Accuracy for Lung Condition Detection.

Model	Feature	Class	Bronchiectasis	COPD	Healthy	LRTI	Pneumonia	URTI	W. AVG
FDC-1	Spec.	Ori.	92%	100%	67%	87%	87%	97%	91%
		Aug.	81 %	100 %	94 %	86 %	100 %	88 %	99%
	MFCC	Ori.	100%	89%	100%	76%	95%	88%	90%
		Aug.	91 %	100 %	95 %	100 %	94 %	91 %	99.3%
	Chroma	Ori.	79%	83%	100%	74%	86%	93%	86%
		Aug.	84 %	100 %	71 %	100 %	81 %	77 %	97%
FDC-2	Spec.	Ori.	73%	78%	62%	92%	84%	95%	87%
		Aug.	91 %	99 %	86 %	100 %	100 %	98 %	98.6%
	MFCC	Ori.	78%	88%	100%	71%	100%	96%	93%
		Aug.	81%	100%	88%	94%	92%	77%	98%
	Chroma	Ori.	100 %	80 %	40%	75%	94%	80%	83%
		Aug.	85 %	100 %	80 %	75 %	88 %	77 %	97%
FDC-3	Spec.	Ori.	86%	64%	100%	79%	100%	83%	84%
		Aug.	94 %	99 %	100 %	100 %	100 %	90 %	98.3%
	MFCC	Ori.	67%	85%	60%	77%	95%	79%	83%
		Aug.	69 %	100 %	59 %	50 %	77 %	74 %	98.2%
	Chroma	Ori.	86%	87%	80%	88%	98%	79%	89%
		Aug.	78 %	97 %	78 %	100 %	82 %	70 %	95%
FDC-FS	Spec.	Ori.	100%	100%	100%	99%	94%	93%	97%
		Aug.	95 %	100 %	90 %	100 %	100 %	96 %	99.1%
	MFCC	Ori.	75%	82%	67%	87%	100%	92%	91%
		Aug.	92 %	100 %	96 %	80 %	93 %	100 %	99%
	Chroma	Ori.	100%	100%	100%	97%	96%	89%	95%
		Aug.	90 %	100 %	88 %	100 %	89 %	91 %	98.4%

Table 11. Class Wise Accuracy for Heart Condition Detection.

Model	Feature	Class	Extrastole	Murmur	Noisy Murmur	Noisy Normal	Normal	Unlabeled	W. AVG
FDC-1	Spec.	Ori.	69%	89%	50%	97%	85%	79%	85%
		Aug.	94%	88%	87%	93%	95%	95%	93%
	MFCC	Ori.	83%	79%	83%	75%	98%	87%	89%
		Aug.	99%	93%	96%	96%	98%	90%	95%
	Chroma	Ori.	100%	67%	78%	100%	97%	92%	89%
		Aug.	95%	94%	95%	93%	99%	89%	94%
FDC-2	Spec.	Ori.	75%	55%	75%	90%	89%	76%	81%
		Aug.	93%	91%	89%	94%	93%	91%	92%
	MFCC	Ori.	75%	69%	67%	92%	100%	93%	91%
		Aug.	93%	91%	77%	96%	96%	90%	93%
	Chroma	Ori.	88 %	71 %	86%	78%	93%	92%	89%
		Aug.	91%	90%	83%	96%	95%	90%	93%
FDC-3	Spec.	Ori.	82%	70%	75%	81%	70%	68%	73%
		Aug.	97%	96%	100%	99%	96%	98%	92%
	MFCC	Ori.	67%	62%	88%	96%	98%	82%	89%
		Aug.	95%	96%	100%	96%	97%	95%	96%
	Chroma	Ori.	88%	100%	75%	66%	84%	89%	84%
		Aug.	97%	96%	96%	97%	100%	96%	95%
FDC-FS	Spec.	Ori.	94%	78%	100%	97%	83%	84%	89%
		Aug.	99%	87%	96%	95%	96%	94%	97%
	MFCC	Ori.	67%	82%	100%	92%	96%	95%	93%
		Aug.	97%	94%	96%	97%	98%	92%	96%
	Chroma	Ori.	67%	100%	100%	88%	92%	98%	92%
		Aug.	94%	98%	98%	96%	96%	91%	97%

5. Comparison with State-of-the-Art Research

For the comparative evaluation of our frameworks, we considered the state-of-the-art research published in reputed journals and conferences between 2018 and 2021, commonly used benchmark datasets from the ICBHI [27] and the heart challenge [57]. First, we conducted a comparative evaluation of the proposed framework (FDC) with different lung sound classification approaches [32,35–38,40]. Second, we conducted a comparative evaluation of the proposed framework (FDC) with different heart sound classification approaches [41–43,45,46,58–60].

5.1. Lung Sound Classification

A comprehensive evaluation of the lung sound classification models has been conducted regarding feature selection and representation, network architecture design, accuracy, and the number of trainable parameters on the lung and heart sound datasets. The best state-of-the-art approach for lung classification that has obtained the highest accuracy of 98.20% is by [60]. However, they have mixed the ICHBI dataset with their own recorded sounds from a local hospital, and another factor is that they are using shallow learning models. Ref. [38] proposed methodology obtained 98.70% accuracy, their number of trainable parameters was 3.8 M. To train their model, they needed more computational power and time. Similarly, ref. [35] used different features using the ResNet-50 model, which is a massive model with over 23 M trainable parameters. It can be seen from Table 12 that our model has shallow trainable parameters, i.e., 1.48 M, which is the lowest as compared to all state-of-the-art research. Thus, it requires very minimum resources (we mainly used CoLab for training and testing) and low epochs of only 50 for training our models. The accuracy performance is also slightly better than other approaches. FDC model also achieved the highest accuracy of approximately 99.1%. The overall comparison of our model performance for the lung sound classification with state-of-the-art research is shown in Table 12.

Table 12. State-of-the-art Lung Classification Models.

Work	Method	Network	Class#	Data	Para#	Aug	Feature	Results
Dalal (2018) [32]	Ensemble	SVM, KNN, GMM, CNN	7	R.A.L.E data	NA	✓	MFCC, LBP	ACC: 95.56%
Hai (2019) [35]	NA	ResNet50	3	489	+23 M		Sp	ACC: 98.79%
Fatih (2020) [36]	Ensemble	CNN	4	920	NA		Sp Images, Deep Features	ACC: 71.15%
Demir (2020) [37]	NA	CNN, SVM	4	6898	138 M		Sp	ACC: 65.9%
Demir (2020) [37]	Transfer learning	CNN, SVM	4	6898	138 M		Sp Images	ACC: 63.09%
Samiul (2020) [38]	NA	CNN	6	917	3.8 M	✓	Hybrid Scalogram	98.70%
Luay (2021) [40]	Ensemble	SVM, KNN, DT, KNN	6	308/1176	NA		Entropy features	ACC: 98.20%
FDC-FS (Ours)	Fusion	DCNN	6	Original (Augmented): 919 (10,109)	**1.48 M**	✓	SP, MFCC, CH	**ACC: 99.1%**

5.2. Heart Sound Classification

Similarly, we conducted a comprehensive evaluation of the heart sound classification models. Based on the number of parameters for FDC-1, the total trainable parameters are 0.24 M, and we obtained an accuracy of 93%. In contrast, for FDC-3, we received an accuracy of 96%, and the total parameters are 0.36 M. After applying the fusion technique, the parameters increased to 1.48 M with an accuracy of 97%. However, our accuracy for the fused model is near that of the state-of-the-art (approximately 98%). Still, some works did not report the trainable parameters of their proposed models [46]. Furthermore, they used the dataset with additional samples equally balanced. Therefore, it can be assumed that their trainable parameters may slightly be higher due to their network architecture of paralleling recurrent convolutional neural network (CNN), i.e., input shape, the number of layers, max-pooling, strides, the output classification size, etc. However, our accuracy is comparable to Shuvo et al. [38], whose accuracy is 97% with a model with 0.32 M trainable parameters. The overall comparison of our model performance for the heart sound classification with state-of-the-art research is shown in Table 13.

Table 13. State-of-the-art Heart Classification Models.

Work	Method	Network	Class#	Data	Para#	Aug	Features	Results
Potes (2016) [41]	Ensemble	CNN	2	Normal (Abnormal): 2575 (665)	NA		MFCC	ACC: 85%
Zhang (2017) [42]	NA	CNN+SVM	3/4	Heart sounds 1 & 2	NA		SP	Precision: 77%/71%
Bozkurt (2018) [43]	NA	CNN	4	PhysioNet: Abnormal (Normal)	NA	✓	MFCC, Mel-SP	ACC: 81.50%
Wu (2019) [58]	Ensemble	CNN	2	Normal (Abnormal): 2575 (665)	61 M		Sp, Mel-SP, MFCC	ACC: 86%
Shu (2020) [45]	NA	WaveNet	5	1000	0.32 M		Multiple features	Training ACC: 97%
Xiao (2020) [59]	Transition	1D CNN	4	PhysioNet: 3153	0.19M		Raw signal w/t band filter	ACC: 93%
Muqing (2020) [46]	Concat.	CRNN, PRCNN	4	PhysioNet: 3240	NA		MFCC	ACC: 98%
Koike (2020) [61]	Pre-train.	PANN	2	PhysioNet:	80.7M	NA	Log-Mel	UAR: 89.7%
Mehmat (2021) [60]	NA	1D CNN	4	PhysioNet	NA		LBP+LTP	ACC: 91%
FDC-FS (Ours)	Fusion	DCNN	6	Original (Augmented): 656 (7216)	**1.48 M**	✓	SP, MFCC, CH	**ACC: 97%**

5.3. Discussion

Our proposed framework demonstrated superior performance compared to the state-of-the-art research both in lung and heart sound classification. We summarize the primary reasons had such good performance in lung or heart condition detection and why it consistently achieves such high performance. (i) Selection of compelling audio features to maximize the characteristics of lung or heart sounds. (ii) Application of data augmentation techniques effectively to overcome the audio data issues such as the low quality and unbalanced datasets. (iii) Transformation of the selected audio features (Spectrogram, MFCC, and Chromagram) to visual feature vectors to maximize the learning performance from deep learning. (iv) Design three unique deep neural network models (FDC-1, FDC-2, FDC-3) to discover new image patterns of audio features involved in a specific disease in lung or heart domains. (v) The fusion model (FDC-FS) is based on the transfer learning from the three different models (FDC-1, FDC-2, FDC-3) from three unique features (Spectrogram, MFCC, and Chromagram) in the lung or heart sound domains.

The limitations of the proposed framework are (i) The proposed framework performs well in two domain lung and heart sound domains; however, there is a lack of generalization.

Nevertheless, we will investigate well enough to offer scientific evidence to explain why some models or specific features are better than others. (ii) We will develop suitable pattern mining methods and practices for automatic network design according to the given datasets. (iii) We will incorporate more effective transfer learning or subsequent knowledge distillation through the fusion networks that might be further optimized for the excellent balance between conciseness (fusion) and detail (specific features). (iv) We will improve pre-processing or data augmentation methods to help to overcome the data issues (noise and data imbalance), which are common in medical research, resulting in poor performance and sometimes bias in network design and parameter estimates. (v) We maintained the size of the floating window constant to maximize model efficiency. However, we can take into account the size of the floating window and then compare the output of each model.

Time is critical for our inquiry, as time-frequency images may vary between subjects due to subject-specific features and heart rate variability. As previously stated, a spectrogram is a graphical representation of a time-frequency domain signal. The signal's frequency and sequence, as well as its temporal variations, were determined using Short Time Fourier transform (STFT). Using STFT, we were able to construct characteristics that could be used to discriminate across conditions but were unaffected by subject variance. Rather of concentrating exclusively on individual differences, we sought to discover broad characteristics that may help in correct categorization. Temporal elements are decreased when the medium changes from audio to video. By and large, our technique achieved exceptional results for a variety of reasons, including the successful extraction of audio features, their transfer to visuals, and the novel design of a deep neural network for the visual representation of heart and lung disorders.

6. Conclusions

In this paper, we developed the feature-based fusion network FDC-FS for the heart and lung disease classification. We used the two publicly available sound datasets with different numbers of samples and class imbalance ratios for this study. In addition, we performed our experimentation with the original dataset to compare our results with the current state-of-the-art research. The experimental results confirmed the superiority of FDC-FS that is a fusion network by combines the three unique models, i.e., FDC-1, FDC-2, and FDC-3, built with the images of specific audio features of Spectrogram, MFCC, and Chromagram. The accuracy reported for the lung dataset is 97% for Spectrogram, 91% for MFCC, and 95% for Chromagram. In contrast, for the heart data, the accuracy reported is 89% for Spectrogram, 93% for MFCC, and 92% for Chromagram.

We further improved the results by applying the data augmentation techniques to the audio clips rather than the images. We used three types of audio augmentation techniques, i.e., noise, pitch shifting, and time stretching, carefully selecting the ranges of values. As a result, the accuracy reported for the augmented lung dataset is 99.1% for Spectrogram, 99% for MFCC, and 98.4% for Chromagram. For the heart dataset, the reported accuracy is based on the accuracy of the dataset% augmentation is 97% for Spectrogram, 96% for MFCC, and 97% for Chromagram. We will further apply the proposed models and techniques to more various datasets. Moreover, we will take our research toward the multi-tasks classification by combining lung and heart models. Finally, we will extend the work for interpretable deep learning and explainable AI by providing evidence of unique patterns discovered for specific conditions.

Author Contributions: Conceptualization, Z.T., S.K.S. and Y.L.; methodology, Z.T., S.K.S. and Y.L.; software, Z.T. and S.K.S.; validation, Z.T., S.K.S. and Y.L.; formal analysis, Z.T., S.K.S. and Y.L.; investigation, Z.T., S.K.S. and Y.L.; resources, Z.T., S.K.S. and Y.L.; data curation, Z.T. and S.K.S.; writing—original draft preparation, Z.T., S.K.S. and Y.L.; writing—review and editing, Z.T., S.K.S. and Y.L.; visualization, Z.T. and S.K.S.; supervision, Y.L.; project administration, Y.L.; funding acquisition, Y.L. All authors have read and agreed to the published version of the manuscript.

Funding: This research was partially funded by NSF grant number 1935076.

Institutional Review Board Statement: Not applicable.

Informed Consent Statement: Not applicable.

Data Availability Statement: Not applicable.

Acknowledgments: The co-author, Yugyung Lee, would like to acknowledge the partial support of the NSF, USA Grant No. 1747751, 1935076, and 1951971.

Conflicts of Interest: The authors declare no conflict of interest. The funders had no role in the design of the study; in the collection, analyses, or interpretation of data; in the writing of the manuscript, or in the decision to publish the results.

References

1. WHO. WHO's Global Health Estimates: The Top 10 Causes of Death. 2020. Available online: https://www.who.int/news-room/fact-sheets/detail/the-top-10-causes-of-death (accessed on 2 July 2021).
2. Ajufo, E.; Rao, S.; Navar, A.M.; Pandey, A.; Ayers, C.R.; Khera, A. US population at increased risk of severe illness from COVID-19. *Am. J. Prev. Cardiol.* **2021**, *6*, 100156. [CrossRef] [PubMed]
3. Hartman, M.; Martin, A.B.; Benson, J.; Catlin, A.; National Health Expenditure Accounts Team. National Health Care Spending In 2018: Growth Driven By Accelerations In Medicare And Private Insurance Spending: US health care spending increased 4.6 percent to reach $3.6 trillion in 2018, a faster growth rate than that of 4.2 percent in 2017 but the same rate as in 2016. *Health Affairs* **2020**, *39*, 8–17. [PubMed]
4. Kahya, Y.P.; Guler, E.C.; Sahin, S. Respiratory disease diagnosis using lung sounds. In Proceedings of the 19th Annual International Conference of the IEEE Engineering in Medicine and Biology Society. 'Magnificent Milestones and Emerging Opportunities in Medical Engineering' (Cat. No. 97CH36136), Chicago, IL, USA, 30 October–2 November 1997; Volume 5, pp. 2051–2053.
5. Arts, L.; Hartono, E.; Lim, T.; van de Ven, P.M.; Heunks, L.; Tuinman, P.R. The diagnostic accuracy of lung auscultation in adult patients with acute pulmonary pathologies: A meta-analysis. *Sci. Rep.* **2020**, *10*, 7347. [CrossRef] [PubMed]
6. Mangione, S.; Nieman, L.Z. Pulmonary auscultatory skills during training in internal medicine and family practice. *Am. J. Respir. Crit. Care Med.* **1999**, *159*, 1119–1124. [CrossRef] [PubMed]
7. Hu, X.J.; Ma, X.J.; Zhao, Q.M.; Yan, W.L.; Ge, X.L.; Jia, B.; Liu, F.; Wu, L.; Ye, M.; Liang, X.C.; et al. Pulse oximetry and auscultation for congenital heart disease detection. *Pediatrics* **2017**, *140*, e20171154. [CrossRef] [PubMed]
8. Mishra, M.; Singh, A.; Dutta, M.K.; Burget, R.; Masek, J. Classification of normal and abnormal heart sounds for automatic diagnosis. In Proceedings of the 2017 40th International Conference on Telecommunications and Signal Processing (TSP), Barcelona, Spain, 5–7 July 2017; pp. 753–757.
9. Brown, C.; Chauhan, J.; Grammenos, A.; Han, J.; Hasthanasombat, A.; Spathis, D.; Xia, T.; Cicuta, P.; Mascolo, C. Exploring automatic diagnosis of COVID-19 from crowdsourced respiratory sound data. In Proceedings of the 26th ACM SIGKDD International Conference on Knowledge Discovery & Data Mining, Virtual Event, 6–10 July 2020; pp. 3474–3484.
10. Nogueira, D.M.; Zarmehri, M.N.; Ferreira, C.A.; Jorge, A.M.; Antunes, L. Heart sounds classification using images from wavelet transformation. In Proceedings of the EPIA Conference on Artificial Intelligence, Vila Real, Portugal, 3–6 September 2019; pp. 311–322.
11. Cobos, M.; Perez-Solano, J.; Berger, L. Acoustic-based technologies for ambient assisted living. *Introd. Smart Ehealth Ecare Technol.* **2016**, 159–180.
12. Dimitrievski, A.; Zdravevski, E.; Lameski, P.; Trajkovik, V. A survey of Ambient Assisted Living systems: Challenges and opportunities. In Proceedings of the IEEE 12th International Conference on Intelligent Computer Communication and Processing (ICCP), Cluj-Napoca, Romania, 8–10 September 2016; pp. 49–53.
13. Doukas, C.; Maglogiannis, I. Advanced patient or elder fall detection based on movement and sound data. In Proceedings of the 2008 Second International Conference on Pervasive Computing Technologies for Healthcare, Tampere, Finland, 1 February 2008; pp. 103–107.
14. Hegde, S.; Shetty, S.; Rai, S.; Dodderi, T. A survey on machine learning approaches for automatic detection of voice disorders. *J. Voice* **2019**, *33*, 947.e11–947.e33. [CrossRef]
15. Dwivedi, A.K.; Imtiaz, S.A.; Rodriguez-Villegas, E. Algorithms for automatic analysis and classification of heart sounds—A systematic review. *IEEE Access* **2018**, *7*, 8316–8345. [CrossRef]
16. Deng, L.; Yu, D. Deep learning: Methods and applications. *Found. Trends® Signal Process.* **2014**, *7*, 197–387. [CrossRef]
17. Alhussein, M.; Muhammad, G.; Hossain, M.S. EEG pathology detection based on deep learning. *IEEE Access* **2019**, *7*, 27781–27788. [CrossRef]
18. Fattah, S.A.; Rahman, N.M.; Maksud, A.; Foysal, S.I.; Chowdhury, R.I.; Chowdhury, S.S.; Shahanaz, C. Stetho-phone: Low-cost digital stethoscope for remote personalized healthcare. In Proceedings of the 2017 IEEE Global Humanitarian Technology Conference (GHTC), San Jose, CA, USA, 19–22 October 2017; pp. 1–7.
19. Dimoulas, C.A. Audiovisual spatial-audio analysis by means of sound localization and imaging: A multimedia healthcare framework in abdominal sound mapping. *IEEE Trans. Multimed.* **2016**, *18*, 1969–1976. [CrossRef]

20. Zhu, H.; Luo, M.D.; Wang, R.; Zheng, A.H.; He, R. Deep audio-visual learning: A survey. *Int. J. Autom. Comput.* **2021**, *18*, 351–376. [CrossRef]
21. Nogueira, D.M.; Ferreira, C.A.; Gomes, E.F.; Jorge, A.M. Classifying heart sounds using images of motifs, mfcc and temporal features. *J. Med. Syst.* **2019**, *43*, 1–13. [CrossRef] [PubMed]
22. Zhu, Z.; Yin, H.; Chai, Y.; Li, Y.; Qi, G. A novel multi-modality image fusion method based on image decomposition and sparse representation. *Inf. Sci.* **2018**, *432*, 516–529. [CrossRef]
23. Luz, J.S.; Oliveira, M.C.; Araújo, F.H.; Magalhães, D.M. Ensemble of handcrafted and deep features for urban sound classification. *Appl. Acoust.* **2021**, *175*, 107819. [CrossRef]
24. Sun, D.; Wang, M.; Li, A. A multimodal deep neural network for human breast cancer prognosis prediction by integrating multi-dimensional data. *IEEE/ACM Trans. Comput. Biol. Bioinform.* **2018**, *16*, 841–850. [CrossRef]
25. Nanni, L.; Maguolo, G.; Brahnam, S.; Paci, M. An Ensemble of Convolutional Neural Networks for Audio Classification. *arXiv* **2020**, arXiv:2007.07966.
26. Bagley, J.A.; Reumann, D.; Bian, S.; Lévi-Strauss, J.; Knoblich, J.A. Fused cerebral organoids model interactions between brain regions. *Nat. Methods* **2017**, *14*, 743–751. [CrossRef]
27. Rocha, B.; Filos, D.; Mendes, L.; Vogiatzis, I.; Perantoni, E.; Kaimakamis, E.; Natsiavas, P.; Oliveira, A.; Jácome, C.; Marques, A.; et al. A respiratory sound database for the development of automated classification. In Proceedings of the International Conference on Biomedical and Health Informatics, Thessaloniki, Greece, 18–21 November 2017; pp. 33–37.
28. Mikołajczyk, A.; Grochowski, M. Data augmentation for improving deep learning in image classification problem. In Proceedings of the 2018 International Interdisciplinary PhD Workshop (IIPhDW), Swinoujscie, Poland, 12 May 2018; pp. 117–122.
29. Nguyen, T.; Pernkopf, F. Lung Sound Classification Using Snapshot Ensemble of Convolutional Neural Networks. In Proceedings of the 2020 42nd Annual International Conference of the IEEE Engineering in Medicine & Biology Society (EMBC), Montreal, QC, Canada, 20–24 July 2020; pp. 760–763.
30. Lella, K.K.; Pja, A. Automatic COVID-19 disease diagnosis using 1D convolutional neural network and augmentation with human respiratory sound based on parameters: Cough, breath, and voice. *AIMS Public Health* **2021**, *8*, 240. [CrossRef]
31. Kochetov, K.; Filchenkov, A. Generative Adversarial Networks for Respiratory Sound Augmentation. In Proceedings of the 2020 International Conference on Control, Robotics and Intelligent System, Xiamen, China, 27–29 October 2020; pp. 106–111.
32. Bardou, D.; Zhang, K.; Ahmad, S.M. Lung sounds classification using convolutional neural networks. *Artif. Intell. Med.* **2018**, *88*, 58–69. [CrossRef]
33. Ward, J.J. R.A.L.E Lung Sounds 3.1 Profesional Edition. *Respir. Care* **2005**, *50*, 1385–1388.
34. Dubey, R.; M Bodade, R. A Review of Classification Techniques Based on Neural Networks for Pulmonary Obstructive Diseases. In Proceedings of the Recent Advances in Interdisciplinary Trends in Engineering & Applications (RAITEA), Indore, Inde, 14–17 February 2019.
35. Chen, H.; Yuan, X.; Pei, Z.; Li, M.; Li, J. Triple-classification of respiratory sounds using optimized s-transform and deep residual networks. *IEEE Access* **2019**, *7*, 32845–32852. [CrossRef]
36. Demir, F.; Ismael, A.M.; Sengur, A. Classification of Lung Sounds with CNN Model Using Parallel Pooling Structure. *IEEE Access* **2020**, *8*, 105376–105383. [CrossRef]
37. Demir, F.; Sengur, A.; Bajaj, V. Convolutional neural networks based efficient approach for classification of lung diseases. *Health Inf. Sci. Syst.* **2020**, *8*, 1–8. [CrossRef]
38. Shuvo, S.B.; Ali, S.N.; Swapnil, S.I.; Hasan, T.; Bhuiyan, M.I.H. A lightweight cnn model for detecting respiratory diseases from lung auscultation sounds using emd-cwt-based hybrid scalogram. *IEEE J. Biomed. Health Inform.* **2020**, *25*, 2595–2603. [CrossRef]
39. Messner, E.; Fediuk, M.; Swatek, P.; Scheidl, S.; Smolle-Jüttner, F.M.; Olschewski, H.; Pernkopf, F. Multi-channel lung sound classification with convolutional recurrent neural networks. *Comput. Biol. Med.* **2020**, *122*, 103831. [CrossRef]
40. Fraiwan, L.; Hassanin, O.; Fraiwan, M.; Khassawneh, B.; Ibnian, A.M.; Alkhodari, M. Automatic identification of respiratory diseases from stethoscopic lung sound signals using ensemble classifiers. *Biocybern. Biomed. Eng.* **2021**, *41*, 1–14. [CrossRef]
41. Potes, C.; Parvaneh, S.; Rahman, A.; Conroy, B. Ensemble of feature-based and deep learning-based classifiers for detection of abnormal heart sounds. In Proceedings of the 2016 Computing in Cardiology Conference (CinC), Vancouver, BC, Canada, 11–14 September 2016; pp. 621–624.
42. Zhang, W.; Han, J. Towards heart sound classification without segmentation using convolutional neural network. In Proceedings of the 2017 Computing in Cardiology (CinC), Rennes, France, 24–27 September 2017; pp. 1–4.
43. Bozkurt, B.; Germanakis, I.; Stylianou, Y. A study of time-frequency features for CNN-based automatic heart sound classification for pathology detection. *Comput. Biol. Med.* **2018**, *100*, 132–143. [CrossRef]
44. Clifford, G.D.; Liu, C.; Moody, B.; Springer, D.; Silva, I.; Li, Q.; Mark, R.G. Classification of normal/abnormal heart sound recordings: The PhysioNet/Computing in Cardiology Challenge 2016. In Proceedings of the 2016 Computing in cardiology conference (CinC), Vancouver, BC, Canada, 11–14 September 2016; pp. 609–612.
45. Oh, S.L.; Jahmunah, V.; Ooi, C.P.; Tan, R.S.; Ciaccio, E.J.; Yamakawa, T.; Tanabe, M.; Kobayashi, M.; Acharya, U.R. Classification of heart sound signals using a novel deep wavenet model. *Comput. Methods Programs Biomed.* **2020**, *196*, 105604. [CrossRef]
46. Deng, M.; Meng, T.; Cao, J.; Wang, S.; Zhang, J.; Fan, H. Heart sound classification based on improved MFCC features and convolutional recurrent neural networks. *Neural Netw.* **2020**, *130*, 22–32. [CrossRef]

47. Chen, W.; Sun, Q.; Chen, X.; Xie, G.; Wu, H.; Xu, C. Deep Learning Methods for Heart Sounds Classification: A Systematic Review. *Entropy* **2021**, *23*, 667. [CrossRef] [PubMed]
48. Acharya, U.R.; Fujita, H.; Oh, S.L.; Hagiwara, Y.; Tan, J.H.; Adam, M. Application of deep convolutional neural network for automated detection of myocardial infarction using ECG signals. *Inf. Sci.* **2017**, *415*, 190–198. [CrossRef]
49. Oh, S.L.; Ng, E.Y.; San Tan, R.; Acharya, U.R. Automated diagnosis of arrhythmia using combination of CNN and LSTM techniques with variable length heart beats. *Comput. Biol. Med.* **2018**, *102*, 278–287. [CrossRef] [PubMed]
50. Rajpurkar, P.; Hannun, A.Y.; Haghpanahi, M.; Bourn, C.; Ng, A.Y. Cardiologist-level arrhythmia detection with convolutional neural networks. *arXiv* **2017**, arXiv:1707.01836 .
51. Wyse, L. Audio spectrogram representations for processing with convolutional neural networks. *arXiv* **2017**, arXiv:1706.09559.
52. McFee, B.; Humphrey, E.J.; Bello, J.P. *A Software Framework for Musical Data Augmentation*; ISMIR: Izmir, Turkey, 2015; Volume 2015, pp. 248–254.
53. Wei, S.; Xu, K.; Wang, D.; Liao, F.; Wang, H.; Kong, Q. Sample mixed-based data augmentation for domestic audio tagging. *arXiv* **2018**, arXiv:1808.03883.
54. Cohen, L. *Time-Frequency Analysis*; Prentice Hall: Hoboken, NJ, USA, 1995; Volume 778.
55. Semmlow, J.L.; Griffel, B. *Biosignal and Medical Image Processing*; CRC Press: Boca Raton, FL, USA, 2014.
56. Molau, S.; Pitz, M.; Schluter, R.; Ney, H. Computing mel-frequency cepstral coefficients on the power spectrum. In Proceedings of the 2001 IEEE International Conference on Acoustics, Speech, and Signal Processing, Proceedings (Cat. No. 01CH37221), Salt Lake City, UT, USA, 7–11 May 2001; Volume 1, pp. 73–76.
57. Bentley, P.; Nordehn, G.; Coimbra, M.; Mannor, S. The PASCAL Classifying Heart Sounds Challenge 2011 (CHSC2011) Results. Available online: http://www.peterjbentley.com/heartchallenge/index.html (accessed on 13 February 2022).
58. Wu, J.M.T.; Tsai, M.H.; Huang, Y.Z.; Islam, S.H.; Hassan, M.M.; Alelaiwi, A.; Fortino, G. Applying an ensemble convolutional neural network with Savitzky–Golay filter to construct a phonocardiogram prediction model. *Appl. Soft Comput.* **2019**, *78*, 29–40. [CrossRef]
59. Xiao, B.; Xu, Y.; Bi, X.; Zhang, J.; Ma, X. Heart sounds classification using a novel 1-D convolutional neural network with extremely low parameter consumption. *Neurocomputing* **2020**, *392*, 153–159. [CrossRef]
60. Bilal, E.M. Heart sounds classification using convolutional neural network with 1D-local binary pattern and 1D-local ternary pattern features. *Appl. Acoust.* **2021**, *180*, 108152.
61. Koike, T.; Qian, K.; Kong, Q.; Plumbley, M.D.; Schuller, B.W.; Yamamoto, Y. Audio for audio is better? an investigation on transfer learning models for heart sound classification. In Proceedings of the 2020 42nd Annual International Conference of the IEEE Engineering in Medicine & Biology Society (EMBC), Montreal, QC, Canada, 20–24 July 2020; pp. 74–77.

sensors

MDPI

Article

A New Framework for Precise Identification of Prostatic Adenocarcinoma

Sarah M. Ayyad [1], Mohamed A. Badawy [2], Mohamed Shehata [3], Ahmed Alksas [3], Ali Mahmoud [3], Mohamed Abou El-Ghar [2], Mohammed Ghazal [4], Moumen El-Melegy [5], Nahla B. Abdel-Hamid [1], Labib M. Labib [1], H. Arafat Ali [1,6] and Ayman El-Baz [3,*]

1 Computers and Systems Department, Faculty of Engineering, Mansoura University, Mansoura 35511, Egypt; sarah_ayyad@mans.edu.eg (S.M.A.); nahla_bishri@mans.edu.eg (N.B.A.-H.); labib_essa@mans.edu.eg (L.M.L.); h.arafat_ali@mans.edu.eg (H.A.A.)
2 Radiology Department, Urology and Nephrology Center, Mansoura University, Mansoura 35516, Egypt; mohammed.ali.badawy@gmail.com (M.A.B.); maboelghar@mans.edu.eg (M.A.E.-G.)
3 BioImaging Laboratory, Bioengineering Department, University of Louisville, Louisville, KY 40292, USA; mnsheh01@louisville.edu (M.S.); ammost01@louisville.edu (A.A.); ahmahm01@louisville.edu (A.M.)
4 Department of Electrical and Computer Engineering, College of Engineering, Abu Dhabi University, Abu Dhabi 59911, United Arab Emirates; mohammed.ghazal@adu.ac.ae
5 Department of Electrical Engineering, Assiut University, Assiut 71511, Egypt; moumen@aun.edu.eg
6 Faulty of Artificial Intelligence, Delta University for Science and Technology, Mansoura 35516, Egypt
* Correspondence: aselba01@louisville.edu

Citation: Ayyad, S.M.; Badawy, M.A.; Shehata, M.; Alksas, A.; Mahmoud, A.; Abou El-Ghar, M.; Ghazal, M.; El-Melegy, M.; Abdel-Hamid, N.B.; Labib, L.M.; et al. A New Framework for Precise Identification of Prostatic Adenocarcinoma. *Sensors* **2022**, *22*, 1848. https://doi.org/10.3390/s22051848

Academic Editor: Loris Nanni

Received: 8 December 2021
Accepted: 24 February 2022
Published: 26 February 2022

Abstract: Prostate cancer, which is also known as prostatic adenocarcinoma, is an unconstrained growth of epithelial cells in the prostate and has become one of the leading causes of cancer-related death worldwide. The survival of patients with prostate cancer relies on detection at an early, treatable stage. In this paper, we introduce a new comprehensive framework to precisely differentiate between malignant and benign prostate cancer. This framework proposes a noninvasive computer-aided diagnosis system that integrates two imaging modalities of MR (diffusion-weighted (DW) and T2-weighted (T2W)). For the first time, it utilizes the combination of functional features represented by apparent diffusion coefficient (ADC) maps estimated from DW-MRI for the whole prostate in combination with texture features with its first- and second-order representations, extracted from T2W-MRIs of the whole prostate, and shape features represented by spherical harmonics constructed for the lesion inside the prostate and integrated with PSA screening results. The dataset presented in the paper includes 80 biopsy confirmed patients, with a mean age of 65.7 years (43 benign prostatic hyperplasia, 37 prostatic carcinomas). Experiments were conducted using different well-known machine learning approaches including support vector machines (SVM), random forests (RF), decision trees (DT), and linear discriminant analysis (LDA) classification models to study the impact of different feature sets that lead to better identification of prostatic adenocarcinoma. Using a leave-one-out cross-validation approach, the diagnostic results obtained using the SVM classification model along with the combined feature set after applying feature selection (88.75% accuracy, 81.08% sensitivity, 95.35% specificity, and 0.8821 AUC) indicated that the system's performance, after integrating and reducing different types of feature sets, obtained an enhanced diagnostic performance compared with each individual feature set and other machine learning classifiers. In addition, the developed diagnostic system provided consistent diagnostic performance using 10-fold and 5-fold cross-validation approaches, which confirms the reliability, generalization ability, and robustness of the developed system.

Keywords: prostate cancer; MRI; texture analysis; shape features; functional features; computer-aided diagnosis; PSA

1. Introduction

In the United States (US), as well as worldwide, prostate cancer (PCa) is one of the most common male malignancies, and the second most common cancer type in the US with a death rate of about 2.4% among male patients [1,2]. It is considered a serious disease because of the danger of its metastasis into other parts of the body, such as the bladder, bones, and rectum. By 2030, it is expected that there will be up to 1.7 M PCa patients worldwide, with nearly half a million corresponding deaths each year [3]. Fortunately, early detection of PCa leads to better treatment and a lower mortality rate. Throughout this paper, PCa refers specifically to prostatic adenocarcinoma, the pathological subtype responsible for 99% of prostate malignancies.

Multiple screening and diagnostic tests are used to search for symptoms of prostate cancer including prostate-specific antigen (PSA) blood test [4], digital rectal examination (DRE) [5], needle biopsy [6], and magnetic resonance imaging (MRI) [7]. All these methods have recognized shortcomings. For instance, because PSA levels are measured in the blood, situations such as inflamed prostate can produce a high PSA value and may lead to treatments that are not needed [8,9]. In the DRE test, the physician checks the prostate manually to feel the surface of the prostate for regions of hardness. This approach can only identify peripheral zone tumors and cannot identify transitional zone and central zone tumors, or tumor regions that are too small to be felt [3,8]. Transrectal ultrasound (TRUS) guided biopsy [8] is the gold standard diagnostic technique, where the doctor takes a set of small tissue samples from the prostate to investigate under a microscope for cancerous cells. However, it is a painful and expensive procedure, and has adverse effects, such as bleeding and infection [8,10].

Over the past decade, prostate MRI has come to be widely used for cancer detection, especially to discover and locate intraprostatic lesions [11,12]. As a result, large numbers of MR examinations need to be processed. There is general consensus that the MRI submodalities best suited for examination of PCa include T2 weighted (T2W), dynamic contrast-enhanced (DCE), and diffusion-weighted (DW). T2W is the most common type of MRI that employs the transverse magnetization time T2 to create a grayscale image of the scanned area of the body [13]. The idea behind DW-MRI is that it generates images with contrast that reflects differences in the microscopic movement of water molecules within tissues [14]. It can distinguish between benign and suspicious prostatic lesions according to apparent diffusion coefficient (ADC) values from the signal intensity in images obtained using different *b*-values [7]. Several studies employed apparent diffusion coefficient (ADC) maps, which are quantitative maps calculated from DW-MRI, for PCa diagnosis [3,7,12]. Moreover, the acquisition of DW images does not involve injecting a human with a contrast agent, unlike DCE-MRI [15]. DW- and T2W-MRI have acquired popularity as non-invasive imaging techniques for detecting prostate cancer and may overcome many of the flaws of other methods [9]. It is worth mentioning that a few studies have tried to advanced modeling using intra-voxel incoherent motion (IVIM) MR imaging for PCa diagnosis [16]. IVIM emerged as a different approach for obtaining of perfusion information. Significant limitations of the IVIM analysis include the influence of the *b*-values used in the measurements and lack of standardization of calculation of IVIM parameters.

Over the last two decades, computer-aided diagnosis (CAD) has become a key technology in healthcare with the potential to enhance diagnosis and detection of diseases and then improvements in treatment [17–19]. Incorporating artificial intelligence (AI) into CAD systems can help clinicians avoid subjective decisions and reducing reading time. A typical AI-based CAD system takes MR images, locates the prostate, detects tumors within the prostate, and then classifies which of those tumors are likely to be malignant [11]. In recent years, abundant research studies on CAD systems were published employing a variety of AI techniques [12,13,15,17–19]. CAD systems employing AI can be largely classified into handcrafted feature-based CAD and deep learning-based CAD. Our proposed framework falls under the category of handcrafted feature-based CAD. Handcrafted feature-based CAD has attained more popularity in texture classification than deep learning-based techniques [20], owing to the fact that texture data tend to occupy much higher dimensional manifolds compared to object recognition data. Furthermore, deep learning techniques require a huge number of images for training models. Many of the effective CAD systems created for PCa use a group of handcrafted features that were applied for medical and non-medical images.

2. Related Works

There are many works of prostate cancer CAD systems in the literature. CADs that rely on handcrafted features have become popular in the medical image analysis field. For example, the work in [19] employed only 215 texture features extracted from T2W-MRI images and combines the prediction results of 11 classifiers. A noteworthy contribution was the work on many different texture features. This implies that their work investigates many features that have not been used before in common CAD systems. This work is limited in several aspects. For one, it examines the peripheral zone only. It also used the default parameter setting for each classifier. Moreover, only voxels within the malignant areas that are observable in T2W-MR images were considered cancerous voxels, this implies that voxels in the cancerous areas, which did not appear in T2W, were deemed normal. In [17], the authors introduced a CAD system based on texture, spatial, and intensity features extracted from DW (b = 2000 s/mm^2), ADC, and T2W images on 244 patients. The total number of features was 17. They applied random forest (RF) classifier and compared their model to previous CAD models based on support vector machine (SVM) assessed on the same test data. However, their model has some limitations in that they use high b-value of 2000 s/mm^2, where many institutes may not have the equipment to acquire such images. In addition, they used an endorectal coil MRI (ERC) when ERC is not available in all institutions.

A new voxel-based classification CAD system was proposed in [21], where each voxel in the prostate gland will be classified as normal or cancerous by the means of four modalities of MRI. Their goal was to produce a probabilistic map of cancer location in the prostate. They extracted a set of texture, intensity, edge, and anatomical features. These features were further decreased to provide a group of significant features that accurately detect malignancies. The random forest was chosen as their base classifier. However, this study is limited in that authors used a small cohort of patients (only 17 patients). Another machine learning (ML) framework was introduced in [22], where authors tested seven different classifiers to identify the classification model that most correctly differentiates between high-risk prostate cancer patients and low-risk patients. They used 55 texture features for both ADC and T2W images on 121 patients.

Recently, authors in [9] created a model based on auto-fixed segmentation through identical VOIs automatically generated a spherical VOI with the center of the lesion image for quantifying the phenotype of clinically significant (CS) peripheral zone lesions. They used two different datasets and extracted 92 quantitative radiomics features. They showed that adding DCE-MR imaging features enhanced the AUC value from 0.81 to 0.87. This model has a limitation that is only applicable to peripheral zone lesions. In addition, many institutions are reluctant in applying contrast agent to the patients. Other researchers, such as those in [23], developed a predictive ML model based on manual segmentation of T2 images on 191 patients. They extracted 367 radiomic features including the features suggested by the radiologist. Moreover, they applied the maximum relevance minimum redundancy technique to elect a subset of correlated features. Four classifiers were applied to evaluate the model and the model was compared with radiologist assessments. The model is concerned with two tasks: (1) normal vs. cancerous prostate lesion and (2) clinically significant prostate cancer vs. clinically insignificant prostate cancer.

In recent years, the breakthrough of deep learning in the field of image processing has radically altered prostate cancer detection and grading using MRI images [24,25]. In the literature, different related attempts on PCa were published [13,26–29]. The prostate CAD in [13] deployed a fully automatic mono-parametric MRI malignant PCa identification and localization system, where authors proposed a new 3D sliding window technique, that preserved the 2D domain complexity while utilizing 3D information. Although there are available four different modalities in their public dataset, the authors used only the

T2W sequence on 19 patients. A first attempt to produce probability maps for prostate cancer detection by applying deep learning was introduced in [26]. The authors enhanced the holistically nested edge detection (HED) deep CNN. The main advantage of their work was in collecting their dataset from six institutions worldwide. One limitation of the study, however, was that the selected patient cohorts comprised high and intermediate risk patients only. In the same context, the authors of [27] introduced another model that also utilized CNN to evaluate predefined regions on prostate MRI. Lesions were manually segmented by a radiologist. They used three independent cohorts to reduce overfitting for the neural network. A four-class CNN was trained using the fastai library. They utilized Cohen's kappa to measure the agreement of the model with the radiologist and found a rather low agreement (kappa = 0.40) between the model-driven and radiologist scoring.

Recently, the authors of [28] introduced a new classification framework, which was trained using patient-level labels only applied for two datasets. Features extracted by employing seven 3D ResNet CNN architectures from DW images, T2W images, and ADC maps. Then, a two-level SVM classifier scheme was applied to integrate the selected feature vectors and normalized clinical features to obtain a final result of classification. However, there was a big difference in performance evaluation between radiologist and their CAD. Another recent study [29], proposed a Retina U-Net detection framework to locate the lesions and expected their most likely Gleason grade. They worked on both the lesion level and the patient level on two different datasets. On the lesion level, they reported a sensitivity of 100%, specificity of 79% and an AUC of 0.96 on the first dataset and a sensitivity of 100%, specificity of 80% and an AUC of 0.96 on the second dataset. However, at the patient level, they found a noticeably reduced performance on the first dataset (AUC = 0.87, sensitivity = 100%, and specificity = 37.5%) and on the second dataset as well (AUC = 0.91, sensitivity = 100%, and specificity = 76.2%). However, their model has two limitations. First, it needs additional validation to evaluate histological results of targeted biopsies to the lesions detected by the model. Second, the authors successfully trained their model on two different datasets, but it still performed differently with each of them. This shows that CAD for prostate MRI is a very challenging area of study. Table 1 reports a brief recapitulation of the reviewed CAD studies.

Table 1. A brief comparison between previous prostate MRI CAD studies.

Reference	Year	Type of Approach	Features Type	Classes	Images Sequences	No. of Patients Involved	Accuracy Result
[17]	2017	Handcrafted features-based CAD	Spatial, intensity, and texture	Benign, Gleason 6, Gleason 7, Gleason 8, Gleason 9, Gleason 10	B2000, ADC, and T2W	224	SVM model achieved an AUC value of 0.86, while Random Forest achieved an AUC of 0.93
[19]	2016		Texture	Malignant or benign	T2W	45	It has a value of 0.93 AUC
[21]	2017		Texture, intensity, edge, and anatomical	Voxel-based classification	DWI, T2W, DCE, and MRSI	17	Classification performance of an average AUC of 0.836 ± 0.083 is achieved
[22]	2019		Texture	High risk patients and low risk patients	T2WI and ADC	121	Quadratic kernel based SVM is the best model with an accuracy of 0.92
[9]	2020		Texture and intensity	Benign and/or cs PCa vs. non-cs PCa	B50, b400, b800, b1400, T2WI, DCE, and ADC	206	It has an average AUC value of 0.838
[23]	2020		Shape, texture, and statistical texture	Normal vs. cancerous prostate lesion and clinically significant PCa vs. clinically insignificant PCa	ADC and T2WI	191	AUC value for normal vs. cancerous classification is 0.889, while the AUC value for clinically significant PCa vs. clinically insignificant PCa is 0.844
[13]	2019	Deep learning-based CAD		Produces a voxel probability map	T2WI	19	The model attained an AUC value of 0.995, a recall of 0.928, and an accuracy of 0.894.

Table 1. *Cont.*

Reference	Year	Type of Approach	Features Type	Classes	Images Sequences	No. of Patients Involved	Accuracy Result
[26]	2018		Deep learning-based CAD	Produces probability maps to detect prostate cancer	T2WI, ADC, and high *b*-value (b1500 for cases imaged without ERC insertion, and b-2000 with ERC insertion)	186	The model attained an average AUC value of 0.94 in the peripheral zone and an average AUC value of 0.92 in transition zone.
[27]	2020			Gives a PI-RADS score to a lesion detected and segmented by a radiologist	T2WI, T1WI, ADC, and (b1500 or b2000)	687	Kappa = 0.40, sensitivity = 0.89, and specificity = 0.73.
[28]	2021			Probability that patient has prostate cancer	T2WI, b200, ADC in the first dataset, T2WI, ADC in the second dataset	249 patients in the 1st dataset and 282 patients in the 2nd dataset	AUC value for the first dataset was 0.79, and for the second dataset was 0.86.
[29]	2021			Predicting the Gleason grade group and classifying benign vs. csPCa	T1WI and T2WI	490 cases for training and 75 cases for testing from 2 different datasets	On the lesion level, AUC of 0.96 for both the first and second datasets. On the patient level, AUC of 0.87 and 0.91, for the first and second datasets, respectively.

To overcome the drawbacks of the aforementioned studies, we developed a new comprehensive framework (shown in Figure 1) for early identification of prostatic adenocarcinoma. The developed CAD system has the following main contributions: (i) it calculates functional features represented using cumulative distribution functions (CDFs) of 3D apparent diffusion coefficients (ADCs), estimated from segmented DW-MR images of the whole prostate. The proposed framework employs DW-MRI data gathered at nine different *b*-values (b = 0, 100, 200, 300, 400, 500, 600, 700, and 1400 s/mm^2); thus, it is not sensitive to a specific choice of *b*-value and accounts for blood perfusion and water diffusion at both low and high *b*-values. (ii) The system extracts first and second order textural features that best describe the malignancy status of the prostate by applying novel rotation invariant techniques. (iii) It estimates best discriminating shape features by applying novel spherical harmonics analysis. (iv) Lastly, it integrates of functional, textural, shape features from two modalities of MRI (DW and T2W) with clinical biomarker (PSA) to produce a new comprehensive CAD system for the early identification of prostatic adenocarcinoma.

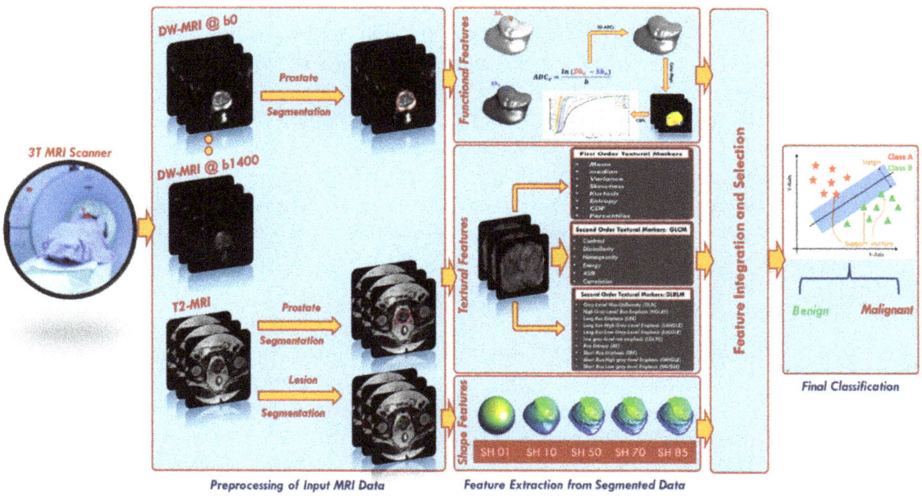

Figure 1. The proposed framework for early detection of prostatic adenocarcinoma.

3. Material and Methods

The steps of the proposed framework are fully illustrated below and depicted in Figure 1.

3.1. Patient Population

A total of 92 patients, who were evaluated for prostate cancer, had undergone T2W-MR and DW-MR imaging at Urology and Nephrology Center, Mansoura University, Egypt, in the period between 2019 and 2021, were included. Inclusion criteria were: (a) high PSA (>4 ng/mL), (b) prostatic adenocarcinoma, and (c) physically and clinically fit for biopsy. Exclusion criteria were: (a) claustrophobia, (b) metallic implants and cardiac pace marker not suitable for MRI, or (c) abnormal coagulation. Twelve patients who had prostatitis and/or refused to participate in the study were then excluded. At the end, we were left with 80 patients with a mean age of 65.7 years, 43 diagnosed with benign prostatic hyperplasia, 37 with prostatic carcinomas). MRI imaging was performed on a 3T scanner (Ingenia, Philips Medical Systems, Best, Holland) with the following settings: number of signals averaging (NSA) = 4, flip angle = 90°, echo time (TE) = 88 ms, fasting imaging mode = echo planner imaging (EPI), and repetition time (TR) = 4734 ms, fat suppression = spectral attenuated inversion recovery (SPAIR), folder-over-suppression = over sampling. Our study was approved by the IRB (Code Number: R.21.04.1289), and all experiments were carried out according to the related rules and instructions, and all patients submitted informed consent to create the original dataset. An experienced radiologist with more than 10 years of hands-on-experience performed the manual segmentation of the prostate and all detected lesions using the Photoshop software tool.

3.2. Extracting Features

Extracting discriminative features from an area of interest is a fundamental characteristic of an efficient CAD system [8,30]. Common features for medical images include texture, topological, color, morphological, intensity, and various features [18,31,32]. Designing an efficient image feature set has a vital role in an accurate CAD system. In this framework, we extracted 266 image feature descriptors for the segmented regions of interest (ROIs) of lesion and prostate, and their extraction was primarily motivated by functional, textural, and morphological points of view. This implies that each voxel can be represented in a 266-dimensional feature space.

3.2.1. Functional Features

Relying on the observations that the ADC measures the degree of molecular mobility and that tumors limit water motion because of the low permittivity of their cell membranes in comparison with the healthy tissue, a high-grade tumor has a smaller ADC value than a low-grade tumor, and a malignant tumor has a smaller ADC value than a benign one [33,34]. Hence, ADC maps could be used as discriminative functional features to enhance the diagnostic performance of PCa. To generate each ADC map, two DW-MR images are required; the first image is acquired at the baseline (b_0), whereas the other image is acquired at a higher b-value. It is calculated at the voxel level as follows:

$$ADC(x,y,z) = \frac{\ln \frac{s_0(x,y,z)}{s_n(x,y,z)}}{b_n - b_0} \quad (1)$$

where s_0 and s_n are the signal intensity acquired at the baseline ($b = 0$) and a higher b-value $b_n \in \{100, 200, 300, 400, 500, 600, 700, 1400\}$ s/mm^2, for the voxel at position x, y, z. Then, ADC maps were calculated at eight different b-values for all cases. Yet applying the voxel-wise ADCs of the whole prostate volume as discriminatory features faces two challenges. The main challenge is the data truncation or zero padding for small or bigger prostate volumes, because of the variable size of input data. The other challenge is that the needed training time to classify large data volumes is very high. We avoided these challenges through constructing the cumulative distribution functions (CDFs) of the 3D ADC maps at different *b*-values for each case. The smallest and largest ADCs are estimated for all datasets. After that, the ADCs are split into one hundred steps, so that all ADC values are maintained as coherent with a unified size without missing any information. Finally, CDFs of the 3D ADC map at different *b*-values are created and employed as discriminative features. Figure 2 shows the different steps to extract the functional features and Figure 3 shows an illustration for the estimated CDF of two cases (benign and malignant).

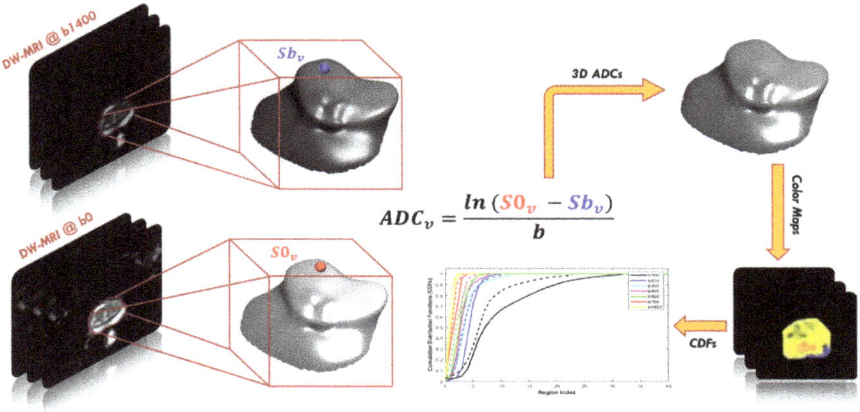

Figure 2. Calculations of voxel-wise apparent diffusion coefficients (ADC) for PCa and the cumulative distribution functions (CDFs) at different *b*-values from b100 to b1400.

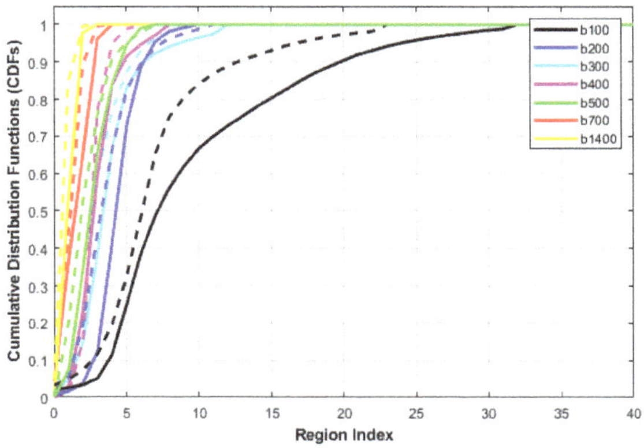

Figure 3. CDFs of ADC values for a benign case (solid) vs. a malignant case (dotted) for ADC maps obtained using different *b*-values from b100 to b1400. Note that region index indicates the different regions where the ADC values within the same range falls into.

3.2.2. Texture Features

Texture analysis (TA) is a significant field of study in medical imaging applications. TA has been utilized in the diagnosis of a variety of cancers [31,35–37]. There is no precise definition of TA, however, it can be described as the analysis of the spatial distribution of patterns that gives the visual appearance of roughness, randomness, smoothness, fluency, etc. [36]. It has been proven that MR images have various textural patterns that are often invisible to the human eye. Accordingly, texture analysis methods were utilized in our framework on the segmented region of interests (ROIs) of the whole prostate gland to precisely extract first and second order texture features that best characterize the homogeneity and heterogeneity between benign and malignant carcinomas. Usage of such extensive texture features depends on the fact that malignant carcinoma usually has high textural heterogeneity when compared to benign carcinoma. Figure 4 shows an illustrative example to compare benign cases and different grades of malignant cases in terms of texture differences.

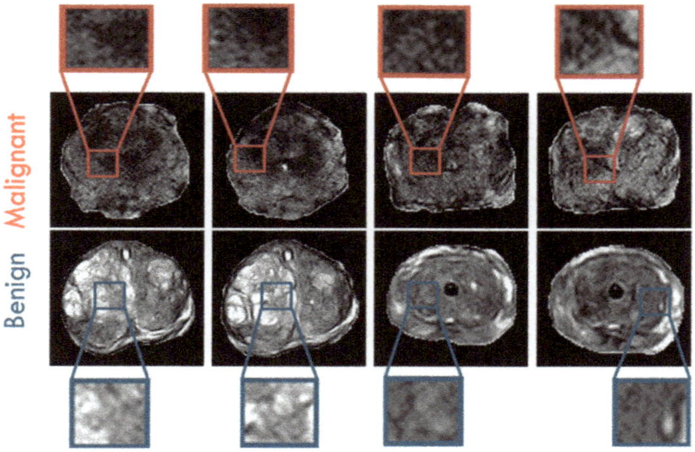

Figure 4. Illustrative examples of prostatic texture differences showing high gray level heterogeneity in four different malignant cases (first row) and low gray level heterogeneity in four different benign cases (second row).

Statistical TA methods can be largely classified into first-order and second-order texture features, based on the manner the gray levels are distributed over the pixels as follows.

First-order texture features: These texture features investigate the frequency distribution in the ROI through a histogram. Specifically, mean, median, variance, standard deviation, kurtosis, skewness, entropy, CDFs (N = 10), descriptive (mean, variance, Nobs, kurtosis), the number of points in each bin, size of bins, lower limit, bin width, cumulative frequency, and the gray level percentiles were calculated; from the 10th to the 100th percentiles with a step of 10%. A total of 36 first-order textural features were calculated. These features do not depend on the pixel's location nor on the gray levels of other pixels in its immediate neighborhood (Figure 5).

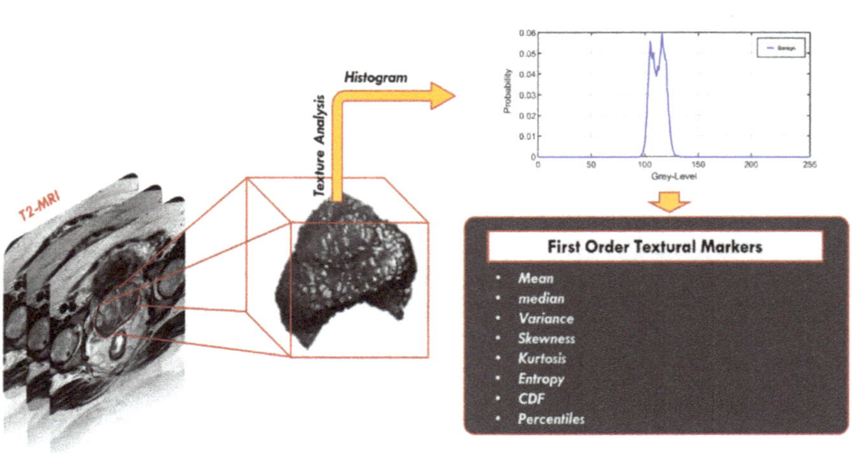

Figure 5. First-order textural features extraction.

Second-order texture features: These features depend on the probability that a pair of gray levels are selected at random distances and directions over the whole image [37]. In our framework, we used the gray level co-occurrence matrix (GLCM) [38] and gray level run length matrix (GLRLM) [39] as follows:

GLCM is based on computing how many times pairs of pixels with similar values and in a specified spatial relationship happen in a prostate object. The process starts with identifying the range of the original gray level of the prostate object and tumor object and normalizing these gray values to be in the range of 0 to 255 bringing on a GLCM matrix with a dimension of 256 × 256. After that, all possible pair combinations are specified to constitute the GLCM columns and rows. Finally, the value of each element within the matrix is estimated by determining the differences between each voxel and its neighbors. The neighborhood block is defined by a distance and an angle (the next voxel with the specified angle). Our neighborhood block has a distance of 1 in the Z-Plane (between different layers) and 1 in the XY plane (within the same layer). We worked with angles of zero, $\frac{\pi}{2}$, $\frac{\pi}{4}$, and $\frac{3\pi}{4}$. Thus, each voxel in our 3D object has a total of 26 neighbors (8 in the same layer, 9 in the upper layer and 9 in the lower layer). After creating the GLCM, it is normalized to have a sum of one to have the ability to extract the texture features depending on it. After each stage, a number of representative texture features (N = 6), specifically; contrast, correlation, angular second moment (ASM), dissimilarity, homogeneity, and energy were extracted as a summary of the GLCM (Figure 6).

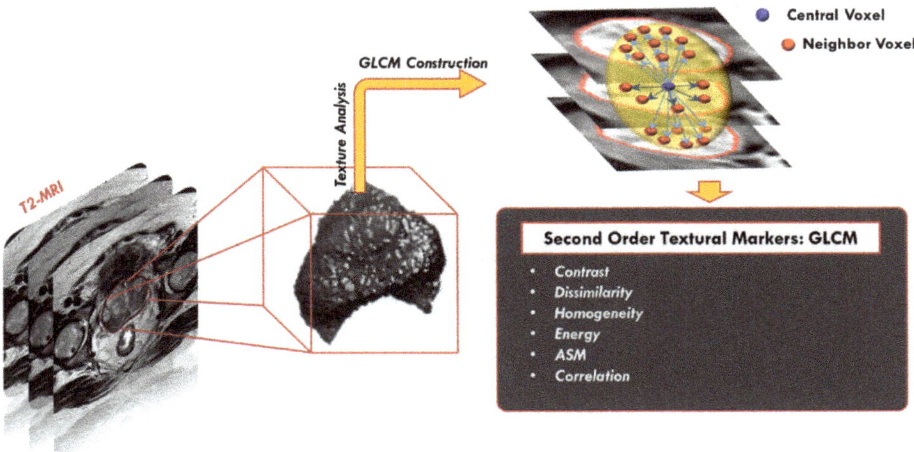

Figure 6. Second-order GLCM textural features extraction, where the central voxel of interest is shown in blue and the 26-neighbors are shown in red. The spatial relationship in the neighborhood block is obtained at different angles of zero, $\frac{\pi}{2}$, $\frac{\pi}{4}$, and $\frac{3\pi}{4}$.

GLRLM can be expressed as a set of pixels in a specific orientation having the same intensity value [40]. The number of such pixels specifies the length of the gray level run. GLRLM is a two-dimensional matrix, where each item $p(i,j\,|\,\theta)$ represents the number of elements (j) having an intensity (i). The normalized gray level matrix in our system has 256 rows with different numbers of columns between our objects. Herein, we searched for groups of sequential horizontal voxels in the XY plane and searched for vertical groups of voxels in the Z plane. Next, we estimated 16 features of the GLRLM, specifically: gray level non-uniformity, gray level non-uniformity normalized, high gray level run emphasis, gray level variance, long run emphasis, long run high gray level emphasis, long run low gray level emphasis, low gray level run emphasis, run length non-uniformity, run entropy, run length non-uniformity normalized, run variance, run percentage, short run emphasis, short run low gray level emphasis, and short run high gray level emphasis (Figure 7).

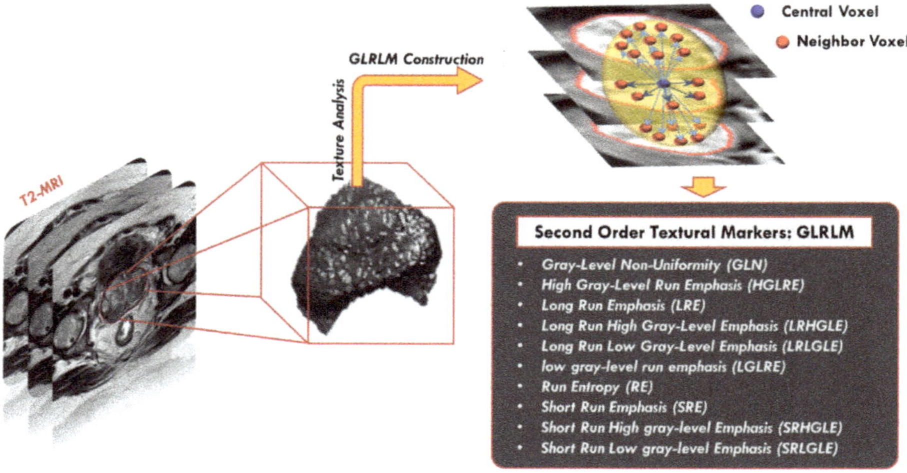

Figure 7. Second-order GLRLM textural features extraction, where the central voxel of interest is shown in blue and the 26-neighbors are shown in red. The spatial relationship is investigated to detect groups of sequential horizontal or vertical voxels with the same gray level.

3.2.3. Shape Features

For prostate cancer diagnosis and classification using T2W images, radiologists and researchers agree that morphological features are significant [23,41,42]. In the proposed framework, a number of shape features (morphological features) were also calculated to depict the morphology of the tumor candidate region. Shape features are extracted by capturing the structural information for the segmented region of interest of the lesion. The motivation for using shape features in our framework is based on the hypothesis that benign lesion has a less complex shape and a smaller growth rate than the malignant lesion. Figure 8 shows an illustrative example to compare between benign cases and malignant cases in terms of shape differences. In our work, we utilized the spectral spherical harmonics (SH) analysis [43] for extracting shape features for PCa diagnosis. A random point inside the region, or precisely in the interior of its convex kernel, was chosen to be the origin point (0, 0, 0). In this coordinate system, the surface of the region can be deemed a function of the polar and azimuth angle, $f(\theta, \varphi)$, which can be expressed as a linear set of base functions $Y_{\tau\beta}$ specified in the unit sphere. The modeling of spherical harmonics constructs a triangulated mesh approximating the surface of the lesion, afterwards maps it to the unit sphere by employing the attraction–repulsion technique [44].

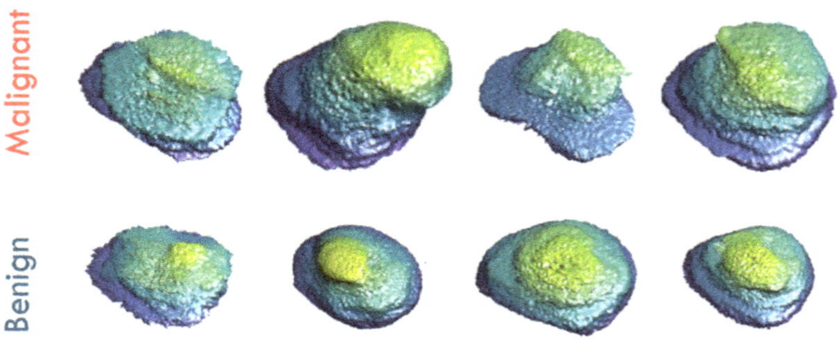

Figure 8. Visualization 3D shape differences between four malignant cases in the first row, and four benign cases in the second row.

Each cycle (α) of the attraction–repulsion approach operates as follows. Assume that $\mathbf{C}_{\alpha,i}$ represents the coordinates of the node on the unit sphere corresponding to mesh vertex i at the beginning of cycle α. Let $d_{\alpha,ji} = C_{\alpha,j} - C_{\alpha,i}$ represent the vector from node i to node j; then, the Euclidean distance between nodes i and j is $d_{\alpha,ji} = ||d_{\alpha,ji}||$. Assume that J_i represents the index group of neighbors of vertex i in the triangulated mesh. Next, the attraction step updates the node's locations to maintain it in the center with its neighbors according to Equation (2).

$$C'_{\alpha+1,i} = C_{\alpha,i} + C_{A,1} \sum_{j\epsilon J_i} \left(d_{\alpha,ji}\, d^2_{\alpha,ji} + C_{A,2} \frac{d_{\alpha,ji}}{d_{\alpha,ji}} \right) \tag{2}$$

where $C_{A,1}$ and $C_{A,2}$ are parameters which specify the strength of the attractive force, $j = 1, 2, 3, \ldots, J-1, J$, and $i = 1, 2, 3, \ldots, I-1, I$. After that, the repulsion step enlarges the spherical mesh to hinder it from deteriorating according to Equation (3).

$$C''_{\alpha+1,i} = C'_{\alpha+1,i} + \frac{C_R}{2I} \sum_{j=1; j\neq i}^{I} \frac{d_{\alpha,ji}}{d^2_{\alpha,ji}} \tag{3}$$

where C_R is a repulsion parameter that determines the shift incurred due to each other surface node and maintains a balance between the processing time and the accuracy. A small value of C_R (e.g., $0.3 \leq C_R \geq 0.7$) maintains a higher accuracy at the cost of increasing processing time. After that, the nodes are projected back onto the unit sphere through giving them the unit norm, and these are their coordinates at the start of the subsequent cycle according to Equation (4).

$$C_{\alpha+1,i} = \frac{C''_{\alpha+1,i}}{\|\, C''_{\alpha+1,i} \,\|} \tag{4}$$

In the final cycle, α_f, of the attraction–repulsion approach, the surface of the lesion is in a one-to-one correspondence with the unit sphere. Every point $C_i = (x_i,\ y_i,\ z_i)$ of the initial mesh has been mapped to a corresponding point $C_{\alpha_f,i} = (\sin\theta_i\ \cos\varphi_i,\ \sin\theta_i \sin\varphi_i,\ \cos\theta_i)$ with polar angle $\theta_i \in [0,\ \pi]$ and azimuth angle $\varphi_i \in [0,\ 2\pi]$. At this time, it is possibly to represent the lesion by a spherical harmonics series ($Y_{\tau\beta}$). Generating SH series is through solving an equation of isotropic heat for the surface that is considered a function on the unit sphere. The $Y_{\tau\beta}$ of degree τ with order β is identified according to Equation (5).

$$Y_{\tau\beta} = \begin{cases} c_{\tau\beta}\, G_\tau^{|\beta|} \cos\theta\ \sin(|\beta|\varphi) & -\tau \leq \beta \geq -1 \\ \frac{c_{\tau\beta}}{\sqrt{2}}\, G_\tau^{|\beta|} \cos\theta & \beta = 0 \\ c_{\tau\beta}\, G_\tau^{|\beta|} \cos\theta\ \cos(|\beta|\varphi) & 1 \leq \beta \geq \tau \end{cases} \tag{5}$$

where $c_{\tau\beta}$ is the spherical harmonics factor and $G_\tau^{|\beta|}$ represents the relevant Legendre polynomial of degree τ with order β. Benign lesions are described by a lower-order integration of spherical harmonic series, since their shapes are homogenous and less complex, whilst malignant lesions are described by a higher-order integration of spherical harmonic series since their shapes are heterogeneous and more complex. Subsequently, the overall number of markers measuring the shape complexity of the identified lesions is the number of the spherical harmonics. In our framework, a total number of 85 is sufficient to properly rebuild any lesion shape. Figure 9 shows the reconstruction errors differences at different harmonics between a malignant and a benign case.

3.3. Feature Integration and Selection

After functional and texture feature extraction from whole prostate gland, and shape feature extraction from lesion part, the features were integrated with the PSA clinical biomarker to produce a combined feature set (FS5) to be used for precise identification of prostatic adenocarcinoma.

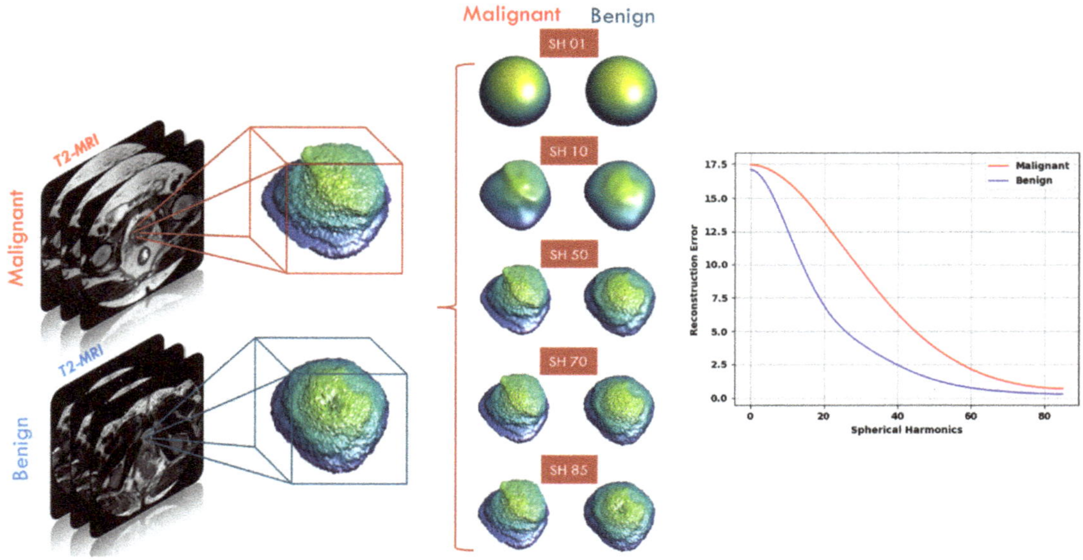

Figure 9. Reconstruction errors differences at different spherical harmonics (SH 01, 10, 50, 70, 85) between a malignant case and a benign case.

A feature selection method generally aims to select the best features subset for correctly classifying objects to different classes in the dataset. Hence, an effective selection method of relevant and redundant features for PCa classification is required to increase classification accuracy, precision, and to minimize complexity. Many feature selection techniques have been developed in the domain of ML. They can be generally categorized into three approaches: filter, wrapper, and embedded [45–49]. A wrapper approach is applied in this framework. Generally, the wrapper-based feature selection approach uses learning procedures to determine which features are beneficial. It follows a greedy search strategy through the space of possible markers. In this study, we performed a bi-directional stepwise procedure [50] to find the optimal set of markers while taking into consideration the dependencies between features.

A bi-directional stepwise procedure is a combination of forward selection and backward elimination. As with forward selection, the procedure starts with no features and adds features using a pre-specified criterion. After adding each new feature, remove any features that no longer provide an improvement in the model fit (like backward selection). We applied the bi-directional algorithm with two thresholds of significance (0.05 and 0.1) on the combined feature sets (FS5) to obtain FS6 and FS7, respectively. A summary of the different feature sets is shown in Table 2.

Table 2. Details of the extracted feature sets. Let ST denote the significance threshold.

Feature Set No.	Representation	Number of Extracted Features
FS1	Functional features for whole prostate	122
FS2	Texture features for whole prostate	58
FS3	Shape features for lesion only	85
FS4	Prostatic-specific antigen (PSA)	1
FS5	Combined features (FS1 + FS2 + FS3 + FS4)	266
FS6	Selected features of FS5 with ST = 0.05	101
FS7-Proposed	Selected features of FS5 with ST = 0.1	162

3.4. Cancer Classification

Following feature extraction and feature selection, our framework proceeds with a classification stage to classify the input images as either benign tumors or malignant tumors. In the training stage, we used four different machine learning classifiers to attain the best possible results (e.g., support vector machine (SVM) [51], random forest (RF) [52], the C4.5 decision tree algorithm (DT) [53] and linear discriminant analysis (LDA) [54]). We chose these classifiers because of their popularity and strength in CAD systems. SVM is a kernel-based learner that is robust regarding the sparsity of data. RF has been highly successful as a general-purpose classifier and is considered as an ensemble of decision trees. DT is fairly robust in the presence of noise and most effective in CAD systems. On the other hand, we used the LDA classifier that permits the fast processing of data samples.

To better highlight the advantage of the feature integration process, we first assessed the performance of each feature set separately. Then, the individual feature sets are combined using a concatenation way, and utilized the aforementioned classifiers to get the final diagnosis. It should be noted that, for each classifier, a grid search algorithm was used to search for the optimal parameters, with the classification accuracy as the improvement criterion, for each of the classifier techniques being tested. In the Section 4, more details about the performance of feature integration will be provided.

3.5. Performance Evaluation

The new framework was tested on the datasets mentioned in Section 3.1. Performance evaluation of the new framework was performed using four accuracy metrics: (I) specificity, (II) sensitivity, (III) accuracy, and (IV) AUC. More details about these metrics can be found in Figure 10. For assessing the performance of the proposed framework, K-fold cross-validation was implemented for numerical evaluation. Three validation procedures were implemented: 5-fold, 10-fold, and leave-one-out cross validation. In order to mitigate accuracy variations, all the experiments were executed 10 times and the mean and standard deviation for the accuracy, sensitivity, specificity, and AUC were calculated for each feature set.

		Actual health condition		
		Diseased	Healthy	
Predicted health condition	Diseased	True Positive (TP)	False Positive (FP)	
	Healthy	False Negative (FN)	True Negative (TN)	
		Sensitivity = $\frac{TP}{(TP+FN)}$	Specificity = $\frac{TN}{(TN+FP)}$	Accuracy = $\frac{TP+TN}{(TP+FP+FN+TN)}$

Figure 10. Performance metrics for evaluation of the proposed framework.

To investigate the added value of our framework, the developed CAD system was also compared to the clinical diagnosis made by an expert radiologist (10 years of experience in prostate MRI) for each patient on the basis of the Prostate Imaging Reporting and Data System (PIRADS) version 2 [55]. PIRADS can be used as a decision support system for targeting suspicious lesions. A radiologist scores each suspicious lesion on a scale from 1 to 5. Table 3 shows the scores that compose the PIRADS score system and their meaning in terms of the risk of the cancer being clinically significant. The radiologist was blinded to the respective PSA levels and pathological classification of tumors. PIRADS uses a dominant MRI sequence, including T2W, DWI, and ADC images.

Table 3. PIRADS scores.

PIRADS Score	Definition
1	Most probably benign (normal)
2	Probably benign tumor
3	Intermediate (the presence of clinically significant cancer is equivocal)
4	Probably malignant tumor
5	Most probably malignant tumor

4. Experimental Results

In order to validate and better highlight the effectiveness of the proposed framework, we first evaluated the proposed CAD system using each individual feature set (descriptions of each feature set are shown in Table 2). Furthermore, we evaluated the proposed CAD system using the combined features after applying feature selection, resulting in a notably improved classification performance. All the seven feature sets were evaluated and compared their performance using SVM, RF, DT, and LDA classifiers. For the purpose of applying the grid search algorithm, we created models for various combinations of parameters, assess the model for each combination and saved the results. We considered the best sets of parameters for each classifier as follows: For SVM we choose the gaussian kernel function for FS2, FS4, and FS6, linear kernel for FS1, and polynomial kernel of order 2 for other feature sets. For RF we set the number of learning cycles to 30. For DT we used Gini diversity index as the split criterion, and the number of splits varied according to feature set (10 for FS1, FS5, FS6, and FS7, 1 for FS2 and FS4, and 4 for FS3). For LDA, the Discriminant type was assumed to be diagLinear for FS1 and FS2 and Linear to other feature sets.

Tables 4–7 present the classification performance using SVM, RF, DT, or LDA classifier, respectively, under the three validation schemas. Overall, the obtained results showed that the performance based on feature set FS7 is much better than all other individual feature sets and this highlights the advantage of the features integration and selection process in the proposed framework. It also showed that using a significance threshold = 0.1 provides better results than using a significance threshold = 0.05. In the three validation schemas, the SVM classifier outperformed all other classifiers. Since SVM demonstrated the best diagnostic capabilities, it was selected for the proposed framework. SVM is also well-known for its great regularization capabilities preventing overfitting. In terms of assessing the individual feature sets, the best results were achieved reassuringly by the functional features (FS1) and this for almost all classifiers. As shown in Table 5, functional features achieved the best classification performance for all experiments running in 5-fold cross validation with 86.67% $\pm$ 1.56% of accuracy, 76.58% $\pm$ 1.27% of sensitivity, 95.35% $\pm$ 2.68% of specificity, and 0.8603% $\pm$ 0.0152% of AUC. The second-ranking performance was achieved by texture features (FS2). PSA alone attained the lowest performance.

It can be noted from comparing the performance metrics of the four classifiers for the different validation schemas, that we can find that there is a low variance between the results in the same classifier and this is a good indicator of a good fit model of ML. It should be pointed out that the implementation of *k*-fold cross-validation was guaranteed to achieve a balanced reduction of variance and bias in classifier performance estimation.

Table 4. Comparison of experimental results of classification accuracy (%), sensitivity (%), specificity (%), and AUC (in terms of mean ± standard deviation) using the proposed SVM classification model, where ϵ indicates 1.0×10^{-5}.

Feature Set	Validation	Accuracy	Sensitivity	Specificity	AUC
FS1	5-fold	81.81 ± 2.13	71.17 ± 3.6	90.96 ± 3.18	0.8106 ± 0.0215
	10-fold	83.75 ± 2.00	72.59 ± 2.25	93.35 ± 2.89	0.8297 ± 0.0197
	Leave-one-out	82.50 ± ϵ	67.57 ± ϵ	95.35 ± ϵ	0.8146 ± ϵ
FS2	5-fold	75.83 ± 1.72	61.26 ± 2.01	88.37 ± 3	0.7482 ± 0.0166
	10-fold	74.82 ± 2.26	61.39 ± 3.45	86.38± 2.3	0.7389 ± 0.0231
	Leave-one-out	77.50 ± ϵ	64.86 ± ϵ	88.37 ± ϵ	0.7662 ± ϵ
FS3	5-fold	74.28 ± 1.87	81.46 ± 2.25	68.11 ± 2.97	0.7479 ± 0.0183
	10-fold	74.58 ± 2.00	**80.63 ± 3.63**	69.38 ± 2.48	0.75 ± 0.0206
	Leave-one-out	77.50 ± ϵ	86.49 ± ϵ	69.77 ± ϵ	0.7813 ± ϵ
FS4	5-fold	72.50 ± ϵ	51.35 ± ϵ	90.70 ± ϵ	0.7102 ± ϵ
	10-fold	72.50 ± ϵ	51.35 ± ϵ	90.70 ± ϵ	0.7102 ± ϵ
	Leave-one-out	72.50 ± ϵ	51.35 ± ϵ	90.70 ± ϵ	0.7102 ± ϵ
FS5	5-fold	84.37 ± 2.01	75.23 ± 4.25	92.25 ± 2.57	0.8373 ± 0.021
	10-fold	84.50 ± 1.27	76.49 ± 2.72	91.39 ± 2.56	0.8394 ± 0.0127
	Leave-one-out	87.50 ± ϵ	81.08 ± ϵ	93.02 ± ϵ	0.8705 ± ϵ
FS6	5-fold	**85.42 ± 0.93**	73.87 ± 1.28	**95.35 ± 1.34**	0.8461 ± 0.0092
	10-fold	85.94 ± 0.83	74.33 ± 1.36	**95.93 ± 1.00**	0.8513 ± 0.0084
	Leave-one-out	86.25 ± ϵ	75.68 ± ϵ	95.35 ± ϵ	0.8551 ± ϵ
FS7	**5-fold**	85.18 ± 1.04	**78.38 ± 1.44**	91.03 ± 1.49	**0.8471 ± 0.0103**
	10-fold	**87.63 ± 1.53**	80.27 ± 2.11	93.95 ± 1.54	**0.8711 ± 0.0155**
	Leave-one-out	**88.75 ± ϵ**	**81.08 ± ϵ**	**95.35 ± ϵ**	**0.8821 ± ϵ**

Table 5. Comparison of experimental results of classification accuracy (%), sensitivity (%), specificity (%), and AUC (in terms of mean ± standard deviation) using a RF classification model, where ϵ indicates 1.0×10^{-5}.

Feature Set	Validation	Accuracy	Sensitivity	Specificity	AUC
FS1	5-fold	86.67 ± 1.56	76.58 ± 1.27	95.35 ± 2.68	0.8603 ± 0.0152
	10-fold	86.09 ± 1.59	77.03 ± 1.35	93.9 ± 2.31	0.8546 ± 0.0154
	Leave-one-out	85.78 ± 1.24	76.35 ± 1.79	93.9 ± 2.83	0.8512 ± 0.0115
FS2	5-fold	76.25 ± 2.28	63.97 ± 4.03	86.82 ± 2.89	0.7539 ± 0.0234
	10-fold	76.67 ± 1.38	65.76 ± 4.03	86.05 ± 2.68	0.7591 ± 0.0148
	Leave-one-out	76.75 ± 1.00	65.4 ± 2.02	86.51 ± 3.08	0.7596 ± 0.0087
FS3	5-fold	73.25 ± 0.61	75.68 ± 1.71	71.16 ± 1.14	0.7342 ± 0.0065
	10-fold	72.68 ± 1.45	75.68 ± 1.45	70.1 ± 1.94	0.7289 ± 0.0153
	Leave-one-out	72.50 ± ϵ	75.68 ± ϵ	69.77 ± ϵ	0.7272 ± ϵ
FS4	5-fold	73.75 ± ϵ	51.35 ± ϵ	93.02 ± ϵ	0.7219 ± ϵ
	10-fold	73.57 ± 0.44	50.96 ± 0.94	93.02 ± ϵ	0.72 ± 0.0047
	Leave-one-out	73.75 ± ϵ	51.35 ± ϵ	93.02 ± ϵ	0.7219 ± ϵ
FS5	5-fold	84.82 ± 1.82	77.22 ± 1.97	91.36 ± 2.05	0.8429 ± 0.0182
	10-fold	87.32 ± 1.56	79.54 ± 1.97	94.02 ± 1.69	0.8678 ± 0.0157
	Leave-one-out	86.13 ± 1.42	77.30 ± 1.32	93.72 ± 2.09	0.8551 ± 0.0138
FS6	5-fold	83.75 ± 0.95	75.29 ± 1.73	91.03 ± 2.30	0.8316 ± 0.0089
	10-fold	84.58 ± 1.56	76.58 ± 3.12	91.47 ± 1.09	0.8402 ± 0.0165
	Leave-one-out	86.38 ± 1.42	78.65 ± 2.24	93.02 ± 1.80	0.8584 ± 0.0144
FS7	5-fold	84.86 ± 1.5	77.78 ± 2.47	90.96 ± 2.31	0.8437 ± 0.015
	10-fold	85.63 ± 1.53	77.67 ± 1.31	92.73 ± 2.44	0.8505 ± 0.0147
	Leave-one-out	86.25 ± 1.48	77.30 ± 1.32	93.95 ± 2.59	0.8564 ± 0.0141

Table 6. Comparison of experimental results of classification accuracy (%), sensitivity (%), specificity (%), and AUC (in terms of mean ± standard deviation) using a DT classification model, where ϵ indicates 1.0×10^{-5}.

Feature Set	Validation	Accuracy	Sensitivity	Specificity	AUC
FS1	5-fold	75.45 ± 2.86	76.35 ± 4.22	84.71 ± 6.62	0.7553 ± 0.0266
	10-fold	75.50 ± 1.27	77.30 ± 1.32	73.95 ± 1.74	0.7563 ± 0.0125
	Leave-one-out	77.50 ± ϵ	72.97 ± ϵ	81.40 ± ϵ	0.7718 ± ϵ
FS2	5-fold	70.63 ± 1.88	53.60 ± 4.25	85.27 ± 4.58	0.6944 ± 0.0182
	10-fold	71.00 ± 0.94	54.59 ± 3.15	85.12 ± 3.78	0.6978 ± 0.0082
	Leave-one-out	70.00 ± ϵ	45.95 ± ϵ	90.70 ± ϵ	0.6832 ± ϵ
FS3	5-fold	66.79 ± 1.13	61.78 ± 4.88	71.10 ± 3.90	0.6644 ± 0.0122
	10-fold	65.00 ± 2.85	62.16 ± 2.96	67.44 ± 3.89	0.6480 ± 0.0280
	Leave-one-out	66.25 ± ϵ	70.27 ± ϵ	62.79 ± ϵ	0.6653 ± ϵ
FS4	5-fold	66.88 ± 3.59	61.71 ± 2.88	71.32 ± 5.48	0.6652 ± 0.0347
	10-fold	67.50 ± 1.12	58.38 ± 2.76	75.35 ± 1.86	0.6686 ± 0.0117
	Leave-one-out	65.00 ± ϵ	56.76 ± ϵ	72.09 ± ϵ	0.6442 ± ϵ
FS5	5-fold	78.44 ± 2.32	79.39 ± 3.56	77.62 ± 4.93	0.7851 ± 0.0221
	10-fold	80.25 ± 3.10	79.46 ± 2.16	80.93 ± 5.58	0.8019 ± 0.0293
	Leave-one-out	82.50 ± ϵ	83.78 ± ϵ	81.40 ± ϵ	0.8259 ± ϵ
FS6	5-fold	79.84 ± 3.09	76.01 ± 4.95	83.14 ± 4.15	0.7958 ± 0.0312
	10-fold	79.82 ± 1.82	79.92 ± 4.30	79.73 ± 3.67	0.7983 ± 0.0185
	Leave-one-out	83.75 ± ϵ	83.78 ± ϵ	83.72 ± ϵ	0.8375 ± ϵ
FS7	5-fold	81.46 ± 1.97	77.93 ± 2.88	84.50 ± 3.72	0.8121 ± 0.019
	10-fold	80.36 ± 1.10	80.31 ± 2.78	80.40 ± 2.44	0.8035 ± 0.0112
	Leave-one-out	83.75 ± ϵ	83.78 ± ϵ	83.72 ± ϵ	0.8375 ± ϵ

Table 7. Comparison of experimental results of classification accuracy (%), sensitivity (%), specificity (%), and AUC (in terms of mean ± standard deviation) using an LDA classification model, where ϵ indicates 1.0×10^{-5}.

Feature Set	Validation	Accuracy	Sensitivity	Specificity	AUC
FS1	5-fold	79.38 ± 0.88	72.97 ± ϵ	84.88 ± 1.64	0.7893 ± 0.0082
	10-fold	79.75± 0.94	72.97 ± ϵ	85.58 ± 1.74	0.7928 ± 0.0087
	Leave-one-out	80.00 ± ϵ	72.97 ± ϵ	86.05 ± ϵ	0.7951 ± ϵ
FS2	5-fold	73.03 ± 1.13	58.69 ± 1.89	85.38 ± 1.05	0.7203 ± 0.0116
	10-fold	72.92 ± 0.59	59.01 ± 1.86	84.89 ± 1.17	0.7195 ± 0.0064
	Leave-one-out	71.25 ± ϵ	56.76 ± ϵ	83.72 ± ϵ	0.7024 ± ϵ
FS3	5-fold	72.29 ± 0.86	74.33 ± 1.36	70.54 ± 2.19	0.7243 ± 0.0078
	10-fold	71.50 ± 1.22	74.6 ± 1.33	68.84 ± 1.86	0.7172 ± 0.0119
	Leave-one-out	72.50 ± ϵ	75.68 ± ϵ	69.77 ± ϵ	0.7272 ± ϵ
FS4	5-fold	73.13 ± 0.88	50 ± 1.91	93.02 ± ϵ	0.7151 ± 0.0095
	10-fold	73.39 ± 0.56	50.58 ± 1.22	93.02 ± ϵ	0.718 ± 0.0061
	Leave-one-out	73.75 ± ϵ	51.35 ± ϵ	93.02 ± ϵ	0.7219 ± ϵ
FS5	5-fold	81.56 ± 0.54	73.99 ± 1.31	88.08 ± 0.77	0.8103 ± 0.0057
	10-fold	81.75 ± 0.83	74.87 ± 1.24	87.67 ± 1.06	0.8127 ± 0.0083
	Leave-one-out	82.50 ± ϵ	75.68 ± ϵ	88.37 ± ϵ	0.8202 ± ϵ
FS6	5-fold	82.92 ± 0.59	73.42 ± 1.01	91.09 ± 0.86	0.8226 ± 0.0059
	10-fold	82.32 ± 0.8	72.97 ± 2.04	90.37 ± 0.82	0.8167 ± 0.0087
	Leave-one-out	82.50 ± ϵ	72.97 ± ϵ	90.70 ± ϵ	0.8184 ± ϵ
FS7	5-fold	83.00 ± 0.93	75.68 ± ϵ	89.30 ± 1.54	0.8249 ± 0.0077
	10-fold	82.29 ± 0.47	75.68 ± ϵ	87.98 ± 0.87	0.8183 ± 0.0043
	Leave-one-out	82.50 ± ϵ	75.68 ± ϵ	88.37 ± ϵ	0.8202 ± ϵ

To highlight the advantages of the proposed feature set (FS7), we provided a summary of comparison between the different classifiers using the three validation schemas applied on FS7 only in Table 8. From this table, the best results were achieved for FS7 by the SVM classifier using leave-one-out cross validation with 88.57% ± 0.00% of accuracy, 81.08% ± 0.00% of sensitivity, 95.35% ± 0.00% of specificity, and 0.8821 ± 0.00 of AUC. The second highest performance results were also achieved for FS7 by the RF classifier using leave-one-out cross validation with 86.25% ± 1.48% of accuracy and 93.95% ± 2.59% of specificity, and 0.8564 ± 0.0141 of AUC, while the DT achieved the highest sensitivity of 83.78% ± 0.00%. This suggests that using SVM classifier for classification is a promising one.

Table 8. Comparison of experimental results of classification accuracy (%), sensitivity (%), specificity (%), and AUC (in terms of mean ± standard deviation) using the different classifiers for only our proposed feature set (FS7), where ϵ indicates 1.0×10^{-5}.

Classifier	Validation	Accuracy	Sensitivity	Specificity	AUC
SVM	5-fold	**85.18 ± 1.04**	**78.38 ± 1.44**	**91.03 ± 1.49**	**0.8471 ± 0.0103**
	10-fold	**87.63 ± 1.53**	80.27 ± 2.11	**93.95 ± 1.54**	**0.8711 ± 0.0155**
	Leave-one-out	**88.75 ± ϵ**	81.08 ± ϵ	**95.35 ± ϵ**	**0.8821 ± ϵ**
RF	5-fold	84.86 ± 1.5	77.78 ± 2.47	90.96 ± 2.31	0.8437 ± 0.015
	10-fold	85.63 ± 1.53	77.67 ± 1.31	92.73 ± 2.44	0.8505 ± 0.0147
	Leave-one-out	86.25 ± 1.48	77.3 ± 1.32	93.95 ± 2.59	0.8564 ± 0.0141
DT	5-fold	81.46 ± 1.97	77.93 ± 2.88	84.50 ± 3.72	0.8121 ± 0.019
	10-fold	80.36 ± 1.1	**80.31 ± 2.78**	80.40 ± 2.44	0.8035 ± 0.0112
	Leave-one-out	83.75 ± ϵ	**83.78 ± ϵ**	83.72 ± ϵ	0.8375 ± ϵ
LDA	5-fold	83.00 ± 0.93	75.68 ± ϵ	89.3 0± 1.54	0.8249 ± 0.0077
	10-fold	82.29 ± 0.47	75.68 ± ϵ	87.98 ± 0.87	0.8183 ± 0.0043
	Leave-one-out	82.50 ± ϵ	75.68 ± ϵ	88.37 ± ϵ	0.8202 ± ϵ

In a clinical setting, the AUC value is grouped into three grades: (1) acceptable when the score ranges from 0.7 to 0.8, (2) excellent when the score ranges from 0.8 to 0.9, and (3) outstanding when the score is over 0.9 [21,49]. In this regard, the proposed framework upgrades the CAD system from an acceptable grade to an excellent grade using the proposed feature set (FS7). The AUC reached in leave-one-out cross validation using SVM classifier was an average of 0.88 with FS7, while it was an average of 0.87 with FS5. This confirms that the results provided here constitute strong evidence to support the proposed feature integration hypothesis and feature selection method.

The receiver operating characteristics (ROC) curves for SVM using leave-one-out cross validation for all feature sets and the proposed FS7 using the three validation schemas in all classifiers are visualized in Figure 11. ROC shows the trade-off between true positive rate (sensitivity) and false negative rate (1—specificity). As shown in this figure, the ROC area of the proposed FS7 is the maximum when compared to other feature sets and this highlights the advantages of using the proposed feature set (FS7) over other feature sets. Furthermore, the functional features demonstrated a potential in identifying the malignancy status of a given prostate tumor. Moreover, SVM classifier is optimal in comparison to other classifiers evidenced by the highest AUC, as shown in Figure 11.

The PIRADS v2 scores resulted in the correct classification of 47 of 51 lesions (17 benign prostatic hyperplasia cases and 30 prostatic carcinomas cases). The four lesions that were not detected were benign lesions. The counts of PIRADS 3 were 29 from 80 cases that were undecided and this is considered high, more specifically the number of PIRADS 3 was 22 for benign prostatic hyperplasia cases and 6 for prostatic carcinomas. For a fair comparison, we can say that PIRADS missed 33 cases and there is a large degree of subjectivity. It is worth mentioning that there were no cases given a score of PIRADS 1 by the radiologist as PIRADS 1 lesions were generally not biopsied and therefore are only partially included in this study. These results stress the need for our CAD system to distinguish these equivocal lesions further into insignificant and significant tumors and to be more objective.

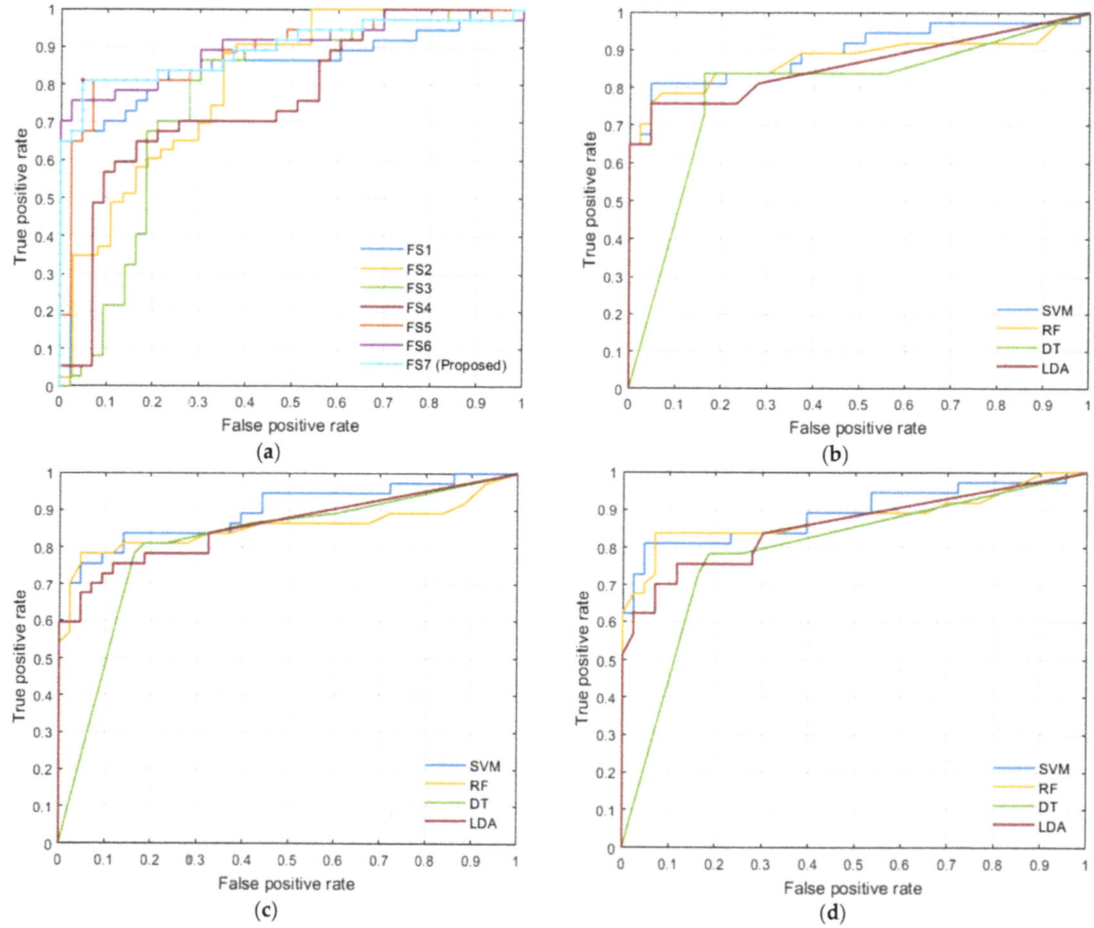

Figure 11. ROC curves of (**a**) SVM comparing various feature sets using leave-one-out cross validation, (**b**) different classifiers comparison using FS7 along with leave-one-out cross validation, (**c**) different classifiers comparison using FS7 along with 5-fold cross validation, and (**d**) comparison of classifiers using FS7 along with 10-fold cross validation.

5. Discussion

With a high mortality rate, prostate cancer is considered as one of the worldwide leading cancerous causes of death. Precisely detecting prostate cancer at early stages could enhance the survival opportunities of the patients.

In this study, we introduce a new comprehensive framework to precisely differentiate between malignant and benign prostate cancer. The classification results of the developed CAD system that combined different imaging markers and clinical biomarkers showed high accuracy, sensitivity, specificity, and AUC. These results revealed the feasibility and efficacy of the developed CAD system to non-invasively identify prostatic adenocarcinoma at an early stage. Classification results attained using individual features (functional or texture or shape or PSA) had lower accuracy, sensitivity, specificity, and AUC compared to using combined features. Validation schema experiments further reinforce the reliability of our accuracy findings.

It is worth noting that this high diagnostic accuracy of the developed CAD system is obtained by SVM classifier due to its ability to handle non-planar class boundaries in an efficient and stable manner by using kernels [51]. Throughout this study, we have extracted functional features from the whole prostate ROI, textural feature from the whole prostate ROI, and shape features from the lesion ROI only. This can be justified in part by the fact that the prostate gland as a whole is more informative in terms of functionality analysis to study the motion of water molecules quantified by 3D ADCs and in terms of texture analysis by providing a larger area to study the spatial relationship between the neighboring voxels using various first and second order texture features. On the other hand, lesion ROI is more informative in terms of the lesion shape, size, and complexity of the surface.

Most of the clinical research calculates the ADC at a few select b-values [9,14,17,26,27], typically one of the lower b-values and one of the higher b-values along with the baseline ($b = 0$). This study utilized nine different b-values to accurately differentiate between malignant and benign cases.

There are several other studies that designed to extract different features from DW MRI and T2 MRI that check the existence of PCa [9,17,21,23,42]. Few have investigated using clinical features for PCa detection [56]. To the best of our knowledge, there is no work in the literature that was conducted a fusion of texture, functional, shape imaging features and clinical features for PCa detection. This implies that our study could be a base for further studies using a combination of imagery and clinical MRI derived features to discriminate between benign and malignant PCa. A direct comparison between our study and other literature would not be objective as the other studies incorporate different data sets and variations in imaging protocols. However, our results are in line with the findings of other studies [9,17,21,23], showing that the combination of different features attained higher classification results than using textural features or morphological features alone. Moreover, our developed CAD system achieved AUC of 0.882, an improvement over the study done of Lemaitre et al. [21] that produced an AUC of 0.838, despite using more imaging modalities than used our study. Additionally, our performance is greater than the study done by Bleker et al. [9], as they attained an AUC of 0.838, in spite of using greater sample size in their study (206 patients).

Adding this superiority of the developed system (compared to the literature) to our experimental findings (Tables 4–8), reflect the accuracy of our methodology and the potential clinical utility of these provided approaches when used with MR imaging in computer-aided diagnosis of prostate cancers.

6. Conclusions

In this study, a new CAD system for the precise identification of prostate cancer in multiple modalities of MRI is presented. The paper depicts the complete design of the proposed framework to assess the potential role of integrating functional, textural, shape features combined with PSA and provides a detailed diagnostic performance analysis. The proposed framework achieved a high classification accuracy of 88.75%, a sensitivity of 81.08%, a specificity of 95.35%, an AUC of 0.8821, in differentiating benign tumor from malignant tumor using SVM along with the selected features set (FS7) outperforming the diagnostic abilities of individual and combined feature sets and other well-known ML classification models (e.g., LDA, RF, and DT). We have also included three validation schemas (5-fold, 10-fold, and leave-one-out cross validation). These results highlight the advantage of integrating clinical biomarker with DW-MRI and T2W-MRI for prostate cancer diagnosis.

Our framework is not devoid of limitations. Firstly, it needs manual lesion segmentation, that supposes that the tumor can be discovered and segmented accurately. Secondly, we studied DW-MRI and T2W-MRI acquired from one hospital and using only one type of scanner. The focus of the future work will be on validating our framework on a large dataset to verify the robustness of the proposed system. Further research is also needed to investigate whether we can reduce the number of *b*-values that are not informative enough. In addition, we plan to investigate the potential capabilities of the IVIM model in early and precise identification of prostatic adenocarcinoma. Moreover, a deep learning-based CAD will be established for the fully automated extraction of imagery features.

Author Contributions: Conceptualization, S.M.A., M.S., A.A., M.A.E.-G., M.E.-M., H.A.A. and A.E.-B.; data curation, M.A.B., M.A.E.-G., M.G., M.E.-M. and A.E.-B.; formal analysis, S.M.A., M.A.B., M.S. and H.A.A.; investigation, S.M.A., M.S., A.M., M.G., N.B.A.-H., L.M.L., H.A.A. and A.E.-B.; methodology, S.M.A., M.S., A.A., A.M. and A.E.-B.; project administration, A.E.-B.; resources, M.A.B., M.A.E.-G., M.G. and M.E.-M.; supervision, N.B.A.-H., L.M.L., H.A.A. and A.E.-B.; validation, M.A.B., M.A.E.-G., M.G., M.E.-M., N.B.A.-H., L.M.L., H.A.A. and A.E.-B.; visualization, S.M.A., M.S. and A.A.; writing—original draft, S.M.A., M.A.B., M.S. and A.A.; writing—review and editing, S.M.A., M.S., A.A., A.M., N.B.A.-H., L.M.L., H.A.A. and A.E.-B. All authors have read and agreed to the published version of the manuscript.

Funding: This research received external funding from the Academy of Scientific Research and Technology (ASRT) in Egypt (Project No. JESOR 1046).

Institutional Review Board Statement: The study was conducted according to the guidelines of the Declaration of Helsinki, and approved by the Institutional Review Board of Mansoura University (R.21.04.1289).

Informed Consent Statement: Informed consent was obtained from all subjects involved in the study.

Data Availability Statement: Data can be made available upon a reasonable request to the corresponding author.

Conflicts of Interest: The authors declare no conflict of interest.

References

1. Siegel, R.L.; Miller, K.D.; Fuchs, H.E.; Jemal, A. Cancer statistics, 2021. *CA Cancer J. Clin.* **2021**, *71*, 7–33. [CrossRef] [PubMed]
2. American Cancer Society. Key Statistics for Prostate Cancer. Available online: http://www.cancer.org/cancer/prostate-cancer/about/key-statistics.html (accessed on 7 December 2021).
3. Reda, I.; Khalil, A.; Elmogy, M.; El-Fetouh, A.A.; Shalaby, A.; El-Ghar, M.A.; Elmaghraby, A.; Ghazal, M.; El-Baz, A. Deep Learning Role in Early Diagnosis of Prostate Cancer. *Technol. Cancer Res. Treat.* **2018**, *17*, 1533034618775530. [CrossRef]
4. Partin, A.W.; Catalona, W.J.; Southwick, P.C.; Subong, E.N.; Gasior, G.H.; Chan, D.W. Analysis of percent free prostate-specific antigen (PSA) for prostate cancer detection: Influence of total PSA, prostate volume, and age. *Urology* **1996**, *48*, 55–61. [CrossRef]
5. Okotie, O.T.; Roehl, K.A.; Han, M.; Loeb, S.; Gashti, S.N.; Catalona, W.J. Characteristics of prostate cancer detected by digital rectal examination only. *Urology* **2007**, *70*, 1117–1120. [CrossRef] [PubMed]
6. Pepe, P.; Aragona, F. Saturation prostate needle biopsy and prostate cancer detection at initial and repeat evaluation. *Urology* **2007**, *70*, 1131–1135. [CrossRef]
7. Javadrashid, R.; Olyaei, A.S.; Tarzamni, M.K.; Razzaghi, R.; Jalili, J.; Hashemzadeh, S.; Mirza-Aghazadeh-Attari, M.; Nazarlou, A.K.; Zarrintan, A. The diagnostic value of diffusion-weighted imaging in differentiating benign from malignant hepatic lesions. *Egypt. Liver J.* **2020**, *10*, 13. [CrossRef]
8. Wang, S.; Burtt, K.; Turkbey, B.; Choyke, P.; Summers, R.M. Computer aided-diagnosis of prostate cancer on multiparametric MRI: A technical review of current research. *BioMed Res. Int.* **2014**. [CrossRef]
9. Bleker, J.; Kwee, T.C.; Dierckx, R.A.; de Jong, I.J.; Huisman, H.; Yakar, D. Multiparametric MRI and auto-fixed volume of interest-based radiomics signature for clinically significant peripheral zone prostate cancer. *Eur. Radiol.* **2020**, *30*, 1313–1324. [CrossRef]
10. Lopes, P.M.; Sepúlveda, L.; Ramos, R.; Sousa, P. The role of transrectal ultrasound in the diagnosis of prostate cancer: New contributions. *Radiol. Bras.* **2015**, *48*, 7–11. [CrossRef]
11. O'Connor, L.; Wang, A.; Walker, S.M.; Yerram, N.; Pinto, P.A.; Turkbey, B. Use of multiparametric magnetic resonance imaging (mpMRI) in localized prostate cancer. *Expert Rev. Med. Devices* **2020**, *17*, 435–442. [CrossRef]
12. Sunoqrot, M.R.; Nketiah, G.A.; Selnæs, K.M.; Bathen, T.F.; Elschot, M. Automated reference tissue normalization of T2-weighted MR images of the prostate using object recognition. *Magn. Reson. Mater. Physics Biol. Med.* **2021**, *34*, 309–321. [CrossRef]
13. Alkadi, R.; Taher, F.; El-Baz, A.; Werghi, N. A deep learning-based approach for the detection and localization of prostate cancer in T2 magnetic resonance images. *Digit. Imaging* **2019**, *32*, 793–807. [CrossRef] [PubMed]
14. Nguyen, V.T.; Rahbar, H.; Olson, M.L.; Liu, C.L.; Lehman, C.D.; Partridge, S.C. Diffusion-weighted imaging: Effects of intravascular contrast agents on apparent diffusion coefficient measures of breast malignancies at 3 tesla. *J. Magn. Reson. Imaging* **2015**, *42*, 788–800. [CrossRef] [PubMed]

15. McClure, P.; Khalifa, F.; Soliman, A.; Abou El-Ghar, M.; Gimelfarb, G.; Elmagraby, A.; El-Baz, A. A novel NMF guided level-set for DWI prostate segmentation. *J. Comput. Sci. Syst. Biol.* **2014**, *7*, 1. [CrossRef]
16. Freidlin, R.Z.; Agarwal, H.K.; Sankineni, S.; Brown, A.M.; Mertan, F.; Bernardo, M.; Daar, D.; Merino, M.; Citrin, D.; Wood, B.J.; et al. Application of an unsupervised multi-characteristic framework for intermediate-high risk prostate cancer localization using diffusion-weighted MRI. *Magn. Reson. Imaging* **2016**, *34*, 1227–1234. [CrossRef]
17. Lay, N.S.; Tsehay, Y.; Greer, M.D.; Turkbey, B.; Kwak, J.T.; Choyke, P.L.; Pinto, P.; Wood, B.J.; Summers, R.M. Detection of prostate cancer in multiparametric MRI using random forest with instance weighting. *J. Med. Imaging* **2017**, *4*, 24506. [CrossRef]
18. Ayyad, S.M.; Shehata, M.; Shalaby, A.; El-Ghar, A.; Ghazal, M.; El-Melegy, M.; Abdel-Hamid, N.B.; Labib, L.M.; Ali, H.A.; El-Baz, A. Role of AI and Histopathological Images in Detecting Prostate Cancer: A Survey. *Sensors* **2021**, *21*, 2586. [CrossRef]
19. Rampun, A.; Zheng, L.; Malcolm, P.; Tiddeman, B.; Zwiggelaar, R. Computer-aided detection of prostate cancer in T2-weighted MRI within the peripheral zone. *Phys. Med. Biol.* **2016**, *61*, 4796–4825. [CrossRef]
20. Basu, S.; Mukhopadhyay, S.; Karki, M.; DiBiano, R.; Ganguly, S.; Nemani, R.; Gayaka, S. Deep neural networks for texture classification—A theoretical analysis. *Neural Netw.* **2018**, *97*, 173–182. [CrossRef]
21. Lemaitre, G.; Marti, R.; Rastgoo, M.; Meriaudeau, F. Computer-aided detection for prostate cancer detection based on multi-parametric magnetic resonance imaging. In Proceedings of the 2017 39th Annual International Conference of the IEEE Engineering in Medicine and Biology Society (EMBC), Jeju, Korea, 11–15 July 2017; pp. 3138–3141. [CrossRef]
22. Varghese, B.; Chen, F.; Hwang, D.; Palmer, S.L.; De Castro Abreu, A.L.; Ukimura, O.; Aron, M.; Aron, M.; Gill, I.; Duddalwar, V.; et al. Objective risk stratification of prostate cancer using machine learning and radiomics applied to multiparametric magnetic resonance images. In Proceedings of the 11th ACM International Conference on Bioinformatics, Computational Biology and Health Informatics, Online, 21 September 2020; pp. 1–10. [CrossRef]
23. Woźnicki, P.; Westhoff, N.; Huber, T.; Riffel, P.; Froelich, M.F.; Gresser, E.; von Hardenberg, J.; Mühlberg, A.; Michel, M.S.; Schoenberg, S.O.; et al. Multiparametric MRI for prostate cancer characterization: Combined use of radiomics model with PI-RADS and clinical parameters. *Cancers* **2020**, *12*, 1767. [CrossRef]
24. Hasan, A.M.; Jalab, H.A.; Meziane, F.; Kahtan, H.; Al-Ahmad, A.S. Combining deep and handcrafted image features for MRI brain scan classification. *IEEE Access* **2019**, *7*, 79959–79967. [CrossRef]
25. Burt, J.R.; Torosdagli, N.; Khosravan, N.; RaviPrakash, H.; Mortazi, A.; Tissavirasingham, F.; Hussein, S.; Bagci, U. Deep learning beyond cats and dogs: Recent advances in diagnosing breast cancer with deep neural networks. *Br. J. Radiol.* **2018**, *91*, 20170545. [CrossRef] [PubMed]
26. Sumathipal, Y.; Lay, N.S.; Turkbey, B.; Smith, C.; Choyke, P.L.; Summers, R.M. Prostate cancer detection from multi-institution multiparametric MRIs using deep convolutional neural networks. *J. Med. Imaging* **2018**, *5*, 044507. [CrossRef]
27. Sanford, T.; Harmon, S.A.; Turkbey, E.B.; Kesani, D.; Tuncer, S.; Madariaga, M.; Yang, C.; Sackett, J.; Mehralivand, S.; Yan, P.; et al. Deep-Learning-Based Artificial Intelligence for PI-RADS Classification to Assist Multiparametric Prostate MRI Interpretation: A Development Study. *J. Magn. Reson. Imaging* **2020**, *52*, 1499–1507. [CrossRef] [PubMed]
28. Mehta, P.; Antonelli, M.; Ahmed, H.U.; Emberton, M.; Punwani, S.; Ourselin, S. Computer-aided diagnosis of prostate cancer using multiparametric MRI and clinical features: A patient-level classification framework. *Med. Image Anal.* **2021**, *73*, 102153. [CrossRef]
29. Pellicer-Valero, O.J.; Jiménez, J.L.; Gonzalez-Perez, V.; Ramón-Borja, J.L.; García, I.M.; Benito, M.B.; Gómez, P.P.; Rubio-Briones, J.; Rupérez, M.J.; Martín-Guerrero, J.D. Deep Learning for fully automatic detection, segmentation, and Gleason Grade estimation of prostate cancer in multiparametric Magnetic Resonance Images. *arXiv* **2021**, arXiv:2103.12650. [CrossRef]
30. Ragab, D.A.; Sharkas, M.; Attallah, O. Breast cancer diagnosis using an efficient CAD system based on multiple classifiers. *Diagnostics* **2019**, *9*, 165. [CrossRef]
31. Giambelluca, D.; Cannella, R.; Vernuccio, F.; Comelli, A.; Pavone, A.; Salvaggio, L.; Galia, M.; Midiri, M.; Lagalla, R.; Salvaggio, G. PI-RADS 3 lesions: Role of prostate MRI texture analysis in the identification of prostate cancer. *Curr. Probl. Diagn. Radiol.* **2021**, *50*, 175–185. [CrossRef]
32. Aboubakr, N.; Popova, M.; Crowley, J. Color-based Fusion of MRI Modalities for Brain Tumor Segmentation. In *Medical Imaging and Computer Aided Diagnosis*; Springer: Singapore, 2021; pp. 89–97. [CrossRef]
33. Lim, H.K.; Kim, J.K.; Kim, K.A.; Cho, K.S. Prostate cancer: Apparent diffusion coefficient map with T2-weighted images for detection—A multireader study. *Radiology* **2009**, *250*, 145–151. [CrossRef]
34. Tamada, T.; Huang, C.; Ream, J.M.; Taffel, M.; Taneja, S.S.; Rosenkrantz, A.B. Apparent diffusion coefficient values of prostate cancer: Comparison of 2D and 3D ROIs. *Am. J. Roentgenol.* **2018**, *210*, 113–117. [CrossRef]
35. Wanamaker, M.W.; Vernau, K.M.; Taylor, S.L.; Cissell, D.D.; Abdelhafez, Y.G.; Zwingenberger, A.L. Classification of neoplastic and inflammatory brain disease using MRI texture analysis in 119 dogs. *Vet. Radiol. Ultrasound* **2021**, *62*, 445–454. [CrossRef] [PubMed]
36. Larroza, A.; Bodí, V.; Moratal, D. Texture Analysis in Magnetic Resonance Imaging: Review and Considerations for Future Applications. In *Assessment of Cellular and Organ Function and Dysfunction Using Direct and Derived MRI Methodologies*; BoD—Books on Demand: Norderstedt, Germany, 2016; Volume 26, pp. 75–106. [CrossRef]
37. Nailon, W.H. Texture analysis methods for medical image characterisation. In *Biomedical Imaging*; IntechOpen: London, UK, 2010; pp. 75–100, ISBN 978-953-307-071-1.

38. Preethi, G.; Sornagopal, V. MRI image classification using GLCM texture features. In Proceedings of the 2014 International Conference on Green Computing Communication and Electrical Engineering (ICGCCEE), Coimbatore, India, 6–8 March 2014; pp. 1–6. [CrossRef]
39. Loh, H.H.; Leu, J.G.; Luo, R.C. The analysis of natural textures using run length features. *IEEE Trans. Ind. Electron.* **1988**, *35*, 323–328. [CrossRef]
40. Kairuddin, W.N.; Mahmud, W.M. Texture feature analysis for different resolution level of kidney ultrasound images. In *IOP Conference Series*: Materials Science and Engineering; IOP Publishing: Bristol, UK, 2017; Volume 226, p. 012136. [CrossRef]
41. Cameron, A.; Modhafar, A.; Khalvati, F.; Lui, D.; Shafiee, M.J.; Wong, A.; Haider, M. Multiparametric MRI prostate cancer analysis via a hybrid morphological-textural model. In Proceedings of the 2014 36th Annual International Conference of the IEEE Engineering in Medicine and Biology Society, Chicago, IL, USA, 26 August 2014; pp. 3357–3360. [CrossRef]
42. Hussain, L.; Ahmed, A.; Saeed, S.; Rathore, S.; Awan, I.A.; Shah, S.A.; Majid, A.; Idris, A.; Awan, A.A. Prostate cancer detection using machine learning techniques by employing combination of features extracting strategies. *Cancer Biomark.* **2018**, *21*, 393–413. [CrossRef] [PubMed]
43. El-Baz, A.; Nitzken, M.; Khalifa, F.; Elnakib, A.; Gimel'farb, G.; Falk, R.; El-Ghar, M.A. 3D shape analysis for early diagnosis of malignant lung nodules. In *Biennial International Conference on Information Processing in Medical Imaging*; Springer: Berlin/Heidelberg, Germany, 2011; pp. 772–783. [CrossRef]
44. Nitzken, M.J. Shape Analysis of the Human Brain. Ph.D. Thesis, University of Louisville, Louisville, KY, USA, 2015.
45. Mandal, M.; Singh, P.K.; Ijaz, M.F.; Shafi, J.; Sarkar, R. A tri-stage wrapper-filter feature selection framework for disease classification. *Sensors* **2021**, *21*, 5571. [CrossRef]
46. Ayyad, S.M.; Saleh, A.I.; Labib, L.M. A new distributed feature selection technique for classifying gene expression data. *Int. J. Biomath.* **2019**, *12*, 1950039. [CrossRef]
47. Barone, S.; Cannella, R.; Comelli, A.; Pellegrino, A.; Salvaggio, G.; Stefano, A.; Vernuccio, F. Hybrid descriptive-inferential method for key feature selection in prostate cancer radiomics. *Appl. Stoch. Model. Bus. Ind.* **2021**, *37*, 961–972. [CrossRef]
48. Shehab, N.; Badawy, M.; Ali, H.A. Toward feature selection in big data preprocessing based on hybrid cloud-based model. *J. Supercomput.* **2021**, *78*, 3226–3265. [CrossRef]
49. Lemaitre, G. Computer-Aided Diagnosis for Prostate Cancer Using Multi-Parametric Magnetic Resonance Imaging. Ph.D. Thesis, Universitat de Girona, Girona, Spain, 2016.
50. Devakumari, D.; Thangavel, K.; Sarojini, K. Unsupervised bidirectional feature selection based on contribution entropy for medical databases. *Int. J. Health Technol. Manag.* **2011**, *12*, 364. [CrossRef]
51. Schölkopf, B.S.; Burges, C.J.C.; Smola, A.J. *Advances in Kernel Methods: Support Vector Learning*; MIT press: Cambridge, MA, USA, 1999.
52. Breiman, L. Random forests. *Mach. Learn.* **2001**, *45*, 5–32. [CrossRef]
53. Dietterich, T.G.; Kong, E.B. *Machine Learning Bias, Statistical Bias, and Statistical Variance of Decision Tree Algorithms*; Technical Report; Department of Computer Science; Oregon State University: Corvallis, OR, USA, 1995. Available online: https://citeseerx.ist.psu.edu/viewdoc/download?doi=10.1.1.38.2702&rep=rep1&type=pdf (accessed on 7 December 2021).
54. Balakrishnama, S.; Ganapathiraju, A. Linear discriminant analysis-a brief tutorial. *Inst. Signal Inf. Process.* **1998**, *18*, 1–8. Available online: https://www.zemris.fer.hr/predmeti/kdisc/bojana/Tutorial-LDA-Balakrishnama.pdf (accessed on 7 December 2021).
55. Barentsz, J.O.; Weinreb, J.C.; Verma, S.; Thoeny, H.C.; Tempany, C.M.; Shtern, F.; Padhani, A.R.; Margolis, D.; Macura, K.J.; Haider, M.A.; et al. Synopsis of the PI-RADS v2 guidelines for multiparametric prostate magnetic resonance imaging and recommendations for use. *Eur. Urol.* **2016**, *69*, 41. [CrossRef] [PubMed]
56. Mehta, P.; Antonelli, M.; Singh, S.; Grondecka, N.; Johnston, E.W.; Ahmed, H.U.; Emberton, M.; Punwani, S.; Ourselin, S. AutoProstate: Towards Automated Reporting of Prostate MRI for Prostate Cancer Assessment Using Deep Learning. *Cancers* **2021**, *13*, 6138. [CrossRef] [PubMed]

sensors

MDPI

Article

Effect of Strength Training Protocol on Bone Mineral Density for Postmenopausal Women with Osteopenia/Osteoporosis Assessed by Dual-Energy X-ray Absorptiometry (DEXA)

Iulian Ștefan Holubiac [1], Florin Valentin Leuciuc [1,*], Daniela Maria Crăciun [1] and Tatiana Dobrescu [2]

[1] Department of Physical Education and Sport, Stefan cel Mare University, 720229 Suceava, Romania; holubiac.iulianstefan@usm.ro (I.Ș.H.); daniela.craciun@usm.ro (D.M.C.)

[2] Department of Physical Education and Sport Performance, Vasile Alecsandri University, 600115 Bacau, Romania; tatiana.dobrescu@ub.ro

* Correspondence: florin.leuciuc@usm.ro

Abstract: This study aims to introduce a resistance training protocol (6 repetitions × 70% of 1 maximum repetition (1RM), followed by 6 repetitions × 50% of 1RM within the same set) specifically designed for postmenopausal women with osteopenia/osteoporosis and monitor the effect of the protocol on bone mineral density (BMD) in the lumbar spine, assessed by dual-energy X-ray absorptiometry (DEXA). The subjects included in the study were 29 postmenopausal women (56.5 ± 2.8 years) with osteopenia or osteoporosis; they were separated into two groups: the experimental group (n = 15), in which the subjects participated in the strength training protocol for a period of 6 months; and the control group (n = 14), in which the subjects did not take part in any physical activity. BMD in the lumbar spine was measured by DEXA. The measurements were performed at the beginning and end of the study. A statistically significant increase (Δ% = 1.82%) in BMD was observed at the end of the study for the exercise group (0.778 ± 0.042 at baseline vs. 0.792 ± 0.046 after 6 months, p = 0.018, 95% CI [−0.025, −0.003]); while an increase was observed for the control group (Δ% = 0.14%), the difference was not statistically significant (0.762 ± 0.057 at baseline vs. 0.763 ± 0.059, p = 0.85, 95% CI [−0.013, 0.011]). In conclusion, our strength training protocol seems to be effective in increasing BMD among women with osteopenia/osteoporosis and represents an affordable strategy for preventing future bone loss.

Keywords: osteoporosis; strength training; osteopenia; bone mass; DEXA

Citation: Holubiac, I.Ș.; Leuciuc, F.V.; Crăciun, D.M.; Dobrescu, T. Effect of Strength Training Protocol on Bone Mineral Density for Postmenopausal Women with Osteopenia/Osteoporosis Assessed by Dual-Energy X-ray Absorptiometry (DEXA). *Sensors* **2022**, 22, 1904. https://doi.org/10.3390/s22051904

Academic Editors: Ayman El-baz, Ahmed Shalaby, Guruprasad A. Giridharan, Ali H. Mahmoud and Mohammed Ghazal

Received: 1 February 2022
Accepted: 27 February 2022
Published: 28 February 2022

1. Introduction

The introduction of the bone mass assessment method using dual-energy X-ray absorptiometry (DEXA) measurement is an important step for clinical trials aimed at assessing bone density. DEXA has certain advantages, such as increased accuracy and the low radiation dose to which the subject is exposed. DEXA investigation can measure bone mass for the spine, hip, and forearm, thereby helping in the diagnosis of osteopenia or osteoporosis. DEXA is a non-invasive diagnostic technique used to determine bone density and it is a reference method in this domain [1].

The combination of bone density and bone quality (obtained from bone mass assessment) mainly reflects bone strength. When talking about bone quality, several variables are considered, such as structural changes, the relationship between osteolysis and osteogenesis, collagen structure, possible bone damage (e.g., fractures or microfractures), and the level of bone mineralisation. Osteoporosis can be the result of lack of calcium, as well as other minerals in bones, and these deficiencies can make bone weaker, more fragile, and more prone to injuries and fractures, even following minor trauma [2,3]. Osteoporosis can be classified according to the causative factor; however, in the case of primary osteoporosis, it affects about 80% of women and about 60% of men. Primary osteoporosis includes idiopathic osteoporosis (i.e., the cause of osteoporosis is unknown), Type I osteoporosis (which is caused by a lack of oestrogen, a common condition in postmenopausal women), and Type II (degenerative) osteoporosis. Osteoporosis caused by oestrogen deficiency is characterised by loss of bone density, which may be accompanied by fractures in the femoral neck, lumbar spine, and distal radius. Oestrogen plays a protective role in the bone system, and when women enter the postmenopausal period and oestrogen levels drop significantly, osteolysis becomes more pronounced compared with osteogenesis because the lack of oestrogen tends to cause an imbalance between osteogenesis and osteolysis (in favour of osteolysis), making bones more fragile. In other words, osteoclasts (the bone cells responsible for osteolysis) become more active than osteoblasts (the bone cells responsible for osteogenesis). Loss of cortical and trabecular bone, as well as proximal fractures of the humerus and tibia, femoral neck, and pelvis, are specific to Type II osteoporosis. Oestrogen plays a critical role in regulating several factors that are responsible for osteogenesis, such as RANKL (nuclear activator receptor kappa-B ligand factor) in osteoblasts, IL-1, IL-6, TNF-α, and M-CSF. Oestrogen also stimulates osteoprotegerin activity in osteoblasts, an action that results in the apoptosis of osteoclasts and prevents the apoptosis of osteocytes (bone cells). When oestrogen levels decrease (as in the case of menopause), the rate of osteolysis increases and the rate of osteogenesis decreases, which leads to a decrease in bone mass. To improve mobility, bone strength, and physical function, and to prevent fractures (as a consequence of falls), resistance training should be practiced along with balance exercises and weight-bearing activities [4]. Resistance exercises seem to be effective even amongst older women when it comes to bone mass [5], with recommended intensities between 70% and 80% of one maximum repetition (1RM), performed two to three times a week being an affordable and efficient solution for increasing bone mass amongst postmenopausal women [6,7].

This study aims to evaluate the influence of a resistance training protocol for lumbar spine bone mineral density (BMD) amongst women with postmenopausal osteopenia/osteoporosis assessed by DEXA.

2. Materials and Methods

Twenty-nine non-smoking women with postmenopausal osteopenia/osteoporosis, a body mass index (BMI) of $\leq$25, and no physical exercise contraindications were included in the study. The subjects had not participated in any exercise program in the last 3 months, and all of them were sedentary people (less than 60 min of exercise per week). BMD was measured using DEXA analysis (Hologic Horizon, Santa Clara, CA, USA) and radiological examination (see Figures 1 and 2). Skeletal BMD can be measured using DEXA, which is considered by some authors to be one of the most effective methods of diagnosing osteoporosis or osteopenia [8]. Currently, DEXA is the standard reference for diagnosing osteoporosis [9,10]. It is a precise evaluation method that involves exposing the areas to be evaluated to a small amount of X-rays and allows the areas of interest to be objectively measured. In this method, the two X-rays are absorbed differently in the bone, and the BMD is calculated in g/cm^2 using simultaneous equations. Among the results offered by DEXA investigation is some information on bone mineral content (BMC) given in g, area measured in cm^3, and BMD given in g/cm^2 [11]. The measurement was compared with two reference values: one for young adults (30 years, which gives a T-score) and one for people of the same age as the evaluated person (which gives a Z score) [12]. DEXA has certain strengths, such as not exposing the patient to a high dose of radiation (1–6 μSv) and having a short time scan (1–2 min). Following the DEXA investigation, the software recorded the values obtained and displayed them on the screen. The T-score obtained by the subject being examined refers to her bone mass, taking as reference an individual of the same gender with peak bone mass. A classification was established depending on the score obtained: normal bone mass density (score between -1 and 0 or higher), osteopenia (between -1.1 and -2.4), and osteoporosis (a score of -2.5 or less). The Z score obtained refers to the BMD of the scanned subject compared with a subject of the same age and weight (see Figure 2).

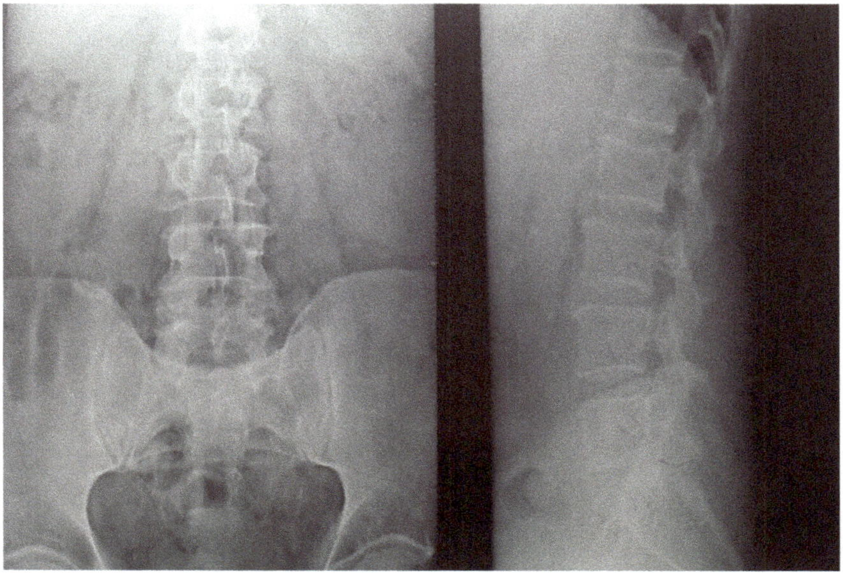

Figure 1. Radiological image of the subjects included in the study (X-ray of the lumbar spine). (**Left side**) an image in the frontal plane; (**right side**) an image in the sagittal plane (profile). Using radiography as an auxiliary method provides information on the height of the vertebrae, the intervertebral spaces, and on other possible associated problems that could be contraindications for participating in the training protocol.

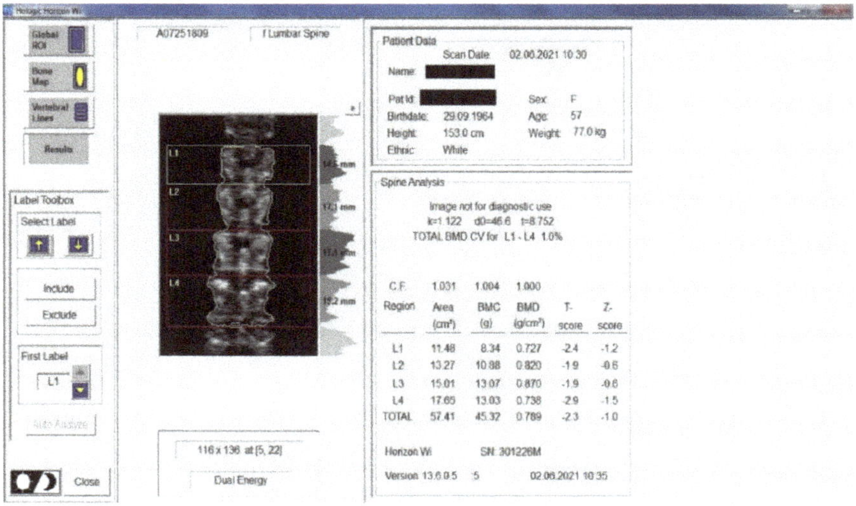

Figure 2. Measurement of BMD for the subjects included in the study. The results are displayed planimetrically, relating the BMC to the surface being evaluated (g/cm^2). This also gives us a total T-score expressing whether the person has normal BMD (T-score between −1 and 0 or above), osteopenia (T-score between −1.1 and −2.4), or osteoporosis (T-score of −2.5 or less). The results in the image show us that the subject has osteopenia (but is extremely close to osteoporosis).

Medical investigations (DEXA and radiographs) were conducted by a technician and the radiographs was interpreted by a specialist. The T-score provided information on whether the subject could be included in the study (the condition being that the subjects had osteopenia or osteoporosis), and the lumbar spine BMD was the quantitative information we used to make pre- and post-test comparisons. Tables 1 and 2 and Figure 2 present information on BMD in each vertebra, but the last and the most important result is the total BMD, which is the reference result. With the help of radiography, we used visual information about the body and height of the vertebrae, the presence or absence of vertebral fractures, and the height of the intervertebral spaces. We could also observe if the subject had a history of other pathologies that would be a contraindication to performing the training protocol. Different from the DEXA investigation, which was made at the beginning and at the end of the study, the X-ray was used only at the beginning of the study to rule out the possibility of other pathologies in the lumbar area that could prevent the subjects from participating in the program.

Table 1. Baseline characteristics of the participants.

	Exercise (n = 15)	Control (n = 14)	p (Between Groups)
Age (years)	56.2 ± 3.2	56.8 ± 2.3	0.77
Weight (kg)	65.8 ± 7.4	63.2 ± 7.5	0.36
Height (cm)	161 ± 6.3	157.6 ± 4.7	0.12
BMI	25.4 ± 2.6	25.4 ± 2.1	0.99
BMD L_1	0.754 ± 0.057	0.750 ± 0.072	0.87
BMD L_2	0.780 ± 0.050	0.764 ± 0.067	0.46
BMD L_3	0.785 ± 0.054	0.786 ± 0.064	0.97
BMD L_4	0.789 ± 0.058	0.750 ± 0.070	0.11
BMD TOTAL	0.778 ± 0.042	0.762 ± 0.057	0.39

Note: results are represented as mean and standard deviation (±); BMI = body mass index; BMD = bone mineral density (g/cm^2).

Table 2. Intra-group and inter-group comparison after 6 months.

	Exercise (n = 15)			Control (n = 14)			
	Pre	Post	p (Intra-Group)	Pre	Post	p (Intra-Group)	p (Inter-Groups)
Weight (kg)	65.8 ± 7.4	64.5 ± 7.4	0.008 *	63.2 ± 7.5	63.9 ± 7.6	0.065	0.85
Height (cm)	161 ± 6.3	160.8 ± 6.3	0.082	157.6 ± 4.7	157.5 ± 4.6	0.17	0.12
BMI	25.4 ± 2.6	24.9 ± 2.4	0.017 *	25.4 ± 2.1	25.7 ± 2.1	0.062	0.37
BMD L_1	0.754 ± 0.057	0.777 ± 0.055	0.079	0.750 ± 0.072	0.743 ± 0.061	0.26	0.12
BMD L_2	0.780 ± 0.050	0.791 ± 0.061	0.24	0.764 ± 0.067	0.777 ± 0.067	0.11	0.55
BMD L_3	0.785 ± 0.054	0.805 ± 0.057	0.053	0.786 ± 0.064	0.776 ± 0.066	0.38	0.21
BMD L_4	0.789 ± 0.058	0.794 ± 0.057	0.65	0.750 ± 0.070	0.755 ± 0.073	0.62	0.12
BMD TOTAL	0.778 ± 0.042	0.792 ± 0.046	0.018 *	0.762 ± 0.057	0.763 ± 0.059	0.85	0.15

* Statistical significance.

The study involved women with osteopenia/postmenopausal osteoporosis who were separated into two groups, as shown in Figure 3. The exercise group was formed by volunteer women; the control group was formed by women who did not want to participate in the training protocol. All the subjects received the same treatment (0.5 µg of alfacalcidol daily). The subjects gave their written consent to the use of the data obtained and the study was conducted according to the guidelines of the Declaration of Helsinki. The flowchart of patient registration is shown in Figure 3.

The training protocol was designed by two physical therapists and two sports training specialists. The training program lasted 6 months; the duration of each training session was about 60 min and took place in the gym of Stefan cel Mare University of Suceava. Exercises included in the training protocol (seated hip abduction, seated machine dip, seated back extension, standing hip flexion, standing hip extension, seated hip adduction, horizontal leg press, prone hamstring curls, seated knee extension, and bicep curls) were performed on the machines. Only bodyweight squats were not performed on the machine. The first six exercises were performed in the first training session of the week and the other five exercises were performed in the second training session of the week. All exercises were performed in two sets of 12 repetitions (6 repetitions with an intensity of 70% of 1RM, followed by 6 repetitions with an intensity of 50% of 1RM). The only exception was bodyweight squats, where no extra weights were used to avoid overloading the lower limb joints. The pause between sets was 90 s. The subjects had two weeks to familiarise themselves with the exercises and learn the correct execution technique. Three days before the start of the training protocol, the subjects were tested for 1RM for each exercise, such that we could determine the 70% and 50% of 1RM. The 1RM represents the weight with which the subject can perform only one repetition. This test was repeated every 4 weeks, such that the future estimates of 70% and 50% could be made according to the new maximum repetition (1RM). The strength exercises were performed with an intensity of 40% of 1RM in the first two weeks with 12–15 repetitions per series, followed by 50% of 1RM in the third week. Starting in the fourth week, we switched to a method involving six repetitions with an intensity of 50% of 1RM followed by six repetitions with an intensity of 70% of 1RM within the same set. Given that fractures of the wrist, vertebral body, and femoral neck are the fractures that warn of the presence of osteoporosis, the exercises proposed in this protocol focused muscle groups that are involved in the movement of wrist, spine, and hip joints. Seated hip abduction targets the gluteus medius and gluteus minimus muscles. Standing hip flexion targets the iliopsoas and quadriceps femoris muscles (more precisely, rectus femoris muscles). The psoas major muscle originates in the adjacent margins of the bodies of the vertebrae (T_{12}–L_5) and intervening intervertebral disc, such that its contraction acts on the vertebral bodies. Standing hip extension is an exercise that strengthens the gluteus maximus muscle. Seated hip adduction mainly targets the adductor magnus, adductor longus, and adductor brevis muscles. Prone hamstring curls target the biceps femoris, semitendinosus, and semimembranosus muscles. Horizontal leg press targets the gluteus maximus, quadriceps femoris, and triceps surae muscles. Seated knee extension involves an isolated movement of the knee joint with excellent effect on the quadriceps femoris muscle. Seated machine dips stimulate the muscles of the upper limbs, shoulder, and thorax (pectoralis major, anterior deltoid, and triceps brachii). Bicep curls strengthen the muscles of the front of the arm and forearm (especially the biceps brachii, brachialis, and brachioradialis). Seated back extension exercises strengthen the back muscles. The muscles that are involved in this movement are the erectores spinae (iliocostalis, longissimus, and spinalis), aided by the quadratus lumborum and latissimus dorsi. With age, especially in women with osteopenia/osteoporosis, thoracic curvature (kyphosis) increases due to vertebral deformities. Thus, we selected the above exercise because it strengthens the back extensors to maintain a correct posture.

SPSS version 26 was used for statistical analysis. To determine the statistical significance, a paired sample *t* test was applied for within-group comparisons and an independent sample *t* test was applied for between-group comparisons. The Mann–Whitney U test was applied to the variable 'age' to determine if there existed significant differences between the two groups. A p value < 0.05 was considered statistically significant. The equation used for the paired sample *t* test is

$$t = \frac{\overline{X_D}}{S_D/\sqrt{n}} \tag{1}$$

- $\overline{X_D}$ = mean difference between the two groups (control and exercise groups for each variable: BMD_{L1}, BMD_{L2}, BMD_{L3}, BMD_{L4} and BMD_{total}); S_D = standard deviation of the difference scores; and n = number of subjects. The equation for S_D calculation is

$$S_D = \sqrt{\frac{\sum_x 2 - (\sum_x)2/n}{n-1}} \tag{2}$$

The equation used for the independent sample *t* test is

$$t_{test} = \frac{M_x - M_y}{\sqrt{\frac{(\sum X^2 - (\sum X)^2/N_x) + (\sum Y^2 - (\sum Y)^2/N_y) * \left(\frac{1}{N_x} + \frac{1}{N_{xy}}\right)}{N_x + N_y - 2}}} \quad (3)$$

- M_x = mean score for exercise group; M_y = mean score for control group; $\sum X^2$ = sum of the squared X (control group) scores; $(\sum X)^2$ = sum of the X (control group) scores squared; $\sum Y^2$ = sum of the squared Y (exercise group) scores; $(\sum Y)^2$ = sum of the Y (exercise group) scores squared; N_x = number of control group subjects; and N_y = number of exercise group subjects.

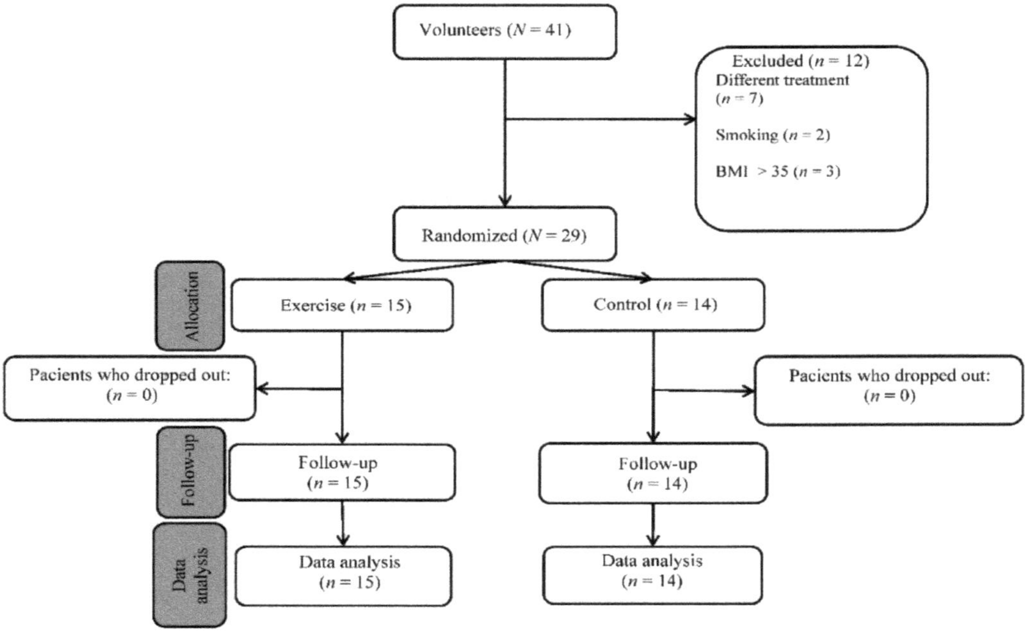

Figure 3. Flow diagram of study participants.

3. Results

The baseline characteristics of the participants are shown in Table 1. For the exercise group, the weight of the subjects showed a significant decrease (Δ% = −1.93%) at the end of the study (64.5 ± 7.9 vs. 65.8 ± 7.4, t(14) = 3.11, p = 0.008, 95% CI [0.39, 2.14]). Within the control group, the weight of the subjects increased (Δ% = 1.13%) after 6 months (M = 63.9, SD = 7.6) compared with the initial results (M = 63.2, SD = 7.5, t(13) = −2.02, p = 0.065, 95% CI [0.05, −2.02]). Although a difference existed between the two groups, the statistical analysis showed that it was not statistically significant (t(27) = 0.21, p = 0.84, 95% CI [−5.31, 6.52]). The height of the subjects who participated in the weight training program decreased (Δ% = −0.12) after 6 months (160.8 ± 6.3 vs. 161.0 ± 6.3, t(14) = 1.87, p = 0.082, 95% CI [−0.03, 0.43]). No significant differences (Δ% = −0.09) were observed at the end of the study in the control group (M = 157.5, SD = 4.6) compared with the initial test (M = 157.6, SD = 4.7, t(13) = 1.47, p = 0.17, 95% CI [−0.07, 0.35]). The intergroup differences were not statistically significant (t(27) = 1.60, p = 0.12, 95% CI [−0.93, 7.53]).

BMI decreased (Δ% = −1.79) within the exercise group at the end of the study (24.9 ± 2.4 vs. 25.4 ± 2.6, t(14) = 2.71, p = 0.017, 95% CI [0.10, 0.81]); within the control group, there was an increase by 1.27% at the end of the study (M = 25.7, SD = 2.1) compared with the baseline (M = 25.4, SD = 2.1, t(13) = −2.04, p = 0.062, 95% CI [−0.66, 0.02]), but the differences were insignificant at the end of the study between the two groups (t(27) = −0.90, p = 0.37, 95% CI [−2.48, 0.96]; see Figure 4 and Table 2).

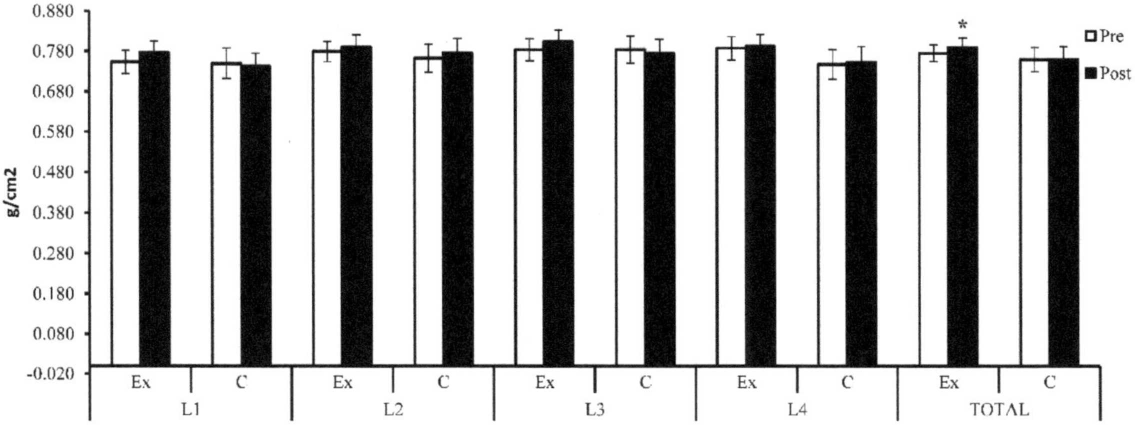

Figure 4. Lumbar spine BMD (g/cm^2)—initial and baseline results; Ex = exercise group; C = control group. The symbol (*) indicates intra-group difference (p < 0.05).

BMD showed an increase (Δ% = 3.01%) at the L_1 lumbar spine after 6 months (M = 0.777, SD = 0.055) compared with the baseline (M = 0.754, SD = 0.057), but the difference was not statistically significant (t(14) = −1.90, p = 0.079, 95% CI [−0.048, 0.003]). For the same area, the subjects who did not participate in the weight training program showed a decrease (Δ% = −1.01%) after 6 months compared with the initial results (0.743 ± 0.061 vs. 0.750 ± 0.072, t(13) = 1.17, p = 0.26, 95% CI [−0.006, 0.022]). Although there existed a difference between the groups, the difference was not statistically significant (t(27) = 1.59, p = 0.12, 95% CI [−0.010, 0.078]).

At the L_2 level, BMD showed an increase (Δ% = 1.44%) within the exercise group after 6 months (0.791 ± 0.061 vs. 0.780 ± 0.050), but the increase was not statistically significant (t(14) = −1.24, p = 0.24, 95% CI [−0.031, 0.008]). Within the control group, an increase (Δ% = 1.70%) was also observed at the end of the research compared with the baseline (t(13) = −1.74, p = 0.11, 95% CI [−0.029, 0.003]). Between the two groups, the difference was not statistically significant at the end of the study (t(27) = 0.61, p = 0.55, 95% CI [−0.034, 0.063]). At the end of the study, the exercise group showed an increase (Δ% = 2.55%) at the L_3 level, but the increase was not statistically significant (0.805 ± 0.057 vs. 0.785 ± 0.054, t(14) = −2.11, p = 0.053, 95% CI [−0.040, 0.000]). At the same level, the control group showed a decrease in bone mass at the end of the study (Δ% = −1.29%) compared with the initial results (0.776 ± 0.066 vs. 0.786 ± 0.064, t(13) = 0.91, p = 0.38, 95% CI [−0.014, 0.034]). However, the difference was insignificant between the two groups (t(27) = 1.28, p = 0.21, 95% CI [−0.018, 0.076]). Both groups registered an extremely close increase in value at the level of the L_4 lumbar spine (exercise group: Δ% = 0.68%, t(14) = −0.47, p = 0.65 and 95% CI [−0.030, 0.019]; control group: Δ% = 0.69%, t(13) = −0.51, p = 0.62, 95% CI [−0.027, 0.017]), but the difference not being statistically significant between the two groups (t(27) = 1.63, p = 0.12, 95% CI [−0.010, 0.089]). Total lumbar spine BMD showed a statistically significantly increase (Δ% = 1.82%) in the exercise group after 6 months (0.792 ± 0.046 vs. 0.778 ± 0.042, t(14) = −2.68, p = 0.018, 95% CI [−0.025, −0.003]). The control group also showed an improvement (Δ% = 0.14%) after 6 months (M = 0.763, SD = 0.059) compared with the initial results (M = 0.762, SD = 0.057), but the difference was not statistically significant (t(13) = −0.20, p = 0.85, 95% CI [−0.013, 0.011]). Although the experimental group showed a higher increase compared with the control group, the difference was not statistically significant at the end of the study (t(27) = 1.49, p = 0.15, 95% CI [−0.011, 0.069]).

4. Discussion

Radiological evaluation is still used in the diagnosis of osteoporosis, although it records at a low sensitivity. The changes that we can observe on the radiograph are represented by osteopenia, fractures, and the consequences of these deformities. Thus, a decrease of the vertebrae height is a consequence of the fractures, a particularly important aspect in the diagnosis of osteoporosis. In the case of radiographic investigations, for a person's bones to show osteopenic signs, they have to lose about 20–30% of their bone mass, which is a fairly high percentage [13]. Therefore, this condition is a limitation of radiographic investigations. Some features of the osteoporotic bone, visible on radiographic investigations, are represented by the thinning of the cortical bone and deformities of the spine vertebrae [14,15]. However, one study found that hand radiographs are not as accurate compared with DEXA (dual X-ray) measurements [16]. The diagnosis of osteopenia or osteoporosis using radiographic imaging is not highly accurate because it is influenced by the position of the patient's body during the investigation. The diagnosis depends on the level of training and experience of the doctor who interprets the X-ray. Identifying people at increased risk of a fracture within a year or two of the assessment data (imminent risk of fracture) is a new concept that can be useful in selecting people to receive immediate treatment and a program of fall prevention [17].

DEXA investigation is used to measure the BMC of the human skeleton or certain areas considered vulnerable to fracture (hip, spine, and forearm). DEXA can help determine the strength and strength of bone, which are influenced by bone size. The best anatomical area to measure BMD is at the hip joint (hip).

The BMD resulting from this investigation is closely related to the thickness of the bone trabeculae, but also to their number. Cortical bone thickness and bone section area are also related to BMD, these parameters being in turn subject to hormonal influences, lifestyle, physical activity, hereditary antecedents, and constituting factors that interfere with the evaluation and interpretation of DEXA. The areas of interest used in this technique are at the hip joint and at the lumbar spine (L_1–L_4). Investigation of the hip joint is preferred in patients, especially after the age of 65 when other degenerative diseases progress and may interfere with the bone mass present in the spine. Other areas of interest are represented by the middle and distal radius. According to the National Osteoporosis Foundation, the indications for DEXA investigation are: (a) women aged 65 and over and men aged 70 and over; (b) postmenopausal women and men ≥50 years of age with other risk factors involved; (c) postmenopausal women and men ≥50 years of age who have suffered a fracture at or after the age of 50; and (d) adults who suffer from rheumatoid arthritis or who use medications, such as glucocorticoids, and who have low bone mass or bone loss [18,19]. This routine investigation is not recommended for premenopausal woman. DEXA has some limitations, although it is a quick and an inexpensive method of diagnosing osteoporosis. This technology cannot produce 3D images and cannot distinguish between cortical and trabecular bones [20]. During the DEXA investigation, the operator may be exposed to a low dose of radiation [20–22].

The effect of resistance training on BMD depends on the duration of the program, the intensities used, and the treatment followed.

A study conducted in 2013 on 21 women with osteopenia/osteoporosis reported positive results for the experimental group (61.9 ± 5.0 years; n = 10) compared with the group control (66.7 ± 7.4 years; n = 11) at the end of 12 weeks of weight training, with the program performed three times a week. The program started with two warm-up series of 8–12 repetitions with an intensity of 50% of 1RM, followed by four series of 3–5 repetitions with an intensity of 85–90% of 1RM, with the rest between the series being 2–3 min. At the level of the experimental group, BMC registered a significant increase in the lumbar spine (Δ% = 2.9, p = 0.012) [23]. The intensities used in this study were extremely high (85–90%);

in our case, we used lower intensities to avoid the risk of injury. Given that overloading the joints by using extremely heavy weights can increase the risk of bone cartilage damage, our decision to use lower intensities is understandable. Although the improvement observed in that study is more obvious, with an increase 1% higher compared with our work, the subjects underwent a treatment based on Vitamin D and calcium; however, the dosage is unspecified, which can explain greater increase in BMD. In 2009, a 12-month study of 59 women with postmenopausal osteoporosis/osteopenia assessed the effect of resistance exercise on BMD in the femur and lumbar spine. The experimental group (57.5 ± 5.1 years) participated in a training program (divided in four stages), with the exercises performed in a closed kinematic chain. The exercises were divided into four stages; each stage lasted months and the number of repetitions progressively increased from 10 repetitions (in the first month) to 12 repetitions (the second month) to 15 (in the third month), with 1 min rest between sets and exercises. The control group (56.6 ± 4.6 years) did not participate in any exercise program during the 12 months and no group received drug treatment during the study. At the end of the 12 months, the experimental group recorded an increase (Δ% = 1.17) in BMD compared with the initial results in the lumbar spine (0.845 ± 0.09 vs. 0.855 ± 0.09, $p = 0.22$), whereas the control group recorded a statistically significant decrease in BMD in the lumbar spine (Δ% = −2.26, $p = 0.019$). The changes (post-test–pre-test) regarding the BMD (g/cm^2) at the level of the lumbar spine were significantly different between the experimental group (0.010 ± 0.043) and the control group (−0.018 ± 0.039, $p < 0.013$) [24]. In the case of our implemented protocol, higher increases in lumbar spine BMD were observed compared with the study mentioned above (+1.17% vs. +1.82% in our case). We specify that the duration of the program used by Matos et al. was twice as long as ours, but the subjects did not receive Vitamin D treatment. Moreover, only weights of 1, 2, 3, and 4 kg were used, but the intensities used are not mentioned, meaning that we cannot make a comparison regarding this factor.

A one-year study conducted in 2013 separated the participants (postmenopausal women) into three groups: a control group (52 ± 3.4 years), a group participating in the resistance training (51.4 ± 2.7 years), and a group involved in a water exercise program (54.5 ± 3.3 years). BMD was assessed before the study and at its end. The resistance training program was performed three times a week, with a number of repetitions between 10–15 for each exercise. All the subjects underwent a hormone-based treatment, and at the end of the study, the group that followed the resistance training program recorded an increase in the lumbar spine L_2–L_4 of 16.40% ($p < 0.05$). Between the control group and the group participating in the resistance training program, the differences were significant in the lumbar spine (1283 ± 0.169 vs. 1070 ± 0.030, $p < 0.001$) [25]. Although increases in BMD are more evident in this study, the subjects in the group participating in strength training had been on a hormone-based treatment for 3 years (3.0 ± 1.7 years). The subjects of this study already registered a high BMD (because none of the subjects in the group who participated in the strength exercise program had osteopenia or osteoporosis; all of them had normal BMD).

Basat et al. conducted a 6-month study and compared the effects of training programs on BMD in postmenopausal women. In this study, one group participated in a resistance training program (55.9 ± 4.9 years; $n = 11$), one group participated in a program of exercises involving movements with high impact on bone-jumping (55.6 ± 2.9 years; $n = 12$), and a control group (56.2 ± 4.0 years; $n = 12$) did not exercise throughout the study; all groups received treatment with Vitamin D (800 IU) and calcium (1200 mg) daily. The training programs were conducted three times a week with 60 min session durations; after 15 min of warm-up, the subjects performed the isometric training program lasting 45–60 min, in which they performed one series of 10 repetitions for each exercise. At the end of the study, the group that participated in the resistance exercise program had an increase in BMD in the lumbar spine L_1–L_4 (Δ% = 1.3) compared with a decrease in BMD observed in the control group (Δ% = −2.5). Between the two groups, the differences were significant at the end of the study in the lumbar spine ($p = 0.032$) [26]. However, in this study, the subjects also underwent calcium-based treatment (and not just Vitamin D-based treatment, as in our case). The increase in lumbar spine BMD in our study is higher (+1.82%) compared to the increase (+1.3%) observed in the study conducted by Basat et al., although the duration of the intervention program was identical (6 months).

Exercise programs that do not involve weight training may also be effective in increasing BMD. Angin et al. showed significant differences after 6 months of practicing tai chi exercises compared with initial results on the BMD in the lumbar spine L_2–L_4 (0.673 ± 0.09 vs. 0.714 ± 0.09, $p = 0.002$), recording an increase of 0.04 ± 0.06 g/cm^2, which is a 6.1% increase in BMD. However, in this study, the subjects were treated with bisphosphonates, which was also a criterion for including the subjects in the study [27].

5. Conclusions

This study shows the effect that our strength training protocol has on postmenopausal women with osteopenia or osteoporosis. Therefore, alternating loads of 70% of 1RM with loads of 50% of 1RM within the same set and performing the exercise protocol twice a week may lead to an increase in lumbar spine BMD for postmenopausal women with osteopenia/osteoporosis.

The method is also safe because the intensities do not exceed 70% of 1RM. Comparing the costs of drugs for treating osteopenia or osteoporosis with the costs involved in adopting such a training program indicates that this proposed method is an affordable strategy for the prevention of osteopenia or osteoporosis. In the future, we aim to evaluate the BMD and body composition of subjects (using bioimpedance devices) included in such a strength training protocol, as well as use specific dynamometers to measure muscle strength in order to assess to what extent muscle strength and muscle mass influence BMD for women with osteopenia or osteoporosis. We also want to evaluate the effect that this strength training protocol has on BMD in the hip, and its relationship to fat mass and lean mass for women with postmenopausal osteopenia/osteoporosis.

Author Contributions: Conceptualisation, I.Ș.H., F.V.L., T.D. and D.M.C.; methodology, I.Ș.H., F.V.L., T.D. and D.M.C.; software, I.Ș.H.; validation, F.V.L. and T.D.; formal analysis, I.Ș.H. and D.M.C.; investigation, F.V.L.; resources, F.V.L. and D.M.C.; data curation, I.Ș.H.; writing—original draft preparation, I.Ș.H. and T.D.; writing—review and editing, F.V.L. and D.M.C.; visualisation, D.M.C.; supervision, F.V.L.; project administration, I.Ș.H. All authors have read and agreed to the published version of the manuscript.

Funding: The APC was funded by Stefan cel Mare University of Suceava.

Institutional Review Board Statement: The study was conducted according to the guidelines of the Declaration of Helsinki and approved by the Institutional Review Board of Stefan cel Mare University of Suceava (protocol code 35 from 28 May 2021).

Informed Consent Statement: Informed consent was obtained from all subjects involved in the study. Written informed consent was obtained from the patient(s) to publish this paper.

Conflicts of Interest: The authors declare no conflict of interest.

References

1. Blake, G.M.; Fogelman, I. Technical principles of dual energy x-ray absorptiometry. *Semin. Nucl. Med.* **1997**, *27*, 210–218. [CrossRef]
2. Chun, K.J. Bone densitometry. *Semin. Nucl. Med.* **2011**, *41*, 220–228. [CrossRef] [PubMed]
3. Miller, A.J.; Jones, C.; Liss, F.; Abboudi, J.; Kirkpatrick, W.; Beredjiklian, P. Qualitative Evaluation of Digital Hand X-rays Is Not a Reliable Method to Assess Bone Mineral Density. *Arch. Bone Jt. Surg.* **2017**, *5*, 10–13. [PubMed]
4. Guerri, S.; Gómez, M.P.; Mercatelli, D.; Napoli, A.; Guglielmi, G.; Battista, G.; Bazzocchi, A. Quantitative imaging techniques for the assessment of osteoporosis and sarcopenia. *Quant. Imaging Med. Surg.* **2018**, *8*, 60–85. [CrossRef]
5. Coronado-Zarco, R.; León, A.O.G.; García-Lara, A.; Quinzaños-Fresnedo, J.; Nava-Bringas, T.I.; Macías-Hernández, S.I. Nonpharmacological interventions for osteoporosis treatment: Systematic review of clinical practice guidelines. *Osteoporos. Sarcopenia* **2019**, *5*, 69–77. [CrossRef]

6. Beck, B.R.; Daly, R.M.; Singh, M.A.; Taaffe, D.R. Exercise and Sports Science Australia (ESSA) position statement on exercise prescription for the prevention and management of osteoporosis. *J. Sci. Med. Sport* **2017**, *5*, 438–445. [CrossRef]
7. Pellikaan, P.; Giarmatzis, G.; Sloten, J.V.; Verschueren, S.; Jonkers, I. Ranking of osteogenic potential of physical exercises in postmenopausal women based on femoral neck strains. *PLoS ONE* **2018**, *13*, e0195463. [CrossRef]
8. Johansson, H.; Siggeirsdóttir, K.; Odén, N.C.A.; Gudnason, V.; McCloskey, E.; Kanis, J.A. Imminent risk of fracture after fracture. *Osteoporos. Int.* **2017**, *28*, 775–780. [CrossRef]
9. Bruyere, O.; Reginster, J.Y. Monitoring of osteoporosis therapy. *Best Pract. Res. Clin. Endocrinol. Metab.* **2014**, *28*, 835–841. [CrossRef]
10. Manhard, M.K.; Nyman, J.S.; Does, M.D. Advances in imaging approaches to fracture risk evaluation. *Transl. Res.* **2017**, *181*, 1–14. [CrossRef]
11. Schultz, K.; Wolf, J.M. Emerging Technologies in Osteoporosis Diagnosis. *Hand Surg. Landsc.* **2019**, *44*, 240–243. [CrossRef]
12. Adams, J.E. Advances in bone imaging for osteoporosis. *Nat. Rev. Endocrinol.* **2013**, *9*, 28–42. [CrossRef] [PubMed]
13. Daly, R.M.; Via, J.D.; Duckham, R.L.; Fraser, S.F.; Helge, E.W. Exercise for the prevention of osteoporosis in postmenopausal women: An evidence-based guide to the optimal prescription. *Braz. J. Phys. Ther.* **2019**, *23*, 170–180. [CrossRef]
14. Ardran, G.M. Bone destruction not demonstrable by radiography. *Br. J. Radiol.* **1951**, *24*, 107–109. [CrossRef] [PubMed]
15. Daphne Theodorou, J.; Stavroula Theodorou, J.; Timothy Duncan, D.; Steven Garfin, R.; Wade Wong, H. Percutaneous balloon kyphoplasty for the correction of spinal deformity in painful vertebral body compression fractures. *Clin. Imaging* **2002**, *26*, 1–5. [CrossRef]
16. Bouxsein, M.; Seeman, E. Quantifying the material and structural determinants of bone strength. *Best Pract. Res. Clin. Rheumatol.* **2009**, *23*, 741–753. [CrossRef]
17. Roux, C.; Briot, K. Imminent fracture risk. *Osteoporos. Int.* **2017**, *28*, 1765–1769. [CrossRef]
18. Eastell, R. Identification and management of osteoporosis in older adults. *Med. Older Adults* **2016**, *45*, 55–61.
19. Cosman, F.; Beur, S.J.; LeBoff, M.S.; Lewiecki, E.M.; Tanner, B.; Randall, S.; Lindsay, R. Clinician's Guide to Prevention and Treatment of Osteoporosis. *Osteoporos. Int.* **2014**, *25*, 2359–2381, Erratum in *Osteoporos. Int.* **2015**, *26*, 2045–2047. [CrossRef]
20. Nishiyama, K.K.; Shane, E. Clinical Imaging of Bone Microarchitecture with HR-pQCT. *Curr. Osteoporos. Rep.* **2013**, *11*, 147–155. [CrossRef]
21. Thomas, L.D. Osteoporosis Imaging: State of the Art and Advanced Imaging. *Radiology* **2012**, *263*, 3–17.
22. Choksi, P.; Jepsen, K.J.; Clines, G.A. The challenges of diagnosing osteoporosis and the limitations of currently available tools. *Clin. Diabetes Endocrinol.* **2018**, *4*, 1–13. [CrossRef] [PubMed]
23. Mosti, M.; Kaehler, N.; Stunes, A.; Hoff, J.; Syversen, U. Maximal strength training in postmenopausal women with osteoporosis or osteopenia. *J. Strength Cond. Res.* **2013**, *27*, 2879–2886. [CrossRef] [PubMed]
24. Matos, O.D.; Silva, D.J.; Oliveira, J.M.; Castelo-Branco, C. Effect of specific exercise training on bone mineral density in women with postmenopausal osteopenia or osteoporosis. *Gynecol. Endocrinol.* **2009**, *25*, 616–620. [CrossRef] [PubMed]
25. Sandor, B.; Licia, M.H.M.; Frederico, S.S.; Dahan, C.N.; Lidia, M.A.B.; Denise, O.C.B.; João, L.C.B.; Ana, P.P.; Martim, B. Resistance training versus weight-bearing aquatic exercise: A cross-sectional analysis of bone mineral density in postmenopausal women. *Rev. Basileira De Reumatol. (Engl. Ed.)* **2013**, *53*, 193–198.
26. Basat, H.; Esmaeilzadeh, S.; Eskiyurt, N. The effects of strengthening and high-impact exercises on bone metabolism and quality of life in postmenopausal women: A randomized controlled trial. *J. Back Musculoskelet. Rehabil.* **2013**, *26*, 427–435. [CrossRef]
27. Angin, E.; Erden, Z.; Can, F. The effects of clinical pilates exercises on bone mineral density, physical performance and quality of life of women with postmenopausal osteoporosis. *J. Back Musculoskelet. Rehabil.* **2015**, *28*, 849–858. [CrossRef]

sensors

MDPI

Article

Automated Diagnosis of Optical Coherence Tomography Angiography (OCTA) Based on Machine Learning Techniques

Ibrahim Yasser [1], Fahmi Khalifa [2], Hisham Abdeltawab [2], Mohammed Ghazal [3], Harpal Singh Sandhu [2] and Ayman El-Baz [2,*]

1 Faculty of Engineering, Mansoura University, Mansoura 35516, Egypt; ibrahim_yasser@mans.edu.eg
2 Department of Bioengineering, University of Louisville, Louisville, KY 40292, USA; fakhal01@louisville.edu (F.K.); hisham.abdeltawab@louisville.edu (H.A.); harpal.sandhu@gmail.com (H.S.S.)
3 Electrical and Computer Engineering Department, Abu Dhabi University, Abu Dhabi P.O. Box 59911, United Arab Emirates; mohammed.ghazal@adu.ac.ae
* Correspondence: ayman.elbaz@louisville.edu

Abstract: Diabetic retinopathy (DR) refers to the ophthalmological complications of diabetes mellitus. It is primarily a disease of the retinal vasculature that can lead to vision loss. Optical coherence tomography angiography (OCTA) demonstrates the ability to detect the changes in the retinal vascular system, which can help in the early detection of DR. In this paper, we describe a novel framework that can detect DR from OCTA based on capturing the appearance and morphological markers of the retinal vascular system. This new framework consists of the following main steps: (1) extracting retinal vascular system from OCTA images based on using joint Markov-Gibbs Random Field (MGRF) model to model the appearance of OCTA images and (2) estimating the distance map inside the extracted vascular system to be used as imaging markers that describe the morphology of the retinal vascular (RV) system. The OCTA images, extracted vascular system, and the RV-estimated distance map is then composed into a three-dimensional matrix to be used as an input to a convolutional neural network (CNN). The main motivation for using this data representation is that it combines the low-level data as well as high-level processed data to allow the CNN to capture significant features to increase its ability to distinguish DR from the normal retina. This has been applied on multi-scale levels to include the original full dimension images as well as sub-images extracted from the original OCTA images. The proposed approach was tested on in-vivo data using about 91 patients, which were qualitatively graded by retinal experts. In addition, it was quantitatively validated using datasets based on three metrics: sensitivity, specificity, and overall accuracy. Results showed the capability of the proposed approach, outperforming the current deep learning as well as features-based detecting DR approaches.

Keywords: diabetic retinopathy (DR); optical coherence tomography angiography (OCTA); convolutional neural networks (CNN); image encryption; security analysis

Citation: Yasser, I.; Khalifa, F.; Abdeltawab, H.; Ghazal, M.; Sandhu, H.S.; El-Baz, A. Automated Diagnosis of Optical Coherence Tomography Angiography (OCTA) Based on Machine Learning Techniques. *Sensors* **2022**, *22*, 2342. https://doi.org/10.3390/s22062342

Academic Editor: Sheryl Berlin Brahnam

Received: 4 January 2022
Accepted: 14 March 2022
Published: 18 March 2022

1. Introduction

Diabetic retinopathy (DR) is among several retinal diseases that represent major public health threats, which can lead to vision loss [1,2]. Diabetes mellitus is a metabolic disease characterized by hyperglycemia, and diabetic retinopathy is one of the cardinal late-stage organic manifestations of the disease. Persistent hyperglycemia causes microvascular damage in the retina through a number of mechanisms, leading to pericyte loss, endothelial damage, and ultimately capillary permeability and/or dropout. As a result, the eye develops vascularanomalies, such as neovascularization on the surface of retina in the advanced form of the disease, called proliferative diabetic retinopathy (PDR); however, these new vessels are incompetent and tend to haemorrhage or scar [3]. Although there are no vision alterations in the early stages of DR, it eventually leads to vision loss [4,5]. As a result, early detection and treatment of DR can delay or prevent diabetic-related blindness [6].

In the International Clinical Diabetic Retinopathy Disease Severity Scale, DR is classified as either proliferative (PDR) or non-proliferative (NPDR). The non-proliferative DR (NPDR) kind is divided into categories: (a) mild NPDR, in which there is no alteration in vision and the retina has fewer microaneurysms; (b) moderate NPDR, which has more microaneurysms than mild NPDR but is less severe than Severe NPDR; and (c) severe NPDR, in which patients have obvious intraretinal microvascular abnormalities (IRMA), confirmed venous bleeding in two or more quadrants, and multiple intraretinal haemorrhages in all four quadrants. Many blood vessels are blocked in severe NDPR, which induces abnormal growth factor production. In proliferative DR (PDR), patients with vitreous/preretinal and neovascularization disease are at high risk of irreversible blindness without sufficient treatment, hence its designation as advanced disease [7].

The algorithms for diagnosis are dependent on the retinal medical imaging techniques, that can be categorized as non-invasive or invasive image techniques. Indocyanine green angiography (ICGA) and fluorescein angiography (FA) are invasive methods that require 10–30 min of imaging and intravenous dye administration. They show dynamic imaging of blood flow through retinal vessels in 2D images [8,9]. Non-invasive approaches, on the other hand, include OCT angiography (OCTA) and optical coherence tomography (OCT) [10,11]. OCTA is a technique that is used to acquire angiographic information non-invasively without the need to use dye [12]. In most cases, to correctly portray vessels through different segmented parts of the eye, OCTA uses the backscatter of laser light from the surface of moving red blood cells, and that may be more accurate in detecting microvascular changes in retinal disorders than standard FA [13].

Several studies in the literature have investigated using FA to diagnose diseases in the posterior segment of the eye [12]. Despite that, FA has some limitations, such as its inability to visualize different levels of major capillary networks separately. This is because FA is unable to differentiate deep capillary plexus (DCP) from superficial capillary plexus (SCP). Additionally, it is hard to use FA in obtaining enhanced images of perifoveal capillaries because it has a challenge in focusing images when macular edema is present [10]. Moreover, FA is an invasive, time-consuming and relatively expensive modality, which makes it not ideal for regular use in clinical settings. Fluorescein dye is known to be safe; however, its side effects include nausea, allergic reactions and anaphylaxis in some rare cases [14].

Artificial intelligence (AI) consists of a set of branches, including the machine learning (ML) branch, where based on frequent exposure to labelled datasets, algorithms learn to classify data, such as medical images. Medical imaging offers a plethora of applications for ML, and the area has recently flourished in ophthalmology, with a retinal imaging focus. Image analysis and diagnosis, on the other hand, are not the most important aspects of machine learning in medicine. These methods can be used to analyze a variety of data types, including clinical data and demographic. This paper's goal was to utilize ML techniques and OCTA image data to build a computer-aided diagnostic (CAD) that automates DR diagnosis. The following are the most important contributions of this work:

- We propose a novel CNN model for OCTA scans, for tissue classification by exploiting multiple contrasts of OCTA.
- The method is based on a combination of three channels between gray, binary, and distance map to enhance the DL system ability to to capture both appearance and morphological markers of the retinal vascular system.
- Our system employs multi-scale levels to include the original full dimension images as well as sub-images extracted from the original OCTA images. This allow the CNN to capture significant features and increases its ability to distinguish DR from the normal retina.
- Evaluation has been conducted using in-vivo data and has been compared with DL-based methods as well as hand-crafted based approaches.

This paper is structured as follows: In Section 2, a general overview of existing OCTA classification is discussed followed by details of the proposed OCTA classification system in Section 3. In Section 4, experimental results for the proposed OCTA model are presented including classification performance metrics. Finally, the concluding remarks and suggested future works are given is Section 5.

2. Related Work

Computerized image analysis of retinal images is a hot topic in the scientific community. Many strategies for automatically classifying the severity of DR have been presented. Deep learning (DL) is a class of ML techniques which allows computational models made up of different processing layers to learn to represent data. DL has proven its superiority in providing a huge workforce and financial resources, and achieving high accuracy in many areas compared to traditional methods [15–18]. Through its strong diagnostic performance in detecting various pathological conditions, deep learning has been applied, mainly fundus images and to the examination of major eye diseases such as DR, age-related macular degeneration and glaucoma, which either depend on well-established guidelines or require long-term follow-up [19–25]. The convolutional neural network (CNN) has become the most extensively used technique for retinal images in particular and image classification problems in general. Most prior research used color fundus images to segment retinal blood vessels because there were few studies on OCTA image processing, OCTA being a relatively new modality. Heisler et al. [26] for example, used single data types to build the component of neural networks, which were fine-tuned using pretrained DenseNet, ResNet50, and VGG19 architectures. They studied the role of ensemble deep learning in classifying DR from OCTA images and co-registered OCT images of the retinal layers. For the stacking and majority soft voting approaches, ensemble networks built with the four fine-tuned VGG19 architectures obtained accuracies about 0.90 and 0.92, respectively. This research supports CNN's ability to accurately diagnose DR in OCTA, but it does have several drawbacks, as using ensemble learning methods, for example, considerably increases the computational cost because it necessitates the training of several networks.

Eladawi et al. [27] developed a CAD system for DR diagnosis utilizing OCTA that includes retinal vessel (RV) segmentation, image–derived markers, and an SVM-based classification. Based on a stochastic approach, the system describes the appearance of blood vessels at different levels ("deep" and "superficial") for diabetic and normal cases using a joint Markov-Gibbs random field (MGRF) model. Based on the biomarkers extracted from OCTA scans, their approach can diagnose various pathologies of choroid and retina. The image without the GGMRF and RDHE models has an AUC of 56.71%, a VVD of 58.33%, and a DSC of 54.56. While AUC was 96.18 percent, VVD was 7.95% and DSC was 96.04% for the image with enhancing stage. Le et al. [28] employed a deep-learning CNN architecture and VGG16 for automated OCTA classification using transfer learning. For training and cross-validation, a dataset of 131 images (75 DR, 24 diabetic without DR [non-DR], and 32 healthy) was employed. With the last nine layers retrained, the CNN architecture produced the greatest results. The retrained classifier's cross-validation specificity, sensitivity, and accuracy for distinguishing between DR, non-DR, and healthy eyes were 90.82%, 83.7%, and 87.27%, respectively. The CNN can provide a prediction, but a physician will have no idea how the CNN arrived at that prediction. Thus, the lack of interpretability is one of this study's flaws.

Nagasato et al. [29] utilized SVM and DL with a radial basis function kernel to create a nonperfusion area (NPA) automatic detection of retinal vein occlusion (RVO) in OCTA images. They examined the diagnostic ability of the seven ophthalmologists, SVM, and DNN (average required time, specificity and sensitivity). For discriminating NPA from normal OCTA images with RVO-OCTA images using the DNN, the mean specificity, sensitivity and AUC were 97.3%, 93.7%, and 98.6%, respectively. Average time to produce a diagnosis was 176.9 s. However, the study had some drawbacks, the 3×3 mm scan area was insufficient to detect the full NPA associated with RVO. Furthermore, they solely compared OCTA images between RVO and normal eyes, excluding the other diseases of the retina. Alam et al. [30] developed a DL-based framework for automated artery-vein (AV) classification in OCTA. On the test data, the AV-Net had an average accuracy of about

86.75 percent (86.71% for artery and 86.80% for vein), an F1-score of 82.81% and a mean IOU of 70.72 %. Because there are substantial areas of misclassification, such as at vessel cross points, this study suffers from some limitations. Díaz et al. [31] utilized a variety of morphological operators to select the FAZ candidates on the images of OCTA projection using FOVs two types. The method uses a combination of image processing algorithms to first identify the region in which the FAZ is located, then extract its precise contour. The proposed approach obtained an accuracy (Jaccard index) for diabetic OCTA images about 0.93 (0.83) and for healthy participants about 0.93 (0.82). Patients lacking various important illnesses that impact retinal vascularity are one of the drawbacks of design the research that include image datasets.

Kim et al. [32] used wide-field swept source OCTA (SS-OCTA) to construct the usefulness of semiautomated diagnostic for microvascular parameters for rating the DR severity with a perspectives variety. This study categorized 235 diabetic eyes into five categories: proliferative DR (PDR), severe NPDR, moderate NPDR, mild non-proliferative retinopathy (NPDR), and diabetes with no retinopathy (no-DR). The capillary NPA, vessel density (VD), and FAZ metrics were all measured. For grading severe NPDR from PDR, moderate from severe NPDR, mild from moderate NPDR, and no-DR, the NPA cutoff values were 21.4% (AUC: 0.90), 9.3% (AUC: 0.94), 4.7% (AUC: 0.94), and 3.7 percent (AUC: 0.91), respectively. The fundamental disadvantage of this study is that projection artefacts induced by bleeding or vitreous opacity might obscure normal microvasculature, resulting shadowing of the NPA. Ong et al. [33] developed a strategy based on the length of DCP skeletonized vessels. The deep capillary plexus (DCP), middle (MCP), and superficial (SCP) segments of OCTA slabs were segmented and thresholded using a new approach depending on DCP skeletonized vessel length. After adjusting for imaging quality and age, the adjusted flow index (AFI), parafoveal VD, and FAZ area from the vascular length density (VLD) of the SCP, as well as all three capillary layers, were compared between each DR severity category. The results showed that the values of AUC were moderate (0.731—0.752), with specificity ranging from 57.1% to 64.3% and sensitivity ranging from 83.3% to 88.9%. One of the study's drawbacks is the large racial differences between study groups as well as its insufficient powering for the DCP, which may have reduced the ability to resolve real variations in DCP parameters across groups. Alibhai et al. [34] proposed a semiautomatic, custom software method for eye scans with various degrees of DR or without DR for quantifying regions of nonperfusion capillary for OCTA classification. In eyes with proliferative DR, the mean percentage of nonperfused region was 8.5% (with 95% confidence interval CI: 5.0–14.3), in nonproliferative DR eyes, 2.1 percent (95 percent CI: 1.2–3.7), and in eyes without DR was 0.1 percent (with 95 percent CI: 0.0–0.4). The limitation of this study was that the sample size was modest, with only a few individuals having NPDR severe or moderate, necessitating that all eyes with NPDR be combined for statistical analysis purposes.

In summary, various algorithms and techniques have been developed and introduced for OCTA classification. Most of the previous techniques in the literature, however, have some limitations, such as: (1) Current discriminative methods suffer from insufficient features that can represent the OCTA problem, leading to lower accuracies. (2) Current generative methods suffer from the computationally expensive registration tasks. In addition, the built atlas may not represent well the image population. (3) Current deep learning methods suffer from the computationally expensive cost for training the CNN layers. In addition, the selection of the best number of layers and the best number of neurons per each layer is still an open research problem.

According to current surveys of DR works and the above literature survey, practically all examinations of retinal blood vessels are conducted using fundus imaging, a technique that lacks depth information. Furthermore, generality present DR-CAD systems begin with a threshold-based segmentation method, that may limit the diagnostic system's specificity and sensitivity due to the error of segmentation. Furthermore, most of the published studies concentrated on examining retinal layers in OCTA images without taking into consideration in the retinal vascular system changes. Finally, several present DR-CAD systems make decisions based on widely extracted features, that may not be sensitive enough to detect DR early on.

To address the aforementioned problems, we present a comprehensive DR-CAD system that relies its diagnosis on newly derived features from the retinal blood vessels' spatial structure and appearance. This improvement allows us to collect more imaging features of the retina, which improves classification accuracy and reduces noise. On the same cohort dataset, the overall framework was evaluated and compared to comparable studies.

3. The Proposed Classification Systems

A non-invasive, automated, early DR classification system from OCTA images is developed, and Figure 1 summarizes the proposed system's essential steps. The proposed pipeline is composed of four parallel analysis phases. Essentially, we propose a multi-scale framework at which the OCTA images are analyzed at different scales. DR affects the width of vessels, thus it is in our best interest to present this for the network, because it is a direct feature correlated to DR disease. The input to the system contains three sources of information from which a multi-layer input image is constructed as an input to the classification system: the original superficial OCTA images, the original greyscale image, a binary map of its segmented retinal vasculature (RV) network and a distance map of blood vessels. The purpose of the segmented RV and its distance map is to introduce some sort of network's attention as indicated by the reviewer to help improving the performance. Furthermore, we have used multi-scaled input (different input size) to help the network extract more local features from the greyscale channel. The retinal blood vessel structure is segmented using our previously developed segmentation approach [27].

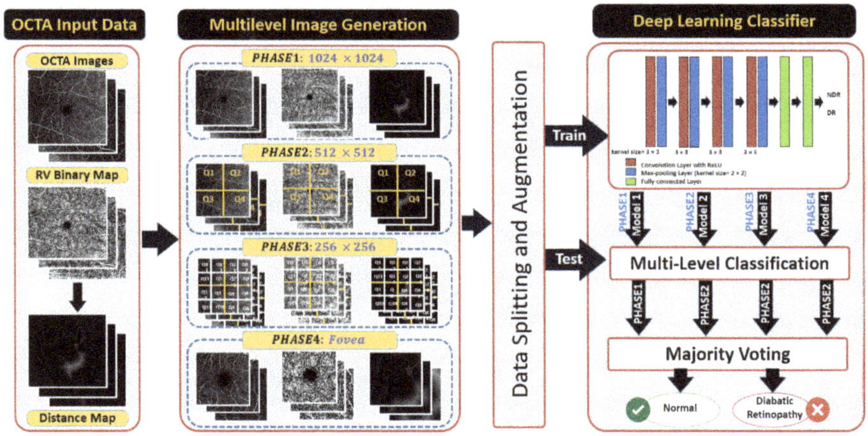

Figure 1. A schematic diagram of deep learning-based optical coherence tomography angiography pipeline.

From the combined images, multiscale inputs are constructed as inputs for different phases in the pipeline. Namely; the first phase provides a more global retinal features using full-sized images (i.e., 1024 × 1024) that is fed to a deep fully CNN. Smaller-sized images are used in the other phases for more local features extractions. Particularly, the full-sized OCTA image is split into equally-sized four quarters (i.e., 512 × 512 each) in the second phase, and into sixteen equally-sized parts (i.e., 256 × 256 each) in the third one. The last phase of our system is dedicated to extracting deep features around the fovea as a 512 × 512 window centered around the fovea is extracted and used to train and test another CNN. Individual CNN outputs are combined, and a soft voting method is utilized to combine the prediction scores of the individual networks for obtaining the final diagnosis.

3.1. RV Segmentation

The input to the CNN is a 3-channel image in which the second channel contains the binary map of the RV. As a result, for diabetic and normal instances, our pipeline first segments blood vessels in the deep and superficial compartments. Preprocessing, i.e. contrast enhancement and noise reduction, is first applied to the OCTA scans. This is achieved by using the RDHE algorithm [35] to ensure that the image's grey levels are regularly distributed by altering each pixel's intensity (grayscale) value based on the values of nearby pixels. After that, the generalized Gauss-Markov random field (GGMRF) model is used to reduce noise while preserving image detail [27]. Second, the vasculature was segmented from background using a combined Markov-Gibbs random field (MGRF) model. This combines a probabilistic "prior appearance" model of OCTA with spatial interaction (smoothness) and intensity distribution of different image segments. To overcome the poor contrast blood vessels and certain other retinal or choroidal tissue, the 1st-order intensity model, in addition to the higher order MGRF is employed to consider spatial information. Lastly, we enhanced the segmentation by applying a 2D connectivity filter to extract connected regions. Figure 2b,e shows two example RV Binary Map images with inadvertent contrast changes in various image regions.

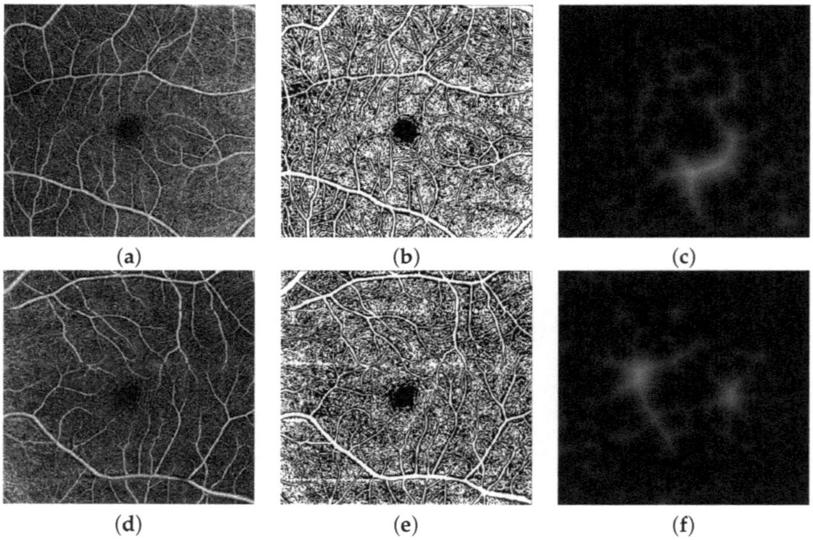

Figure 2. OCTA image example input data for DR and NDR: (**a**,**d**) the original superficial OCTA, (**b**,**e**) a binary map of the retinal vessels (RV), and (**c**,**f**) distance map of OCTA images.

In addition to the grayscale values and the RV binary maps, we also incorporate a distance-map-based image descriptor as the third channel of the input image to be analyzed. Namely, a signed distance map for the points of an object-background, or binary image, and is represented by the zero-level set , $B_t = \{\mathbf{p} : \mathbf{p} \in \mathbf{R}; \Phi(\mathbf{p}, t) = 0\}$, of higher-dimensional function, $\Phi(\mathbf{p}, t)$, on the lattice $\mathbf{R}$, as follows:

$$\Phi(\mathbf{p}, t) = \begin{cases} d(\mathbf{p}, B_t) & \text{if } \mathbf{p} \text{ in the interior of } B_t, \\ 0 & \text{if } \mathbf{p} \in B_t, \text{ and} \\ -d(\mathbf{p}, B_t) & \text{if } \mathbf{p} \text{ exterior to } B_t \end{cases}$$

where $d(\mathbf{p}, B_t) = \min_{\mathbf{b} \in B_t} \|\mathbf{p} - \mathbf{b}\|$ is the distance from the point $\mathbf{p}$ to the surface B_t, as shown in Figure 2c,f.

3.2. Multilevel Image Generation

The second stage of our proposed pipeline is generation of multi-scale images i.e., 512 × 512, and 256 × 256, shown in Figures 3 and 4. The main idea behind this is that with smaller size will (1) avoid the inclusion of redundant surrounding vessel pixels and (2) emphasis local features and thus enhance the CNN learning process. According to previous research, the foveal region and FAZ are affected by various retinal diseases [36]. Thus, the area around the fovea includes features that can discriminate between normal and diseased subjects. To benefit from this and provide more accurate diagnosis, a more focused image around the center of the original image that includes the fovea is extracted, cropped (zone with size 512 × 512), and used as another level for diagnosis. Figure 5 shows cropping of the fovea in a diabetic patient versus a healthy control.

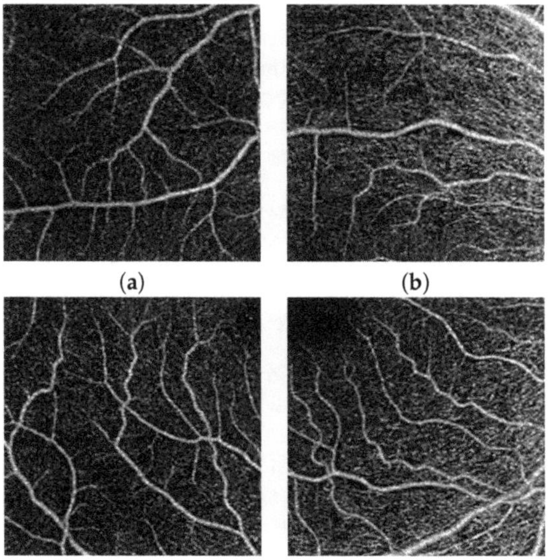

(a) (b) (c) (d)

Figure 3. The four parts of OCTA image with equal size (512 × 512): (**a**) upper left, (**b**) upper right, (**c**) lower left, and (**d**) lower right quarter.

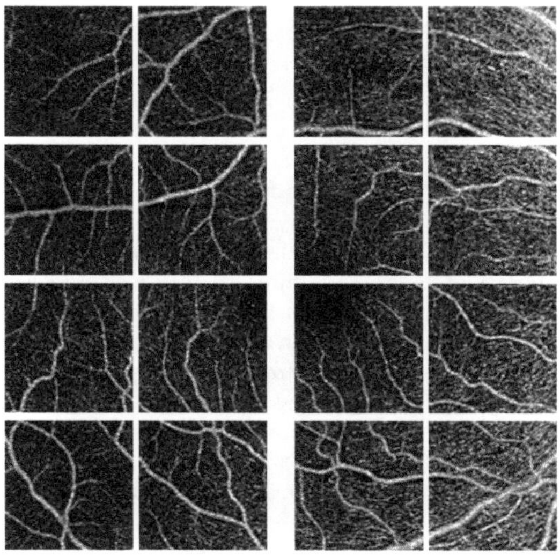

Figure 4. Normal OCTA image splitting for 16 equal size (256 × 256) sub-images.

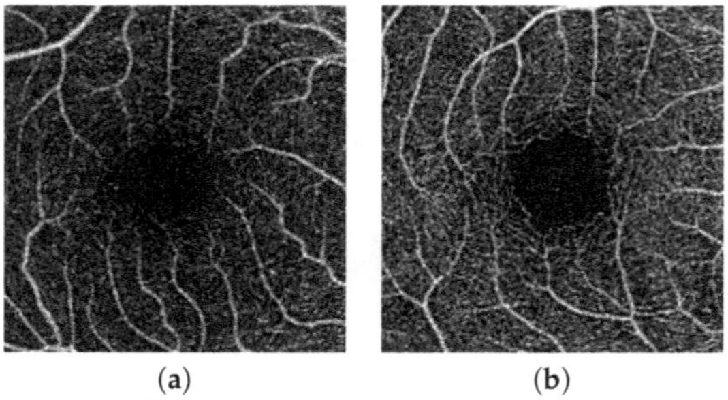

Figure 5. OCTA fovea zone with size (512 × 512); (**a**) DR, and (**b**) NDR.

3.3. *Deep Learning Classifier*

Our CNN architectures in Figure 6 were built using a succession of convolutional blocks, each of which had two convolutional layers followed by a max-pooling layer. Subsequent to these was a pair of fully connected layers and finally a soft-max output layer. The convolutional layers extract low-level feature maps comprising the trainable kernels' responses to the input objects. Because we employed a filter group, each convolutional layer created a large number of feature maps. Filters with a size of 33, a stride of 1, and rectified linear unit (ReLU) activation functions were used in our design. In max-pooling layers, the feature maps spatial dimensions were lowered by a factor of two. The most significant features were maintained in the max-pooling layers, while the less important ones were removed. Additionally, max-pooling layers lowered computational cost and training time. In max-pooling layers, we used a stride of 2. In total, each CNN had four max-pooling layers and eight convolutional layers. For the four-way classification, the two fully connected layers had twelve and four neurons, respectively. The soft-max output layer translates the fully connected layer's activation into class membership probabilities. The input patch is labeled with the class corresponding to the output neuron with the greatest probability. Our CNN model, with a total of 63,095,922 trainable parameters, is summarized in Table 1. Training used a 0.3 dropout rate and 0.001 learning rate. To find the optimal set of hyper-parameters, such as the number of layers, the nodes number in each layer (range: 10–100), L2 regularisation (range: 103–106), sparseness control parameters (range: 1–20), and the sparsity parameter (range: 0.05–0.9), grid search algorithm was used with the reconstruction error as the metric to optimise. The same principles can be applied to different patch sizes as well. Each CNN was trained by minimizing cross-entropy loss between ground truth labels and predicted class probabilities. The following is the definition of cross-entropy loss:

$$LBCE = -\sum_{i=0}^{2N_b-1} y_{o,i} \log P_{o,i} \tag{1}$$

where N is the number of classes, $y_{o,i}$ is a binary indicator (0 or 1) which indicates the correct classification that observation o belongs to class i. The probability that observation o belongs to class i is given by $P_{o,i}$. In the convolutional and fully connected layers, a drop out with a rate of 0.2 was utilized to avoid network overfitting.

The usage of these architectures has two significant advantages, as we have shown in this paper. First, fine-tuning the network's weights using the newly labeled images and pre-trained deep CNNs could result in enhanced performance metrics and a potential reduction in training resources such as memory, compute operations, and time. Second, even in a training from scratch scheme, the improved architecture and design of these CNNs may ensure greater performance ratios. For grading, we used a multi-level classification for classifying the inflammation of vitreous region into two classes (DR, NDR).

With the image's distribution, the entire data set was separated randomly into two groups: training set and testing set, in addition to using the validation set to keep track of training process epochs. Table 1 shows the number of epochs that outperformed the in terms of accuracy in DR and NDR classes with the validation set. After the selection of the hyper-parameters, the proposed system was trained and tested using 91 cases of 55 DR and 36 NDR using a five-fold cross validation. The data sets are divided into 80% for training and 20% for testing. Throughout all the multi-level experiments, the test sets were identical.

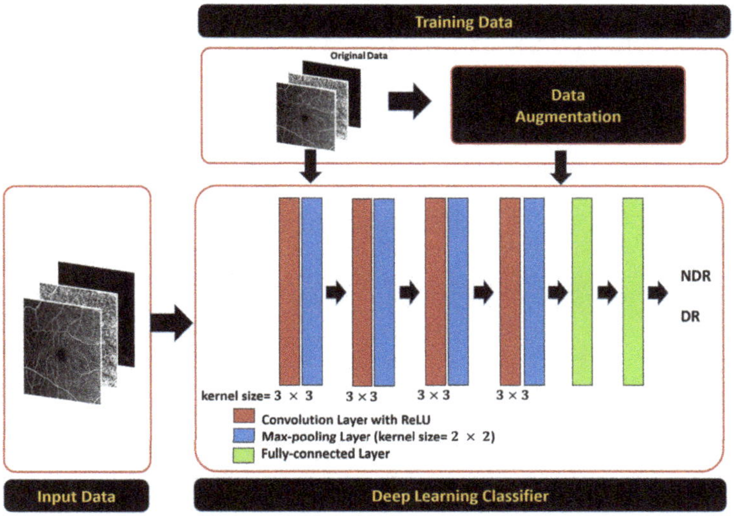

Figure 6. Schematic diagram of the proposed CNN with multi-input with size 1024 × 1024 that shows the design and the layers.

Table 1. Summary of our proposed system parameters setting for input size 1024 × 1024.

Layer	Depth	kernel	Stride	Spatial Size	Param.
Input	3	-	-	1024 × 1024 × 3	0
1. Conv	16	3 × 3	1 × 1	1022 × 1022 × 16	432
2. Max-pool	16	2 × 2	2 × 2	511 × 511 × 16	0
3. Conv	32	3 × 3	1 × 1	509 × 509 × 32	4608
4. Max-pool	32	2 × 2	2 × 2	254 × 254 × 32	0
5. Conv	64	3 × 3	1 × 1	252 × 252 × 64	18,432
6. Max-pool	64	2 × 2	2 × 2	126 × 126 × 9	0
7. Conv	128	3 × 3	1 × 1	124 × 124 × 128	73,728
8. Max-pool	128	2 × 2	2 × 2	62 × 62 × 128	0
9. Concat	1	-	-	492,032 × 1	0
10. Full	1	-	-	128 × 1	62,980,096
11. Full	1	-	-	128 × 1	16,384
12. Softmax	1	-	-	128 × 1	0
Batch Size	32				
Learning Rate	0.001				
Optimizer	Adam				
No. of Epochs	50				
Total Parameters	63,095,922				
Trainable Parameters	63,094,930				
Non-Trainable Parameters	992				

4. Experimental Results

The OCTA scans were collected using a ZEISS AngioPlex OCT angiography machine. The AngioPlex OCT produces five different blood vessel maps. The deep and superficial retinal maps with pixels size of 1024 × 1024 were used to test our proposed CAD system. The images were captured on sections of 512 × 512 and are centered on the fovea. Every image was classified as to DR severity by a board-certified ophthalmologist. We considered two categories, DR and normal or non-DR (NDR).

We used a data augmentation method by using systematically transformed images to augment the class size because of the limited number of data sets. The transformations employed often have to keep the original image's classification. Each image in the batch could be transformed by operations of random combination in DR and NDR groups in each iteration: (a) horizontal and vertical flips in the case of a random combination of flips and normal images, (b) random small rotations by 90, 180, and 270 degrees, which inherently augment the size of class. In all the network sizes, we used data augmentation during training. Experiments have been conducted utilizing an Intel Core i5-2400 machine running Windows 10 with 4 GB RAM, 160 GB HDD and a Python programming environment.

Many performance indicators were used to assess the system, such as sensitivity (Sens), accuracy (Acc), specificity (Spec), and F1-score. The number of images with DR that were correctly recognized are the number of true positives (TP), divided by the total of TP and false negatives (FP), or images wrongly classified as normal, is represent the sensitivity (recall, or true positive rate). As a result, the sensitivity indicates the percentage of correctly diagnosed DR cases by the system. On the other hand, the normal cases number that is correctly detected or the number of true negatives (TN) and false positives (FP), i.e., images mistakenly classified as DR, divided by the total number of TN and FP are represent the specificity. As a result, specificity is a proportion indicating the percentage of normal cases correctly diagnosed. Precision is the number of correctly predicted positive class values divided by the total number of positive predictions. Finally, the weighted average of recall and precision is the F1-Score. As a result, the F1-score takes into account both FP and FN. F1 is frequently more useful than accuracy, even though it is not as intuitive as accuracy, especially if the class distribution is unequal. When the cost of FP and FN are similar, accuracy works best. If the cost difference between FP and FN is significant, it is best to consider recall and precision [37,38].

The results of individual CNN and their fusion are summarized in Table 2. The overall accuracies of DR classification on our dataset for different levels, i.e., 1024 × 1024, 512 × 512, 256 × 256, Fovea (512 × 512), and overall fusion are 72.2%, 83.3%, 88.8%, 88.8% and 94.4%, respectively. The CNN system of fused multi-input outperforms all independent CNN systems in terms of diagnostic accuracy, as shown in Table 2. The results show that employing a smaller number of CNN layers can improve the accuracy of diagnostic, and that is a benefit of the proposed approach over previous CNN techniques. During model training (i.e., 1024 × 1024), Figure 7 shows loss curves and training vs accuracy of the validation. Overall, the results showed that the validation accuracy can achieve 100% with small loss after a few epochs, implying that multi-input CNNs can improve the CAD system's diagnostic accuracy.

Table 2. The ACC(%), Sen(%), Spec(%), and F1-score(%) for the proposed DR classifier with multiple size. ACC = accuracy, Sen = sensitivity, and Spec = specificity

Phases	Acc(%)	Sen(%)	Spec(%)	F1-Score(%)
1024 × 1024	72.2	75.0	66.6	78.3
512 × 512	83.3	83.3	83.3	86.9
256 × 256	88.8	90.9	85.7	90.9
Fovea (512 × 512)	88.8	84.6	100	91.6
Fusion	94.4	91.7	100	95.6

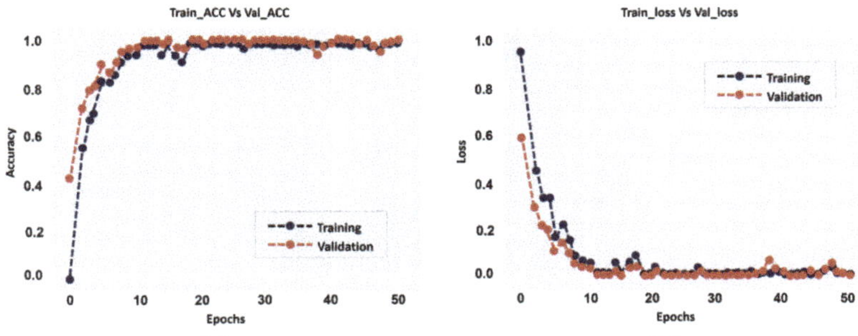

(a) (b)

Figure 7. Progression of training and validation set accuracy (**a**) and loss (**b**) during network training.

In addition to accuracy metrics, Figure 8 shows the confusion matrices of the classification results at different input levels. DR cases are easy to distinguish at all input image levels, even though most NDR images are correctly identified. Furthermore, the classification accuracy for NDR and DR is greater when using fovea images, which demonstrates the advantage of a wider visual degree of the retinal range. The original fovea images achieved an accuracy with 88.8% while the images with 1024, 512 and 256 achieved 72.2%, 83.3% and 88.8%, respectively. Since our dataset is not balanced with respect to class size, balanced accuracy is calculated as a weighted kappa. Further, Figure 9 visualises the proposed network attention maps using the visualization model proposed in [39]. The figure clearly shows the difference between the OCTA classes, i.e., DR and DR.

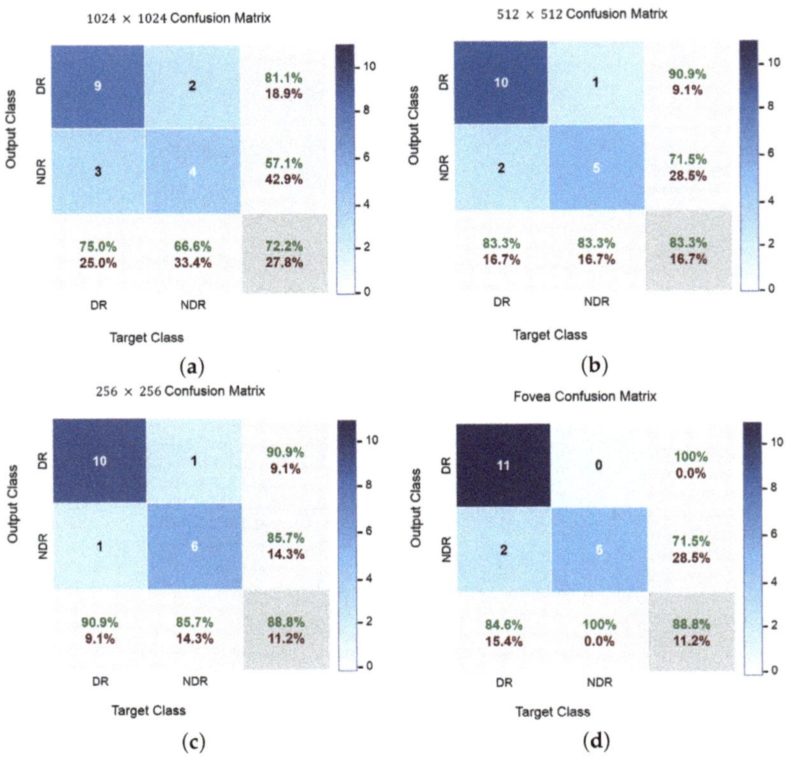

Figure 8. The grading details confusion matrix. The grades DR and NDR respectively correspond to the classes 1 and 2. (**a**) Phase 1: 1025 × 1024; (**b**) Phase 2: 512 × 512; (**c**) Phase 3: 256 × 256; and (**d**) Phase 4: Fovea. Please note that the green and dark-red colored-numbers represent the percentage of correctly and incorrectly classified instances, respectively.

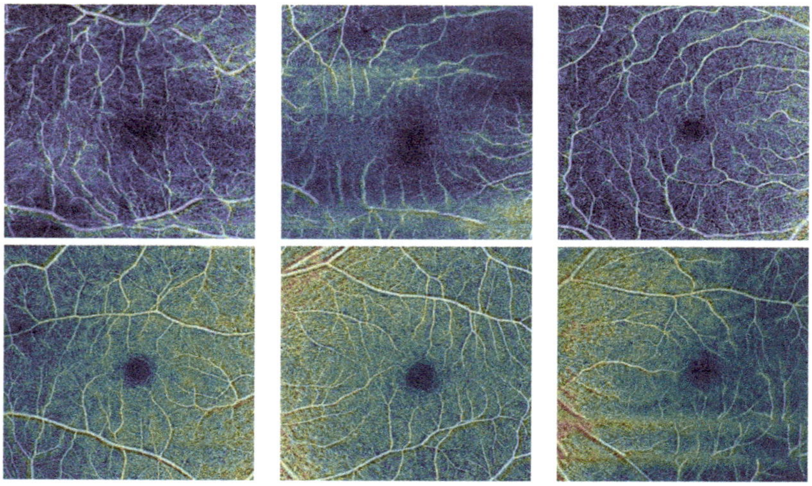

Figure 9. Network attention maps showing the difference between the DR and NDR cases, in the first and second row, respectively.

We also used the receiver operating characteristic (ROC) curve to assess the whole system's accuracy in comparison to the classification threshold setting. This step is necessary to ensure that the used classifier is reliable. The ROC curves for the utilized classifiers at various image levels, as well as their fusion, are shown in Figure 10. The area under a classifier's respective curve is commonly used to assess its quality (a.k.a. area under the curve or AUC). The classifier is better when AUC is closer to unity. As shown in Figure 10, the AUCs were 70.83%, 83.33%, 88.31%, 92.3%, and 95.83% for the 1024 × 1024, 512 × 512, 256 × 256, Fovea, and total fusion between all classifiers, respectively.

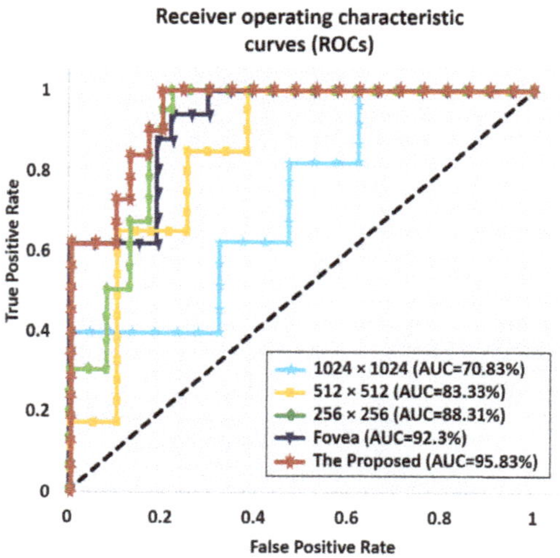

Figure 10. The ROC curves of the proposed CNN classifier for the model cross-validation in all image sizes.

To highlight the advantage of the multi-scale pipeline, comparisons with handcrafted-based ML models, in addition to comparisons with other state-of-the-art CNN approaches for diagnosis of DR have been performed. The results are summarized in in Table 3. As can be seen, our approach achieved an accuracy value of 94.4 compared to 72, 61, 81, 90, 93, 90, 90, 89, and 89 obtained with AlexNet, ResNet 18, random forest (RF), classification tree,

K-nearest neighborhood (KNN), support vector machine (SVM Linear), SVM (Polynomial), and SVM (RBF) respectively. In addition, it achieved a sensitivity of 91.7, a specificity of 100, and an AUC of 95.83.

Table 3. The proposed DR classification system comparative performance and other related works. Using the ACC (%), Sens (%), Spec (%), and AUC (%).

Tested Systems	ACC (%)	Sens (%)	Spec (%)	AUC (%)
AlexNet	72	80	62	71
ResNet 18	61	70	50	60
RF	81	83	78	87
Classification tree	90	96	78	87
KNN	93	94	91	93
SVM (Linear)	90	96	78	87
SVM (Polynomial)	90	89	91	90
SVM (RBF)	89	96	74	85
Proposed system	94.4	91.7	100	95.83

Furthermore, the other state-of-the-art CNN approaches, the methods introduced by Le et al. [28], Alam et al. [30], and Ong et al. [33], tested on their respective dataset, are used for comparison. The proposed CAD system has the best diagnostic performance, according to the comparative results. It is worth noting that, in comparison to the other models, our system has a comparatively low number of layers. It achieved a 94.4(%) overall accuracy, compared with 87.27, 86.75, and 75.2, as shown in Table 4.

Table 4. Comparisons with the previous works for DR diagnosis.

Study	Data Set Size	Validation (Train:Test)	Technique	ACC
Le et al. [28]	131	(80%:20%)	VGG16	87.27%
Alam et al. [30]	50	(80%:20%)	AV-Net	86.75%
Ong et al. [33]	117	-	DCP VLD-based	75.2%
Proposed model	91	(80%:20%)	Shallow CNN	94.4%

5. Conclusions and Suggested Future Work

We proposed a novel CAD algorithm to differentiate between DR and NDR. A framework that can detect DR from OCTA based on capturing the appearance and morphological markers of the retinal vascular system. The proposed system's main contributions are the use of a CNN multi-input that can recognize texture patterns from each input separately. Our CNN model captures significant features to increase its ability to distinguish DR from the normal retina. The proposed approach was tested on in vivo data using 91 patients, which were qualitatively graded by retinal experts. We compared our system's classification accuracy to that of other deep learning and machine learning methodologies. Our system's results outperform those produced by competing algorithms. The ultimate goal of our research is to integrate a variety of data types (e.g., OCTA, OCTA, FA, and Funds images), demographic data and standard clinical markers, in order to build a more comprehensive diagnostic system that automates DR grading and diagnosis.

Author Contributions: I.Y., F.K., M.G., H.S.S. and A.E.-B.: conceptualization and formal analysis. I.Y., F.K., H.A. and A.E.-B.: methodology. I.Y. and H.A.: Software development. I.Y., F.K., H.A. and A.E.-B. validation and visualization. I.Y. and F.K.: Initial draft. M.G., H.S.S. and A.E.-B.: Resources, data collection, and data curation. I.Y., F.K., H.A., M.G., H.S.S. and A.E.-B.: review and editing. H.S.S. and A.E.-B.: Project Administration. H.S.S. and A.E.-B.: Project Directors. All authors have read and agreed to the published version of the manuscript.

Funding: This work is supported, in part, by ASPIRE Award for Research Excellence 2019 under the Advanced Technology Research Council—ASPIRE.

Institutional Review Board Statement: The study was conducted according to the guidelines of the Declaration of Helsinki, and approved by the Institutional Review Board of the University of Louisville (IRB #18.0010).

Informed Consent Statement: Informed consent was obtained from all subjects involved in the study.

Data Availability Statement: Data could be made available upon a reasonable request to the corresponding author.

Conflicts of Interest: The authors declare no conflict of interest.

References

1. Wang, W.; Lo, A.C. Diabetic retinopathy: Pathophysiology and treatments. *Int. J. Mol. Sci.* **2018**, *19*, 1816. [CrossRef] [PubMed]
2. Romero-Aroca, P.; Baget-Bernaldiz, M.; Pareja-Rios, A.; Lopez-Galvez, M.; Navarro-Gil, R.; Verges, R. Diabetic macular edema pathophysiology: Vasogenic versus inflammatory. *J. Diabetes Res.* **2016**, *2016*. [CrossRef]
3. Brownlee, M. The pathobiology of diabetic complications: A unifying mechanism. *Diabetes* **2005**, *54*, 1615–1625. [CrossRef] [PubMed]
4. Bek, T. Diameter changes of retinal vessels in diabetic retinopathy. *Curr. Diabetes Rep.* **2017**, *17*, 1–7. [CrossRef] [PubMed]
5. Stewart, M.W. Pathophysiology of diabetic retinopathy. *Diabet. Retin.* **2010**, *2013*, 343560.
6. Kern, T.S.; Antonetti, D.A.; Smith, L.E. Pathophysiology of diabetic retinopathy: Contribution and limitations of laboratory research. *Ophthalmic Res.* **2019**, *62*, 196–202. [CrossRef]
7. Wong, T.Y.; Sun, J.; Kawasaki, R.; Ruamviboonsuk, P.; Gupta, N.; Lansingh, V.C.; Maia, M.; Mathenge, W.; Moreker, S.; Muqit, M.M.; et al. Guidelines on diabetic eye care: The international council of ophthalmology recommendations for screening, follow-up, referral, and treatment based on resource settings. *Ophthalmology* **2018**, *125*, 1608–1622. [CrossRef]
8. Windisch, R.; Windisch, B.K.; Cruess, A.F. Use of fluorescein and indocyanine green angiography in polypoidal choroidal vasculopathy patients following photodynamic therapy. *Can. J. Ophthalmol.* **2008**, *43*, 678–682. [CrossRef]
9. Teussink, M.M.; Breukink, M.B.; van Grinsven, M.J.; Hoyng, C.B.; Klevering, B.J.; Boon, C.J.; de Jong, E.K.; Theelen, T. OCT angiography compared to fluorescein and indocyanine green angiography in chronic central serous chorioretinopathy. *Investig. Ophthalmol. Vis. Sci.* **2015**, *56*, 5229–5237. [CrossRef] [PubMed]
10. De Carlo, T.E.; Romano, A.; Waheed, N.K.; Duker, J.S. A review of optical coherence tomography angiography (OCTA). *Int. J. Retin. Vitr.* **2015**, *1*, 5. [CrossRef]
11. Tey, K.Y.; Teo, K.; Tan, A.C.; Devarajan, K.; Tan, B.; Tan, J.; Schmetterer, L.; Ang, M. Optical coherence tomography angiography in diabetic retinopathy: A review of current applications. *Eye Vis.* **2019**, *6*, 1–10. [CrossRef] [PubMed]
12. Witmer, M.T.; Parlitsis, G.; Patel, S.; Kiss, S. Comparison of ultra-widefield fluorescein angiography with the Heidelberg Spectralis® noncontact ultra-widefield module versus the Optos® Optomap®. *Clin. Ophthalmol.* **2013**, *7*, 389. [CrossRef]
13. Abdelsalam, M.M. Effective blood vessels reconstruction methodology for early detection and classification of diabetic retinopathy using OCTA images by artificial neural network. *Inform. Med. Unlocked* **2020**, *20*, 100390. [CrossRef]
14. Spaide, R.F.; Klancnik, J.M.; Cooney, M.J. Retinal vascular layers imaged by fluorescein angiography and optical coherence tomography angiography. *JAMA Ophthalmol.* **2015**, *133*, 45–50. [CrossRef] [PubMed]
15. Wang, Z.; Keane, P.A.; Chiang, M.; Cheung, C.Y.; Wong, T.Y.; Ting, D.S.W. Artificial intelligence and deep learning in ophthalmology. *Artif. Intell. Med.* **2020**, *20*, 3469–3473._200-1. [CrossRef]
16. LeCun, Y.; Bengio, Y.; Hinton, G. Deep learning. *Nature* **2015**, *521*, 436–444. [CrossRef]
17. Sheikh, H.R.; Sabir, M.F.; Bovik, A.C. A statistical evaluation of recent full reference image quality assessment algorithms. *IEEE Trans. Image Process.* **2006**, *15*, 3440–3451. [CrossRef]
18. Lakhani, P.; Sundaram, B. Deep learning at chest radiography: Automated classification of pulmonary tuberculosis by using convolutional neural networks. *Radiology* **2017**, *284*, 574–582. [CrossRef]
19. Ran, A.R.; Cheung, C.Y.; Wang, X.; Chen, H.; Luo, L.Y.; Chan, P.P.; Wong, M.O.; Chang, R.T.; Mannil, S.S.; Young, A.L.; et al. Detection of glaucomatous optic neuropathy with spectral-domain optical coherence tomography: A retrospective training and validation deep-learning analysis. *Lancet Digit. Health* **2019**, *1*, e172–e182. [CrossRef]
20. Balyen, L.; Peto, T. Promising artificial intelligence-machine learning-deep learning algorithms in ophthalmology. *Asia-Pac. J. Ophthalmol.* **2019**, *8*, 264–272.
21. Ting, D.S.W.; Cheung, C.Y.L.; Lim, G.; Tan, G.S.W.; Quang, N.D.; Gan, A.; Hamzah, H.; Garcia-Franco, R.; San Yeo, I.Y.; Lee, S.Y.; et al. Development and validation of a deep learning system for diabetic retinopathy and related eye diseases using retinal images from multiethnic populations with diabetes. *JAMA* **2017**, *318*, 2211–2223. [CrossRef] [PubMed]
22. Keenan, T.D.; Dharssi, S.; Peng, Y.; Chen, Q.; Agrón, E.; Wong, W.T.; Lu, Z.; Chew, E.Y. A deep learning approach for automated detection of geographic atrophy from color fundus photographs. *Ophthalmology* **2019**, *126*, 1533–1540. [CrossRef] [PubMed]

23. Milea, D.; Najjar, R.P.; Jiang, Z.; Ting, D.; Vasseneix, C.; Xu, X.; Aghsaei Fard, M.; Fonseca, P.; Vanikieti, K.; Lagrèze, W.A.; et al. Artificial intelligence to detect papilledema from ocular fundus photographs. *N. Engl. J. Med.* **2020**, *382*, 1687–1695. [CrossRef] [PubMed]
24. Owais, M.; Arsalan, M.; Choi, J.; Park, K.R. Effective diagnosis and treatment through content-based medical image retrieval (CBMIR) by using artificial intelligence. *J. Clin. Med.* **2019**, *8*, 462. [CrossRef]
25. Shen, C.; Yan, S.; Du, M.; Zhao, H.; Shao, L.; Hu, Y. Assessment of capillary dropout in the superficial retinal capillary plexus by optical coherence tomography angiography in the early stage of diabetic retinopathy. *BMC Ophthalmol.* **2018**, *18*, 1–6. [CrossRef]
26. Heisler, M.; Karst, S.; Lo, J.; Mammo, Z.; Yu, T.; Warner, S.; Maberley, D.; Beg, M.F.; Navajas, E.V.; Sarunic, M.V. Ensemble deep learning for diabetic retinopathy detection using optical coherence tomography angiography. *Transl. Vis. Sci. Technol.* **2020**, *9*, 20. [CrossRef]
27. Eladawi, N.; Elmogy, M.; Helmy, O.; Aboelfetouh, A.; Riad, A.; Sandhu, H.; Schaal, S.; El-Baz, A. Automatic blood vessels segmentation based on different retinal maps from OCTA scans. *Comput. Biol. Med.* **2017**, *89*, 150–161. [CrossRef]
28. Le, D.; Alam, M.; Yao, C.K.; Lim, J.I.; Hsieh, Y.T.; Chan, R.V.; Toslak, D.; Yao, X. Transfer learning for automated OCTA detection of diabetic retinopathy. *Transl. Vis. Sci. Technol.* **2020**, *9*, 35. [CrossRef]
29. Nagasato, D.; Tabuchi, H.; Masumoto, H.; Enno, H.; Ishitobi, N.; Kameoka, M.; Niki, M.; Mitamura, Y. Automated detection of a nonperfusion area caused by retinal vein occlusion in optical coherence tomography angiography images using deep learning. *PLoS ONE* **2019**, *14*, e0223965. [CrossRef]
30. Alam, M.; Le, D.; Son, T.; Lim, J.I.; Yao, X. AV-Net: Deep learning for fully automated artery-vein classification in optical coherence tomography angiography. *Biomed. Opt. Express* **2020**, *11*, 5249–5257. [CrossRef]
31. Díaz, M.; Novo, J.; Cutrín, P.; Gómez-Ulla, F.; Penedo, M.G.; Ortega, M. Automatic segmentation of the foveal avascular zone in ophthalmological OCT-A images. *PLoS ONE* **2019**, *14*, e0212364. [CrossRef]
32. Kim, K.; You, J.I.; Park, J.R.; Kim, E.S.; Oh, W.Y.; Yu, S.Y. Quantification of retinal microvascular parameters by severity of diabetic retinopathy using wide-field swept-source optical coherence tomography angiography. *Graefe's Arch. Clin. Exp. Ophthalmol.* **2021**, *259*, 2103–2111. [CrossRef]
33. Ong, J.X.; Kwan, C.C.; Cicinelli, M.V.; Fawzi, A.A. Superficial capillary perfusion on optical coherence tomography angiography differentiates moderate and severe nonproliferative diabetic retinopathy. *PLoS ONE* **2020**, *15*, e0240064.
34. Alibhai, A.Y.; De Pretto, L.R.; Moult, E.M.; Or, C.; Arya, M.; McGowan, M.; Carrasco-Zevallos, O.; Lee, B.; Chen, S.; Baumal, C.R.; et al. Quantification of retinal capillary nonperfusion in diabetics using wide-field optical coherence tomography angiography. *Retina* **2020**, *40*, 412–420. [CrossRef] [PubMed]
35. Iwanami, T.; Goto, T.; Hirano, S.; Sakurai, M. An adaptive contrast enhancement using regional dynamic histogram equalization. In Proceedings of the 2012 IEEE International Conference on Consumer Electronics (ICCE), Las Vegas, NV, USA, 12–15 January 2012; pp. 719–722.
36. Kim, D.Y.; Fingler, J.; Zawadzki, R.J.; Park, S.S.; Morse, L.S.; Schwartz, D.M.; Fraser, S.E.; Werner, J.S. Noninvasive imaging of the foveal avascular zone with high-speed, phase-variance optical coherence tomography. *Investig. Ophthalmol. Vis. Sci.* **2012**, *53*, 85–92. [CrossRef] [PubMed]
37. Joshi, R. Accuracy, precision, recall & f1 score: Interpretation of performance measures. *Retr. April* **2016**, *1*, 2016.
38. Das, H.; Pattnaik, P.K.; Rautaray, S.S.; Li, K.C. *Progress in Computing, Analytics and Networking: Proceedings of ICCAN 2019*; Springer: Berlin/Heidelberg, Germany, 2020; Volume 1119.
39. Selvaraju, R.R.; Cogswell, M.; Das, A.; Vedantam, R.; Parikh, D.; Batra, D. Grad-cam: Visual explanations from deep networks via gradient-based localization. In Proceedings of the IEEE International Conference on Computer Vision, Venice, Italy, 22–29 October 2017; pp. 618–626.

sensors

Article

Brain MRI Analysis for Alzheimer's Disease Diagnosis Using CNN-Based Feature Extraction and Machine Learning

Duaa AlSaeed * and Samar Fouad Omar

College of Computer and Information Sciences, King Saud University, Riyadh 11451, Saudi Arabia; samar.fouad.omar@gmail.com
* Correspondence: dalsaeed@ksu.edu.sa

Abstract: Alzheimer's disease is the most common form of dementia and the fifth-leading cause of death among people over the age of 65. In addition, based on official records, cases of death from Alzheimer's disease have increased significantly. Hence, early diagnosis of Alzheimer's disease can increase patients' survival rates. Machine learning methods on magnetic resonance imaging have been used in the diagnosis of Alzheimer's disease to accelerate the diagnosis process and assist physicians. However, in conventional machine learning techniques, using handcrafted feature extraction methods on MRI images is complicated, requiring the involvement of an expert user. Therefore, implementing deep learning as an automatic feature extraction method could minimize the need for feature extraction and automate the process. In this study, we propose a pre-trained CNN deep learning model ResNet50 as an automatic feature extraction method for diagnosing Alzheimer's disease using MRI images. Then, the performance of a CNN with conventional Softmax, SVM, and RF evaluated using different metric measures such as accuracy. The result showed that our model outperformed other state-of-the-art models by achieving the higher accuracy, with an accuracy range of 85.7% to 99% for models with MRI ADNI dataset.

Keywords: Alzheimer's disease; deep learning; convolutional neural network (CNN); MRI; brain imaging

Citation: AlSaeed, D.; Omar, S.F. Brain MRI Analysis for Alzheimer's Disease Diagnosis Using CNN-Based Feature Extraction and Machine Learning. *Sensors* **2022**, *22*, 2911. https://doi.org/10.3390/s22082911

Academic Editors: Guruprasad A. Giridharan, Ali H. Mahmoud, Ahmed Shalaby, Ayman El-baz and Mohammed Ghazal

Received: 6 February 2022
Accepted: 1 April 2022
Published: 11 April 2022

1. Introduction

The brain is one of the most significant and complex organs in the human body. It has several vital functions, such as idea formation, problem-solving, thinking, decision-making, imagination, and memory. Memory can save and retrieve information or experiences. Our physical memory stores the whole record of our lives and plays an essential role in defining our character and identity. Memory loss caused by dementia and the inability to recognize our environment are terrifying experiences. Alzheimer's disease (AD) is the most common form of dementia. Becoming older increases people's fears of developing Alzheimer's. Alzheimer's disease gradually kills brain cells and, as a result of that, patients end up disconnecting from everything around them and losing loving memories, childhood memories, the ability to recognize their family members, and even the ability to follow simple instructions. They also lose the ability to swallow, cough, and breathe in advanced stages. Approximately 50 million people worldwide are affected by dementia, and the cost of providing health and social care for them is equivalent to the world's 18th largest economy [1]. In addition, the annual number of new cases of AD and other dementias is projected to triple by 2050, reaching 152 million cases, which means one new case of dementia every 3 seconds. Diagnosis of AD is complicated by its overlapping symptoms with normal ageing or vascular dementia (VD) [2,3]. Early and accurate diagnosis of AD plays an essential role in prevention, treatment, and patient care through tracking its development. The focus of several research projects is to detect Alzheimer's disease using brain imaging, including MRI. It can measure the size and number of cells in the brain. Also, it can show the parietal atrophy for AD cases [4].

Images play an essential role in many scientific fields. In addition, medical imaging has become a powerful tool to understand brain functions. Brain imaging/neuroimaging, such as magnetic resonance imaging (MRI), has been used in the medical diagnosis of brain conditions to enable visualization of the structure and functionality of the brain. Physicians evaluate AD signs and symptoms, as well as perform several tests to diagnose AD dementia. Doctors may order additional laboratory tests, brain imaging tests, or memory testing for patients. These tests can help doctors make diagnoses by ruling out other conditions that cause similar symptoms. MRI can detect brain abnormalities associated with mild cognitive impairment (MCI) and can be used to predict which MCI patients will develop AD in the future. They will be looking in MRI images for any abnormalities, such as a decrease in the size of different areas of the brain (mainly affecting the temporal and parietal lobes).

With the evolution of technology and the growth of data generated by brain-imaging techniques, machine learning (ML) and deep learning (DL) are becoming increasingly crucial for extracting accurate and relevant information and making accurate predictions of AD from brain-imaging data.

Several machine-learning methods have been applied for the classification of AD, and the results of the models show good performance. In general, the conventional learning-based methods consist of three stages: 1—the predetermination of the regions of interest (ROIs) of the brain, 2—features selection from the ROIs, and 3—the classification models are built and evaluated. The main issue with conventional learning-based methods is the process of features engineering (i.e., manual selection and extraction), which has a great influence on the performance of the model. Compared with traditional ML methods, DL has become a revolutionizing methodology in recent decades [5]. Instead of extracting the features manually and in a separate process from the classifier, DL has automated the process without the engagement of human experts for feature extraction because it can learn directly from images through the neural networks. Recently, convolutional neural networks (CNNs) have achieved very high accuracy and precision on image classifications [5].

Based on the excellent performance of DL and convolutional neural network methods in various image classification tasks, this paper aims at evaluating CNN-based MRI feature extraction for the automatic classification of Alzheimer's diseases. CNN-based models are developed as a DL method to diagnose Alzheimer's diseases on MRI images with three different classifiers (Softmax, SVM, and RF) and the model's performance was compared between fully connected layers. The research objectives are to answer the following research questions. (1) Is the pre-train DL CNN approach ResNet50 used in this study useful for the classification of Alzheimer's diseases in MRI brain images? (2) Which classifier used with pre-trained CNN will give us better classification performance: Softmax, SVM, or RF?

The rest of this paper is organized as follows: Section 2 reviews the previous studies of AD diagnosis and classification, Section 3 presents the methodology, describing how to build and evaluate the proposed CNN model, Section 4 provides the experimental and evaluation results, and, finally, Section 5 concludes the paper and discusses future work.

2. Related Work

Several studies have proposed AD diagnosis and detection systems that utilize a variety of classification techniques. This section contains a review of recent studies that used conventional ML and DL approaches in AD diagnosis and detection systems.

Some of the previous studies on Alzheimer's disease diagnosis have applied conventional machine-learning techniques. They are focused on developing models to analyze the anatomical or structural brain images such as MRI and brain functionality to detect any defect or disorders. In addition, it considered segmentation tasks as classification issues and heavily depended on manually designed features and feature representations as to the voxel, region, or patch-based methods. It required several expert segmented images to train classification models, and that takes a longer time.

Liu et al. (2016) [6] proposed an inherent structure-based multiview learning (ISML) method for AD/MCI classification. The proposed method consists of three stages: (1) multiview feature extraction using multiple templates and using gray matter (GM) tissues as tissue-segmented brain image for feature extraction, (2) subclass clustering-based feature selection through using voxel selection that improving the power of features, and (3) using SVM-based ensemble classification. They evaluated the efficiency of the proposed method on the MRI baseline dataset consisting of 549 subjects (70 AD and 30 Normal Control—NC) provided by the ADNI (http://adni.loni.usc.edu/, accessed on 5 February 2022) database [7]. The experiment result shows that the proposed ISML method obtains an accuracy of 93.83% and specificity of 95.69%, and sensitivity of 92.78% for AD vs. NC.

In another study, Krashenyi et al. (2016) [8] proposed an AD classification approach based on fuzzy logic. Their classification technique is based on multimodal data PET and MRI data. The dataset consists of 70 AD, 111 MCI, and 68 NC subjects provided by the ADNI database. The proposed approach consists of three stages: (1) image pre-processing, including MRI/PET normalization and MRI data segmented into white matter (WM) and grey matter (GM), then they used a voxel selection procedure to reduce low-activated voxels; (2) feature selection is based on ROI, and then they apply t-test as statistical tests for feature ranking and selection to reduce the number of ROI; and (3) do a fuzzy classification using the c-means algorithm. The classification performance of the proposed approach has been used under the receiver operating characteristic (AUC), while the regions with the highest AUC area should be defined in the PET and MRI images as the optimal number of regions. The highest classification performance achieved with a combination of features (7 MRI and 35 PET) is AUC = 94.01%. The experiment result shows that the proposed approach obtains 89.59% accuracy, 92.2% specificity, and 93.27% sensitivity for AD vs. NC.

Lazli et al. (2018) [9] proposed an AD computer-aided diagnosis (CAD) system to distinguish between AD cases and normal control cases and evaluate the tissue volume of MRI and PET images. The proposed approach consists of two processes: segmentation and classification. First, they used fuzzy possibilistic tissue segmentation as a hybrid of the fuzzy c-means (FCM) and a possibilistic c-means (PCM) segmentation processes. Then in the classification process, they used SVM classifiers with different types of kernels (linear, polynomial, and RBF) to decide the final diagnosis (AD or NC). The proposed approach was tested on MRI and PET images that consisted of 45 AD subjects and 50 healthy subjects provided by the ADNI database. The classification performance of the proposed approach has been evaluated with the leave-one-out cross-validation method. The experiment showed that the proposed solution obtains better accuracy, sensitivity, and specificity compared to the other three approaches, FCM, PCM, and VAF [10] (Voxels-As-Features), and achieved a higher accuracy rate of 75% for MRI and 73% for PET images.

The similar work by Thulasi N P and Varghese (2018) [11] proposed a diagnosis system of Alzheimer's disease based on image processing techniques and SVM classifiers. The proposed approach was trained and tested on a small MRI scanning dataset consisting of 100 subjects (70 AD and 30 NC) provided by the ADNI database. The proposed solution consisted of two phases: feature extraction/selection and classification. In the first phase, the authors used speeded-up robust features (SURF) to extract the key points of the corresponding MRI images, then the gray level co-occurrence matrix (GLCM) was used for feature extraction. In the classification phase, they used the support vector machines (SVM) to classify MRI images to AD or normal controls.

Recently, many improvements have been observed in the research field of AD diagnoses/classification using DL techniques. In opposition to conventional ML methods, DL methods are able to extract/select special features automatically from a raw dataset with higher performance results achieved. Liu et al. (2015) [12] studied Alzheimer's disease classification using multi-modality data MRI and PET scans from the ADNI dataset. They proposed a novel diagnostic framework to aid AD diagnosis by using DL architecture. To extract complementary information from multimodal neuroimaging data (MRI and PET), their framework uses a stacked auto-encoder SAE and a zero-mask strategy for data fusion. It also uses a Softmax logistic regressor as a classifier. The results show that based on MRI and PET ADNI, this framework outperformed with 91.4% accuracy. However, when PET data is not available and MRI is the only input, this percentage reduces to 82.6%.

Korolev et al. (2017) [13] apply two different 3D CNN approaches (3D-VGGNet and 3D-ResNet) with Softmax nonlinearity for classification. They use the ADNI dataset of 3D structural MRI brain scans. The result shows that the accuracy of AD/CN classification reaches 79% for Voxnet and 80% for ResNet. In addition, their algorithms are simpler to implement and do not need the manual extraction step.

In recent evidence, Gunawardena et al. (2017) [14] proposed a simple, convolutional neural network for AD pre-detection. Their study consists of two experiments that use MRI scans provided by ADNI. First, they use the SVM classifier as the most common detection method. This decision is based on their assumption that a successful AD detection method can be successfully applied to AD pre-detection. The SVM classifier obtains 84.41% accuracy, 95.3% sensitivity, and 71.4% specificity in the first experiment. For the second experiment, they utilized the proposed CNN model. They tested the CNN model with different datasets and different image segmentation methods through the six evaluation processes. The best image segmentation method was extended ROI without detecting edges, which obtained the best and highest accuracy rate (96%), with 96% sensitivity and 98% specificity.

Lan Lin et al. (2018) [15] proposed a new classification method that automatically differentiates patients with AD from HC based on MRI data. The feature was extracted from the pre-trained convolutional neural network (CNN) using AlexNet, as well as feature selection based on principal component analysis (PCA) and sequential feature selection (SFS). While they adopt a support vector machine (SVM) to evaluate the classification accuracy, the results show that a high classification accuracy for AD/CN classification reaches 90%.

Another related work is found in the study elaborated by Bäckström et al. (2018) [16]. Their work was focused on proposing a novel and effective three-dimensional convolutional network (3D ConvNet) architecture to achieve high performance for the detection of AD. The proposed 3D ConvNet consisted of five convolutional layers for feature extraction, followed by three fully connected layers for AD/NC classification. In addition, the study focused on the impact of the following factors on the performance of AD classification: hyper-parameter selection, pre-processing, data partitioning, and dataset size. They obtained a dataset from ADNI consisting of 430 subjects (199 AD and 141 NC). MRI scans were randomly partitioned into three subsets, with 60% in the training set, 20% in the validation set, and 20% in the test set. The results showed that the proposed method achieved a 98.74% accuracy rate for detecting AD vs. CN.

On the other hand, Huanhuan et al. (2019) [5] proposed an ensemble learning method for the early diagnosis of AD by using convolutional neural networks (ConvNets) as a DL technique based on MRI scans. They obtained a dataset consisting of 615 MRI images that were split into 179 AD, 254 MCI, and 182 NC in NifTI format from ADNI. They resized the MRI images to 224×224 and grouped them into WM and GM. Only 20 slices were selected as the data from GM and WM and sent to the DL model ConvNet for training. To enhance the classification process, the researchers used ensemble learning methods after the convolutional operations. They selected ResNet50, NASNet, and MobileNet as the combined base classifiers for the early diagnosis of AD. The results show that the proposed method obtained accuracy rates of 98.59 % for AD vs. NC, 97.65% for AD vs. MCI, and 88.37% for MCI vs. NC.

The study by Rallabandi et al. (2020) [17] proposed a model for early diagnosis and classification of AD and MCI from elderly cognitive normal, as well as the prediction and diagnosis of early and late MCI individuals. The dataset consists of 1167 whole-brain magnetic resonance imaging subjects, 371 NC, 328 early MCI, 169 late MCI, and 284 AD, provided by the ADNI database. They used FreeSurfer analysis for each individual scan to extract 68 features of the cortical thickness and utilized these features for building the model. They further tested scans using various machine learning methods (non-linear SVM (RBF kernel), naive Bayesian, K-nearest neighborhood, random forest, decision tree, and linear SVM). The non-linear SVM classifier with radial basis function showed the highest specificity, sensitivity, F-score, Matthew's correlation coefficient, and kappa-statistic, receiver operating characteristic area under the curve (ROC AUC), as well as 75% accuracy in classifying all four groups using 10-fold cross-validation.

Table 1 below summarizes the reviewed studies and shows a comparison between them based on (1) dataset (dataset name, image modality, and size of the dataset that was used), (2) methodology (feature selection and classifier), and (3) performance evaluation results.

Table 1. Summary and comparison of the selected recent research.

References	Dataset			Methodology		Evaluation Result
	Name	Modality	Size	Feature Selection	Classifier	
Liu et al. (2016) [6]	ADNI	MRI	549 subjects 70 AD 30 NC	Multiview learning using GM	SVM	AD vs. NC. Accuracy: 93.83% specificity: 95.69% sensitivity: 92.78%
Krashenyi et al. (2016) [8]	ADNI	MRI PET	249 subjects 70 AD 111 MCI 68 NC	ROI + statistical tests (t test)	fuzzy logic using: c-means algorithm	AD vs. NC Accuracy: 89.59% specificity: 92.2% sensitivity: 93.27% AUC= 94.01%.
Lazli et al. (2018) [9]	ADNI	MRI PET	95 subjects 45 AD 50 NC	Fuzzy-Possibilistic Tissue Segmentation	SVM (Linear, Polynomial, and RBF)	AD vs. NC Accuracy: 75% (for MRI), 73% (for PET)
Thulasi N P and Varghese (2018) [11]	ADNI	MRI	100 subjects 70 AD 30 NC	Speeded Up Robust Features (SURF) Gray Level Co-Occurrence Matrix (GLCM)	SVM	-
Liu et al. (2015) [12]	ADNI	MRI PET	758 MRIsubjects 180 AD 160 cMCI 214 ncMCI 204 NC 331 subject Both MR & PET data 85 AD 67 cMCI 102 ncMCI 77 NC	stacked auto-encoder SAE	Softmax logistic regressor	AD vs. NC Accuracy: 91.40% specificity: 90.42% sensitivity: 92.32% MCI vs. NC. Accuracy: 82.10% specificity: 92.32% sensitivity: 60.00%
Korolev et al. (2017) [13]	ADNI	MRI	231 Subjects 50 AD 43 LMCI 77 EMCI 61 NC	3D CNN (VoxCNN & ResNet)	Softmax	AD vs. NC Accuracy: 79% VoxCNN 80% ResNet AUC: 88% VoxCNN 87% ResNet
Gunawardena et al. (2017) [14]	ADNI	MRI	D1: 36 subjects (AD 7, MCI 14, NC 15) > 1615 2D images generated D2: 36 subjects (AD 9, MCI 16, NC 11) > 1743 2D images generated from 3D	CNN	SVM	The best classification accuracy (96%) with (Extended ROI without detecting edges) among the other segmentation methods
Lan Lin et al. (2018) [15]	ADNI	MRI	422 subjects 105 AD 123 MCI 194 NC	CNN (AlexNet)	SVM	AD vs. NC Accuracy: 90% specificity: 91% sensitivity: 87% AD vs. MCI Accuracy: 81% specificity: 88% sensitivity: 70% MCI vs. NC Accuracy: 72% specificity: 74% sensitivity: 69%
Bäckström et al. (2018) [16]	ADNI	MRI	340 subjects 199 AD 141 NC 1198 MRI Scans	3D ConvNet	Softmax	AD vs. NC Accuracy: 98%
Huanhuan et al. (2019) [5]	ADNI	MRI	615 subjects 179 AD 254 MCI 182 NC	ConvNet	ResNet50, NASNet, and MobileNet	AD vs. NC Accuracy: 98.59% AD vs. MCI Accuracy: 97.65% MCI vs. NC Accuracy: 88.37
Rallabandi et al. (2020) [17]	ADNI	MRI	1167 subjects 371 NC 328 EMCI, 169 LMCI 284 AD	FreeSurfer	Non-linear SVM (RBF kernel) Naive Bayesian K-Nearest Neighborhod Random Forest Decision Tree Linear SVM	non-linear SVM classifier showed the highest result in classifying all four groups 77% specificity 75% sensitivity 72% F-score 71% Matthew's correlation coefficient 69% kappa-statistic 76% (ROC AUC) 75% accuracy

Considering the above, to the best of our knowledge no study has focused on evaluating CNN-based MRI feature extraction using different classifiers. Thus, the aim of this paper is to analyze CNN-based MRI feature extraction for automatic classification of patients with Alzheimer's disease using pretrained CNN ResNet-50 with SVM, RF, and Softmax.

3. Materials and Methods

The main aim of this paper is to investigate and enhance the classification performance of MRI images for the early diagnosis of AD through DL and CNN. Thus, this paper proposes to build and evaluate a disease diagnosis approach based on a CNN DL technique based on MRI feature extraction for the automatic classification of AD using three different classifiers, SVM, RF, and Softmax. Figure 1 shows the general structure of the proposed approach.

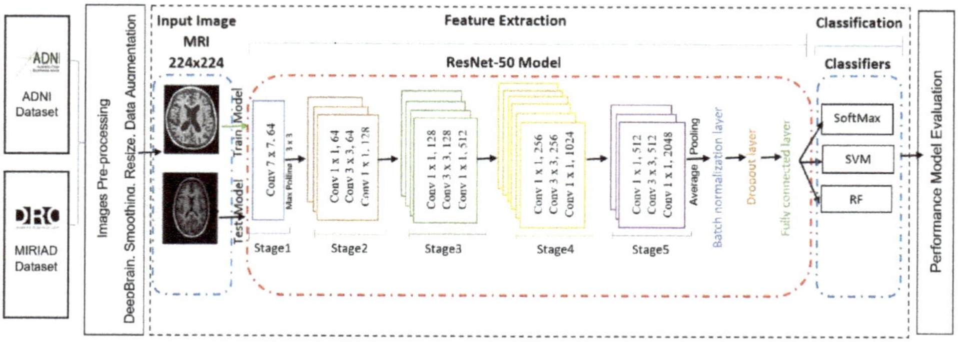

Figure 1. The general structure of the proposed approach.

In this work, we will start by building and validating a CNN model for feature extraction and classification. The validated model will then be used in experiments to evaluate the model through analyzing the features extracted by CNN (ResNet) from the fully connected layer. Three of the most well-known conventional ML classifiers will be applied (SVM, RF, and Softmax) for each set of features and for evaluating the results, where SVM and RF are the most common classification techniques used for AD classification based on our literature review. To build an AD diagnosis approach, the methodology goes through the following stages: first, the MRI data collection stage. In the second stage, the image pre-processing, we resized each MRI image to a suitable size for the CNN model. After that, we employed the pre-trained convolution neural networks ResNet50 to extract MRI image features and utilize them in the following classification stage in the feature's extraction stage. We use three different classifiers, SoftMax, SVM, and RF, in the classification stage. Finally, we looked at the different results, analyzed the efficiency and the effectiveness of each approach using the evaluation metrics, and compared our results with recent studies results. Figure 2 illustrates the detailed steps of the solution.

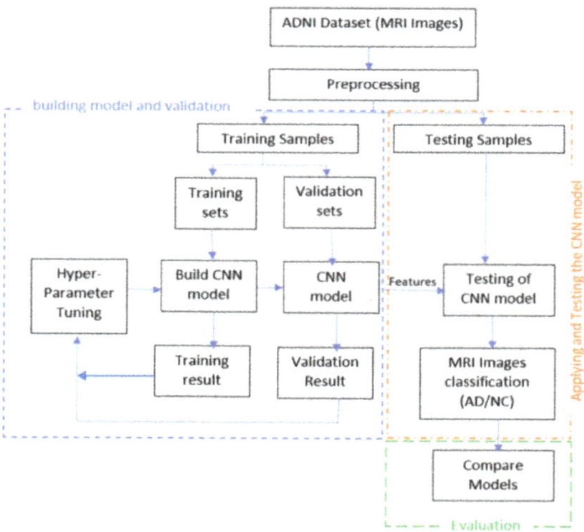

Figure 2. The detailed steps of the proposed solution.

3.1. MRI Dataset

This study will use two public datasets, the Alzheimer's Disease Neuroimaging Initiative (ADNI) [7] and Minimal Interval Resonance Imaging in Alzheimer's Disease (MIRIAD) [18]. The ADNI [7] was launched in 2003 by the National Institute of Biomedical Imaging and Bioengineering as a non-profit organization led by principal investigator Michael W. Weiner, MD. The initial goal of ADNI is to evaluate the progression of early Alzheimer's disease. The ADNI-1 Dataset consists of 1.5 T T1-weighted MRI images with 128 sagittal slices, typically 256 × 256 matrices with a voxel size of approximately 1.33 mm × 1 mm × 1 mm). The dataset is encompassing 741 subjects divided into Alzheimer's disease (AD) and normal control (NC). This dataset consists of 314 AD scans and 427 NC [7]. The MIRIAD dataset is a publicity available scan database of MRI brain scans consisting of 46 Alzheimer's patients and 23 normal control cases. Many scans were collected from each participant at intervals between 2 weeks and 2 years, and the study was designed to examine the feasibility of using MRI scans as an outcome measure for clinical trials of Alzheimer's therapies. It includes a total of 708 scans. Three-dimensional T1-weighted images were acquired with an IR-FSPGR (inversion recovery prepared fast spoiled gradient recalled) sequence, field of view 24 cm, 256 × 256 matrix, 124 1.5 mm coronal partitions, TR 15 ms, TE 5.4 ms, flip angle 15°, and TI 650 ms [18]. In both datasets, images from AD patients did not specify AD degrees. In our experiments, multiple images from one patient are treated independently, as if for different patients.

The data format is NIFTI and the file extension is (.nii). MRI data provide details of the brain and visualize the anatomy in all three planes: axial, sagittal, and coronal (see Figure 3 below). Figure 4 shows a comparison between a healthy brain (NC brain) and an AD brain of axial planes [18].

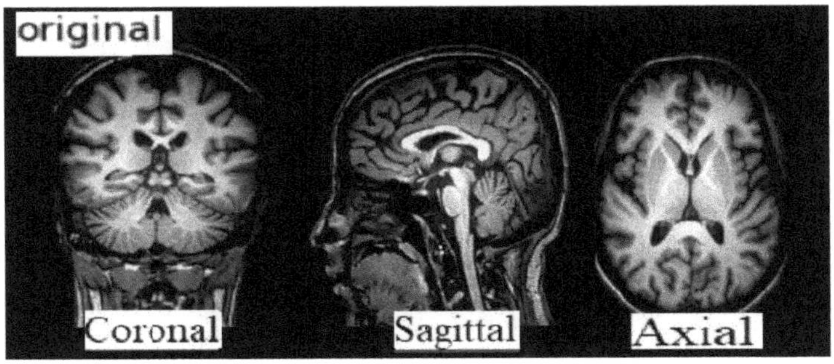

Figure 3. MRI Imaging Planes.

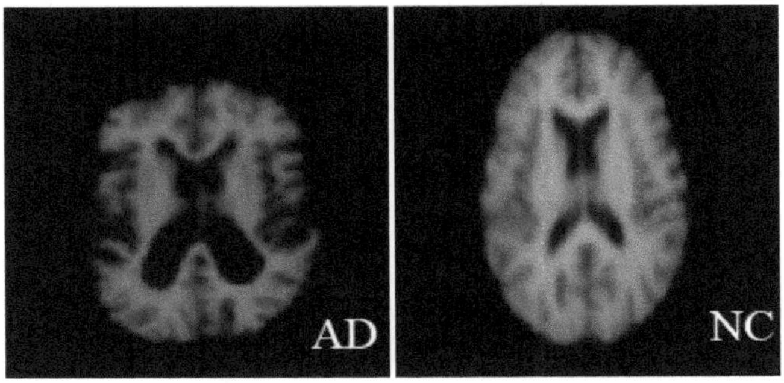

Figure 4. Normal brain vs. brain affected with Alzheimer's.

3.2. Data Pre-Processing

The pre-processing phase of the MRI datasets aims to transform the data into a more optimal representation to match the pre-trained CNN's input size requirements. First, we extracted the brain from MRI 3D images by removing the skull from the image and eliminating noise for improving the model performance. Then, applying the smoothing technique of MRI is often used to reduce noise within an image and produce a less pixelated image. We have smoothed our MRI images with a 4 mm FWHM Gaussian filter, while FWHM is the width of the kernel. Moreover, the ResNet architecture uses input images 224 × 224 pixels in size, meaning that each input MRI image in our CNN model resized to 224 × 224 pixels before being fed into the model.

3.3. CNN Model

The architecture of the proposed pre-trained CNN model (ResNet-50 [19]) consists of five Conv blocks stages, pooling layers, and the fully connected (FC) layer. Convolutional and pooling layers are used for feature extraction, while the fully connected layers are used for the image classification stage. Feature extraction in CNN uses local connections for local features detected and pooling for merging similar local features to be one feature. Meanwhile, FC layers are used to compute the output for each input MRI image. In addition, for optimizing the classification task, the FC layers can be replaced by other classifiers, such as SVM or RF.

After the data collection and image pre-processing stage, the dataset is divided into three sets: training, validation, and a testing set. Since we have small datasets, we used the data augmentation technique, which helps to increase the number of samples in our training dataset and this has expanded the number of images to 741 for ADNI [7] and 708 for MIRIAD [18]. The training set (a labeled dataset) trains the CNN model on a particular task, such as feature extraction, where the CNN model will generate MRI features vectors from the fully connected layer. After that, the features vectors are entered into three different classifiers. The validation set provides an impartial evaluation of a model fit on the training dataset while tuning the model. The test set was used to evaluate the ResNet50-Softmax, ResNet50-SVM, and ResNet50-RF model approaches.

We apply a pre-trained CNN called ResNet-50 using Tensorflow [20] and Keras [21] applications to the MRI images instead of training a CNN from scratch, which requires a huge dataset. In addition, this helps to avoid the overfitting problem caused by the small dataset. We selected the ResNet-50 model because it is arguably the most groundbreaking work in the computer vision/DL community in the last 5 years. ResNet makes it possible to train hundreds of layers that go deeper and deeper and still achieve good performance. It won the 2015 ImageNet Large Scale Visual Recognition Challenge (ILSVRC) and it outperformed all prior competitors and won the challenge by reducing the top-five error to 3.57%. Our study used ResNet-50 with three classifiers, Softmax, SVM, and RF, to determine which one performs better with the ResNet-50 model.

In the following paragraphs, there will be a brief description of the methodology CNN model of each set of layers.

3.3.1. Convolutional Layer

The convolutional layer is the essential part and the core building block of the DL CNN. It is responsible for the feature extraction process, while its output sets of 2D matrices are called feature maps. Each convolutional layer consists of a fixed number of filters that act as feature detectors and extract the features by convolving the input image with these filters. The size of the filters is chosen in ResNet50 (7 × 7), (1 × 1), and (3 × 3). During the training process, each filter acquires the ability to detect the analyzed images' low-level features, such as colors, edges, blobs, and corners.

3.3.2. Pooling Layer

The pooling layers [22] are places after the convolutional layers (Conv). The subsampling layer is responsible for decreasing the size of the feature maps that produce the convolutional layers. Max pooling is the most popular pooling operation that reduces the feature maps by reducing the small region in the image with the maximum value in the region. The max-pooling process is based on the partition of the images into sets of 2×2 non-overlapping regions. The maximum value from every region is taken. The 2×2 pooling layer reduces the size of the feature map by four times.

The process of max pooling is performed to avoid overfitting by providing an abstract of the image representation regions. In addition, it minimizes the computational cost by decreasing the number of parameters. Furthermore, the average pooling layer is another type of pooling. This layer acts as max pooling, but it calculates 2×2 rectangles' averages to create a subsampled image instead of taking the maximum value.

3.3.3. Batch Normalization Layer

The batch normalization layer [23] is used to normalize the convolution layer's output by setting the batch's mean to 0 and the variance to 1. This technique speeds up the training process, using higher learning rates. Moreover, it prevents the gradients of the model from vanishing during backpropagation. In addition, DL models with batch normalization layers are more robust against improper weights initialization.

3.3.4. Dropout Layer

The dropout layer [24] is used to avoid overfitting phenomena. This technique is based on a mechanism where, during the training, neurons are randomly removed. The dropout rate parameter controls the number of removed neurons, which decides the likelihood of neuron removal. The neurons are removed only during the training process.

3.3.5. Fully Connected Layer

The fully connecting layer is the last layer in the ResNet50 network. It acts as a classifier, and its function is to connect the layers in the network and give the final result of the classification. Usually, it is followed by the final layer with a normalized exponential function (Softmax). This layer has been modified to fine-tune the ResNet50 for the classification of Alzheimer's disease.

3.4. MRI Image Classification

The FC layers of CNN can be replaced by other classifiers, for example, based on logistic regression or SVMs, which are optimized for the task of classification. In this project, we will evaluate CNN with Softmax, SVM, and RF classifier.

3.4.1. Softmax Classification Layer

In general, in the last layer of CNN architecture is the Softmax function used to classify the labeled data and calculate the probability of each ground-truth label of outputs between 0 and 1, and output values converted to perceptible values. The formula of the Softmax function is given by the following equation [25]:

$$f(x)i = \frac{e^{zj}}{\sum_{n=1}^{N} e^{zk}} for\ j = 1, \ldots\ldots, N, \tag{1}$$

where N is denoted as the dimension of random values (x), which are converted to the meaningful values between 0 and 1 by the Softmax function $f(x)$.

3.4.2. SVM Classification

We will replace the final FC layers by SVM classifier with a number of splits (folds number = 10 and seed = 7). SVMs are often used for binary image classification, AD vs. NC, and they have achieved noteworthy results in real-life problems. In addition, using the RBF kernel, the SVM classifier generates a nonlinear classifier that can map the original dataset to the higher dimensional space by generating linear data. This is shown in the equation below, where input vectors are shown by x and y, the squared Euclidean distance between x and y vectors is shown by $||x-y||^2$, and the kernel parameter is shown by σ^2 [25]:

$$k(x,y) = \exp\left(-\frac{||x-y||^2}{2\sigma^2}\right), \tag{2}$$

3.4.3. Random Forest

Random forest (RF) is a technique for reducing the variance of an estimated prediction function. RF is a substantial modification of bagging that builds a large collection of de-correlated trees and then averages them. The essential idea in bagging is to average many noisy but approximately unbiased models and reduce the variance. Trees are ideal candidates for bagging since they can capture complex interactions [26]. It can be used for classification and regression. When used for classification, a random forest obtains a class vote from each tree and then classifies using a majority vote. When used for regression, the predictions from each tree at target point x are simply averaged. In our study, we used RF for classification with number estimator = 20 while the default = 100 and it can be change from 1–100 after trying several values 20 gives us the best result.

On many problems, random forests' performances are much like boosting, and they are simpler to train and tune. Consequently, random forests are popular, and are implemented in a variety of packages [26].

3.5. Performance Evaluation Metrics

The most important performance indicator (accuracy, ACC) of the AD diagnosis is used to measure the ResNet50-Softmax, ResNet-SVM, and ResNet-RF performance models. In addition, sensitivity (*SEN*) and specificity (*SPE*) are performance indicators. The true positives (*TP*) refer to the classifier's positive tuples that were correctly labeled. Let TP be the number of true positives. The false positives (*FP*) are the negative tuples that were incorrectly labeled as positive. Let FP be the number of false positives. The true negative (*TN*) are the negative tuples that the classifier correctly labeled. Let TN be the number of true negatives. The false negatives (*FN*) are the positive tuples that were mislabeled as negative. Let FN be the number of false negatives.

- Accuracy (*ACC*): the percentage of the number of records classified correctly versus the total records shown in the equation below:

$$ACC = (TP + TN)/(TP + TN + FP + FN), \tag{3}$$

- Sensitivity (*SEN*)/Recall shows the percentage of the number of records identified correctly over the total number of AD subjects, as shown in the equation below:

$$SEN = TP/(TP + FN), \tag{4}$$

- Specificity (*SPE*): the percentage of the number of records. Normal control is divided by the total number of normal nodes, as shown in the equation below:

$$SPE = TP/(TP + FP), \tag{5}$$

- $F_{measure}$: a measure of a test's accuracy:

$$F_{measure} = 2 * \frac{(precision * recall)}{(precision + recall)} \tag{6}$$

4. Experiments and Results

This section describes the conducted experiment and its setup, followed by our experiment's results. We will first give a brief description of the experiment's setup, which includes software and hardware settings, followed by the results of model training and validation. The third subsection is related to the obtained results when applying the CNN model for feature extraction with the three classifiers (Softmax, SVM, and RF). Finally, we will compare the obtained results in the proposed approach with those of other methods.

4.1. Experimental Setup

The experiments were conducted using the Google Colaboratory Pro [27] platform (Colab Pro) as a Python development environment. It is a cloud service provided by Google that allows users to write and execute Python codes in a hosted GPU. We used DL Python libraries TensorFlow [20], Keras [21], Scikit-learn [21], Numpy [21], and OpenCV [28] for developing the proposed solution. In addition, we used Nibabel [29], Nilearn [30], and DeepBrain [31] as Python libraries for neuroimaging data (MRI) analysis. This study employed an ADNI [7] dataset with the NIFTI format of MRI scans and focused on coronal plane visualization of brain anatomy. A coronal plane is an x-z plane perpendicular to the ground, which (in humans) separates the anterior from the posterior. Studies show that using the coronal plane is more effective [32].

The dataset consists of 741 subjects [AD:427 and, NC: 314]. As a pre-processing stage, for ResNet-50 we needed to resize all MRI images to 224 × 224 and convert them to RGB.

4.2. The Results of Model Training and Validation

In our study, the dataset was randomly partitioning into 75:15:10, 75% for the training, 15% for validation, and 10% for testing. Table 2 below shows the details of the dataset.

Table 2. Datasets details.

Data Set	Size	Training (75%)	Validation (15%)	Testing (10%)
ADNI [7]	741 [AD:427, NC:314]	555	111	75
MIRIAD [18]	708 [AD:466, NC:243]	530	105	73

The proposed CNN model structure is the same as that of the ResNet50 model, with some modifications that were made to avoid overfitting and enhancing the model performance. After the last convolution layer and after each fully connected layer, a batch normalization layer was added to normalize the output. One dropout layer was added before the classifier and after the last fully connected layer to avoid overfitting phenomena, while the dropout rate was set to 0.5. The ResNet-50 network was trained using the stochastic gradient descent (SGD) optimizer with the learning rate to 0.0004 and momentum to 0.9. The batch size was set to 10 for training and validation sets, while batch size equals sample number in the testing set. We set epoch to 100, while it is a hyperparameter predefined before training a model.

We evaluated the model based on the accuracy and categorical cross-entropy (loss) of classification AD and normal MRI images. Loss functions are intended to compute the quantity that a model should seek to minimize during training. Figure 5 shows the performance of the proposed pretrained CNN model ResNet-50 from training and validation for the ADNI and MIRIAD datasets. Top graphs show loss vs. epochs; meanwhile, down graphs show accuracy vs. epochs; red from training and orange from validation results, while epochs equal 100.

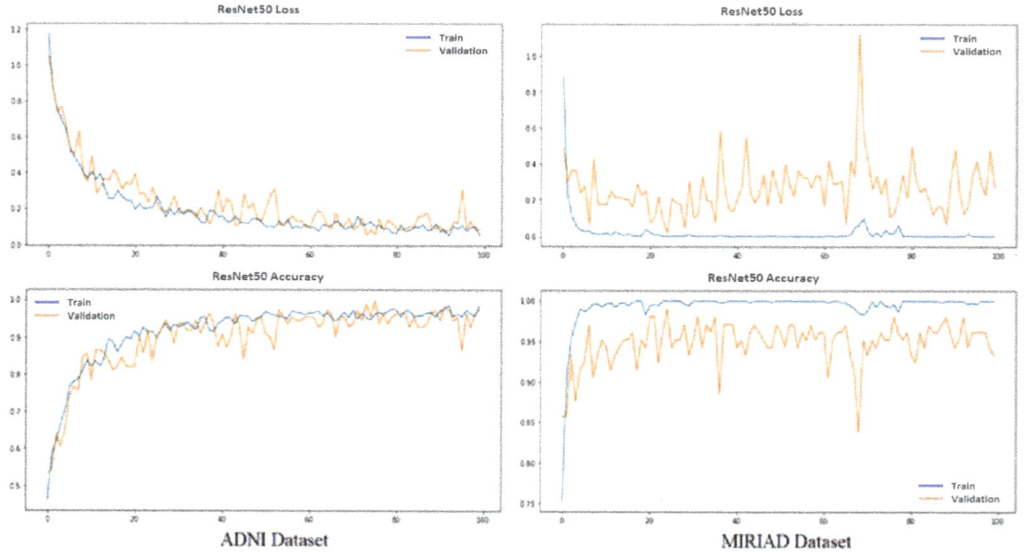

Figure 5. Training and validation performance of ResNet50-Softmax.

4.3. Classification Result Evaluation or Performance Analysis

To answer our first and second research questions, different experiments were conducted using three different classifiers (Softmax, SVM, and RF). Thus, in our experiments, we evaluated the proposed model's classification performance using Softmax, SVM, and RF classifiers with the ADNI [7] dataset and MIRIAD [18] dataset.

The experiment aims at determining the most accurate approach for the AD diagnostic pre-train model ResNet50. First, we apply transfer learning on ResNet50 using Softmax in the classifier layer. After that, the proposed approaches (ResNet50-Softmax, ResNet50-SVM, and ResNet50-RF) were tested on the ADNI and MIRIAD datasets. Results showed that the model with the Softmax classifier outperforms SVM and RF in all performance measures. Table 3 below shows the accuracy, specificity, sensitivity, and F-measure of each classifier on both datasets.

Table 3. Performance of the three classifiers in the proposed model.

Dataset	Classifier Used with ResNet50	Accuracy	Specificity	Sensitivity	F-Measure
ADNI [7]	Softmax	**99%**	**98%**	**99%**	**98%**
	SVM	92%	91%	87%	89%
	RF	85.7%	88%	79%	84%
MIRIAD [18]	Softmax	**96%**	**95%**	**96%**	**97%**
	SVM	90%	91%	87%	87%
	RF	84.8%	84%	73%	79%

Since Softmax has the best results over the other classifiers (RF and SVM) for both datasets, we will investigate more in evaluating this classifier's performance in terms of individual classes [AD and NC]. Figure 6 below shows the confusion matrix for the Softmax classifier on the ADNI and MIRIAD datasets. Tables 4 and 5 show the classification performance results of Softmax in precision, recall, f1-measure, and support, where support represents the number of samples.

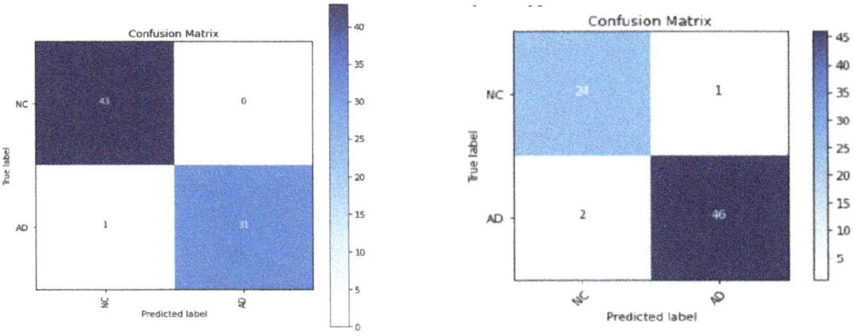

ADNI Dataset MIRIAD Dataset

Figure 6. Confusion matrix obtained on the test dataset with Resnet50-Softmax.

Table 4. Resnet50-Softmax experiment results with the ADNI dataset.

	Precision	Recall	F1-Score	Support
NC	98%	100%	99%	43
AD	100%	97%	98%	32
Accuracy			99%	75
Macro avg	99%	98%	99%	75
Weighted avg	99%	99%	99%	75

Table 5. Resnet50-Softmax experiment results with the MIRIAD dataset.

	Precision	Recall	F1-Score	Support
NC	92%	96%	94%	25
AD	98%	96%	97%	48
Accuracy			96%	73
Macro avg	95%	96%	95%	73
Weighted avg	96%	96%	96%	73

From Figure 6 and Tables 4 and 5, it can be clearly observed that the proposed AD diagnosis model has been shown to be effective, with a favorable AD classification rate (96.875%) and a low false alarm of 3.125% for the ADNI dataset, and with an AD classification rate (95.83%) with a low false alarm of 4.16% for the MIRIAD dataset.

Results also show that the performance is consistent in the three classifiers. This is demonstrated by the accuracy achieved by the Softmax classifiers being the highest. Likewise, SVM comes as the second-best classifier, and RF comes third. This shows that performance of the proposed model is not affected by the dataset.

4.4. Comparison with the State-of-the-Art Models

As shown in the previous sections, the proposed model has shown promising results on the ADNI [7] and MIRIAD [18] datasets with three different classifiers, with accuracy, specificity, sensitivity, and F-measure. It gave good results, answering our first research question about the effectiveness of the proposed model needs and evaluating its classification performance compared to other approaches in the literature to assess its effectiveness. To achieve that, we need to compare its performance against some of the state-of-the-art approaches discussed in our literature review. The approaches in the related work section were tested on the MRI of the ADNI [7] dataset. We compared the obtained results on ADNI with our proposed method in all three approaches (ResNet-50 + Softmax, ResNet-50 + SVM, and ResNet-50 + RF). Table 6 shows the results of our proposed model on the ADNI dataset in comparison to the results obtained by other approaches. From the results, it can be clearly seen that the proposed ResNet50-Softmax approach achieved very high performance of 99%, close to the approach result proposed by Huanhuan et al. [5], which combines three pre-trained models, including ResNet50, and achieves 98.59%. In addition, the proposed approach using different techniques such as MRI image smoothing, add batch normalization, and dropout layers that improve the network performance, compared with the ResNet50-Softmax approach proposed by Korolev et al. [13], is one of the proposed approaches using the same pre-train model ResNet50 without add batch normalization, or dropout and achieves only 80%. On the other hand, ResNet50 + SVM obtains a good result compared with [6,9,13,16]; it achieves 92% accuracy. In addition, ResNet + RF outperform three approaches that are the fuzzy-possibilistic tissue segmentation + SVM approach [9], VoxCNN + Softmax, and ResNet50 + Softmax proposed by [13]. Figure 7 below represents the results in the flow chart.

Table 6. Comparison of our test performance with eight existing state-of-the-art methods.

Models	Used Approach	Accuracy	Specificity	Sensitivity
Liu et al. (2016) [6]	Multiview learning using GM + SVM	93.83%	95.69%	92.78%
Lazli et al. (2018) [9]	Fuzzy-Possibilistic Tissue Segmentation + SVM	73%	-	-
Liu et al. (2015) [12]	stacked auto-encoder SAE + Softmax	91.40	90.42%	92.32%
Korolev et al. (2017) [13]	VoxCNN + Softmax	79%	-	-
	ResNet + Softmax	80%	-	-
Lan Lin et al. (2018) [15]	AlexNet + SVM	90%	91%	87%
Bäckström et al. (2018) [16]	3D ConvNet + Softmax	96%		
Huanhuan et al. (2019) [5]	ResNet50, NASNet, and MobileNet + Softmax	98.59	-	-
Rallabandi et al. (2020) [17]	Non-linear SVM (RBF kernel)	75%	79%	75%
Proposed model ADNI [7]	ResNet50 + Softmax	99%	98%	99%
	ResNet50 + SVM	92%	91%	87%
	ResNet50 + RF	85.7%	88%	79%

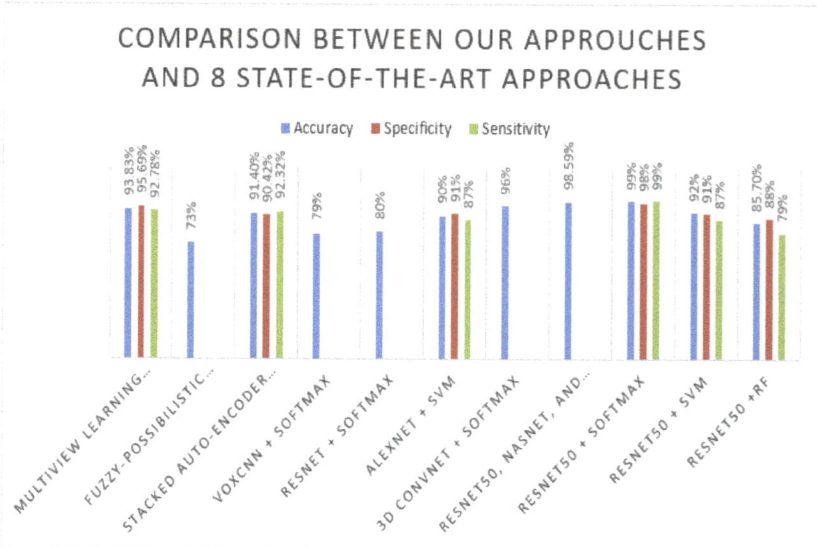

Figure 7. Comparison between our approaches and eight state-of-the-art approaches.

5. Conclusions

To conclude, in this paper an Alzheimer's disease classification model was developed for MRI. The pre-trained convolution neural network (CNN) architecture ResNet-50 was applied for an AD diagnoses system with different approaches (ResNet50 + Softmax,

ResNet50 + SVM, and ResNet50 + RF). First, we evaluated the performance for transfer learning from pre-trained CNN ResNet-50 for the classification task using Softmax. After that, we evaluated the performance for ResNet-50 for extracting features and using a support vector machine (SVM) and random forest (RF) for the classification task. This study was conducted on the ADNI MRI and MIRIAD datasets. The results show an accuracy of 99% for ResNet + Sofmax, 92% for ResNet50+SVM, and 85.7% for ResNet50 + RF with the ADNI dataset, while the results of the MIRIAD dataset showed accuracy of 96% for ResNet + Sofmax, 90% for ResNet50 + SVM, and 84.4% for ResNet50 + RF. We compared our model with the state-of-the-art models using the ADNI dataset and the results show that our model ResNet50 + Softmax achieved a higher accuracy than most of the state-of-the-art models.

Author Contributions: Conceptualization, D.A.; Funding acquisition, D.A.; Investigation, S.F.O.; Methodology, D.A.; Project administration, D.A.; Resources, D.A.; Software, S.F.O.; Supervision, D.A. All authors have read and agreed to the published version of the manuscript.

Funding: This research project was supported by a grant from the Research Supporting Program Project Number (RSP2022R281), King Saud University, Riyadh, Saudi Arabia.

Institutional Review Board Statement: Not applicable.

Informed Consent Statement: Not applicable.

Data Availability Statement: Not applicable.

Acknowledgments: Data collection and sharing for this project was funded by the Alzheimer's Disease Neuroimaging Initiative (ADNI) (National Institutes of Health Grant U01 AG024904) and DOD ADNI (Department of Defense award number W81XWH-12-2-0012). ADNI is funded by the National Institute on Aging, the National Institute of Biomedical Imaging and Bioengineering, and through generous contributions from the following: AbbVie, Alzheimer's Association; Alzheimer's Drug Discovery Foundation; Araclon Biotech; BioClinica, Inc.; Biogen; Bristol-Myers Squibb Company; CereSpir, Inc.; Cogstate; Eisai Inc.; Elan Pharmaceuticals, Inc.; Eli Lilly and Company; EuroImmun; F. Hoffmann-La Roche Ltd. and its affiliated company Genentech, Inc.; Fujirebio; GE Healthcare; IXICO Ltd.; Janssen Alzheimer Immunotherapy Research & Development, LLC.; Johnson & Johnson Pharmaceutical Research & Development LLC.; Lumosity; Lundbeck; Merck & Co., Inc.; Meso Scale Diagnostics, LLC.; NeuroRx Research; Neurotrack Technologies; Novartis Pharmaceuticals Corporation; Pfizer Inc.; Piramal Imaging; Servier; Takeda Pharmaceutical Company; and Transition Therapeutics. The Canadian Institute of Health Research is providing funds to support ADNI clinical sites in Canada. Private sector contributions are facilitated by the Foundation for the National Institutes of Health (www.fnih.org). The grantee organization is the Northern California Institute for Research and Education, and the study is coordinated by the Alzheimer's Therapeutic Research Institute at the University of Southern California. ADNI data are disseminated by the Laboratory for Neuro Imaging at the University of Southern California. This research project was supported by a grant from the Research Supporting Program Project Number (RSP2022R281), King Saud University, Riyadh, Saudi Arabia.

Conflicts of Interest: The authors declare no conflict of interest.

References

1. *World Alzheimer Report 2018—The State of the Art of Dementia Research: New Frontiers. New Frontiers*; Alzheimer's Disease International: London, UK, 2018; Volume 48.
2. Huang, J.; van Zijl, P.C.M.; Han, X.; Dong, C.M.; Cheng, G.W.Y.; Tse, K.-H.; Knutsson, L.; Chen, L.; Lai, J.H.C.; Wu, E.X.; et al. Altered d-glucose in brain parenchyma and cerebrospinal fluid of early Alzheimer's disease detected by dynamic glucose-enhanced MRI. *Sci. Adv.* **2020**, *6*, eaba3884. [CrossRef] [PubMed]
3. Castellazzi, G.; Cuzzoni, M.G.; Cotta Ramusino, M.; Martinelli, D.; Denaro, F.; Ricciardi, A.; Vitali, P.; Anzalone, N.; Bernini, S.; Palesi, F.; et al. A Machine Learning Approach for the Differential Diagnosis of Alzheimer and Vascular Dementia Fed by MRI Selected Features. *Front. Neuroinform.* **2020**, *14*, 25. [CrossRef]
4. How MRI Is Used to Detect Alzheimer's Disease. Available online: https://www.verywellhealth.com/can-an-mri-detect-alzheimers-disease-98632 (accessed on 12 September 2019).
5. Ji, H.; Liu, Z.; Yan, W.Q.; Klette, R. Early Diagnosis of Alzheimer's Disease Using Deep Learning. In Proceedings of the 2nd International Conference on Control and Computer Vision, Jeju, Korea, 15–18 June 2019; ACM: New York, NY, USA, 2019; pp. 87–91.

6. Liu, M.; Zhang, D.; Adeli, E.; Shen, D. Inherent Structure-Based Multiview Learning With Multitemplate Feature Representation for Alzheimer's Disease Diagnosis. *IEEE Trans. Biomed. Eng.* **2016**, *63*, 1473–1482. [CrossRef] [PubMed]
7. Jack, C.R.; Bernstein, M.A.; Fox, N.C.; Thompson, P.; Alexander, G.; Harvey, D.; Borowski, B.; Britson, P.J.; Whitwell, L.J.; Ward, C.; et al. The Alzheimer's Disease Neuroimaging Initiative (ADNI): MRI methods. *J. Magn. Reson. Imaging* **2008**, *27*, 685–691. [CrossRef]
8. Krashenyi, I.; Popcv, A.; Ramirez, J.; Gorriz, J.M. Fuzzy computer-aided diagnosis of Alzheimer's disease using MRI and PET statistical features. In Proceedings of the 2016 IEEE 36th International Conference on Electronics and Nanotechnology (ELNANO), Kyiv, Ukraine, 19–21 April 2016; pp. 187–191.
9. Lazli, L.; Boukadoum, M.; Mohamed, O.A. Computer-Aided Diagnosis System for Alzheimer's Disease Using Fuzzy-Possibilistic Tissue Segmentation and SVM Classification. In Proceedings of the 2018 IEEE Life Sciences Conference (LSC), Montreal, QC, Canada, 28–30 October 2018; pp. 33–36.
10. Ortiz, A.; Lozano, F.; Peinado, A.; Garía-Tarifa, M.J.; Górriz, J.M.; Ramírez, J. PET Image Classification Using HHT-Based Features Through Fractal Sampling. In Proceedings of the Natural and Artificial Computation for Biomedicine and Neuroscience, Corunna, Spain, 19–23 June 2017; Ferrández Vicente, J.M., Álvarez-Sánchez, J.R., de la Paz López, F., Toledo Moreo, J., Adeli, H., Eds.; Springer International Publishing: Cham, Switzerland, 2017; pp. 314–323.
11. NP, K.T.; Varghese, D. A Novel Approach for Diagnosing Alzheimer's Disease Using SVM. In Proceedings of the 2018 2nd International Conference on Trends in Electronics and Informatics (ICOEI), Tirunelveli, India, 11–12 May 2018; pp. 895–898.
12. Liu, S.; Liu, S.; Cai, W.; Che, H.; Pujol, S.; Kikinis, R.; Feng, D.; Fulham, M.J. ADNI Multimodal neuroimaging feature learning for multiclass diagnosis of Alzheimer's disease. *IEEE Trans. Biomed. Eng.* **2015**, *62*, 1132–1140. [CrossRef]
13. Korolev, S.; Safiullin, A.; Belyaev, M.; Dodonova, Y. Residual and plain convolutional neural networks for 3D brain MRI classification. In Proceedings of the 2017 IEEE 14th International Symposium on Biomedical Imaging (ISBI 2017), Melbourne, VIC, Australia, 18–21 April 2017; pp. 835–838.
14. Gunawardena, K.A.N.N.P.; Rajapakse, R.N.; Kodikara, N.D. Applying convolutional neural networks for pre-detection of alzheimer's disease from structural MRI data. In Proceedings of the 2017 24th International Conference on Mechatronics and Machine Vision in Practice (M2VIP), Auckland, New Zealand, 21–23 November 2017; pp. 1–7.
15. Lin, L.; Zhang, B.; Wu, S. Hybrid CNN-SVM for Alzheimer's Disease Classification from Structural MRI and the Alzheimer's Disease Neuroimaging Initiative (ADNI). *Age* **2018**, *72*, 199–203.
16. Bäckström, K.; Nazari, M.; Gu, I.Y.-H.; Jakola, A.S. An efficient 3D deep convolutional network for Alzheimer's disease diagnosis using MR images. In Proceedings of the 2018 IEEE 15th International Symposium on Biomedical Imaging (ISBI 2018), Washington, DC, USA, 4–7 April 2018; pp. 149–153.
17. Rallabandi, V.P.S.; Tulpule, K.; Gattu, M. Automatic classification of cognitively normal, mild cognitive impairment and Alzheimer's disease using structural MRI analysis. *Inform. Med. Unlocked* **2020**, *18*, 100305. [CrossRef]
18. UCL Minimal Interval Resonance Imaging in Alzheimer's Disease (MIRIAD). Available online: https://www.ucl.ac.uk/drc/research/methods/minimal-interval-resonance-imaging-alzheimers-disease-miriad (accessed on 7 May 2020).
19. He, K.; Zhang, X.; Ren, S.; Sun, J. Deep Residual Learning for Image Recognition. *arXiv* **2015**, arXiv:1512.03385.
20. TensorFlow. Available online: https://www.tensorflow.org/?hl=ar (accessed on 1 March 2020).
21. Costa, C.D. Best Python Libraries for Machine Learning and Deep Learning. Available online: https://towardsdatascience.com/best-python-libraries-for-machine-learning-and-deep-learning-b0bd40c7e8c (accessed on 29 February 2020).
22. Deep Learning in Neural Networks: An Overview—Science Direct. Available online: https://www.sciencedirect.com/science/article/abs/pii/S0893608014002135 (accessed on 7 May 2020).
23. Ioffe, S.; Szegedy, C. Batch Normalization: Accelerating Deep Network Training by Reducing Internal Covariate Shift. *Int. Conf. Mach. Learning. PMLR* **2015**, *37*, 448–456.
24. Srivastava, N.; Hinton, G.E.; Krizhevsky, A.; Sutskever, I.; Salakhutdinov, R. Dropout: A simple way to prevent neural networks from overfitting. *J. Mach. Learn. Res.* **2014**, *15*, 1929–1958.
25. Polat, H.; Danaei Mehr, H. Classification of Pulmonary CT Images by Using Hybrid 3D-Deep Convolutional Neural Network Architecture. *Appl. Sci.* **2019**, *9*, 940. [CrossRef]
26. Hastie, T.; Tibshirani, R.; Friedman, J. *The Elements of Statistical Learning: Data Mining, Inference, and Prediction*, 2nd ed.; Springer Series in Statistics; Springer: New York, NY, USA, 2009; ISBN 978-0-387-84857-0.
27. Google Colaboratory. Available online: https://colab.research.google.com/notebooks/pro.ipynb#scrollTo=BJW8Qi-pPpep (accessed on 29 April 2020).
28. About OpenCV. Available online: https://opencv.org/about/ (accessed on 3 May 2020).
29. Neuroimaging in Python—NiBabel 3.1.0+3.g1660b1a1 Documentation. Available online: https://nipy.org/nibabel/ (accessed on 30 April 2020).
30. Nilearn: Machine Learning for NeuroImaging in Python—Machine Learning for NeuroImaging. Available online: https://nilearn.github.io/introduction.html (accessed on 30 April 2020).
31. Iitzco/Deepbrain: Deep Learning Tools for Brain Medical Images. Available online: https://github.com/iitzco/deepbrain (accessed on 5 February 2022).
32. Park, M.; Moon, W.J.; Structural, M.R. Imaging in the Diagnosis of Alzheimer's Disease and Other Neurodegenerative Dementia: Current Imaging Approach and Future Perspectives. *Korean J. Radiol.* **2016**, *17*, 827–845. [CrossRef] [PubMed]

sensors

MDPI

Article

A Model for Predicting Cervical Cancer Using Machine Learning Algorithms

Naif Al Mudawi * and Abdulwahab Alazeb

Department of Computer Science, College of Computer Science and Information System, Najran University, Najran 55461, Saudi Arabia; afalazeb@nu.edu.sa
* Correspondence: naalmudawi@nu.edu.sa

Abstract: A growing number of individuals and organizations are turning to machine learning (ML) and deep learning (DL) to analyze massive amounts of data and produce actionable insights. Predicting the early stages of serious illnesses using ML-based schemes, including cancer, kidney failure, and heart attacks, is becoming increasingly common in medical practice. Cervical cancer is one of the most frequent diseases among women, and early diagnosis could be a possible solution for preventing this cancer. Thus, this study presents an astute way to predict cervical cancer with ML algorithms. Research dataset, data pre-processing, predictive model selection (PMS), and pseudo-code are the four phases of the proposed research technique. The PMS section reports experiments with a range of classic machine learning methods, including decision tree (DT), logistic regression (LR), support vector machine (SVM), K-nearest neighbors algorithm (KNN), adaptive boosting, gradient boosting, random forest, and XGBoost. In terms of cervical cancer prediction, the highest classification score of 100% is achieved with random forest (RF), decision tree (DT), adaptive boosting, and gradient boosting algorithms. In contrast, 99% accuracy has been found with SVM. The computational complexity of classic machine learning techniques is computed to assess the efficacy of the models. In addition, 132 Saudi Arabian volunteers were polled as part of this study to learn their thoughts about computer-assisted cervical cancer prediction, to focus attention on the human papillomavirus (HPV).

Keywords: machine learning (ML); cervical cancer; human papillomavirus (HPV); gradient boosting; support vector machine (SVM)

Citation: Al Mudawi, N.; Alazeb, A. A Model for Predicting Cervical Cancer Using Machine Learning Algorithms. *Sensors* **2022**, *22*, 4132. https://doi.org/10.3390/s22114132

Academic Editors: Ayman El-baz, Guruprasad A. Giridharan, Ahmed Shalaby, Ali H. Mahmoud and Mohammed Ghazal

Received: 5 May 2022
Accepted: 26 May 2022
Published: 29 May 2022

1. Introduction

Human life is plagued with difficulties because it is difficult to predict when problems arise. In general, women usually experience several difficulties in their lifetime. One of the most critical ailments they may face is cervical cancer, which causes many problems [1]. The elevated mortality age of uterine cancer is due to women's lack of knowledge about the importance of early detection [2]. Cervical cancer is a dangerous cancer, which threatens women's health worldwide, and its early signs are relatively difficult to detect [3]. It is responsible for damaging deep tissues of the cervix and can gradually reach other areas of the human body, such as the lungs, liver, and vagina, which can increase the difficulties involved [4]. However, while cervical cancer is a slow-growing malignancy, precancerous advances have made early detection, prevention, and therapy possible. Cervical cancer has been reduced in most nations over past decades as detection technologies have improved. This year, 4290 people are predicted to die from cervical cancer [5]. The fatality rate has dropped by roughly half since the mid-1970s, thanks in part to enhanced screening, which has resulted in the early identification of cervical cancer. The death rate has reduced from over 4% per year in 1996–2003 to less than 1% in 2009–2018 [6]. The pre-invasive stages of cervical cancer of the uterus last for a long time. Screening tests can provide successful treatment of precancerous-stage lesions, so that cancer can be prevented. Nonetheless, it has been determined that the death rate in underdeveloped nations is exceptionally high, since they do not benefit from state-provided preventive strategies, such as free immunization programs and national assessment programs.

When the cervix's human papillomavirus (HPV) infection is left untreated, cervical cancer develops [7]. Because it causes neoplastic development, the human papillomavirus (HPV) is the most common infectious agent in cervical cancer. The improper proliferation of cervical cancer cells and the multiplication of abnormal cells as a result of a malignant phase is referred to as neoplastic progression [8]. The healthcare industry regularly generates massive amounts of data that can be used to extract information for forecasting future sickness based on a patient's treatment history and health data. Furthermore, these areas can be enhanced by leveraging crucial data in healthcare. Machine learning helps individuals process vast amounts of complex medical data in healthcare and then analyze it for therapeutic insights. Doctors can then use this information to provide medical care. As a result, patient satisfaction can be improved when machine learning (ML) is employed in healthcare.

Cervical cancer is one of the most common malignancies among women worldwide. Recently, many studies have been conducted on cervical cancer using modern techniques that provide prediction in the early stage. Using machine learning has contributed to early prediction [9]. Therefore, the most important causes of this disease among female populations are lack of awareness, lack of access to resources and medical centers, and the expense of undergoing regular examination in some countries [10]. Machine learning has improved the performance of analyses and the generation of accurate patient data. One researcher [11] employed text mining, machine learning, and econometric tools to determine which core and enhanced quality attributes and emotions are more relevant in forecasting clients' satisfaction in different service scenarios. Their paper presents findings related to health product marketing and services, and proposes an automated and machine-learning-based technique for generating insights. It also aids healthcare/health product e-commerce managers improve the design and execution of e-commerce services. Moreover, the importance of continuous quality improvement in the performance of machine learning algorithms from a health care management and management information technologies point of view is demonstrated in this paper by describing different kinds of machine learning algorithms and analyzing healthcare data utilizing machine learning algorithms [12]. This study identified algorithms that are better suited for the categorization of negative and positive cervical cancer for clinical use. Cervical cancer can be diagnosed with the help of such algorithms. Deep learning has shown a significant impact on health and medical imaging, which helps evaluate the diagnostic accuracy of deep learning (DL) algorithms in identifying pathologies in medical imaging [13].

The objectives of this study are as follows:

- To analyze and classify cervical cancer using machine learning algorithms that will help doctors accurately diagnose the cancer.
- To identify the correlations between the parameters that are likely to be responsible for cervical cancer.
- To conduct a survey that identifies women's concerns about cervical cancer, and provides a message to the readers as well as the research community.

Section 2 provides a literature review, Section 3 describes the research methodology, and Section 4 includes the results and discussion.

2. Literature Review

This section provides the literature selection criteria (LSC) and the papers that have been collected to review the literature from all the databases. The literature selection criteria (LSC) section shows how we selected related papers based on the selection criteria, after collecting the articles from the databases. Looking at papers published between 2010 and November 2020, this research has explored several electronic databases, such as Institute of Electrical and Electronics Engineers (IEEE) Xplore, PubMed, National Center for Biotechnology Information (NCBI), Springer, Google Scholar, and Elsevier. Based on the selected articles, the literature review is provided in detail below.

Literature Selection Criteria

The advantage of selection criteria is that it is possible to work according to a plan, especially when downloading the papers. According to the time duration set, articles can be searched, and fake journals can be skipped. In terms of search criteria, the research paper must be a conference paper or journal article, and it must use a machine-learning-based model or program intended solely for cervical cancer prediction. In addition, the following conditions must be met:

- Purposes must be included in the research paper.
- The time frame being surveyed is from 2010 to 30 November 2021. It is important to analyse the previous studies' insights
- We do not include any research work that has not yet been printed, or is not peer reviewed.

In [14], the authors conducted a survey-based study on cervical cancer detection, including performance analysis to determine the accuracy of various distinctive types of architecture in an artificial neural network (ANN), where the ANN was used for identifying cancerous, normal, and abnormal cells. The authors of [15] used cervigram images to illustrate a method of screening cervical cancer with the oriented local histogram technique (OLHT), which can increase edges, and the dual-tree complex wavelet transform (DT-CWT), which can help achieve multi-resolution images. Using a UCI data repository and six machine learning (ML) classifiers, ref. [16] proposed a model that can predict the exact level of cervix infection. Data pre-processing was carried out with physician verification to extract some features and to perform validation. To complete the study, 10-fold cross-validation is utilized to assess the performance of the suggested model. Another key study was published in [16], which used machine learning classifiers (SVM, QUEST, C&R tree, and MLP). The investigation examined distinct metrics such as accuracy, sensitivity, specificity, and area under the curve (AUC). The QUEST parameters were 95.55%, 90.48%, 100%, and 95.20%, respectively. This research proposed a federated learning method for machinery malfunction diagnostics to address the data island problem. Each participant's model training is implemented on a local level, and a self-supervised learning scheme is provided to improve learning performance [17].

Five different machine learning algorithms are used by [18], including random forest, KNN, C5.0, SVM, and RPart. After finishing the training and evaluating the performance of all of the classifiers (C5.0, RF, RPART, SVM, and KNN), the best options in terms of accuracy were investigated, showing values of 97%, 96.9%, 96%, 88%, and 88%. Machine learning (ML) algorithms such as decision tree, random forest, and logistic regression were used in conjunction with the voting model. In [19], cervical cancer was detected using a dataset containing four target parameters (biopsy, cytology, Schiller, and Hinselmann), as well as 32 risk factors, collected from the University of California (UCI). Machine learning (ML) algorithms were applied, including the the decision tree and decision jungle approaches. The study observed that the decision tree algorithm showed a higher value (98.5%). In another study using the Microsoft Azure ML tool, an appropriate data mining technique was developed from the boosted decision tree, decision forest, and decision jungle algorithms to detect cervical cancer [20]. The models' performances were measured in terms of accuracy, area under the receiver operating characteristic (AUROC) curve, specificity, and sensitivity, with 10-fold cross-validation applied to the outputs to improve the decision tree algorithm's performance, reaching a value of 97.8% on the AUROC curve. The authors of [21] presented a survey-based study on cervical cancer prevention from the perspective of women in Bug, IRI, and Mayuge in Eastern Uganda, using a questionnaire to collect data from 900 women aged 25 to 49 years. After measuring and scoring the women's knowledge and statements about cervical cancer treatment, the data was analyzed using Stata 12.0 software. After doing bivariate and multivariate analysis, the authors discovered that 794 women, or roughly 88.2%, had heard of the condition. A majority of 557 women

(70.2%) acquired their information from the radio, while a minority of 120 women (15.1%) got their information from health care organizations.

The authors of [22] analyzed various machine learning approaches used from 2006 to 2017 to diagnose cervical cancer. In this research, a comparison was made using existing relevant works based on cervical cancer medical data, to determine the benefits and drawbacks of different approaches. Most studies had used unbalanced medical image datasets. The survey also mentioned employing deep learning to predict cervical cancer. Furthermore, the goal of [23] was to see how well the Cox proportional hazard regression model and the deep learning neural network model predicted survival in cervical cancer patients. A dataset from the University of California, Irvine, was used in the study [23], which included age, number of pregnancies, contraceptive use, smoking habits, and chronological records of sexually transmitted infections (STDs). The study's essential purpose was to use Hinslemann screening methods to predict cervical cancer. With 10-fold validation, a data mining strategy was used with the boosted decision tree, decision forest, and decision jungle approaches. Moreover, on the AUROC (area under receiver operating characteristic) curve, the boosted decision tree method achieved a forecast precision of 98%. The best example of using electronic health record (EHR) data to predict cervical cancer is [24]. Four machine learning classifiers were used to predict cancer. The random forest algorithm produced the best results, with an AUC (area under the curve) of 0.97 one day before diagnosis, up from 0.70 a year before diagnosis. The primary purpose of [25] was to create a method that can anticipate the early effects of radiation on bone metastases in cervical cancer patients. The researchers employed class imbalance learning (CIL) in data mining to tackle the challenge of an imbalanced dataset. To deal with the issue of imbalanced data categorization, many models, such as ant-miner, RIPPER, Ridor, PART, ADTree, C4.5, ELM, and weighted ELM, with the synthetic minority over-sampling approach (SMOTE) were used. The study aimed to assist in the early detection of cervical cancer. The study showed the use of machine learning in defining a data validation mechanism to improve the performance of cervical cancer prediction. The study also suggested genetic assistance as an optional strategy to enhance the validity of the prediction. Additionally, [26] has presented a method based on machine learning approaches for identifying cardiac disease. Classification algorithms were used to construct the system. The model suggested a conditional mutual information feature selection method to overcome the feature selection problem. Feature selection methods are utilized to improve classification accuracy and shorten the time it takes to develop a classification system.

Furthermore, the fundamental purpose of [27] was to examine how big data analytics and machine-learning-based approaches may be used for diabetes. The results demonstrate that the proposed machine-learning-based system might score as high as 86% on the diagnostic accuracy of DL. Health specialists and other stakeholders collaborated to create classification models that would assist in diabetes prediction and the design of prevention measures. Based on the findings, the authors review the literature on machine models and propose an intelligent framework for diabetes prediction. Anther study has been conducted [28] where a methodology for heart disease was developed using the UCI repository dataset and healthcare monitors to estimate the public's risk of heart disease. In addition, classification algorithms were employed to classify patient data to detect cardiac disease, such as doosted decision tree and decision forest. The classification was performed using data from the benchmark dataset during the training phase. At the testing stage, accurate patient data was used to determine whether illness existed. The results demonstrate that the proposed model based on machine learning could score as high as 92% on the diagnostic accuracy of DL. Comparative analysis of existing research are provided in Table 1.

Table 1. Comparative analysis of existing research.

Source	Used Dataset	Classifiers	Evaluation Matrix	Findings
[14]	UCL-858 patients and 36 attributes	ROC-AUC	ML method	Cervical cancer diagnosis
[15]	Patient demographics	N/A	Neural network	Applied Cox proportional techniques
[16]	UCL repository	ROC-AUC	Decision tree	Hinslemann screening methods
[17]	EHRs	AUC	Random forest	Traditional approaches
[18]	N/A	G-mean and F-measure	ADTree	Handling the data imbalance
[19]	Dataset collected from the University of California (UCI)	Using four target parameters: biopsy, cytology, Schiller, and Hinselmann, as well as 32 risk factors	Machine learning (ML) algorithms are applied, such as decision tree and decision jungle approaches.	Decision tree algorithm shows a higher value of 98.5%.
[20]	Data mining technique	(AUROC)	The Microsoft Azure ML tool	Decision tree algorithm, a higher value range of 97.8% on the AUROC curve.
[21]	A survey-based study on cervical cancer to collect data from 900 women aged 25 to 49 years	N/A	Using Stata 12.0 software.	A majority of 557 women (70.2%) acquired their information from the radio, while a minority of 120 women (15.1%) got their information from health care organizations.
[22]	Unbalanced medical image dataset	Assisted in determining cervical cancer, and benefits and drawbacks of different approaches	Machine learning approaches	Employing deep learning to predict cervical cancer with high probability.
[23]	A dataset from the University of California, Irvine	Used Hinslemann screening methods to forecast cervical cancer	Deep-learning neural network	Boosted decision tree, decision forest, and decision jungle approaches.
[24]	Electronic health record (EHR) data	Four machine learning classifiers	Random forest algorithm	The boosted decision tree method produced a precise forecast of 98%.
[25]	Data radiation on bone metastases in cervical cancer patients	Ant-miner, RIPPER, Ridor, PART, ADTree, C4.5, ELM, and Weighted ELM	Class imbalance learning (CIL)	Suggested genetic assistance as an optional strategy to enhance the validity of the prediction.
[26]	N/A	Classification algorithms are used to construct the system	Method based on machine learning approaches	Utilized to improve classification accuracy and shorten the time it takes to develop a classification system.
[27]	Data related to diabetes	Health specialists and other stakeholders collaborate	Big data analytics and machine-learning-based approaches may be used for diabetes.	Machine learning-based system might score as high as 86% on the diagnostic accuracy Of DL.
[28]	UCI repository dataset	Classify patient data to detect cardiac disease	Boosted decision tree, decision forest	Score as high as 92% on the diagnostic accuracy of DL.

Based on the above review, it can be stated that several traditional algorithms have been used to predict cervical cancer; still, the models do not achieve a satisfactory level, because the selection of important features is the most crucial part of machine learning, and the authors have not specified how the chosen features were selected. In addition, just using traditional deep learning algorithms does not indicate that a model is suitable for practical implementation in the healthcare sector; rather, model customization is required to remove the overfitting and make it faster for a clinical application. Nonetheless, this research has come up with an effective solution. Various state-of-the-art techniques are used in this study to take this research to a satisfactory level and assist doctors in diagnosing cervical disease.

3. Methodology

The proposed research methodology is classified into several segments: research dataset, data preprocessing, predictive model selection (PMS), and training method. Figure 1 depicts an architectural diagram of the proposed research; by looking at Figure 1, it can be clearly observed that the architectural diagram has been separated into four phases, because the model presented in this research performs some essential tasks in each stage. Details on research data collection are described in the Research Dataset section. The Data

Preprocessing section mentions how to remove noise from the dataset and make it useful for feeding in machine learning. The type of predictive model selected to predict cervical cancer in this research is shown in the PMS portion. The requisites for model training are shown in the Training Methods section. Finally, we design the platform to provide an overall pipeline of cervical cancer prediction using the Python programming language. This research implements an algorithm that is better suited for the categorization of negative and positive cervical cancer diagnoses for clinical use. Cervical cancer can be diagnosed with the help of algorithms including decision tree, logistic regression, support vector machine (SVM), K-nearest neighbours (KNN), adaptive boosting, dradient boosting, random forest, and XGBoost. The sequence and consequences are presented in the following sections.

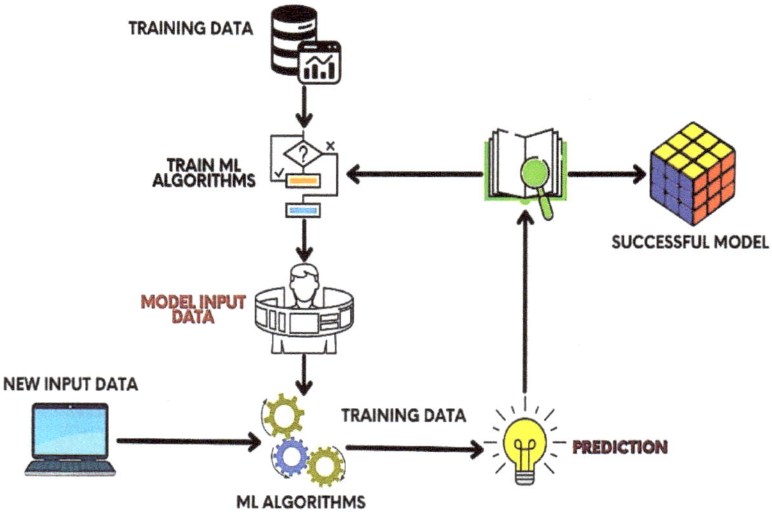

Figure 1. Proposed research model for classifying cervical cancer.

The proposed ML-based model is depicted in Figure 1. The training data will be fed to the system at the beginning of the model training. Then, ML algorithms are adopted. After that, model input data and new input data are applied to the scheme to train the architecture properly. Finally, prediction is performed on the newly accumulated data.

3.1. Research Dataset

The UCI repository contributed to the dataset "Cervical Cancer Risk Factors for Biopsy" [29]. The collection contains information about 858 people's activities, demographics, and medical history. Multiple missing values occur in this dataset for hospital patients as a result of several patients declining to answer questions due to privacy concerns [30]. The collection has 858 instances, each with 32 properties. The dataset includes 32 variables and the histories of 858 female patients [30]. The dataset includes 32 variables and the histories of 858 female patients, including factors such as age, IUD, smokes, STDs, and so on. The research dataset's attributes are provided in Table 2.

3.2. Data Preprocessing

Data preprocessing is divided into three sections, which are as follows: data cleaning, data transformation, and data reduction. Data preprocessing is critical since it directly impacts project success. Data impurity occurs when attributes or attribute values contain noise or outliers, and redundant or missing data [30]. We have removed the missing values and outliers from this dataset. The data transformation stage is kept in place to change the data into suitable forms for the mining process. This research combines normalization, attribute selection, discretization, and concept hierarchy generation. When dealing with a huge amount of data, analysis becomes more difficult when the data dimension is large. The data reduction approach is employed in this research to overcome this. It seeks to improve storage efficiency, while lowering the cost of data storage and processing. We have applied the dimension reduction technique because it is another useful technique that can be used to mitigate overfitting in machine learning models. For that, we have applied the principal component analysis (PCA) technique.

Table 2. Attributes of the research dataset.

No.	Attribute	Type
1	Age	Int
2	Number of sexual partners	Int
3	First sexual intercourse	Int
4	Number of pregnancies	Int
5	Smokes	Bool
6	Smokes (years)	Bool
7	Smokes (pack/year)	Bool
8	Hormonal contraceptives	Bool
9	Hormonal contraceptives (years)	Int
10	IUD	Bool
11	IUD (years)	Int
12	STDs	Bool
13	STDs (number)	Int
14	STDs: condylomatosis	Bool
15	STDs: cervical condylomatosis	Bool
16	STDs: vaginal condylomatosis	Bool
17	STDs: vulvo-perineal condylomatosis	Bool
18	STDs: syphilis	Bool
19	STDs: pelvic inflammatory	Bool
20	STDs: genital herpes	Bool
21	STDs: molluscum contagiosum	Bool
22	STDs: AIDS	Bool
23	STDs: HIV	Bool
24	STDs: hepatitis B	Bool
25	STDs: HPV	Bool
26	STDs: number of diagnoses	Int
27	STDs: time since first diagnosis	Int
28	STDs: time since last diagnosis	Int
29	Dx: cancer	Bool
30	Dx: CIN	Bool
31	Dx: HPV	Bool
32	Dx	Bool

3.3. Predictive Model Selection (PMS)

Several machine learning classification algorithms have been used in the PMS, namely support vector machine (SVM), decision tree classifier (DTC), random forest (RF), logistic regression (LR), gradient boosting (GB), XGBoost, adaptive boosting (AB), and K-nearest neighbor (KNN). This section has highlighted some of the algorithms that have achieved a satisfactory level of accuracy on the adopted research dataset. Thus, we have illustrated the theoretical interpretation of these algorithms in the following subsections.

3.3.1. Decision Tree (Dt)

Both classification and regression problems can be solved with the classification and regression tree or CART algorithm, which is also called the DT. The DT looks a lot like the branches of a tree, which is why the word 'tree' is included in its name. The decision tree starts from the 'root node' just as the tree starts from the root. From the root node, the branches of this tree spread through different decision conditions; such nodes are called decision nodes (and called leaf nodes after making a final decision).

3.3.2. Random Forest (Rf)

Ensemble learning enhances model performance by using multiple learners. RF is also a kind of ensemble learning. Following the RF bagging method reduces the chances of results being affected by outliers. This works well for both categorical and continuous data. Datasets do not need to be scaled, and the higher the number of learners, the more computational resources are required for complex models. In this algorithm, the decision is made by voting. Such an algorithm is called ensemble learning. Random forests are made up of many trees or shrubs. Just as there are many trees in the forest, random forests also have many decision trees. The decision that most trees make is considered the final decision.

3.3.3. Adaptive Boosting (AB)

The adaptive boosting technique creates a powerful learner by combining the knowledge of a number of weak learners. In this scenario, every single weak learner utilizes the exact same input, often known as a training set. Every initial input or piece of training data is given the same amount of importance. The responsibility for correcting the incorrect predictions made by the first weak learner is passed on to the next weak learner, who is given greater weight on the predictions made by the first weak learner and is turned over to the next weak learner. As a result, the errors that the second weak learner made in its predictions are passed on to the following weak learner in the same fashion, but with increased weight. The same process is continued until the number of inaccurate forecasts is reduced to a manageable level. In the end, a powerful learner is developed via the combined efforts of all the weak learners. In this way, the amount of inaccuracy in the forecast is reduced.

3.3.4. Support Vector Machine (SVM)

The support vector machine algorithm can be used for classification and regression problems. However, SVMs are quite popular for relatively complex types of small or medium classification datasets. In this algorithm, data points are separated by a hyperplane, and the kernel determines what the hyperplane will look like. If we plot multiple variables in a normal scatter plot, in many cases, that plot cannot separate two or more data classes. The kernel of an SVM is a significant element, which can convert lower-dimensional data into higher-dimensional space, and thus differentiate between types [31]. The following equations are used in the case of SVM (1) and (2) [32]:

$$\vec{w} \cdot \vec{x} + b = 0 \tag{1}$$

In this case, w is the (possibly normalized) average vector to the hyperplane. These two specific hyperplanes bound the "margin" in the region or area, and the maximum hyperplane lies halfway between them. These hyperplanes can be defined by equations using a normalized or standardized dataset.

$$\text{Plus} - \text{plane } = \vec{w} \cdot \vec{x} + b = 0$$

$$\text{Minus} - \text{plane } = \vec{w} \cdot \vec{x} - b = 0$$

Therefore, the width or the margin of the two hyperplanes for data classification can be written as follows:

$$width = \frac{\vec{W}}{abs(\vec{W})} \tag{2}$$

3.4. Radial Basis Function (RBF) Kernel Support Vector Machine (SVM)

The support vector machine (SVM) performs well on linear and nonlinear data. This method of classifying nonlinear data includes the radial base function. Putting data in the function space relies heavily on the kernel function [33]. When plotting many variables in a typical scatter plot, it is often impossible to distinguish between various sets of data. An SVM's kernel is a technique for transforming lower-dimensional input into higher-dimensional space and identifying different classes. In addition, the radial basis function is a nonlinear function. The support vector machine's most popular feature is its ability to classify objects automatically. Infinite-dimensional space can be mapped to any input with this kernel.

$$\mathrm{K}(x_1, x_2) = \exp\left(-\frac{|x_1 - x_2|^2}{2\sigma^2}\right) \tag{3}$$

After utilizing Equation (1), we can obtain the following:

$$f(X) = \sum_i^N \alpha_i y_i k(X_i, X) + b \tag{4}$$

By applying Equation (3) in (4), we get a new function, where N represents the trained data.

$$f(X) = \sum_i^N \alpha_i y_i \exp\left(-\frac{|x_1 - x_2|^2}{2\sigma^2}\right) + b \tag{5}$$

Gradient Boosting

The gradient boosting algorithm also follows the sequential ensemble learning method. Through loss optimization, weak learners gradually become better than previous weak learners. For example, the second weak learner is better than the first, the third weak learner is better than the second, and so on. As the weak learner periodicity increases, the amount of error in the model decreases, and the model becomes a stronger learner. The gradient boosting algorithm works relatively well for regression-type problems [34].

The difference between gradient boosting and adaptive boosting is that in adaptive boosting, error is gradually reduced by updating the weight of the wrong predictive samples. In gradient boosting, the loss function is optimized, and each loss is optimized [35]. The amount of error also decreases. To optimize this loss function, each weak learner changes its alternative weak learner model, so that the next weak learner is better than the previous one. Gradient boosting consists of three components: weak learner, loss function optimization, and additive model. The following Equations (6)–(11) show the working procedure of the gradient boosting algorithm mathematically [36]:

1. "Reconfigure the function estimate with a constant value"

$$\hat{f}(x) = \hat{f}_0, \hat{f}_0 = \gamma, \gamma \in \mathbb{R}, \hat{f}_0 = \underset{\gamma}{\operatorname{argmin}} \sum_{i=1}^n L(y_i, \gamma) \tag{6}$$

2. "For each iteration "t = 1, . . . ,T":"

$$\text{Compute pseudo} - \text{residuals } r_t, r_{it} = -\left[\frac{\partial L(y_i, f(x_i))}{\partial f(x_i)}\right]_{f(x) = \hat{f}(x)} \quad \text{for } i = 1, \ldots, n \tag{7}$$

Include the latest function g_t (x) (it can be any model, but here we are applying decision trees) as regression on pseudo-residuals.

$$\{(x_i, r_{it})\}_{i=1,\ldots,n} \tag{8}$$

"Determine optimal coefficient "ρ_t" at "g_t (x)" about the initial loss function"

$$\rho_t = \underset{\rho}{\operatorname{argmin}} \sum_{i=1}^n L\left(y_i, \hat{f}(x_i) + \rho \cdot g_t(x_i, \theta)\right) \tag{9}$$

"Improve current approximation"

$$\begin{aligned}\hat{f}(x)\text{where}\hat{f}_t(x) = \rho_t \cdot g_t(x) \\ \hat{f}(x) \leftarrow \hat{f}(x) + \hat{f}_t(x) = \sum_{i=0}^{t} \hat{f}_i(x)\end{aligned} \tag{10}$$

3. The ultimate GBM model will be the addition of the elementary constant and the entire following function update:

$$\hat{f}(x) = \sum_{i=0}^{T} \hat{f}(x) \tag{11}$$

4. Result Analysis

This section is categorized into four parts: empirical consequence report (ECP), exploratory cervical data analysis (ECDA), computational complexity analysis (CCA), comparative analysis, and survey data analysis (SDA).

4.1. Empirical Consequence Report (ECP)

The accuracy of predictions from the classification algorithms is estimated by applying a classification report. The report demonstrates the precision, recall, and f1 score of the key classification metrics on a per-class basis. By using true positive (TP), false positive (FP), true negative (TN), and false negative (FN), the metrics are computed [37]. Table 3 demonstrates the classification reports of the several traditional machine learning algorithms where the precision, recall, and F1 scores are denoted by "P", "R", and "F1". Precision is the ratio of the model's correct positive estimates to the total (correct and incorrect) positive estimates; recall is the ratio of being able to predict positive as positive; and F1 is the weighted average of precision and recall (this score considers both false positives and false negatives). A classification report has been included in the table, where 0 means negative class and 1 means positive class.

Table 3. Classification report of the machine learning algorithms for classifying cervical cancer.

Algorithm	For the Case of "0"				For the Case of "1"			
	Purpose	P	R	F1	P	R	F1	Accuracy Score
Logistic Regression	Cervical cancer prediction	0.98	1.00	0.99	1.00	0.77	0.87	0.98
SVM		0.99	1.00	1.00	1.00	0.92	0.96	0.99
Random Forest		1.00	1.00	1.00	1.00	1.00	1.00	1.00
Decision Tree		1.00	1.00	1.00	1.00	1.00	1.00	1.00
Adaptive Boosting		1.00	1.00	1.00	1.00	1.00	1.00	1.00
KNN		0.95	1.00	0.97	1.00	0.31	0.47	0.95

To obtain the classification report [38], the following Equations (12)–(15) are used.

P: The relationship between the accurate positive estimate generated by the model and the overall (correct and inaccurate) positive estimate. It is articulated as:

$$P = \frac{TP}{TP + FN} \tag{12}$$

Recall/sensitivity: Positivity is represented by the ratio of accurate to inaccurate predictions. It is written in mathematical notation as follows:

$$F2 = 2 \cdot \frac{TP}{TP + FN} \tag{13}$$

F1: This is the harmonic mean of precision and recall, and it provides a more accurate estimate of the amount of misclassification cases than the accuracy metric. It can be expressed numerically as:

$$F2 = \frac{Precision \cdot Recall}{Precision + Recall} \quad (14)$$

Accuracy: It is the measure of all the instances correctly predicted. It is given as:

$$\text{Accuracy} = \frac{TP + TN}{TP + TN + FP + FN} \quad (15)$$

The mean squared error (MSE), mean absolute error (MAE), root mean squared error (RMSE), and R-squared (R2) are frequently used to measure a model's effectiveness in terms of regression analysis. The accuracy of gradient boosting and XGBoost is obtained with the performance metrics, as shown in Table 3. The MAE illustrates the commonality of clearly distinguishing between specific and predicted values within the dataset. Similarly, the MAE shows the traditional square difference between main and anticipated standards. The RMSE also computes the standard deviation of the residuals. Finally, the R-squared (R2) represents the fraction of variation inside the variable quantity defined by the regression toward the mean model [38]. We have interpreted different algorithms with the corresponding evaluation matrices. From the finding in Table 3, the highest classification scores have been achieved with random forest (RF), decision tree (DT), and adaptive boosting. In contrast, XGBoost provides a higher level of regularization for the gradient boosting algorithm. Advanced regularization (L1 and L2) is utilized in XGBoost to increase model generalization. In terms of performance, XGBoost is superior to the gradient boosting algorithm. Its training is quite fast, and it may be dispersed across numerous clusters if necessary. Because we need to determine the distinction between a classification model, XGBoost, and gradient boosting, we have separated these models into a separate table (Table 4) to survey the accuracy measurements of each of them, and found the highest accuracy of 100 with gradient boosting.

Table 4. Accuracy measurement of gradient boosting and XGradient boosting.

Algorithm	MAE	MSE	RMSE	Accuracy	R2
Gradient Boosting	$7.330935195811098 \times 10^{-165}$	0.0	0.0	1.00	1.00
XGBoost	0.04847228	0.021919228	0.14805144	0.68628035	0.68628035

4.2. Exploratory Cervical Data Analysis (ECDA)

Figure 2 shows the correlation graph. Correlation describes how two or more variables are connected [39]. These variables may be input data features used to forecast our target variable. Correlation is a mathematical method used to evaluate how one variable moves or shifts in relation to another. It informs us about the intensity of the relationship between the two variables. It is a bivariate analysis measure that defines the relationship between various variables [39]. Moreover, finding the correlation is significant in cervical analysis because essential factors can be identified by finding the relationship between each variable. Two characteristics (variables) may be positively correlated with one another.

In the same way, two features (variables) can be negatively correlated with one another. This implies that as the value of one variable rises, the other variable(s) falls. On the other hand, if one variable's value increases or decreases, but the value of the other variable(s) does not, this indicates no correlation. The correlations are illustrated in Figure 2.

Figures 3 and 4 visualize the count measurement regarding the number of pregnancies, the number of sexual partners, and age, and a comparison between biopsy and number of pregnancies. The cervix is the uterus's lower, narrowest portion. It creates a canal that leads to the vaginal opening. Cervical biopsies can be performed in a variety of ways. As shown in Figure 4, it is evident that a relationship between biopsy and pregnancy exists, but occasionally fluctuates.

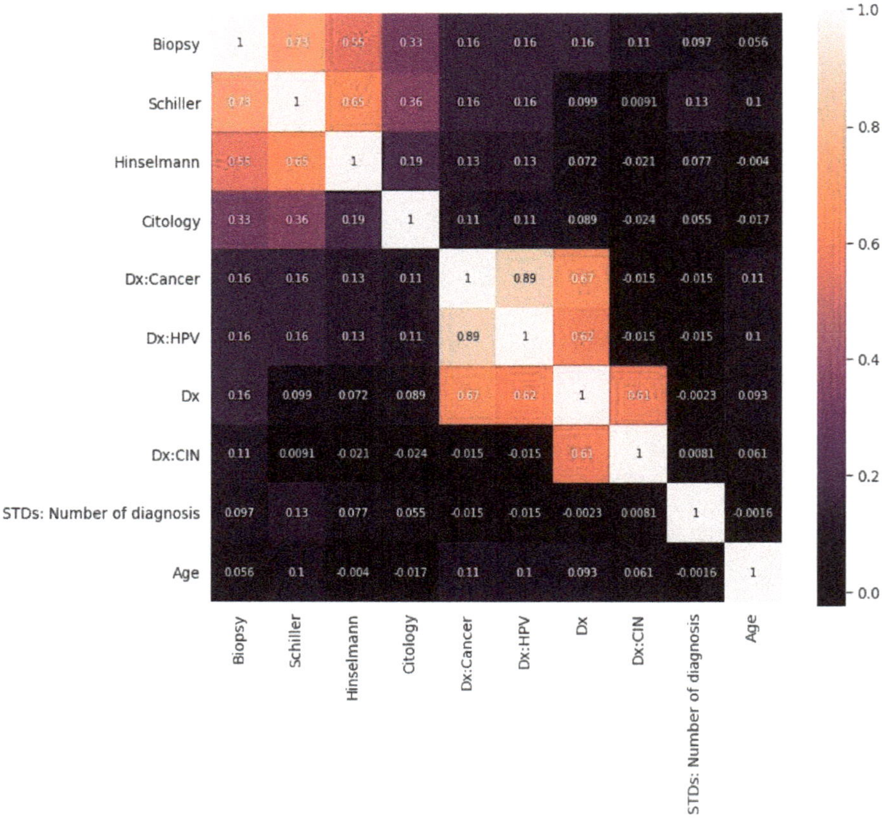

Figure 2. Correlations between different variables of cervical cancer.

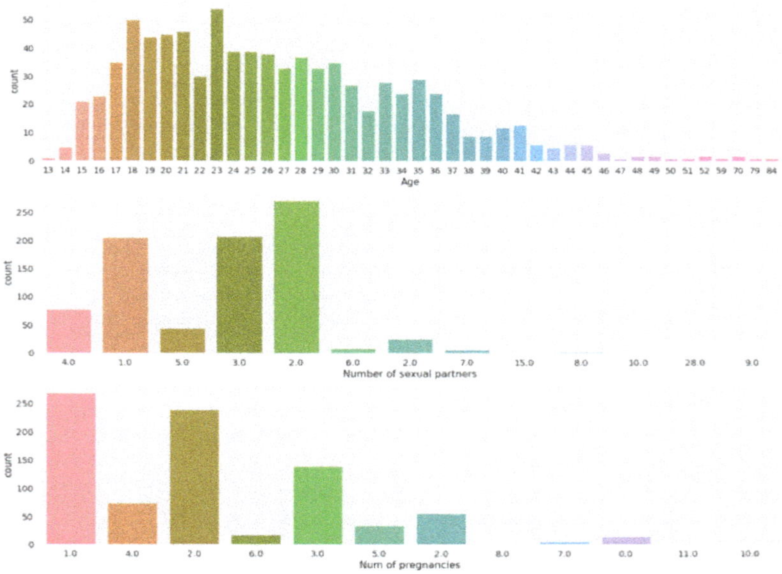

Figure 3. Count measurement in terms of the number of pregnancies, number of sexual partners, and age.

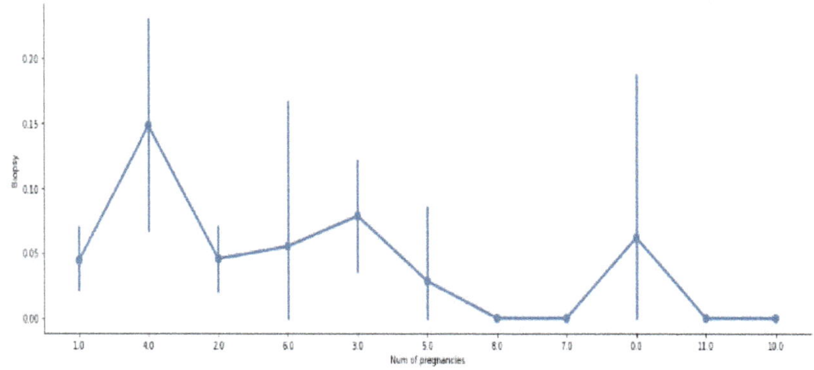

Figure 4. Visualization of comparison between biopsy and number of pregnancies.

4.3. Computational Complexity Analysis (CCA)

Machine learning computational complexity is a quantitative examination of the possibilities for effective computer learning [40]. It is focused on successful and general learning algorithms and works within recently deployed machine inference models based on computational complexity theory. We conducted a complexity analysis of various classic algorithms because these types of algorithms have previously been utilized to identify cervical cancer. Researchers confront numerous challenges regarding algorithm selection, so determining the computational complexity before creating a model is critical. Table 5 shows a short summary of different algorithms, indicating the complexity analysis of regression, dataset training, and prediction.

Table 5. Computational complexity of machine learning algorithms.

Algorithm	Classification/Regression	Training	Prediction
Decision Tree	C + R	$O(n^2p)$	$O(p)$
Random Forest	C + R	$O(n^2pn_{\text{trees}})$	$O(pn_{\text{trees}})$
Gradient Boosting (n_{trees})	C + R	$O(npn_{\text{trees}})$	$O(pn_{\text{trees}})$
SVM (Kernel)	C + R	$O(n^2p+n^3)$	$O(n_{sv}p)$
k-Nearest Neighbours	C + R	-	$O(np)$

4.4. Validation

This research has applied cross-validation, which is a method that examines the research model to achieve better residuals [41]. The problem with validation is that it does not indicate how good data will be when it is used to make new estimates for a new result. The better solution to this problem is not applying the entire dataset when we run data training, which requires removing some of the data before training starts. Then, when we finish training with the data, we can use the data removed in the assessment to show how the model fits on "new" data. We have applied five-fold cross validation, and we did a resampling method that uses different portions of the data to test and train a model on various iterations. This model achieved satisfactory performance, and as the data size is not large, we aim to apply these validation indicators in the next phase as our research is still ongoing.

4.5. Survey Data Analysis (SDA)

Another part of our research is conducting survey data analysis. To determine how many people are aware of cervical cancer, we have completed survey questionnaires based on the aim of this research. In this research, a stratified sampling technique has been used; stratified sampling is a similar or homogenous group-based sampling method [42].

Our priority for this survey was to analyze the number of women who are less aware of cervical cancer. It is certainly true that many women often feel too shy to talk about the mentioned diseases with their parents, so in this research, we have highlighted this issue, so that essential steps can be taken to raise awareness. In addition, the core biopsy test is significant, and many are not familiar with this test. This was the primary reason for taking a survey and analyzing the data. All members of the same group usually have the same characteristics; such groups are called strata. Table 6 shows some major survey questions (number of responses: N = 132; 94.69% answered all questions correctly).

Table 6. Some major survey questions for investigating cervical cancer.

Some Major Survey Questions that Match Survey Goal	Response N = 132		
	Yes/Agree	No/Disagree	Maybe/No Idea
Have you done a biopsy test or any other cervical cancer (uterus)-related test before?	68%	26%	6%
Is everyone in your family aware of cervical cancer?	76%	20%	4%
Do you agree with the statement that the rate of being affected by this cancer is becoming higher than before?	73%	10%	17%
Do you know about human papillomavirus (HPV)?	62%	31%	7%
Does living in a city or urban area affect how conscious people are of this cancer?	71%	21%	8%
Have you had a biopsy or any other cervical cancer (uterus)-related test before?	54%	35%	11%

Figure 5 illustrates the number of responses in terms of awareness of human papillomavirus (HPV). By looking at Figure 5, it can be clearly seen that 31% of the participants are not aware of HPV, while 62% are aware of the virus. Only 7% of respondents were unsure.

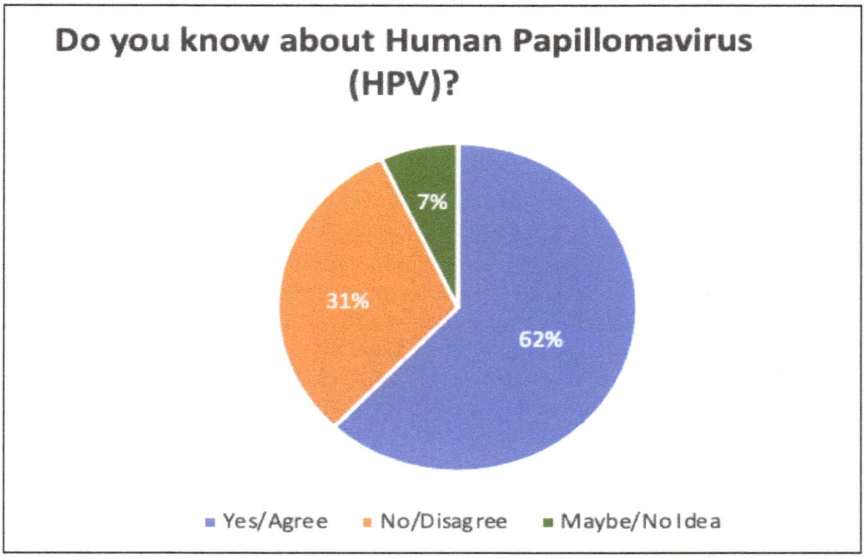

Figure 5. Number of responses regarding the awareness of human papillomavirus (HPV).

In addition, Figure 6 compares the responses in terms of whether or not the rate of being affected by cervical cancer is becoming higher than before. It is noticeable that 73%

of participants agreed with this statement, while 17% disagreed. A minority of participants (around 10%) were unsure.

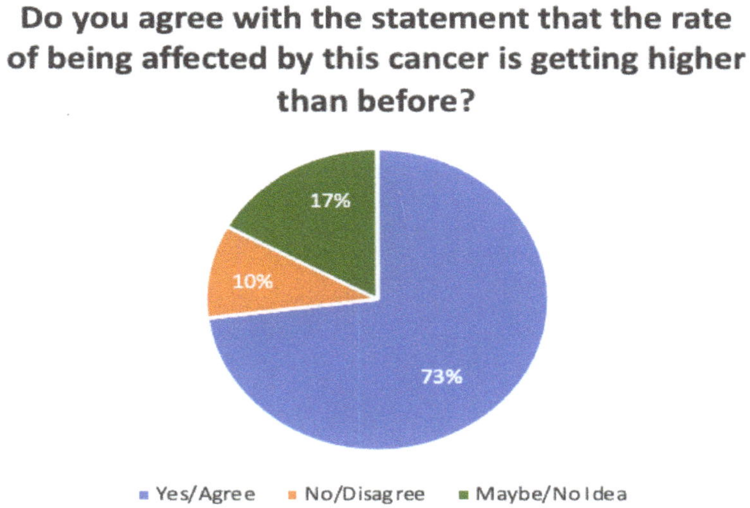

Figure 6. Survey responses regarding whether or not the rate of being affected by cervical cancer is becoming higher than before.

Figures 7 and 8 compare the proportions of biopsy tests and awareness levels in rural vs. urban areas. A total of 132 responses were recorded during the survey. Of these, 26% of all participants had not yet undergone a biopsy test, while 6% of participants were unsure. According to the survey, those who live in cities are more aware (71%) than those in rural areas (21%). Another 8% of participants said both are equivalently aware of cervical cancer.

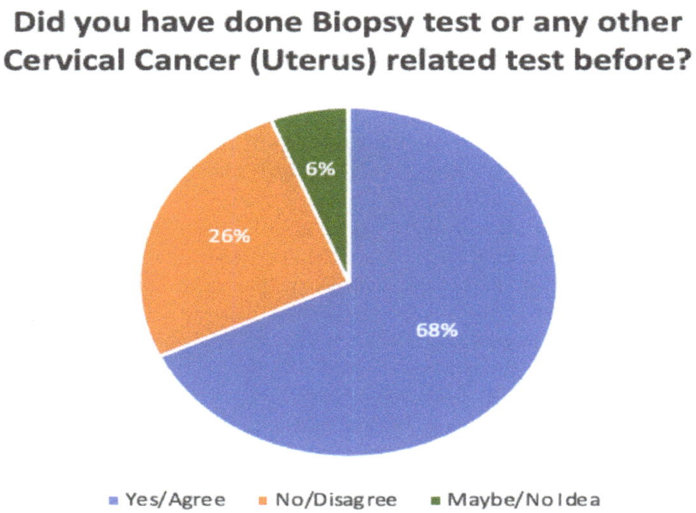

Figure 7. Total percentage of individuals who have undergone a biopsy test or another cervical cancer (uterus)-related test before.

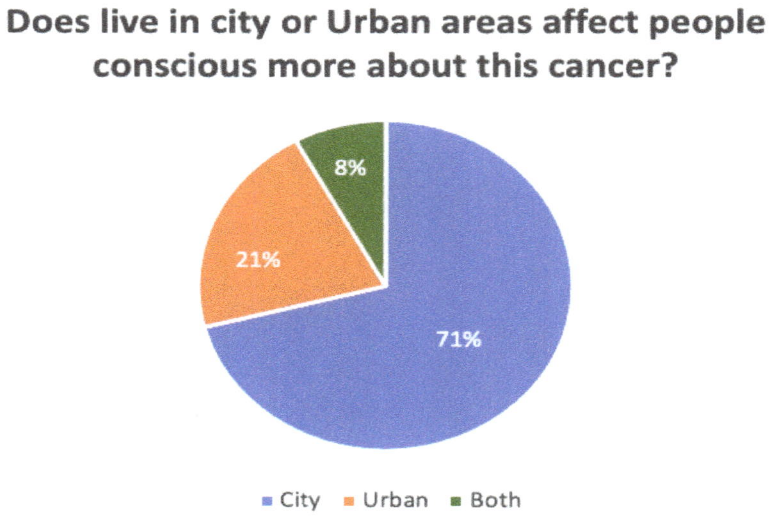

Figure 8. The awareness level in rural and urban areas regarding cervical cancer.

5. Discussion

Based on the findings of this research, it can be stated that the objectives of this paper have been achieved. Its research methodology was enriched with a set of algorithms including decision tree (DT), logistic regression (LR), support vector machine (SVM), K-nearest neighbors (KNN), adaptive boosting, gradient boosting, random forest (RF), and XGBoost. The research has reached a satisfactory result for both predictions and classification. This investigation also observed that the DT and RF algorithms were used in conjunction with the Microsoft Azure machine learning (ML) method to achieve a proper data mining technique for predicting cervical cancer. The study has further noticed that the performances of the traditional algorithms used in previous research are comparatively low. It is important to use data scaling, conduct missing value removal, and select a suitable algorithm in the case of disease analysis and prediction. Still, previous research has not shown the details of this pipeline. It is a matter of great concern that this work has not been accomplished much in previous research using gradient boosting algorithms. Since the gradient boosting algorithm also follows the sequential ensemble learning method, the wave learners gradually get better than their previous wave learners through this method of loss optimization.

It is essential to point out that the researchers did not restrict their effort to simply developing the model; rather, they also validated and evaluated the model's performance. Several validation strategies, including ROC-AUC, confusion matrix, and cross-validation, were applied by the researchers, and the researchers found that the efficacy with respect to cervical cancer is adequate. In addition, the current research investigated the most important predictors and the algorithms that are most frequently utilized for the purpose of cervical cancer prediction. During the preprocessing phase, some aspects of the patients' samples, such as the length of time they drank alcohol and their HIV and HSV2 infection status, revealed that factors whose samples had undergone modest variations could not be considered accurate predictors. Fewer predictors may need to be analyzed in subsequent studies because of the potential importance of a given characteristic for the community or the patient's social status. This may make it easier to conduct the research more quickly. However, with the help of this machine learning model, women have the opportunity to benefit from knowing more about cervical cancer and what effect it has on the human body. This study will focus on women in order to identify which symptoms or parameters are important for identifying for cervical cancer, as well as the causes and effects of these symptoms and parameters.

This study has further performed a survey with 132 participants in Saudi Arabia to explore cervical cancer awareness, focusing on the human papillomavirus (HPV). This data is mainly gathered to identify individuals' thoughts and comments regarding HPV and cervical cancer. By conducting survey-based data analysis, the study has evaluated and rated the women's awareness and behaviors regardings cervical cancer care. It is notable that the authors did not address why HPV is responsible for cervical cancer; also, the survey did not show how much women knew about the biopsy test.

While working with the proposed models and algorithms, a number of limitations have been observed. First of all, the DT algorithm is very unstable, which means that a slight change in the data will significantly change the layout of the best decision tree. It is insufficiently reliable. With similar data, several other predictors perform better. Second, this study faced massive problems while dealing with the dataset, because numerous data have been enumerated and interpreted in the data pre-processing stage. The model will provide an optimum result only if a considerable number of data-processing techniques have been adopted. Third, the survey data have been preserved to apply machine learning to conduct sentiment analysis regarding cervical cancer, but in this study, the researchers could not accommodate different data-processing techniques to apply the ML models.

6. Conclusions

Early detection increases the likelihood of successful treatment in the pre-cancer and cancer stages. Being aware of any signs and symptoms of cervical cancer can also aid in avoiding diagnostic delays. This research has focused on cervical cancer using conventional machine learning (ML) principles and several traditional machine learning algorithms, such as decision tree (DT), logistic regression (LR), support vector machine (SVM), and K-nearest neighbors (KNN). In terms of cervical cancer prediction, the highest classification score of 100% has been achieved with the random forest (RF), decision tree (DT), adaptive boosting, and gradient boosting algorithms. In contrast, 99% accuracy has been found with SVM. The results of these algorithms are applied to identify the most relevant predictors. We have received satisfactory accuracy compared to the support vector machine algorithm. The findings of this study revealed that the SVM model could be used to find the most important predictors. As the number of essential predictors for analysis decreases, the computational cost of the proposed model decreases. The disease can be predicated more accurately with the use of machine learning. Furthermore, boosting patients' personal health and socio-cultural status can lead to cervical cancer prevention.

In addition, this research conducted a survey in Saudi Arabia, with 250 participants, to learn their thoughts in response to the investigation of cervical cancer; risk factors have also been identified through some data analyses. In the future, this research will experiment with many datasets, analyze various deep learning algorithms and their computational complexity, and show a pipeline that can extract more important insights through statistical analysis in further research.

Author Contributions: Conceptualization, N.A.M. and A.A.; methodology, N.A. and A.A.; software, A.A. and N.A.M.; validation, N.A.M. and A.A.; formal analysis, N.A.M. and A.A.; investigation, A.A.; resources, N.A.M. and A.A.; writing—original draft preparation, N.A.M. and A.A.; writing—review and editing, N.A. and A.A.; supervision, N.A.M. and A.A.; project administration, N.A.M. All authors have read and agreed to the published version of the manuscript.

Funding: The funding for this work was provided by the Research Groups Funding program, grant code (NU/RG/SERC/11/8).

Institutional Review Board Statement: Not applicable.

Informed Consent Statement: Not applicable.

Data Availability Statement: Data of Cervical cancer Availability Statement: dataset was obtained from the open-access Cervical cancer (Risk Factors) Data Set database of Cervical Cancer Risk Factors for Biopsy and are available at https://archive.ics.uci.edu/ml/datasets/Cervical+cancer+%28Risk+Factors%29 (accessed on 24 March 2022).

Acknowledgments: The authors are thankful to the Dean of Scientific Research at Najran University for funding this work under the Research Groups Funding program, grant code (NU/RG/SERC/11/8).

Conflicts of Interest: The authors declare no conflict of interest.

References

1. Martin, C.M.; Astbury, K.; McEvoy, L.; Toole, S.; Sheils, O.; Leary, J.J. Gene expression profiling in cervical cancer: Identification of novel markers for disease diagnosis and therapy. In *Inflammation and Cancer*; Springer: Berlin, Germany, 2009; Volume 511, pp. 333–359.
2. Purnami, S.; Khasanah, P.; Sumartini, S.; Chosuvivatwong, V.; Sriplung, H. Cervical cancer survival prediction using hybrid of SMOTE, CART and smooth support vector machine. *AIP Conf. Proc.* **2016**, *1723*, 030017.
3. Yang, X.; Da, M.; Zhang, W.; Qi, Q.; Zhang, C.; Han, S. Role of lactobacillus in cervical cancer. *Cancer Manag. Res.* **2018**, *10*, 1219–1229. [CrossRef] [PubMed]
4. Ghoneim, A.; Muhammad, G.; Hossain, M.S. Cervical cancer classification using convolutional neural networks and extreme learning machines. *Future Gener. Comput. Syst.* **2020**, *102*, 643–649. [CrossRef]
5. Rehman, O.; Zhuang, H.; Muhamed Ali, A.; Ibrahim, A.; Li, Z. Validation of miRNAs as breast cancer biomarkers with a machine learning approach. *Cancers* **2019**, *11*, 431. [CrossRef] [PubMed]
6. Ashok, B.; Aruna, P. Comparison of Feature selection methods for diagnosis of cervical cancer using SVM classifier. *Int. J. Eng. Res.* **2016**, *6*, 94–99.
7. Kable, A.K.; Pich, J.; Maslin-Prothero, S.E.A. Structured approach to documenting a search strategy for publication: A 12 step guideline for authors. *Nurse Educ. Today* **2012**, *32*, 878–886. [CrossRef]
8. Chatterjee, S.; Divesh, G.; Prakash, A.; Sharma, A. Exploring healthcare/health-product ecommerce satisfaction: A text mining and machine learning application. *J. Bus. Res.* **2021**, *131*, 815–825. [CrossRef]
9. Osuwa, A.; Öztoprak, H. Importance of Continuous Improvement of Machine Learning Algorithms From A Health Care Management and Management Information Systems Perspective. In Proceedings of the 2021 International Conference on Engineering and Emerging Technologies (ICEET), Istanbul, Turkey, 29–30 September 2021; pp. 1–5.
10. Prabhpreet, K.; Gurvinder, S.; Parminder, K. Intellectual detection and validation of automated mammogram breast cancer images by multi-class SVM using deep learning classification. *Inform. Med. Unlocked* **2019**, *16*, 100151.
11. Sharif-Khodaei, Z.; Ghajari, M.; Aliabadi, M.H.; Apicella, A. SMART Platform for Structural Health Monitoring of Sensorised Stiffened Composite Panels. *Key Eng. Mater.* **2012**, *52*, 581–584. [CrossRef]
12. Devi, M.A.; Ravi, S.; Vaishnavi, J.; Punitha, S. Classification of cervical cancer using artificial neural networks. *Procedia Comput. Sci.* **2016**, *89*, 465–472. [CrossRef]
13. Mao, Y.J.; Lim, H.J.; Ni, M.; Yan, W.H.; Wong, D.W.C.; Cheung, J.C.W. Breast Tumour Classification Using Ultrasound Elastography with Machine Learning: A Systematic Scoping Review. *Cancers* **2022**, *14*, 367. [CrossRef] [PubMed]
14. Singh, J.; Sharma, S. Prediction of Cervical Cancer Using Machine Learning Techniques. *Int. J. Appl. Eng. Res.* **2019**, *14*, 2570–2577.
15. Asadi, F.; Salehnasab, C.; Ajori, L. Supervised Algorithms of Machine Learning for the Prediction of Cervical Cancer. *J. Biomed. Phys. Eng.* **2020**, *10*, 509–513.
16. Nithya, B.; Ilango, V. Evaluation of machine learning based optimized feature selection approaches and classification methods for cervical cancer prediction. *SN Appl. Sci.* **2019**, *1*, 641. [CrossRef]
17. Lu, L.; Song, E.; Ghoneim, A.; Alrashoud, M. Machine learning for assisting cervical cancer diagnosis: An ensemble approach. *Future Gener. Comput. Syst.* **2020**, *106*, 199–205. [CrossRef]
18. Alam, T.M.; Khan, A.; Iqbal, A.; Abdul, W.; Mushtaq, M. Cervical cancer prediction through different screening methods using data mining. *Int. J. Adv. Comput. Sci. Appl.* **2019**, *10*, 346–357. [CrossRef]
19. Mukama, T.; Ndejjo, R.; Musabyimana, A.; Halage, A.; Musoke, D. Women's knowledge and attitudes towards cervical cancer prevention: A cross sectional study in Eastern Uganda. *BMC Women's Health* **2017**, *17*, 9. [CrossRef]
20. Shetty, A.; Shah, S. Survey of cervical cancer prediction using machine learning: A comparative approach. In Proceedings of the 2018 9th International Conference on Computing, Communication and Networking Technologies (ICCCNT), Bengaluru, India, 10–12 July 2018; pp. 1–6.
21. Bahad, P.; Saxena, P. Study of adaboost and gradient boosting algorithms for predictive analytics. In Proceedings of the Intelligent Computing and Smart Communication, Singapore, 20 December 2019.
22. Weegar, R.; Sundström, K. Using machine learning for predicting cervical cancer from Swedish electronic health records by mining hierarchical representations. *PLoS ONE* **2020**, *15*, e0237911. [CrossRef]
23. Dokduang, K.; Chiewchanwattana, S.; Sunat, K.; Tangvoraphonkchai, V. A comparative machine learning algorithm to predict the bone metastasis cervical cancer with imbalance data problem. *Recent Adv. Inf. Commun. Technol.* **2014**, *10*, 93–102.
24. Šarenac, T.; Mikov, M. Cervical cancer, different treatments and importance of bile acids as therapeutic agents in this disease. *Front. Pharmacol.* **2019**, *10*, 484–513. [CrossRef]

25. Vos, D.; Verwer, S. Efficient Training of Robust Decision Trees Against Adversarial Examples. In Proceedings of the International Conference on Machine Learning—PMLR 2021, Virtual, 18–24 July 2021; Volume 139, pp. 10586–10595.
26. Wang, L. *Support Vector Machines: Theory and Applications*; Springer Science & Business Media: Berlin, Germany, 2015; Volume 177.
27. Shankar, K.; Lakshmanaprabu, S.K.; Gupta, D.; Maseleno, A.; Albuquerque, V.H. Optimal feature-based multi-kernel SVM approach for thyroid disease classification. *J. Supercomput.* **2020**, *76*, 1128–1143. [CrossRef]
28. González-Recio, O.; Jiménez-Montero, J.; Alenda, R. The gradient boosting algorithm and random boosting for genome-assisted evaluation in large data sets. *J. Dairy Sci.* **2013**, *96*, 614–624. [CrossRef] [PubMed]
29. Fernandes, K.; Jaime, S.; Cardoso, G.; Fernandes, J. Transfer Learning with Partial Observability Applied to Cervical Cancer Screening. In Proceedings of the Iberian Conference on Pattern Recognition and Image Analysis, Faro, Portugal, 20–23 June 2017; Springer International Publishing: Berlin, Germany, 2017. Available online: https://archive.ics.uci.edu/ml/datasets/Cervical+cancer+%28Risk+Factors%29 (accessed on 24 March 2022).
30. Bentéjac, C.; Csörgő, A.; Martínez-Muñoz, G. A comparative analysis of gradient boosting algorithms. *Artif. Intell.* **2021**, *54*, 1937–1967. [CrossRef]
31. Novaković, D.; Veljović, A.S.; Ilić, S.; Papić, Ž; Tomović, M. Evaluation of classification models in machine learning. *Theory Appl. Math. Comput. Sci.* **2017**, *7*, 39–46.
32. Raschka, S. *Model Evaluation, Model Selection, and Algorithm Selection in Machine Learning*; University of Wisconsin: Madison, WI, USA, 2018.
33. Sadrawi, M.; Lin, Y.T.; Lin, C.H.; Mathunjwa, B.; Fan, S.Z.; Abbod, M.F.; Shieh, J.S. Genetic Deep Convolutional Autoencoder Applied for Generative Continuous Arterial Blood Pressure via Photoplethysmography. *Sensors* **2020**, *20*, 3829. [CrossRef]
34. Hall, M.A. *Correlation-Based Feature Selection for Machine Learning*; The University of Waikato: Hamilton, New Zealand, 1999.
35. Kondratenko, Y.; Atamanyuk, I.; Sidenko, I.; Kondratenko, G.; Sichevskyi, S. Machine Learning Techniques for Increasing Efficiency of the Robot's Sensor and Control Information Processing. *Sensors* **2022**, *22*, 1062. [CrossRef]
36. Żelasko, D.; Książek, W.; Pławiak, P. Transmission Quality Classification with Use of Fusion of Neural Network and Genetic Algorithm in Pay&Require Multi-Agent Managed Network. *Sensors* **2021**, *21*, 4090.
37. Scribber, A. *How to Use Stratified Sampling*; 2020; Volume 21, pp. 234–248.
38. Li, J.P.; Haq, A.U.; Din, S.U.; Khan, J.; Khan, A.; Saboor, A. Heart Disease Identification Method Using Machine Learning Classification in E-Healthcare. *IEEE Access* **2020**, *8*, 107562–107582. [CrossRef]
39. Krishnamoorthi, R.; Joshi, S.; Almarzouki, H.Z.; Shukla, P.K.; Rizwan, A.; Kalpana, C.; Tiwari, B. A Novel Diabetes Healthcare Disease Prediction Framework Using Machine Learning Techniques. *J. Healthc. Eng.* **2022**, *2*, 37–45. [CrossRef]
40. Ganesan, M.; Sivakumar, N. IoT based heart disease prediction and diagnosis model for healthcare using machine learning models. In Proceedings of the 2019 IEEE International Conference on System, Computation, Automation and Networking (ICSCAN), Pondicherry, India, 29–30 March 2019; pp. 1–5.
41. Matsuo, K.; Purushotham, S.; Jiang, B.; Mandelbaum, R.S.; Takiuchi, Y.; Liu, T. Survival outcome prediction in cervical cancer: Cox models vs deep-learning model. *Am. J. Obstet. Gynecol.* **2019**, *220*, 38–381. [CrossRef]
42. Zhang, W.; Li, X.; Ma, H.; Luo, Z.; Li, X. Federated learning for machinery fault diagnosis with dynamic validation and self-supervision. *Knowl.-Based Syst.* **2021**, *213*, 106679. [CrossRef]

sensors

MDPI

Article

On the Automatic Detection and Classification of Skin Cancer Using Deep Transfer Learning

Mohammad Fraiwan *and Esraa Faouri

Department of Computer Engineering, Jordan University of Science and Technology, Irbid 22110, Jordan; enfaouri@just.edu.jo
* Correspondence: mafraiwan@just.edu.jo

Abstract: Skin cancer (melanoma and non-melanoma) is one of the most common cancer types and leads to hundreds of thousands of yearly deaths worldwide. It manifests itself through abnormal growth of skin cells. Early diagnosis drastically increases the chances of recovery. Moreover, it may render surgical, radiographic, or chemical therapies unnecessary or lessen their overall usage. Thus, healthcare costs can be reduced. The process of diagnosing skin cancer starts with dermoscopy, which inspects the general shape, size, and color characteristics of skin lesions, and suspected lesions undergo further sampling and lab tests for confirmation. Image-based diagnosis has undergone great advances recently due to the rise of deep learning artificial intelligence. The work in this paper examines the applicability of raw deep transfer learning in classifying images of skin lesions into seven possible categories. Using the HAM1000 dataset of dermoscopy images, a system that accepts these images as input without explicit feature extraction or preprocessing was developed using 13 deep transfer learning models. Extensive evaluation revealed the advantages and shortcomings of such a method. Although some cancer types were correctly classified with high accuracy, the imbalance of the dataset, the small number of images in some categories, and the large number of classes reduced the best overall accuracy to 82.9%.

Keywords: deep learning; skin lesions; skin cancer; melanoma; image classification

Citation: Fraiwan, M.; Faouri, E. On the Automatic Detection of Skin Cancer Using Deep Transfer Learning. *Sensors* **2022**, *22*, 4963. https://doi.org/10.3390/s22134963

Academic Editors: Ayman El-baz, Guruprasad A. Giridharan, Ahmed Shalaby, Ali H. Mahmoud and Mohammed Ghazal

Received: 4 June 2022
Accepted: 29 June 2022
Published: 30 June 2022

1. Introduction

Skin cancer is considered one of the most dangerous types of cancer in the world [1,2], and the number of deaths is increasing daily as a result of this disease [3,4]. Moreover, it is one of the fastest spreading types of cancer [5]. However, treatment is possible if it is detected in its early stages [6]. According to recent statistics, it was reported that 20% of skin cancer reached a point where survival is not possible due to the disease progression [7]. Worldwide, approximately 50,000 people die each year from skin cancer [7,8], which represents 0.7 of the death rate due to cancer [8]. The estimated cost of treatment is approximately USD 30 million, which is prohibitive for treatment [5].

Doctors use multiple methods to detect skin cancer [9]. Visual detection is the initial way to identify the possibility of the disease [10,11]. The American Center for the Study of Dermatology developed a guide for the possible shape of melanoma, which is called ABCD (asymmetry, border, color, diameter) [2,12,13] and is used by doctors for initial screening of the disease. If a suspected skin lesion is found, the doctor takes a biopsy of the visible lesion on the skin [14], and examines it microscopically for a benign or malignant diagnosis and the type of skin cancer [15]. Dermoscopy is a technique that doctors use to diagnose skin cancer [16]. It involves taking bright pictures of the shape of the skin lesion, which comes in the form of dark spots [17]. However, this method faces many difficulties, the most important of which is the inability to determine the nature of the lesion due to the surrounding conditions such as the presence of hair, blood vessels, correct lighting, inability to take the correct shape of the spot, and the similarity of the shape of the spots among cancerous and non-cancerous diseases [18,19]. Moreover, some people may ignore skin lesions due to poverty, lack of access to proper healthcare, or misdiagnosis. Given an image of a skin lesion, the goal of this work to easily and automatically classify this image into benign or possible cancer. Such a system can be deployed as an easy-to-use smartphone application.

The contributions of this paper are as follows:

1. Develop an artificial intelligence-based screening system for skin cancer (melanoma and non-melanoma) using dermoscopic images of the skin lesions as input. Such a system can aid in clinical screening tests, reduce errors, and improve early diagnosis;
2. Implement transfer learning of 13 deep convolutional neural networks models for the classification of skin lesion images into seven categories, including melanoma, benign keratosis-like lesions, and five other non-melanoma cancers;
3. Evaluate classification performance using common relevant metrics for all models. In addition, the training behavior and time requirements were also included.

The remainder of this paper is organized as follows: the related work is discussed in Section 2, the dataset, deep learning models, and performance evaluation metrics and setup are explained in detail in Section 3, Section 4 presents the performance evaluation results along with a comparison to the related literature and discussion of the models, and we conclude in Section 5.

2. Related Work

Recent advances in artificial intelligence (AI) during the past decade and specifically in the field of deep learning and convolutional neural networks (CNNs) have opened the door for the development of reliable screening and diagnosis image-based medical systems [20]. The research landscape has recently witnessed a shift from image segmentation (i.e., separation of relevant areas in the image) and feature extraction toward automated classification using deep learning. The literature in the context of skin cancer detection/screening followed a similar trajectory with the traditional approach of image processing to remove irrelevant artifacts (e.g., hair) being overcome by using sophisticated deep learning artificial intelligence. Such recent techniques do not require explicit feature extraction and are generally immune to noise factors that affect images (e.g., light intensity, color, translation, reflection, etc.) [21]. However, they tend to be computationally intensive [22].

Li et al. [1] proposed digital hair removal (DHS) to filter the hair out of the skin lesion image, and analyzed the effect of hair removal using intra-structural similarity (Intra-SSIM). In another study, Liu et al. [23] developed a new method using deep learning to segment lesion images according to regions of interest (ROI). They used a new mid-level feature representation, where pre-trained neural networks (e.g., ResNet and DenseNet) were used to extract information from the ROI. Similarly, Pour and Seker [24] used convolutional neural networks for the segmentation of lesions and dermoscopic features. They used the CIELAB color space in addition to RGB color channels instead of excessive augmentation or using a pertained model. Almansi et al. [25] proposed a new segmentation methodology using full-resolution convolutional networks (FrCN). They worked on the image without pre/post-processing, and their results showed that the proposed method (FrCN) yielded better results than the other deep learning segmentation approaches. Dash et al. [26] proposed a new segmentation method based on a deep fully convolutional network comprised of 29 layers. Xie et al. [27] proposed the segmentation of dermoscopy images based on a convolutional neural network with an attention mechanism, which can preserve edge details. Serte and Demirel [28] proposed a novel Gabor wavelet-based deep learning model for the classification of melanoma and seborrheic keratosis. This model builds on an ensemble of seven Gabor wavelet-based CNN models. Furthermore, their model fuses the Gabor wavelet-based model and an image-based CNN model. The performance evaluation results showed that an ensemble of the image and Gabor wavelet-based models outperformed the individual separate image and Gabor wavelet-based models. This ensemble also outperformed the group of only Gabor wavelet-based CNN models.

Deep transfer learning has been widely deployed in the medical imaging literature for powerful, automatic, and internal (i.e., implicit) feature extraction. In this regard, Manzo et al. [29] employed a three-step approach for melanoma detection. In the first step, the images are converted into the proper size and the dataset is balanced. After that, deep transfer learning is used for feature extraction. These features feed an ensemble of traditional classification algorithms, including support-vector machine (SVM), logistic label propagation (LLP), and k-nearest neighbors (KNN). Jain et al. [30] compared six different transfer learning networks for multiclass lesion classification. However, their reported results relied upon increasing the size of the dataset by augmentation. Augmentation is typically used to introduce changes into the input images without duplication. Thus, making several augmented copies of the same image in the dataset will result in biased results that do not represent the actual performance [21].

3. Materials and Methods

Figure 1 shows the steps used to develop the skin cancer classification system using images of skin lesions. The methods used in this work do not need any feature extraction, nor does it perform any segmentation (i.e., separation of lesions from the rest of the image). All of these are automatically handled by the complexities of the deep learning model layers and operations. The next few subsections explain each part in detail.

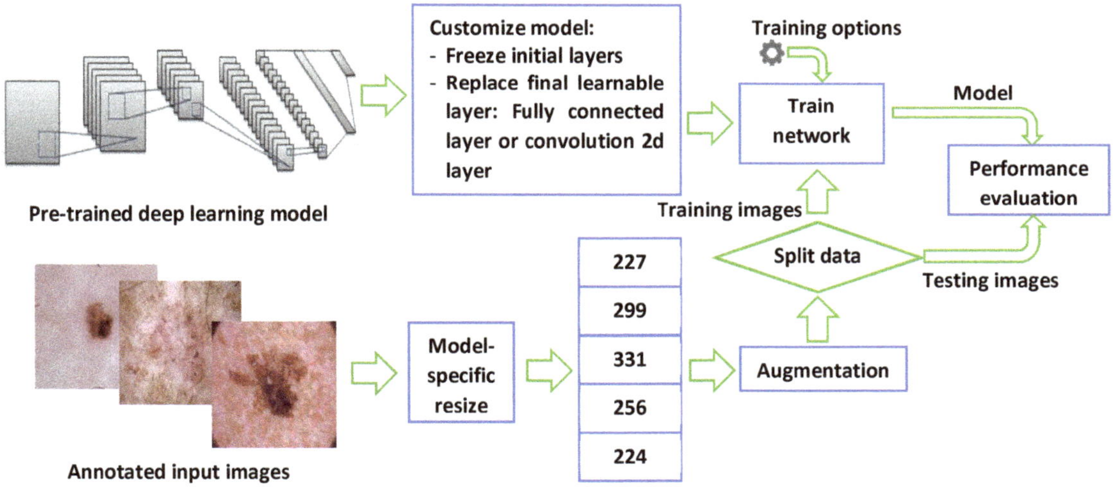

Figure 1. A graphical abstract of the general steps used in this paper.

3.1. Dataset

This work uses the dataset called HAM1000 (Human Against Machine) [2], which is comprised of 10,015 dermatoscopic images of the most common skin cancers. The images are divided into seven categories: 327 actinic keratosis and intraepithelial carcinoma (AKIEC), 514 basal cell carcinoma (BCC), 1099 benign keratosis-like lesions (BLS), 115 dermatofibroma (DF), 1113 melanoma (Mel), 6705 melanocytic nevi (NV), and 142 vascular lesions (VASC). Two augmentation operations were applied: random x-y scaling in the range (0.9, 1.1), and random x-y translation in the pixel range (−30, 30).

3.2. Deep Learning Models

Transfer learning has been found to be extremely effective in many image-based medical applications [31]. It replaces ad hoc deep convolutional neural network (CNN) designs with pre-trained, well-designed, and extensively-tested models. The initial layers of such models are trained to detect generic image features such as color, contrast, etc. On the other hand, later layers toward the output need to be customized and retrained on specific task-related features. Such methodology has proved its worth in a wide range of studies [20,22,32]. In this paper, 13 deep learning models were customized, retrained, evaluated individually, and compared on their ability to classify skin lesions into the seven aforementioned categories in the HAM1000 dataset. These were: SqueezeNet [33], GoogLeNet [34], Inceptionv3 [35], DenseNet-201 [36], MobileNetv2, ResNet18, Rest-Net50, ResNet101, Xception [37], Inception-ResNet, ShuffleNet [38], DarkNet-53 [39], and EfficientNet-b0 [40]. These models require input images to be of a certain size. More specifically, these models require the input to be of size 224 × 224 × 3, 227 × 227 × 3, 256 × 256 × 3, 299 × 299 × 3, or 331 × 331× 3. However, all of them were pre-trained using ImageNet [41].

3.3. Performance Evaluation Metrics and Setup

The performance was evaluated using five metrics [42]: accuracy, precision, recall, specificity, and F1 score. The accuracy measures the ratio of true positive plus true negatives for all the images. Precision measures the ratio of true positives to all elements identified as positives (including false positives). Recall (i.e., sensitivity) measures the ratio of true positives to all relevant elements (i.e., the actual positives). Specificity (i.e., selectivity) measures the ratio of true negatives to all images that are actually negative, and the F1 score is the harmonic mean of the recall and precision and expresses the accuracy of classification in unbalanced datasets. The five measures are defined in Equations (1)–(5). The reported results refer to the mean overall value when each separate class is considered as the positive case.

The model parameters were commonly set for all models as follows: minimum batch size = 16 (higher values are more computationally efficient but require significantly more memory), maximum number of epochs = 10 (no need to do further training if the loss/validation curve flattens out after a certain number of epochs with no improvement), initial learning rate = 0.0003, and the network solver = stochastic gradient descent with momentum (SGDM). Three strategies for data splitting into training and validation were used (i.e., 70/30, 80/20, and 90/10), which will measure the models' improvement if more input images were available and their ability to generalize without overfitting the input images. Input images were augmented to increase their variety by using standard image processing operations as follows: random axis translation (i.e., image movement over the x and y axes) = (−30, 30), and random scaling using the range (0.9, 1.1).

The implementation and evaluation of the models was conducted using MATLAB R2021a software running on an HP OMEN 30L desktop GT13 with 64 GB RAM, an NVIDIA GeForce RTX 3080 GPU, an Intel Core i7-10700K CPU @ 3.80 GHz, and a 1TB SSD.

$$Accuracy = \frac{TP + TN}{P + N} \tag{1}$$

$$Precision = \frac{TP}{TP + FP} \tag{2}$$

$$Recall = \frac{TP}{TP + FN} \tag{3}$$

$$Specificity = \frac{TN}{TN + FP} \tag{4}$$

$$F1 = 2 \times \frac{Recall \times Precision}{Recall + Precision} \tag{5}$$

where TP represents the number of correctly classified images, FP represents the number of wrongly classified images as another class, FN indicates the number of images missed by the classifier, P indicates the number of all images considered as the positive class, and N is the number of all images other than the positive class.

4. Results and Discussion

The related work in the literature has already established that high performance is achievable in binary (i.e., benign vs. melanoma) or ternary (i.e., benign vs. melanoma vs. non-melanoma) classification of skin lesion images. The goal of the experiments was to evaluate the ability of transfer learning of the deep convolutional network models to correctly classify skin lesion images into one of the seven aforementioned categories in the dataset. Moreover, the training was repeated for 10 times to account for variability in the random data split of images into training and validation, and the mean values were reported. In addition, due to the high computational cost of deep learning models, the training and validation times were also included in the results.

Table 1 shows the mean overall performance metrics over 10 runs of each of the 13 deep learning models and using 70% of the data for training. All models achieved comparable accuracy values, with Resnet101 performing the best with 76.7%. The sample confusion matrix with row and column summaries in Figure 2 provides further insight into the results. First, due to the imbalanced number of images in each class and with smaller-sized classes achieving lower accuracies, the F1 score numbers are lower than the accuracy values. The NV class with the largest number of images achieved the highest precision (92.5%; see the NV column summary) and highest recall (82.5%; see the NV row summary). In comparison, the melanoma class was detected with 71% sensitivity (i.e., recall) but 43.1% precision. However, the other classes show less precision/recall variation.

Figure 3 shows a sample training/validation progress curve for Resnet101 and a 70/30 data split. This figure shows two possible observations: first, the model is unable to achieve consistently reduced loss and produce high testing accuracy, even when the number of epochs is increased (not reported here), and second, due to the small number of images in most classes (deep learning requires large datasets [43]), there is an obvious gap between the validation vs testing performance (i.e., overfitting or inability to generalize to the validation data).

Table 2 shows the mean overall performance metrics over 10 runs of each of the 13 deep learning models using 80% of the data for training. The 10% increase in the size of the training set did not have a significant effect on the performance metrics, with the best F1 score being 66.1% (DenseNet201 model). The confusion matrix in Figure 4 shows that a major source for errors was the misclassification of NV images as melanoma. Most classes achieved relatively high precision but low recall. Moreover, the same training and overfitting trends appear in Figure 5.

Table 1. The mean overall Accuracy, F-score, Precision, Recall, and Specificity for each deep learning model and 70/30 data split.

Model	F1 Score	Precision	Recall	Specificity	Accuracy
SqueezeNet	51.2%	63.1%	49.6%	93.8%	71.7%
GoogLeNet	55.4%	63.2%	53.4%	94.3%	74.0%
Inceptionv3	61.5%	65.5%	60.7%	94.5%	74.2%
DenseNet201	64.8%	70.9%	62.7%	94.7%	75.8%
MobileNetv2	61.0%	67.2%	58.4%	94.1%	75.6%
Resnet101	64.3%	67.6%	63.8%	95.0%	76.7%
Resnet50	63.4%	68.5%	62.4%	94.7%	74.4%
Resnet18	59.3%	64.7%	57.8%	94.6%	75.3%
Xception	60.9%	66.5%	59.2%	94.7%	75.4%
Inception-ResNet-v2	61.4%	65.3%	60.8%	94.4%	75.5%
ShuffleNet	60.6%	64.9%	58.7%	93.5%	74.6%
DarkNet-53	61.9%	66.8%	61.9%	94.5%	71.6%
EfficientNetb0	57.6%	70.3%	53.7%	94.1%	73.8%

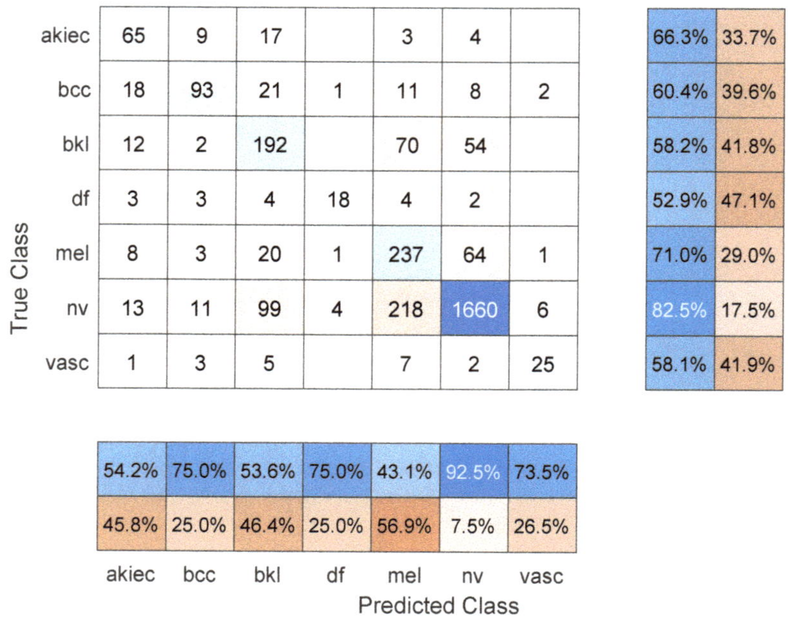

Figure 2. Sample confusion matrix for Resnet101 model and 70/30 data split.

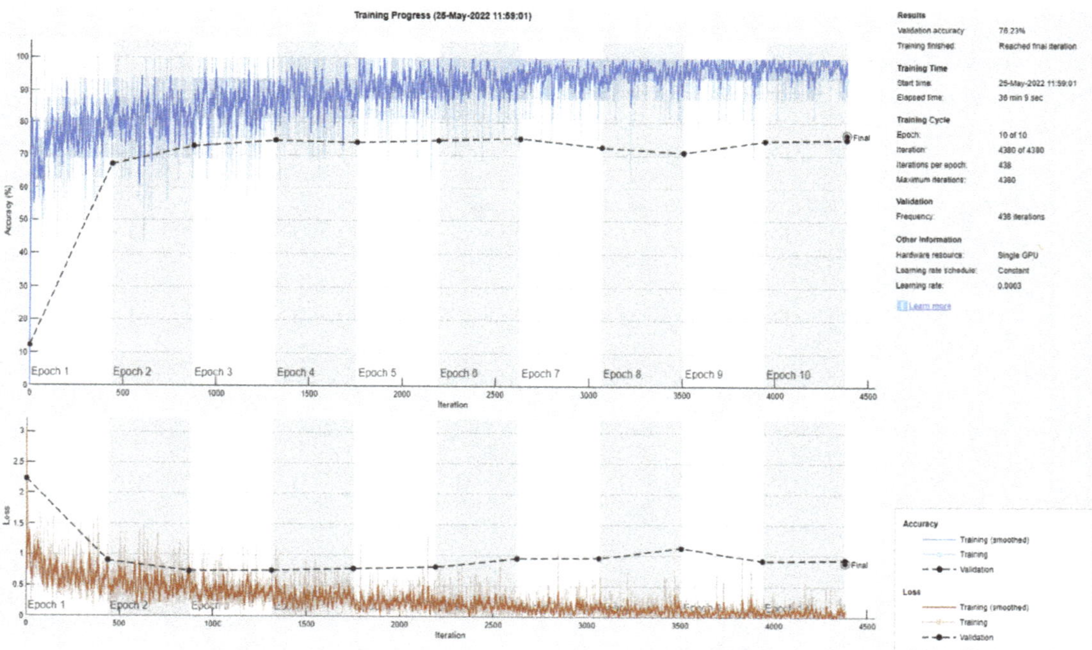

Figure 3. Sample training/validation progress curve for Resnet101 and 70/30 data split.

Table 2. The mean overall accuracy, F-score, precision, recall, and specificity for each deep learning model and an 80/20 data split.

Model	F1 Score	Precision	Recall	Specificity	Accuracy
SqueezeNet	52.6%	64.0%	50.8%	93.4%	68.0%
GoogLeNet	56.2%	70.0%	53.8%	93.4%	68.5%
Inceptionv3	61.1%	64.2%	62.6%	94.0%	68.8%
DenseNet201	66.1%	74.7%	63.3%	94.3%	73.5%
MobileNetv2	61.5%	65.9%	60.2%	93.9%	73.0%
Resnet101	62.3%	69.0%	62.2%	94.2%	70.2%
Resnet50	63.2%	71.7%	61.8%	93.9%	67.7%
Resnet18	62.2%	64.7%	63.2%	93.8%	69.6%
Xception	56.1%	61.3%	55.9%	94.0%	70.2%
Inception-ResNet-v2	58.5%	63.9%	59.7%	93.8%	67.4%
ShuffleNet	61.2%	70.2%	57.8%	93.3%	70.0%
DarkNet-53	61.4%	70.7%	58.5%	93.6%	70.2%
EfficientNetb0	56.0%	69.8%	52.6%	93.6%	72.2%

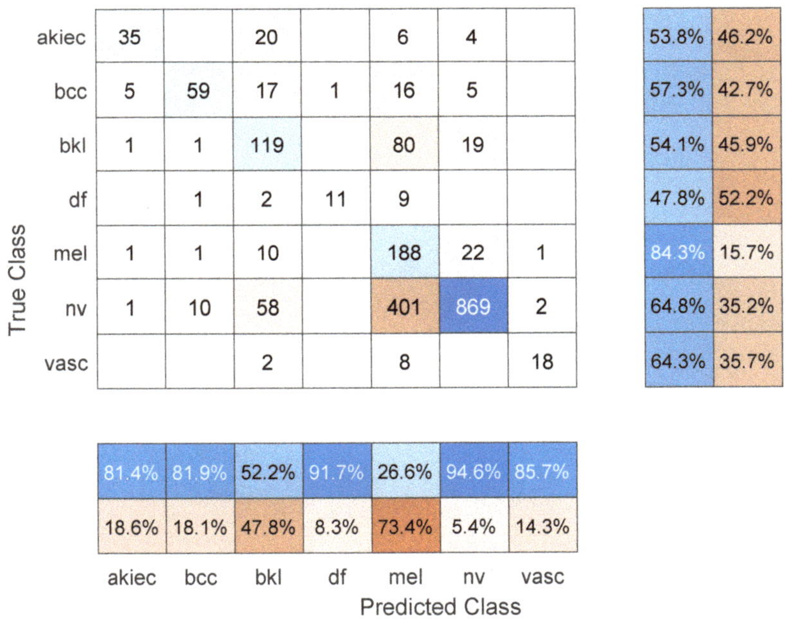

Figure 4. Sample confusion matrix for DenseNet201 model and 80/20 data split.

A further 10% increase in training data made the percentage of testing images 90% of the dataset. Table 3 shows the mean overall performance metrics over 10 runs of each of the 13 deep learning models. Three of the models (i.e., DenseNet201, DarkNet53, and ResNet101) achieved an accuracy above 80% with a corresponding F1 score of 74.4% for DenseNet201. The table shows steady improvement for most models with a larger set of training data over all metrics, except for the small model SqueezeNet. Generally, deep learning models, unlike traditional machine learning, benefit from larger datasets [44], which may be the reason for improved performance. The sample confusion matrix for DarkNet-53 in Figure 6 shows considerably better performance in terms of entries with one or fewer false misclassifications. However, the training/validation progress curve in Figure 7 still shows signs of overfitting.

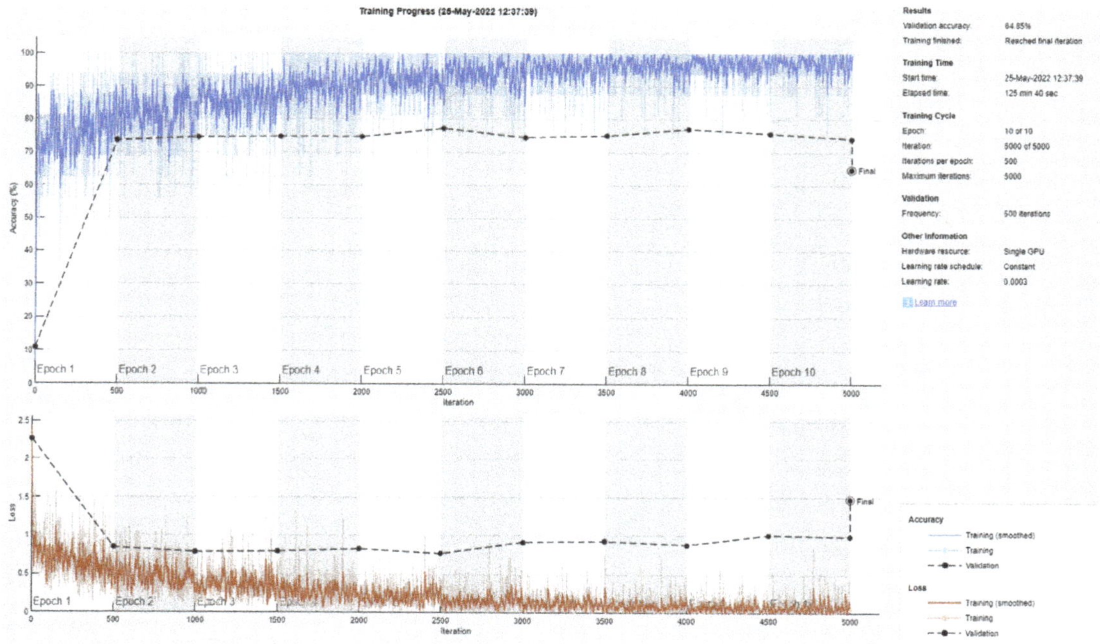

Figure 5. Sample training/validation progress curve for DenseNet201 and 80/20 data split.

Although an increased size of the training dataset showed signs of promise, much is still desired to reach a reliable diagnosis system that surpasses screening requirements. However, some of the results were affected by the small number of images in each class. For example, in Figure 6, the class DF had 11 images, VASC had 14 images, and AKIEC had 32 images. Such numbers are extremely low for an effective deep learning model, and single errors will have a profound effect on overall performance indices.

Table 3. The mean overall accuracy, F-score, precision, recall, and specificity for each deep learning model and 90/10 data split.

Model	F1 Score	Precision	Recall	Specificity	Accuracy
SqueezeNet	52.7%	67.1%	48.0%	92.7%	75.0%
GoogLeNet	54.5%	64.2%	53.1%	94.5%	73.4%
Inceptionv3	67.9%	69.9%	70.1%	95.3%	79.3%
DenseNet201	74.4%	78.5%	73.6%	96.0%	82.9%
MobileNetv2	63.5%	68.8%	63.4%	94.8%	74.9%
Resnet101	71.7%	71.1%	74.5%	96.3%	81.2%
Resnet50	67.8%	72.6%	68.3%	95.5%	77.8%
Resnet18	67.9%	72.3%	68.3%	95.1%	79.0%
Xception	59.5%	65.0%	58.5%	94.4%	72.1%
Inception-ResNet-v2	64.4%	66.6%	66.8%	94.8%	73.9%
ShuffleNet	65.8%	74.0%	61.8%	94.3%	79.0%
DarkNet-53	66.3%	70.0%	66.1%	95.1%	80.8%
EfficientNetb0	61.3%	73.4%	57.0%	94.7%	76.7%

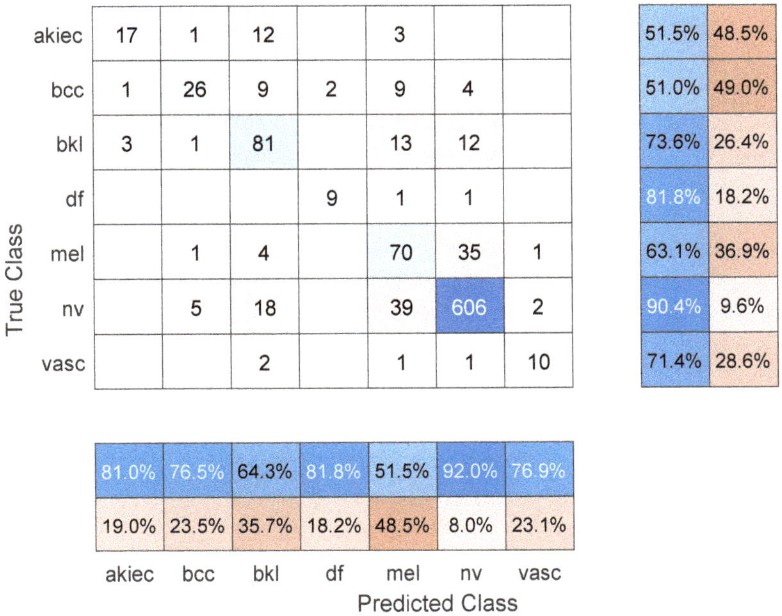

Figure 6. Sample confusion matrix for DarkNet-53 model and 90/10 data split.

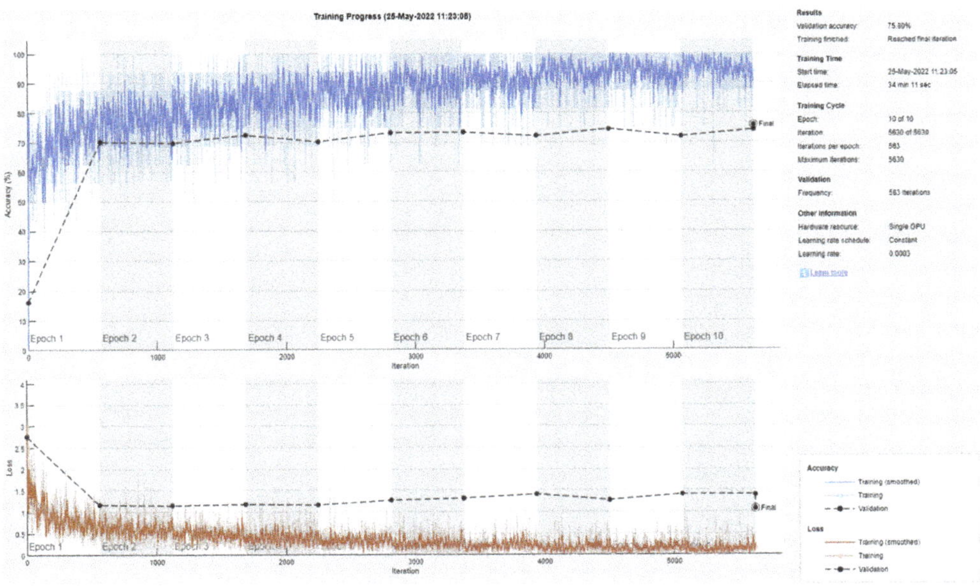

Figure 7. Sample training/validation progress curve for DarkNet-53 and 90/10 data split.

To assess the computational cost of training the deep learning models, the time required for each model was reported for each strategy of data split; see Table 4. In general, the required time increases linearly in less than 10% increments with each increase in the size of the training dataset. SqueezeNet is the fastest model, but DarkNet-53 is the best model that combines classification prowess with speed of training, followed by Resnet101.

Table 4. The mean training and validation times for all algorithms and data split strategies. All times are in seconds.

Data Split / Model	70/30	80/20	90/10
SqueezeNet	377.0	400.4	422.6
GoogLeNet	726.8	795	855.0
Inceptionv3	2182.9	2419.9	2655.2
DenseNet201	7190.8	7884.7	8686.6
MobileNetv2	3266.3	3678.5	4028.5
Resnet101	2196.5	2449.5	2682.7
Resnet50	992.2	1100.0	1192.9
Resnet18	413.6	439.9	470.0
Xception	9076.2	10,111.1	11,094.8
Inception-ResNet-v2	6698.0	7495.4	8254.3
ShuffleNet	2386.9	2641.0	2916.0
DarkNet-53	1761	1974.6	2126.3
EfficientNet-b0	5432.4	6028.4	6737.5

A comparison to the related literature is shown in Table 5. Although the referenced studies achieve high performance values, they tackle a far easier problem in classifying fewer number of classes (two or three). Moreover, some of these studies require explicit feature extraction, which is not needed by deep transfer learning. Others, including Pezhman Pour and Seker [24] and Lie et al. [1], do not address the classification problem directly but rather on processing techniques for lesion segmentation (i.e., separation of lesion from other artifacts in the image) and hair removal from lesion images, respectively.

Table 5. A summary of the latest literature in automatic skin lesion classification.

Study	Objective	Dataset	Approach	Performance
Li et al. (2020) [23]	Two-class classification: melanoma and seborrheic keratosis	600 images	Mid-level features and segmentation according to ROI	Area under the receiver-operating characteristic curve, ResNet (89.00%), DenseNet (88.85%), Fusion(90.67%)
Pezhman Pour and Seker [24]	Lesion segmentation	3879 images	Dermoscopic feature segmentation using CNN	2% and 7% improvement in Jaccard index and sensitivity, respectively
Al-masni et al. [25]	Three-class classification: melanoma, benign, and seborrheic keratosis	2950 images	Segmentation using FrCN	Segmentation accuracy of 95.62% (clinical benign cases), 90.78% (melanoma, and 91.29% (seborrheic keratosis)
Dash et al.[26]	Three-class classification: moderate, severe, and very severe	6267 images	Segmentation using modified U-Net architecture	93.03% Dice coefficient, 94.8% accuracy, 89.6% sensitivity, and 97.60% specificity
Xie et al. [27]	Segmentation into two semantic classes: lesion and background	1479 images	Segmentation of dermoscopy images preserving edge details	Jaccard indices of 0.783, 0.858, and 0.857
Serte et al. [28]	Two-class classification: melanoma and seborrheic keratosis	2000 images	Gabor wavelet-based deep learning model for melanoma and seborrheic keratosis	Average area under the receiver-operating characteristic curve, 91%
Li et al. [1]	Optimal hair removal (reduce over/under removal)	1751 dermoscopic images with hair occlusion	Digital hair removal from images of skin lesion using CNN	Accuracy (99.08%), Specificity (99.85%), F1 score (94.43%), precision (99.09%), sensitivity (95.74%)
This work	Seven-class classification	10015 dermoscopic images	Deep transfer learning of a CNN	Accuracy (82.9%)

Special Cases

Further investigation of the classification performance and training behavior was conducted in order to shed light on shortcomings, as follows:

- Maximum number of epochs. Increasing the number of epochs will require more training time and may achieve better performance if the model has more room to learn, especially in large datasets. However, an exaggerated value for this hyper-parameter may lead to overfitting. Three models were retrained with a maximum number of epochs = 50. These were: Resnet101 with a 70/30 data split, DenseNet201 with an 80/20 data split, and DarkNet-53 with a 90/10 data split. In comparison to the values in Tables 1–3, the F1 score for Resnet101 improved slightly to 67.2% (was 64.3%), DenseNet201 performed a little worse with an F1-score of 63.7%, down from 66.1% in Table 2 (i.e., the model started to overfit the training data), and Darknet-53 improved to an F1-score of 83.1%. The other performance metrics showed similar trends to the F1 score. Figures 8–10 show the corresponding confusion matrices;
- Classifying a lesser number of skin cancer types. Since the dataset is highly imbalanced with some classes having a significantly smaller number of images in the dataset (e.g., 115 DF and 142 VASC), it is worthwhile to explore several subsets of the classification problem as follows:
  - Eliminate the DF and VASC classes and perform 5-class classification. The same three models and corresponding data split as in the previous case with a maximum number of epochs = 10 were used. Surprisingly, in comparison to Tables 1–3, the F1 score displayed very small change (Resnet101: 64.8%, DenseNet201: 65.2%, and DarkNet-53: 67.1%), which was similar to the trend in the other performance metrics;
  - Eliminate the BCC (514 images), AKIEC (327 images), DF, and VASC classes and perform 3-class classification. The Resnet101 (70/30 data split), DenseNet201 (80/20 data split), and DarkNet-53 (90/10) were used with a maximum number of epochs =10. An easier classification problem has resulted in an improved F1 score for Resnet101 and DarkNet-53 of 71.1% and 72.8%, respectively. However, DenseNet201 performed worse at 62.3%, probably due to overfitting;
  - Using the same setup as above, perform pair-wise 2-class classification on the three classes, NV, MEL, and BKL. For the MEL vs. BKL classification, the F1 score of Resnet101 = 80.6%, DenseNet = 73.44%, and DarkNet201 = 83.7%. For the NV vs. MEL classification, all models performed badly. The F1 score for Resnet101 = 58.8%, DenseNet201 = 55.13%, and DarkNet-53 = 63.4%. Although the two classes have a good number of images, it seems like the similarities between the two types are too difficult to spot. Moreover, the lack of proper image cropping (i.e., elimination of useless parts of the images and keeping the lesion) contributed to this factor as it consumes a significant part of the image representation, especially that these algorithms require a scaled-down copy of the input, as mentioned in Section 3. The last pair-wise classification problem is NV vs. BKL, for which Resnet 101 achieved an F1 score = 72.8% (93% accuracy), DenseNet201 reported a 71.8% F1 score and 91.9% accuracy, and DarkNet-53 managed a 70.0% F1 score and 89.9% accuracy.

Surprisingly, lowering the number of classes did not result in improved performance in general. Although deep transfer learning has been effective in many medical and image-based applications, it seems like its application in this scenario requires more investigation and probably larger datasets.

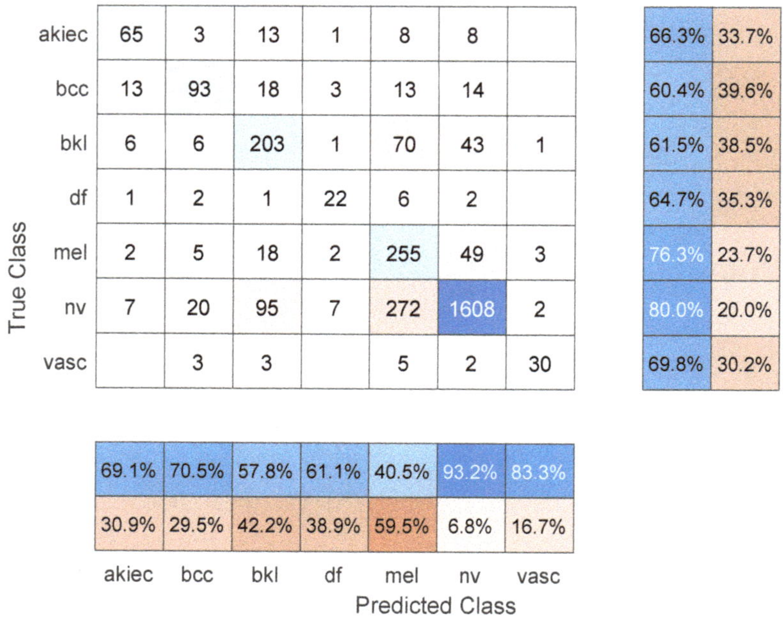

Figure 8. Sample confusion matrix for Resnet101 model, 70/30 data split and 50 epochs of training.

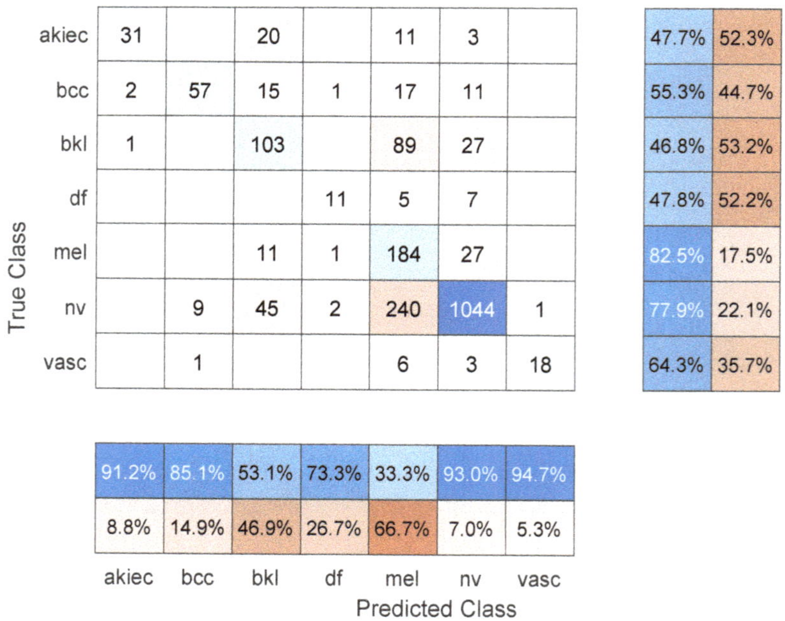

Figure 9. Sample confusion matrix for DenseNet201 model, 80/20 data split and 50 epochs of training.

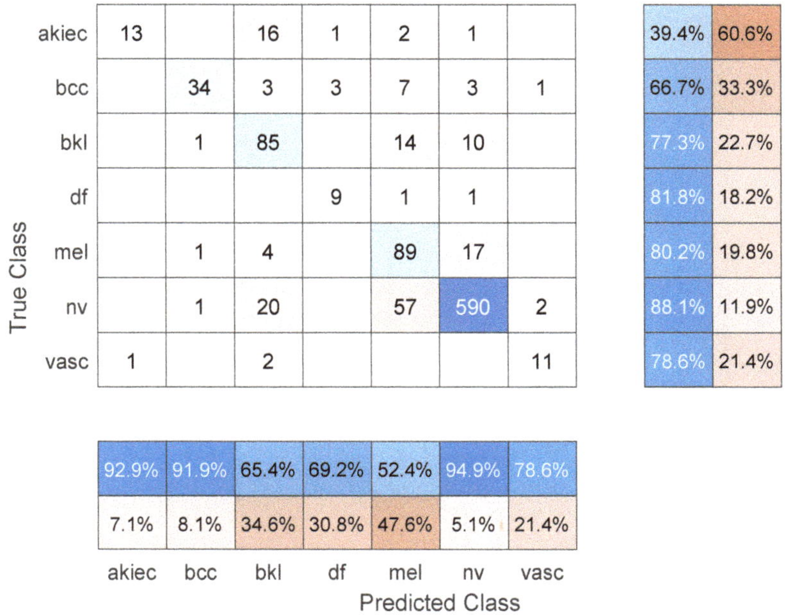

Figure 10. Sample confusion matrix for DarkNet-53 model, 90/10 data split and 50 epochs of training.

5. Conclusions

Skin cancer in both melanoma and non-melanoma types is common and leads to many yearly deaths worldwide. Early diagnosis has been show to drastically reduce therapy time, cost, and suffering from the prolonged traditional treatment methods (e.g., chemotherapy). However, accurate screening/diagnosis requires specialist knowledge of the different types of cancers and how they appear in the form of skin lesions. Some people may ignore such lesions due to ignorance, indifference, cost, or doctor appointment scheduling delays. Recently, the field of deep learning and artificial intelligence has opened the door for the development of reliable image-based medical systems for screening and diagnosis. In this paper, we have used a well-known dermoscopy dataset of seven common types of cancerous skin lesions, utilized recent advances in the design of deep convolutional neural networks, and applied deep transfer learning to the application of screening/diagnosing skin lesion images. Such an approach has the capability to achieve high accuracies that reduce the burden on specialists. Moreover, it can be easily implemented and used in real-life applications due to the elimination of explicit feature extraction or manual image processing. Future work will focus on improving the balance of the dataset by collecting specific dermoscopy images of underrepresented skin lesion types and making those publicly available in the research domain.

Author Contributions: Conceptualization, M.F.; methodology, M.F. and E.F.; software, M.F. and E.F.; validation, M.F. and E.F.; formal analysis, M.F.; investigation, M.F. and E.F.; resources, M.F.; data curation, M.F. and E.F.; writing—original draft preparation, M.F.; writing—review and editing, M.F.; supervision, M.F.; project administration, M.F.; funding acquisition, M.F. All authors have read and agreed to the published version of the manuscript.

Funding: This research is supported by the Deanship of Scientific Research at Jordan University of Science and Technology, Jordan, grants No. 20210047.

Institutional Review Board Statement: Not applicable.

Informed Consent Statement: Not applicable.

Data Availability Statement: Not applicable.

Conflicts of Interest: The authors declare no conflict of interest.

Abbreviations

The following abbreviations are used in this manuscript:

ABCD	Asymmetry, border, color, diameter
AI	Artificial intelligence
CNN	Convolutional neural networks
DHS	Digital hair removal
Intra-SSIM	Intra-structural similarity
ROI	Regions of interest
CIELAB	International Commission on Illumination Lightness A, B
RGB	Red, green, blue
FrCN	Full-resolution convolutional networks
SVM	Support-vector machine
LLP	Logistic label propagation
KNN	K-nearest neighbors
HAM	Human against machine
AKIEC	Actinic keratoses and intraepithelial carcinoma
BCC	Basal cell carcinoma
BLS	Benign keratosis-like lesions
DF	Dermatofibroma
Mel	Melanoma
NV	Melanocytic nevi
VASC	Vascular lesions
TP	True positive
TN	True negative
FN	False negative
FP	False positive
N	Negatives
P	Positives
SGDM	Stochastic gradient descent with momentum

References

1. Li, W.; Raj, A.N.J.; Tjahjadi, T.; Zhuang, Z. Digital hair removal by deep learning for skin lesion segmentation. *Pattern Recognit.* **2021**, *117*, 107994. [CrossRef]
2. Tschandl, P.; Rosendahl, C.; Kittler, H. The HAM10000 dataset, a large collection of multi-source dermatoscopic images of common pigmented skin lesions. *Sci. Data* **2018**, *5*, 180161. [CrossRef]
3. Arora, R.; Raman, B.; Nayyar, K.; Awasthi, R. Automated skin lesion segmentation using attention-based deep convolutional neural network. *Biomed. Signal Process. Control* **2021**, *65*, 102358. [CrossRef]
4. Esteva, A.; Kuprel, B.; Novoa, R.A.; Ko, J.; Swetter, S.M.; Blau, H.M.; Thrun, S. Dermatologist-level classification of skin cancer with deep neural networks. *Nature* **2017**, *542*, 115–118. [CrossRef] [PubMed]
5. Zhang, X. Melanoma segmentation based on deep learning. *Comput. Assist. Surg.* **2017**, *22*, 267–277. [CrossRef] [PubMed]
6. Oliveira, R.B.; Filho, M.E.; Ma, Z.; Papa, J.P.; Pereira, A.S.; Tavares, J.M.R. Computational methods for the image segmentation of pigmented skin lesions: A review. *Comput. Methods Programs Biomed.* **2016**, *131*, 127–141. [CrossRef]
7. das Chagas, J.V.S.; Ivo, R.F.; Guimarães, M.T.; de A. Rodrigues, D.; de S. Rebouças, E.; Filho, P.P.R. Fast fully automatic skin lesions segmentation probabilistic with Parzen window. *Comput. Med. Imaging Graph.* **2020**, *85*, 101774. [CrossRef]
8. Mahbod, A.; Schaefer, G.; Wang, C.; Dorffner, G.; Ecker, R.; Ellinger, I. Transfer learning using a multi-scale and multi-network ensemble for skin lesion classification. *Comput. Methods Programs Biomed.* **2020**, *193*, 105475. [CrossRef]
9. Borges, A.L.; Nicoletti, S.; Dufrechou, L.; Centanni, A.N. Dermatoscopy in the Public Health Environment. In *Dermatology in Public Health Environments*; Springer International Publishing: Berlin/Heidelberg, Germany, 2017; pp. 1157–1188. [CrossRef]
10. Amin, J.; Sharif, A.; Gul, N.; Anjum, M.A.; Nisar, M.W.; Azam, F.; Bukhari, S.A.C. Integrated design of deep features fusion for localization and classification of skin cancer. *Pattern Recognit. Lett.* **2020**, *131*, 63–70. [CrossRef]
11. Pathan, S.; Prabhu, K.G.; Siddalingaswamy, P. Techniques and algorithms for computer aided diagnosis of pigmented skin lesions—A review. *Biomed. Signal Process. Control* **2018**, *39*, 237–262. [CrossRef]
12. Chatterjee, S.; Dey, D.; Munshi, S.; Gorai, S. Extraction of features from cross correlation in space and frequency domains for classification of skin lesions. *Biomed. Signal Process. Control* **2019**, *53*, 101581. [CrossRef]

13. Premaladha, J.; Ravichandran, K.S. Novel Approaches for Diagnosing Melanoma Skin Lesions Through Supervised and Deep Learning Algorithms. *J. Med. Syst.* **2016**, *40*, 96. [CrossRef]
14. Kasmi, R.; Mokrani, K. Classification of malignant melanoma and benign skin lesions: Implementation of automatic ABCD rule. *IET Image Process.* **2016**, *10*, 448–455. [CrossRef]
15. Yu, Z.; Jiang, F.; Zhou, F.; He, X.; Ni, D.; Chen, S.; Wang, T.; Lei, B. Convolutional descriptors aggregation via cross-net for skin lesion recognition. *Appl. Soft Comput.* **2020**, *92*, 106281. [CrossRef]
16. Celebi, M.E.; Kingravi, H.A.; Uddin, B.; Iyatomi, H.; Aslandogan, Y.A.; Stoecker, W.V.; Moss, R.H. A methodological approach to the classification of dermoscopy images. *Comput. Med. Imaging Graph.* **2007**, *31*, 362–373. [CrossRef]
17. Goel, N.; Yadav, A.; Singh, B.M. Breast Cancer Segmentation Recognition Using Explored DCT-DWT based Compression. *Recent Patents Eng.* **2022**, *16*, 55–64. [CrossRef]
18. Hosny, K.M.; Kassem, M.A.; Foaud, M.M. Classification of skin lesions using transfer learning and augmentation with Alex-net. *PLoS ONE* **2019**, *14*, e0217293. [CrossRef]
19. Oliveira, R.B.; Pereira, A.S.; Tavares, J.M.R. Skin lesion computational diagnosis of dermoscopic images: Ensemble models based on input feature manipulation. *Comput. Methods Programs Biomed.* **2017**, *149*, 43–53. [CrossRef]
20. Khasawneh, N.; Fraiwan, M.; Fraiwan, L.; Khassawneh, B.; Ibnian, A. Detection of COVID-19 from Chest X-ray Images Using Deep Convolutional Neural Networks. *Sensors* **2021**, *21*, 5940. [CrossRef]
21. Shorten, C.; Khoshgoftaar, T.M. A survey on Image Data Augmentation for Deep Learning. *J. Big Data* **2019**, *6*. [CrossRef]
22. Kim, H.E.; Cosa-Linan, A.; Santhanam, N.; Jannesari, M.; Maros, M.E.; Ganslandt, T. Transfer learning for medical image classification: A literature review. *BMC Med. Imaging* **2022**, *22*, 69. [CrossRef]
23. Liu, L.; Mou, L.; Zhu, X.X.; Mandal, M. Automatic skin lesion classification based on mid-level feature learning. *Comput. Med. Imaging Graph.* **2020**, *84*, 101765. [CrossRef]
24. Pour, M.P.; Seker, H. Transform domain representation-driven convolutional neural networks for skin lesion segmentation. *Expert Syst. Appl.* **2020**, *144*, 113129. [CrossRef]
25. Al-masni, M.A.; Al-antari, M.A.; Choi, M.T.; Han, S.M.; Kim, T.S. Skin lesion segmentation in dermoscopy images via deep full resolution convolutional networks. *Comput. Methods Programs Biomed.* **2018**, *162*, 221–231. [CrossRef]
26. Dash, M.; Londhe, N.D.; Ghosh, S.; Semwal, A.; Sonawane, R.S. PsLSNet: Automated psoriasis skin lesion segmentation using modified U-Net-based fully convolutional network. *Biomed. Signal Process. Control* **2019**, *52*, 226–237. [CrossRef]
27. Xie, F.; Yang, J.; Liu, J.; Jiang, Z.; Zheng, Y.; Wang, Y. Skin lesion segmentation using high-resolution convolutional neural network. *Comput. Methods Programs Biomed.* **2020**, *186*, 105241. [CrossRef]
28. Serte, S.; Demirel, H. Gabor wavelet-based deep learning for skin lesion classification. *Comput. Biol. Med.* **2019**, *113*, 103423. [CrossRef]
29. Manzo, M.; Pellino, S. Bucket of Deep Transfer Learning Features and Classification Models for Melanoma Detection. *J. Imaging* **2020**, *6*, 129. [CrossRef] [PubMed]
30. Jain, S.; Singhania, U.; Tripathy, B.; Nasr, E.A.; Aboudaif, M.K.; Kamrani, A.K. Deep Learning-Based Transfer Learning for Classification of Skin Cancer. *Sensors* **2021**, *21*, 8142. [CrossRef] [PubMed]
31. Fraiwan, M.; Audat, Z.; Fraiwan, L.; Manasreh, T. Using deep transfer learning to detect scoliosis and spondylolisthesis from X-ray images. *PLoS ONE* **2022**, *17*, e0267851. [CrossRef] [PubMed]
32. Fraiwan, M.; Fraiwan, L.; Alkhodari, M.; Hassanin, O. Recognition of pulmonary diseases from lung sounds using convolutional neural networks and long short-term memory. *J. Ambient. Intell. Humaniz. Comput.* **2021**. [CrossRef]
33. Iandola, F.N.; Moskewicz, M.W.; Ashraf, K.; Han, S.; Dally, W.J.; Keutzer, K. SqueezeNet: AlexNet-level accuracy with 50x fewer parameters and <1MB model size. *arXiv* **2016**, arXiv:1602.07360.
34. Szegedy, C.; Liu, W.; Jia, Y.; Sermanet, P.; Reed, S.; Anguelov, D.; Erhan, D.; Vanhoucke, V.; Rabinovich, A. Going deeper with convolutions. In Proceedings of the 2015 IEEE Conference on Computer Vision and Pattern Recognition (CVPR), Boston, MA, USA, 7–12 June 2015; pp. 1–9. [CrossRef]
35. Szegedy, C.; Ioffe, S.; Vanhoucke, V.; Alemi, A.A. Inception-v4, Inception-ResNet and the Impact of Residual Connections on Learning. In Proceedings of the Thirty-First AAAI Conference on Artificial Intelligence, AAAI'17, San Francisco, CA, USA, 4–9 February 2017; AAAI Press: Menlo Park, CA, USA, 2017; pp. 4278–4284.
36. Huang, G.; Liu, Z.; Van Der Maaten, L.; Weinberger, K.Q. Densely Connected Convolutional Networks. In Proceedings of the 2017 IEEE Conference on Computer Vision and Pattern Recognition (CVPR), Honolulu, HI, USA, 21–26 July 2017; pp. 2261–2269. [CrossRef]
37. Chollet, F. Xception: Deep Learning with Depthwise Separable Convolutions. In Proceedings of the 2017 IEEE Conference on Computer Vision and Pattern Recognition (CVPR), Honolulu, HI, USA, 21–26 July 2017; pp. 1800–1807. [CrossRef]
38. Zhang, X.; Zhou, X.; Lin, M.; Sun, J. ShuffleNet: An Extremely Efficient Convolutional Neural Network for Mobile Devices. In Proceedings of the 2018 IEEE/CVF Conference on Computer Vision and Pattern Recognition, Salt Lake City, UT, USA, 18–23 June 2018; pp. 6848–6856. [CrossRef]
39. Redmon, J. Darknet: Open Source Neural Networks in C, 2013–2016. Available online: https://pjreddie.com/darknet (accessed on 21 June 2022).

40. Tan, M.; Le, Q. EfficientNet: Rethinking Model Scaling for Convolutional Neural Networks. In Proceedings of the 36th International Conference on Machine Learning, Long Beach, CA, USA, 10–15 June 2019; Chaudhuri, K., Salakhutdinov, R., Eds.; PMLR: London, UK, 2019; Volume 97, pp. 6105–6114.
41. Deng, J.; Dong, W.; Socher, R.; Li, L.J.; Li, K.; Fei-Fei, L. ImageNet: A large-scale hierarchical image database. In Proceedings of the 2009 IEEE Conference on Computer Vision and Pattern Recognition, Miami, FL, USA, 20–25 June 2009; pp. 248–255. [CrossRef]
42. Tharwat, A. Classification assessment methods. *Appl. Comput. Inform.* **2020**, *17*, 168–192. [CrossRef]
43. Najafabadi, M.M.; Villanustre, F.; Khoshgoftaar, T.M.; Seliya, N.; Wald, R.; Muharemagic, E. Deep learning applications and challenges in big data analytics. *J. Big Data* **2015**, *2*, 1. [CrossRef]
44. Bailly, A.; Blanc, C.; Francis, É.; Guillotin, T.; Jamal, F.; Wakim, B.; Roy, P. Effects of dataset size and interactions on the prediction performance of logistic regression and deep learning models. *Comput. Methods Programs Biomed.* **2022**, *213*, 106504. [CrossRef]

sensors

MDPI

Article

A New Approach for Detecting Fundus Lesions Using Image Processing and Deep Neural Network Architecture Based on YOLO Model

Carlos Santos [1,2,*], Marilton Aguiar [2], Daniel Welfer [3] and Bruno Belloni [4]

1 Computer Center, Federal Institute of Education, Science and Technology Farroupilha, Alegrete 97555-000, Brazil
2 Postgraduate Program in Computing (PPGC), Federal University of Pelotas, Pelotas 96010-610, Brazil
3 Postgraduate Program in Computer Science (PPGCC), Departament of Applied Computing (DCOM), Federal University of Santa Maria, Santa Maria 97105-900, Brazil
4 Federal Institute of Education, Science and Technology Sul-Rio-Grandense, Passo Fundo 99064-440, Brazil
* Correspondence: carlos.santos@iffarroupilha.edu.br

Abstract: Diabetic Retinopathy is one of the main causes of vision loss, and in its initial stages, it presents with fundus lesions, such as microaneurysms, hard exudates, hemorrhages, and soft exudates. Computational models capable of detecting these lesions can help in the early diagnosis of the disease and prevent the manifestation of more severe forms of lesions, helping in screening and defining the best form of treatment. However, the detection of these lesions through computerized systems is a challenge due to numerous factors, such as the characteristics of size and shape of the lesions, noise and the contrast of images available in the public datasets of Diabetic Retinopathy, the number of labeled examples of these lesions available in the datasets and the difficulty of deep learning algorithms in detecting very small objects in digital images. Thus, to overcome these problems, this work proposes a new approach based on image processing techniques, data augmentation, transfer learning, and deep neural networks to assist in the medical diagnosis of fundus lesions. The proposed approach was trained, adjusted, and tested using the public DDR and IDRiD Diabetic Retinopathy datasets and implemented in the PyTorch framework based on the YOLOv5 model. The proposed approach reached in the DDR dataset an mAP of 0.2630 for the IoU limit of 0.5 and F1-score of 0.3485 in the validation stage, and an mAP of 0.1540 for the IoU limit of 0.5 and F1-score of 0.2521, in the test stage. The results obtained in the experiments demonstrate that the proposed approach presented superior results to works with the same purpose found in the literature.

Keywords: Diabetic Retinopathy; fundus images; lesions detection; deep learning; YOLO

Citation: Santos, C.; Aguiar, M.; Welfer, D.; Belloni, B. A New Approach for Detecting Fundus Lesions Using Image Processing and Deep Neural Network Architecture Based on YOLO Model. *Sensors* **2022**, 22, 6441. https://doi.org/10.3390/s22176441

Academic Editor: Enrico G. Caiani

Received: 9 July 2022
Accepted: 23 August 2022
Published: 26 August 2022

1. Introduction

Vision is one of the most essential and complex senses; through it, it is possible to see and interact with the world around us. Vision is based on the absorption of light by the photoreceptor cells of the eye [1]. Unfortunately, various diseases can harm the eyes. Thus, taking care of this organ is essential to prevent or even reduce the severity of these diseases. Furthermore, eye health is associated with a better quality of life, so it is necessary to maintain a healthy vision. The human retina is the most complex of eye tissues, having a highly organized structure. The retina receives the visual image produced by the eye's optical system and converts the light energy into an electrical signal, which, after initial processing, is transmitted through the optic nerve to the visual cortex [2]. It is a thin, semitransparent, multi-layered layer of nervous tissue that lines the inside of the posterior two-thirds of the eyeball wall. It is sensitive to light and can be compared to a film in a photographic camera, being like a screen to project the images seen, which retains the images, translating to the brain through the electrical impulses sent by the optic nerve to the brain [3].

In patients with diabetes, the retina can be affected by the pathology known as Diabetic Retinopathy (DR) [2,4], which occurs when abnormal material is deposited on the blood vessel walls of the retina, which is the known region as the fundus of the eye, causing narrowing and sometimes blockage of the blood vessel, in addition to weakening of the vessel wall and the appearance of fundus lesions [3]. In the United States, between 40 and 45% for people with diabetes have retinopathy. Type 1 diabetics develop a severe form of retinopathy within 20 years in about 60 to 75% cases, even with reasonable diabetes control. In patients with diabetes type 2, generally older, the most frequent retinopathy is non-proliferative [2]. The early stages of DR can be clinically asymptomatic, and if the disease is detected in advanced stages, the treatment can become difficult [5].

Depending on the presence of clinical features, researchers classify DR as Mild Non-Proliferative Diabetic Retinopathy (NPDR); moderate NPDR; severe NPDR; Proliferative Diabetic Retinopathy (PDR); and Diabetic Macular Edema (DME) [6–9]. DR is usually identified through ophthalmologic examinations that aim to identify retinal lesions, including hard exudate (EX), soft exudate (SE), microaneurysms (MA), and hemorrhages (HE). Microaneurysms are small lesions in the form of small circular red dots that appear on the retina, in saccular shape, caused by a leak from vascular weakness at a certain point and represent the first signs of DR [10,11]. According to the International Council of Ophthalmology [12], microaneurysms are red, isolated spherical dots of varying sizes, which may reflect an abortive attempt to form a new vessel or maybe a weakness of the capillary vessel wall due to loss of normal structural integrity. On the other hand, hemorrhages can occur in the pre-retinal layer, retina, or vitreous and may have a different appearance depending on where they occur [13]. Hard exudates are lipoproteins and other proteins that leak through abnormal retinal vessels [6], being irregularly shaped yellow lesions [10], and may also have a whitish-yellow color, with a shiny appearance and well-defined margins [7], appearing in different dispositions: isolated, in clusters, in confluent trails or a partial or complete ring [13]. Soft exudates are retinal microinfarcts resulting from diabetes, hypertension, retinal vein occlusion, papilledema, collagen diseases, anemia, and leukemia [13], having the form of spots and having a pale appearance, usually in greyish-white tones, and with blurred and irregular edges.

Detection of retinal lesions associated with DR in the early stages is essential for preventing more severe forms of this disease that can cause irreversible vision loss. However, screening patients in the early stages of DR remains challenging as this eye disease is asymptomatic and progresses at a very high rate [14]. Another challenge is the availability of adequate numbers of specialized professionals and infrastructure, especially in developing regions [15], which cannot meet the growing demand due to the increase in diabetes cases in the last two decades [16]. While conventional approaches to identifying DR are effective, their resource demands are high. The level of experience of the health professional who will care for patients and the equipment needed to perform the tests are often insufficient in regions where the rate of diabetes in the local population is high; thus, the detection of DR is more necessary.

Due to these limitations, the severity of DR, and also the impact of this disease on health and quality of life over the people, it is opportune to propose the creation or optimization of procedures, approaches, and computational tools capable of providing fast and accurate support for medical diagnosis, with minimal human intervention. In the literature, approaches based on deep learning have been presented to classify, segment, and detect retinal lesions associated with DR. These works aim to assist in diagnosing DR through deep neural networks, such as [17–21]. However, although these works have achieved promising results, detecting retinal lesions has presented limited results. The limitations are due to the complexities of retinal fundus images (low contrast, irregular lighting, blurred lesion boundaries, shape, and size) and the few examples of the lesions, which cause problems in feature extraction and training approaches based on deep neural networks.

In this context, this work aims to present a state-of-the-art approach based on a pre-trained deep neural network model that, through image pre-processing and data augmentation techniques, can detect fundus lesions and assist in the medical diagnosis and treatment of Diabetic Retinopathy.

The contributions of this work concerning the state-of-the-art can be summarized as follows: (i) presentation of a convolutional neural network structure based on YOLO version 4 and 5 architectures to improve fundus lesions detection and performing real-time inferences on low-cost GPUs; (ii) implementation of a pre-processing block to reduce *outliers* and improve enhancement, to provide a more efficient extraction of features from retinal lesions; and, (iii) method for partial *cropping* of the black background of the fundus images in order to minimize the generation of false positives pixels and the creation of blocks (*tiles*) to increasing the receptive field of the input images and minimizing the loss of information caused by the reduction of the images used at the entrance of the network, especially in the case of small lesions, such as in the case of microaneurysms.

The article is structured as follows. Section 2 describes related works. Section 3 presents the materials and methods used for this work. Section 4 will describe the results obtained through the proposed approach. Section 5 presents the discussions about the results obtained in this work. Finally, in Section 6 we will describe the final considerations.

2. Related Work

Li et al. [17] presented a new Diabetic Retinopathy dataset titled *Dataset for Diabetic Retinopathy* (DDR) and evaluated state-of-the-art deep learning models for classification, segmentation, and detection of lesions associated with Diabetic Retinopathy. To evaluate these methods in clinical situations, 13,673 fundus images were collected from 9598 patients. These images were divided into six classes and evaluated by seven specialists to identify the stage of Diabetic Retinopathy. In addition, the authors selected 757 images with Diabetic Retinopathy to annotate the fundus lesions: Microaneurysms, Hemorrhages, Hard Exudates, and Soft Exudates.

The authors used the DDR dataset to evaluate ten deep learning models, including five classification models, two segmentation models, and three detection models. Experimental results demonstrate that research must improve the model performance for microlesion recognition to apply deep learning models to clinical practice. To perform the classification of DR, the authors used the models VGG-16 [22], ResNet-18 [23], GoogLeNet [24], DenseNet-121 [25] and SE-BN-Inception [26]. To perform the segmentation of DR lesions, the authors used the HED [27] and DeepLab-v3+ [28] models, while they used the SSD [29] and YOLO [30] models for the detection single-stage. The authors evaluated the models with the metrics *mean Average Precision* and the mean Intersection over Union (*mIoU*) [31], obtained in the set of validation and testing of the DDR dataset. Although the authors obtained an accuracy of 0.8284 in Accuracy with the SE-BN-Inception model for the classification of Diabetic Retinopathy, the detection and segmentation models performed poorly in detecting fundus lesions.

The work by Porwal et al. [18] presents results of deep learning models used for segmentation, classification, and detection of fundus lesions during the *IDRiD: Diabetic Retinopathy—Segmentation and Grading Challenge*. The main contribution was the availability of the set of public images of Diabetic Retinopathy called IDRiD. Most of the teams participating in the challenge explored the U-Net architecture for segmenting (microaneurysms, hemorrhages, hard exudates, and soft exudates) [32]. The U-Net architecture is an extended version of the fully convolutional networks (FCN), providing more precise segmentation, even in small training sets [33]. In the classification challenge, they categorized the fundus images according to the severity level of DR and Diabetic Macular Edema. The team that achieved the best results presented a method based on a ResNet [23] architecture and Deep Layer Aggregation (DLA) [34]. Finally, the detection challenge aimed to obtain the location of the Optical Disc and the Fovea. The winning team presented a method based on the Mask R-CNN model to locate and segment the Optical Disc and Fovea simultaneously.

First, the authors pre-processed the fundus images to a fixed size to use them as neural network input. Then, they performed a scan on the image to generate the region proposals. Then, the authors classified proposals into different classes and created a binary mask for each object. Next, they used a ResNet-50 architecture to extract features from the images and a Feature Pyramid Network (FPN) to generate feature maps at different scales and extract regions of interest from the images. A Region Proposal Network (RPN) then traverses the feature maps and locates regions that contain objects. Finally, architectural branches are employed to obtain the label, mask, and bounding box for each region of interest. Transfer learning technique was applied to train the model. The authors started with a learning rate of 0.001 and a *momentum* of 0.9. They trained the network with 20 epochs. In the Optical Disc and Fovea segmentation and detection task, the team that obtained the best result in the test dataset achieved a Jaccard coefficient equal to 0.9338.

Mateen et al. [19] proposed a pre-trained framework based on a convolutional neural network to detect exudates in fundus images through transfer learning. In the proposed structure, the authors combined three pre-trained network architectures to perform the fusion of features since, according to the authors, different architectures could capture various features. The three models used to compose the framework proposed by the authors are Inception-v3 [35], VGG-19 [22] and ResNet-50 [23]. In addition, the collected features are treated as input in the fully connected layers to perform further actions, such as classification, performed through the *Softmax* function. When using the e-Ophtha dataset, the highest accuracy obtained individually by the Inception-v3, ResNet-50, and VGG-19 architectures was 93.67%, 97.80%, and 95.80%, respectively, while the approach proposed by the authors reached a classification accuracy of 98.43%. Moreover, using the DIARETDB1 dataset, the highest accuracy obtained individually by the Inception-v3, ResNet-50, and VGG-19 architectures was 93.57%, 97.90% and 95.50%, respectively, while the approach proposed by the authors reached a classification accuracy of 98.91%

The work by Alyoubi et al. [20] presented a DR diagnostic system that classifies fundus images into five stages (no DR, mild DR, moderate DR, severe DR, and proliferative DR) and the location of lesions on the retinal surface. The system is composed of two models based on deep learning. The first model used is a CNN512, in which the images are used to classify in one of the five stages of DR. The public datasets DDR and Kaggle APTOS 2019 [36] were used. The second model was a YOLOv3 [37], adopted to detect DR lesions. Finally, both proposed frameworks, CNN512 and YOLOv3, were combined to classify DR images and locate DR lesions. The data balancing of the data sets used when performing the training of the models was not performed. In classifying the type of DR, the CNN512 model achieved an accuracy of 88.6% and 84.1% in the DDR and APTOS Kaggle 2019 public datasets, respectively, while the YOLOv3 model, adopted to detect the DR lesions, obtained a mAP of 0.216 in the detection of lesions in the DDR dataset.

The main limitation of the work was not performing the balancing in the retinal image datasets to perform the training of the models, which may have generated a bias in the detection of lesions. For example, there are lesions with a significantly higher number of examples concerning the others, as in the case of hard exudates. This imbalance in the training of models can make the deep neural network tend to classify objects in the majority classes, causing the model to have its generalization ability impaired. In future work, the authors claim that it is necessary to balance the number of examples in the data sets to train the models and conduct experiments with the YOLOv4 and YOLOv5 models to verify the performance of these models in the detection of fundus lesions.

The work by Dai et al. [21] presented a deep learning system, called DeepDR, to detect early and late stages of Diabetic Retinopathy using 466,247 fundus images of 121,342 patients with diabetes. The DeepDR system architecture had three subnetworks: an image quality assessment subnetwork, the subnet for lesion recognition, and the subnet for DR classification. These subnets were developed based on a ResNet [23] architecture and a Mask R-CNN [38] architecture, responsible for performing the detection of lesions in 2 stages:

a preliminary stage, in which regions of interest (RoI) are selected and then, in a second stage, check for the presence of lesions in the regions verified in the previous step [39–41].

First, the authors used 466,247 images to train the image quality assessment subnet to check for quality problems in terms of artifacts in the retinal images. After this analysis, 415,139 images were used to train the DR classification subnet to classify the images: no DR, mild nonproliferative DR, moderate nonproliferative DR, severe nonproliferative DR, or proliferative DR. The subnetwork for detecting and segmenting the lesions was trained using 10,280 images with annotations of retinal lesions: microaneurysms, soft exudates, hard exudates, and hemorrhages. For microaneurysms, the value obtained from *IoU* (*Intersection Over Union*) [42,43] was not presented. For soft exudates, hard exudates, and hemorrhages, *IoU* of 0.941, 0.954, and 0.967 were obtained.

The study had limitations. The first one was using only a private DR dataset to train the deep learning models, making it difficult to reproduce the results obtained by the authors using the same method. In the validation step, the authors used the Kaggle eyePACS [44] public DR dataset only. The second limitation is that the subnet that detects the lesions was tested only on the local validation dataset due to the lack of lesion annotations in the public dataset that the authors used. Therefore, in future work, the authors claim that further validation through public datasets is necessary to assess the proposed deep learning system's performance in classifying DR and detecting fundus lesions.

The works in the literature applied deep neural networks to identify DR, but the deep learning models presented limitations. The work by Porwal et al. [18] showed results in detecting only the fovea and the optical disc, while the work by Mateen et al. [19] only exudates. The work by Li et al. [17] showed promising results in the classification of DR but limited results in the detection of fundus lesions. The work by Alyoubi et al. [20] showed promising results in detecting lesions but did not balance the datasets used, which possibly impacted the results presented. The work proposed by Dai et al. [21] used a private dataset for training and validating the model responsible for detecting lesions, which makes a fair comparison and validation with the models we propose impossible. Furthermore, the model used by Dai et al. [21] is based on a model that performs the detection of objects in 2 stages, unlike the conception of our work, which performs the *Single-Stage* detection after pre-processing and augmentation of image data. A summarized comparison between related works is presented in Table 1.

Table 1. Comparison between related work that use deep learning to classify, segment and detect objects in diabetic retinopathy images.

Ref.	Dataset	# Images	# of Images with Lesions Annotated				Data Augmentation	Unbalanced Data	Model	Performance Measure	Limitations
			MA	HE	EX	SE					
[18]	IDRiD	516	81	80	81	40	Applied	Yes	Mask R-CNN	IoU = 0.9338	EX, MA, SE e HE not detected
[17]	DDR	12,522	570	601	486	239	Not applied	Yes	SSD, YOLO	mAP = 0.0059 mAP = 0.0035	Low performance in detecting MA and SE
[20]							Applied	Yes	YOLOv3	mAP = 0.216	Imbalance of data used in training
[19]	DIARETDB1	89	80	54	48	36	Applied	Yes	CNN	Accuracy = 98.91%	MA e HE not detected
[21]	Private dataset	666,383	-	-	-	-	Not applied	Yes	Mask R-CNN	AUC = 0.954 AUC = 0.901 AUC = 0.941 AUC = 0.967	The dataset with fundus images used for training is private Validation of detection of lesions performed only in images from the private dataset

Definitions in Table 1: MA, microaneurysms; HE, hemorrhages; EX, hard exudates; SE, soft exudates; IDRiD, Indian Diabetic Retinopathy Image Dataset; DDR, Dataset for Diabetic Retinopathy; DIARETDB1, Standard Diabetic Retinopathy Database Calibration level 1; Mask R-CNN, Mask Regions with Convolutional Neural Network features; SSD, Detector MultiBox Single Shot; YOLO, You Only Look Once; YOLOv3, You Only Look Once version 3; CNN, Convolutional Neural Network; IoU, Intersection Over Union; mAP, mean Average Precision; AUC, Area Under The Curve.

3. Materials and Methods

The *pipeline* of the proposed approach is presented in the form of a block diagram in Figure 1. The proposed approach was based on the YOLOv5 [45–51] deep neural network model and implemented through the open-source machine learning library PyTorch (https://pytorch.org, accessed on 25 August 2022). The model was trained with 8000 epochs and 32 batches per epoch, with a learning rate of 0.01 and a *momentum* rate of 0.937. The size of the bounding box anchors was adaptively calculated [52], through a genetic algorithm, which optimizes the anchors after a scan performed by the unsupervised K-means algorithm [53] before the step of training.

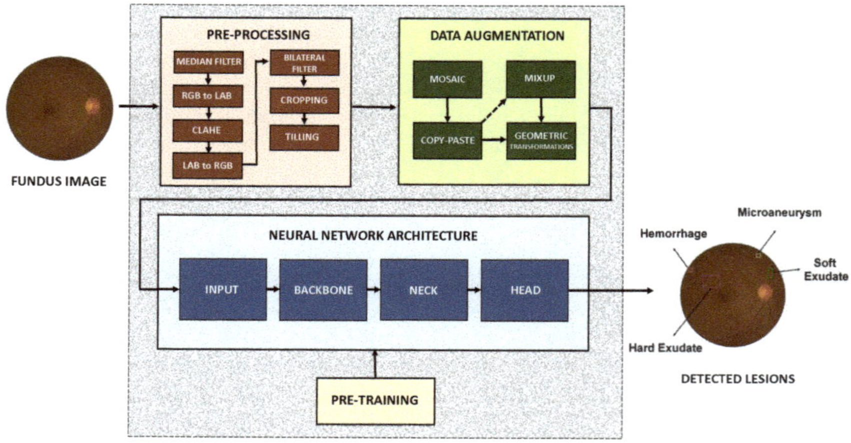

Figure 1. Block diagram of the proposed approach. First, the images are passed to the Pre-processing block for noise filtering, contrast improvement, partial elimination of the black background of the images, and creation of *tiles*. Then, the pre-processed images are transferred to the Data Augmentation block, where sub-images are artificially created that will be used in the neural network input layer for training the proposed approach, which will be carried out after a pre-stage step training the network with the weights fitted to the Common Objects in Context (COCO) dataset.

An anchor set more adjusted improves detection accuracy and speed [54]. Anchors are the initial sizes (width, height) of bounding boxes that will be adjusted to the size closest to the object to be detected using some neural network output (final feature maps). In this way, the network will not predict the final size of the object but only adjust the size of the anchor closest to the object's size. For this reason, YOLO is regarded as a method that treats object detection as a regression problem, in which a single neural network predicts the bounding boxes and class occurrence probabilities directly on the complete image being evaluated. Moreover, as all detection is performed in one network (*Single-Stage*), the neural network model can be directly optimized end-to-end [30].

In the proposed approach, detection is performed in the final layers and at three scales, as proposed in the YOLOv3 [37] model, allowing learning objects in different sizes, the scales being: 19×19, specialized in object detection of large size; 38×38, which specializes in detecting medium-sized objects; and, 76×76, which specializes in detecting small objects. Each of these outputs or detection "heads" has a separate set of anchor scales. In YOLOv3, 9 anchor sizes are used, with 3 anchors per detection head. After detection, the confidence percentage was reached for each identified lesion. To carry out the experiments a Core i7-7700K 8×4.6 GHz device, 32 GB of RAM and an NVIDIA Titan Xp GPU with 12 GB of VRAM were used.

YOLOv5 is a single-stage detection model capable of detecting objects without a preliminary step, as in the case of two-stage detectors, which use a preliminary stage where regions of importance are then classified to check if objects have been detected in those areas. The advantage of a single-stage detector is the speed at which it can make real-time inferences. Furthermore, another feature of this model type is the possibility of working on edge devices and with low-cost hardware, whose training can be performed with just one GPU [55]. Therefore, we intend to present an approach that achieves greater precision than approaches with the same purpose presented in the literature. Next, we methodologically detail each step that makes up the pipeline of the proposed approach.

3.1. Dataset

The DDR image dataset was used in this work, which has 757 images labeled in JPEG format with variable sizes. Second [17] to capture these images 45 TRC NW48, Nikon D5200, and Canon CR 2 cameras were used. In addition, the lesions contained in these fundus images contain annotations (*Ground Truth*), as illustrated in Figure 2.

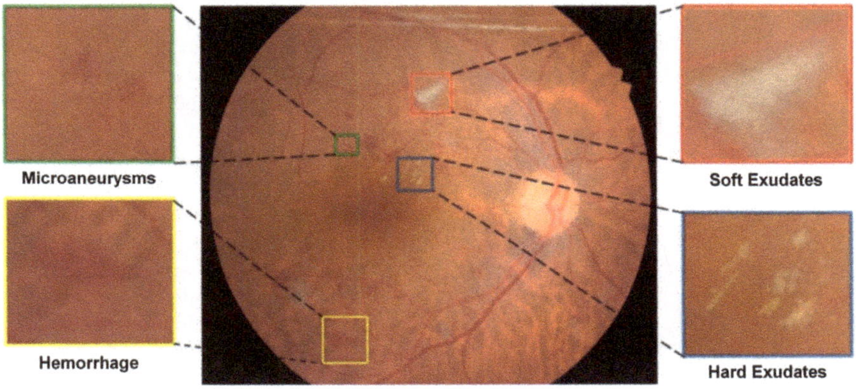

Figure 2. Representation of fundus image with the lesions annotated: Microaneurysms, Hemorrhages, Soft Exudates, and Hard Exudates.

Table 2 presents attributes of the DDR dataset, such as the number of images, the resolution of the images, the type of annotations, the number of images with annotations for MA, HE, EX, and SE, and the total amount of annotations by lesion type before the data augmentation step.

Table 2. Number of annotated images for Microaneurysms, Hemorrhages, Hard Exudates, and Soft Exudates and the total amount of annotations by lesion type in the Dataset for Diabetic Retinopathy (DDR) before the data augmentation step.

# Images	Resolution	MA	HE	EX	SE	Notes of Lesions at *Pixel*	Multiple Experts
12,522	Variable	**# of images with lesion annotations**				Yes	Yes
		570	601	486	239		
		# of lesion annotations					
		10,388	13,093	23,713	1558		

Definitions in the Table 2: MA, microaneurysms; HE, hemorrhages; EX, hard exudates; SE, soft exudates.

Data were collected using single-view images. The bounding box annotations were generated automatically from the *pixel* level annotations of the lesions [17]. Although the DDR dataset is of good quality, training the deep neural network of the proposed approach has challenges, such as the small number of annotated fundus lesions and the variability in size and shape of these lesions. Another factor that generates problems in training deep learning models to detect retinal lesions is the reduced size of some types of lesions, as in the case of microaneurysms. Data augmentation was performed to circumvent problems related to the sub-sampling of the data set due to the small number of examples by creating artificial images derived from the original images and annotations of the fundus lesions. This data augmentation and the other techniques applied to overcome the challenges mentioned above will be discussed in the following sections.

3.2. Pre-Processing and Image Preparation

The use of a pre-processing block aims to (i) improve the quality of images through the elimination of periodic or random patterns through the application of filters and (ii) increase the image enhancement to improve and accentuate the characteristics of the lesions that will be used for training the deep neural network. The treatment of the images aims at (i) filtering noise generated during the capture of fundus images, (ii) correcting lighting deformities, and (iii) improving the contrast and enhancement of the images [56].

For image smoothing, the median filter of size 5×5 was used. The median filter is non-linear and very effective in removing impulsive noise (irregular pulses of large amplitudes), such as *Salt & Pepper* [57,58] noise. Moreover, the contrast-limited histogram adaptive equalization technique (CLAHE) [20,59] was used to enhance the images. This technique was initially developed for low contrast image enhancement and is an evolution of the histogram equalization method [60], and has been used as part of pre-processing *pipelines* to improve image quality. medical images [61]. However, before applying the CLAHE algorithm to the fundus images of the dataset, it was necessary to define the most suitable color space to perform the image enhancement (i.e., RGB, HSV, or LAB).

The background suppression was performed as the last step in the pre-processing and image preparation stage. As the works by El abbadi and Hammod [62] and Alyoubi et al. [20], a pre-processing step for partial *cropping* of the black background of the retinal images was performed, as illustrated in the Supplementary Materials. According to El abbadi and Hammod [62], the importance of removing the black background from the retinal image is related to the generation of false positives during the detection of lesions, especially at the retina border, where there is a similarity of the retinal border with the blood vessels. Furthermore, in the case of fundus images, only the *pixels* of the retina have significant information; the rest is considered the background. Therefore, it is essential to locate the area of interest and remove unwanted features related to the image's background.

Details about the median filter, CLAHE, and the suppression of the useless retinal background are presented in the Supplementary Materials attached to this article. It is important to note that this additional document presents images where these pre-processing methods are tested and where the used measures are clearly presented and discussed.

Pre-processing techniques were explored to improve the performance of the proposed approach, especially in detecting microlesions for better smoothing and enhancement of the fundus images. In addition, the black background that caused the generation of false positives was partially removed, and the Tilling of the original images was applied to use the resulting image blocks in the training of the deep neural network. Finally, a Data Augmentation step was applied after pre-processing the fundus images, as we will explain in the next section.

3.3. Data Augmentation

In the proposed approach, a data augmentation was performed from the images and labeled lesions available in the DDR dataset. Then, for each training batch, the model was configured to pass the images through a data loader that creates the artificial images while they are accessed. The data loader did the following types of augmentations: *Mosaic*, *MixUp*, *Copy-Paste* and Geometric Transformations.

This technique works in real-time, i.e., *on-the-fly* [63,64], and new examples are not generated in advance (before training). Thus, at each training performed, a random number of artificially created examples are generated and passed on for training the neural network. Each data augmentation technique is applied to all images in the batch, except the Mix-Up, which was set to randomly apply to 50% of the images in the batch. Details on the methods applied in the data augmentation block of the fundus images are presented in the

Supplementary Materials attached to this article. It is important to note that this additional document discusses the methods used and the images with the results obtained in this step.

After performing the data increase, we also had to deal with the problem related to data imbalance. Models based on deep learning generally try to minimize the number of errors when classifying new data. Therefore, the cost of different errors must be equal. However, the costs of different errors are often unequal in real-world applications. For example, in the area of medical diagnosis, the cost of misdiagnosing a sick patient as healthy (False Negative) can be much higher than accidentally diagnosing a healthy person as sick (False Positive) since the former type of error can result in the loss of a life [65].

There are cases in which data imbalance causes biases in the training of models, including generating uncertainties about the results obtained [66,67]. In the case of eye fundus lesions, an imbalance in the number of examples of different fundus lesions was verified, as shown in Table 2. This imbalance can become even more significant after the application of the data increase step since the number of new examples created after this step is random, and it is impossible to accurately predict the number of new examples generated for each lesion.

To balance the number of examples of each lesion, during training the method *Threshold-Moving* [68–70] was used through the parameter `image-weights`, in which the samples of training set images are weighted by their *mean Average Precision* (mAP) inverse of the previous epoch test. Unlike uniformly sampling the images during training, as in conventional training, sampling during training is based on the weighted images based on the result obtained by a certain evaluation metric calculated in the test of the previous epoch. of training. This method moves the decision boundary so that minority class examples can easily predict correctly [71,72].

The *Threshold-Moving* method was used to minimize the imbalance of the dataset and reduce the possibility of biases during the classification due to the presence of classes with a significantly larger number of examples. Due to the need for many examples to obtain more accurate results, we chose not to use the subsampling technique of the majority classes. Likewise, the oversampling of minority classes was also discarded because the number of examples of these classes to equate them to the majority classes would not reflect the natural incidence of fundus lesions.

Our approach used a method to minimize the imbalance problem in the number of examples of lesions to avoid possible overfitting of the model associated with misclassification of lesions in the majority class. After the step of increasing and balancing the data, our method was trained to perform the detection of fundus lesions. The next section will discuss the architecture of the deep neural network used in our proposed approach.

3.4. Deep Neural Network Architecture

After the pre-processing and data augmentation steps described above, the image set of the DDR dataset was split into a training set (50%), validation set (20%), and test set (30%), the same proportion performed in the work by Li et al. [17]. The images of one set are not present in the others to avoid bias during the evaluation of the proposed approach. A validation step to fine-tune the hyperparameters of the architecture and a test step to assess the generalization capability of the neural network was used. In addition, the public Diabetic Retinopathy dataset IDRiD [18] was also used to validate our proposed approach.

In our approach, we used the architecture of the YOLOv5 [20,45–50,53,73] model as a basis. This model currently has four versions: s (*small*), m (*medium*), l (*large*) and x (*extra-large*). Each version has different features. Before choosing the YOLOv5 s as the base architecture for our proposed approach, different versions of YOLOv5 have been tried. The quantities of depth (*depth*) and scale (*width*) multipliers of convolutional cores of the adopted model are 0.33 and 0.50, respectively. According to Iyer et al. [74], YOLOv5s achieves precision equivalent to YOLOv3 (https://pjreddie.com/darknet/yolo/, accessed on 25 August 2022), but with superior performance in performing real-time inferences at a lower computational cost.

The YOLOv5 *s* was used because it achieved the best results in detecting fundus lesions and at a lower computational cost compared to other versions. The explanation for the shorter version of YOLOv5 to have obtained the best results lies in the fact that the fundus microlesions present a gradient dissipation problem when training the versions of YOLOv5 with greater depth and number of parameters. Thus, using a model with a smaller number of parameters allowed us to use fewer hardware resources, thus enabling the detection of fundus lesions through low-cost GPUs without impacting the precision of the proposed approach. The deep neural network structure used in our approach has a total of 283 layers, 7.2 million parameters, and 17.1 GFLOPs. According to Yu et al. [75], GFLOPs represent the 1 billion worth of FLOPs (floating-point math operations). Another advantage of using the YOLOv5 model as the basis of this approach is the possibility of integration and portability with different types of projects, including mobile devices. This feature is associated with the fact that this model has been implemented natively in PyTorch.

The network Backbone was used as a pre-trained feature extractor on an image classification dataset, useful for detecting objects in the last layers of the network. The *Backbone* used in the experiments is composed of a CSP-Darknet-53. The convolutional neural network Darknet-53 was initially used as *Backbone* of the YOLOv3 [37] model, replacing its predecessor Darknet-19 [30], as it includes the use of residual connections as well as more layers since it has 53 depth layers [37]. Furthermore, its architecture is built by consecutive layers of convolution 3×3 and 1×1 followed by a jump connection, which helps activations propagate through deeper layers without gradient dissipation.

The CSP proposed by Wang et al. [76] can be applied in different architectures, such as ResNet [23], ResNeXt [77], DenseNet [25], YOLOv4 [55] and YOLOv5 [45,46] as it not only produces a reduction in computational cost and memory usage of these networks but also brings benefits such as improved inference speed and increased precision. These goals are achieved by partitioning the base layer feature map into two parts. Then, the parts are merged through a hierarchy of crossed stages, whose main idea is to make the gradient propagate through different network paths.

The block diagram of the neural network architecture that composes the proposed approach, responsible for detecting fundus lesions, is illustrated in Figure 3. As shown in, the network architecture is based on the structure of YOLOv5 version small [45,46,74] and is divided into three main blocks: *Backbone*, *Neck* and *Head*. The network input layer size is $640 \times 640 \times 3$, where the first two values correspond to the height and width in *pixels*, and the third value corresponds to the number of channels in the input image. The DDR dataset makes the bounding box annotations of fundus lesions available for deep neural network training. These bounding boxes were used to calculate the initial anchor sizes. In the architectures of the YOLO family, we usually configure the sizes of the initial anchors before training the model.

In training the proposed approach, we produced bounding boxes with predictions based on the lengths of the initial anchors. Then a comparison of the bounding box of the detected object is performed with the bounding box of the object annotated (*Ground Truth*). Then we used the result of this comparison to update the neural network weights during the training stage. Therefore, defining the initial size of the anchors is essential, especially when training the neural network on objects with sizes different from the standard dimensions of anchors, which are typically calculated based on objects from datasets such as COCO, for example. The YOLOv5 model repository has a function that performs the adaptive calculation of the anchors, in which, when training the neural network, it is possible to enable the "`auto-anchor`" option so that the best values for the docking boxes automatically. This function was used before training the proposed approach to ensure that the anchors were adjusted according to the sizes of fundus lesions present in the dataset used in the experiment.

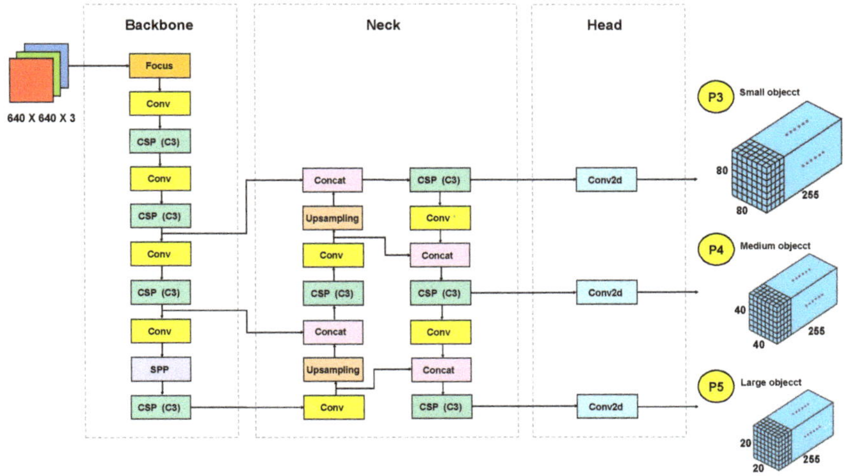

Figure 3. The neural network architecture block diagram composes the proposed approach for detecting fundus lesions. The structure is divided into three main blocks: *Backbone*, *Neck* and *Head*. The *Backbone* block consists of a Focus module, four Conv modules, four CSP modules (C3), and an SPP module. The *Neck* block consists of four Conv modules and four CSP modules (C3). The network input receives images of size 640 × 640 × 3, and the output is composed of three detection heads: the P3 layer, responsible for detecting small objects; layer P4, responsible for detecting medium objects; and, finally, the P5 layer, responsible for detecting large objects. CSP (C3), Cross Stage Partial Network C3; SPP, Spatial Pyramid Pooling; Conv, Convolution module; Concat, concatenation; Conv2d, 2D convolution layer.

The *Backbone* structure of the neural network starts with the *Focus* module, responsible for performing a slicing operation. In the case of the neural network structure of the proposed approach, when we insert an image of size 640 × 640 × 3 in the module *Focus*, a slicing operation is performed on this image to generate a map of size features 304 × 304 × 64. Still in *Backbone*, the modules *Conv* are composed of a 2d convolution, followed by a batch normalization. The batch normalization reduces the number of training cycles needed to train deep networks, providing a regularization and reducing generalization error [78]. After batch normalization, the activation function *Sigmoid Linear Unit* (SiLU) [79], derived from the function *Rectified Linear* (ReLU) [80] is applied.

In network architecture, the CSP module (C3) is used both in the *Backbone* and in the *Neck* of the network. These CSPs were used to connect the front and back layers of the network, aiming to improve the model inference speed without compromising its precision. Also, they allow better integration of different parts that make up the neural network, in addition to a reduction in the size of the model [45]. These C3 modules have in their structure three Conv modules and a *Bottleneck* [23] module. The module *Bottleneck* consists of two Conv modules followed by an addition operation (*add*), responsible for adding tensors without expanding the image dimension.

The *Backbone* of the proposed approach is composed of four CSP modules (C3). After *Bottleneck* module, each C3 module, there is a concatenation module (*Concat*) so that the features that were divided at the beginning of the C3 block are regrouped, expanding the dimensions of the tensors. The flow and constitution of the various modules that make up the *Backbone* were illustrated in Figure 3. Another *Backbone* component of the proposed approach is the SPP module (*Spatial Pyramid Pooling*) [81]. With SPP, it is possible to introduce multiple variable-scale *pools* concatenated to form a 1 dimension vector for the FC layer. As in He et al. [81], the MaxPool method was used with groupings of size equal to 1 × 1, 5 × 5, 9 × 9 and 13 × 13, followed by the *Concat* operation to concatenate feature maps at different scales.

The *Backbone* structure is responsible for extracting feature maps of different sizes from the input image through multiple convolutions and clusters [82]. The *Neck* structure, in turn, is responsible for merging these feature maps obtained from different levels of the architecture to obtain more contextual information and reduce problems related to information loss during the process of extracting features from the images [45]. In the process of merging the feature maps from the *Backbone*, the *Feature Pyramid Network* (FPN) [83] and the PAN (*Path Aggregation Network*) [84] are used as illustrated in Figure 4. The structure of the FPN itself can be extensive, as the spatial information may need to be propagated to hundreds of layers. In this context, an FPN in conjunction with a PAN was used. The PAN structure follows an additional upward path than the downward path taken by the FPN, helping to shorten this path by using lateral connections as a shortcut.

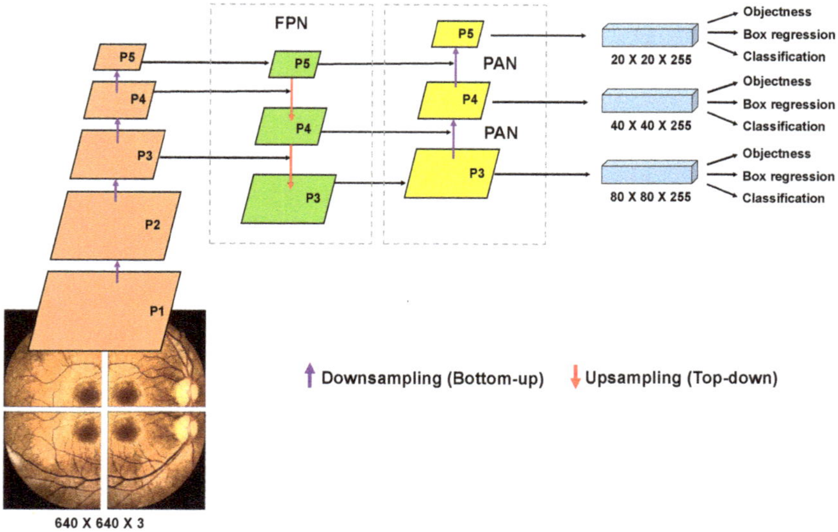

Figure 4. FPN+PAN structure used in the *Neck* of the neural network architecture of the proposed approach. FPN has a *Top-Down* structure and lateral connections that enable it to build feature maps with high-level semantic meaning, which are used to detect objects at different scales. The PAN architecture conveys strong localization features from the lower-feature maps to the upper-feature maps (*Bottom-up*). The two structures combined to reinforce the ability to merge characteristics of the *Neck* structure. The detection of lesions is performed in layers P3, P4 and P5 of the FPN+PAN structure, having outputs with sizes of $80 \times 80 \times 255$, $40 \times 40 \times 255$ and $20 \times 20 \times 255$, respectively. FPN, Feature Pyramid Network; PAN, Path Aggregation Network.

In the structure of *Neck* four CSP modules (C3) were used, as illustrated in Figure 3. These C3 modules were adopted to strengthen the ability to integrate the characteristics extracted from the lesions during the propagation of this information in the neural network. In Figure 4 it is possible to observe that the detection of lesions is performed in layers P3 (small objects), P4 (medium objects) and P5 (large objects), with sizes of $80 \times 80 \times 255$, $40 \times 40 \times 255$ and $20 \times 20 \times 255$, respectively.

Finally, the *Head* part of the neural network is responsible for making the dense prediction (final prediction). This part is composed of a vector that contains the predicted bounding box (central coordinates, height, width), the confidence score of the prediction, and the label of the class to which the detected object belongs. The prediction mechanism used in the *Head* of the deep neural network architecture of the proposed approach is equivalent to the one used in YOLOv3 [37]. A bounding box predicts each object, and in case several bounding boxes are detected for the same object, then we apply the NMS technique, which allows us to discard bounding boxes with an IoU below a predefined threshold as shown in Table 3. The *Head* structure used in our approach is composed of 3 layers responsible for performing the detection of fundus lesions, each of these layers dividing the image into grid cells of sizes $20 \times 20 \times 255$, $40 \times 40 \times 255$ and $80 \times 80 \times 255$, as illustrated in Figures 3 and 4. The smaller the size of feature maps, the larger the image area to which each grid unit in the feature map corresponds, indicating that it is suitable for detecting large objects from feature maps of size $20 \times 20 \times 255$. In contrast, feature maps of size $80 \times 80 \times 255$ are better suited for detecting small objects.

Table 3. Hyperparameters adjusted during the validation step using the Dataset for Diabetic Retinopathy (DDR).

Parameters	Value
Batch Size	32
Number of Epochs	8000
Learning Rate	0.01
Momentum	0.937
Activation Function	SiLU
Optimizer	SGD and Adam
Weight Decay	0.0005
Dropout	10%
Threshold IoU NMS	0.45
Confidence Limit	0.25
Size of initial anchors (COCO)	(10, 13), (16, 30), (33, 23)—P3 (30, 61), (62, 45), (59, 119)—P4 (116, 90), (156, 198), (373, 326)—P5
Adjusted anchor size	(3, 3), (4, 4), (7, 7)—P3 (10, 10), (15, 15), (23, 28)—P4 (33, 24), (44, 49), (185, 124)—P5
Early Stopping	*Patience value* = 100

Definitions in Table 3: SiLU, Sigmoid Linear Unit; SGD, Stochastic Gradient Descent; IoU NMS, Intersection Over Union Non-max Suppression; COCO, Common Objects in Context.

The final loss function used in the proposed approach is calculated based on the confidence score (*Objectness*), the classification score (*Class Probability*) and the bounding box regression score (*Bounding Box Regression*), according to Equation (1). *Objectness* determines whether there are objects in the grid cell, *Class Probability* determines which category objects that are in a grid cell belong to, and *Bounding Box Regression* is just calculated when the box predicted contains objects. In this case, the *Bounding Box Regression* calculation is performed by comparing the predicted box with the box associated with the *Ground Truth* of the detected object.

$$Loss = L_{Objectness} + L_{ClassProbability} + L_{BoundingBoxRegression} \tag{1}$$

To calculate the confidence score loss (*objecteness*) and classification score (*class probability*) functions, the *Binary Cross-Entropy* with the PyTorch Logits function [85] was used. To calculate the loss function referring to the bounding box regression, the loss function *Generalized Intersection over Union* (GIoU) [86–88] was used.

In the post-processing of the detection of fundus lesions, it was necessary to perform the screening and removal of duplicated bounding boxes representing the same object. The NMS technique was used for that, which keeps the bounding box detected with a higher precision index. Therefore, the NMS method used is based on the obtained *IoU* values (`IoU_nms`), in which a threshold of 0.45 [48] was set for the training step.

3.5. Pre-Training

Transfer learning is a method employed in the area of machine learning that consists of reusing information learned in a given task as a starting point for the solution of a new task [89]. This method is often used when it is not possible to obtain a large-scale dataset with labeled objects to solve a particular Computer Vision task [90]. In this context, as the public DR datasets do not contain a large number of labeled lesions, in addition to a data augmentation step, the proposed approach has a pre-training step. In this step, the *Transfer Learning* with pre-trained weights on the COCO [91] followed by the *Fine-Tuning* dataset from the last layers of the neural network were applied. To fine-tune the proposed approach, we kept the weights of the first layers and changed only the weights of the last layers of the neural network.

COCO provides a large dataset with labeled images for object detection tasks. The neural network output of the proposed approach was modified to suit the problem of detecting fundus lesions, preserving the knowledge (weights) of the initial layers. The reuse of information from these initial layers is essential to obtain the most basic characteristics of fundus lesions, such as contours, edges, etc. In addition, pre-training enabled a reduction in computational cost and training time of the proposed approach. The method adopted to carry out the transfer of learning was based on the work proposed by Franke et al. [92] and consists of the four steps presented below:

1. The initial layers of the architecture of the proposed approach, focused on detecting the most fundamental characteristics of objects, were pre-trained with the weights of the COCO dataset, composed of 80 categories.
2. The last three layers (out of a total of 283) that make up the *Head* of the architecture of the proposed approach are cut and replaced by new layers.
3. The new layers added are adjusted by training the neural network on the DR dataset, while the weights of the initial layers are frozen.
4. After fine-tuning the *Head* layers of the architecture, the entire neural network is unfrozen and retrained so that minor adjustments to the weights are performed across the entire network.

The fine-tuning of the neural network aimed to optimize the proposed approach to achieve more accurate results. So, hyperparameters, such as batch size, number of epochs, and learning rate, were adjusted. According to Franke et al. [92], the optimization of hyperparameters aims to find a set of values that produces an ideal model in which a predefined loss function is minimized. As in work proposed by Franke et al. [92], the methodology adopted to fine-tune the proposed approach consisted of the following steps:

1. For each adjustment performed, a hyperparameter value is varied, and the proposed approach is retrained, keeping the other hyperparameter values constant.
2. The effect of this change is analyzed through the performance evaluation of the proposed approach with the metrics *Average Precision* (AP) and *mean Average Precision* (mAP), which will be presented and discussed in the next section of this article.
3. If there is an improvement in the metric values, the hyperparameter value is further adjusted (increased or decreased) until the local maximum is reached.
4. The exact process is carried out for the other hyperparameters until an optimal set of values is obtained that produces the maximum results of AP and mAP for the detection of the investigated fundus lesions.

After performing these steps using the validation dataset from the DDR, the ideal fit for hyperparameters was found, as shown in Table 3. With the hyperparameter values adequately adjusted, the next step was to evaluate the proposed approach in the test set of the dataset used in the experiments. In the next section, the metrics used to evaluate the performance of the proposed approach will be presented and discussed.

3.6. Performance Metrics

Typically, these models are evaluated by their performance on a dataset's validation/test set, measured using different metrics. The metrics adopted to evaluate a model must follow the type of task being investigated so that it is possible to adequately and quantitatively compare the performance of this model. For example, quantitative evaluation is performed for object detection tasks in images by estimating overlapping regions between detected images and annotating bounding boxes of objects in original images (*Ground Truth*).

Metrics typically used to evaluate problems involving object detection and segmentation of instances in images are the Intersection over Union (IoU) [31,86], the *Average Precision* (AP) [38,55,93,94] and the *mean Average Precision* (mAP) [30,31,37,40]. The IoU, also identified by the similarity coefficient of Jaccard [42,43] is a statistic to estimate the similarity between two sets of samples. The Intersection over Union is obtained by the ratio between the Area of Overlap and the Area of Union of the predicted bounding boxes and the Ground Truth bounding boxes.

The *Average Precision* corresponds to the *Area Under the Curve* (AUC) of *Precision* × *Recall*, also called the PR [95] curve. With the Precision and Recall values, it is possible to plot a graph, where the y axis is the *Precision* and the x axis is the *Recall*. Recall, and Precision are then calculated for each class by applying the formulas for each image, as shown in Equations (2) and (3), respectively:

$$Recall = \frac{TP}{TP + FN} = \frac{\text{Objects detected correctly}}{\text{All Ground Truth objects}} \tag{2}$$

$$Precision = \frac{TP}{TP + FP} = \frac{\text{Objects detected correctly}}{\text{All objects detected}} \tag{3}$$

Precision and *Recall* are useful measures to assess the efficiency of a model in predicting classes when they are unbalanced. The Precision×Recall (PR curve) presents the trade-off between *Precision* and *Recall* for different thresholds. The PR curve is an important tool for analyzing the results of a predictor. The PR curve is an important tool for analyzing the results of a predictor.

The same approach used in the COCO [96] challenge were used to perform the AP calculation, a range of threshold values of IoU, calculate the average of the AP for each IoU, and then obtain a final average of AP. Another critical aspect of calculating the AP in the COCO challenge is that 101 recovery points are used in the PR [96] curve.

Another way to evaluate models that perform object detection is through mAP, a metric widely used to evaluate deep learning models [30,31,37,40]. Its main feature is the ability to compare different models, contrasting precision with recall. The definition of the mAP metric for object detection was first formalized in the PASCAL VOC challenge. To calculate mAP, just average the *Average Precision* calculated for all object classes [95], as shown in Equation (4). Although it is not simple to quantify and interpret the results of a model, mAP is a metric that helps evaluate deep learning models that perform object detection.

$$mAP = \frac{1}{N}\sum_{i=1}^{N} AP_i \tag{4}$$

4. Experiments and Results

The performance evaluation of the proposed approach experiments was performed using the public DDR Diabetic Retinopathy dataset. To avoid biasing the results, divided the data set into training, validation, and test sets in a proportion of 50%, 20%, and 30%, respectively. The architecture was implemented and trained based on the YOLOv5 model. First, we perform transfer learning based on the pre-trained weights in the COCO dataset, then fine-tune the detection layers of the architecture, and finally, we retrain the entire neural network.

During the training of the proposed approach was used the regularization method *Early Stopping* [97]. With this technique, it was not necessary to statically define the number of epochs necessary for training the proposed approach since the classification precision is calculated in the validation data at the end of each epoch. When the precision stops improving, the training is finished. Therefore, with the use of *Early Stopping*, it was possible to avoid problems such as *underfitting*, in which the neural network cannot extract enough features from the images during training due to an insufficient number of epochs; and, *overfitting*, where the neural network overfits the training data due to an excessive amount of epochs [98]. To do so, a parameter was defined to terminate training if the classification precision has not improved during the last 100 epochs, as shown in Table 3.

In addition to the *Early Stopping* method, the *Dropout* [99] technique was used to help regularize the proposed approach. This technique is widely used to regularize the training of deep neural networks [100]. *Dropout* helps to regularize the model [101], without modifying the cost function. Also, with the use of *Dropout* some hidden neurons of the neural network are randomly and temporarily turned off without changing the input and output neurons. Therefore, this technique causes some neurons not to function according to a certain probability during training.

Dropout helps regularization because it reduces complex co-adaptations of neurons, causing some neurons to be forced to learn features that *a priori* would be learned by other neurons in the architecture. In short, the main idea is to drop units (neurons) randomly (along with their connections) from the neural network during training, preventing the units from adapting too much to the data [99], reducing the possibility of problems related to *overfitting* of the neural network after data augmentation, for example. The parameter defined in the proposed approach for using *Dropout* is shown in Table 3.

The proposed approach was evaluated with the AP and mAP metrics to compare the results. These metrics are often used to measure the precision of deep learning algorithms that perform object detection [29,37]. The proposed approach was compared with related approaches found in the literature, including, SSD [17], YOLO [17], YOLOv3 [20], YOLOv4 [59] and YOLOv5 (unmodified) as shown in Table 4. After the experiments carried out during the validation step of the proposed approach in the DDR dataset using the Stochastic Gradient Descent (SGD) optimizer, the best result was obtained using the *Tilling* method, with a mAP of 0.2490 (indicated in bold font) and values of AP with a limit of IoU of 0.5 equal to 0.2290, 0.3280, 0.1050 and 0.3330, for Hard Exudates (EX), Soft Exudates (SE), Microaneurysms (MA) and Hemorrhages (HE), respectively, as shown in Table 4.

To investigate the results of our proposed approach, the PR curve instead of the ROC curve (*Receiver Operating Characteristic*) [102] was chosen to be analyzed. It is important to observe that the ROC curve is not recommended for situations where the dataset presents an imbalance in the number of examples among the investigated classes. In these cases, the ROC curve usually presents a very high AUC due to the predictor correctly classifying the class with the highest number of examples (majority class) [103,104].

Precision and *Recall* were used to evaluate the results obtained, which are performance metrics commonly used to evaluate image classification and information retrieval systems. Generally speaking, Precision and Recall are not discussed in isolation, and some issues may require a higher *Recall* over *Precision*, or vice versa, depending on the importance given to false positives versus false negatives. In classification problems involving medical images, for example, what is generally desired is to minimize the incidence of false negatives; therefore, a high *Recall* becomes more important than a high *Precision* since a false negative can imply a wrong medical diagnosis and, therefore, patient risks.

Table 4. Results obtained by the proposed approach with SGD optimizer compared to works related to the metrics AP and mAP for the limit of Intersection over Union of 0.5 in the validation set of the Dataset for Diabetic Retinopathy (DDR).

Models	*AP*				*mAP*
	EX	**SE**	**MA**	**HE**	
SSD [17]	0	0.0227	0	0.0007	0.0059
YOLO [17]	0.0039	0	0	0.0101	0.0035
YOLOv3+SGD [20]	-	-	-	-	0.1100
YOLOv3+SGD+*Dropout* [20]	-	-	-	-	0.1710
YOLOv4 [59]	0.0370	0.1493	0.0193	0.0849	0.0716
YOLOv5 (unmodified)	0.0306	0.2500	0.0047	0.1300	0.1040
Proposed Approach+SGD without *Tilling*	0.1490	0.4060	0.0454	0.2780	0.2200
Proposed Approach+SGD with *Tilling*	0.2290	0.3280	0.1050	0.3330	**0.2490**

Definitions in Table 4: AP, Average Precision; EX, hard exudates; SE, soft exudates; MA, microaneurysms; HE, hemorrhages; mAP, mean Average Precision; SSD, Single Shot MultiBox Detector; YOLO, You Only Look Once; YOLOv3, You Only Look Once version 3; YOLOv4, You Only Look Once version 4; YOLOv5, You Only Look Once version 5; SGD, Stochastic Gradient Descent.

Figure 5 presents the graph referring to the PR curve with a limit of IoU of 0.5 obtained during the validation stage using the proposed approach with the SGD optimizer and *Tilling* in the DDR dataset. The AP values obtained by the fundus lesions are plotted on the graph, according to the results presented in Table 4, whose *mean Average Precision* value obtained by all the classes corresponds to 0.249.

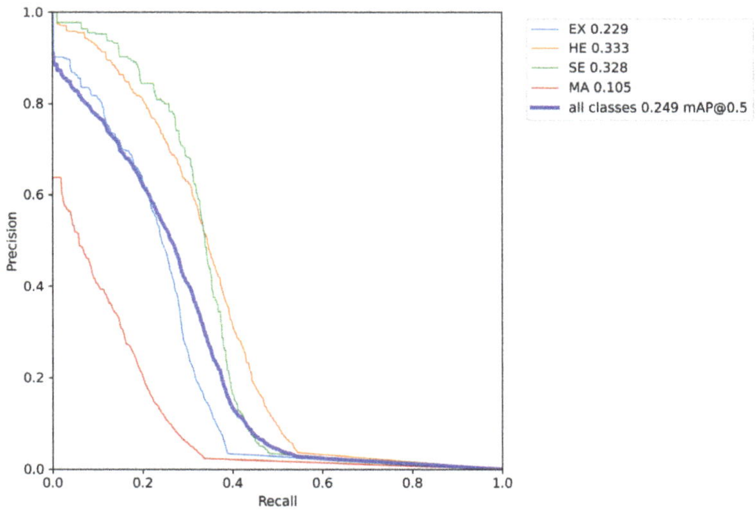

Figure 5. Graph with Precision×Recall curve with a limit of Intersection over Union of 0.5 obtained during the validation step of the proposed approach with Stochastic Gradient Descent (SGD) optimizer and *Tilling* in the Dataset for Diabetic Retinopathy (DDR). EX, hard exudates; HE, hemorrhages; SE, soft exudates; MA, microaneurysms; mAP, mean Average Precision.

The x axis of the PR curve represents *Recall* while the y axis represents *Precision*. This curve mainly focuses on the performance of positive classes, which is critical when dealing with unbalanced classes. Thus, in the PR space, the goal is to be in the upper right corner $(1, 1)$, meaning that the predictor classified all positives as positive ($Recall = 1$) and that everything that was classified as positive is true positive ($Precision = 1$).

It is possible to verify, based on the analysis of the PR curve graph, that the proposed approach found greater difficulty in predicting Microaneurysms (MA) (red curve) followed by Hard Exudates (EX) (cyan curve), with the best results obtained with the prediction of Soft Exudates (SE) (green curve) and Hemorrhages (HE) (orange curve), respectively. The low precision obtained in the detection of MA is mainly related to the size of these microlesions and the gradient dissipation of these objects when the neural network is trained, causing a high rate of errors. This fact can be noted in the confusion matrix (as shown in Figure 6), with 79% of *background* FN and 38% of *background* FP, second only to hard exudates, with 40%. The fact that the proposed approach has achieved better results in predicting SE is associated with the morphological characteristics of these lesions since they generally have larger sizes than other lesions.

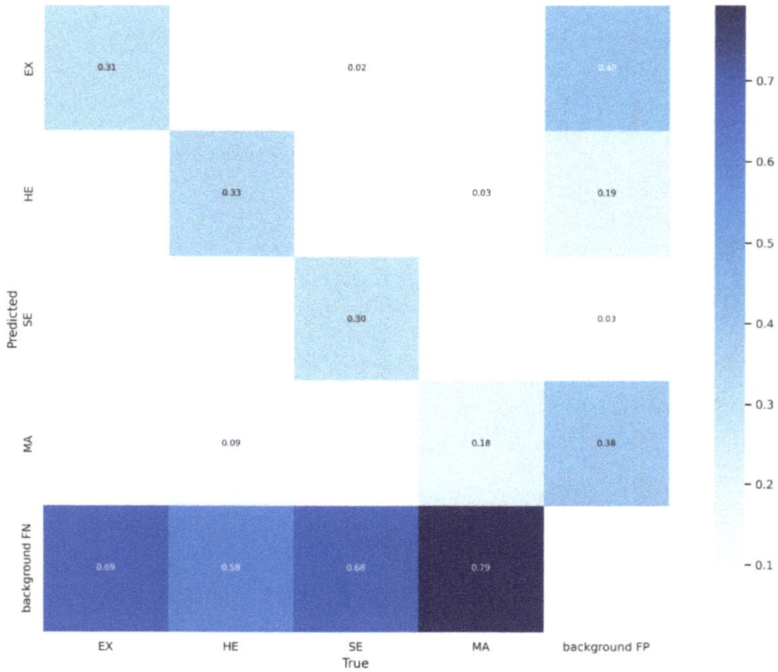

Figure 6. Confusion matrix obtained by the proposed approach with the Stochastic Gradient Descent (SGD) optimizer and *Tilling* during the validation step on the Dataset for Diabetic Retinopathy (DDR). EX, hard exudates; HE, hemorrhages; SE, soft exudates; MA, microaneurysms; FN, False Negative; FP, False Positive.

The confusion matrix is a table containing data from experiments with the proposed approach. Based on these data, it was possible to summarize the information related to the performance of the proposed approach and compare it with the results obtained with similar works in state-of-the-art. Figure 6 presents the confusion matrix obtained by the proposed approach with the SGD optimizer and *Tilling* during the validation step on the DDR dataset. It should be noted that the confusion matrix resulting from the detection of objects presents different characteristics when compared to problems that only involve the classification of objects in images since most model errors are associated with the background class and not with the other classes. In addition, the results presented in the confusion matrix will vary according to the defined confidence limit.

When detecting objects, it is common for information regarding false positives (FP) and false negatives (FN) to be presented in the confusion matrix (*background*). In this sense, the confidence limit established for detecting objects present in these images will directly impact the results obtained from *background* FP and *background* FN.

Therefore, the last row of the confusion matrix refers to *Ground Truth* objects that were not detected by the approach (*background* FN) and therefore considered as background. The last column of the confusion matrix is the detections performed by the approach that does not have any corresponding label in the *Ground Truth* (*background* FP), that is, the image background detected as a lesion.

A confidence limit is applied to filter the bounding boxes of a possible object to eliminate bounding boxes with low confidence scores through a Non-Maximum Suppression algorithm, which disregards detected objects with IoU less than the defined threshold. Thus, if a high confidence limit is defined, such as 0.90, there will be little confusion between the classes and low *background* FP results, but there will be a marked elimination of correctly detected fundus lesions (although with a low confidence limit), but with a confidence limit lower than 0.90. On the other hand, if a confidence limit of 0.25 is defined, there will be a more significant generation of *background* FP and *background* FN since it increases the probability of the model detecting the background as a lesion and vice versa.

Therefore, as the confidence limit tends to 1, the fund FPs will tend to 0. The results presented in the confusion matrix were calculated using a fixed confidence limit of 0.25, which is in line with the default inference configuration contained in the `detect.py` file of the proposed approach. In summary, with lower confidence limits, the results of mAP will be improved but will also produce a more significant amount of *background* FP that will appear in the confusion matrix, while if you increase the confidence limit, there will be a decrease in *background* FP in the confusion matrix, however, with a loss in mAP since more lesions are lost.

Cells with darker shades of blue indicate a greater number of samples. The confusion matrix presents the hits in the prediction of fundus lesions on the main diagonal, while the values off the main diagonal correspond to prediction errors. It is possible to verify that the highest incidence of *background* FN occurred in Microaneurysms (with 79%), followed by Hard Exudates (with 69%), Soft Exudates (with 68%), and Hemorrhages (with 58%). As for FP *background* errors, the highest incidence occurred in Hard Exudates (with 40%), followed by Microaneurysms (with 38%), Hemorrhages (with 19%), and Soft Exudates (with 3%). Also, it can be seen that 9% of Hemorrhages were incorrectly detected as Microanerysms, 2% of Soft Exudates were incorrectly detected as Hard Exudates, and 3% of Microaneurysms were incorrectly detected as Hemorrhages.

Thus, the results presented in the confusion matrix cannot be directly compared with the results of AP presented in this work, because the values are associated with the area under the PR curve, as shown in Figure 5. A good mAP produced by a low confidence limit, for example, will necessarily contain thousands of FPs, pushed to the lower right corner of the PR curve, with trends from *Recall* to 1 and *Precision* to 0, as shown in Figure 5.

During the test stage of the proposed approach in the DDR dataset using the SGD optimizer, the best result obtained reached a mAP of 0.1430 (indicated in bold font) and values of AP with a limit of IoU of 0.5 equal to 0.2100, 0.1380, 0.0530 and 0.1710, for Hard Exudates (EX), Soft Exudates (SE), Microaneurysms (MA) and Hemorrhages (HE), respectively, as presented in Table 5. Furthermore, both results obtained by the proposed approach, with and without the use of *Tilling*, achieved superior results to related works, which also detected fundus lesions in images from the test set of the DDR dataset.

Experiments were carried out during the validation stage of the proposed approach in the DDR dataset using the Adam optimizer, in which the best result was obtained using the *Tilling* method, with a mAP of 0.2630, and AP amounts with a IoU limit of 0.5 equal to 0.2240, 0.3650, 0.1110 and 0.3520, for Hard Exudates (EX), Soft Exudates (SE), Microaneurysms (MA) and Hemorrhages (HE), respectively, as shown in Table 6.

Table 5. Results obtained by the proposed approach with SGD optimizer compared to works related to the metrics AP and mAP for the limit of Intersection over Union of 0.5 in the test set of the Dataset for Diabetic Retinopathy (DDR).

Models	AP				mAP
	EX	SE	MA	HE	
SSD [17]	0.0002	0	0.0001	0.0056	0.0015
YOLO [17]	0.0012	0	0	0.0109	0.0030
YOLOv5 (unmodified)	0.0342	0.1000	0.0028	0.0590	0.0511
Proposed Approach+SGD without *Tilling*	0.1430	0.2040	0.0280	0.1480	0.1310
Proposed Approach+SGD with *Tilling*	0.2100	0.1380	0.0530	0.1710	**0.1430**

Definitions in Table 5: AP, Average Precision; EX, hard exudates; SE, soft exudates; MA, microaneurysms; HE, hemorrhages; mAP, mean Average Precision; SSD, Single Shot MultiBox Detector; YOLO, You Only Look Once; YOLOv5, You Only Look Once version 5; SGD, Stochastic Gradient Descent.

Table 6. Results obtained by the proposed approach with Adam optimizer compared to works related to the metrics AP and mAP for the Intersection over Union limit of 0.5 in the validation set of the Dataset for Diabetic Retinopathy (DDR).

Models	AP				mAP
	EX	SE	MA	HE	
SSD [17]	0	0.0227	0	0.0007	0.0059
YOLO [17]	0.0039	0	0	0.0101	0.0035
YOLOv3+Adam+*Dropout* [20]	-	-	-	-	0.2160
Proposed Approach+Adam without *Tilling*	0.1640	0.4020	0.0610	0.3290	0.2390
Proposed Approach+Adam with *Tilling*	0.2240	0.3650	0.1110	0.3520	**0.2630**

Definitions in Table 6: AP, Average Precision; EX, hard exudates; SE, soft exudates; MA, microaneurysms; HE, hemorrhages; mAP, mean Average Precision; SSD, Single Shot MultiBox Detector; YOLO, You Only Look Once; YOLOv3, You Only Look Once version 3.

The use of the Adam optimizer resulted in a higher mAP than the result obtained by the proposed approach with the SGD optimizer, presented in Table 4. The proposed approach presented results superior to all works with the same purpose found in the literature. Figure 7 presents the graph of the PR curve with a limit of IoU of 0.5 obtained during the validation step using the proposed approach with the optimizer Adam and *Tilling* in the DDR dataset. The AP values obtained by the fundus lesions are plotted on the graph, according to the results presented in Table 6, whose *mean Average Precision* value obtained for all classes corresponds to 0.2630 (indicated in bold font). Analyzing the PR curve, it appears that using the Adam optimizer, the proposed approach presented similar results to those obtained using the SGD optimizer, i.e., there was a high rate of errors in detecting Microaneurysms (MA) (curve in red).

The best results were achieved in the prediction of Soft Exudates (SE) (curve in green color) and Hemorrhages (HE) (curve in orange color), respectively. It is possible to verify in the confusion matrix (as shown in Figure 8) the high rate of *background* FN (89%) and high rate of *background* FP (34%) of microaneurysms. The rate of *background* FP of hard exudates also stands out from the other classes of lesions, reaching 44%. The reasons that led to the high rates of FN and FP, both in detecting microaneurysms and hard exudates, have already been discussed.

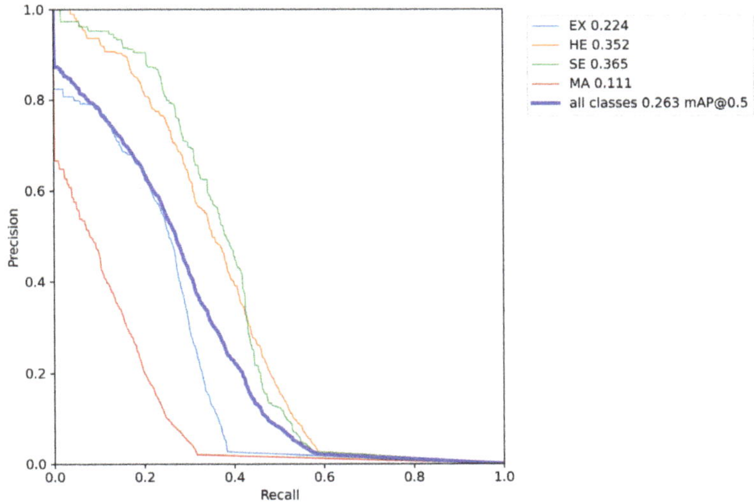

Figure 7. Graph of the Precision × Recall curve with a limit of Intersection over Union of 0.5 obtained during the validation step of the proposed approach with Adam optimizer and *Tilling* in the Dataset for Diabetic Retinopathy (DDR). EX, hard exudates; HE, hemorrhages; SE, soft exudates; MA, microaneurysms; mAP, mean Average Precision.

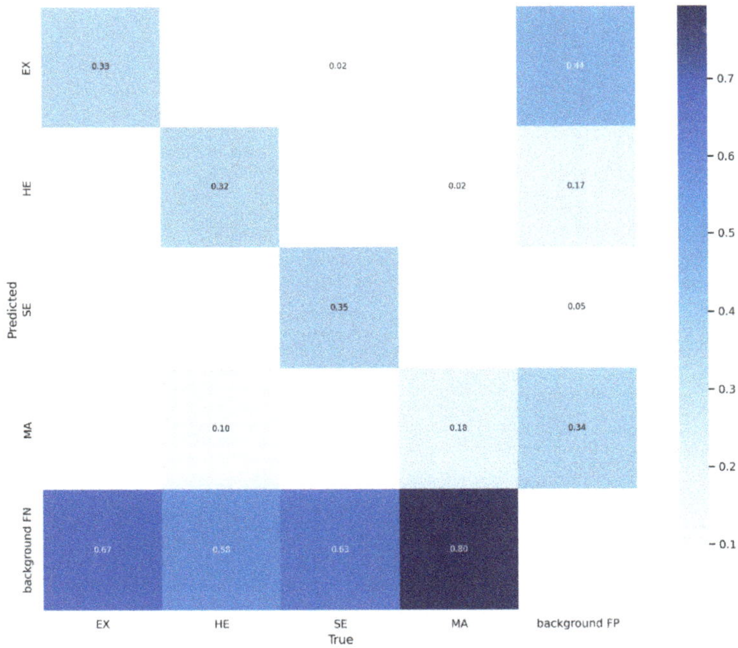

Figure 8. Confusion matrix obtained by the proposed approach with the Adam optimizer and *Tilling* during the validation step on the Dataset for Diabetic Retinopathy (DDR). EX, hard exudates; HE, hemorrhages; SE, soft exudates; MA, microaneurysms; FN, False Negative; FP, False Positive.

Figure 8 presents the confusion matrix obtained by the proposed approach with the Adam optimizer and *Tilling* during the validation step on the DDR dataset. It is possible to verify that the highest incidence of *background* FN occurred in Microaneurysms (with 80%), followed by Hard Exudates (with 67%), Soft Exudates (with 63%), and Hemorrhages (with 58%). As for FP *background* errors, the highest incidence occurred in Hard Exudates (with 44%), followed by Microaneurysms (with 34%), Hemorrhages (with 17%), and Soft Exudates (with 5%). Also, it can be seen that 10% of Hemorrhages were incorrectly detected as Microaneurysms, 2% of Soft Exudates were incorrectly detected as Hard Exudates, and 2% of Microaneurysms were incorrectly detected as Hemorrhages.

Figure 9 presents a batch with fundus images from the DDR dataset along with annotations (*Ground Truth*) of the fundus lesions after the preprocessing steps and augmentation of data that were used to validate the proposed approach using Adam optimizer and *Tilling*. Figure 10 shows the detections of fundus lesions performed on the same batch of fundus images described above.

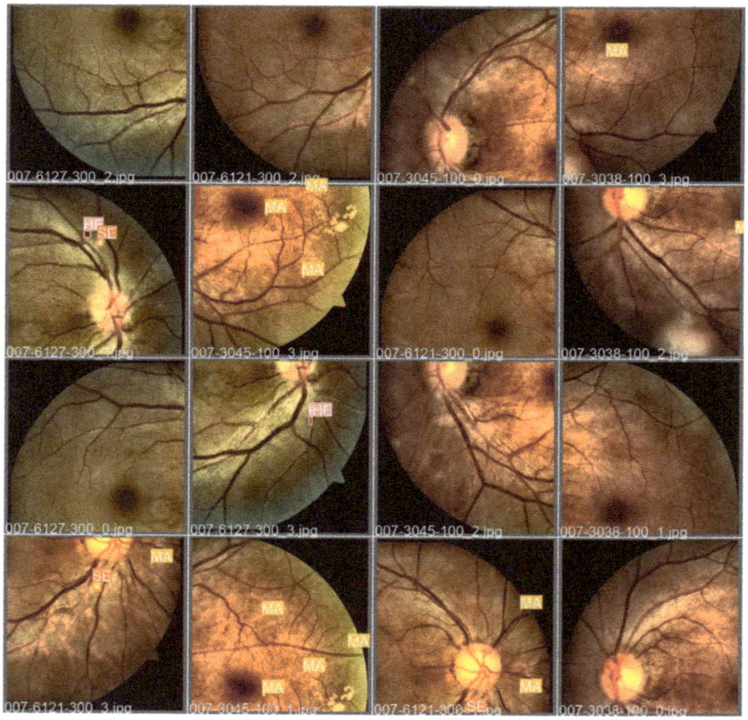

Figure 9. Batch example with fundus images of the Dataset for Diabetic Retinopathy (DDR) along with annotations (*Ground Truth*) of the fundus lesions after the pre-processing and data augmentation steps that were used to validate the proposed approach. MA, microaneurysms; HE, hemorrhages; SE, soft exudates.

The proposed approach was able to satisfactorily detect fundus lesions, such as the microaneurysm located in the image "007-3038-100_3.jpg", or the hemorrhage and soft exudate in the image "007-6127-300_1.jpg", or the microaneurysm and soft exudate in the image "007-6121-300_3.jpg", and microaneurysms in the image "007-6121-300_1.jpg". However, there were cases in which the proposed approach failed to detect the lesions or detected them wrongly, as in the case of one of the microaneurysms not located in the image "007-3045-100_3.jpg", the hemorrhage in the image "007 -6127-300_3.jpg", and two microaneurysms from image "007-3045-100_1.jpg".

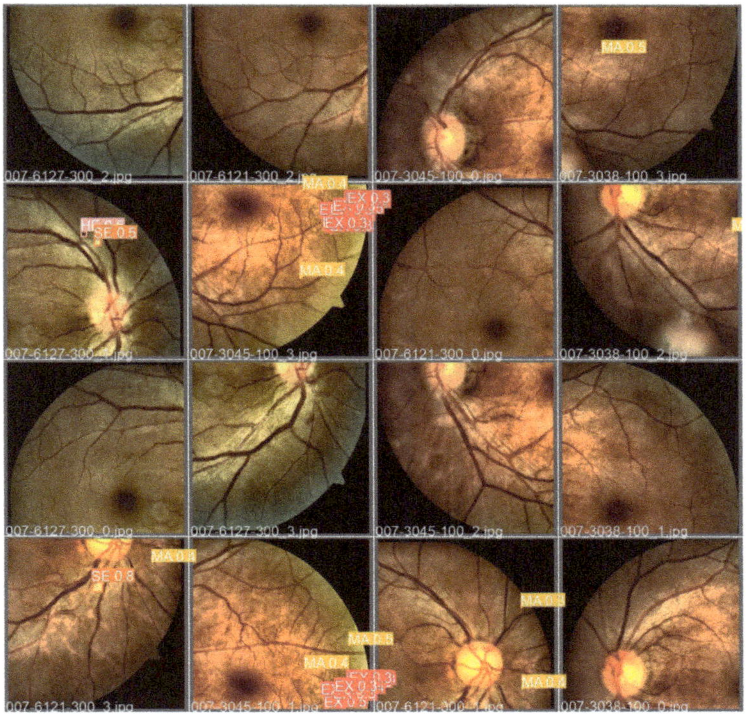

Figure 10. Batch with fundus images from the Dataset for Diabetic Retinopathy (DDR) with fundus lesions detected by the proposed approach during the validation step. MA, microaneurysms; HE, hemorrhages; SE, soft exudates; EX, hard exudates.

Even so, there were also situations where the proposed approach detected objects in the "007-3045-100_3.jpg" image as hard exudates, even though there were no annotations of these lesions in the *Ground Truth* of the DDR dataset. As this image presents microaneurysms in the same sector as the localized hard exudates, it is possible that these exudates were correctly detected, even though they were not originally located in the dataset. However, there is no way to confirm this information since only by verifying the absence of luminescence in these lesions, confirmed by image angiography (not available in the dataset), would it be possible to be sure about the diagnosis. In any case, based on the lesions detected and the generalization capacity verified after the predictions made on unknown images *a priori*, the proposed approach proved to be an essential tool to aid in medical diagnosis.

During the test stage of the proposed approach in the DDR dataset using the Adam optimizer, the best result obtained reached a mAP of 0.1540 (indicated in bold font) and values of AP with a limit of IoU of 0.5 equal to 0.2210, 0.1570, 0.0553 and 0.1840, for Hard Exudates (EX), Soft Exudates (SE), Microaneurysms (MA) and Hemorrhages (HE), respectively, as shown in Table 7. As in the validation set, the proposed approach (with and without the use of *Tilling*) obtained better results than the related works tested in the test set of the DDR dataset.

It is possible to verify that the optimization method that presented the best results was Adam. Thus, we can conclude that this optimizer has excellent potential for application in problems involving the detection of fundus lesions. However, in future works, we intend to conduct experiments with other optimization methods in state-of-the-art using different variations of hyperparameters.

Table 7. Results obtained by the proposed approach with Adam optimizer compared to works related to the *AP* and *mAP* metrics for the Intersection over Union limit of 0.5 in the test set of the DDR (Dataset for Diabetic Retinopathy).

Models	*AP*				*mAP*
	EX	**SE**	**MA**	**HE**	
SSD [17]	0.0002	0	0.0001	0.0056	0.0015
YOLO [17]	0.0012	0	0	0.0109	0.0030
Proposed Approach+Adam without *Tilling*	0.1540	0.2110	0.0296	0.1590	0.1380
Proposed Approach+Adam with *Tilling*	0.2210	0.1570	0.0553	0.1840	**0.1540**

Definitions in Table 7: AP, Average Precision; EX, hard exudates; SE, soft exudates; MA, microaneurysms; HE, hemorrhages; mAP, mean Average Precision; SSD, Single Shot MultiBox Detector; YOLO, You Only Look Once.

The results obtained with the metrics are presented below: *Precision*, which considers, among all the positive classifications made by the model, how many are correct; the *Recall*, which assumes, among all situations of the positive class as expected value, how many are correct; and, the F1-*score*, which calculates the harmonic mean between Precision and Recall.

The best results achieved by the approach proposed in the DDR dataset were obtained using the Adam optimizer and the *Tilling* method, according to the F1-*score* metric obtained in the Validation and Testing stages, with values of 0.3485 (indicated in bold font) and 0.2521 (indicated in bold font), respectively, as shown in Table 8.

Table 8. Results obtained with the metrics: *Precision*, *Recall* and F1-*score* with the Stochastic Gradient Descent (SGD) and Adam optimizers during the validation and testing steps using the Dataset for Diabetic Retinopathy (DDR).

Models	*Precision* Validation	*Recall* Validation	*F1-Score* Validation	*Precision* Test	*Recall* Test	*F1-Score* Test
Proposed Approach+SGD without *Tilling*	0.4533	0.2233	0.2992	0.3270	0.1540	0.2094
Proposed Approach+Adam without *Tilling*	0.4618	0.2484	0.3231	0.3060	0.1710	0.2194
Proposed Approach+SGD com *Tilling*	0.4775	0.2653	0.3411	0.3390	0.1820	0.2368
Proposed Approach+Adam with *Tilling*	0.4462	0.2859	**0.3485**	0.3410	0.2000	**0.2521**

The mean inference time to detect fundus lesions per image in the DDR dataset in the Validation and Testing steps of the proposed approach is presented in Table 9. The approach proposed without *Tilling* had the lowest average inference time per image with the Adam optimizer, with 14.1 *ms*, while with *Tilling* the lowest average inference time per image was achieved with the SGD optimizer, with 4.6 *ms* (indicated in bold font). However, the highlight is the inference time of the proposed approach using *Tilling*, which was around 3 times faster than the inference time of the proposed approach applied to the images without performing from *Tilling*. Therefore, in addition to increasing the precision of the proposed approach in detecting fundus lesions, the *Tilling* method made the prediction process faster.

Table 9. Mean inference time to detect fundus lesions per image in the Dataset for Diabetic Retinopathy (DDR) in the Validation and Testing stages of the proposed approach.

Models	Inference Time (ms) Validation	Inference Time (ms) Test
Proposed Approach+SGD without *Tilling*	15.7	13.0
Proposed Approach+Adam without *Tilling*	14.1	21.1
Proposed Approach+SGD with *Tilling*	**4.6**	5.9
Proposed Approach+Adam with *Tilling*	5.5	7.5

Definitions in Table 9: ms, millisecond; SGD, Stochastic Gradient Descent.

To assess the precision of the proposed approach in different public DR datasets, we also performed experiments with the Diabetic Retinopathy image set IDRiD [18]. During the validation step on the IDRiD dataset, the best result obtained by the proposed approach was using the SGD optimizer with the *Tilling* method, with a mAP of 0.3280 (indicated in bold font) and values of AP with a limit of IoU of 0.5 equal to 0.2630, 0.5340, 0.2170 and 0.2980, for Hard Exudates (EX), Soft Exudates (SE), Microaneurysms (MA) and Hemorrhages (HE), respectively, as shown in Table 10.

Table 10. Results obtained by the proposed approach with *Tilling* and the SGD and Adam optimizers with the metrics AP and mAP for the Intersection over Union limit of 0.5 in the validation set of the Indian Diabetic Retinopathy Image Dataset (IDRiD).

Models	AP				mAP
	EX	SE	MA	HE	
Proposed Approach+SGD without *Tilling*	0.1030	0.2940	0.0601	0.2460	0.1760
Proposed Approach+Adam without *Tilling*	0.1040	0.1810	0.0723	0.1350	0.1230
Proposed Approach+SGD with *Tilling*	0.2630	0.5340	0.2170	0.2980	**0.3280**
Proposed Approach+Adam with *Tilling*	0.2670	0.2740	0.2100	0.3200	0.2680

Definitions in Table 10: AP, Average Precision; EX, hard exudates; SE, soft exudates; MA, microaneurysms; HE, hemorrhages; mAP, mean Average Precision; SGD, Stochastic Gradient Descent.

The best result of mAP obtained by the proposed approach during the validation using the IDRiD dataset surpassed the results obtained in the DDR dataset, thus attesting to the generalization capacity of the method adopted by the proposed approach for the detection of fundus lesions.

In the test stage of the proposed approach using the IDRiD dataset, the best result was obtained with the Adam optimizer and the use of *Tilling*, reaching a mAP of 0.2950 (indicated in bold font), and values of AP with a limit of IoU of 0.5 equal to 0.2530, 0.4090, 0.2210 and 0.2970, for Hard Exudates (EX), Soft Exudates (SE), Microaneurysms (MA) and Hemorrhages (HE), respectively, as shown in Table 11. The results obtained by the proposed approach in the test set of the IDRiD dataset were superior to those obtained in the test set of the DDR dataset.

Figure 11a corresponds to the fundus image "007-3711-200.jpg" from the test set of the DDR dataset, along with the annotations (*Ground Truth*) of fundus lesions; Figure 11b is the segmentation mask of hard exudates; Figure 11c is the hemorrhage segmentation mask; and, Figure 11d is the segmentation mask of microaneurysms. It is important to note that there is no presence of soft exudates in this fundus image.

Table 11. Results obtained by the proposed approach with *Tilling* and the SGD and Adam optimizers with the metrics AP and mAP for the Intersection over Union threshold of 0.5 in the test set of the Indian Diabetic Retinopathy Image Dataset (IDRiD).

Models	AP				mAP
	EX	SE	MA	HE	
Proposed Approach+SGD without *Tilling*	0.1260	0.3000	0.0787	0.2630	0.1920
Proposed Approach+Adam without *Tilling*	0.0993	0.2640	0.0661	0.1380	0.1420
Proposed Approach+SGD with *Tilling*	0.2390	0.3940	0.2010	0.2890	0.2810
Proposed Approach+Adam with *Tilling*	0.2530	0.4090	0.2210	0.2970	**0.2950**

Definitions in Table 11: AP, Average Precision; EX, hard exudates; SE, soft exudates; MA, microaneurysms; HE, hemorrhages; mAP, mean Average Precision; SGD, Stochastic Gradient Descent.

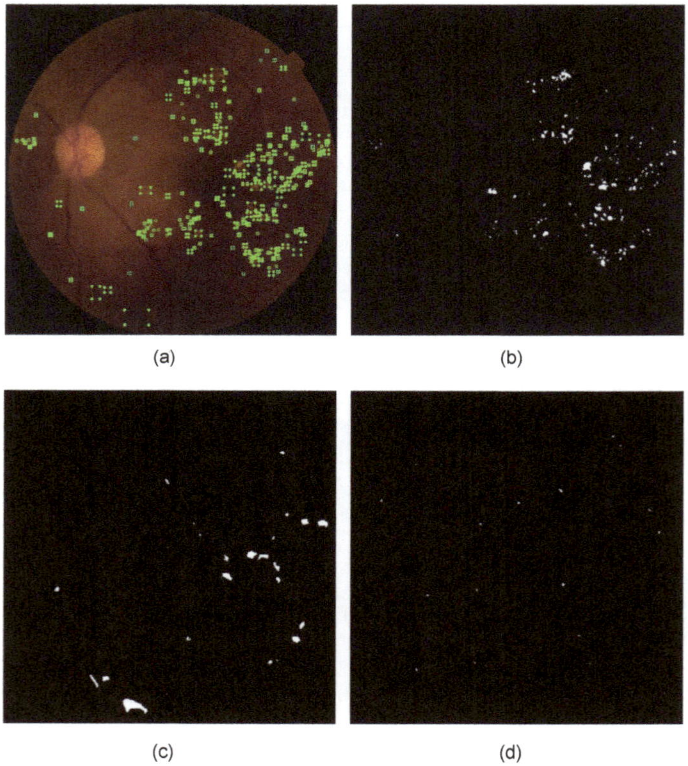

Figure 11. Example of fundus image of the dataset accompanied by the segmentation masks of the lesions present in the image. In (**a**), the fundus image "007-3711-200.jpg" of the test set from the Dataset for Diabetic Retinopathy (DDR), along with annotations (*Ground Truth*) of the fundus lesions; (**b**) segmentation mask of hard exudates; (**c**) hemorrhage segmentation mask; and (**d**) microaneurysm segmentation masks.

Figure 12 demonstrates the detection of fundus lesions performed by the proposed approach and the percentage of confidence obtained in each object located in the fundus image "007-3711-200.jpg" of the set test of the DDR dataset. This retinal image has a darker background, a recurrent feature in several fundus images of the investigated public datasets, which frequently causes problems in detecting lesions (mainly microaneurysms and hemorrhages). In addition, this feature generates high rates of errors during classification, in which a lesion is erroneously considered as background (*background* FN) or, conversely, where the background is erroneously considered as a lesion (*background* FP). For these cases, the image processing techniques applied in the pre-processing block of the proposed approach play an important role, as they aim to minimize these problems by reducing noise and improving the contrast of these images, for example.

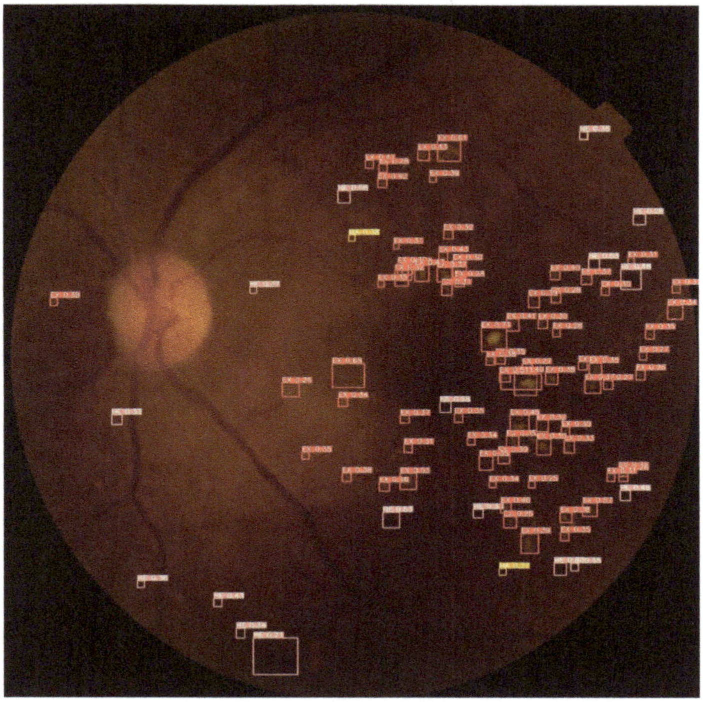

Figure 12. Detection of fundus lesions performed by the proposed approach and the percentage of confidence obtained in each object located in the fundus image "007-3711-200.jpg" of the test set of the Dataset for Diabetic Retinopathy (DDR). EX, hard exudates; HE, hemorrhages; MA, microaneurysms.

Another aspect that can also be seen in this fundus image is the identified microlesions, as in the case of microaneurysms. These are extremely small lesions that end up making them challenging to detect. For these cases, the importance of, for example, the application of the *Tilling* method (pre-processing block of the proposed approach), the application of geometric transformations (data enhancement block of the proposed approach) and the architectural characteristics of the neural network of the proposed approach, such as the use of CSPs integrating *Backbone* and *Neck*, which aim to minimize problems of gradient dissipation of these microlesions during neural network training. Even so, with all these characteristics observed in this fundus image that make it challenging to identify the lesions, it is possible to verify that the proposed approach accurately performed the detection of most fundus lesions, localizing hard exudates (EX), hemorrhages (HE) and microaneurysms (MA) present in the image.

Figure 13 shows the detection of fundus lesions in the "007-3892-200.jpg" image of the test set of the DDR dataset. With a higher level of detail, it is possible to observe the different morphological aspects of some identified lesions, such as hard exudates and Hemorrhages (that often produce classification errors due to similarities with microaneurysms). How shown the results presented in the confusion matrices of the experiments (Figures 6 and 8).

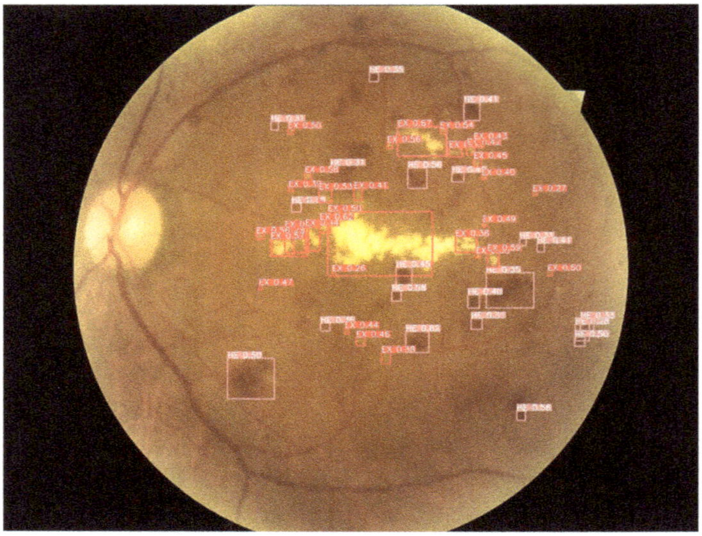

Figure 13. Detection of fundus lesions in the "007-3892-200.jpg" image of the test set of the Dataset for Diabetic Retinopathy (DDR). It is possible to observe different morphological aspects of the identified lesions, as in the case of hard exudates in the image's central region and distributed in other regions of the retina, or hemorrhages, which, like the hard exudates detected. Also, they assume different shapes and sizes, in addition to being able to manifest themselves in different regions of the retina. EX, hard exudates; HE, hemorrhages.

5. Discussion

The works proposed by Alyoubi et al. [20] and Dai et al. [21] presented results in the validation set. Unlike these works, the same methodology as the work proposed by Li et al. [17] was adopted, which evaluated the proposed approach through the analysis of the results obtained both in the validation stage and in the test stage using the public dataset of DDR Diabetic Retinopathy. This method was adopted to avoid the evaluation of the proposed approach being carried out only in the validation set since this evaluation could give a false impression that the proposed approach is accurate in detecting fundus lesions.

Evaluating the approach on a validation set (where the neural network model is fitted) and then on a test set (where the data is not known *a priori*) allowed the generalization capability of the proposed approach to be properly verified, without the risk of biases produced by possible overfitting of the model during the validation. To validate the predictive capacity of the proposed approach regarding the detection of fundus lesions, we also evaluated it in the IDRiD dataset, in which we achieved results equivalent to those obtained in the DDR dataset.

The work by Dai et al. [21] was not compared with the proposed approach, as the authors used a 2-stage architecture while we used a single-stage architecture. The authors did not present the results of AP or mAP, unlike other works with a similar purpose found in the literature, which makes an adequate comparison impossible. In addition, the authors used a private DR dataset to train the deep learning models, which makes it difficult to reproducible the results obtained using the same method.

In the work proposed by Li et al. [17], the best results obtained regarding the detection of fundus lesions in the DDR dataset, using a Single-Stage model, was 0.0059 of mAP in the validation step with SSD and 0.0030 in the test step with YOLO. Santos et al. [59], using the DDR dataset, obtained a mAP of 0.0716 with the YOLOv4 model in the validation step. In work presented by Alyoubi et al. [20], the best result obtained by the authors in the validation step with the DDR dataset was a mAP of 0.1710, using the YOLOv3 model.

The approach based on the YOLOv5 model proposed in this work, obtained a mAP of 0.2630 in the validation step and 0.1540 in the test step, both in DDR dataset.

With a confidence limit set at 0.25, the lesions were identified with their respective confidence percentages. The experimental results showed that the proposed approach obtained greater precision than similar works found in the literature. Another aspect observed during the experiments is that the proposed approach obtained greater precision in detecting Soft Exudates, Hemorrhages, and Hard Exudates, and, in contrast, a lower precision in detecting Microaneurysms was reached.

The detection of these lesions through computerized systems is a challenge due to numerous factors, among which: are the characteristics of size and shape of these lesions; noise and image contrast available in public DR datasets; the number of annotated examples of these lesions available in public DR datasets; and, the difficulty of deep learning algorithms in detecting very small objects. These problems were reported in the literature and observed during the experiments performed. Thus, a new image processing-based approach techniques and a state-of-the-art *Single-Stage* deep neural network architecture were proposed to overcome some of these problems to detect lesions in fundus images.

For the problem related to the shape and size of objects, in which very small lesions such as microaneurysms are more challenging to detect, techniques were applied to increase the receptive field of these lesions, such as partial *Cropping* of the black background of the images, and the *Tilling* of the input images for training the neural network. Also, a data augmentation technique based on the *Scale* geometric transformation was applied. In this case, a 50% zoom is randomly performed on the input images so that new images are artificially created for training. Thus, the neural network can extract more features, making it more efficient in detecting microlesions. A pre-processing block was developed in which we first filter the images to remove *outliers* from capturing these images and then apply the contrast-limited adaptive histogram equalization method to increase the local contrast of fundus images and improve lesion enhancement.

A block responsible for data augmentation was developed to minimize the problem of the small number of lesion examples noted in the public DR datasets. In this block, different state-of-the-art methods were applied, such as *Mosaic*, *MixUp*, *Copy-Paste* and geometric transformations (*flipping*, *scaling*, *perspective*, *translation* and *shearing*). The purpose of this step was to artificially create a greater number of example images with annotated lesions for training the proposed approach, to allow the deep neural network to extract a greater amount of lesion characteristics and, consequently, to increase the generalization capacity of the proposed approach.

In comparison to similar works found in the literature, it is essential to highlight the contributions of the proposed approach related to the structure of the deep neural network used, such as the use of CSP modules (C3) in the *Backbone* and *Neck* of the architecture, which minimized gradient dissipation problems, caused by the number of dense layers. In addition, through these modules, there was an improvement in inference speed and precision in lesion detection, as well as a reduction in computational cost and memory usage. Another innovation in the proposed approach's structure was using the SiLU activation function throughout the neural network to simplify the architecture and reduce the number of hyperparameters. The *Threshold-Moving* method was applied during neural network training so that the image samples were weighed using a precision metric to minimize the imbalance in the number of examples of the different classes of lesions investigated and avoid classification biases in significant classes. Finally, the adjustments and tests were performed on the proposed approach through different public datasets on Diabetic Retinopathy. These datasets were split into Training, Validation, and Testing to evaluate the proposed approach according to the results of the different performance metrics.

The main limitation of our proposed approach focuses on identifying some lesions, as in the case of hard exudates, which have characteristics similar to drusen other than ocular signs caused by DR, for example. For this reason, the proposed approach made classification errors considering these drusen as hard exudates. Thus, a public dataset, with a broader range of eye signals, with lesions labeled and with a reasonable number of examples, associated or not with Diabetic Retinopathy, could support the training of deep learning models and the distinction more accurate of these different types of eye signals.

Another limitation observed during the experiments is associated with detecting microaneurysms. Although the results are better than similar works found in the literature, they are still low due to the size of these microlesions and have gradient dissipation problems. In this sense, we aimed to increase the detection accuracy of these microlesions by exploring architectures that perform the detection in two stages. Furthermore, we intend to explore different strategies, namely: (1) augmenting data to increase the number of examples of these microlesions; (2) improving the process of creating tiles from fundus images to provide the neural network images with the highest possible level of detail for extracting features from fundus lesions.

6. Conclusions

This article presented a new approach to fundus lesion detection using image processing techniques and a deep neural network based on a state-of-the-art YOLO architecture. Two public datasets of Diabetic Retinopathy images were used to train and evaluate the proposed approach's precision: DDR and IDRiD. Only the images with annotated lesions in the datasets were used to perform the training and evaluation of the proposed approach. These datasets were partitioned into training, validation, and testing sets in a ratio of 50:20:30, respectively. The best results were achieved in the DDR dataset using the Adam optimizer and the *Tilling* method, reaching in the validation stage the mAP of 0.2630 for the limit of IoU of 0.5 and F1-*score* of 0.3485, and in the test step the mAP of 0.1540 for the limit of IoU of 0.5 and F1-*score* of 0.2521. The results obtained in the experiments demonstrate that the proposed approach presented results superior to equivalent works found in the literature.

The deep neural network architecture was implemented based on the YOLOv5 framework and the framework PyTorch, reaching 22.4% in the validation stage *Average Precision* for Hard Exudates, 36.5% for Soft Exudates, 11.1% for Microaneurysms, and 35.2% for Hemorrhages, in the DDR dataset. Different state-of-the-art image processing and data augmentation techniques were explored, such as CLAHE, *Tilling*, *Mosaic*, *Copy-Paste* and *MixUp*. In this way, it was possible to increase the precision of the proposed approach in detecting fundus lesions because, with the help of these techniques, the deep neural network architecture extracted a greater and more representative amount of characteristics of the lesions investigated during the training stage.

The experiments achieved state-of-the-art results, surpassing related works found in the literature with similar purpose and application and demonstrating that the detection of fundus lesions can be performed effectively through a deep learning-based approach. Furthermore, for the problem related to the size of objects, in which very small lesions are more difficult to detect, techniques were applied to increase the receptive field of these lesions, such as partial *Cropping* of the black background of the images and *Tilling* of the input images for training the neural network. However, the results presented in this work indicate that detecting microlesions such as microaneurysms in fundus images remains challenging for future research.

In future work, we intend to explore state-of-the-art architectures that perform instance segmentation to investigate and compare the trade-off between the precision and inference speed of these architectures with the approach proposed in this work. Furthermore, we intend to explore new data augmentation strategies and structures for the *Backbone*, *Neck* and *Head* of the deep neural network architecture implemented in the proposed approach, as well as to carry out experiments with other sets of public data on Diabetic Retinopathy.

Supplementary Materials: The following supporting information can be downloaded at: https://www.mdpi.com/article/10.3390/s22176441/s1, Supplementary Materials: Pre-Processing, Image Preparation, and Data Augmentation in Details. References [105–161] are cited in Supplementary Materials File.

Author Contributions: For this research, C.S., M.A. and D.W. carried out the conceptualization of the research; C.S. and B.B. conducted the experiments and data analysis; C.S. wrote the draft of the article; M.A. and D.W. reviewed and edited the entire article. All authors have read and agreed to the published version of the manuscript.

Funding: This study was financed in part by the Coordenação de Aperfeiçoamento de Pessoal de Nível Superior—Brasil (CAPES)—Finance Code 001.

Institutional Review Board Statement: Not applicable.

Informed Consent Statement: Not applicable.

Data Availability Statement: We used publicly available datasets in this study. DDR dataset at https://doi.org/10.1016/j.ins.2019.06.011, accessed 9 May 2020 and IDRiD at https://ieee-dataport.org/open-access/indian-diabetic-retinopathy-image-dataset-idrid (accessed 5 August 2020).

Conflicts of Interest: The authors declare no conflict of interest.

References

1. Delgado-Bonal, A.; Martín-Torres, J. Human vision is determined based on information theory. *Sci. Rep.* **2016**, *6*, 36038. [CrossRef] [PubMed]
2. Riordan-Eva, P.; Augsburger, J.J. *General Ophthalmology*, 19th ed.; Mc Graw Hill Education: New York, NY, USA, 2018.
3. IORJ. O que é Retina. 2021. Available online: https://iorj.med.br/o-que-e-retina/ (accessed on 15 June 2021).
4. Mookiah, M.R.K.; Acharya, U.R.; Chua, C.K.; Lim, C.M.; Ng, E.Y.; Laude, A. Computer-aided diagnosis of diabetic retinopathy: A review. *Comput. Biol. Med.* **2013**, *43*, 2136–2155. [CrossRef] [PubMed]
5. Yen, G.G.; Leong, W.F. A sorting system for hierarchical grading of diabetic fundus images: A preliminary study. *IEEE Trans. Inf. Technol. Biomed.* **2008**, *12*, 118–130. [CrossRef] [PubMed]
6. Alghadyan, A.A. Diabetic retinopathy—An update. *Saudi J. Ophthalmol.* **2011**, *25*, 99–111. [CrossRef] [PubMed]
7. ETDRSR. Grading Diabetic Retinopathy from Stereoscopic Color Fundus Photographs—An Extension of the Modified Airlie House Classification. *Ophthalmology* **1991**, *98*, 786–806. [CrossRef]
8. Philip, S.; Fleming, A.D.; Goatman, K.A.; Fonseca, S.; Mcnamee, P.; Scotland, G.S.; Prescott, G.J.; Sharp, P.F.; Olson, J.A. The efficacy of automated "disease/no disease" grading for diabetic retinopathy in a systematic screening programme. *Br. J. Ophthalmol.* **2007**, *91*, 1512–1517. [CrossRef]
9. ETDRSR. Classification of Diabetic Retinopathy from Fluorescein Angiograms. *Ophthalmology* **1991**, *98*, 807–822. [CrossRef]
10. Hendrick, A.M.; Gibson, M.V.; Kulshreshtha, A. Diabetic Retinopathy. *Prim. Care-Clin. Off. Pract.* **2015**, *42*, 451–464. [CrossRef]
11. Williams, R.; Airey, M.; Baxter, H.; Forrester, J.; Kennedy-Martin, T.; Girach, A. Epidemiology of diabetic retinopathy and macular oedema: A systematic review. *Eye* **2004**, *18*, 963–983. [CrossRef]
12. International Council of Ophthalmology. Updated 2017 ICO Guidelines for Diabetic Eye Care. In *ICO Guidelines for Diabetic Eye Care*; International Council of Ophthalmology: Brussels, Belgium, 2017; pp. 1–33.
13. Cardoso, C.d.F.d.S. Segmentação Automática do Disco óptico e de vasos Sanguíneos em Imagens de Fundo de Olho. Ph.D. Thesis, Universidade Federal de Uberlândia, Uberlândia, Brazil, 2019.
14. Lecaire, T.J.; Palta, M.; Klein, R.; Klein, B.E.; Cruickshanks, K.J. Assessing progress in retinopathy outcomes in type 1 diabetes. *Diabetes Care* **2013**, *36*, 631–637. [CrossRef]
15. Chakrabarti, R.; Harper, C.A.; Keeffe, J.E. Diabetic retinopathy management guidelines. *Expert Rev. Ophthalmol.* **2012**, *7*, 417–439. [CrossRef]
16. Vocaturo, E.; Zumpano, E. The contribution of AI in the detection of the Diabetic Retinopathy. In Proceedings of the—2020 IEEE International Conference on Bioinformatics and Biomedicine, BIBM 2020, Seoul, Korea, 16–19 December 2020; pp. 1516–1519. [CrossRef]
17. Li, T.; Gao, Y.; Wang, K.; Guo, S.; Liu, H.; Kang, H. Diagnostic assessment of deep learning algorithms for diabetic retinopathy screening. *Inf. Sci.* **2019**, *501*, 511–522. [CrossRef]
18. Porwal, P.; Pachade, S.; Kokare, M.; Deshmukh, G.; Son, J.; Bae, W.; Liu, L.; Wang, J.; Liu, X.; Gao, L.; et al. IDRiD: Diabetic Retinopathy—Segmentation and Grading Challenge. *Med. Image Anal.* **2020**, *59*, 101561. [CrossRef]
19. Mateen, M.; Wen, J.; Nasrullah, N.; Sun, S.; Hayat, S. Exudate Detection for Diabetic Retinopathy Using Pretrained Convolutional Neural Networks. *Complexity* **2020**, *2020*, 5801870. [CrossRef]
20. Alyoubi, W.L.; Abulkhair, M.F.; Shalash, W.M. Diabetic Retinopathy Fundus Image Classification and Lesions Localization System Using Deep Learning. *Sensors* **2021**, *21*, 3704. [CrossRef]
21. Dai, L.; Wu, L.; Li, H.; Cai, C.; Wu, Q.; Kong, H.; Liu, R.; Wang, X.; Hou, X.; Liu, Y.; et al. A deep learning system for detecting diabetic retinopathy across the disease spectrum. *Nat. Commun.* **2021**, *12*, 3242. [CrossRef]
22. Simonyan, K.; Zisserman, A. Very deep convolutional networks for large-scale image recognition. In Proceedings of the 3rd International Conference on Learning Representations, ICLR 2015—Conference Track Proceedings, San Diego, CA, USA, 7–9 May 2015; pp. 1–14.

23. He, K.; Zhang, X.; Ren, S.; Sun, J. Deep residual learning for image recognition. In Proceedings of the IEEE Computer Society Conference on Computer Vision and Pattern Recognition, Las Vegas, NV, USA, 27–30 June 2016; Volume 2016-Decem, pp. 770–778. [CrossRef]
24. Szegedy, C.; Liu, W.; Jia, Y.; Sermanet, P.; Reed, S.; Anguelov, D.; Erhan, D.; Vanhoucke, V.; Rabinovich, A. Going deeper with convolutions. In Proceedings of the 2015 IEEE Conference on Computer Vision and Pattern Recognition (CVPR), Boston, MA, USA, 7–12 June 2015; pp. 1–9. [CrossRef]
25. Huang, G.; Liu, Z.; Van Der Maaten, L.; Weinberger, K.Q. Densely connected convolutional networks. In Proceedings of the—30th IEEE Conference on Computer Vision and Pattern Recognition, CVPR 2017, Honolulu, HI, USA, 21–26 July 2017; pp. 2261–2269. [CrossRef]
26. Hu, J.; Shen, L.; Sun, G. Squeeze-and-Excitation Networks. In Proceedings of the 2018 IEEE/CVF Conference on Computer Vision and Pattern Recognition, Salt Lake City, UT, USA, 18–23 June 2018; pp. 7132–7141. [CrossRef]
27. Xie, S.; Tu, Z. Holistically-nested edge detection. In Proceedings of the IEEE International Conference on Computer Vision, Santiago, Chile, 7–13 December 2015; pp. 1395–1403. [CrossRef]
28. Chen, L.C.; Zhu, Y.; Papandreou, G.; Schroff, F.; Adam, H. Encoder-decoder with atrous separable convolution for semantic image segmentation. *Lect. Notes Comput. Sci.* **2018**, *11211 LNCS*, 833–851. [CrossRef]
29. Konishi, Y.; Hanzawa, Y.; Kawade, M.; Hashimoto, M. SSD: Single Shot MultiBox Detector. *Eccv* **2016**, *1*, 398–413. [CrossRef]
30. Redmon, J.; Divvala, S.; Girshick, R.; Farhadi, A. You only look once: Unified, real-time object detection. In Proceedings of the IEEE Computer Society Conference on Computer Vision and Pattern Recognition, Las Vegas, NV, USA, 27–30 June 2016; pp. 779–788. [CrossRef]
31. Melo, R.; Lima, G.; Corrêa, G.; Zatt, B.; Aguiar, M.; Nachtigall, G.; Araújo, R. Diagnosis of Apple Fruit Diseases in the Wild with Mask R-CNN. In *Intelligent Systems;* Cerri, R., Prati, R.C., Eds.; BRACIS 2020. Lecture Notes in Computer Science; Springer: Cham, Switzerland, 2020; Volume 12319, pp. 256–270. [CrossRef]
32. Ronneberger, O.; Fischer, P.; Brox, T. U-net: Convolutional networks for biomedical image segmentation. *Lect. Notes Comput. Sci.* **2015**, *9351*, 234–241. [CrossRef]
33. Shelhamer, E.; Long, J.; Darrell, T. Fully Convolutional Networks for Semantic Segmentation. *IEEE Trans. Pattern Anal. Mach. Intell.* **2017**, *39*, 640–651. [CrossRef]
34. Yu, F.; Wang, D.; Shelhamer, E.; Darrell, T. Deep Layer Aggregation. In Proceedings of the IEEE Computer Society Conference on Computer Vision and Pattern Recognition, Salt Lake City, UT, USA, 18–23 June 2018; pp. 2403–2412. [CrossRef]
35. Szegedy, C.; Vanhoucke, V.; Ioffe, S.; Shlens, J.; Wojna, Z. Rethinking the Inception Architecture for Computer Vision. In Proceedings of the IEEE Computer Society Conference on Computer Vision and Pattern Recognition, Las Vegas, NV, USA, 27–30 June 2016; pp. 2818–2826. [CrossRef]
36. Tsiknakis, N.; Theodoropoulos, D.; Manikis, G.; Ktistakis, E.; Boutsora, O.; Berto, A.; Scarpa, F.; Scarpa, A.; Fotiadis, D.I.; Marias, K. Deep learning for diabetic retinopathy detection and classification based on fundus images: A review. *Comput. Biol. Med.* **2021**, *135*, 104599. [CrossRef] [PubMed]
37. Redmon, J.; Farhadi, A. YOLOv3: An Incremental Improvement. *arXiv* **2018**, arXiv:1804.02767.
38. He, K.; Gkioxari, G.; Dollár, P.; Girshick, R. Mask R-CNN. *IEEE Trans. Pattern Anal. Mach. Intell.* **2020**, *42*, 386–397. [CrossRef] [PubMed]
39. Ramcharan, A.; McCloskey, P.; Baranowski, K.; Mbilinyi, N.; Mrisho, L.; Ndalahwa, M.; Legg, J.; Hughes, D. Assessing a mobile-based deep learning model for plant disease surveillance. *arXiv* **2018**, arXiv:1805.08692.
40. Ren, S.; He, K.; Girshick, R.; Sun, J. Faster R-CNN: Towards Real-Time Object Detection with Region Proposal Networks. *IEEE Trans. Pattern Anal. Mach. Intell.* **2017**, *39*, 1137–1149. [CrossRef]
41. Ojha, A.; Sahu, S.P.; Dewangan, D.K. Vehicle Detection through Instance Segmentation using Mask R-CNN for Intelligent Vehicle System. In Proceedings of the 5th International Conference on Intelligent Computing and Control Systems (ICICCS), Madurai, India, 6–8 May 2021; pp. 954–959. [CrossRef]
42. Iacovacci, J.; Wu, Z.; Bianconi, G. Mesoscopic structures reveal the network between the layers of multiplex data sets. *Phys. Rev.-Stat. Nonlinear Soft Matter Phys.* **2015**, *92*, 42806. [CrossRef]
43. Bertels, J.; Eelbode, T.; Berman, M.; Vandermeulen, D.; Maes, F.; Bisschops, R.; Blaschko, M.B. Optimizing the Dice Score and Jaccard Index for Medical Image Segmentation: Theory and Practice. *Lect. Notes Comput. Sci.* **2019**, *11765 LNCS*, 92–100. [CrossRef]
44. Kaggle. Diabetic Retinopathy Detection. 2015. Available online: https://www.kaggle.com/c/diabetic-retinopathy-detection (accessed on 11 June 2021).
45. Zhu, L.; Geng, X.; Li, Z.; Liu, C. Improving YOLOv5 with Attention Mechanism for Detecting Boulders from Planetary Images. *Remote Sens.* **2021**, *13*, 3776. [CrossRef]
46. Xu, R.; Lin, H.; Lu, K.; Cao, L.; Liu, Y. A forest fire detection system based on ensemble learning. *Forests* **2021**, *12*, 217. [CrossRef]
47. Qi, D.; Tan, W.; Yao, Q.; Liu, J. YOLO5Face: Why Reinventing a Face Detector. *arXiv* **2021**, arXiv:2105.12931.
48. Zhu, X.; Lyu, S.; Wang, X.; Zhao, Q. TPH-YOLOv5: Improved YOLOv5 Based on Transformer Prediction Head for Object Detection on Drone-captured Scenarios. In Proceedings of the IEEE/CVF International Conference on Computer Vision, Montreal, QC, Canada, 10–17 October 2021.

49. Rahman, R.; Azad, Z.B.; Hasan, M.B. Densely-Populated Traffic Detection using YOLOv5 and Non-Maximum Suppression Ensembling. In Proceedings of the International Conference on Big Data, IoT, and Machine Learning, Cox's Bazar, Bangladesh, 23–25 September 2021.
50. Zheng, Z.; Zhao, J.; Li, Y. Research on Detecting Bearing-Cover Defects Based on Improved YOLOv3. *IEEE Access* **2021**, *9*, 10304–10315. [CrossRef]
51. Xie, J.; Zheng, S. ZSD-YOLO: Zero-Shot YOLO Detection using Vision-Language KnowledgeDistillation. *arXiv* **2021**, arXiv:2109.12066.
52. Solawetz, J. YOLOv5: The Latest Model for Object Detection. YOLOv5 New Version—Improvements and Evaluation. 2020. Available online: https://blog.roboflow.com/yolov5-improvements-and-evaluation/ (accessed on 31 May 2021).
53. Couturier, R.; Noura, H.N.; Salman, O.; Sider, A. A Deep Learning Object Detection Method for an Efficient Clusters Initialization. *arXiv* **2021**, arXiv:2104.13634
54. Li, Jichao.; Guo, Shengyu.; Kong, Liulin.; Tan, Siqi.; Yuan, Yican. An improved YOLOv3-tiny method for fire detection in the construction industry. *E3S Web Conf.* **2021**, *253*, 03069. [CrossRef]
55. Bochkovskiy, A.; Wang, C.Y.; Liao, H.Y.M. YOLOv4: Optimal Speed and Accuracy of Object Detection. *arXiv* **2020**, arXiv:2004.10934.
56. Walter, T.; Klein, J.C.; Massin, P.; Erginay, A. A contribution of image processing to the diagnosis of diabetic retinopathy—Detection of exudates in color fundus images of the human retina. *IEEE Trans. Med. Imaging* **2002**, *21*, 1236–1243. [CrossRef]
57. Jasim, M.K.; Najm, R.; Kanan, E.H.; Alfaar, H.E.; Otair, M. Image Noise Removal Techniques: A Comparative Analysis. 2019. Available online: http://www.warse.org/IJSAIT/static/pdf/file/ijsait01862019.pdf (accessed on 25 August 2022).
58. Gonzalez, R.; Woods, R. *Processamento Digital de Imagens*, 3rd ed.; Pearson Prentice Hall: São Paulo, Brazil, 2010.
59. Santos, C.; De Aguiar, M.S.; Welfer, D.; Belloni, B. Deep Neural Network Model based on One-Stage Detector for Identifying Fundus Lesions. In Proceedings of the 2021 International Joint Conference on Neural Networks (IJCNN), Shenzhen, China, 18–22 July 2021; pp. 1–8. [CrossRef]
60. Rai, R.; Gour, P.; Singh, B. Underwater Image Segmentation using CLAHE Enhancement and Thresholding. *Int. J. Emerg. Technol. Adv. Eng.* **2012**, *2*, 118–123.
61. Horry, M.J.; Chakraborty, S.; Paul, M.; Ulhaq, A.; Pradhan, B.; Saha, M.; Shukla, N. COVID-19 Detection Through Transfer Learning Using Multimodal Imaging Data. *IEEE Access* **2020**, *8*, 149808–149824. [CrossRef]
62. El abbadi, N.; Hammod, E. Automatic Early Diagnosis of Diabetic Retinopathy Using Retina Fundus Images Enas Hamood Al-Saadi-Automatic Early Diagnosis of Diabetic Retinopathy Using Retina Fundus Images. *Eur. Acad. Res.* **2014**, *2*, 1–22.
63. Nguyen, T.S.; Stueker, S.; Niehues, J.; Waibel, A. Improving sequence-to-sequence speech recognition training with on-the-fly data augmentation. In Proceedings of the IEEE International Conference on Acoustics, Speech and Signal Processing (ICASSP), Brighton, UK, 12–17 May 2019. [CrossRef]
64. Lam, T.K.; Ohta, M.; Schamoni, S.; Riezler, S. On-the-Fly Aligned Data Augmentation for Sequence-to-Sequence ASR. *arXiv* **2021**, arXiv:2104.01393. [CrossRef]
65. Liu, C.; Jin, S.; Wang, D.; Luo, Z.; Yu, J.; Zhou, B.; Yang, C. Constrained Oversampling: An Oversampling Approach to Reduce Noise Generation in Imbalanced Datasets with Class Overlapping. *IEEE Access* **2020**, 1–13. [CrossRef]
66. Japkowicz, N. Learning from imbalanced data sets: A comparison of various strategies. In Proceedings of the AAAI Workshop on Learning from Imbalanced Data Sets, Austin, TX, USA, 31 July 2000; Volume 68, pp. 10–15.
67. Provost, F. Machine learning from imbalanced data sets 101. In Proceedings of the AAAI'2000 Workshop on Imbalanced Data Sets, Austin, TX, USA, 31 July 2000; p. 3.
68. Zhou, Z.H.; Liu, X.Y. Training cost-sensitive neural networks with methods addressing the class imbalance problem. *IEEE Trans. Knowl. Data Eng.* **2006**, *18*, 63–77. [CrossRef]
69. Buda, M.; Maki, A.; Mazurowski, M.A. A systematic study of the class imbalance problem in convolutional neural networks. *Neural Netw.* **2018**, *106*, 249–259. [CrossRef]
70. Zhang, X.; Gweon, H.; Provost, S. Threshold Moving Approaches for Addressing the Class Imbalance Problem and their Application to Multi-label Classification. *Pervasivehealth Pervasive Comput. Technol. Healthc.* **2020**, *169255*, 72–77. [CrossRef]
71. He, H.; Garcia, E.A. Learning from Imbalanced Data. *IEEE Trans. Knowl. Data Eng.* **2009**, *21*, 1263–1284. [CrossRef]
72. Fernández, A.; García, S.; Galar, M.; Prati, R.C. *Learning from Imbalanced Data Sets*; Springer: Berlin, Germany, 2019; pp. 1–377.
73. Ge, Z.; Liu, S.; Wang, F.; Li, Z.; Sun, J. YOLOX: Exceeding YOLO Series in 2021. *arXiv* **2021**, arXiv:2107.08430.
74. Iyer, R.; Shashikant Ringe, P.; Varadharajan Iyer, R.; Prabhulal Bhensdadiya, K. Comparison of YOLOv3, YOLOv5s and MobileNet-SSD V2 for Real-Time Mask Detection Comparison of YOLOv3, YOLOv5s and MobileNet-SSD V2 for Real-Time Mask Detection View project Comparison of YOLOv3, YOLOv5s and MobileNet-SSD V2 for Real-Time Mask Detection. *Artic. Int. J. Res. Eng. Technol.* **2021**, *8*, 1156–1160.
75. Yu, Y.; Zhao, J.; Gong, Q.; Huang, C.; Zheng, G.; Ma, J. Real-Time Underwater Maritime Object Detection in Side-Scan Sonar Images Based on Transformer-YOLOv5. *Remote Sens.* **2021**, *13*, 3355. [CrossRef]
76. Wang, C.Y.; Mark Liao, H.Y.; Wu, Y.H.; Chen, P.Y.; Hsieh, J.W.; Yeh, I.H. CSPNet: A new backbone that can enhance learning capability of CNN. In Proceedings of the IEEE Computer Society Conference on Computer Vision and Pattern Recognition Workshops, Seattle, WA, USA, 14–19 June 2020; pp. 1571–1580. [CrossRef]

77. Xie, S.; Girshick, R.; Dollár, P.; Tu, Z.; He, K. Aggregated residual transformations for deep neural networks. In Proceedings of the 30th IEEE Conference on Computer Vision and Pattern Recognition, CVPR 2017, Salt Lake City, UT, USA, 19–21 June 2018; pp. 5987–5995. [CrossRef]
78. Ioffe, S.; Szegedy, C. Batch Normalization: Accelerating Deep Network Training by Reducing Internal Covariate Shift. In Proceedings of the International Conference on Machine Learning, Lille, France, 6–11 July 2015.
79. Elfwing, S.; Uchibe, E.; Doya, K. Sigmoid-Weighted Linear Units for Neural Network Function Approximation in Reinforcement Learning. *Neural Netw.* **2017**, *107*, 3–11. [CrossRef]
80. Agarap, A.F. Deep Learning using Rectified Linear Units (ReLU). *arXiv* **2019**, arXiv:1803.08375.
81. He, K.; Zhang, X.; Ren, S.; Sun, J. Spatial Pyramid Pooling in Deep Convolutional Networks for Visual Recognition. *Lect. Notes Comput. Sci.* **2014**, *8691*, 346–361. [CrossRef]
82. Zeiler, M.D.; Taylor, G.W.; Fergus, R. Adaptive deconvolutional networks for mid and high level feature learning. In Proceedings of the 2011 International Conference on Computer Vision, Washington, DC, USA, 6–13 November 2011; pp. 2018–2025. [CrossRef]
83. Li, X.; Lai, T.; Wang, S.; Chen, Q.; Yang, C.; Chen, R. Feature Pyramid Networks for Object Detection. In Proceedings of the 2019 IEEE International Conference on Parallel and Distributed Processing with Applications, Big Data and Cloud Computing, Sustainable Computing and Communications, Social Computing and Networking, ISPA/BDCloud/SustainCom/SocialCom 2019, Xiamen, China, 16–18 December 2019; pp. 1500–1504. [CrossRef]
84. Liu, S.; Qi, L.; Qin, H.; Shi, J.; Jia, J. Path Aggregation Network for Instance Segmentation. In Proceedings of the IEEE Computer Society Conference on Computer Vision and Pattern Recognition, Salt Lake City, UT, USA, 18–23 June 2018; pp. 8759–8768. [CrossRef]
85. Jadon, S. A survey of loss functions for semantic segmentation. In Proceedings of the 2020 IEEE Conference on Computational Intelligence in Bioinformatics and Computational Biology, CIBCB 2020, Virtual, 27–29 October 2020. [CrossRef]
86. Rezatofighi, H.; Tsoi, N.; Gwak, J.; Sadeghian, A.; Reid, I.; Savarese, S. Generalized intersection over union: A metric and a loss for bounding box regression. In Proceedings of the IEEE Computer Society Conference on Computer Vision and Pattern Recognition, Long Beach, CA, USA, 15–20 June 2019; pp. 658–666. [CrossRef]
87. Lin, K.; Zhao, H.; Lv, J.; Zhan, J.; Liu, X.; Chen, R.; Li, C.; Huang, Z. Face Detection and Segmentation with Generalized Intersection over Union Based on Mask R-CNN. In *Advances in Brain Inspired Cognitive Systems, Proceedings of the 10th International Conference, BICS 2019, Guangzhou, China, 13–14 July 2019*; Springer: Berlin/Heidelberg, Germeny, 2019; pp. 106–116. [CrossRef]
88. Oksuz, K.; Cam, B.C.; Kahraman, F.; Baltaci, Z.S.; Kalkan, S.; Akbas, E. Mask-aware IoU for Anchor Assignment in Real-time Instance Segmentation. *arXiv* **2021**, arXiv:2110.09734.
89. Pan, S.J.; Yang, Q. A survey on transfer learning. *IEEE Trans. Knowl. Data Eng.* **2010**, *22*, 1345–1359. [CrossRef]
90. Blitzer, J.; Dredze, M.; Pereira, F. Biographies, Bollywood, Boom-boxes and Blenders: Domain Adaptation for Sentiment Classification. In Proceedings of the 45th Annual Meeting of the Association of Computational Linguistics, Prague, Czech Republic, 23–30 June 2007; Association for Computational Linguistics: Prague, Czech Republic, 2007; pp. 440–447.
91. Lin, T.Y.; Maire, M.; Belongie, S.; Hays, J.; Perona, P.; Ramanan, D.; Dollár, P.; Zitnick, C.L. Microsoft COCO: Common objects in context. *Lect. Notes Comput. Sci.* **2014**, *8693 LNCS*, 740–755. [CrossRef]
92. Franke, M.; Gopinath, V.; Reddy, C.; Ristić-Durrant, D.; Michels, K. Bounding Box Dataset Augmentation for Long-Range Object Distance Estimation. In Proceedings of the IEEE/CVF International Conference on Computer Vision (ICCV) Workshops, Montreal, QC, Canada, 11–17 October 2021; pp. 1669–1677.
93. Mamdouh, N.; Khattab, A. YOLO-Based Deep Learning Framework for Olive Fruit Fly Detection and Counting. *IEEE Access* **2021**, *9*, 84252–84262. [CrossRef]
94. Dewi, C.; Chen, R.C.; Liu, Y.T.; Jiang, X.; Hartomo, K.D. Yolo V4 for Advanced Traffic Sign Recognition with Synthetic Training Data Generated by Various GAN. *IEEE Access* **2021**, *9*, 97228–97242. [CrossRef]
95. Freitas, G.A.d.L. *Aprendizagem Profunda Aplicada ao Futebol de Robôs : Uso de Redes Neurais Convolucionais para Detecção de Objetos Universidade Estadual de Londrina Centro de Tecnologia e Urbanismo Departamento de Engenharia Elétrica Aprendizagem Profunda Aplicada ao Fute*; Trabalho de conclusão (curso de engenharia elétrica); Universidade Estadual de Londrina: Londrina, Brazil, 2019.
96. COCO. Detection Evaluation Metrics Used by COCO. 2021. Available online: https://cocodataset.org/#detection-eval (accessed on 25 August 2022).
97. Prechelt, L. *Early Stopping—But When?*; Springer: Berlin/Heidelberg, Germany, 1998; pp. 55–69. [CrossRef]
98. Zhang, C.; Bengio, S.; Hardt, M.; Recht, B.; Vinyals, O. Understanding deep learning requires rethinking generalization. *arXiv* **2017**, arXiv: cs.LG/1611.03530.
99. Srivastava, N.; Hinton, G.; Krizhevsky, A.; Sutskever, I.; Salakhutdinov, R. Dropout: A Simple Way to Prevent Neural Networks from Overfitting. *J. Mach. Learn. Res.* **2014**, *15*, 1929–1958.
100. Liang, X.; Wu, L.; Li, J.; Wang, Y.; Meng, Q.; Qin, T.; Chen, W.; Zhang, M.; Liu, T.Y. R-Drop: Regularized Dropout for Neural Networks. *Adv. Neural Inf. Process. Syst.* **2021**, *34*, 10890–10905.
101. Labach, A.; Salehinejad, H.; Valaee, S. Survey of Dropout Methods for Deep Neural Networks. *arXiv* **2019**, arXiv:1904.13310.
102. Davis, J.; Goadrich, M. The relationship between Precision-Recall and ROC curves. In Proceedings of the ICML 2006—Proceedings of the 23rd International Conference on Machine Learning, Pittsburgh, PL, USA, 25–29 June 2006; pp. 233–240.
103. Manning, C.D.; Raghavan, P.; Schütze, H. *Introduction to Information Retrieval*; Cambridge University Press: Cambridge, MA, USA, 2008.

104. Flach, P.A.; Kull, M. Precision-Recall-Gain curves: PR analysis done right. *Adv. Neural Inf. Process. Syst.* **2015**, *28*, 838–846.
105. Asamoah, D.; Ofori, E.; Opoku, S.; Danso, J. Measuring the Performance of Image Contrast Enhancement Technique. *Int. J. Comput. Appl.* **2018**, *181*, 6–13. [CrossRef]
106. Bodla, N.; Singh, B.; Chellappa, R.; Davis, L.S. Soft-NMS - Improving Object Detection with One Line of Code. In Proceedings of the IEEE International Conference on Computer Vision, Venice, Italy, 22–29 October 2017; pp. 5562–5570. [CrossRef]
107. Carratino, L.; Cissé, M.; Jenatton, R.; Vert, J.P. On Mixup Regularization. *arXiv* **2020**, arXiv:2006.06049.
108. Castro, D.J.L. Garra Servo-Controlada com Integração de Informação táCtil e de Proximidade. Master's Thesis, Universidade de Coimbra, Coimbra, Portugal, 1996.
109. Chandrasekar, L.; Durga, G. Implementation of Hough Transform for image processing applications. In Proceedings of the 2014 International Conference on Communication and Signal Processing, Bangkok, Thailand, 10–12 October 2014; pp. 843–847. [CrossRef]
110. Claro, M.; Vogado, L.; Santos, J.; Veras, R. Utilização de Técnicas de Data Augmentation em Imagens: Teoria e Prática. 2020. Available online: https://sol.sbc.org.br/livros/index.php/sbc/catalog/view/48/224/445-1 (accessed on 1 November 2021).
111. Li, F.-F.; Krishna, R.; Xu, D. cs231n, Lecture 15—Slide 4, Detection and Segmentation. 2021. Available online: http://cs231n.stanford.edu/slides/2021/lecture_15.pdf (accessed on 26 December 2021).
112. Li, F.-F.; Deng, J.; Li, K. ImageNet: Constructing a large-scale image database. *J. Vis.* **2010**, *9*, 1037–1037. [CrossRef]
113. Dai, F.; Fan, B.; Peng, Y. An image haze removal algorithm based on blockwise processing using LAB color space and bilateral filtering. In Proceedings of the 2018 Chinese Control And Decision Conference (CCDC), Shenyang, China, 9–11 June 2018; pp. 5945–5948.
114. Dai, J.; Li, Y.; He, K.; Sun, J. R-FCN: Object Detection via Region-Based Fully Convolutional Networks. *arXiv* **2016**, arXiv:1605.06409.
115. dos Santos, J.R.V. Avaliação de Técnicas de Realce de Imagens Digitais Utilizando Métricas Subjetivas e Objetivas. Master's Thesis, Universidade Federal do Ceará, Fortaleza, Brazil, 2016.
116. Dvornik, N.; Mairal, J.; Schmid, C. Modeling Visual Context is Key to Augmenting Object Detection Datasets. *arXiv* **2018**, arXiv:1807.07428.
117. Dwibedi, D.; Misra, I.; Hebert, M. Cut, Paste and Learn: Surprisingly Easy Synthesis for Instance Detection. *arXiv* **2017**, arXiv:1708.01642.
118. Erfurt, J.; Helmrich, C.R.; Bosse, S.; Schwarz, H.; Marpe, D.; Wiegand, T. A Study of the Perceptually Weighted Peak Signal-To-Noise Ratio (WPSNR) for Image Compression. In Proceedings of the 2019 IEEE International Conference on Image Processing (ICIP), Taipei, Taiwan, 22–25 September 2019; pp. 2339–2343. [CrossRef]
119. Fardo, F.A.; Conforto, V.H.; de Oliveira, F.C.; Rodrigues, P.S. A Formal Evaluation of PSNR as Quality Measurement Parameter for Image Segmentation Algorithms. *arXiv* **2016**, arXiv:1605.07116.
120. Faria, D. *Trabalhos Práticos Análise e Processamento de Imagem*; Faculdade de Engenharia da Universidade do Porto: Porto, Portugal, 2010.
121. Ghiasi, G.; Cui, Y.; Srinivas, A.; Qian, R.; Lin, T.Y.; Cubuk, E.D.; Le, Q.V.; Zoph, B. Simple Copy-Paste is a Strong Data Augmentation Method for Instance Segmentation. *arXiv* **2021**, arXiv:2012.07177.
122. Girshick, R.; Donahue, J.; Darrell, T.; Malik, J. Rich feature hierarchies for accurate object detection and semantic segmentation. In Proceedings of the IEEE Computer Society Conference on Computer Vision and Pattern Recognition, Columbus, OH, USA, 23–28 June 2014; pp. 580–587. [CrossRef]
123. Girshick, R. Fast R-CNN. In Proceedings of the IEEE International Conference on Computer Vision, ICCV 2015, Santiago, Chile, 7–13 December 2015; pp. 1440–1448. [CrossRef]
124. Gonzalez, R.C.; Woods, R.E.; Eddins, S.L. *Digital Image Processing Using MATLAB*; Prentice-Hall, Inc.: Upper Saddle River, NJ, USA, 2003.
125. Guo, H.; Mao, Y.; Zhang, R. Augmenting Data with Mixup for Sentence Classification: An Empirical Study. *arXiv* **2019**, arXiv:1905.08941.
126. Guo, H.; Mao, Y.; Zhang, R. MixUp as Locally Linear Out-Of-Manifold Regularization. *arXiv* **2018**, arXiv:1809.02499.
127. Hao, R.; Namdar, K.; Liu, L.; Haider, M.A.; Khalvati, F. A Comprehensive Study of Data Augmentation Strategies for Prostate Cancer Detection in Diffusion-weighted MRI using Convolutional Neural Networks. *arXiv* **2020**, arXiv:2006.01693.
128. Hawas, A.R.; Ashour, A.S.; Guo, Y. 8—Neutrosophic set in medical image clustering. In *Neutrosophic Set in Medical Image Analysis*; Guo, Y., Ashour, A.S., Eds.; Academic Press: Cambridge, MA, USA, 2019; pp. 167–187. [CrossRef]
129. Huynh-The, T.; Le, B.V.; Lee, S.; Le-Tien, T.; Yoon, Y. Using weighted dynamic range for histogram equalization to improve the image contrast. *EURASIP J. Image Video Process.* **2014**, *2014*, 44. [CrossRef]
130. Illingworth, J.; Kittler, J. The Adaptive Hough Transform. *IEEE Trans. Pattern Anal. Mach. Intell.* **1987**, *PAMI-9*, 690–698. [CrossRef]
131. Kim, J.H.; Choo, W.; Jeong, H.; Song, H.O. Co-Mixup: Saliency Guided Joint Mixup with Supermodular Diversity. *arXiv* **2021**, arXiv:2102.03065.
132. Liu, Z.; Chen, W.; Zou, Y.; Hu, C. Regions of interest extraction based on HSV color space. In Proceedings of the IEEE 10th International Conference on Industrial Informatics, Beijing, China, 25–27 July 2012; pp. 481–485. [CrossRef]

133. Ma, J.; Fan, X.; Yang, S.X.; Zhang, X.; Zhu, X. Contrast Limited Adaptive Histogram Equalization-Based Fusion in YIQ and HSI Color Spaces for Underwater Image Enhancement. *Int. J. Pattern Recognit. Artif. Intell.* **2018**, *32*, 1–26. [CrossRef]
134. Marroni, L.S. Aplicação da Transformada de Hough Para Localização dos Olhos em Faces Humanas. Master's Thesis, Universidade de São Paulo, São Carlos, Brazil, 2002.
135. McREYNOLDS, T.; BLYTHE, D. CHAPTER 12—Image Processing Techniques. In *Advanced Graphics Programming Using OpenGL*; McReynolds, T., Blythe, D., Eds.; The Morgan Kaufmann Series in Computer Graphics; Morgan Kaufmann: San Francisco, CA, USA, 2005; pp. 211–245. [CrossRef]
136. Mukhopadhyay, S.; Mandal, S.; Pratiher, S.; Changdar, S.; Burman, R.; Ghosh, N.; Panigrahi, P.K. A comparative study between proposed Hyper Kurtosis based Modified Duo-Histogram Equalization (HKMDHE) and Contrast Limited Adaptive Histogram Equalization (CLAHE) for Contrast Enhancement Purpose of Low Contrast Human Brain CT scan images. *arXiv* **2015**, arXiv:1505.06219.
137. Nixon, M.S.; Aguado, A.S. 5—High-level feature extraction: fixed shape matching. In *Feature Extraction and Image Processing for Computer Vision*, 4th ed.; Nixon, M.S., Aguado, A.S., Eds.; Academic Press: Cambridge, MA, USA, 2020; pp. 223–290. [CrossRef]
138. Paris, S.; Durand, F. A Fast Approximation of the Bilateral Filter Using a Signal Processing Approach. In Proceedings of the Computer Vision—ECCV 2006, Graz, Austria, 7–13 May 2006; Leonardis, A., Bischof, H., Pinz, A., Eds.; Springer: Berlin/Heidelberg, Germany, 2006; pp. 568–580.
139. Park, G.H.; Cho, H.H.; Choi, M.R. A contrast enhancement method using dynamic range separate histogram equalization. *IEEE Trans. Consum. Electron.* **2008**, *54*, 1981–1987. [CrossRef]
140. Peixoto, C.S.B. Estudo de Métodos de Agrupamento e Transformada de Hough para Processamento de Imagens Digitais. Master's Thesis, Universidade Federal da Bahia, Salvador, Spain, 2003.
141. Pujari, J.; Pushpalatha, S.; Padmashree, D. Content-Based Image Retrieval using color and shape descriptors. In Proceedings of the 2010 International Conference on Signal and Image Processing, Chennai, India, 15–17 December 2010; pp. 239–242. [CrossRef]
142. Rong, F.; Du-wu, C.; Bo, H. A Novel Hough Transform Algorithm for Multi-objective Detection. In Proceedings of the 2009 Third International Symposium on Intelligent Information Technology Application, NanChang, China, 21–22 November 2009; Volume 3, pp. 705–708. [CrossRef]
143. Schettini, R.; Gasparini, F.; Corchs, S.; Marini, F.; Capra, A.; Castorina, A. Contrast image correction method. *J. Electron. Imaging* **2010**, *19*, 023005. [CrossRef]
144. Setiawan, A.W.; Mengko, T.R.; Santoso, O.S.; Suksmono, A.B. Color retinal image enhancement using CLAHE. In Proceedings of the International Conference on ICT for Smart Society 2013: "Think Ecosystem Act Convergence", ICISS 2013, Jakarta, Indonesia, 13–14 June 2013; pp. 215–217. [CrossRef]
145. Shene, C.K. Geometric Transformations. 2018. Available online: https://pages.mtu.edu/~shene/COURSES/cs3621/NOTES/geometry/geo-tran.html (accessed on 1 November 2021).
146. Shiao, Y.H.; Chen, T.J.; Chuang, K.S.; Lin, C.H.; Chuang, C.C. Quality of compressed medical images. *J. Digit. Imaging* **2007**, *20*, 149–159. [CrossRef]
147. Shorten, C.; Khoshgoftaar, T.M. A survey on Image Data Augmentation for Deep Learning. *J. Big Data* **2019**, *6*, 60. [CrossRef]
148. Singh, P.K.; Tiwari, V. Normalized Log Twicing Function for DC Coefficients Scaling in LAB Color Space. In Proceedings of the International Conference on Inventive Research in Computing Applications, ICIRCA 2018, Coimbatore, India, 11–12 July 2018; pp. 333–338. [CrossRef]
149. Sun, K.; Wang, B.; Zhou, Z.Q.; Zheng, Z.H. Real time image haze removal using bilateral filter. *Trans. Beijing Inst. Technol.* **2011**, *31*, 810–814.
150. Unel, F.O.; Ozkalayci, B.O.; Cigla, C. The Power of Tiling for Small Object Detection. In Proceedings of the 2019 IEEE/CVF Conference on Computer Vision and Pattern Recognition Workshops (CVPRW), Long Beach, CA, USA, 16–17 June 2019; pp. 582–591. [CrossRef]
151. Wang, K.; Fang, B.; Qian, J.; Yang, S.; Zhou, X.; Zhou, J. Perspective Transformation Data Augmentation for Object Detection. *IEEE Access* **2020**, *8*, 4935–4943. [CrossRef]
152. Wang, S.; Zheng, J.; Hu, H.M.; Li, B. Naturalness Preserved Enhancement Algorithm for Non-Uniform Illumination Images. *IEEE Trans. Image Process.* **2013**, *22*, 3538–3548. [CrossRef]
153. Warner, R. Measurement of Meat Quality | Measurements of Water-holding Capacity and Color: Objective and Subjective. In *Encyclopedia of Meat Sciences*, 2nd ed.; Dikeman, M., Devine, C., Eds.; Academic Press: Oxford, UK, 2014; pp. 164–171. [CrossRef]
154. Yadav, G.; Maheshwari, S.; Agarwal, A. Contrast limited adaptive histogram equalization based enhancement for real time video system. In Proceedings of the 2014 International Conference on Advances in Computing, Communications and Informatics (ICACCI), Delhi, India, 24–27 September 2014; pp. 2392–2397. [CrossRef]
155. Yang, Q.; Tan, K.H.; Ahuja, N. Real-time O(1) bilateral filtering. In Proceedings of the 2009 IEEE Conference on Computer Vision and Pattern Recognition, Miami, FL, USA, 20–25 June 2009; pp. 557–564. [CrossRef]
156. Ye, H.; Shang, G.; Wang, L.; Zheng, M. A new method based on hough transform for quick line and circle detection. In Proceedings of the 2015 8th International Conference on Biomedical Engineering and Informatics (BMEI), Shenyang, China, 14–16 October 2015; pp. 52–56. [CrossRef]

157. Ye, Z.; Mohamadian, H.; Ye, Y. Discrete Entropy and Relative Entropy Study on Nonlinear Clustering of Underwater and Arial Images. In Proceedings of the 2007 IEEE International Conference on Control Applications, Singapore, 1–3 October 2007; pp. 313–318. [CrossRef]
158. Yuen, H.; Princen, J.; Illingworth, J.; Kittler, J. Comparative study of Hough Transform methods for circle finding. *Image Vis. Comput.* **1990**, *8*, 71–77. [CrossRef]
159. Zhang, H.; Cisse, M.; Dauphin, Y.N.; Lopez-Paz, D. MixUp: Beyond empirical risk minimization. In Proceedings of the 6th International Conference on Learning Representations, ICLR 2018—Conference Track Proceedings, Vancouver, BC, Canada, 30 April–3 May 2018; pp. 1–13.
160. Zhao, H.; Li, Q.; Feng, H. Multi-Focus Color Image Fusion in the HSI Space Using the Sum-Modified-Laplacian and a Coarse Edge Map. *Image Vis. Comput.* **2008**, *26*, 1285–1295. [CrossRef]
161. D. D. Silva, A.; B. P. Carneiro, M.; F. S. Cardoso, C. Realce De Microaneurimas Em Imagens De Fundo De Olho Utilizando Clahe. In *Anais do V Congresso Brasileiro de Eletromiografia e Cinesiologia e X Simpósio de Engenharia Biomédica*; Even3: Uberlândia, Brazil, 2018; pp. 772–775. [CrossRef]

MDPI
St. Alban-Anlage 66
4052 Basel
Switzerland
www.mdpi.com

Sensors Editorial Office
E-mail: sensors@mdpi.com
www.mdpi.com/journal/sensors

www.ingramcontent.com/pod-product-compliance
Lightning Source LLC
Chambersburg PA
CBHW041014270926
51850CB00024B/40
9783036595320